Acquiring Medical Language

Second Edition

Steven L. Jones, PhD
Rice University
Houston Baptist University

Andrew Cavanagh, MD
Texas A&M College of Medicine

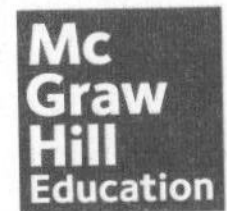

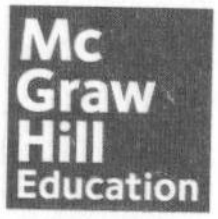

ACQUIRING MEDICAL LANGUAGE, SECOND EDITION

Published by McGraw-Hill Education, 2 Penn Plaza, New York, NY 10121.

Some ancillaries, including electronic and print components, may not be available to customers outside the United States.

This book is printed on acid-free paper.

4 5 6 7 8 9 LMN 21 20

ISBN 978-1-259-63816-9
MHID 1-259-63816-2

Senior Portfolio Manager: *William Mulford*
Senior Product Developer: *Yvonne Lloyd*
Marketing Manager: *Valerie Kramer*
Content Project Manager: *Ann Courtney*
Buyer: *Susan K. Culbertson*
Design: *Tara McDermott*
Content Licensing Specialist: *Lorraine Buczek*
Cover Image: *Getty Images*
Compositor: *Lumina Datamatics, Inc.*

All credits appearing on page or at the end of the book are considered to be an extension of the copyright page.

Library of Congress Cataloging-in-Publication Data

Jones, Steven L., 1975- author.
Acquiring medical language / Steven L. Jones, PhD, Houston Baptist University, Andrew Cavanagh, MD, Texas A & M College of Medicine.
Second edition. | New York, NY : McGraw-Hill Education, [2019] |
Includes index.
LCCN 2017049794 | ISBN 9781259638169 (alk. paper)
LCSH: Medicine–Terminology.
LCC R123 .J686 2018 | DDC 610.1/4–dc23 LC record
https://lccn.loc.gov/2017049794

mheducation.com/highered

brief contents

Table of Contents

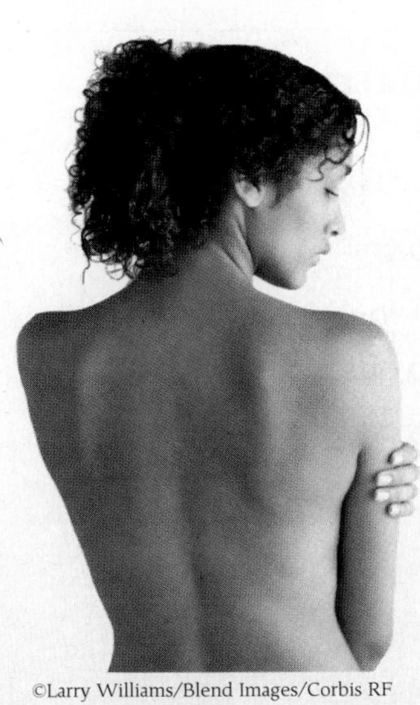
©Larry Williams/Blend Images/Corbis RF

CHAPTER 4 The Musculoskeletal System–Orthopedics 182

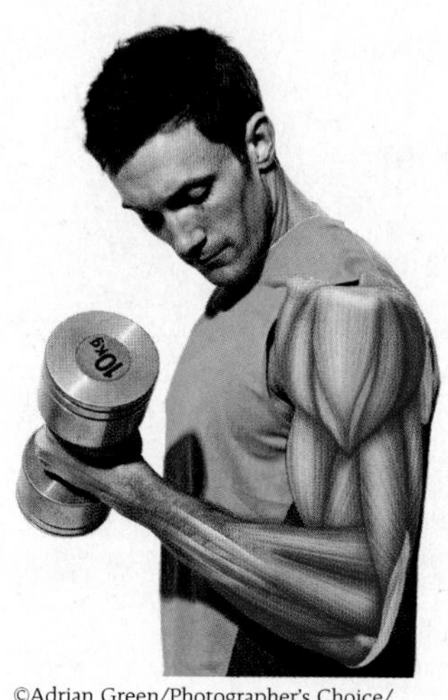

©Adrian Green/Photographer's Choice/ Getty Images

CHAPTER 5 The Nervous System–Neurology and Psychiatry 247

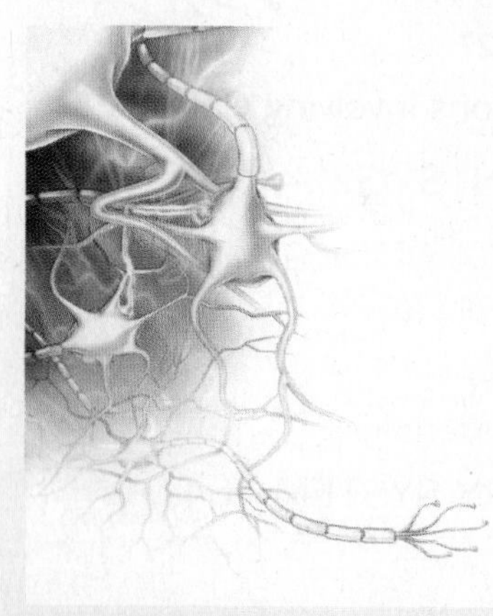

CHAPTER 6 The Sensory System–Ophthalmology and Otolaryngology 314

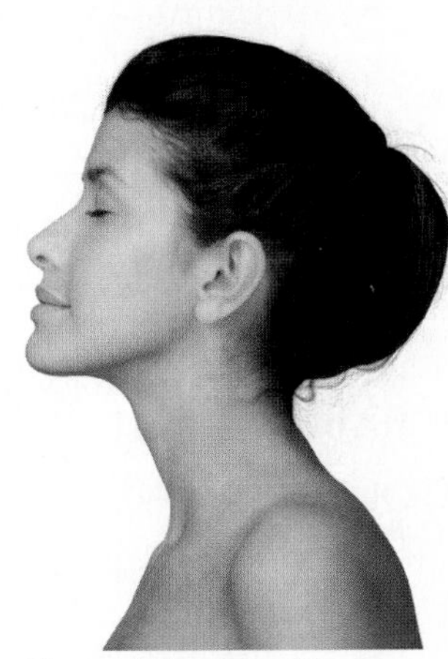
©Fotosearch/Getty Images RF

CHAPTER 7 The Endocrine System–Endocrinology 389

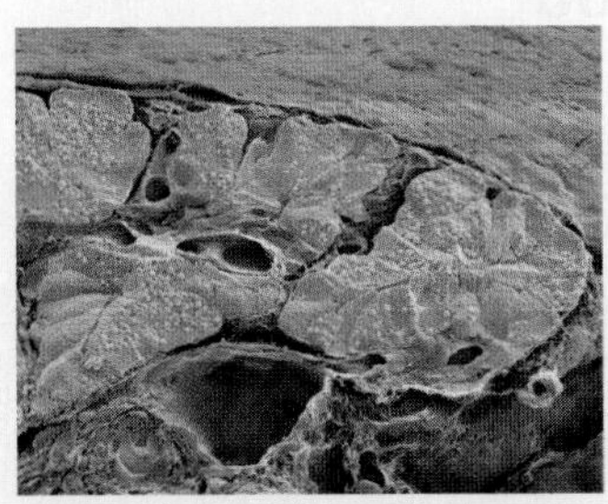
©Steve Gschmeissner/Science Source

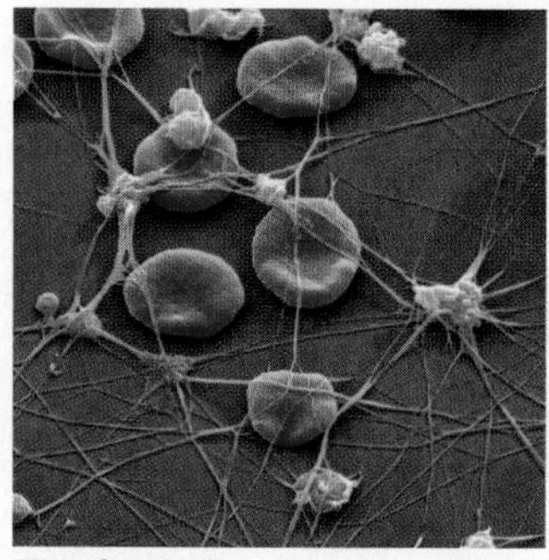
©Eye of Science/Science Source

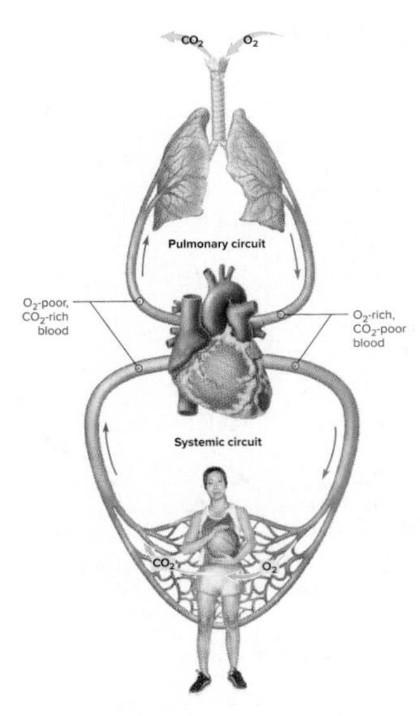

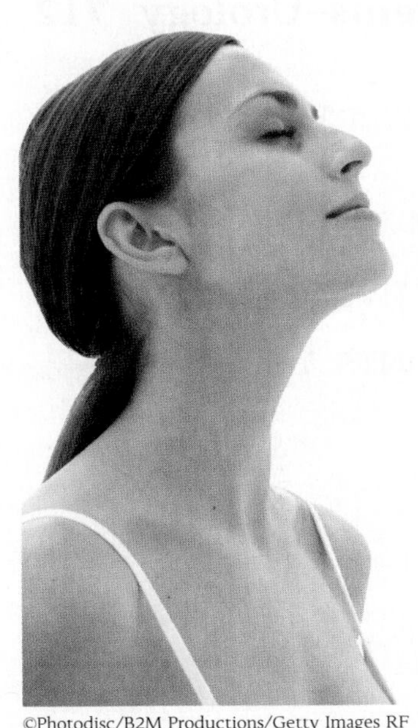
©Photodisc/B2M Productions/Getty Images RF

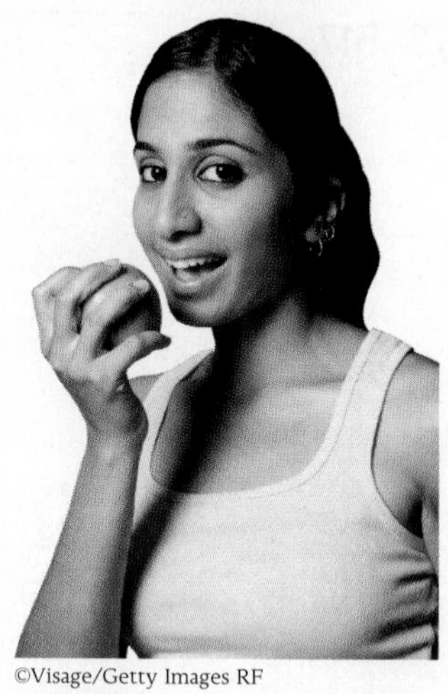

©Visage/Getty Images RF

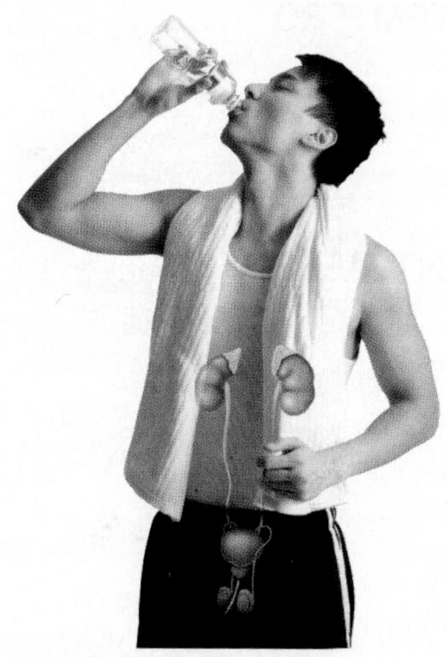

©Asia selects/Getty Images RF

CHAPTER 13 The Female Reproductive System–Gynecology, Obstetrics, and Neonatology 802

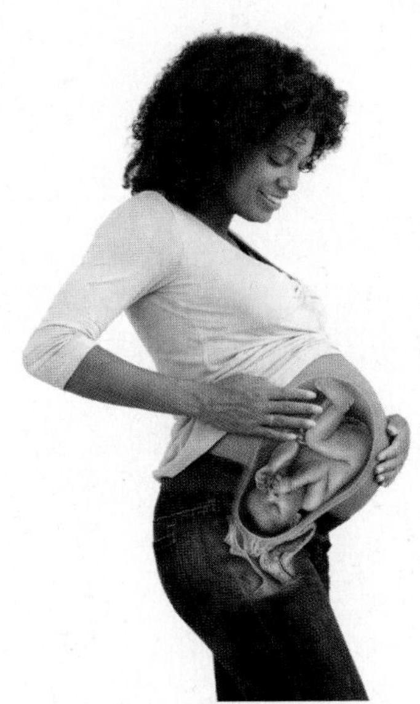
©Larry Williams/Corbis/Getty Images

Appendixes

dedication

To our wives:

Tamber Jones

and

Ashley Cavanagh.

Your devotion, support, encouragement, and assistance made this book possible.

Steven L. Jones, PhD

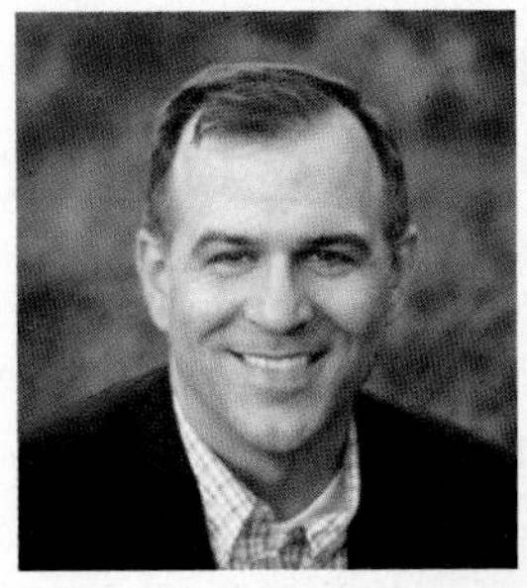
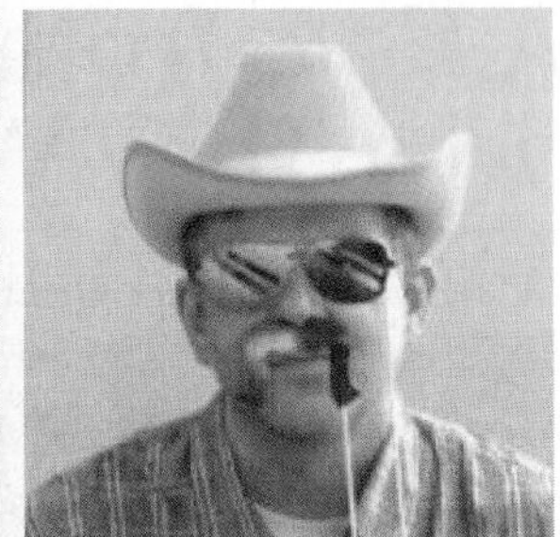
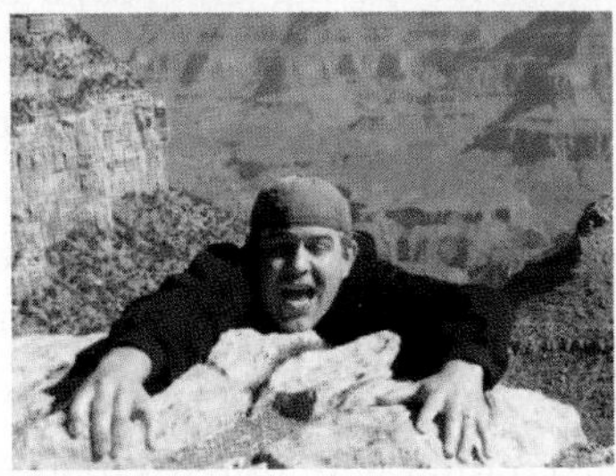

(top left): ©Steve L. Jones; (top right): ©Tamber Jones; (bottom): ©Tamber Jones

Steve holds a BA in Greek and Latin from Baylor University, an MA in Greek, Latin, and Classical Studies from Bryn Mawr College, and a PhD in Classics from the University of Texas at Austin. Steve has held previous faculty appointments at Trinity University, the University of Texas at Austin, and Baylor University. Currently he is Associate Professor of Classics at Houston Baptist University in Houston, where he also serves as chair of the Department of Classics & Biblical Languages and as director of the Master of Arts in Biblical Languages Program. He teaches courses on Latin, Greek, classical civilization, early Christianity, and the classical roots of medical language. He also teaches Medical Terminology at Rice University in Houston, Texas.

When not breaking down medical words, Steve enjoys taking road trips with his wife and five children, watching baseball, eating tacos, drinking ice-cold Dr Pepper, and showing off his parallel-parking skills.

Andrew Cavanagh, MD

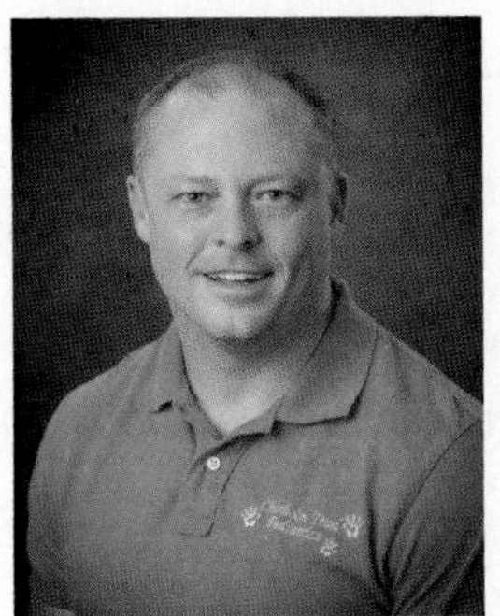
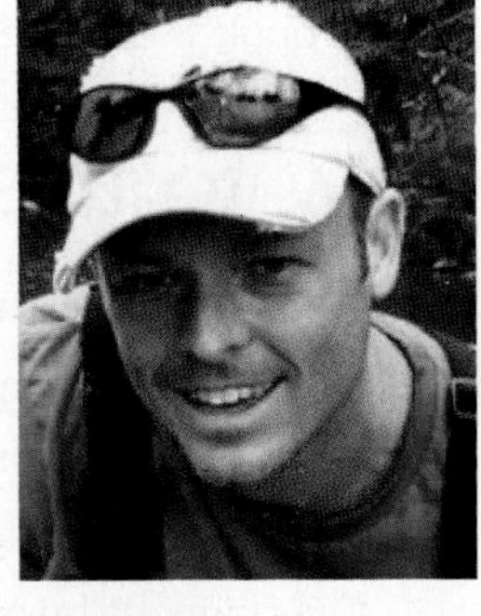
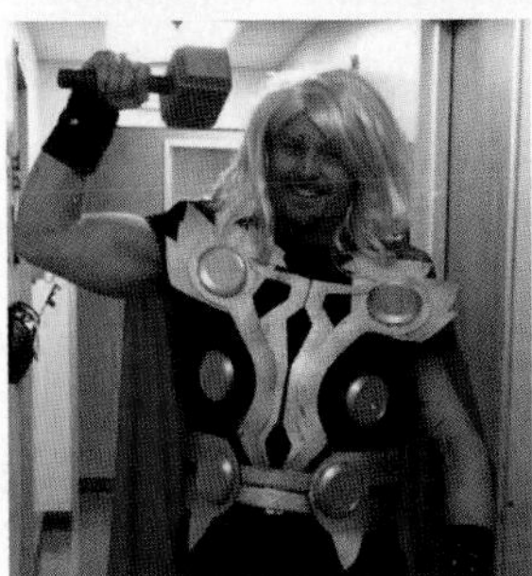

(top left): ©Shane Littleton; (top right): ©Andy Cavanagh; (bottom): ©Andy Cavanagh

Andy holds a BS in Genetics from Texas A&M University and an MD from Texas A&M College of Medicine. After completing his residency at Palmetto Health Children's Hospital, he moved to the Austin area. He is currently owner and Chief Medical Officer of Chisholm Trail Pediatrics in Georgetown, Texas. In addition to being board-certified in pediatrics, Andy has served as the pediatric specialty chief for Dell Children's Medical Center and on the board of Dell Children's Medical Center Executive Committee. He currently serves as a clinical assistant professor of pediatrics at the Texas A&M College of Medicine.

When not comforting sick children at work or wrestling with his own three kids at home, Andy enjoys powerlifting, hiking, and making his wife laugh.

A Note from the Authors on Why They Wrote This Book

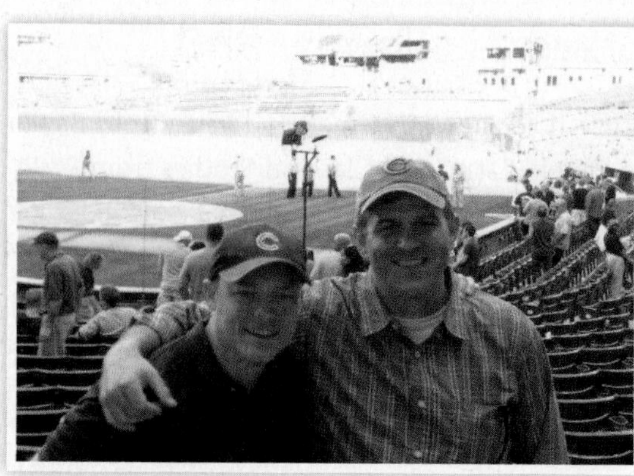
Courtesy of the authors

This book has its beginning in the friendship that Andy and Steve developed while they both lived in Austin, Texas. Andy was beginning his pediatric practice. Steve was completing his doctorate at UT. They had kids the same age and attended the same church. One evening after dinner, while sitting on Andy's back porch, Steve mentioned a new course he had been assigned to teach: Medical Terminology. What started as Steve complaining ended in a game where Andy tried to stump Steve by asking him what various medical words meant. Andy was amazed at how much Steve could figure out just by breaking down words. Steve was astonished to realize that most people–from medical assistants to medical doctors–weren't taught medical language this way. Through this conversation and others like it, Steve and Andy realized three things:

1. Understanding how to break down medical language is an essential skill in the medical field.
2. Having a basic knowledge of the Greek and Latin roots made medical language radically transparent.
3. The current market is lacking a textbook that teaches medical language this way.

This book is their attempt to meet those needs.

New to the Second Edition

1. Updated abbreviations in every chapter
2. Body system chapters contain word tables organized by categories, such as pharmacology, radiology, oncology, and health professions
3. Expanded coverage of the variety of health professions (Ch. 2)
4. Overview of burns (Ch. 3)
5. Expanded coverage of eye conditions, including glaucoma (Ch. 6)
6. Expanded coverage of gastrointestinal diagnoses and hepatitis (Ch. 11)
7. Expanded coverage of sexually transmitted diseases (Ch. 12)
8. Overview of the process of fertilization (Ch. 13)

How to Use the Book

The Approach

Acquiring Medical Language, 2e, approaches medical terminology not as words to be memorized but as a language to be learned. If you treat medical terminology as a language and learn how to read terms like sentences, you will be able to communicate clearly as a health care professional and will be a full participant in the culture of medicine. Memorizing definitions is equal to a traveler memorizing a few phrases in another language to help during a brief vacation: it will help a traveler survive for a few days. But if one is going to live in another culture for an extended period of time, learning to speak and understand the language becomes essential.

Acquiring Medical Language, 2e, teaches students to **break down words into their composite word parts.** Instead of only using a dictionary full of terms that need to be memorized, a student equipped with groups of roots, prefixes, and suffixes can easily understand a vast amount of medical terminology.

Acquiring Medical Language, 2e, bridges the gap between the two somewhat disparate fields that make up medical terminology–medicine and second-language acquisition–by providing assistance in language skills to equip health care professionals with the ability to learn and apply a useful skill and not lists of words. It will also equip language professionals with real-world examples that make their knowledge of languages applicable to working in the world of health care.

The process is best illustrated by considering the following word: *pneumonoultramicroscopicsilicovolcanoconiosis.* Memorizing the definition to words like this would seem like an intimidating task. If you break it into its composite parts, you get:

pneumono / ultra / micro / scopic / silico / volcano / coni / osis
lung extremely small looking sand volcanic dust condition

Through knowledge of roots and word formation, the meaning becomes transparent: "a condition of the lungs caused by extremely small bits of volcanic sand." Instead of having to memorize a long list of even longer words, a student equipped with the knowledge of roots and how to break apart words can tackle–and not be intimidated by–the most complicated sounding medical terms.

Organization and Key Features

Acquiring Medical Language, 2e, begins with two introductory chapters: Chapter 1, Introduction to Medical Language; and Chapter 2, Introduction to Health Records. Chapters 3 through 13 are dedicated to individual systems of the body and review common roots, words, and abbreviations for each system.

1. **"Card-Based" Approach:** Each body system chapter opens with a section on word parts for that particular body system. Students are introduced to roots via "cards" with illustrations of body systems that contain the names of body parts, specific word roots related to those parts, a few examples containing the roots, as well as some interesting facts to make the information more memorable. The student is introduced to all relevant information (the root, its meaning, its use) and sees how each root relates to the other roots in the context of the body system, without ever needing to turn the page.
2. **SOAP Note Organization:** After the student is introduced to the important roots for the chapter using cards, the medical terms relevant to the body system are presented using the SOAP note as an organizational framework. SOAP is an acronym used by many health care professionals to help organize the diagnostic process (SOAP is explained more fully in Chapter 2). The terms will be divided under the following headings:

S Subjective: Patient History, Problems, Complaints

O Objective: Observation and Discovery

A Assessment: Diagnosis and Pathology

P Plan: Treatments and Therapies

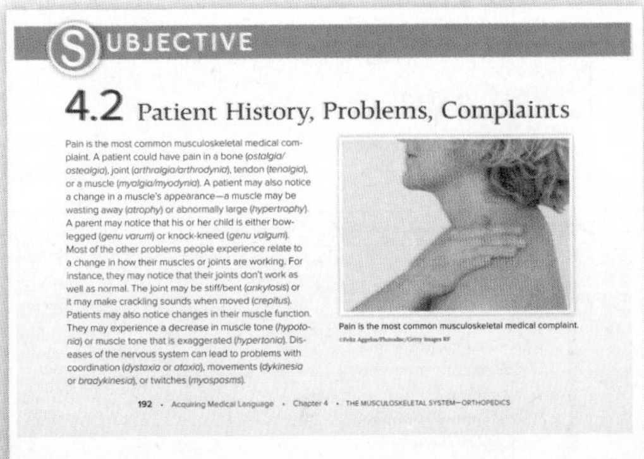
SUBJECTIVE

4.2 Patient History, Problems, Complaints

Pain is the most common musculoskeletal medical complaint. A patient could have pain in a bone (*ostalgia/ostealgia*), joint (*arthralgia/arthrodynia*), tendon (*tenalgia*), or a muscle (*myalgia/myodynia*). A patient may also notice a change in a muscle's appearance—a muscle may be wasting away (*atrophy*) or abnormally large (*hypertrophy*). A parent may notice that his or her child is either bow-legged (*genu varum*) or knock-kneed (*genu valgum*). Most of the other problems people experience relate to a change in how their muscles or joints are working. For instance, they may notice that their joints don't work as well as normal. The joint may be stiff/bent (*ankylosis*) or it may make crackling sounds when moved (*crepitus*). Patients may also notice changes in their muscle function. They may experience a decrease in muscle tone (*hypotonia*) or muscle tone that is exaggerated (*hypertonia*). Diseases of the nervous system can lead to problems with coordination (*dystaxia* or *ataxia*), movements (*dykinesia* or *bradykinesia*), or twitches (*myospasms*).

Pain is the most common musculoskeletal medical complaint.

192 · Acquiring Medical Language · Chapter 4 · THE MUSCULOSKELETAL SYSTEM—ORTHOPEDICS

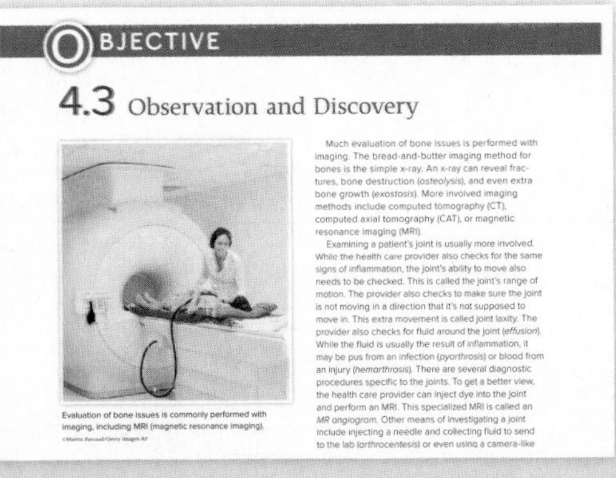
OBJECTIVE

4.3 Observation and Discovery

Evaluation of bone issues is commonly performed with imaging, including MRI (magnetic resonance imaging).

Much evaluation of bone issues is performed with imaging. The bread-and-butter imaging method for bones is the simple x-ray. An x-ray can reveal fractures, bone destruction (*osteolysis*), and even extra bone growth (*exostosis*). More involved imaging methods include computed tomography (CT), computed axial tomography (CAT), or magnetic resonance imaging (MRI).

Examining a patient's joint is usually more involved. While the health care provider also checks for the same signs of inflammation, the joint's ability to move also needs to be checked. This is called the joint's range of motion. The provider also checks to make sure the joint is not moving in a direction that it's not supposed to move in. This extra movement is called joint laxity. The provider also checks for fluid around the joint (*effusion*). While the fluid is usually the result of inflammation, it may be pus from an infection (*pyorthrosis*) or blood from an injury (*hemarthrosis*). There are several diagnostic procedures specific to the joints. To get a better view, the health care provider can inject dye into the joint and perform an MRI. This specialized MRI is called an *MR angiogram*. Other means of investigating a joint include injecting a needle and collecting fluid to send to the lab (*arthrocentesis*) or even using a camera-like

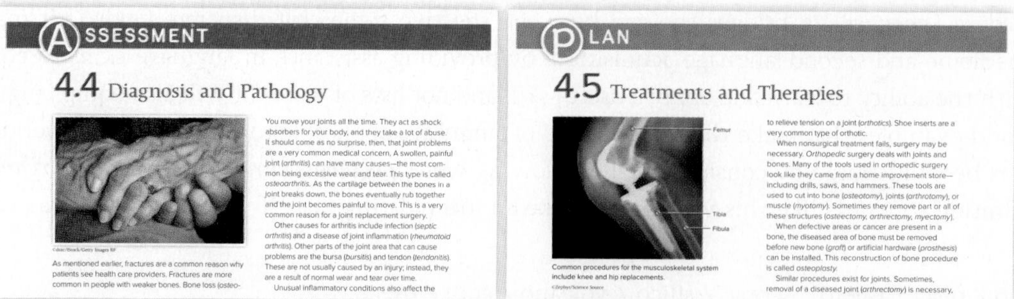

ASSESSMENT

4.4 Diagnosis and Pathology

©duac/Brock/Getty Images RF

As mentioned earlier, fractures are a common reason why patients see health care providers. Fractures are more common in people with weaker bones. Bone loss (osteo-

You move your joints all the time. They act as shock absorbers for your body, and they take a lot of abuse. It should come as no surprise, then, that joint problems are a very common medical concern. A swollen, painful joint (*arthritis*) can have many causes—the most common being excessive wear and tear. This type is called *osteoarthritis*. As the cartilage between the bones in a joint breaks down, the bones eventually rub together and the joint becomes painful to move. This is a very common reason for a joint replacement surgery.

Other causes for arthritis include infection (*septic arthritis*) and a disease of joint inflammation (*rheumatoid arthritis*). Other parts of the joint area that can cause problems are the bursa (*bursitis*) and tendon (*tendonitis*). These are not usually caused by an injury; instead, they are a result of normal wear and tear over time.

Unusual inflammatory conditions also affect the

PLAN

4.5 Treatments and Therapies

Common procedures for the musculoskeletal system include knee and hip replacements.

©Zephyr/Science Source

to relieve tension on a joint (*orthotics*). Shoe inserts are a very common type of orthotic.

When nonsurgical treatment fails, surgery may be necessary. *Orthopedic* surgery deals with joints and bones. Many of the tools used in orthopedic surgery look like they came from a home improvement store—including drills, saws, and hammers. These tools are used to cut into bone (*osteotomy*), joints (*arthrotomy*), or muscle (*myotomy*). Sometimes they remove part or all of these structures (*osteectomy, arthrectomy, myectomy*).

When defective areas or cancer are present in a bone, the diseased area of bone must be removed before new bone (*graft*) or artificial hardware (*prosthesis*) can be installed. This reconstruction of bone procedure is called *osteoplasty*.

Similar procedures exist for joints. Sometimes, removal of a diseased joint (*arthrectomy*) is necessary,

The SOAP note method is a fundamental way of thinking about the language of health care. By building this approach into the framework of the pedagogy, *Acquiring Medical Language, 2e,* prepares future health care professionals to speak the language of medicine.

3. **Realistic Medical Histories:** *Acquiring Medical Language, 2e,* incorporates realistic medical histories in reviewing each chapter's material to expose students to what they can expect in the real world. The student is given an example of an electronic health care record and is asked a series of questions. Though it is not expected that everything in the record will be intelligible to them, the goal is to expose students to the context in which they will see medical terminology. This process will encourage students not to feel intimidated by the prospect of seeing words they are unfamiliar with. We have seen this help students glean information from the chart by using the skills they are acquiring in translating medical terminology.

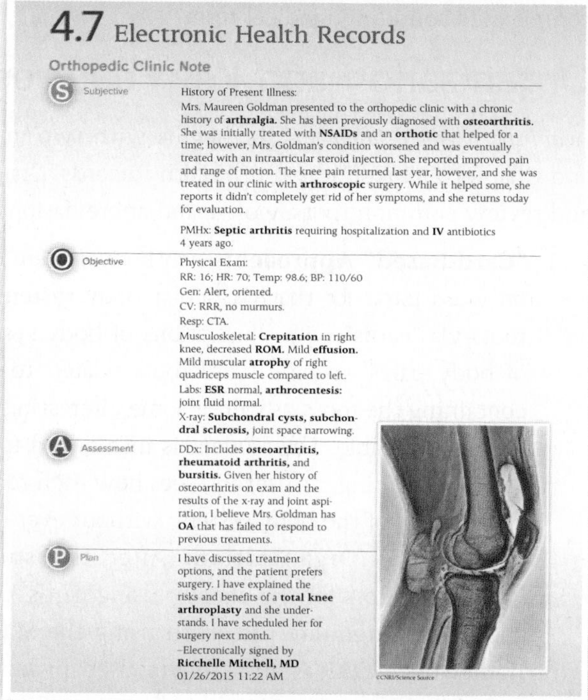

4.7 Electronic Health Records

Orthopedic Clinic Note

S Subjective

History of Present Illness:
Mrs. Maureen Goldman presented to the orthopedic clinic with a chronic history of **arthralgia.** She has been previously diagnosed with **osteoarthritis.** She was initially treated with **NSAIDs** and an **orthotic** that helped for a time; however, Mrs. Goldman's condition worsened and was eventually treated with an intraarticular steroid injection. She reported improved pain and range of motion. The knee pain returned last year, however, and she was treated in our clinic with **arthroscopic** surgery. While it helped some, she reports it didn't completely get rid of her symptoms, and she returns today for evaluation.

PMHx: **Septic arthritis** requiring hospitalization and **IV** antibiotics 4 years ago.

O Objective

Physical Exam:
RR: 16; HR: 70; Temp: 98.6; BP: 110/60
Gen: Alert, oriented.
CV: RRR, no murmurs.
Resp: CTA.
Musculoskeletal: **Crepitation** in right knee, decreased **ROM.** Mild **effusion.** Mild muscular **atrophy** of right quadriceps muscle compared to left.
Labs: **ESR** normal, **arthrocentesis:** joint fluid normal.
X-ray: **Subchondral cysts, subchondral sclerosis,** joint space narrowing.

A Assessment

DDx: Includes **osteoarthritis, rheumatoid arthritis,** and **bursitis.** Given her history of osteoarthritis on exam and the results of the x-ray and joint aspiration, I believe Mrs. Goldman has **OA** that has failed to respond to previous treatments.

P Plan

I have discussed treatment options, and the patient prefers surgery. I have explained the risks and benefits of a **total knee arthroplasty** and she understands. I have scheduled her for surgery next month.
–Electronically signed by
Ricchelle Mitchell, MD
01/26/2015 11:22 AM

©CNRI/Science Source

4. **Practice Exercises:** Each section ends with an abundance of practice exercises, giving students the opportunity to practice and apply what they have just learned. Exercises are grouped into categories: Pronunciation, Translation, and Generation. This progression and repetition allows students to gradually build their skills–and their confidence–as they learn to apply their medical language skills. Abundant Chapter Review exercises, as well as additional labeling and audio exercises, are available through McGraw-Hill Connect®.

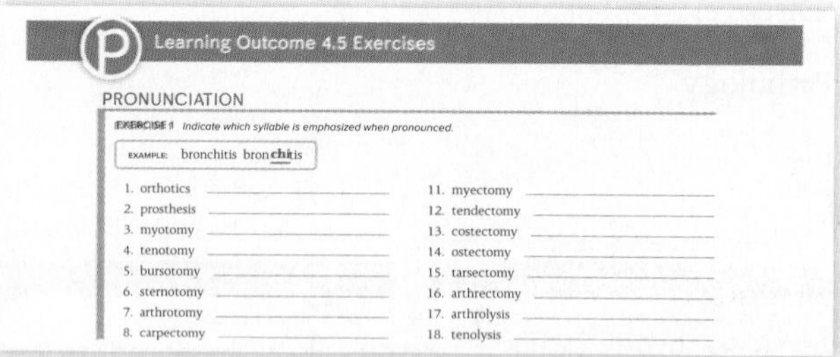

Learning Outcome 4.5 Exercises

PRONUNCIATION

EXERCISE 1 *Indicate which syllable is emphasized when pronounced.*

EXAMPLE: bronchitis bron**chi**tis

1. orthotics ______
2. prosthesis ______
3. myotomy ______
4. tenotomy ______
5. bursotomy ______
6. sternotomy ______
7. arthrotomy ______
8. carpectomy ______
11. myectomy ______
12. tendectomy ______
13. costectomy ______
14. ostectomy ______
15. tarsectomy ______
16. arthrectomy ______
17. arthrolysis ______
18. tenolysis ______

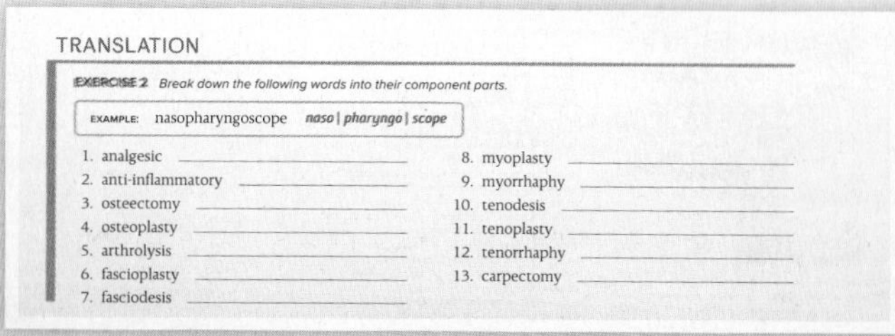

TRANSLATION

EXERCISE 2 *Break down the following words into their component parts.*

EXAMPLE: nasopharyngoscope *naso | pharyngo | scope*

1. analgesic ______
2. anti-inflammatory ______
3. osteectomy ______
4. osteoplasty ______
5. arthrolysis ______
6. fascioplasty ______
7. fasciodesis ______
8. myoplasty ______
9. myorrhaphy ______
10. tenodesis ______
11. tenoplasty ______
12. tenorrhaphy ______
13. carpectomy ______

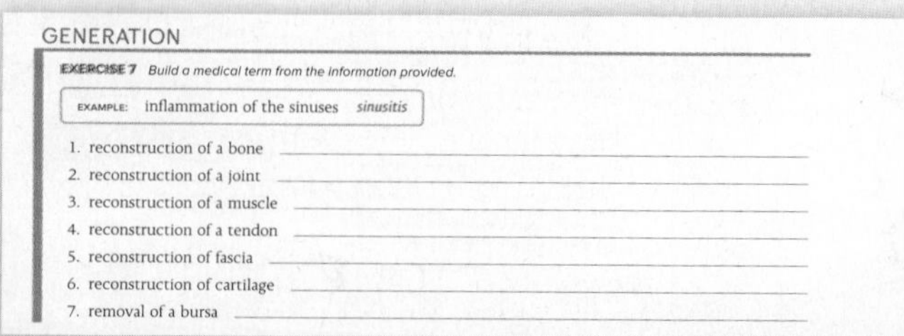

GENERATION

EXERCISE 7 *Build a medical term from the information provided.*

EXAMPLE: inflammation of the sinuses *sinusitis*

1. reconstruction of a bone ______
2. reconstruction of a joint ______
3. reconstruction of a muscle ______
4. reconstruction of a tendon ______
5. reconstruction of fascia ______
6. reconstruction of cartilage ______
7. removal of a bursa ______

To the Instructor

To teach medical terminology as a language, we adopt techniques employed in second-language acquisition. This helps students not just learn the roots, but also adopt a way of thinking and speaking that enables them to communicate using the language of medicine. Cognitive and educational psychologists divide language instruction techniques into two primary categories: contextualized (real-world exercises) and decontextualized (academic/grammar exercises).

Using this framework, some of the techniques employed in *Acquiring Medical Language* include:

1. **Contextualized language techniques (real-world exercises)**
   a. *Link new language to old language.* Pointing out instances of medical terms or roots in everyday use enables the students to connect new information they are studying with information they already possess.
   b. *Use new language in context.* Using the card system to introduce the root words enables students to understand word parts in the context of larger body systems and in relation to other word parts. Using realistic medical charts enables students to see the terms they use not as lists but as parts of a system of communication.
2. **Decontextualized language techniques (academic/grammar exercises)**
   a. *Use repetition.* The students are exposed to roots, prefixes, and suffixes multiple times and in multiple ways. Roots are changed by the addition of prefixes or suffixes. Familiar prefixes and suffixes are applied to new roots. This way, the word components are continuously reinforced.
   b. *Use translation.* Students are asked to provide literal definitions of medical terms, which provides practice in breaking down words into their component parts and determining their meaning.
   c. *Use generation.* Students are asked to produce medical terms based on the literal definition provided. Though this is only an academic exercise, such practice reinforces material learned by reversing the cognitive process of translation.
   d. *Challenge.* Students will be exposed to a handful of longer-than-average terms and asked to break them down into component parts and translate them. A key part of teaching any language is helping students feel comfortable with–not intimidated by–new material. One method is by periodically challenging them to tackle situations that may at first appear overwhelming.

As you use this text, here are some things to keep in mind:

1. **Breakdown Is the Key**–the goals of this approach to medical terminology are to help students internalize the word parts (roots, prefixes, suffixes) and to reinforce the concept that medical terms are not to be memorized but to be translated.
2. **Words Are Practice**–the words in each chapter are a chance to practice breaking down terms into their component parts, identifying the roots, and learning to define the terms using this translation method. Because of that, each chapter contains four classes of words.
   a. *Essential words that break down*–each chapter contains words that are essential for students to know AND that also break down easily using this method. The core of each chapter is words like this. The goal is to show students that the vast majority of medical terms are translatable using the method taught by this book.
   b. *Nonessential words that break down*–each chapter also contains words that are not necessarily essential for students to know or common in the medical field, but break down clearly and are easily translatable using the method taught by this book. We include them as chances to practice the concept of translating medical terms and to show how easy the method is to apply.
   c. *Essential words that it doesn't help to break down*–there are terms that can be broken down but the breakdown doesn't help you understand what the word means. This can happen for a variety of reasons, such as the term describes a symptom rather than the disease, or reflects an outdated way of understanding the disease, or is an ancient term that just means what it means, or is a very recent and technical term and so there are no other words to compare it to. In these cases, even though the method taught by this book may not be ideal in helping to learn these terms, we still provide breakdowns and other notes to help make the information stick in the student's memory.

d. *Essential words that don't break down*–We admit it. This method doesn't work for every word. Some words essential for students to know do not break into word components. They must be memorized. We include those words because they are crucial words for medical professionals to know. Our hope is that the inclusion of these words in the real-life health records and other contextualized learning environments in this book will support students in internalizing these essential terms.

3. **The Use of Roots in Place of Combining Forms**–we understand that it's common practice in medical terminology courses to teach students the difference between roots and combining forms. This is not a part of our approach and you will see that in this book the term *combining form* is absent and the term *root* has been used in its place. Here are the reasons why we decided to do this.

   a. In the real world of medical language, the classifications of root and combining form are nonexistent. The reason for this is that they mean virtually the same exact thing to health care professions in practice. The part of the term that is defined as a combining form can be used interchangeably with root without confusion. Also, word roots are more commonly used outside the world of medical terminology instruction. For our approach, using *root* instead of *combining form* prepares students better by presenting terminology as it is commonly used in broader health professions. If you were to hit Ctrl+F, to find and replace all instances of the word *root* with *combining form* in our text, nothing . . . NOTHING . . . is changed, lost, or unclear to the student.

   b. The importance of combining vowels and forms deals with how they impact pronunciation of terms, not definitions. Some instructors will argue but there is only a minimal difference in meaning, if any. We feel that great confusion is created by insisting on and highlighting the difference, as once a student completes the medical term class, being able to identify a component part as root or combining form is no longer practical. We do recognize this difference between a root and a combining form in Chapter 1 as follows: "When we say that a word part like cardi/o is a root, we aren't speaking precisely. Technically, cardi/o is called a combing form. A combining form is a combination of a root with a combining vowel."

   c. The word *root* is shorter than *combining form* by more than a third of letters (4 letters versus 13 letters). It may sound silly, but to us the purpose of teaching medical terminology is to streamline communication. The use of combining form is an unnecessary complication that doesn't bring value to the learner but may add potential confusion.

4. **Pronunciations Are Challenging for Students.**

   a. *We All Speak Differently*–English is an incredibly diverse language with numerous dialects and accents from all over the globe. One consequence of this is that we all speak in slightly different ways. Some of us break words into syllables at slightly different places or pronounce certain syllables differently. With that in mind, the pronunciation guides given in the book should be viewed as guidelines or directions, not universal laws.

   b. *Phonetic Versus Nonphonetic Syllable Breakdowns*–In the exercises, we frequently ask students to break words into syllables. When that happens, students might ask for guidance in doing this. Though we didn't explicitly break words into syllables, the syllable breakdown can be determined by looking at the phonetic pronunciation guide provided for each word. Encourage students to use critical thinking skills to align letters in the term with syllables in the guides.

   c. *For Example: Consider the Word* Salpingoscope. The phonetic pronunciation guide describes it as: sal-PING-goh-skohp. But how does that translate to syllable breakdown? Why is the *g* used in two syllables? Shouldn't it be either sal-pin-go-scope or sal-pingo-scope? Well, a case can be made for either of those two choices. The truth of the matter is that we all say the word slightly differently. The word is most accurately pronounced by leaving a little bit of the *g* in both syllables. Admit it, when you drop the *g* from PIN, you end up saying PIN a little bit differently. We say this not to complicate things but to encourage you to be flexible. We acknowledge that our pronunciation guides aren't etched in stone . . . more like etched in silly putty.

A Note from the Authors: To the Student

The purpose of this program is to equip you with foundational skills as you prepare for a career in health and medicine. As you enter the culture of medicine, you will need to speak the language to understand what is going on around you and to be understood by your colleagues and patients. Though learning medical language can seem a daunting task, it is our hope that this program reduces some of the anxiety that accompanies learning any new language. We hope this program shows you how clear the language of medicine is to understand as you begin to master some key concepts. As you get started, here are some helpful words of advice:

1. *Don't panic.* Immersing yourself in any new language can be intimidating. On occasion you will probably feel overwhelmed, like you are being bombarded with information you don't understand and don't know how to make sense of. Start by trying not to panic. Things always look intimidating when you begin. The water is always coldest when you first jump in. You will get used to it. Be patient. Follow the steps.
2. *Eat the elephant.* Do you know how to eat an elephant? One bite at a time. One of the easiest ways to keep from panicking is to break down things into easily digestible chunks. Don't focus on the total amount of information you have to learn; rather, focus on the bite in front of you.
3. *Practice makes permanent.* The easiest way to master medical language is to practice. You readily absorb what you are repeatedly exposed to. So practice. Repeat. Do it again. The more you do it, the more you will be able to do it, and the more you will enjoy doing it.
4. *Build bridges.* Medical language is everywhere: on TV shows, in the news, in your own life. Look for it. See if you can figure out the meaning of words you hear. Build connections between what you are learning and the world you live in. See how often you encounter these words. The more you practice it, the more it will be burned into your memory.

In addition to providing innovative approaches to learning medical terminology, McGraw-Hill Education wants to provide the materials you need in order to be successful. We are committed to providing you with high-quality, accurate resources.

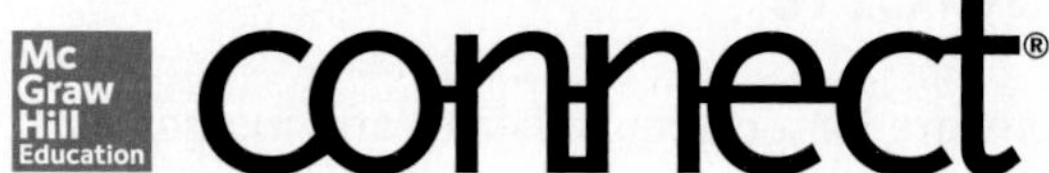

McGraw-Hill Connect® is a highly reliable, easy-to-use homework and learning management solution that utilizes learning science and award-winning adaptive tools to improve student results.

Homework and Adaptive Learning

- Connect's assignments help students contextualize what they've learned through application, so they can better understand the material and think critically.
- Connect will create a personalized study path customized to individual student needs through SmartBook®.
- SmartBook helps students study more efficiently by delivering an interactive reading experience through adaptive highlighting and review.

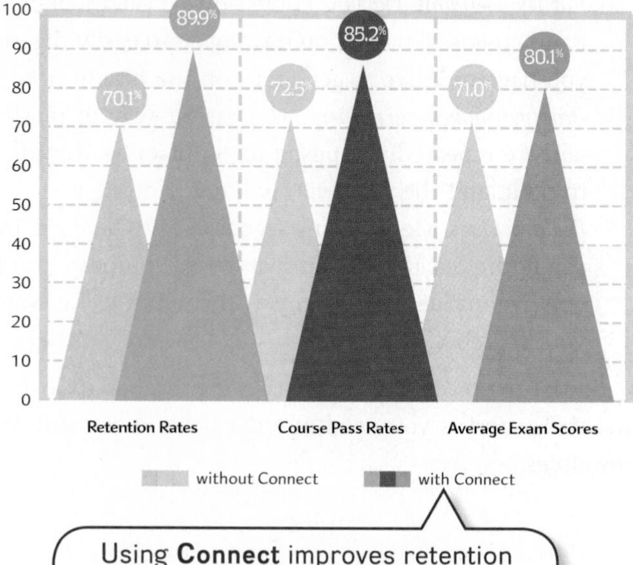

Using **Connect** improves retention rates by **19.8%**, passing rates by **12.7%, and** exam scores by **9.1%**.

Over **7 billion questions** have been answered, making McGraw-Hill Education products more intelligent, reliable, and precise.

73% of instructors who use **Connect** require it; instructor satisfaction **increases** by 28% when **Connect** is required.

Quality Content and Learning Resources

- Connect content is authored by the world's best subject matter experts, and is available to your class through a simple and intuitive interface.
- The Connect eBook makes it easy for students to access their reading material on smartphones and tablets. They can study on the go and don't need internet access to use the eBook as a reference, with full functionality.
- Multimedia content such as videos, simulations, and games drive student engagement and critical thinking skills.

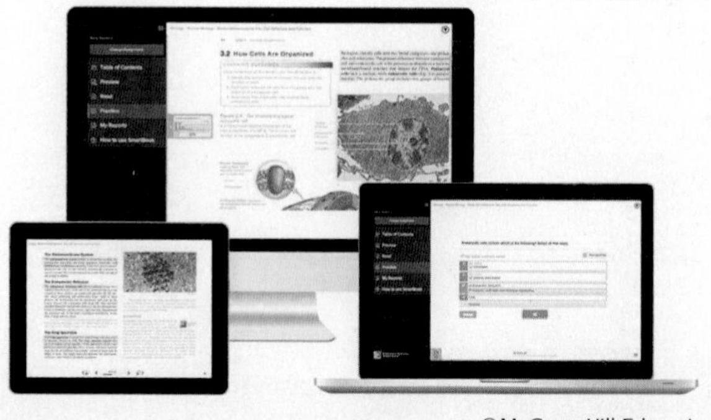

Robust Analytics and Reporting

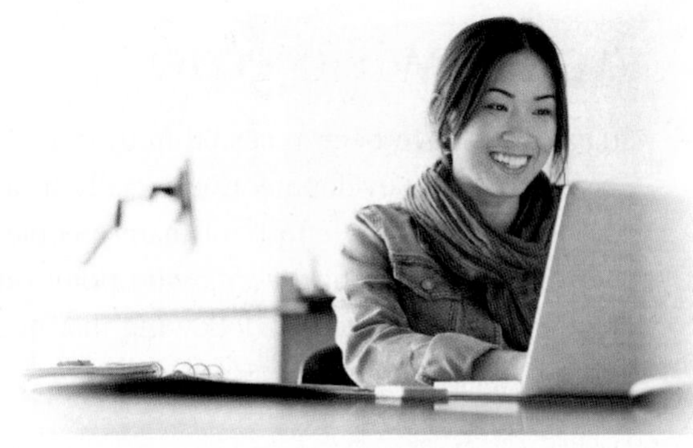

©Hero Images/Getty Images

- Connect Insight® generates easy-to-read reports on individual students, the class as a whole, and on specific assignments.
- The Connect Insight dashboard delivers data on performance, study behavior, and effort. Instructors can quickly identify students who struggle and focus on material that the class has yet to master.
- Connect automatically grades assignments and quizzes, providing easy-to-read reports on individual and class performance.

Impact on Final Course Grade Distribution

without Connect	Grade	with Connect
22.9%	A	31.0%
27.4%	B	34.3%
22.9%	C	18.7%
11.5%	D	6.1%
15.4%	F	9.9%

More students earn **As** and **Bs** when they use **Connect**.

Trusted Service and Support

- Connect integrates with your LMS to provide single sign-on and automatic syncing of grades. Integration with Blackboard®, D2L®, and Canvas also provides automatic syncing of the course calendar and assignment-level linking.
- Connect offers comprehensive service, support, and training throughout every phase of your implementation.
- If you're looking for some guidance on how to use Connect, or want to learn tips and tricks from super users, you can find tutorials as you work. Our Digital Faculty Consultants and Student Ambassadors offer insight into how to achieve the results you want with Connect.

Acknowledgments

Suggestions have been received from faculty and students throughout the country. This is vital feedback that is relied on for product development, especially in a second edition. Each person who has offered comments and suggestions has our thanks. The efforts of many people are needed to develop and improve a product. Among these people are the reviewers and consultants who point out areas of concern, cite areas of strength, and make recommendations for change. In this regard, the following instructors provided feedback that was enormously helpful in preparing the book and related products.

Survey Respondents

Many instructors participated in surveys to help guide the early development of the product.

Kim Bell, RHIA
Edgecombe Community College

Dorisann Halvorsen Brandt, MSPT
Greenville Technical College

Christine Chiappini-Williamson, PhD
Stark State College

Pamela Claybaker
Nashville State Community College

Kari Johnson Cook, MSRS, RT (R)
Northwestern State University

Ellen Stoehr Gallavan, RN, BSN, MA
Lansing Community College

Diana Gardner, MBA-HM, CPC, CMPE
Florence-Darlington Technical College

Jackie Gordon, CMA, NCPT, BS
South Suburban College

Susan Harrison, RN
William Rainey Harper College

Lisa Nowak
Waukesha County Technical College

Nancy Owens, RN, DNP
Somerset Community College

Susan Reading-Martin, MS, RN, CS, FNP, ARNP-BC
Western Nebraska Community College

Julie Schumacher, EdD, RD, LDN
Heartland Community College

Valentina Spencer Holder, RHIA, MEd
Pitt Community College

Susan Sykes Berry, RN, BSN, MLS, MA
University of Missouri–Kansas City

Manuscript Reviewers

Multiple instructors reviewed the manuscript while it was in development, providing valuable feedback that directly impacted the product.

Carole Berube, MA, MSN, BSN, RN
Bristol Community College

Cynthia Boles, CMA, MAN, MSHA
Bradford School–Pittsburgh

Mary Ellen Camier, CFS, MS, PhD
University of Maine

Amanda Campbell, MAT
Dorsey Business School

Steven Carlo, AAS, EMT-I, CI/C, BS
Erie Community College–North Campus

Christine Christensen, CCA
Williston State College

Janie Corbitt, RN, MLS
Central Georgia Technical College

Kelly Coreas, RRT, RRT-NPS, BSRT, MSHS
Mt. San Antonio College

Gerard Cronin, CCA, CCS-P, DC, BS
Salem Community College

Colleen Croxall, BA, MSHA, PhD
Eastern Michigan University

Heather Drake, ADN, BSN
Southern West Virginia Community and Technical College

Sally Erdel, BSN, CNE, MS, RN
Bethel College

Connie Erdmann, MS, CT (ASCP)
Utah Valley University

Robert E. Fanger, BS, MSEd
Del Mar College

Savanna Garrity, MPA
Madisonville Community College

Le'Nita Gilliam, BA, CET, CMA, CPT
Lansdale School of Business

Mandi N. Haynes, BSISM, RT (R), ARRT
South Arkansas Community College

Dolly R. Horton, CMA, MEd
AB Tech Community College

Judy Hurtt, MEd
East Central Community College

Cecelia Jacob, MA, MS
Southwest Tennessee Community College

Mark Jaffe, MHA, DPM
Nova Southeastern University

Susan Jaros, RN, MSN, CNP
Owens Community College

Patti Kalvelage, MS, OTR/L
Governors State University

Judith Karls, RN, BSN, MSEd
Madison Area Technical College

Barbara Klomp, BA, RT (R)
Macomb Community College

Jennifer Lame, RHIT, MPH
Southwest Wisconsin Technical College

Joseph K. LeJeune, CPFT, RRT, MS
University of Arkansas Community College at Hope

Cynthia Lowes, ADN, BSN
Southern West Virginia Community and Technical College

Wanda MacLeod, AHI, CMAA
Ross Medical Education Center

Michelle Maguire McDaniel, HCC, BA, CMA, LPN
Ivy Tech Community College

Amie L. Mayhall, MBA, CCA
Olney Central College

Wilsetta McClain, CPT, RMA, NCICS, PhD
Baker College of Auburn Hills

Charlotte Susie Myers, MA
University of Iowa

Alice Noblin, RHIA, CICS
University of Central Florida

Martha Olson, BSN, MS, RN
Iowa Lakes Community College

Tina Paduhovich, BA
Yorktowne Business Institute

Sally Pestana, BS, MT/PBT
Kapiolani Community College

Tammie Petersen, RNC-OB, BSN
Austin Community College

Stephen Picca, MD
Mandl School, the College of Allied Health

Rose M. Powell, PhD, RN
Stephen F. Austin State University

Adrienne Reaves, RMA
Westwood College

LuAnn Reicks, BC, BS, BSN, MSN, RN
Iowa Central Community College

Lisa Ritchie, EdD, RD, LD
Harding University

Lorinda G. Sipe, MS, RD
Front Range Community College

Angela Stahler, AAS, BS, RMA
Lincoln Technical Institute

Charlene Thiessen, MEd, CMT
Gateway Community College

Judy Truempler, RHIT
Idaho State University

Helen Weeks, MA, RMA
Henry Ford Community College

Kari Williams, BS, DC
Front Range Community College

Lori Warren Woodard, CCP, CPC, MA, RN, CPC-I, CLNC
Spencerian College

Technical Editing/Accuracy Panel

A panel of instructors completed a technical edit and review of the content in the book page proofs to verify its accuracy.

Denise Dedeaux, MBA
Fayetteville Technical Community College

Suzee Gay, LPN
Pinnacle Career Institute

Lori Hogue, CMA, RMA, CPT, LPT, LME
Mohave Community College

Sheila Newberry, PhD, RHIT
St. Petersburg College

Brian Spence, BSRS, RT(R)
Tarrant County College

Barbara Westrick, AAS, CMA (AAMA), CPC
Ross Medical Education Center

Digital Tool Development

Special thanks to the instructors who helped with the development of Connect, LearnSmart, and SmartBook.

Jim Hutchins, PhD
Weber State University

Carrie Mack, AS, CMA
Branford Hall Career Institute

Brian Spence, BSRS, RT(R),
Tarrant County College

Acknowledgments from the Authors

We would like to thank the following individuals who helped develop, critique, and shape our textbook, our digital materials, and our other ancillaries. We are grateful for the efforts of our team at McGraw-Hill Education who made all of this come together. We would especially like to thank Chad Grall, director of health professions; William Mulford, brand manager; Yvonne Lloyd, product developer; Harper Christopher, executive marketing manager; Angie FitzPatrick, program manager; Ann Courtney, Brent dela Cruz, and Mary Jane Lampe, content project managers; Matt Backhaus, designer; Susan Culbertson, buyer; Katherine Ward, digital product analyst; and Lori Hancock, content licensing specialist.

Acknowledgments from Steven L. Jones

Above all, I am grateful for the love and support of my family: my wife, Tamber, and our five children, Bethany, Rachel, Hannah, Madelyn, and Asa. I am also grateful for the support of the colleagues and friends at the universities I have taught at while completing this project. At the University of Texas: Karl Galinsky, my academic mentor; Lesley Dean-Jones, who first introduced me to medical terminology pedagogy; and Stephen White, who first gave me the opportunity to teach Medical Terminology. At Baylor University: Alden Smith for encouraging me to pursue this unusual academic project. At Houston Baptist University: Robert Sloan, president; Christopher Hammons, Micah Mattix, Timothy A. Brookins, Evan J. Getz, Gary Hartenburg, Jerry Walls, and Randy Hatchett. At Rice: Nicholas K. Iammarino, Chair of the Department of Kinesiology; and Jennifer Zinn-Winkler, the program administrator. In addition, I am deeply indebted to my friends for their encouragement: Daniel Benton, Michael Bordelon, Michael Czapla, Nathan Cook, Russell Thompson, Dan Euhus, and Brad Flurry.

Acknowledgments from Andrew Cavanagh

I am most thankful for the loving support of my wife, Ashley, and children, Katie, Nathaniel, and Jack. I owe a great debt of gratitude to my mother, Katherine Cavanagh, who worked tirelessly to provide for me as I grew up and passed on to me her admirable work ethic. I would also like to thank John Blevins for fostering my love of medicine and pediatrics and for being a great role model. I would like to thank Caughman Taylor and the entire residency training program at Palmetto Health Richland, University of South Carolina, for their amazing teaching and dedication to the lives of the residents. I am grateful for Chisholm Trail Pediatrics. It is a true joy to practice medicine in such a positive environment.

Introduction to Medical Language

1

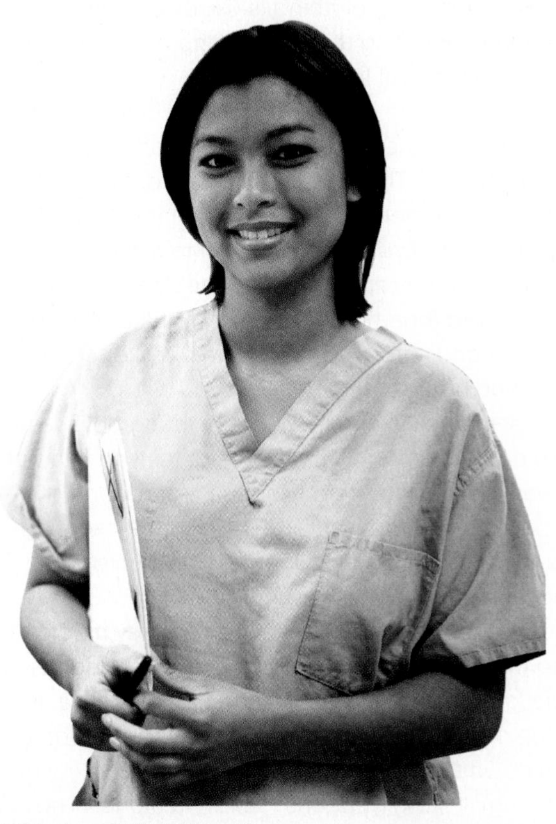

©AbleStock.com/360/GettyImages RF

learning outcomes

Upon completion of this chapter, you will be able to:

1.1 Summarize the purpose of **medical language.**

1.2 Summarize the origins of **medical language.**

1.3 Summarize the principles of **medical language.**

1.4 Summarize how to pronounce terms associated with **medical language.**

1.5 Identify the parts used to build **medical language.**

1.6 Summarize how to put together **medical terms.**

1.7 Describe how **medical terms** are translated.

Introduction

You've probably had conversations with people who like to use big words. Maybe you've responded with a blank expression and a sarcastic phrase—something like, "Say it in English, please!" This happens all the time in health care practices.

When a patient comes in for treatment, he or she is often bombarded with unfamiliar words. The patient leaves bewildered, wondering what the health care professional just said. Sometimes patients do get up the courage to ask what it all means and health care professionals explain in simpler terms. And patients wonder, "Well, why couldn't you have just said that in the first place? Why did you have to use all those big words?"

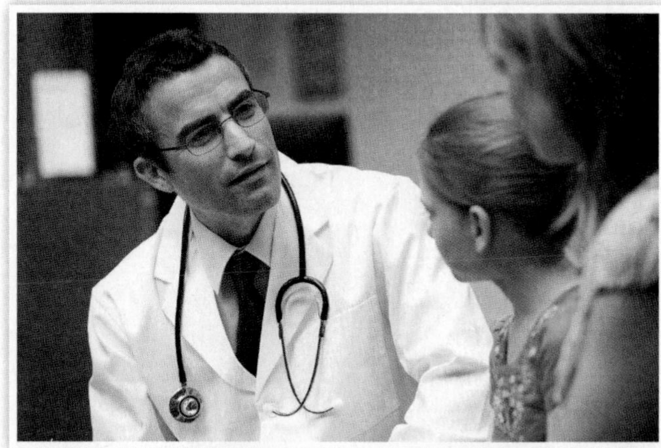

Talking with a doctor, nurse, or other health care professional can sometimes be bewildering or confusing.

©Adie Bush/Cultura/Getty Images RF

1.1 The Purpose of Medical Language

Why Is Medical Language Necessary?

"Why did you have to use all those big words?" is a good question. Why is medical language necessary? Following are a few reasons why medical language is both necessary and useful.

First, medical language allows health care professionals to be **clear**. Ours is a multicultural society. Many languages are spoken, each with their own words for illnesses and body parts. By using medical language, health care professionals are able to communicate and understand one another clearly, no matter what their first language is.

Second, medical language allows health care professionals to communicate **quickly**. Think about how this works in English. Instead of saying "a tall thing in the yard with green leaves," we just use the word "tree." Instead of saying "a meal made up of a few slices of meat and cheese, topped with lettuce, mustard, and mayonnaise, and placed between two slices of bread," we just say "sandwich." Instead of having to use valuable time describing the symptoms of a disease or the findings of an examination, a health care professional uses medical language in order to be clear and easily understandable to other health care professionals.

Third, medical language allows health care professionals to **comfort** patients. This reason might seem kind of odd, but it is true. When patients first enter a health care facility, they often don't feel well and are a little confused and worried about what is going on. Using medical language reassures patients that the health care professionals know what is going on and are in control. Sometimes a patient can be calmed and reassured that everything is OK by a health care professional repeating the same symptoms the patient reported—in medical language.

For example, one of us once saw a doctor about a rapid heart rate. The doctor was very reassuring—it was just "tachycardia." The doctor, however, didn't know he was talking to someone who was familiar with medical language. *Tachycardia* breaks down to *tachy* (fast, as in a car's *tachometer* reports the engine's revolutions per minute) + *card* (heart) + *ia* (condition). It literally means "fast heart condition." The doctor was just repeating what he had heard.

Here's another example. Once, a young boy was sick and his doctors performed a series of tests to find out what was wrong. After receiving the test reports, the boy's parents were reassured. The doctors had diagnosed their child with an "idiopathic blood disorder." The diagnosis was enough for them.

Because the doctor had attached a fancy medical term to their son's condition, the parents figured the doctors knew what was wrong and how to treat it. In truth, the doctor hadn't told them anything. *Idiopathic* breaks down to *idio* (private or alone) + *pathic* (disease or suffering). It literally means "suffering alone." The boy's condition was something the doctors had never seen before.

Medical language enables health care professionals to communicate quickly and easily no matter what their specific speciality or native language.

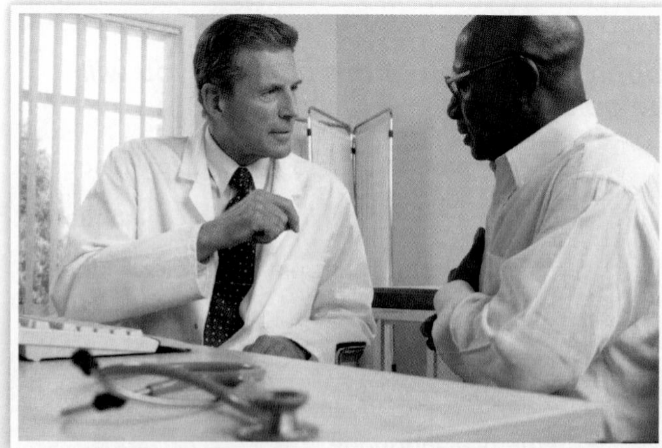

Medical language is able to reassure patients that health care professionals know what is going on and are in control.

Learning Outcome 1.1 Exercises

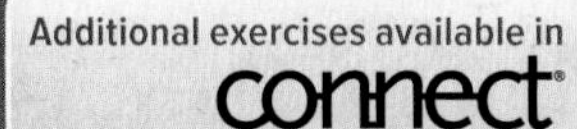

EXERCISE 1 *Multiple-choice questions. Select the correct answer.*

1. Which of the following is NOT a reason why medical language is necessary and useful?
   a. Medical language allows health care professionals to be clear.
   b. Medical language allows health care professionals to comfort patients.
   c. Medical language allows health care professionals to communicate quickly.
   d. Medical language allows health care professionals to intimidate their patients.
2. Medical language allows health care professionals to be clear because:
   a. few people really understand medical terminology, so at least everyone is speaking the same way
   b. health care professionals are in control of the situation and don't want to scare patients with a language that they could understand
   c. we live in a multicultural society with a variety of languages, and medical language is a way of speaking the same way about the same thing despite your native language
   d. none of these
3. Medical language allows health care professionals to communicate quickly because:
   a. it is a quick way to speak to other health care professionals without taking the time to describe symptoms or examine findings
   b. the patients are usually baffled by the terminology and do not ask additional questions
   c. words with many syllables always communicate more information than words with few syllables
   d. none of these
4. Medical language allows health care professionals to comfort patients because:
   a. it communicates a sense that the health care professionals are in control of the situation
   b. it lets the patients know that the health care professionals are not caught off guard by the symptoms at hand
   c. it lets the patients know that the health care professionals know what is going on
   d. all of these

1.2 The Origins of Medical Language

Where Does It Come From?

Medical language is made up primarily (but not exclusively) of words taken from two ancient languages: Greek and Latin. Other words creep in from other sources, but Greek and Latin serve as the foundation of medical language.

Some of these other sources include:

Eponyms. The word *eponym* is derived from the Greek words *epi* (upon) + *onyma* (name). It literally means "to put your name on something." Thus, an eponym is a word formed by including the name of the person who discovered or invented whatever is being described. Sometimes, in the case of diseases, an eponym is named in honor of the disease's first or most noteworthy diagnosed victim.

This reminds us of a great old joke.

A doctor says to a patient, "I have good news and bad news. Which do you want first?"

The patient responds, "The good news."

The doctor replies, "Well, you are about to have a disease named after you."

One famous eponym is Lou Gehrig's disease. The neurological disease was named after the famous New York Yankee first baseman who suffered from the disease. The disease's scientific name is *amyotrophic lateral sclerosis.*

Acronyms. The word *acronym* is derived from the Greek words *acro* (high, end) + *onyma* (name). It literally means "to make a name with the ends." Thus, an acronym is a word made up of the first letters of each of the words that make up a phrase. One example is the diagnostic imaging process called **m**agnetic **r**esonance **i**maging, or MRI. Remember that acronyms are just shorthand—you still need to know what the words mean.

Modern languages. Frequently, words from modern languages creep into the vocabulary of health care professionals. These words tend to come from whatever language happens to be most commonly spoken by the majority of health care professionals. In centuries past, German or French were the most common languages, so they were the foundation of many medical terms. Currently, the fastest-growing and most-used language in the world is English. Thus, English has also contributed a fair number of medical terms.

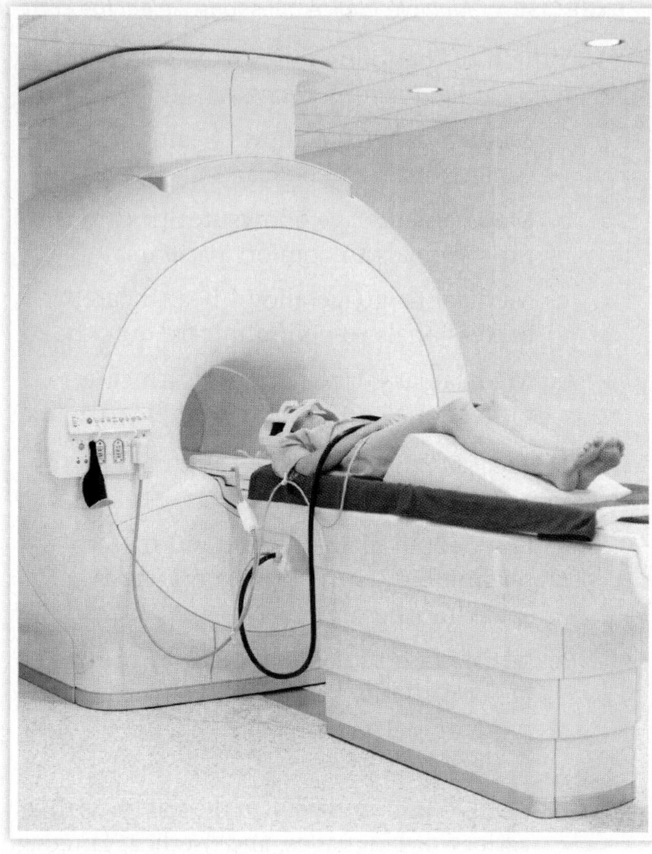

MRI, which stands for **m**agnetic **r**esonance **i**maging, is an example of an acronym.

Why Greek and Latin?

Although the three previously mentioned categories have contributed a significant number of words to the language of medicine, Greek and Latin make up its foundation and backbone. Even *eponym* and *acronym* were derived from Greek! But why are Greek and Latin so prevalent? There are at least three reasons why.

Reason 1: The foundations of Western medicine were in ancient Greece and Rome. The first people to systematically study the human body and develop theories about health and disease were the ancient Greeks. The Hippocratic Oath, the foundation of modern medical ethical codes, is named after and was possibly composed by a man named Hippocrates who lived in Greece from about 460 BC to about 370 BC. Hippocrates is widely considered to be the father of Western medicine.

The development of the health care profession began in ancient Greece and continued in ancient Rome. There, Galen, who lived from AD 129 to about AD 217, made some of the greatest advancements of our understanding of the human body, how disease affects it, and how drugs work.

Medical advances began to occur with greater frequency during the scientific revolution, adding to an already existing body of knowledge based on ancient Greek and Latin. In fact, some of the oldest terms have been in use for more than 2,000 years, such as terms for the skin, because these body parts were more easily viewed and studied.

Reason 2: Latin was the global language of the scientific revolution. The scientific revolution took place from the sixteenth through the eighteenth century. It was a time of enormous discoveries in physics, biology, chemistry, and human anatomy. This period saw a rapid increase in human knowledge thanks to the scientific method, which is a set of techniques developed in this period and still in use today using observation and experimentation for developing, testing, and proving or disproving hypotheses.

Medical research involving many different subjects, people, and places occurred all over Europe. To allow people from England, Italy, Spain, Poland, and elsewhere to talk with one another, Latin became the language of scholarly discussion. It was already the common language of the Holy Roman Empire and Catholic church, so many people already knew it well.

By using Latin to record and spread news of their discoveries, scientists of this time were able to share their new knowledge beyond the borders of their countries. At the same time, the number of medical words that sprang from Latin grew.

Reason 3: Dead languages don't change. "Fine," you think. "The language of medicine is based on Greek and Latin. But why do we keep using it? No one speaks either of these languages anymore. Why don't we just use English?"

The reason we keep using Greek and Latin is exactly that—no one speaks them anymore. All spoken languages change over time. Take the English word *green,* for instance, and its non-color-related meaning. In the past 20 or so years, the word *green* has become understood to mean "environmentally responsible," as in the phrase "green energy." Before that, the term was widely understood to mean something different: "immature or inexperienced," such as "I just started this job, so I am still a little green." Dead languages, which aren't spoken anymore, have an advantage because they don't change. There is no worry that words will change their meaning over time.

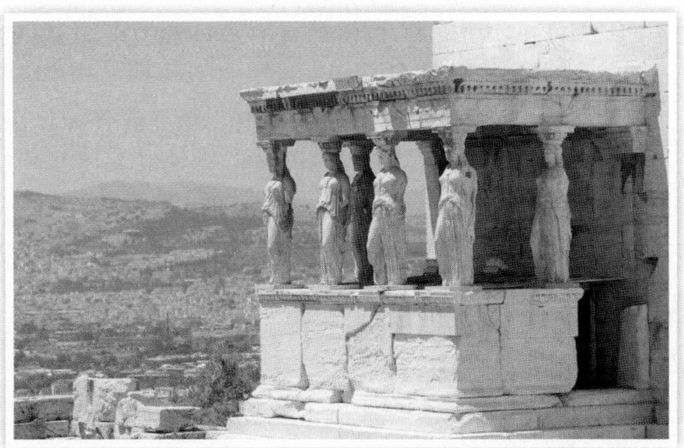

The foundations of Western medicine were laid in Greece and Rome.

Learning Outcome 1.2 Exercises

EXERCISE 1 *True or false questions. Indicate true answers with a T and false answers with an F.*

1. Medical language is made up primarily, but not exclusively, of words taken from two ancient languages: Greek and Latin. ____
2. Some other sources of medical language include eponyms, acronyms, and modern languages. ____
3. An example of an eponym is a medical term named after a famous patient who had the disease. ____
4. MRI is an example of an eponym. ____
5. Acronyms are used to say things more quickly. ____
6. Greek and Latin provide the basis of the language of medicine because Western medicine has its foundations in the Greek and Roman cultures. ____
7. The first people to systematically study the human body and develop theories about health and disease were the ancient Greeks. ____
8. Even though German was the global language of the scientific revolution, the Catholic church forced all academics to use Latin, a language unknown to most people. ____
9. During the scientific revolution, Latin was used as the language of scholarly discussion in order to allow people across Europe to share their knowledge more quickly despite their different native languages. ____
10. A dead language is a language that people do not like to hear or speak anymore because it is no longer useful to a society. ____
11. Latin and Greek provide an excellent basis for medical terminology because dead languages do not change. ____

1.3 The Principles of Medical Language

How Does It Work?

Don't think of medical language as words to be memorized. Instead, they are sentences to be translated.[1]

Each medical word is a description of some aspect of health care. Think of it this way: If you were taking a trip to another country, you might try to memorize a few key words or phrases. It might be useful to know how to say common things like "Where is the bathroom?" or "How much does this cost?" But if you were going to live in that country for a while, you wouldn't just try to memorize a few stock phrases, you would try to learn the language so you could understand what other people were saying.

The same is true of medical language. If you understand the way the language works, you will be able to not only to know the meaning of a few individual words, but also to break down and understand words you have never seen before, and even generate words on your own.

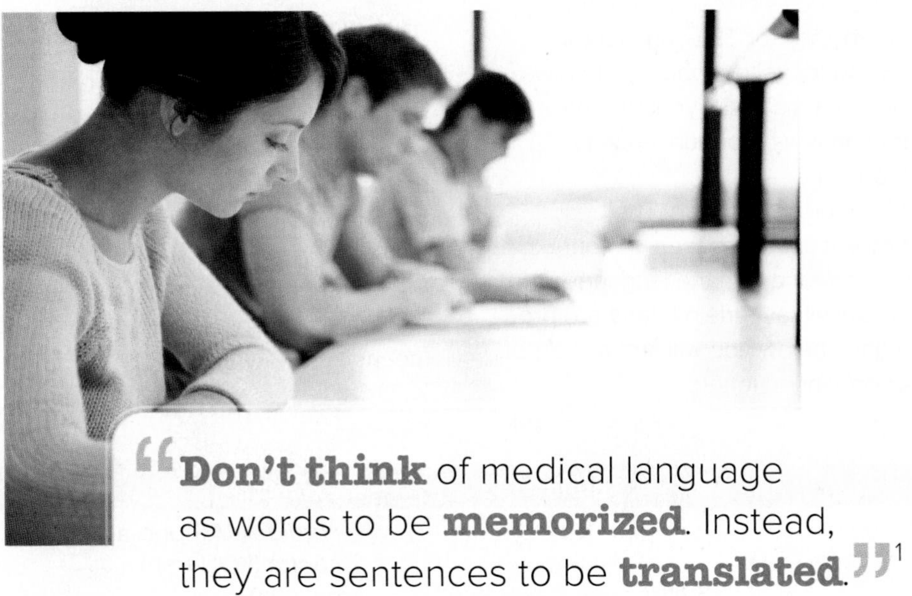

"**Don't think** of medical language as words to be **memorized**. Instead, they are sentences to be **translated**."[1]

©S.Olsson/PhotoAlto RF

[1] For more on this concept, see Lesley A. Dean-Jones, "Teaching Medical Terminology as a Classics Course," *Classical Journal* 93 (1998): 290–96.

1.4 How to Pronounce Terms Associated with Medical Language

The first step in learning any language is learning correct pronunciation. Like any other language, knowing and understanding medical terminology is useless unless you pronounce the terms correctly. With medical terms, the matter is complicated by two facts: First, many of the words come from foreign languages (and not just any foreign languages, but foreign languages no one speaks anymore). Second, some of the words are really long.

You probably have noticed the way native speakers of other languages pronounce certain letters differently. Think of the word *tortilla*. It takes a bit of experience with Spanish to know that two *l*'s placed together (*ll*) is pronounced like a *y*. You say tor-TEE-yah, not tor-TILL-ah. The Spanish word for yellow, *amarillo,* follows this rule. It is pronounced ah-mah-REE-yoh. But the Texas town of the same name is pronounced very differently: am-ah-RIL-oh.

The same is true for medical language. The best way to learn terms is by encountering them in context. Once you get a little experience with the language, you will pick up the unique ways that certain letters are pronounced. In the meantime, below you will find a chart of some commonly mispronounced letters.

Syllable Emphasis

Every medical term is constructed from syllables. Another thing that can affect the way words are pronounced is which syllable or syllables should be stressed, or emphasized. You must always make sure to put the emphasis on the right syllable.

For example, consider that last phrase: *Put the emphasis on the right syllable.* The correct way to pronounce it would be:

PUT the EM-fah-sis on the RAIT SIL-ah-bul.

It would sound funny to say:

PUT the em-FAH-sis on the RAIT si-LAH-bul.

Knowing which syllable to emphasize can seem tricky, but is actually pretty easy. Usually, for the sake of emphasis, the only syllables that you need to focus on are these last three syllables. So, starting at the end of the word, count back three syllables.

Although they are not terribly important to know, there are names for the various syllables in a word:

The last syllable is called the *ultima,* which means "last."

Letter	Sound	Example
c (before *a, o, u*)	k	*cardiac* (KAR-dee-ak) *contra* (KON-trah) *cut* (KUT)
c (before *e, i, y*)	s	*cephalic* (seh-FAL-ik) *cilium* (SIL-ee-um) *cyst* (SIST)
ch	k	*chiropractor* (KAI-roh-PRAK-tor)
g (before *a, o, u*)	g	*gamma* (GAM-ah) *goiter* (GOI-ter) *gutta* (GUT-tah)
g (before e, *i, y*)	j	*genetic* (jeh-NEH-tik) *giant* (JAI-int) *biology* (bai-AW-loh-jee)
ph	f	*pharmacy* (FAR-mah-see)
pn	n	*pneumonia* (noo-MOHN-yah)
pt (initial)	t	*pterigium* (tir-IH-jee-um)
rh, rrh	r	*rhinoplasty* (RAI-noh-PLAS-tee) *hemorrhage* (HEH-moh-rij)
x (initial)	z	*xeroderma* (ZER-oh-DER-mah)

The second-to-last syllable is called the *penult,* which means "almost the last." The prefix *pen-* means "almost." Think of the word *peninsula,* which is a body of land with water on three sides. The word literally translates to "almost an island."

The third-to-last syllable is called the *antepenult.* The literal translation of this word is one of our favorites. *Ante-* means "before," so *antepenult* means "the one before the one that is almost the last." When it comes to emphasizing the right syllable, the basic rule is this: In most words, the emphasis usually falls on the third-to-last syllable (the *antepenult,* if you are keeping track).

> *Cardiac* is split into three syllables: car / di / ac.
>
> Count backward three syllables from the end of the word to figure out which syllable gets emphasized: *car.*
>
> Therefore, the word is pronounced **KAR** / dee / ak.

> *Cardiology* is split into five syllables: car / di / o / lo / gy.
>
> Count backward three syllables from the end of the word to figure out which syllable gets emphasized: *o.*
>
> Therefore, the word is pronounced kar / dee / **AW** / loh / jee.

It gets tricky when a word remains unchanged except for the addition or subtraction of only a few letters. Two good examples are the words *colonoscopy* and *colonoscope.*

> *Colonoscopy* is split into five syllables: co / lon / o / sco / py.
>
> Count backward three syllables from the end of the word to figure out which syllable gets emphasized: *o.*
>
> Therefore, the word is pronounced koh / lon / **AW** / skoh / pee.

> *Colonoscope* is split into four syllables: co / lon / o / scope.
>
> Count backward three syllables from the end of the word to figure out which syllable gets emphasized: *lon.*
>
> Therefore, the word is pronounced koh / **LAWN** / oh / skohp.

Notice how easy it is to spot the pronunciation change if you focus on counting backward from the end of the word?

As with any rule, there are countless exceptions and technicalities. That said, the easiest way to master pronunciation is not to learn countless rules, but instead to *practice pronouncing words.* Learn this one rule—let's call it the three-syllable rule—and make sure you take note of the pronunciations offered throughout the chapters. Don't just read them silently! Pronounce the words out loud. The more times you practice saying a word, the more comfortable and natural you will feel when you have to use it for real.

But make sure you are pronouncing correctly. Practice does *not* make perfect; practice makes permanent. Whatever you do over and over will be cemented in your brain, so make sure you do it right. *Perfect* practice makes perfect.

Learning Outcome 1.4 Exercises

EXERCISE 1 *Identify the correct pronunciation for the underlined syllable.*

EXAMPLES: thora**co**centesis *answer: koh (the c is hard because it is followed by an* ***o****)*
thora**cen**tesis *answer: sin (the c is soft because it is followed by an* ***i****)*

______	1. **gut**	a. jut	b. gut
______	2. di**git**	a. jit	b. git
______	3. **gag** reflex	a. jag	b. gag
______	4. dermatolo**gy**	a. jee	b. gee
______	5. **ge**neticist	a. jen	b. gen
______	6. **go**nad	a. joh	b. goh
______	7. colla**gen**	a. jen	b. gen
______	8. **phar**macist	a. par	b. far
______	9. **cu**ticle	a. kyoo	b. suh
______	10. **cor**nea	a. kor	b. sor
______	11. **cath**eter	a. kath	b. sath
______	12. on**co**logy	a. kaw	b. saw
______	13. geneti**cist**	a. kist	b. sist
______	14. pharma**cist**	a. kist	b. sist
______	15. **cys**tic fibrosis	a. kis	b. sis
______	16. **cho**lera	a. kawl	b. chohl
______	17. psy**cho**sis	a. koh	b. choh
______	18. pneumato**cele**	a. keel	b. seel
______	19. **rheu**matoid arthritis	a. roo	b. rhee-yoo
______	20. **pneu**matocele	a. noo	b. puh-noo
______	21. **pter**ion	a. tir	b. puh-tir
______	22. **xer**osis	a. zer	b. ex-er
______	23. en**cepha**litis	a. kep	b. sef
______	24. **cirrho**sis	a. kir-hoh	b. sir-oh

EXERCISE 2 *Indicate which syllable is emphasized when pronounced.*

EXAMPLE: bronchitis bron**chi**tis

1. cholera ______________________________
2. cornea ______________________________
3. cuticle ______________________________

Learning Outcome 1.4 Exercises

4. catheter ________________
5. collagen ________________
6. anemia ________________
7. oncology ________________
8. optometry ________________
9. rheumatoid ________________
10. geneticist ________________
11. dermatology ________________
12. psychotherapist ________________

1.5 Parts Used to Build Medical Language

Just as any language has nouns, verbs, and adjectives, the language of medicine is made up of three main building blocks: roots, suffixes, and prefixes. Medical language is constructed by combining a root with a suffix and often a prefix.

Root—foundation or subject of the term
Suffix—ending that gives essential meaning to the term
Prefix—added to the beginning of a term when needed to further modify the root

Common Roots

A root is the foundation of any medical term. Roots function like nouns in the language of medicine. It is the base, or subject, of a word—it is what the word is about. Most roots refer to things like body parts, organs, and fluids.

There are a few types of roots in medical language. In the roots that follow, notice that a slash divides the last letter from the rest of the word (as in *arthr/o*). The final letter in these roots is called a *combining vowel*; these are discussed in detail later in the chapter. For now, just know that the final letter occurs in some words and not in others. Whenever possible, the examples provided include both words that use a combining vowel and words that don't. Don't worry about what the example words mean. This is just to get you used to seeing the roots in context.

Some meanings have only one potential root.

Root	Definition	Examples
arthr/o AR-throh	joint	*arthroscope, arthritis*
cardi/o KAR-dee-oh	heart	*cardiology, pericardium*
enter/o EN-ter-oh	small intestine	*enteropathy, dysentery*
gastr/o GAS-tro	stomach	*gastrointestinal, gastritis*

Root	Definition	Examples
hepat/o he-PAH-toh	liver	*hepatology, hepatitis*
neur/o NUR-oh	nerve	*neurology, neuralgia*

Some meanings have a few similar-sounding potential roots. Why? Some suffixes just sound better when attached to another root. Look at the examples in the chart below and switch the roots around—*hematorrhage* and *hemoma*. The meanings are the same, but they sure sound funny.

Root	Definition	Examples
hem/o HEE-moh	blood	*hemorrhage*
hemat/o heh-MAH-toh		*hematoma*

Some meanings have a couple of potential roots that are completely different but mean the same thing. This is because one word comes from Greek and the other comes from Latin. Normally, however, one of the roots is much more commonly used than the other. As shown below, *myo* is used much more often than *musculo.*

Root	Definition	Examples
my/o MAI-oh	muscle	*myocardial, myalgia*
muscul/o MUS-kyoo-loh		*musculoskeletal, muscular*

Some meanings have several potential roots that mean the same thing. Some are similar, and some are completely different. These are basically a combination of the two previous categories. These meanings each have a couple of similar roots *as well as* at least one root from Greek and one from Latin.

Question: Why doesn't each meaning have only one potential root?

Answer: The main reason multiple roots are available is to provide *options*. Some suffixes simply sound better or are easier to say when they are combined with one root rather than another.

Root	Definition	Examples
angi/o AN-gee-oh	vessel (most commonly refers to blood vessel, but can also refer to other types of vessels as well)	*angioplasty, angiectomy* ©BioPhoto Assoc./Science Source
vas/o VAS-oh		*vasospasm, vasectomy*
vascul/o VAS-kyoo-loh		*vasculopathy, vasculitis*
derm/o DER-moh	skin	*dermoscopy, dermis*
dermat/o der-MAT-oh		*dermatology, dermatitis*
cutane/o kyoo-TAY-nee-oh		*subcutaneous*
pneum/o NOO-moh	lung	*pneumotomy*
pneumon/o noo-MAW-noh		*pneumonia, pneumonitis*
pulmon/o PUL-maw-noh		*pulmonologist, cardiopulmonary*

GENERAL-PURPOSE ROOTS

This list contains roots that will recur often in multiple chapters. It is important to learn these roots now.

Root	Definition	Examples
gen/o JIN-oh	creation, cause	*pathogenic*
hydr/o HAI-droh	water	*hydrophobia, dehydration* ©Comstock Images RF
morph/o MOR-foh	change	*morphology*
myc/o MAI-koh	fungus	*dermatomycosis*
necr/o NEK-roh	death	*necrosis*
orth/o OR-thoh	straight	*orthodontist*
path/o PAH-thoh	suffering, disease	*pathology*
phag/o FAY-goh	eat	*aphagia*
plas/o PLAS-oh	formation	*hyperplasia*
py/o PAI-oh	pus	*pyorrhea, pyemia*
scler/o SKLEH-roh	hard	*scleroderma*
sten/o STIH-noh	narrowing	*stenosis* ©Scott Camazine/ScienceSource
troph/o TROH-foh	nourishment, development	*trophology, hypertrophy*
xen/o ZEE-noh	foreign	*xenograft*

Common Suffixes

A *suffix* is a word part placed at the end of a word. The word *suffix* literally means "to attach (fix) after or below (sub, which if you say it fast starts to sound like suff)." As roots function as nouns, so suffixes function as verbs in the language of medicine. They describe something the root is doing, or something that is happening to the root.

There are many types of suffixes in medical language. In general, they can be divided into two basic groups: simple and complex.

SIMPLE SUFFIXES

These suffixes (as their name suggests) are basic and are used to turn a root into a complete word.

Adjective. These suffixes turn the root they follow into an adjective. Thus, they all mean "pertaining to," or something similar to that.

Suffix	Definition	Examples
-ac ak	pertaining to	*cardiac*
-al al		*skeletal*
-ar ar		*muscular*
-ary ar-ee		*pulmonary*
-eal ee-al		*esophageal*
-ic ik		*medic*
-tic tik		*neurotic*
-ous us		*subcutaneous*

Noun. All of these suffixes turn the root they are added to into nouns.

Suffix	Definition	Examples
-ia ee-ah	condition	*pneumonia*
-ism iz-um		*autism*
-ium ee-um	tissue, structure	*pericardium*
-y ee	condition, procedure	*hypertrophy*

Diminutive. When added to a root, these suffixes transform a term's meaning to a smaller version of the root. In English, for example, the suffix *-let* is diminutive. A *booklet* is a "little book." In Spanish, the suffix *-ita* is diminutive. *Señora* is the Spanish word for *lady,* so *señorita* therefore means "little lady."

Suffix	Definition	Examples
-icle ik-el	small	*ventricle*
-ole ohl		*arteriole*
-ule yool		*pustule*
-ula yoo-lah		*uvula*

COMPLEX SUFFIXES

Complex suffixes aren't necessarily more difficult to understand than simple suffixes. They just have more parts. Sometimes, these suffixes are referred to as compound or combination suffixes because the suffixes themselves are put together from other suffixes, roots, and prefixes.

Following is an example.

> The suffix *-y* means "condition" or "procedure." When combined with *tom/o*, a root meaning "to cut," the result is the complex suffix *-tomy*, which means "a cutting procedure" or "incision."
>
> *tom/o* (cut) + *-y* (process) = *-tomy* = a cutting procedure or incision
>
> But you can take it a step further. If you add the prefix *ec-* to *-tomy*, you will create the complex suffix -ectomy, which means "to cut out" or "to surgically remove something."
>
> *ec-* (out) + *tom/o* (cut) + *-y* (process) = *-ectomy* = a cutting out procedure or surgical removal

Though it is useful to understand how complex suffixes are able to be broken down into smaller parts, throughout this book, we will keep the complex suffixes together and provide a single definition for their meaning instead of breaking them down further.

Following are lists of some categories of complex suffixes. Some complex suffixes are professional terms.

Suffix	Definition	Examples
-iatrics ee-AH-triks	medical science	*pediatrics* ©Anna Grigorjeva/123 RF
-iatry AI-ah-tree		*psychiatry*
-iatrist EE-ah-trist	specialist in medicine of	*psychiatrist*
-ist ist	specialist	*dentist*
-logist loh-jist	specialist in the study of	*psychologist* ©Don Hammond/Design Pics RF
-logy loh-jee	study of	*psychology*

Some complex suffixes describe symptoms, diseases, or conditions that are either mentioned by patients or diagnosed by health professionals.

symptoms, diseases, and conditions

Suffix	Definition	Examples
-algia AL-jah	pain	*myalgia*
-dynia DAI-nee-ah		*gastrodynia*
-cele SEEL	hernia (a bulging of tissue into an area where it doesn't belong)	*hydrocele*

symptoms, diseases, and conditions *continued*

Suffix	Definition	Examples
-emia EE-mee-ah	blood condition	*leukemia* ©Science Photo Library RF/Getty Images RF
-iasis AI-ah-sis	presence of	*lithiasis*
-itis AI-tis	inflammation	*arthritis*
-lysis lih-sis	loosen, break down	*hemolysis*
-malacia mah-LAY-shah	abnormal softening	*osteomalacia*
-megaly MEH-gah-lee	enlargement	*hepatomegaly*
-oid OYD	resembling	*keloid*
-oma OH-mah	tumor	*melanoma* Source: National Cancer Institute (NCI)
-osis OH-sis	condition	*thrombosis*
-pathy pah-thee	disease	*myopathy*
-penia PEE-nee-ah	deficiency	*leukopenia*
-ptosis puh-TOH-sis	drooping	*nephroptosis*
-rrhage RIJ	excessive flow	*hemorrhage*
-rrhagia RAY-jee-ah		*menorrhagia*
-rrhea REE-ah	flow	*diarrhea*
-rrhexis REK-sis	rupture	*metrorrhexis*
-spasm SPAZ-um	involuntary contraction	*myospasm*

Some complex suffixes describe tests and treatments performed by health professionals. Although it is convenient to place tests and treatments in the same category and label them as "procedures," it is important to distinguish between the two. A *test* is a *procedure done to gain more information in order to diagnose a problem.* A *treatment* is a *process done after a diagnosis to fix a problem.*

tests

Suffix	Definition	Examples
-centesis sin-TEE-sis	puncture	*amniocentesis*
-gram gram	written record	*cardiogram* ©Stockbyte/PunchStock RF
-graph graf	instrument used to produce a record	*cardiograph*
-graphy grah-fee	writing procedure	*cardiography*
-meter mee-ter	instrument used to measure	*cephalometer*
-metry meh-tree	process of measuring	*cephalometry*
-scope skohp	instrument used to look	*arthroscope*
-scopy skoh-pee	process of looking	*arthroscopy*

treatments

Suffix	Definition	Examples
-desis DEE-sis	binding, fixation	*arthrodesis*
-ectomy EK-toh-mee	removal	*vasectomy*
-pexy PEK-see	surgical fixation	*retinopexy*
-plasty PLAS-tee	reconstruction	*rhinoplasty*
-rrhaphy rah-fee	suture	*herniorrhaphy*
-stomy stoh-mee	creation of an opening	*colostomy*
-tomy toh-mee	incision	*dermotomy*

SINGULARS AND PLURALS

In English, the most common way to turn a word from singular to plural is to add an *s*. The plural of *bag* is *bags*, for example. But there are other ways too. The plural of *goose* is *geese*. The plural of *mouse* is *mice*. The plural of *ox* is *oxen*. The plural of *sheep* is *sheep*.

The same is true for medical terms. Because medical words come from different languages, singular words become plural in a variety of ways.

Singular	Plural	Examples	
-a	*-ae*	*vertebra* *larva*	*vertebrae* *larvae*
-ax	*-aces*	*thorax*	*thoraces*
-ex	*-ices*	*cortex*	*cortices*
-ix	*-ices*	*appendix*	*appendices*
-is	*-es*	*neurosis* *diagnosis*	*neuroses* *diagnoses*
-ma	*-mata*	*sarcoma* *carcinoma*	*sarcomata* *carcinomata*
-on	*-a*	*spermatozoon* *ganglion*	*spermatozoa* *ganglia*
-um	*-a*	*datum* *bacterium* *ovum*	*data* *bacteria* *ova*
-us	*-i*	*nucleus* *alveolus* *thrombus*	*nuclei* *alveoli* *thrombi*
-y	*-ies*	*biopsy* *myopathy*	*biopsies* *myopathies*

Common Prefixes

A *prefix* is a word part placed at the beginning of a word. The word *prefix* literally means "to attach (fix) before (pre)." Prefixes function like adjectives in the language of medicine. They supply additional information as needed. In the same way that not every sentence has an adjective, not every medical term has a prefix.

There are many types of prefixes in medical language. Following are a few examples.

NEGATION PREFIXES

Some prefixes negate things:

negation		
Prefix	**Meaning**	**Examples**
a- ay	not	*aphasia*
an- an		*anemia*
anti- AN-tee	against	*antibiotics*
contra- KON-trah		*contraceptive*
de- dee	down, away from	*dehydration*

TIME OR SPEED PREFIXES

Some prefixes describe time or speed:

time/speed

Prefix	Meaning	Examples
ante- an-tee	before	*antepartum*
pre- pree		*precondition*
pro- proh	before, on behalf of	*probiotic* ©McGraw-Hill Education/Bob Coyle, photographer
brady- brah-dih	slow	*bradycardia*
tachy- tak-ih	fast	*tachycardia*
post- pohst	after	*postpartum*
re- ree	again	*rehabilitation*

DIRECTION OR POSITION PREFIXES

Some prefixes describe direction or position:

direction/position

Prefix	Meaning	Examples
ab- ab	away	*abduct*
ad- ad	toward	*adrenaline*
circum- sir-kum	around	*circumcision*
peri- per-ee		*pericardium*
dia- dai-ah	through	*diagnostic*
trans- tranz		*translate*
e- eh	out	*evoke*
ec- ek		*ectopic*
ex- eks		*exhale*

direction/position *continued*

Prefix	Meaning	Examples
ecto- ek-toh	outside	*ectoderm*
exo- ek-soh		*exoskeleton*
extra- eks-trah		
en- en	in, inside	*enema*
endo- en-doh		*endocrine*
intra- in-trah		*intravenous* ©mmmx/123RF RF
epi- eh-pee	upon	*epididymus*
sub- sub	beneath	*subcutaneous*
inter- in-ter	between	*intercostal*

SIZE OR QUANTITY PREFIXES

Some prefixes describe size or quantity:

size/quantity

Prefix	Meaning	Examples
bi- bai	two	*bilateral*
hemi- heh-mee	half	*hemiplegia*
semi- seh-mee		*semilunar*
hyper- hai-per	over	*hyperthermia*
hypo- hai-poh	under	*hypothermia*
macro- mak-roh	large	*macrotia*
micro- mai-kroh	small	*microdontia*

size/quantity *continued*

Prefix	Meaning	Examples
mono- maw-noh	one	*monocyte*
uni- yoo-nee		*unisex*
oligo- aw-lih-goh	few	*oligomenorrhea*
pan- pan	all	*pancytopenia*
poly- pawlee	many	*polygraph*
multi- mul-tee		*multicellular*

GENERAL PREFIXES

Some prefixes are general:

other

Prefix	Meaning	Examples
con- kon	with, together	*congestion* ©Image Source/DigitalVision/Getty Images RF
syn- sin		*syndrome*
sym- sim		*symmetry*
dys- dis	bad	*dysentery*
eu- yoo	good	*euphoria*

Learning Outcome 1.5 Exercises

EXERCISE 1 *Match the root on the left with its definition on the right.*

_____ 1. neur/o — a. heart
_____ 2. cardi/o — b. joint
_____ 3. arthr/o — c. liver
_____ 4. gastr/o — d. nerve
_____ 5. hepat/o — e. small intestine
_____ 6. enter/o — f. stomach

EXERCISE 2 *Translate the following roots.*

1. neur/o _____
2. cardi/o _____
3. arthr/o _____
4. gastr/o _____
5. hepat/o _____
6. enter/o _____

EXERCISE 3 *Underline and define the root in the following terms.*

1. cardiology _____
2. neurology _____
3. gastroscope _____
4. arthroscopy _____
5. enterology _____
6. hepatology _____

EXERCISE 4 *Identify the roots for the following definitions.*

1. heart _____
2. joint _____
3. nerve _____
4. stomach _____
5. liver _____
6. small intestine _____

EXERCISE 5 *Match the root on the left with its definition on the right. Some definitions will be used more than once.*

_____ 1. muscul/o — a. blood
_____ 2. dermat/o — b. blood vessel
_____ 3. derm/o — c. lung
_____ 4. vascul/o — d. muscle
_____ 5. vas/o — e. skin
_____ 6. pneumon/o
_____ 7. pneum/o
_____ 8. pulmon/o
_____ 9. my/o
_____ 10. angi/o
_____ 11. hemat/o
_____ 12. hem/o
_____ 13. cutane/o

Learning Outcome 1.5 Exercises

EXERCISE 6 *Translate the following roots.*

1. muscul/o ____________________
2. dermat/o ____________________
3. derm/o ____________________
4. vascul/o ____________________
5. vas/o ____________________
6. pneumon/o ____________________
7. pneum/o ____________________
8. pulmon/o ____________________
9. my/o ____________________
10. angi/o ____________________
11. hemat/o ____________________
12. hem/o ____________________
13. cutane/o ____________________

EXERCISE 7 *Underline and define the root in the following terms.*

1. muscular ____________________
2. vascular ____________________
3. pulmonary ____________________
4. dermatology ____________________
5. hematology ____________________
6. myospasm ____________________
7. vasospasm ____________________
8. angiogram ____________________
9. dermopathy ____________________
10. hemostatic ____________________
11. percutaneous ____________________
12. vasectomy ____________________
13. pneumonectomy ____________________
14. cardiomyopathy (2 roots) ____________________
15. cardiopulmonary (2 roots) ____________________

EXERCISE 8 *Identify the roots for the following definitions.*

1. muscle (2 roots) ____________________
2. blood (2 roots) ____________________
3. skin (3 roots) ____________________
4. lung (3 roots) ____________________
5. blood vessel (3 roots) ____________________

Learning Outcome 1.5 Exercises

EXERCISE 9 *Match the root on the left with its definition on the right.*

_____	1. gen/o	a. change
_____	2. necr/o	b. creation, cause
_____	3. xen/o	c. death
_____	4. morph/o	d. nourishment, development
_____	5. troph/o	e. eat
_____	6. plas/o	f. foreign
_____	7. sten/o	g. formation
_____	8. phag/o	h. narrowing

EXERCISE 10 *Translate the following roots.*

1. hydr/o ______________________________
2. orth/o ______________________________
3. necr/o ______________________________
4. myc/o ______________________________
5. py/o ______________________________
6. xen/o ______________________________
7. path/o ______________________________
8. scler/o ______________________________
9. phag/o ______________________________

EXERCISE 11 *Underline and define the roots in the following terms.*

1. morphology ______________________________
2. dysplasia ______________________________
3. hypertrophic ______________________________
4. teratogenic ______________________________
5. mycosis ______________________________
6. craniostenosis ______________________________
7. angiosclerosis (2 roots) ______________________________
8. pyarthrosis (2 roots) ______________________________

Learning Outcome 1.5 Exercises

EXERCISE 12 *Identify the roots for the following definitions.*

1. water ______
2. creation, cause ______
3. pus ______
4. straight ______
5. fungus ______
6. suffering, disease ______
7. hard ______
8. formation ______

EXERCISE 13 *Match the suffix on the left with its definition on the right. Some definitions will be used more than once.*

______	1. -ium	a.	condition
______	2. -icle	b.	pertaining to
______	3. -ous	c.	tissue, structure
______	4. -ac	d.	small
______	5. -ia		
______	6. -eal		

EXERCISE 14 *Translate the following suffixes.*

1. -y ______
2. -ism ______
3. -al ______
4. -ic, -tic ______
5. -ar, -ary ______
6. -ole, -ule, -ula ______

EXERCISE 15 *Break down the following words into their component parts.*

> EXAMPLE: nasopharyngoscope *naso | pharyngo | scope*

1. cardiac ______
2. gastric ______
3. neurotic ______
4. skeletal ______
5. esophageal ______
6. muscular ______
7. pulmonary ______
8. cutaneous ______
9. arteriole ______
10. pneumonia ______
11. cardiovascular ______

Learning Outcome 1.5 Exercises

EXERCISE 16 *Underline and define the suffix in the following terms.*

1. cardiac ______
2. gastric ______
3. neurotic ______
4. skeletal ______
5. esophageal ______
6. muscular ______
7. pulmonary ______
8. cardiovascular ______
9. cutaneous ______
10. arteriole ______
11. ventricle ______
12. pustule ______
13. uvula ______
14. pneumonia ______
15. autism ______
16. pericardium ______
17. hypertrophy ______

EXERCISE 17 *Translate the following terms.*

ROOTS:	skelet/o	*skeleton*	esophag/o	*esophagus*	arteri/o	*artery*

1. cardiac ______
2. gastric ______
3. neurotic ______
4. skeletal ______
5. esophageal ______
6. muscular ______
7. pulmonary ______
8. cutaneous ______
9. arteriole ______
10. pneumonia ______
11. cardiovascular ______

Learning Outcome 1.5 Exercises

EXERCISE 18 *Identify the suffixes for the following definitions.*

1. tissue, structure ______
2. condition, process ______
3. condition (three possible options) ______
4. small or any suffix that makes the root a diminutive, or smaller version, of the root (choose three of the four possible options) ______
5. pertaining to (or any suffix that makes a root into an adjective) (choose four of the eight possible options) ______

EXERCISE 19 *Match the suffix on the left with its definition on the right. Some definitions will be used more than once.*

______	1. -logy	a. medical science
______	2. -logist	b. specialist
______	3. -ist	c. specialist in the medicine of
______	4. -iatrist	d. specialist in the study of
______	5. -iatry	e. study of
______	6. -iatrics	f. medicine of

EXERCISE 20 *Translate the following suffixes.*

1. -logy ______
2. -logist ______
3. -ist ______
4. -iatrist ______
5. -iatry ______
6. -iatrics ______

EXERCISE 21 *Break down the following words into their component parts.*

EXAMPLE: sinusitis *sinus | itis*

1. cardiology ______
2. cardiologist ______
3. pathology ______
4. pathologist ______
5. psychology ______
6. psychologist ______
7. dentist ______
8. psychiatry ______
9. psychiatrist ______
10. pediatrics ______

Learning Outcome 1.5 Exercises

EXERCISE 22 *Underline and define the suffix in the following terms.*

1. cardiology ____________________
2. cardiologist ____________________
3. pathology ____________________
4. pathologist ____________________
5. psychology ____________________
6. psychologist ____________________
7. dentist ____________________
8. psychiatry ____________________
9. psychiatrist ____________________
10. pediatrics ____________________

EXERCISE 23 *Fill in the blanks.*

EXAMPLE: cardiologist *specialist in the study of the heart*

1. **psychiatry:** ____________________ **of the mind (psych/o = mind)**
2. **psychiatrist:** ____________________ **of the mind (psych/o = mind)**
3. **psychology:** ____________________ **of the mind (psych/o = mind)**
4. **psychologist:** ____________________ **of the mind (psych/o = mind)**

EXERCISE 24 *Identify the suffixes for the following definitions.*

1. specialist ____________________
2. specialist in the study of ____________________
3. study of ____________________
4. specialist in the medicine of ____________________
5. medical science (two suffixes) ____________________

EXERCISE 25 *Match the suffix on the left with its definition on the right. Some definitions will be used more than once.*

	Suffix	Definition
_____	1. -oid	a. deficiency
_____	2. -iasis	b. drooping
_____	3. -cele	c. flow
_____	4. -penia	d. hernia
_____	5. -rrhea	e. loosen, break down
_____	6. -lysis	f. presence of
_____	7. -ptosis	g. resembling
_____	8. -rrhexis	h. rupture

Learning Outcome 1.5 Exercises

EXERCISE 26 *Translate the following suffixes.*

1. -spasm ______
2. -megaly ______
3. -oma ______
4. -emia ______
5. -itis ______
6. -osis ______
7. -pathy ______
8. -algia ______
9. -dynia ______
10. -malacia ______
11. -rrhage, -rrhagia ______

EXERCISE 27 *Break down the following words into their component parts.*

EXAMPLE: sinusitis *sinus | itis*

1. myospasm ______
2. myopathy ______
3. cardiomegaly ______
4. gastritis ______
5. gastralgia ______
6. gastrodynia ______
7. gastromalacia ______
8. hematoma ______
9. hemolysis ______
10. hemorrhage ______
11. stenosis ______

EXERCISE 28 *Underline and define the suffix in the following terms.*

1. myospasm ______
2. myopathy ______
3. cardiomegaly ______
4. gastritis ______
5. gastralgia ______
6. gastrodynia ______
7. gastromalacia ______
8. hematoma ______
9. melanoma ______
10. hemolysis ______
11. hemorrhage ______
12. hydrocele ______
13. leukopenia ______
14. stenosis ______

Learning Outcome 1.5 Exercises

EXERCISE 29 *Translate the following terms.*

1. myospasm ______
2. myopathy ______
3. cardiomegaly ______
4. gastritis ______
5. gastralgia ______
6. gastrodynia ______
7. gastromalacia ______
8. hematoma ______
9. hemolysis ______
10. hemorrhage ______
11. stenosis ______

EXERCISE 30 *Identify the suffixes for the following definitions.*

1. tumor ______
2. resembling ______
3. blood condition ______
4. presence of ______
5. deficiency ______
6. hernia ______
7. drooping ______
8. flow ______
9. rupture ______

EXERCISE 31 *Match the suffix on the left with its definition on the right. Some definitions will be used more than once.*

	Suffix	Definition
______	1. -meter	a. instrument used to look
______	2. -metry	b. instrument used to measure
______	3. -scope	c. instrument used to produce a record
______	4. -scopy	d. process of looking
______	5. -graph	e. process of measuring
______	6. -graphy	f. writing procedure
______	7. -gram	g. puncture
______	8. -centesis	h. written record

EXERCISE 32 *Translate the following suffixes.*

1. -meter ______
2. -metry ______
3. -scope ______
4. -scopy ______
5. -graph ______
6. -graphy ______
7. -gram ______
8. -centesis ______

Learning Outcome 1.5 Exercises

EXERCISE 33 *Break down the following words into their component parts.*

EXAMPLE: sinusitis *sinus | itis*

1. audiogram ______
2. audiograph ______
3. audiometer ______
4. gastroscope ______
5. audiography ______
6. audiometry ______
7. gastroscopy ______
8. ovariocentesis ______

EXERCISE 34 *Underline and define the suffix in the following terms.*

1. audiogram ______
2. audiograph ______
3. audiometer ______
4. gastroscope ______
5. audiography ______
6. audiometry ______
7. gastroscopy ______
8. ovariocentesis ______

EXERCISE 35 *Translate the following terms.*

ROOT: trache/o *trachea*

1. audiogram ______
2. audiograph ______
3. audiometer ______
4. gastroscope ______
5. audiography ______
6. audiometry ______
7. gastroscopy ______
8. ovariocentesis ______

EXERCISE 36 *Identify the suffixes for the following definitions.*

1. instrument used to look ______
2. process of looking ______
3. instrument used to measure ______
4. process of measuring ______
5. written record ______
6. instrument used to produce a record ______
7. writing procedure ______
8. puncture ______

Learning Outcome 1.5 Exercises

EXERCISE 37 *Match the suffix on the left with its definition on the right.*

_____	1. -plasty	a. binding
_____	2. -tomy	b. creation of an opening
_____	3. -ectomy	c. incision
_____	4. -stomy	d. reconstruction
_____	5. -pexy	e. removal
_____	6. -desis	f. surgical fixation
_____	7. -rrhaphy	g. suture

EXERCISE 38 *Translate the following suffixes.*

1. -plasty ______________________________
2. -tomy ______________________________
3. -ectomy ______________________________
4. -stomy ______________________________
5. -pexy ______________________________
6. -desis ______________________________
7. -rrhaphy ______________________________

EXERCISE 39 *Break down the following words into their component parts.*

EXAMPLE: sinusitis *sinus | itis*

1. myodesis ______________________________
2. myorrhaphy ______________________________
3. gastropexy ______________________________
4. myoplasty ______________________________
5. gastrectomy ______________________________
6. tracheotomy ______________________________
7. tracheostomy ______________________________

EXERCISE 40 *Underline and define the suffix in the following terms.*

1. myoplasty ______________________________
2. tracheotomy ______________________________
3. tracheostomy ______________________________
4. gastrectomy ______________________________
5. gastropexy ______________________________
6. myodesis ______________________________
7. myorrhaphy ______________________________

Learning Outcome 1.5 Exercises

EXERCISE 41 *Translate the following terms.*

ROOTS: audio *sound* ovario *ovary*

1. myoplasty ______
2. tracheotomy ______
3. tracheostomy ______
4. gastrectomy ______
5. gastropexy ______
6. myodesis ______
7. myorrhaphy ______

EXERCISE 42 *Identify the suffixes for the following definitions.*

1. reconstruction ______
2. removal ______
3. incision ______
4. creation of an opening ______
5. surgical fixation ______
6. binding ______
7. suture ______

EXERCISE 43 *Match the singular suffix on the left with the suffix that will make the same term plural on the right. Some plural suffixes will be used more than once.*

	Singular	Plural
______	1. -ax	a. -a
______	2. -ix	b. -aces
______	3. -ex	c. -ae
______	4. -ma	d. -es
______	5. -is	e. -i
______	6. -a	g. -ies
______	7. -um	f. -ices
______	8. -on	h. -mata
______	9. -y	
______	10. -us	

Learning Outcome 1.5 Exercises

EXERCISE 44 *Indicate whether the suffix is singular or plural.*

1. -aces ____________________
2. -ices ____________________
3. -ax ____________________
4. -ex ____________________
5. -ix ____________________
6. -ma ____________________
7. -mata ____________________
8. -on ____________________
9. -um ____________________
10. -ae ____________________
11. -i ____________________
12. -y ____________________
13. -is ____________________
14. -es ____________________
15. -us ____________________
16. -ies ____________________

EXERCISE 45 *Underline the suffix in the following terms and indicate whether the term is singular or plural.*

EXAMPLE: bacteri<u>um</u> *singular* (suffix *-um* is singular)

1. appendix ____________________
2. appendices ____________________
3. cortex ____________________
4. cortices ____________________
5. thorax ____________________
6. thoraces ____________________
7. myopathy ____________________
8. myopathies ____________________
9. vertebra ____________________
10. vertebrae ____________________
11. ganglion ____________________
12. ganglia ____________________
13. carcinoma ____________________
14. carcinomata ____________________
15. ova ____________________
16. ovum ____________________
17. nucleus ____________________
18. nuclei ____________________
19. diagnosis ____________________
20. diagnoses ____________________
21. biopsy ____________________
22. thrombus ____________________
23. spermatozoon ____________________
24. larvae ____________________
25. sarcoma ____________________
26. neuroses ____________________
27. bacteria ____________________

Learning Outcome 1.5 Exercises

EXERCISE 46 *Match the prefix on the left with its definition on the right. Some definitions will be used more than once.*

_____	1. pre-	a.	after
_____	2. post-	b.	again
_____	3. re-	c.	against
_____	4. contra-	d.	before
_____	5. anti-	e.	before, on behalf of
_____	6. pro-	f.	down, away from
_____	7. de-	g.	fast
_____	8. a-	h.	not
_____	9. an-	i.	slow
_____	10. ante-		
_____	11. tachy-		
_____	12. brady-		

EXERCISE 47 *Translate the following prefixes.*

1. pre- ____________________
2. post- ____________________
3. re- ____________________
4. contra- ____________________
5. anti- ____________________
6. pro- ____________________
7. de- ____________________
8. a- ____________________
9. an- ____________________
10. ante- ____________________
11. tachy- ____________________
12. brady- ____________________

EXERCISE 48 *Break down the following words into their component parts.*

EXAMPLE: sinusitis *sinus | itis*

1. bradypnea ____________________
2. tachypnea ____________________
3. apnea ____________________
4. prenatal (3 parts: prefix, root, suffix) ____________________
5. postnatal (3 parts: prefix, root, suffix) ____________________
6. antibiotic (3 parts: prefix, root, suffix) ____________________
7. probiotic (3 parts: prefix, root, suffix) ____________________

Learning Outcome 1.5 Exercises

EXERCISE 49 *Underline and define the prefix in the following terms.*

1. prenatal ______
2. postnatal ______
3. antepartum ______
4. probiotic ______
5. antibiotic ______
6. contraceptive ______
7. dehydration ______
8. rehabilitation ______
9. bradypnea ______
10. tachypnea ______
11. apnea ______

EXERCISE 50 *Select the correct prefix option for each given translation.*

EXAMPLES: hypoglycemia: *(hypo-)* over/<u>under</u> + *(glyc)* sugar + *(-emia)* blood condition
dysmenorrhea: *(dys-)* not/bad + *(meno)* menstruation + *(-rrhea)* discharge

1. *bradypnea: (brady-)* fast/slow + *(pnea)* breathing
2. *tachypnea: (tachy-)* fast/slow + *(pnea)* breathing
3. *apnea: (a-)* again/not + *(pnea)* breathing
4. *antepartum: (ante-)* after/before + *(partum)* birth
5. *postpartum: (post-)* after/before + *(partum)* birth
6. *amenorrhea: (a-)* not/again + *(meno)* menstruation + *(-rrhea)* discharge
7. *prenatal: (pre-)* after/before + *(nat/o)* birth + *(-al)* condition/pertaining to
8. *probiotic: (pro-)* against/on behalf of + *(bio)* life + *(-tic)* condition/pertaining to
9. *antibiotic: (anti-)* against/on behalf of + *(bio)* life + *(-tic)* condition/pertaining to

EXERCISE 51 *Identify the prefixes for the following definitions.*

1. again ______
2. after ______
3. slow ______
4. fast ______
5. down, away from ______
6. before, on behalf of ______
7. before (2 prefixes) ______
8. not (2 prefixes) ______
9. against (2 prefixes) ______

Learning Outcome 1.5 Exercises

EXERCISE 52 *Match the prefix on the left with its definition on the right. Some definitions will be used more than once.*

______	1. ab-		a. away
______	2. ad-		b. toward
______	3. peri-		c. around
______	4. trans-		d. through
______	5. ec-		e. out
______	6. ecto-		f. outside
______	7. extra-		g. in, inside
______	8. en-		h. upon
______	9. intra-		i. beneath
______	10. epi-		j. between
______	11. sub-		
______	12. inter-		

EXERCISE 53 *Translate the following prefixes.*

1. sub- ______________________
2. inter- ______________________
3. circum- ______________________
4. dia- ______________________
5. ab- ______________________
6. ad- ______________________
7. epi- ______________________
8. e-, ec-, ex- ______________________
9. ecto-, exo-, extra- ______________________
10. en-, endo-, intra- ______________________

EXERCISE 54 *Break down the following words into their component parts.*

EXAMPLE: sinusitis *sinus | itis*

1. exhale ______________________
2. ectoderm ______________________
3. exoskeleton ______________________
4. subcutaneous ______________________
5. epicardium (3 parts) ______________________
6. pericardium (3 parts) ______________________
7. transdermal (3 parts) ______________________
8. intradermal (3 parts) ______________________
9. epidermal (3 parts) ______________________
10. extravascular (3 parts) ______________________
11. pericarditis (3 parts) ______________________

Learning Outcome 1.5 Exercises

EXERCISE 55 *Underline and define the prefix in the following terms.*

1. transdermal ______
2. exhale ______
3. extravascular ______
4. circumcision ______
5. pericardium ______
6. pericarditis ______
7. subcutaneous ______
8. exoskeleton ______
9. ectoderm ______
10. ectopic ______
11. intercostal ______
12. intravenous ______
13. intradermal ______
14. epidermal ______
15. epicardium ______
16. endometrium ______
17. abduct ______
18. evoke ______
19. diuresis ______
20. enuresis ______

EXERCISE 56 *Translate the following terms.*

1. ectoderm ______
2. exoskeleton ______
3. subcutaneous ______
4. epicardium (3 parts) ______
5. pericardium (3 parts) ______
6. transdermal (3 parts) ______
7. intradermal (3 parts) ______
8. epidermal (3 parts) ______
9. extravascular (3 parts) ______
10. pericarditis (3 parts) ______

Learning Outcome 1.5 Exercises

EXERCISE 57 *Identify the prefixes for the following definitions.*

1. beneath ______
2. between ______
3. upon ______
4. away ______
5. toward ______
6. around (2 prefixes) ______
7. through (2 prefixes) ______
8. in, inside (3 prefixes) ______
9. out (3 prefixes) ______
10. outside (3 prefixes) ______

EXERCISE 58 *Match the prefix on the left with its definition on the right. Some definitions will be used more than once.*

	Prefix	Definition
______	1. bi-	a. all
______	2. uni-	b. few
______	3. multi-	c. half
______	4. micro-	d. large
______	5. macro-	e. many
______	6. mono-	f. one
______	7. poly-	g. over
______	8. hyper-	h. small
______	9. hemi-	i. two
______	10. hypo-	j. under
______	11. pan-	
______	12. oligo-	

EXERCISE 59 *Translate the following prefixes.*

1. bi- ______
2. uni- ______
3. multi- ______
4. micro- ______
5. macro- ______
6. mono- ______
7. poly- ______
8. hyper- ______
9. hemi- ______
10. hypo- ______
11. pan- ______
12. oligo- ______

Learning Outcome 1.5 Exercises

EXERCISE 60 *Break down the following words into their component parts.*

EXAMPLE: sinusitis *sinus | itis*

ROOTS: cephal/o *head* cyt/o *cell* nephr/o *kidney* pnea *breathing* uria *urine condition*

1. unisex ______
2. monocyte ______
3. oliguria ______
4. polyuria ______
5. hyperpnea ______
6. hypopnea ______
7. macrocephaly (3 parts) ______
8. microcephaly (3 parts) ______
9. pancytopenia (3 parts) ______
10. heminephrectomy (3 parts) ______

EXERCISE 61 *Underline and define the prefixes in the following terms.*

1. unilateral ______
2. bilateral ______
3. monocyte ______
4. oliguria ______
5. polyuria ______
6. polygraph ______
7. hyperpnea ______
8. hypopnea ______
9. macrocephaly ______
10. microcephaly ______
11. pancytopenia ______
12. heminephrectomy ______
13. panhypopituitarism (2 prefixes) ______

EXERCISE 62 *Translate the following terms.*

ROOTS: cephal/o *head* cyt/o *cell* nephr/o *kidney* pnea *breathing* uria *urine condition*

1. monocyte ______
2. oliguria ______
3. polyuria ______
4. hyperpnea ______
5. hypopnea ______
6. polygraph ______
7. macrocephaly ______
8. microcephaly ______
9. pancytopenia ______
10. heminephrectomy ______

Learning Outcome 1.5 Exercises

EXERCISE 63 *Identify the prefixes for the following definitions.*

1. large ____________________
2. small ____________________
3. over ____________________
4. under ____________________
5. two ____________________
6. all ____________________
7. few ____________________
8. one (2 prefixes) ____________________
9. many (2 prefixes) ____________________
10. half (2 prefixes) ____________________

EXERCISE 64 *Match the prefix on the left with its definition on the right. Some definitions will be used more than once.*

______	1. syn-	a. bad
______	2. sym-	b. good
______	3. con-	c. with, together
______	4. dys-	
______	5. eu-	

EXERCISE 65 *Translate the following prefixes.*

1. syn- ____________________
2. sym- ____________________
3. con- ____________________
4. dys- ____________________
5. eu- ____________________

EXERCISE 66 *Break down the following words into their component parts.*

EXAMPLE: sinusitis *sinus | itis*

ROOTS: dactyl/o *finger* pnea *breathing*

1. dyspnea ____________________
2. eupnea ____________________
3. symmetry ____________________
4. congenital (3 parts) ____________________
5. syndactyly (3 parts) ____________________

Learning Outcome 1.5 Exercises

EXERCISE 67 *Underline and define the prefix in the following terms.*

1. congenital ______________________
2. congestion ______________________
3. dysuria ______________________
4. dyspnea ______________________
5. eupnea ______________________
6. euthyroid ______________________
7. syndrome ______________________
8. symmetry ______________________

EXERCISE 68 *Translate the following terms.*

ROOTS: dactyl/o *finger* pnea *breathing*

1. dyspnea ______________________
2. eupnea ______________________
3. syndactyly ______________________
4. congenital ______________________
5. symmetry ______________________

EXERCISE 69 *Identify the prefixes for the following definitions.*

1. bad ______________________
2. good ______________________
3. with, together (3 prefixes) ______________________

1.6 How to Put Together Medical Terms

Putting It All Together

Now you know about roots, suffixes, and prefixes. There's an additional piece that often goes unnoticed: the *combining vowel.* Take the root *cardio,* which means "heart." That *o* on the end is optional. It is used when needed to make it easier to combine this root with other word parts. But if it is not needed, it can go away.

So when we say that a word part like *cardio* is a root, we're not speaking precisely. Technically, *cardio* is called a combining form. A *combining form* is a combination of a root with a combining vowel.

So in the example above:

cardi would be the root (which doesn't change)

o would be the combining vowel (which can come or go as needed)

cardi/o would be the combining form (the slash is there to help you tell the difference between the root and combining vowel)

Note: O is by far the most common combining vowel. The letter *i* is a distant second.

Do Use a Combining Vowel

To join a root to any suffix beginning with a consonant:

splen/o spleen
-megaly enlargement

Root	CV	Suffix	Word	Definition
splen	o	-megaly	splenomegaly	enlargement of the spleen

To join two roots together:

hepat/o liver

Root	CV	Root	CV	Suffix	Word	Definition
hepat	o	splen	o	-megaly	hepatosplenomegaly	enlargement of the liver and spleen

To join two roots together *even when* the second root begins with a vowel:

gastr/o stomach
enter/o intestine
-logy study of

Root	CV	Root	CV	Suffix	Word	Definition
gastr	o	enter	o	-logy	gastroenterology	study of the stomach and intestine

Don't Use a Combining Vowel

To join a root to a suffix that begins with a vowel:

my/o	*muscle*
splen/o	spleen
cardi/o	heart
-algia	pain
-ectomy	surgical removal
-itis	inflammation

Root	CV	Suffix	Word	Definition
my		-algia	myalgia	muscle pain
splen		-ectomy	splenectomy	surgical removal of the spleen
cardi		-itis	carditis	inflammation of the heart

Note: In the last word, the root ends with the same letter that begins the suffix (*cardi* + *itis*). In cases like this, you do not use a combining vowel, and you also drop the final vowel of the root.

Learning Outcome 1.6 Exercises

EXERCISE 1 *Indicate whether the following terms include a combining vowel by underlining the combining vowel.*

EXAMPLE: Root — Word

splen/o — *splenomegaly CV (suffix begins with a consonant)*

splenectomy no CV (suffix begins with a vowel)

ROOT: cardi/o

1. carditis ____________________
2. cardiology ____________________
3. cardiomegaly ____________________
4. cardiomyopathy ____________________
5. cardiovascular ____________________
6. bradycardia ____________________
7. endocardium ____________________
8. pericardiocentesis ____________________

Learning Outcome 1.6 Exercises

EXERCISE 2 *Indicate whether a combining vowel is necessary, and explain why or why not.*

EXAMPLE:	Root	Suffix	Combining Vowel?
	splen/o	*-megaly*	☒ *Yes (suffix begins with a consonant)* ☐ *No*

Root	Suffix	Combining Vowel?
1. cardi/o	-gram	☐ Yes ______ ☐ No ______
2. gastr/o	-scope	☐ Yes ______ ☐ No ______
3. cardi/o	-logist	☐ Yes ______ ☐ No ______
4. cardi/o	-megaly	☐ Yes ______ ☐ No ______
5. gastr/o	-ic	☐ Yes ______ ☐ No ______
6. gastr/o	-dynia	☐ Yes ______ ☐ No ______
7. cardi/o	-itis	☐ Yes ______ ☐ No ______
8. gastr/o	-itis	☐ Yes ______ ☐ No ______
9. cardi/o + my/o	-tomy	☐ Yes ______ ☐ No ______
10. gastr/o + esophag/o	-al	☐ Yes ______ ☐ No ______

EXERCISE 3 *Build a medical term from the information provided.*

EXAMPLE:	Root	Suffix	Term
	splen/o	*-megaly*	*splenomegaly*

Root	Suffix	Term
1. cardi/o	-gram	
2. gastr/o	-scope	
3. cardi/o	-logist	
4. cardi/o	-megaly	
5. gastr/o	-ic	
6. gastr/o	-dynia	
7. cardi/o	-itis	
8. gastr/o	-itis	
9. cardi/o + my/o	-tomy	
10. gastr/o + esophag/o	-al	

1.7 How Medical Terms Are Translated

Think of Medical Terms as Sentences

You can usually figure out the definition of a term by interpreting the

- suffix first
- then the prefix (if one is present)
- then the root or roots

How to translate:

1. Read the word.
2. Say the word out loud.
3. Break the word into parts (suffixes, roots, and prefixes).
4. Translate the parts.
5. Reassemble the pieces into a statement.

Example:

arthritis

1. Read the word:	arthritis
2. Say the word out loud:	ar-THRAI-tis
3. Break the word into parts (suffixes, roots, prefixes):	arthr / itis
4. Translate the parts:	joint / inflammation
5. Reassemble the pieces into one statement:	inflammation of the joint

Here's how this would look in a chart:

Term	Word Analysis
1. arthritis **2.** ar-THRAI-tis **5. Definition** inflammation of the joint	**3. arthr / itis** **4.** joint/inflammation

Some examples are shown to allow you to see the process at work. Don't worry about trying to learn the words themselves right now. They will be taught in later chapters. Right now, focus on getting comfortable with looking at medical terms, breaking them down, and then translating them. The biggest problem people have with medical terms is that they are intimidated by how long or how foreign they look. But if you don't panic and follow these five simple steps, you will be surprised at how quickly you will become comfortable with the language.

Group 1. This group is made up of relatively simple words. Most have just one root and one suffix and the definition is easily deduced from the word analysis.

Term	Word Analysis
angiectomy an-jee-EK-toh-mee **Definition** surgical removal of a vessel	**angi / ectomy** vessel / removal
arthritis ar-THRAI-tis **Definition** inflammation of the joint	**arthr / itis** joint / inflammation

Term	Word Analysis
cardiology kar-dee-AW-loh-jee **Definition** study of the heart	**cardio / logy** heart / study of
hepatitis heh-pah-TAI-tis **Definition** inflammation of the liver	**hepat / itis** liver / inflammation
myalgia mai-AL-jah **Definition** pain of muscle	**my / algia** muscle / pain
osteotomy AWS-tee-AW-toh-mee **Definition** incision into a bone	**osteo / tomy** bone / incision

Group 2. This group of words contains a more complex words. The words in this section are made up of at least three parts—either multiple roots or a prefix, root, and suffix.

Term	Word Analysis
angiosclerosis AN-jee-oh-skleh-ROH-sis **Definition** hardening of a blood vessel	**angio / scler / osis** vessel / hard / condition
cardiopulmonary KAR-dee-oh-PUL-mon-AR-ee **Definition** pertaining to the heart and lungs	**cardio / pulmon / ary** heart / lung /pertaining to
dermatomycosis der-MAH-toh-mai-KOH-sis **Definition** skin condition caused by fungus	**dermato / myc / osis** skin / fungus / condition
dysentery dis-en-TER-ee **Definition** bad intestine condition **NOTE:** Another name for severe diarrhea.	**dys / enter / y** bad / intestine /condition
hepatosplenomegaly heh-PAH-toh-SPLEH-noh-MEH-gah-lee **Definition** enlargement of the liver and spleen	**hepato / spleno / megaly** liver / spleen / enlargement
hyperplasia hai-per-PLAY-zhah **Definition** overformation condition	**hyper / plas / ia** over / formation /condition
hypoglycemia hai-poh-glai-SEE-mee-ah **Definition** condition characterized by low sugar in the blood (low blood sugar)	**hypo / glyc / emia** under /sugar / blood condition

Term	Word Analysis
osteocarcinoma AW-stee-oh-KAR-sih-NOH-mah **Definition** bone cancer tumor	**osteo / carcin / oma** bone / cancer / tumor
osteomyelitis AW-stee-oh-MAI-eh-LAI-tis **Definition** inflammation of the bone marrow	**osteo / myel / itis** bone / marrow / inflammation
pericardium peh-ree-KAR-dee-um **Definition** tissue around the heart	**peri / card / ium** around / heart / tissue

Learning Outcome 1.7 Exercises

EXERCISE 1 *Underline and define the root in the following terms.*

1. cardiology ____________________
2. arthritis ____________________
3. carditis ____________________
4. osteitis ____________________
5. hepatitis ____________________
6. arthralgia ____________________
7. myalgia ____________________
8. ostealgia ____________________
9. myotomy ____________________
10. osteotomy ____________________
11. arthrectomy ____________________
12. hepatectomy ____________________
13. angiectomy ____________________
14. ostectomy ____________________
15. myectomy ____________________

Learning Outcome 1.7 Exercises

EXERCISE 2 *Underline and define the suffix in the following terms.*

1. cardiology ____________________
2. arthritis ____________________
3. carditis ____________________
4. osteitis ____________________
5. hepatitis ____________________
6. arthralgia ____________________
7. myalgia ____________________
8. ostealgia ____________________
9. myotomy ____________________
10. osteotomy ____________________
11. arthrectomy ____________________
12. hepatectomy ____________________
13. angiectomy ____________________
14. ostectomy ____________________
15. myectomy ____________________

EXERCISE 3 *Fill in the blanks.*

EXAMPLE:	Term	Word Analysis
	arthritis	*arthr/itis*
	ar-THRAI-tis	*joint inflammation*

Term	Word Analysis
1. cardiology	cardio / logy heart / __________
2. carditis	card / itis heart / __________
3. osteitis	oste / itis bone / __________
4. hepatitis	hepat / itis liver / __________
5. arthalgia	arthr / algia joint / __________

Learning Outcome 1.7 Exercises

Term	Word Analysis
6. myalgia	my / algia muscle / ______
7. ostealgia	oste / algia bone / ______
8. myotomy	myo / tomy muscle / ______
9. osteotomy	osteo / tomy bone / ______
10. arthrectomy	arthr / ectomy joint / ______
11. hepatectomy	hepat / ectomy liver / ______
12. angiectomy	angi / ectomy vessel / ______
13. ostectomy	ost / ectomy bone / ______
14. myectomy	my / ectomy muscle / ______

EXERCISE 4 *Translate the following terms.*

EXAMPLE: sinusitis *inflammation of the sinuses*

1. cardiology ______
2. arthritis ______
3. carditis ______
4. osteitis ______
5. hepatitis ______
6. arthralgia ______
7. myalgia ______
8. ostealgia ______
9. myotomy ______
10. osteotomy ______
11. arthrectomy ______
12. hepatectomy ______
13. angiectomy ______
14. ostectomy ______
15. myectomy ______

Learning Outcome 1.7 Exercises

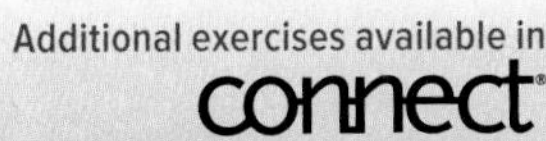

Chapter Review exercises, along with additional practice items, are available in Connect!

review of prefixes, roots, and suffixes

Prefixes	Roots	Suffixes
a- = not	**angi/o** = blood vessel	**-ac** = pertaining to
ab- = away	**arthr/o** = joint	**-al** = pertaining to
ad- = toward	**cardi/o** = heart	**-algia** = pain
an- = not	**derm/o, dermat/o** = skin	**-ar, -ary** = pertaining to
ante- = before	**enter/o** = small intestine	**-cele** = hernia
anti- = against	**gastr/o** = stomach	**-centesis** = puncture
bi- = two	**gen/o** = generation, cause	**-desis** = binding
brady- = slow	**hem/o**, **hemat/o** = blood	**-dynia** = pain
circum- = around	**hepat/o** = liver	**-eal** = pertaining to
con- = with, together	**hydr/o** = water	**-ectomy** = removal
contra- = against	**morph/o** = change	**-emia** = blood condition
de- = down, away from	**muscul/o** = muscle	**-gram** = written record
dia- = through	**my/o** = muscle	**-graph** = instrument used to produce a record
dys- = bad	**myc/o** = fungus	**-graphy** = writing procedure
e- = out	**necr/o** = death	**-ia** = condition
ec- = out	**neur/o** = nerve	**-iasis** = presence of
ecto- = outside	**orth/o** = straight	**-iatrics** = medical science
en- = in, inside	**path/o** = suffering, disease	**-iatrist** = specialist in medicine of
endo- = in, inside	**phag/o** = eat	**-iatry** = medical science
epi- = upon	**plas/o** = formation	**-ic** = pertaining to
eu- = good	**pneum/o, pneumon/o** = lung	**-icle** = small
ex- = out	**pulmon/o** = lung	**-ism** = condition
exo- = outside	**py/o** = pus	**-ist** = specialist
extra- = outside	**scler/o** = hard	**-itis** = inflammation
hemi- = half	**sten/o** = narrowing	**-ium** = tissue, structure
hyper- = over	**troph/o** = nourishment, development	**-logist** = specialist in the study of
hypo- = under	**vas/o, vascul/o** = blood vessel	**-logy** = study of
inter- = between	**xen/o** = foreign	**-lysis** = loosen, break down

review of prefixes, roots, and suffixes *continued*

Prefixes	Roots	Suffixes
intra- = in, inside		**-malacia** = abnormal softening
macro- = large		**-megaly** = enlargement
micro- = small		**-meter** = instrument used to measure
mono- = one		**-metry** = process of measuring
multi- = many		**-oid** = resembling
oligo- = few		**-ole** = small
pan- = all		**-oma** = tumor
peri- = around		**-osis** = condition
poly- = many		**-ous** = pertaining to
post- = after		**-pathy** = disease
pre- = before		**-penia** = deficiency
pro- = before, on behalf of		**-pexy** = surgical fixation
re- = again		**-plasty** = reconstruction
semi- = half		**-ptosis** = drooping
sub- = beneath		**-rrhage, -rrhagia** = excessive flow
sym- = with, together		**-rrhaphy** = suture
syn- = with, together		**-rrhea** = flow
tachy- = fast		**-rrhexis** = rupture
trans- = through		**-scope** = instrument used to look
uni- = one		**-scopy** = process of looking
		-spasm = involuntary contraction
		-stomy = creation of an opening
		-tic = pertaining to
		-tomy = incision
		-ula, -ula = small
		-y = condition, process

Introduction to Health Records

2

Introduction

Medical records save lives. The information they contain can be critical in patient care. For example, documentation of a patient's allergy to a medication can prevent an adverse, potentially fatal, outcome. Whether found in a paper chart or an electronic health record (EHR), the information contained in a patient's records serves as a roadmap to his or her health history detailing previous illnesses and treatments, continuing medical problems, history of family illnesses, and any current medications. These data provide a clearer picture of the best route to take in future treatment of the patient. With an increasingly busy and time-constrained patient culture, seeking care in multiple places such as emergency rooms and urgent care clinics has become more commonplace. This further fuels the need for thorough documentation, because it is the bedrock of solid communication among health care providers.

Medical records are an indispensable component of medicine, so it is prudent to be well acquainted with their general layout. There are countless types of medical documents or records in medicine, from routine wellness visits to hospital discharge summaries. Even x-ray reports are medical notes. To the untrained eye, the layout or sheer volume of information of a medical note may be intimidating. In reality, most medical notes share a consistent, logical organization or layout as well as characteristic language. We addressed the concept of medical language in the first chapter and it will be the main focus of this textbook. In this chapter, we discuss the organization or layout of medical documents. Having a good grasp on the general flow of medical notes allows for successful navigation through the different elements of a patient's chart so you may find any relevant details you seek.

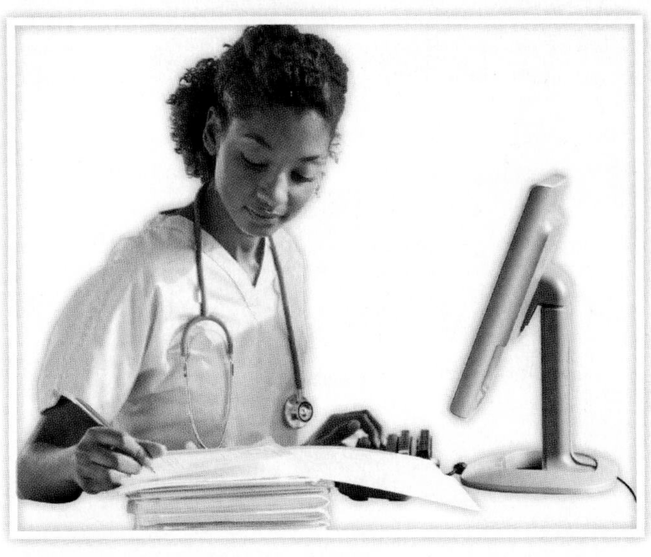

©JGI/Daniel Grill/Blend Images/Getty Images RF

learning outcomes

Upon completion of this chapter, you will be able to:

2.1 Summarize the **SOAP method**.

2.2 Use common terms on **health records**.

2.3 Identify the types of **health records**.

2.4 Use **abbreviations** associated with health care facilities, patient care, and prescriptions.

2.5 Become familiar with different types of **health records**.

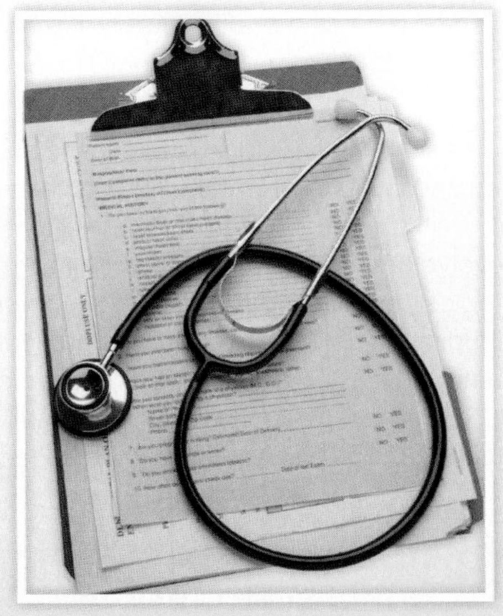

©Creatas/PunchStock RF

2.1 The SOAP Method

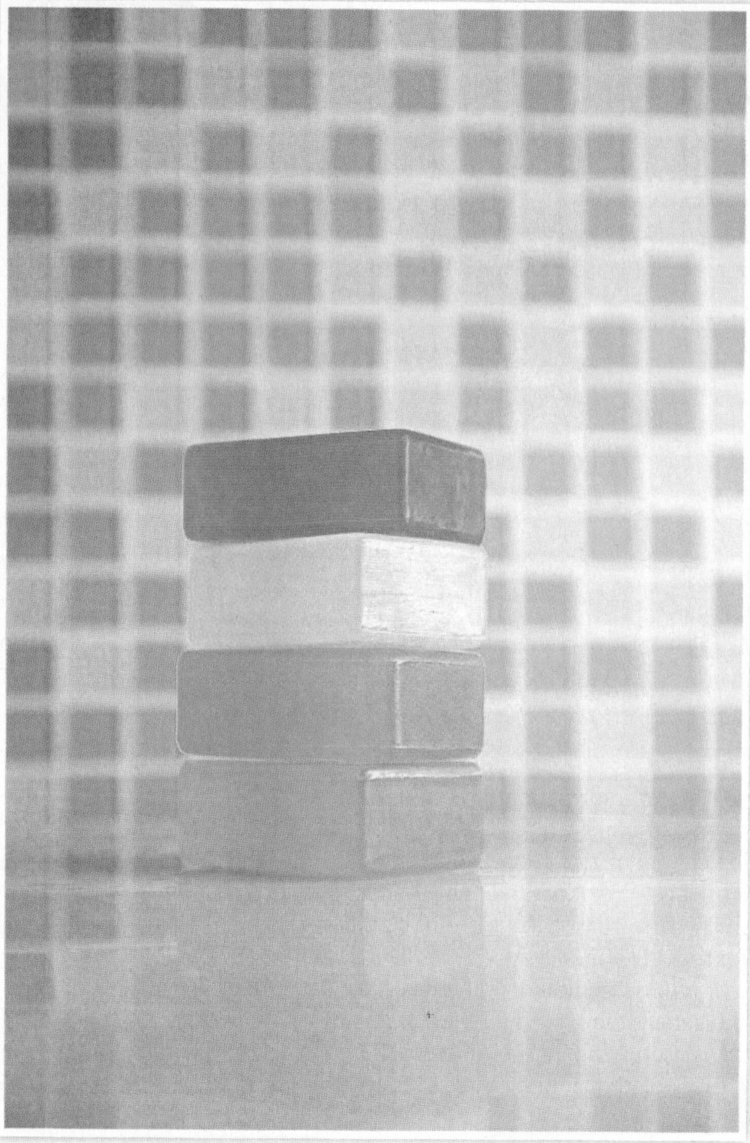

©Randy Faris/Corbis/Jupiter Images RF

Medical notes share a consistent pattern in their organization and layout. This pattern reflects the thought process of health professionals in general. Patient visits typically revolve around addressing a problem. Providers employ a logical approach to solving these problems. In its most rudimentary form, this pattern is presented as what is known as a SOAP note. *SOAP* is an acronym that stands for the four general parts of a medical note: **S**ubjective, **O**bjective, **A**ssessment, and **P**lan.

Diagnostic work in medicine is very similar to the investigative work of a detective. By collecting data and using deductive reasoning, a health care provider can make the most accurate assessment of the patient's problem.

S The first part of the note is the **subjective** part. It is subject to how a patient experiences and personally describes his or her problem as well as personal and family medical histories. Put simply, it is the problem in the patient's own words. The subjective data include the duration of the problem, the quality of the problem, and any exacerbating or relieving factors for that problem.

O The next step in the investigative process involves collecting **objective** data. Objective data comprise the patient's physical exam, any laboratory findings, and imaging studies performed at the visit.

A Upon gathering all the pertinent information, the health care provider formulates a logical analysis. This is known as the **assessment.** An assessment could be a diagnosis, an identification of a problem, or a list of possibilities for the diagnosis, which is known as a differential diagnosis.

P The provider then formulates a **plan,** or a course of action consistent with his or her assessment. The plan could be a treatment with medicine or a procedure. It could also consist of collecting further data to help arrive at a more accurate diagnosis.

The process of collecting subjective history, gathering objective data, formulating an assessment, and developing an action plan is repeated in every health care visit across all disciplines of medicine. It is the baseline of thought in medicine. Consequently, health care records reflect this thought process.

Learning Outcome 2.1 Exercises

Additional exercises available in **connect**

EXERCISE 1 *Multiple-choice questions. Select the correct answer.*

1. The *S* in *SOAP* stands for:
   a. scrutinize
   b. studies
   c. subjective
   d. survey
2. The *O* in *SOAP* stands for:
   a. objective
   b. opinion
   c. order
   d. outline
3. The *A* in *SOAP* stands for:
   a. action
   b. appraisal
   c. arrangement
   d. assessment
4. The *P* in *SOAP* stands for:
   a. plan
   b. procedure
   c. prognosis
   d. purpose
5. A SOAP note is:
   a. a pattern used in writing medical notes
   b. a way of thinking
   c. all of these
   d. none of these
6. A *diagnosis* is:
   a. a list of possible causes of the patient's problem or complaint
   b. ordering of more labs
   c. the identification of the actual problem
   d. treatment with medicine or a procedure
7. A *differential diagnosis* is:
   a. a list of possible causes of the patient's problem or complaint
   b. ordering of more labs
   c. the identification of the actual problem
   d. treatment with medicine or a procedure

EXERCISE 2 *Match the part of the medical SOAP note on the left with its description on the right.*

______	1. subjective	a. cause of the problem
______	2. objective	b. treatment with medicine or a procedure
______	3. assessment	c. a description of the problem in the patient's own words
______	4. plan	d. data collected to assist in understanding the nature of the problem

Learning Outcome 2.1 Exercises

EXERCISE 3 *Identify the part of the SOAP note in which the following information would be found.*

EXAMPLE: Ordering of additional lab work to help arrive at the cause *P (Plan)*

1. scheduling of a surgery ______
2. past medical history, family history ______
3. a diagnosis ______
4. patient's description of the problem or complaint ______
5. treatment with medicine ______
6. an identification of the cause of the problem or complaint ______
7. lab results ______
8. determination of how long the patient has suffered from the same complaint ______
9. information forms provided by the patient prior to the appointment ______
10. initial imaging studies (e.g., an x-ray) ______
11. differential diagnosis ______
12. ordering of more tests or images ______
13. the patient's exam ______
14. list of possible causes that fit the description of the patient's problem ______

EXERCISE 4 *Give an example of what would be found in each part of the SOAP note.*

1. S–Subjective ______
2. O–Objective ______
3. A–Assessment ______
4. P–Plan ______

2.2 Common Terms in Medicine

Your Future Second-Nature Words

Just as various sports have their own special words, such as *rebound*, *home run*, and *touchdown*, health records have special words that are essential to know. While the main purpose of this book is to help you use the roots of ancient words to break down medical words, you must also know many commonly used medical words that are not necessarily based on ancient languages.

When you have been working in the medical field long enough, these words will become second nature to you. You will use them so often that they will become part of your normal vocabulary. This chapter will introduce you to those terms so you will be better able to understand the stories told in health records.

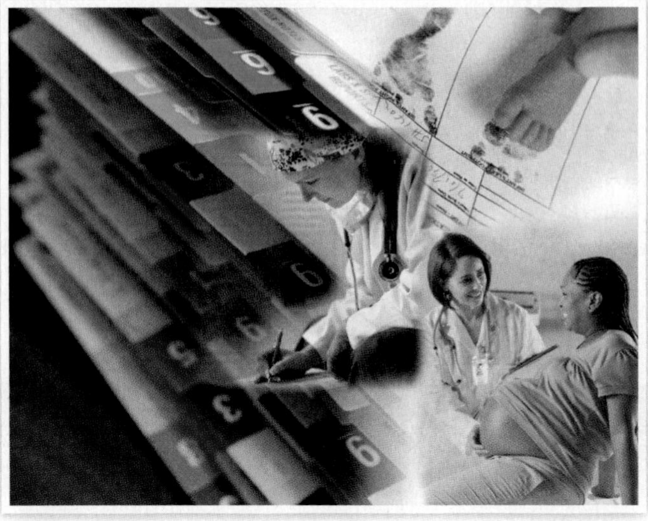

Just like any other specialized field, medicine has a whole host of words that sound strange the first time but become second nature the more you use them.

SUBJECTIVE

As you recall, the subjective section of a health record tells the patient's personal story of his or her health issue. It includes things such as:

- the main reason for the health visit
- the description of his or her problem
- the timing of the problem
- previous medical problems or surgeries
- family health problems that might relate
- current medications and allergies

In describing the chief concern, you may include when the problem began, the severity, any associated problems, and whether anything seems to make the problem better or worse.

general subjective terms

Term	Definition
acute ah-KYOOT	it just started recently or is a sharp, severe symptom
chronic KRAH-nik	it has been going on for a while now
exacerbation ek-SAS-er-BAY-shun	it is getting worse
abrupt ah-BRUPT	all of a sudden
febrile FEH-brail	to have a fever
afebrile AY-FEH-brail	to not have a fever
malaise mah-LAYZ	not feeling well
progressive proh-GREH-siv	more and more each day
symptom SIM-tom	something a patient feels
noncontributory NON-kon-TRIB-yoo-TOH-ree	not related to this specific problem
lethargic lah-THAR-jik	a decrease in level of consciousness; in a medical record, this is generally an indication that the patient is really sick
genetic/hereditary jih-NEH-tik, hah-REH-dih-TEH-ree	it runs in the family

Learning Outcome 2.2 Exercises

PRONUNCIATION

EXERCISE 1 *Indicate which syllable is emphasized when pronounced.*

EXAMPLE: bronchitis bronchitis

1. progressive ______
2. lethargic ______
3. genetic ______
4. febrile ______
5. abrupt ______
6. hereditary ______
7. afebrile ______
8. exacerbation ______
9. noncontributory ______

EXERCISE 2 *Match the term on the left with its definition on the right.*

	Term		Definition
______	1. symptom	a.	something a patient feels
______	2. progressive	b.	a decrease in the level of consciousness
______	3. chronic	c.	symptoms recently began
______	4. febrile	d.	symptoms have been present for a while
______	5. afebrile	e.	to have a fever
______	6. acute	f.	not feeling well
______	7. malaise	g.	to not have a fever
______	8. lethargic	h.	more and more each day

EXERCISE 3 *Translate the following terms.*

1. genetic ______
2. noncontributory ______
3. hereditary ______
4. abrupt ______
5. chronic ______
6. lethargic ______
7. exacerbation ______
8. malaise ______
9. afebrile ______

EXERCISE 4 *Identify the medical term from the definition provided.*

1. a problem that runs in the family ______
2. unrelated to the specific problem ______
3. a problem that recently began ______
4. all of a sudden ______
5. more and more each day ______
6. a problem that is getting worse ______
7. something a patient feels ______
8. to not have a fever ______

OBJECTIVE

The objective part of a health record tells about the data collected during the health care provider's interaction with the patient. What does the provider notice about the patient when he or she examines the patient closely? How does the patient look, sound, feel, smell? It also includes any extra data obtained by tests done in a laboratory or by special images of the patient's body.

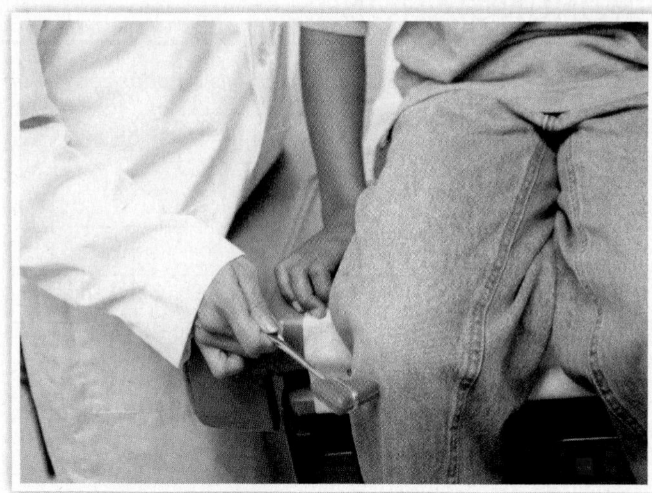

One piece of objective information is measuring a patient's muscle reflexes.

general objective terms

Term	Definition
alert ah-LERT	able to answer questions; responsive; interactive
oriented OR-ee-EN-ted	being aware of who he or she is, where he or she is, and the current time; a patient who is aware of all three is "oriented × 3"
marked MARKT	it really stands out
unremarkable un-ree-MARK-ah-bul	another way of saying normal
auscultation aws-kul-TAY-shun	to listen
percussion per-KUH-shun	to hit something and listen to the resulting sound or feel for the resulting vibration; drums are a percussion instrument
palpation pal-PAY-shun	to feel

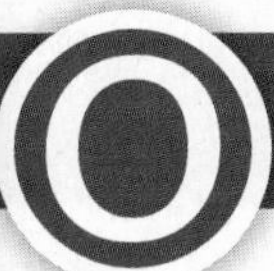

Learning Outcome 2.2 Exercises

EXERCISE 6 *Break down the following words into syllables.*

EXAMPLE: synesthesia *syn | es | the | sia*

1. oriented ______
2. auscultation ______
3. marked ______

EXERCISE 7 *Indicate which syllable is emphasized when pronounced.*

EXAMPLE: bronchitis bronchitis

1. alert ______
2. unremarkable ______
3. palpation ______

EXERCISE 8 *Match the term on the left with its definition on the right.*

	Term		Definition
______	1. unremarkable	a.	able to answer questions; responsive; interactive
______	2. alert	b.	able to identify one's name and location, the time of day, and the date
______	3. marked	c.	something that really stands out
______	4. percussion	d.	normal
______	5. oriented	e.	to listen
______	6. auscultation	f.	to feel
______	7. palpation	g.	to hit something and listen to the sound or feel for the vibration

EXERCISE 9 *Translate the following terms.*

1. marked ______
2. unremarkable ______
3. percussion ______
4. oriented ______
5. auscultation ______
6. palpation ______

EXERCISE 10 *Identify the medical term from the definition provided.*

1. to listen ______
2. to feel ______
3. normal ______
4. something that really stands out ______
5. able to answer questions; responsive; interactive ______
6. to hit something and listen to the sound or feel for the vibration ______

ASSESSMENT

Once the facts from the patient are recorded and data about the patient are collected, it is time to put it all together to reach a conclusion on the nature of the problem. This is known as the diagnosis. Sometimes one exact problem is not so obvious at first. In these cases, a health care provider may list the most likely causes, called a differential diagnosis. In addition to a diagnosis, the provider may offer other opinions, like severity of the problem and the chances for improvement.

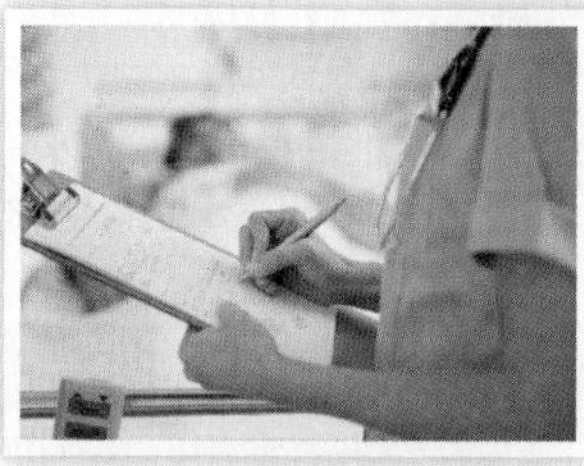

general assessment terms

Term	Definition
impression im-PREH-shun	another way of saying assessment
diagnosis DAI-ag-NOH-sis	what the health care professional thinks the patient has
differential diagnosis dih-fer-EN-shal DAI-ag-NOH-sis	a list of conditions the patient may have based on the symptoms exhibited and the results of the exam
benign beh-NAIN	safe
malignant mah-LIG-nant	dangerous; a problem
degeneration dee-jen-er-AY-shun	to be getting worse
etiology ee-tee-AW-loh-jee	the cause
remission reh-MIH-shun	to get better or improve; most often used when discussing cancer; *remission* does not mean cure
idiopathic ih-dee-oh-PA-thik	no known specific cause; it just happens
localized LOH-kah-LAIZD	stays in a certain part of the body
systemic/generalized sih-STEM-ik, jen-er-ah-LAIZD	all over the body (or most of it)
morbidity mor-BID-ih-tee	the risk for being sick
mortality mor-TA-lih-tee	the risk for dying
prognosis prawg-NOH-sis	the chances for things getting better or worse
occult ah-KULT	hidden
pathogen PATH-oh-jin	the organism that causes the problem
lesion LEE-shun	diseased tissue
recurrent ree-KUR-ent	to have again
sequelae seh-KWEL-ah	a problem resulting from a disease or injury
pending PEN-ding	waiting for

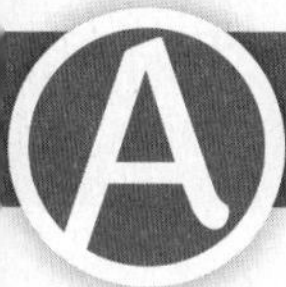

Learning Outcome 2.2 Exercises

EXERCISE 11 *Break down the following words into syllables.*

EXAMPLE: synesthesia *syn | es | the | sia*

1. localized ______
2. diagnosis ______
3. differential diagnosis ______
4. degeneration ______
5. idiopathic ______
6. generalized ______
7. lesion ______
8. recurrent ______

EXERCISE 12 *Indicate which syllable is emphasized when pronounced.*

EXAMPLE: bronchitis bron<u>chi</u>tis

1. impression ______
2. malignant ______
3. remission ______
4. systemic ______
5. morbidity ______
6. mortality ______
7. pathogen ______
8. prognosis ______
9. pending ______

EXERCISE 13 *Match the term on the left with its definition on the right.*

Term	Definition
______ 1. degeneration	a. assessment
______ 2. differential diagnosis	b. what the health care professional thinks the patient has
______ 3. diagnosis	c. a list of conditions the patient may have based on the symptoms exhibited and the results of the exam
______ 4. impression	d. to be getting worse
______ 5. remission	e. the cause
______ 6. mortality	f. to get better or improve; most often used when discussing cancer; does not mean *cure*
______ 7. prognosis	g. no known specific cause; it just happens
______ 8. morbidity	h. the risk for being sick
______ 9. pathogen	i. the risk for dying
______ 10. idiopathic	j. the chances for things getting better or worse
______ 11. etiology	k. the organism that causes the problem
______ 12. sequelae	l. a problem resulting from a disease or injury

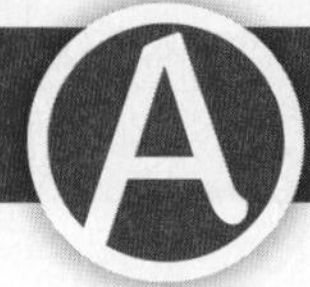

Learning Outcome 2.2 Exercises

EXERCISE 14 *Translate the following terms.*

1. systematic ____________________
2. generalized ____________________
3. localized ____________________
4. occult ____________________
5. lesion ____________________
6. recurrent ____________________
7. pending ____________________
8. benign ____________________
9. malignant ____________________
10. impression ____________________
11. degeneration ____________________
12. remission ____________________
13. pathogen ____________________
14. sequelae ____________________

EXERCISE 15 *Identify the medical term from the definition provided.*

1. safe ____________________
2. dangerous; a problem ____________________
3. stays in a certain part of the body ____________________
4. all over the body ____________________
5. a list of things that the patient may have, based on symptoms and exam ____________________
6. what the medical professional thinks the patient may have ____________________
7. the cause ____________________
8. no known specific cause ____________________
9. the chances for things to get better or worse ____________________
10. risk for being sick ____________________
11. risk for dying ____________________
12. hidden ____________________
13. diseased tissue ____________________
14. to have again ____________________
15. waiting for ____________________

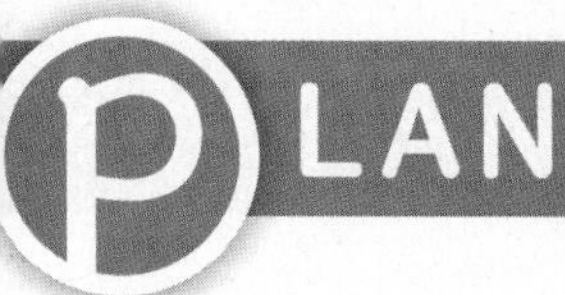

PLAN

In the health record, the plan lays out what the provider recommends to do about the patient's current health status. This may include medicine or home remedies, help from another health provider, surgery, or even waiting to see if the problem will improve on its own. Sometimes the plan is for more data collection to be done in the future to help figure out the true cause of the problem.

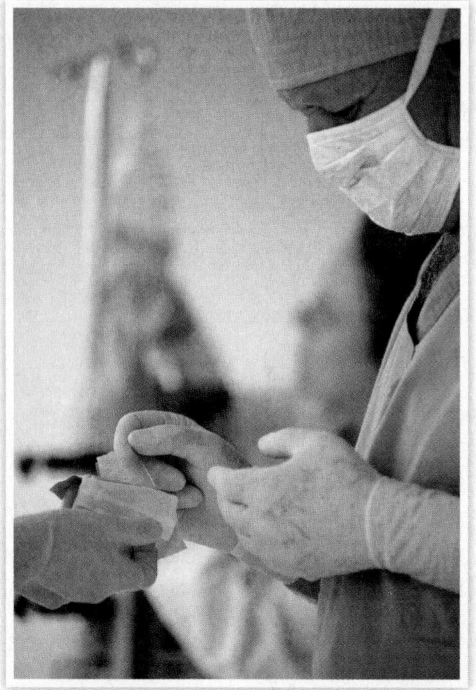

Once an assessment has been made, a course of action is decided upon. This plan can include everything from observation to medication and surgery.

general plan terms

Term	Definition
disposition dis-poh-ZIH-shun	what happened to the patient at the end of the visit; often used at the end of ED notes to reference where the patient went after the visit (home, the ICU, normal hospital bed)
discharge DIS-charj	literally, to *unload*; it has two meanings: 1. to send home (to unload the patient from the health care setting to home) 2. fluid coming out of a part of the body (your body unloading a fluid)
prophylaxis PROH-fuh-LAK-sis	preventive treatment
palliative PA-lee-ah-tiv	treating the symptoms, but not actually getting rid of the cause
observation OB-zer-VAY-shun	watch, keep an eye on
reassurance ree-ah-SHUR-ants	to tell the patient that the problem is not serious or dangerous
supportive care suh-POR-tiv kehr	to treat the symptoms and make the patient feel better
sterile STEH-ril	extremely clean, germ-free conditions; especially important during medical procedures and surgery

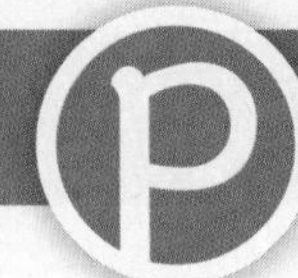

Learning Outcome 2.2 Exercises

EXERCISE 16 *Break down the following words into syllables.*

EXAMPLE: synesthesia *syn | es | the | sia*

1. discharge ______
2. disposition ______
3. observation ______
4. reassurance ______
5. supportive care ______

EXERCISE 17 *Match the term on the left with its definition on the right.*

	Term		Definition
______	1. sterile	a.	what happens to the patient at the end of the visit
______	2. observation	b.	to send home
______	3. disposition	c.	preventive treatment
______	4. discharge	d.	treating the symptoms but not actually getting rid of the cause
______	5. reassurance	e.	keep an eye on
______	6. supportive care	f.	to tell the patient that the problem is not serious or dangerous
______	7. prophylaxis	g.	to treat the symptoms and make the patient feel better
______	8. palliative	h.	extremely clean, germ-free conditions; especially important during medical procedures and surgery

EXERCISE 18 *Translate the following terms.*

1. reassurance ______
2. sterile ______
3. discharge ______
4. observation ______
5. disposition ______
6. supportive care ______
7. palliative ______
8. prophylaxis ______

EXERCISE 19 *Identify the medical term from the definition provided.*

1. to send home ______
2. to keep an eye on ______
3. extremely clean, germ-free conditions ______
4. what happens to the patient at the end of the visit ______
5. preventive treatment ______
6. to treat the symptoms to make the patient feel better ______
7. treating the symptoms but not actually getting rid of the cause ______
8. to tell the patient that the problem is not serious/dangerous ______

Body Planes and Orientation

When giving directions, being more specific leads to greater accuracy. The same goes for describing parts of the body. Often, the words used to describe directions in the body are opposites, like referencing north and south on a compass. This section helps to explain these body-specific opposites. It is important to note when describing the directions on the human body, we use the **anatomic position**. This position is a person standing facing forward, arms at the side with palms forward.

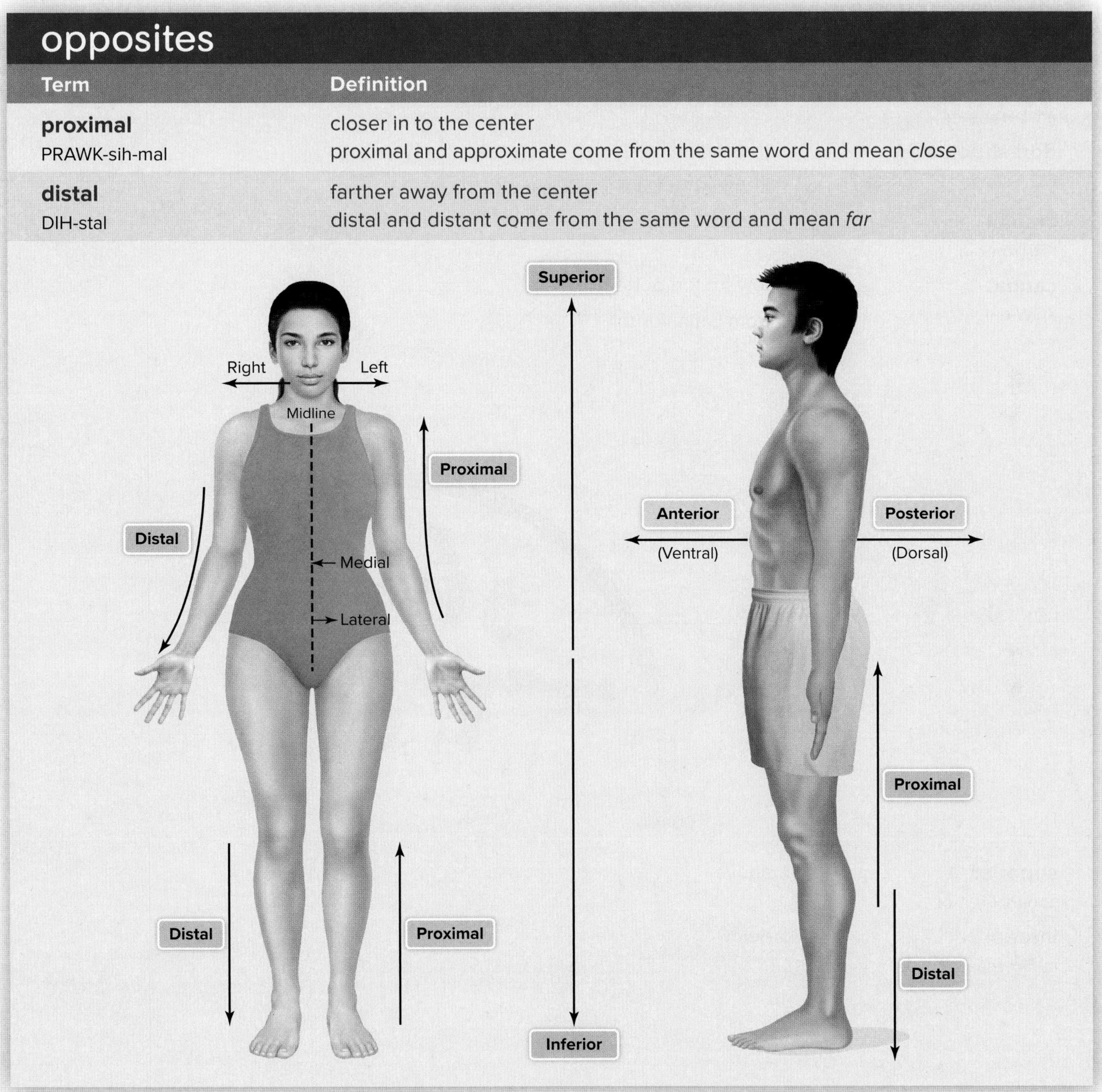

opposites

Term	Definition
proximal PRAWK-sih-mal	closer in to the center proximal and approximate come from the same word and mean *close*
distal DIH-stal	farther away from the center distal and distant come from the same word and mean *far*

opposites *continued*

Term	Definition
lateral LA-ter-al	out to the side think of a quarterback lateraling a football to a running back
medial MEE-dee-al	toward the middle like the median of a highway
ventral/antral/anterior VEN-tral/AN-tral/ an-TIH-ree-or	the front the word *ventral* means "stomach"
dorsal/posterior DOR-sal/pohs-TEER-ee-or	the back a dorsal fin on a shark is on its back
cranial KRAY-nee-al	toward the top
caudal KOW-dal	toward the bottom from Latin, for *tail*

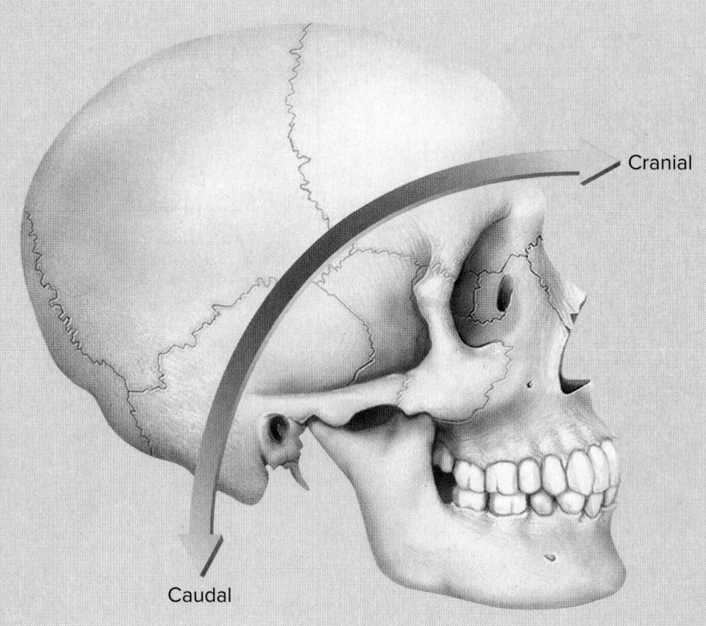

Term	Definition
superior soo-PIH-ree-or	above
inferior in-FIH-ree-or	below

opposites *continued*

Term	Definition
prone PROHN	lying down on belly
supine SOO-pain	lying down on back

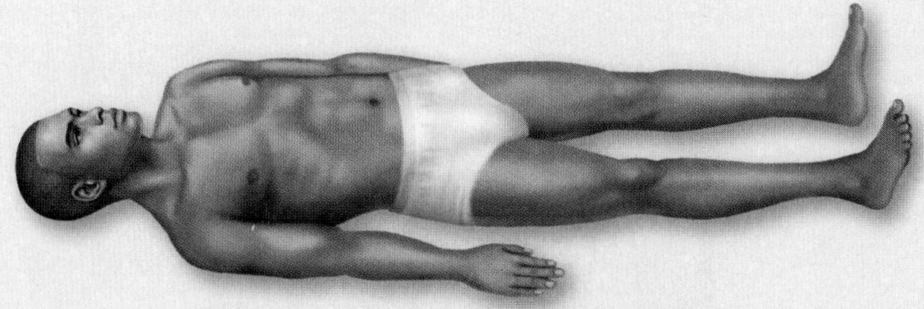

Supine

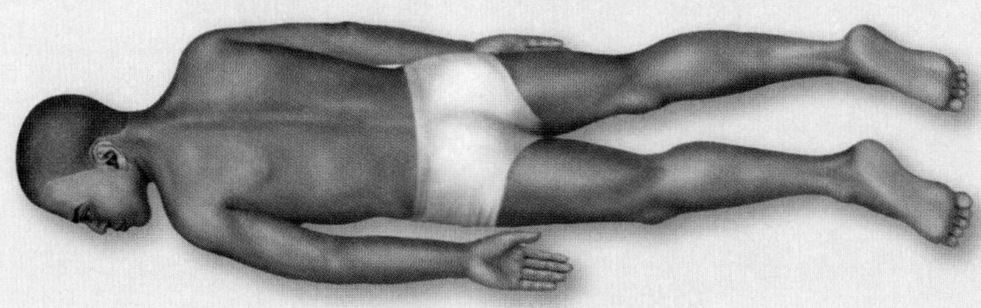

Prone

Term	Definition
contralateral KON-trah-LA-ter-al	opposite side
ipsilateral IP-sih-LA-ter-al	same side

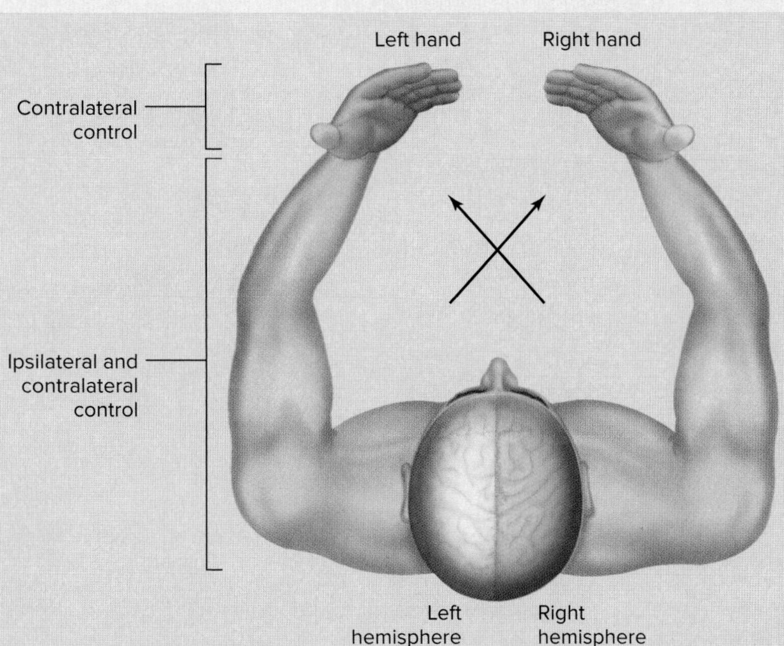

opposites *continued*

Term	Definition
unilateral YOO-nih-LA-ter-al	one side
bilateral BAI-LA-ter-al	both sides

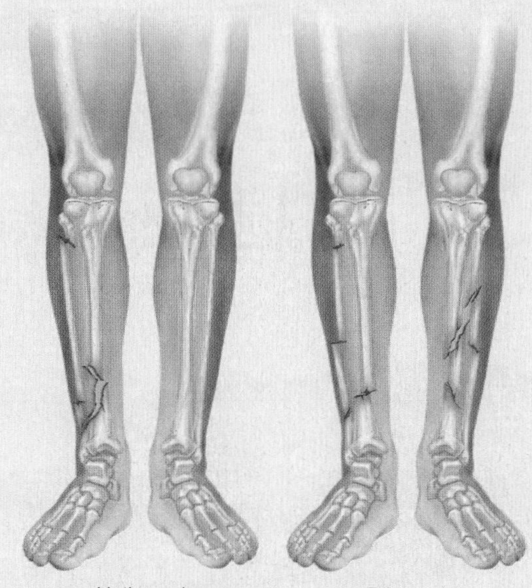

Term	Definition
dorsum DOR-sum	the top of the hand or foot
plantar PLAN-tar	the sole of the foot
palmar PAL-mar	the palm of the hand

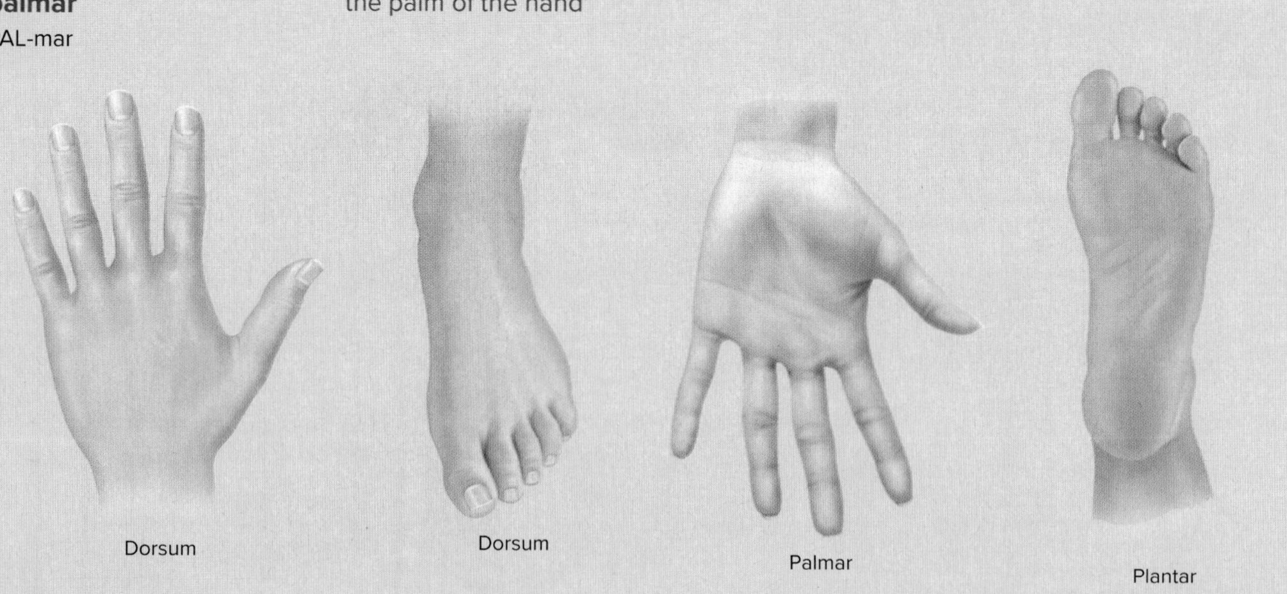

BODY PLANES

Another way of looking at the body is through the three dimensions: right to left (sagittal), front to back (coronal), and top to bottom (transverse). This is especially important in radiology. For instance, a CT scan is actually a series of layered images along one of these dimensions.

body planes

Term	Definition
sagittal SA-jih-tal	divides the body in slices right to left *sagitta* is Latin for *arrow*; think of this as dividing the body in half, as if someone shot an arrow through it
coronal kah-ROH-nal	divides the body into slices from front to back *corona* is Latin for *crown*; this plane divides the body in half from the top of the head down
transverse tranz-VERS	divides the body from top to bottom

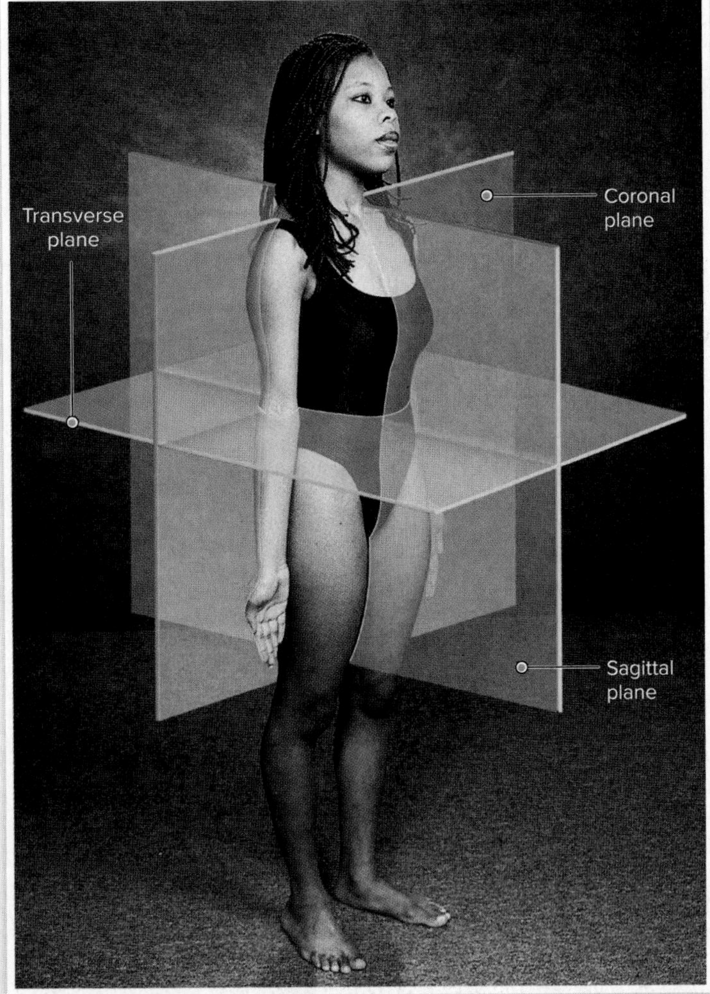

Learning Outcome 2.2 Exercises

EXERCISE 20 *Indicate which syllable is emphasized when pronounced.*

EXAMPLE: bronchitis bron<u>chi</u>tis

1. proximal ______
2. distal ______
3. ventral ______
4. antral ______
5. dorsal ______
6. dorsum ______
7. plantar ______
8. palmar ______
9. coronal ______
10. transverse ______

EXERCISE 21 *Match the term on the left with its definition on the right.*

	Term		Definition
______	1. bilateral	a.	the back
______	2. contralateral	b.	the front
______	3. ipsilateral	c.	lying down on the belly
______	4. unilateral	d.	lying down on the back
______	5. transverse	e.	opposite side
______	6. dorsal	f.	same side
______	7. prone	g.	one side
______	8. coronal	h.	both sides
______	9. supine	i.	divides the body from top to bottom
______	10. antral	j.	divides the body in slices right to left
______	11. sagittal	k.	divides the body in slices from front to back

EXERCISE 22 *Translate the following terms.*

1. posterior ______
2. cranial ______
3. caudal ______
4. superior ______
5. plantar ______
6. palmar ______
7. transverse ______
8. sagittal ______
9. contralateral ______
10. ventral ______

Learning Outcome 2.2 Exercises

EXERCISE 23 *Identify the medical term from the definition provided.*

1. farther away from the center __________
2. closer in to the center __________
3. out to the side __________
4. toward the middle __________
5. toward the top __________
6. the top of the hand or foot __________
7. one side __________
8. divides the body in slices from front to back __________
9. lying down on the back __________
10. below __________

EXERCISE 24 *Identify the opposite for the given term.*

EXAMPLE: cranial *caudal*

1. proximal __________
2. lateral __________
3. ventral __________
4. anterior __________
5. inferior __________
6. prone __________
7. ipsilateral __________
8. bilateral __________
9. palmar __________

Health Professionals

This section introduces some common health care professionals who are referenced throughout this text. Other health professionals will be introduced in the body system chapters.

health professions

Term	Definition
health providers	
physician fuh-ZIH-shun	a skilled health care provider who attended and graduated medical school *There are two types who practice in America: medical doctor (MD) and doctor of osteopathy (DO).*
pediatrician PEE-dee-ah-TRIH-shun	a physician with special training in caring for children
surgeon SIR-jen	a physician qualified to treat patients surgically, that is, by means of operation or invasive procedure
anesthesiologist AN-ehs-THEE-zee-AW-loh-jist	a physician with special training in pain sedation and pain control
physician assistant (PA) fuh-ZIH-shun ah-SIS-tant	a midlevel health care provider who works under the license of a supervising physician; requires postgraduate training
nurse practitioner (NP) NIRS prak-TIH-shuh-ner	a nurse with postgraduate training that serves as a midlevel health care provider; works under the license of a supervising physician
emergency medical technician (EMT) eh-MIR-jen-see MEh-dih-kal tek-NIH-shun	specially trained in the emergency care of a patient before and/or during transport to medical facility
speech therapist SPEECH THEH-rah-pist	specially trained in evaluating and treating problems with speech and/or swallowing
occupational therapist aw-kyoo-PAY-shuh-nal THEH-rah-pist	specially trained in evaluating and treating problems with performing daily activities at home, school, or work
physical therapist FIH-zih-kal THEH-rah-pist	specially trained in evaluating and treating physical impairments including disabilities or recovery from an injury
respiratory therapist reh-sprah-TOR-ee THEH-rah-pist	specially trained in treating patient's respiratory issues under the guidance of a health care provider
dietician dai-ah-TIH-shun	specially trained in evaluating the nutritional status of a patient and developing an appropriate diet plan
licensed practical nurse (LPN) LAI-senzd PRAK-tih-kal NIRS **licensed vocational nurse (LVN)** LAI-senzd voh-KAY-shun-al NIRS	trained and certified to provide basic care to a patient
registered nurse (RN) REH-jis-terd NIRS	an advanced level nurse who has completed an associate's or bachelor's degree; often assists with patient care planning and patient education
medical assistant MEH-dih-kal ah-SIS-tant	trained to carry out basic administrative and clinical tasks under the guidance of a health care provider

health professions *continued*

Term	Definition
laboratory and pathology	
pathologist pah-THAW-loh-jist	a physician with special training in both evaluating the causes and effects of disease and in laboratory medicine
medical laboratory technician meh-DIH-kal LAH-broh-tor-ee tek-NIH-shun	trained in performing laboratory testing on bodily fluids
phlebotomist fleh-BOH-tow-mist	trained in the removal of blood from the body for diagnostic or therapeutic purposes
radiology	
radiologist ray-dee-AW-loh-jist	a physician specially trained in evaluating images of the body to diagnose illness or injury
radiology technician ray-dee-AW-loh-jee tek-NIH-shun	trained to perform radiologic testing or administer radiation therapy under the direction of a health care provider
ultrasonagrapher ul-trah-saw-NAW-grah-fir	trained in performing ultrasound imaging on a patient
pharmacy	
pharmacist FAR-mah-sist	trained and licensed in preparing and dispensing medicine
pharmacy technician FAR-mah-see tek-NIH-shun	trained to assist a pharmacist with pharmacy-related tasks
clinical support	
patient service coordinator PAY-shent SIR-vis coh-OR-dih-nay-tor	handles administrative tasks and coordinates patient care
medical transcriptionist MEH-dih-kal tran-SKRIP-shun-ist	trained in converting the voice-recorded dictations of health care providers into text format

Learning Outcome 2.2 Exercises

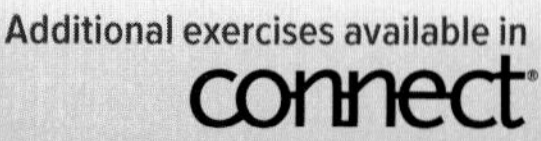

EXERCISE 25 *Match the term on the left with its definition on the right.*

1. anesthesiologist	a. a skilled health care provider who attended and graduated medical school.
2. nurse practitioner	b. a physician with special training in caring for children
3. pharmacist	c. a physician qualified to treat patients by means of operation or invasive procedure
4. pediatrician	d. a physician with special training in pain sedation and pain control
5. registered nurse	e. a physician with special training in both evaluating the causes and effects disease and in laboratory medicine
6. licensed practical nurse/ licensed vocational nurse	f. a health care professional trained and licensed in preparing and dispensing medicine
7. surgeon	g. a physician specially trained in evaluating images of the body to diagnose illness or injury
8. radiologist	h. an advanced-level nurse who has graduated from a graduate-level nursing program
9. pathologist	i. a nurse trained and certified in the basic care of a patient
10. physician	j. a nurse with postgraduate training that serves as a midlevel health care provider

EXERCISE 26 *Match the term on the left with its definition on the right.*

1. physician assistant	a. medical personnel trained in converting the voice-recorded dictations of health care providers into text format
2. emergency medical technician	b. medical personnel who handle administrative tasks and coordinate patient care
3. medical assistant	c. medical personnel trained to assist a pharmacist
4. medical laboratory technician	d. medical personnel trained in performing ultrasound imaging on a patient
5. phlebotomist	e. medical personnel who perform radiologic testing or administer radiation therapy under the direction of a health care provider
6. patient service coordinator	f. medical personnel trained in the removal of blood from the body for diagnostic or therapeutic purposes
7. radiology technician	g. medical personnel trained in performing laboratory testing on bodily fluids
8. ultrasonagrapher	h. medical personnel trained to carry out basic administrative and clinical tasks under the guidance of a health care provider
9. pharmacy technician	i. a health care professional specially trained in the emergency care of a patient before and/or during transport to a medical facility
10. medical transcriptionist	j. a midlevel health care provider who works under the license of a supervising physician; requires postgraduate training

Learning Outcome 2.2 Exercises

EXERCISE 27 *Match the term on the left with its definition on the right.*

1. dietician	a. a health care professional specially trained in evaluating and treating problems with speech and/or swallowing
2. respiratory therapist	b. a health care professional specially trained in evaluating and treating problems with performing daily activities at home, school, or work
3. speech therapist	c. a health care professional specially trained in evaluating and treating physical impairments including disabilities or recovery from an injury
4. physical therapist	d. a health care professional specially trained in treating patient's respiratory issues under the guidance of a health care provider
5. occupational therapist	e. a health care professional specially trained in evaluating the nutritional status of a patient and developing an appropriate diet

2.3 Types of Health Records

From an office setting to the hospital to the operating room, patients receive medical care in many different environments. Consequently, medical documentation of these visits demonstrates differences in their length and format. Regardless of these differences, medical notes continue to follow the same progression, starting from the subjective and ending with the plan. Even radiology and pathology reports exhibit this trend.

Medical records are routinely scoured to find specific information, such as:

- What medicine did the cardiologist prescribe for the patient?
- When is the patient supposed to follow up?
- What did the patient have?

In these instances, subheadings can serve as helpful guideposts. The following table features some common subheadings and their meanings.

The following are descriptions and examples of common types of health care records. As you will notice, they are not complete. The intention is to illustrate how charts are organized. Do not allow yourself to be distracted by any medical terms you have yet to learn. The notes are purposefully color-coded to help emphasize their segment in the SOAP format. The different sections of each note are color-coded in the following manner:

- Subjective: blue
- Objective: red
- Assessment: yellow
- Plan: green (*Note:* Sometimes assessment and plan run together; these instances appear in light green.)

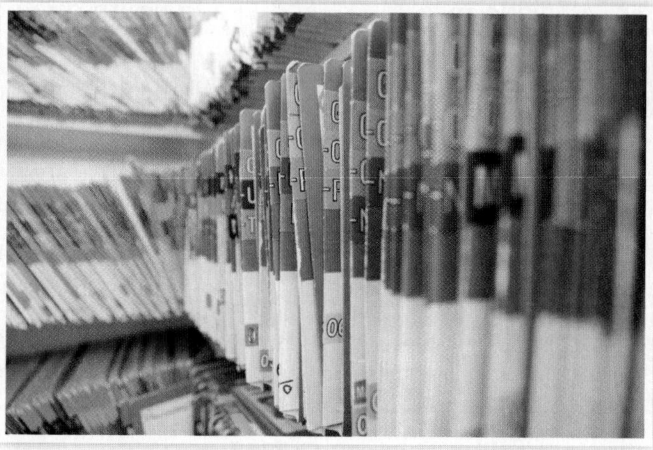

Health records play a vital role in helping organize and document a patient's medical history.

sections of a health record	description
Chief complaint	The main reason for the patient's visit
History of present illness	The story of the patient's problem
Review of systems	Description of individual body systems in order to discover any symptoms not directly related to the main problem
Past medical history	Other significant past illnesses, like high blood pressure, asthma, or diabetes
Past surgical history	Any of the patient's past surgeries
Family history	Any significant illnesses that run in the patient's family
Social history	A record of habits like smoking, drinking, drug abuse, and sexual practices that can impact health

Example Note #1: Clinic Note

Anytime a health care professional sees a patient in an office setting, he or she must document the visit. These notes can be handwritten, dictated, or electronic, or they may involve simply circling the correct words or checking boxes on a template. Regardless of how they are done, these notes always follow the SOAP method. For new patients, there is generally more information in the chart. The SOAP notes for subsequent visits are often more streamlined.

The following is an example of a doctor's office SOAP note.

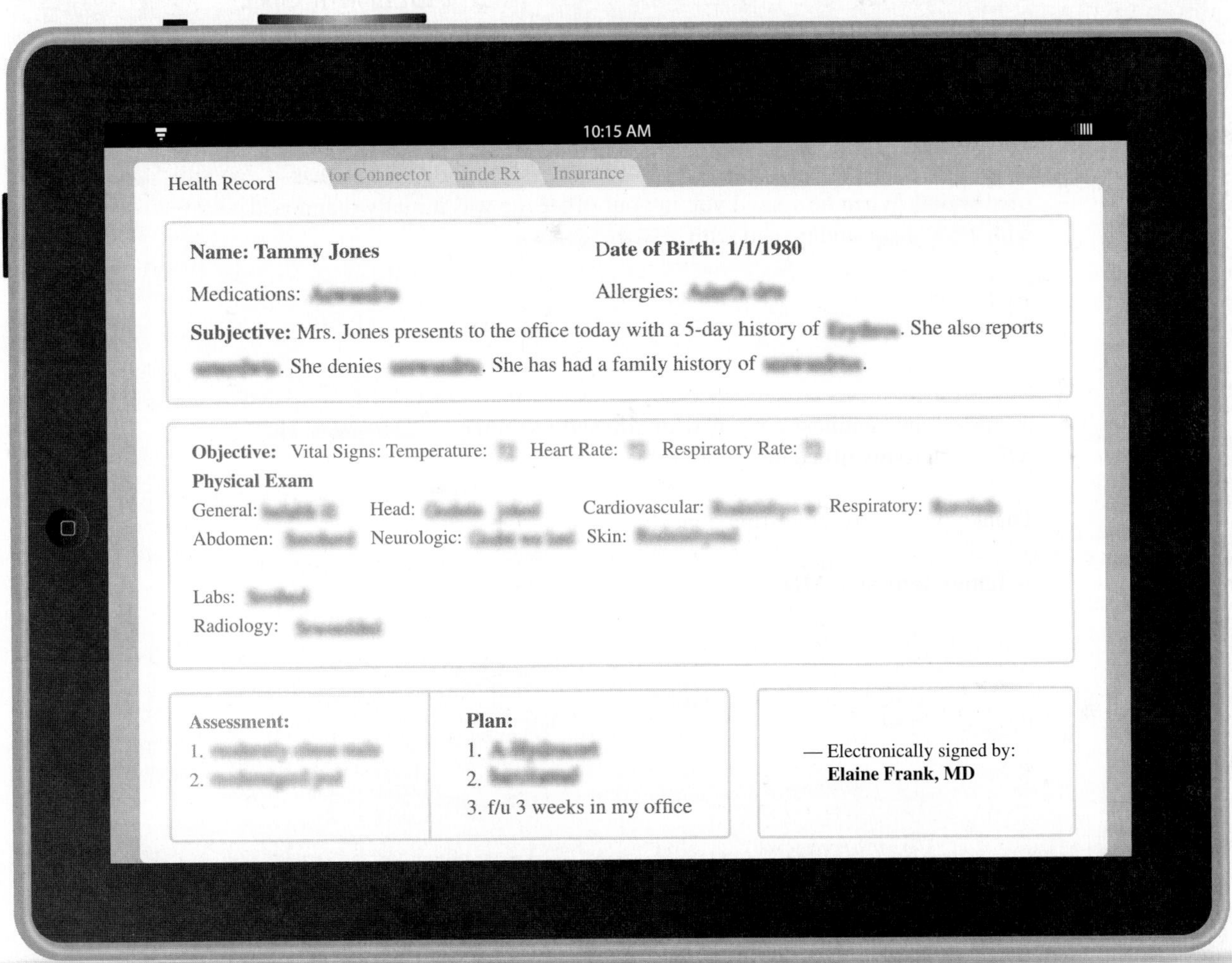

10:15 AM

Health Record | ...tor Connector | ...minde Rx | Insurance

Name: Tammy Jones **Date of Birth: 1/1/1980**

Medications: Allergies:

Subjective: Mrs. Jones presents to the office today with a 5-day history of . She also reports . She denies . She has had a family history of .

Objective: Vital Signs: Temperature: Heart Rate: Respiratory Rate:

Physical Exam

General: Head: Cardiovascular: Respiratory:

Abdomen: Neurologic: Skin:

Labs:

Radiology:

Assessment:

1.

2.

Plan:

1.

2.

3. f/u 3 weeks in my office

— Electronically signed by:
Elaine Frank, MD

Example Note #2: Consult Note

A note from a visit to a specialist or consultant can take two general types of approaches. The most common format is a note similar to the clinic note. Sometimes, however, the specialist may prefer to write the note in the form of a letter to the primary care provider. Even though the example below is in the form of a letter, you should be able to clearly see the SOAP format.

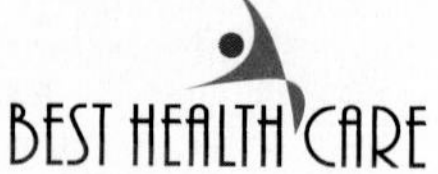

Dear Dr. Passemon,

This letter is in regard to Mr. Robert Meeds, whom you referred to my office for evaluation of [illegible]. The problem began [illegible]. He has tried [illegible]. When he visited you in your office, he was initially diagnosed with [illegible] and treated with [illegible].

On exam today, Mr. Meeds was generally well appearing. His x-rays today revealed [illegible]. I ordered the following labs: [illegible].

Based on Mr. Meeds's clinical picture, I believe he has [illegible]. I discussed the treatment options with him and recommend [illegible]. He will return to my office in 2 months.

Thank you for this interesting consult.

—James Jameson, MD

Example Note #3: Emergency Department Note

Patients seen in emergency departments and urgent care clinics are almost always new to the medical staff. Obtaining a good patient history from an emergency department patient is very important, as information about that patient's past is critical to getting a correct diagnosis in the present. One unique part of these notes is the emergency department (ED) course, which explains what happened to the patient during his or her stay in the ED. The ED course is a mixture of any completed diagnostic tests, the patient assessment, and a plan for the patient that unfolds over time.

CLINIC CORNER

Chief Complaint: Cough.
History of Present Illness: Mr. Stephen Dufresne is a 43-year-old male with a 3-day history of cough with .
Past Medical History: Asthma.
Past Surgical History: None.
Social History: Lives with his wife and two children. Nonsmoker. Drinks 4 glasses of wine a week.

Family History:
Father: Deceased at 68 years of age from stroke.
Mother: Alive, high blood pressure.
Medications: Albuterol, prn.
Allergies: No known drug allergies.

Physical Exam:
Vital Signs: Temperature: Heart Rate: Respiratory Rate:
General:
Head:
Cardiovascular:
Respiratory:
Abdomen:
Neurologic:
Skin:

Emergency Department Course:
Mr. Dufresne arrived to the emergency department in no apparent distress. A chest x-ray showed . We treated him with oxygen and . After two treatments of albuterol, he improved. He was diagnosed with and treated with .

Disposition:
Discharged to home, with follow-up in 3 days with his PCP.

—Christine Christenson, MD

Example Note #4: Admission Summary

Upon admittance to the hospital, patients must provide a medical history and receive a physical exam. Afterward, the attending medical professional writes a detailed admission summary. Detailed admission summaries are usually thorough notes that are very heavy on the subjective and objective parts, because the idea of the summary is to assemble all the facts in one place to help direct the entire hospital course.

- The assessment, which usually describes the thought process behind a patient's diagnosis and a list of possible causes for the patient's problem, is known as a *differential diagnosis*.
- The plan portion of the summary usually involves further testing, as well as care for the patient.

In a problem-based approach, the assessment and plan portions of the summary will be placed together. In such an approach, the patient's problems are numbered. After each number, the problems are described. The description is followed with a plan of what will be done about the problems.

Occasionally, a hospital team will send a courtesy letter to the patient's primary care provider (PCP). This letter can be similar to an admission note, but is usually briefer.

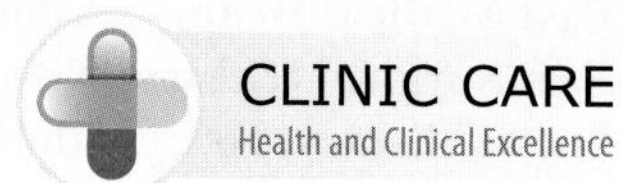

SUBJECTIVE

Chief Complaint: Chest pain.

History of Present Illness: Mr. William Burns is a 45-year-old male with a 2-month history of .
Review of Systems: Positive for .
Medications: None.
Allergies: No known drug allergies.
Past Medical History: .
Past Surgical History: Tonsillectomy/adenoidectomy at 3 years of age.
Social History: 1-pack-per-day smoker, social alcohol intake, divorced. Denies risky sexual behavior.
Family History: Father passed away at .

OBJECTIVE

Vital Signs: Temp: Heart Rate: Respiratory Rate:
Blood Pressure:

Physical Exam:

General:
Head:
Cardiovascular:
Respiratory:
Abdomen:
Neurologic:
Skin:

Labs:

Imaging:

Assessment/Plan:

1. **Chest Pain:** The differential diagnosis includes .
2. **Elevated Blood Sugar:** He did have a large meal .

—Madison Ginger, MD

Example Note #5: Discharge Summary

A discharge summary note details when and why a patient was admitted. It includes how the patient felt when admitted, what happened during the patient's stay in the hospital, and what kind of follow-up the patient will have. Sometimes, the hospital course description of a discharge summary will be broken down into body systems.

A discharge summary can break from the general SOAP pattern in one significant way: Often, the note will lead with the diagnoses—both the initial and also the final—because medical professionals want the most important information to come first. In all other respects it is similar to an emergency department note—but the discharge summary documents a longer stay in the hospital.

CLINIC CARE
Health and Clinical Excellence

DATE OF ADMISSION: [illegible]
DATE OF DISCHARGE: [illegible]

ADMISSION DIAGNOSIS:

1. [illegible]
2. [illegible]

DISCHARGE DIAGNOSIS:

1. [illegible]

DISCHARGE CONDITION: Stable

CONSULTATIONS: Pulmonology

PROCEDURES:

1. [illegible]
2. [illegible]

LABS: [illegible]

IMAGING: Chest x-ray

HPI:

Ms. Regina Klebs is a 28-year-old woman admitted to hospital from the ED with pneumonia. She initially presented with [illegible].

HOSPITAL COURSE:

Ms. Klebs was admitted to the hospital and placed on oxygen and IV antibiotics.

DISCHARGE PHYSICAL EXAMINATION:

Vital Signs: Temperature: [illegible] Heart Rate: [illegible] Respiratory Rate: [illegible]

Physical Exam:

General: [illegible]
Head: [illegible]
Cardiovascular: [illegible]
Respiratory: [illegible]
Abdomen: [illegible]
Neurologic: [illegible]
Skin: [illegible]

ACTIVITY: No restrictions.
DIET: [illegible]
MEDS: Topical penicillin antibiotic ointment.
FOLLOW-UP: Appointment—PCP (Dr. Primo) in 1 week.

—Francis Jerome, MD

Example Note #6: Operative Report

After each surgery, the surgeon completes an operative report that documents in detail the procedure that was performed, the events that transpired during the surgery, and the patient's outcome from the surgery. As with a discharge summary, the diagnosis is presented at the beginning of the note.

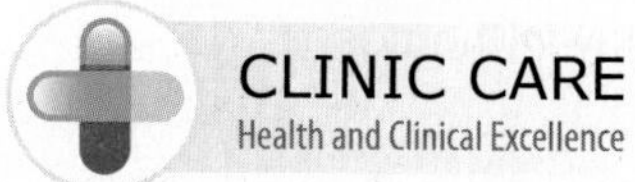

Preoperative Diagnosis: Appendicitis
Postoperative Diagnosis: Appendicitis

Procedure: Appendectomy
Anesthesia: General

Indication: The patient, Wallace Simpson, is a 25-year-old man with acute onset of abdominal pain and fever.

Operative Findings: The patient had a grossly inflamed appendix and local peritonitis.

Description of Procedure: Mr. Simpson was brought to the operating room with suspected appendicitis. Mr. Simpson tolerated the procedure well.

Disposition: Mr. Simpson was sent to the PACU in stable condition.

—James Cutter, MD

Example Note #7: Daily Hospital Note/Progress Note

Every day that a patient is in the hospital, a health care professional must see him or her and document the visit. Usually, the subjective part of these daily hospital notes focuses on how the patient's condition has changed since the previous note. Often, the note's assessment and plan sections will be put together, as with an admission note.

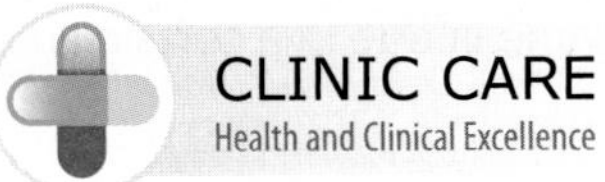

Subjective:

Since yesterday, the patient, Mrs. Penelope Gates, has vomited 3 times.

Objective:

Vital Signs: Temp: Heart Rate: Respiratory Rate:
Intake: Output:

Physical Exam:

General:
Head:
Cardiovascular:
Respiratory:
Abdomen:
Neurologic:
Skin:
Labs:

Assessment/**Plan:**

1. Acute gastroenteritis: No change. Continue IV fluids.
2. Metabolic acidosis: Noticed this AM on lab work. We will begin the patient on .

—Harry Harrison, MD

Example Note #8: Radiology Report

A radiology report note explains the reason for ordering a radiologic image, how the image was performed, what was seen on the image, and the reviewing radiologist's assessment. Sometimes the note provides a recommendation as well. When a recommendation is provided, it is usually a recommendation for a different type of image, or a request to repeat the same image in a certain time frame.

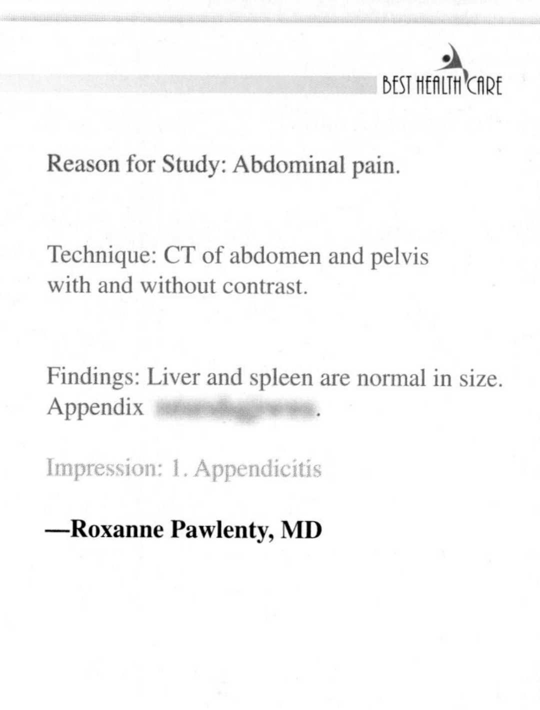

BEST HEALTH CARE

Reason for Study: Abdominal pain.

Technique: CT of abdomen and pelvis with and without contrast.

Findings: Liver and spleen are normal in size. Appendix [illegible].

Impression: 1. Appendicitis

—Roxanne Pawlenty, MD

Example Note #9: Pathology Report

A pathology report note mirrors the same style as the radiology note. This note mentions the reason for the study, what was seen in detail, and the assessment.

CLINIC CORNER

Clinical History: Mrs. Linda Genner, a 48-year-old woman, had a suspicious mass seen on a CT scan.

Specimen: Lung, right upper lobe resection.

Gross Description: A single specimen measuring 2.3 cm × 4.5 cm × 8.2 cm. The surface of the specimen is [illegible].

Diagnosis: Right upper lobe—Adenocarcinoma Grade 1.

—Brendan Kellstrom, MD

Example Note #10: Prescription

This type of note doesn't follow the SOAP note format—because it *is* the plan. A prescription form has a structure all its own:

- The first line is for the name and strength of the medicine. In the name blank, the health care professional may write either the generic name of the actual medicine (e.g., ibuprofen) or a name brand (e.g., Advil).
- The second line, marked "Sig," contains the patient's instructions. On the prescription form, these instructions are written in medical language; it is the pharmacist's job to translate these instructions into lay terms for the patient.
- The third line, usually marked "Dispense," tells the pharmacist how much medicine to give the patient.
- The fourth line mentions how many refills are available for the prescription.
- The prescription form's last line is for the health care provider's signature (either written or electronic). It usually includes a box the health care provider can check to indicate whether the prescribed medication must be a brand name (instead of generic). Please note that with the increasing use of electronic medical records, the use of certain, specific medical terms (such as *BID* or *QHS*) are becoming less common in prescriptions. Nonetheless, it is important to be familiar with these terms as they have not completely disappeared.

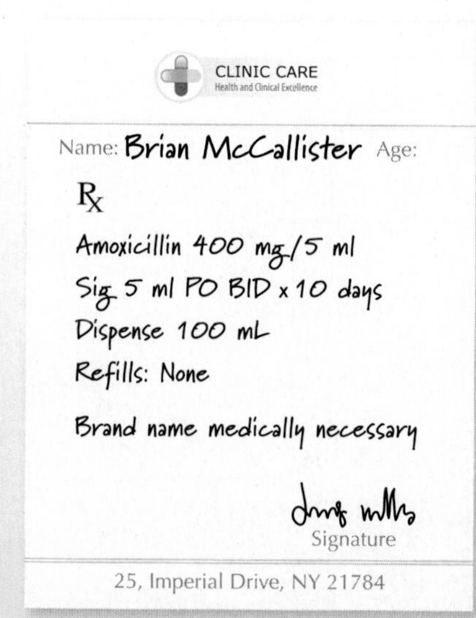

CLINIC CARE
Health and Clinical Excellence

Name: Brian McCallister Age:

℞

Amoxicillin 400 mg/5 ml
Sig 5 ml PO BID x 10 days
Dispense 100 mL
Refills: None
Brand name medically necessary

Signature

25, Imperial Drive, NY 21784

summary of health record notes

	Author	Location	Purpose	Format and Order	Unique Features
1. Clinic note	Medical professional	Clinic	Documents a visit	SOAP	New patient: Includes more history, separate form Repeat patient: Streamlined note
2. Consult note	Physician; usually a specialist	Clinic or hospital	Provides an expert opinion on a more challenging problem	SOAP	Can be in the form of a letter to the PCP
3. Emergency department note	ED medical staff	Emergency department	Documents an emergency department visit	SOAP	The A includes the emergency department course
4. Admission summary	Hospital medical professional	Hospital	Documents the admission of a patient to the hospital	SO A/P	S, O = Very thorough A = Differential diagnosis P = Further testing and care A + P = Problem-based approach
5. Discharge summary	Medical professional	Hospital	Describes when and why the patient was admitted; documents a longer stay	ASOP	Starts with A
6. Operative report	Surgeon		Documents a surgery in detail	ASOP	
7. Daily hospital note/ progress note	Medical professional	Inpatient health care facility	Documents daily hospital visit	SO A/P	S—Focuses on how patient's condition has changed since the previous note A—Sometimes includes a differential diagnosis
8. Radiology report	Radiologist		Explains reason for image, how image was performed, what was seen on image, radiologist's assessment; sometimes a recommendation	SOA	Usually includes only S, O, and A, but may include a P if it recommends that further studies should be performed
9. Pathology report	Pathologist		Provides reasons for test, what was seen on the test, and an assessment	SOA	
10. Prescription	Medical professional		Provides directions for a medication	P	1. Medicine's name 2. Instructions for patient 3. How much medicine should be given 4. Refills, if any 5. Health care professional's signature and whether generic substitution is allowed

Learning Outcome 2.3 Exercises

EXERCISE 1 *Match the health record type on the left with its description on the right.*

_____ 1. prescription
_____ 2. radiology report
_____ 3. pathology report
_____ 4. daily hospital note/progress note
_____ 5. emergency department note
_____ 6. admission summary
_____ 7. operative report
_____ 8. clinic note
_____ 9. consult note
_____ 10. discharge summary

a. documents a patient visit in an office setting
b. document sent to a primary physician, usually by a specialist, to give an opinion on a more challenging problem
c. documents a patient's emergency department visit
d. documents a patient's admission to the hospital
e. documents a patient's admission and hospital stay (usually a longer stay)
f. documents a surgery
g. documents a patient's progress during a daily hospital visit
h. documents an imaging procedure by a radiologist
i. documents a pathology procedure
j. a medical professional's directions for a patient's medication

EXERCISE 2 *Match the term on the left with its definition on the right.*

_____ 1. past surgical history
_____ 2. family history
_____ 3. past medical history
_____ 4. history of present illness
_____ 5. social history
_____ 6. chief complaint
_____ 7. review of systems

a. the main reason for a visit
b. the story of the patient's problem
c. any symptoms not directly related to the main problem
d. other significant past illnesses, like high blood pressure, asthma, or diabetes
e. any past surgeries
f. any significant illnesses that run in the patient's family
g. mainly health habits, like smoking, drinking, drug use, or sexual practices

EXERCISE 3 *Multiple-choice questions. Select the correct answer.*

1. Which health record does NOT follow the SOAP format?
   a. consult note
   b. daily hospital note
   c. emergency department note
   d. prescription
2. Which type of health record is sometimes found in the form of a letter?
   a. clinic note
   b. consult note
   c. daily hospital note
   d. pathology report

Learning Outcome 2.3 Exercises

3. Select the health records that document a type of procedure.
   a. discharge summary
   b. emergency department note
   c. operative report
   d. pathology report
   e. prescription
   f. radiology report
4. Which health record is NOT routinely used in a hospital or inpatient health care facility?
   a. admission summary
   b. clinic note
   c. discharge summary
   d. emergency department note
   e. progress note
5. Which health record would be used to document a routine pediatric wellness exam?
   a. clinic note
   b. consult note
   c. daily hospital note
   d. operative report
6. In a *problem-based approach,* you:
   a. number the problems, describe how the patient's problem has changed, and provide your plan for what to do about the problem
   b. focus on what you are doing wrong and who should take over
   c. try to cause more problems in the patient in the hopes of determining what is really wrong
   d. assume that nothing has been done right so far and redo every test
7. An *emergency department course:*
   a. explains what transpired during the patient's stay in the emergency department; includes any diagnostic tests done, the assessment, and a plan for the patient that unfolds over time
   b. lists the path every patient takes when entering the emergency department for treatment
   c. organizes an emergency department by types of injury
   d. teaches students how to behave in an emergency department

EXERCISE 4 *Identify the author of each of the following types of health records.*

1. pathology report ______________________________
2. operative report ______________________________
3. radiology report ______________________________
4. emergency department note ______________________________
5. consult note ______________________________

Learning Outcome 2.3 Exercises

EXERCISE 5 *Fill in the blanks based on the sample health record.*

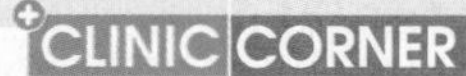

Subjective:

Mrs. Allison Voxenhead is here for a follow-up visit for her schizophrenia. At her last visit, she complained of dystonia on her haloperidol. I changed her to a newer antipsychotic medication at that time, and she is here today to follow up the results. Overall, she is improved and has not had any new hallucinations. Her only concern today is recent insomnia for the past week. She noticed the insomnia started when she began a new job, and she says that learning her new job has been stressful. She has been anxious at night, and that has made it hard for her to sleep.

Objective:

General: Flat affect. Nonagitated. Mood is not dysphoric. Alert, oriented.
HEENT: Pupils equal, round, and reactive to light. Tonsils normal size.
Resp: Clear to auscultation.
CV: RRR without murmur, gallop, rubs.
Neuro: Normal movement. No dyskinesia. Normal tone.

Assessment:

1. Schizophrenia: stable on new medication regimen.
2. Insomnia likely related to new job stress.

Plan:

1. I will begin her short term on an anxiolytic.
2. Continue antipsychotic.
3. Follow-up visit in 2 months.
4. Continue following with psychologist.

Electronically signed by:
Dale Philbert, PA 03/04/2015 9:30 AM

1. The health record type is: ______________________
2. The patient's name is: ______________________
3. The author of the health record is: ______________________
4. The patient has been diagnosed with: ______________ and ______________
5. The format of the health record is: ______________________

Learning Outcome 2.3 Exercises

EXERCISE 6 *Based on the sample health record, fill in the blanks and label parts as noted in Question #5 that follows.*

BEST HEALTH CARE

Dear Dr. Childs,

Thank you for referring Mr. Juan Samuels to my office. I saw him on March 3, 2014. Mr. Samuels has a 4-month history of increasing pain in his right distal femur. He first noticed pain after being kicked in the leg at a soccer game. He was evaluated in your office 3 weeks later for persistent pain. There was a soft tissue mass in his distal femur that was tender to touch. An x-ray was performed to rule out a fracture or chronic osteomyelitis. The x-ray showed both osteolysis of the metaphysis and periosteal new bone formation. Labs were drawn, including CBC, CPK, and ESR. Mr. Samuels was referred to my office for further evaluation of the concerning x-ray findings.

5(a) Health Record Part ______

On exam, Mr. Samuels was a pleasant young man, well developed, well nourished, and in no acute distress. His lungs were clear, and his heart was regular in rate and rhythm. No murmurs were heard. His right leg reveals a significant soft tissue mass over his distal femur on the right. The mass is tender. He did not have any knee effusion. I reviewed the labs and x-ray. His findings were consistent with osteosarcoma.

5(b) Health Record Part ______

I discussed the next steps with the patient and family, including staging the tumor and scheduling a biopsy to confirm the diagnosis. I discussed the surgery with the patient and his family present in the office. His tumor will likely require tumor resection with partial ostectomy of the femur with osteoplasty.

I discussed the benefits of a metal endoprosthesis versus an allograft for the osteoplasty.

5(c) Health Record Part ______

Mr. Samuels is scheduled to return to my office in 1 week after his biopsy to discuss the results.

Thank you for this interesting consult.

—Tara Sanchez, MD, FAAOS

1. The health record type is: ______________________________
2. The patient's name is: ______________________________
3. The author of the health record is: ______________________________
4. Some of the patient's symptoms (reason for the visit) include: ______________________________
5. In the blanks alongside the sample, label the correct parts of the health record using the letter associated with each section.

S–Subjective A–Assessment

O–Objective P–Plan

Learning Outcome 2.3 Exercises

EXERCISE 7 *Based on the sample health record, fill in the blanks and label parts as noted in Question #4 that follows.*

CLINIC CORNER

Discharge Summary

Patient Name: Decker Woolsey

DATE OF ADMISSION: 1/1/15
DATE OF DISCHARGE: 1/4/15

ADMISSION DIAGNOSIS:
1. Hypotonia
2. Scoliosis

4(a) Health Record Part ______

DISCHARGE DIAGNOSIS:
1. Muscular dystrophy
2. Scoliosis

4(b) Health Record Part ______

DISCHARGE CONDITION:
Stable

4(c) Health Record Part ______

CONSULTATIONS:
Neurology
Cardiology
Orthopedic surgery

4(d) Health Record Part ______

PROCEDURES:
1. Electromyography
2. Muscle biopsy

4(e) Health Record Part ______

LABS:
CBC, CMP, CPK, ESR

4(f) Health Record Part ______

IMAGING:
None

4(g) Health Record Part ______

HPI:
Decker Woolsey is an 8-year-old boy admitted directly to the pediatric floor for a workup of chronic progressive hypotonia. His parents report they have noticed progressive weakness. Decker has had increasing difficulty running, jumping, and climbing stairs. Decker's parents initially thought his problems were due to his asthma, but they noticed he also had a waddling gait. They took him to their PCP, who referred him for evaluation. On admission, the patient denied any history of myalgia, arthrodynia, or dystaxia. His problem appeared limited to muscle tone.

4(h) Health Record Part ______

HOSPITAL COURSE:
NEURO: On admission exam, the patient was found to have mild lumbar lordosis, pseudohypertrophy of his calf muscles, and a waddling gait. He did not have any genu varum or genu valgus. No hyporeflexia was noted. The initial concern was a muscular dystrophy. Given a family history of polymyositis, that was considered as well. His labs were consistent with muscular dystrophy.

-1-

continued

Learning Outcome 2.3 Exercises

CLINIC CORNER

An electromyography showed myopathic changes. A muscle biopsy was then performed to help distinguish which of the muscular dystrophies the patient had. The results are pending.
CV: Cardiology was consulted, given the strong risk for developing cardiomyopathy.
RESP: No problems occurred throughout hospital stay. Education was given about breathing exercises and the respiratory problems that are frequently seen later on with this condition.
ORTHO: Orthopedic surgery was consulted for his scoliosis.
SOCIAL: Much of the hospital stay focused on patient education.

4(i) Health Record Part ______

DISCHARGE PHYSICAL EXAMINATION:

Temp 98.6 RR 24 HR 86 BP 100/64
Gen: WDWN. Alert.
CV: RRR.
RESP: CTA.
NEURO: Hypotonia of legs (strength 3/5 bilaterally). Waddling gait. Using assistance to get up from seated position. Normal reflexes. Marked enlargement of calves.

4(j) Health Record Part ______

ACTIVITY:

No restrictions. Referral to PT on discharge. First appointment is next week.

4(k) Health Record Part ______

DIET:

Calcium/vit D supplement to prevent osteoporosis.

4(l) Health Record Part ______

MEDS:

Glucocorticoid.

4(m) Health Record Part ______

FOLLOW-UP:

Appointments:
PCP: Dr. Bening in 1 week
Neurology: Dr. Schwarz in 2 weeks
Cardiology: Dr. Benitez in 6 months
Orthopedic: Dr. Jawarz in 6 months

4(n) Health Record Part ______

-2-

1. The health record type is: ______________________________
2. The patient's name is: ______________________________
3. This health record was written at a(n): ______________________________
4. In the blanks alongside the sample, label the correct parts of the health record using the letter associated with each section.

S–Subjective A–Assessment
O–Objective P–Plan

Learning Outcome 2.3 Exercises

EXERCISE 8 *Based on the sample health record, fill in the blanks, select the correct response, or label parts as noted in Question #3 that follows.*

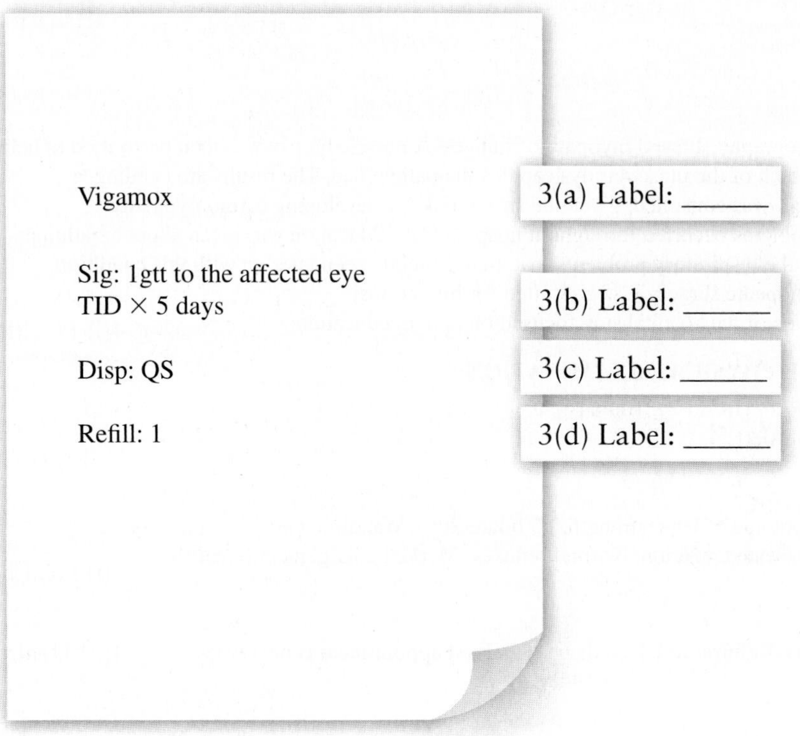

1. The health record type is: ____________________

2. Which part of the SOAP note is included in this health record (select the correct choice)?

   a. S–Subjective
   b. O–Objective
   c. A–Assessment
   d. P–Plan

3. In the blanks alongside the sample, label the correct parts of the health record using the letter associated with each section.

   a. name and strength of the medicine
   b. patient instructions
   c. how much medicine to give the patient
   d. refill information

2.4 Abbreviations

Abbreviations Associated with Health Care Facilities

With more than 82 million people worldwide now sending text messages on a regular basis, it's no wonder that phrases like "LOL," "JK," and "OMG" have become commonly understood abbreviations. Why do people use them? Efficiency.

This love affair with abbreviations was going on in the world of medicine long before text messaging, mobile phones, and even computers arrived on the scene. Whether that's because it is more efficient to cut down a word to a few letters or because it makes these terms somehow seem more important, acronyms and abbreviations are commonplace in health records.

These abbreviations refer to various types of treatment facilities within the medical profession.

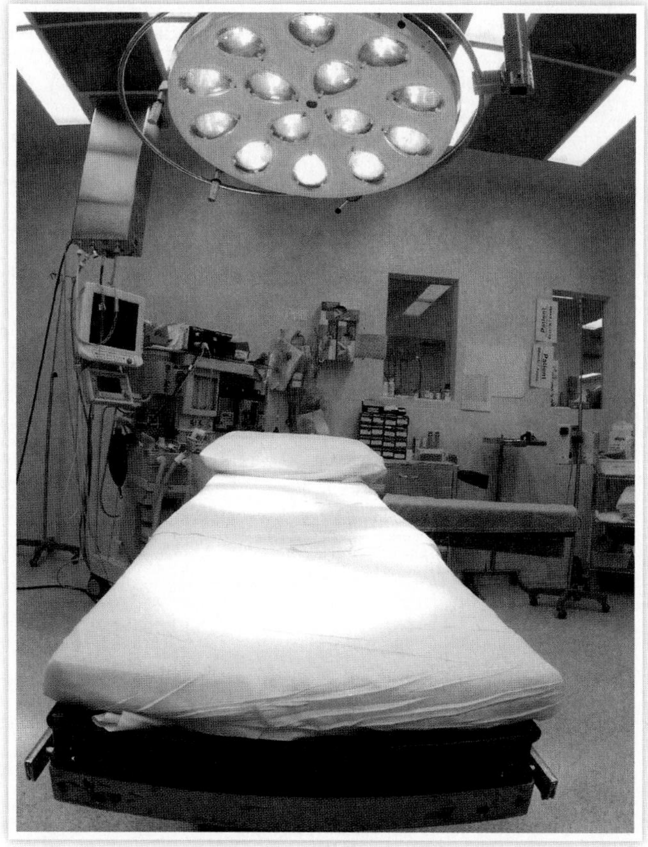

Abbreviations are used to describe a wide variety of health care facilities.

health care facility abbreviations

Abbreviation	Definition
CCU	coronary care unit
ECU	emergency care unit
ER	emergency room
ED	emergency department
ICU	intensive care unit
PICU	pediatric intensive care unit
NICU	neonatal intensive care unit
SICU	surgical intensive care unit
PACU	post-anesthesia care unit
L&D	labor and delivery
OR	operating room
post-op	after surgery
pre-op	before surgery

Learning Outcome 2.4 Exercises

EXERCISE 1 *Match the abbreviation on the left with its definition on the right.*

______	1. pre-op	a. coronary care unit
______	2. post-op	b. emergency room
______	3. ER	c. emergency department
______	4. ICU	d. intensive care unit
______	5. ED	e. neonatal intensive care unit
______	6. CCU	f. surgical intensive care unit
______	7. L&D	g. labor and delivery
______	8. NICU	h. after surgery
______	9. SICU	i. before surgery

EXERCISE 2 *Translate the following abbreviations.*

1. ER ______
2. OR ______
3. ICU ______
4. PICU ______
5. NICU ______
6. SICU ______
7. CCU ______
8. ECU ______
9. PACU ______

EXERCISE 3 *Identify the abbreviation given the information provided.*

1. after surgery ______
2. before surgery ______
3. emergency department ______
4. labor and delivery ______
5. operating room ______
6. emergency care unit ______
7. pediatric intensive care unit ______
8. post-anesthesia care unit ______

Abbreviations Associated with Patient Care

These abbreviations are typical of the ones found on patient charts and other health records.

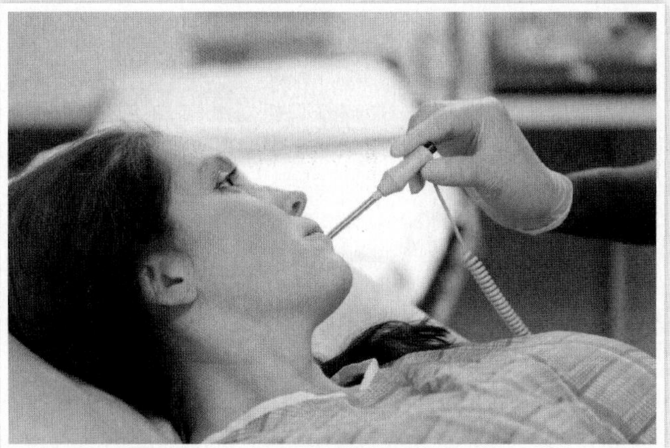

Temperature is one of the many common pieces of information that is abbreviated on health records.

symbols

Abbreviation	Definition
♂	male
♀	female
(R)	right
(L)	left
(B)	bilateral (both sides)
↑	increased
↓	decreased

abbreviations common on health records

Abbreviation	Definition
VS	vital signs
T	temperature
BP	blood pressure
HR	heart rate
RR	respiratory rate
Ht	height
Wt	weight
BMI	body mass index (measurement of body fat based on height and weight)
I/O	intake/output: the amount of fluids a patient has taken in (by IV or mouth) and produced (usually just urine output)

abbreviations common on health records *continued*

Abbreviation	Definition
Dx	diagnosis
DDx	differential diagnosis
Tx	treatment
Rx	prescription
H&P	history and physical
Hx	history
CC	chief complaint (the main reason for the visit)
HPI	history of present illness (the story of the symptoms)
ROS	review of systems (anything else not directly related to the chief complaint)
PMHx	past medical history
FHx	family history
NKDA	no known drug allergies
PE	physical exam
Pt	patient
y/o	years old
h/o	history of
PCP	primary care provider
f/u	follow up

abbreviations used for symptoms or exam findings

Abbreviation	Definition
SOB	while it may mean something outside of medicine, here, it means *shortness* of breath **NOTE:** Because of the negative nonmedical meaning, it has been suggested that SOB should be replaced by other abbreviations like SOA (shortness of air).
HEENT	head, eyes, ears, nose, and throat
PERRLA	pupils are equal, round, and reactive to light and accommodation
NAD	no acute distress (the patient does not display any intense symptoms)
CV	cardiovascular
RRR	regular rate and rhythm (description of a normal heart on exam)
CTA	clear to auscultation (description of normal-sounding lungs)
WDWN	well developed, well nourished (the patient is growing or has grown appropriately and does not appear to be malnourished)
A&O	alert and oriented (the patient can answer questions and is aware of what's going on)

abbreviations used for symptoms or exam findings *continued*

Abbreviation	Definition
WNL	within normal limits
NOS	not otherwise specified
NEC	not elsewhere classified **Note:** NOS and NEC are catch-alls for diagnoses that don't quite fit any specific cause (for example, "rash NOS")

abbreviations associated with orders and administering medicine

Abbreviation	Definition
PO	per os (by mouth)
NPO	nil per os (nothing by mouth)
PR	per rectum (anal)
IM	intramuscular
SC	subcutaneous (under the skin)
IV	intravenous
CVL	central venous line
PICC	peripherally inserted central catheter
Sig	instructions short for *signa,* from Latin, for "label"

Learning Outcome 2.4 Exercises

EXERCISE 4 *Translate each of the following abbreviations or symbols.*

1. (R) ______
2. (L) ______
3. ↓ ______
4. VS ______
5. T ______
6. BP ______
7. HR ______
8. RR ______
9. Dx ______
10. DDx ______
11. Tx ______
12. HPI ______
13. h/o ______
14. PMHx ______
15. FHx ______
16. Pt ______
17. PCP ______
18. f/u ______
19. NAD ______
20. RRR ______
21. NOS ______
22. NKDA ______
23. HEENT ______
24. CV ______

EXERCISE 5 *Match the abbreviation on the left with its definition on the right.*

______	1. CC	a. the patient is growing or has grown properly; is well developed and nourished
______	2. I/O	b. description of a normal heart on an exam
______	3. ROS	c. description of normal-sounding lungs
______	4. PO	d. the patient does not look extremely sick
______	5. WDWN	e. follow up
______	6. BMI	f. catch-all for diagnoses that don't quite fit any specific cause
______	7. NEC	g. the amount of fluid a patient has taken in (by IV or mouth) and produced (usually just urine output)
______	8. f/u	h. measurement of body fat based on height and weight
______	9. NPO	i. the main reason for the visit
______	10. NAD	j. anything else not necessarily directly related to the chief complaint
______	11. CTA	k. nothing by mouth
______	12. SC	l. by mouth
______	13. RRR	m. under the skin

Learning Outcome 2.4 Exercises

EXERCISE 6 *Identify the abbreviation or symbol from the information provided.*

1. body mass index ____________
2. years old ____________
3. shortness of breath ____________
4. clear to auscultation ____________
5. well developed, well nourished ____________
6. ♂ ____________
7. ♀ ____________
8. intake/output ____________
9. CC ____________
10. per os (by mouth) ____________
11. nil per os (nothing by mouth) ____________
12. subcutaneous ____________
13. within normal limits ____________
14. increased ____________
15. pupils are equal, round, and reactive to light and accommodation ____________
16. history and physical ____________
17. physical exam ____________
18. PR ____________
19. follow up ____________
20. intramuscular ____________
21. peripherally inserted central catheter ____________
22. central venous line ____________

EXERCISE 7 *Multiple-choice questions. Select all correct answers that apply.*

1. Select the abbreviations common on health records.
   a. A&O
   b. Ht
   c. Hx
   d. IV
   e. ROS
   f. Sig
   g. Wt
2. Select the abbreviations used for symptoms or exam findings.
   a. A&O
   b. Ht
   c. Hx
   d. IV
   e. ROS
   f. Rx
   g. Sig
   h. Wt
3. Select the abbreviations associated with ordering and administering medicine.
   a. A&O
   b. Ht
   c. Hx
   d. IV
   e. ROS
   f. Sig
   g. Wt
4. Which abbreviation means "both sides"?
   a. B
   b. BS
   c. SOB
   d. SC

Timing- and Frequency-Based Abbreviations

The following abbreviations deal with the frequency of an order. They are also frequently found on prescriptions.

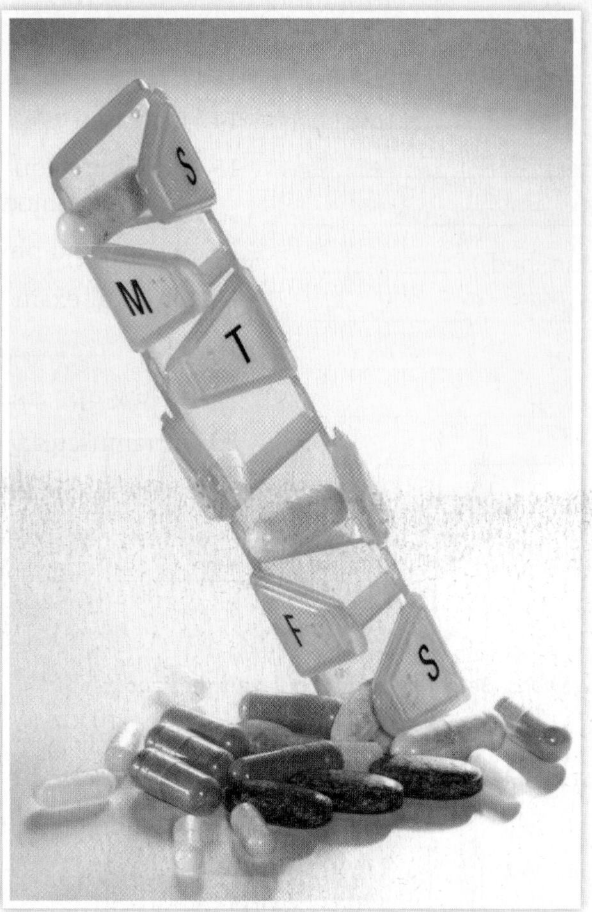

Prescriptions are a major area where doctors use abbreviations.

timing abbreviations

Abbreviation	Definition
BID	twice daily, from the Latin phrase *bis in die*, which means "two in a day"
TID	three times daily, from the Latin phrase *ter in die*, which means "three in a day"
Q	every x, example Q4hr would mean every 4 hours or Q3 days would be every 3 days.
QD*	daily, from the Latin phrase *quaque die*, which means "each day"
QID*	four times daily, from the Latin phrase *quater in die*, which means "four in a day"
QHS	at night, from the Latin phrase *quaque hora somni*, which means "each night at the hour of sleep"
AC	before meals, from the Latin phrase *ante cibum*, which means "before food"
PC	after meals, from the Latin phrase *post cibum*, which means "after food"
prn	as needed, from the Latin phrase *per re nata*, which means "as the need arises"
ad lib	as desired

* The abbreviations *QD* and *QID* are now prohibited in many health care settings because they are easily confused. We've included mention of them in case you come across them, but we *do not* encourage their use.

Learning Outcome 2.4 Exercises

EXERCISE 8 *Match the term on the left with its definition on the right.*

______	1. AC		a. daily
______	2. BID		b. twice daily
______	3. PC		c. three times daily
______	4. prn		d. four times daily
______	5. QD		e. before meals
______	6. QHS		f. after meals
______	7. QID		g. as needed
______	8. TID		h. at night

EXERCISE 9 *Translate the following terms.*

1. BID ______
2. TID ______
3. AC ______
4. PC ______
5. prn ______
6. QD ______
7. QID ______
8. QHS ______

EXERCISE 10 *Identify the medical abbreviation from the information provided.*

1. before meals ______
2. after meals ______
3. at night ______
4. as needed ______
5. daily ______
6. twice daily ______
7. three times daily ______
8. four times daily ______

2.5 Electronic Health Records

Clinic Note

To help you become more familiar with health records, we will include cases at the end of every chapter. Following each case, you will be able to do exercises about the cases to help you practice your medical language skills. Now that you are more familiar with many general medical words and abbreviations, let's reexamine some of the records you saw earlier in the chapter.

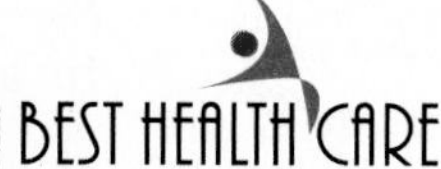

Name: Tammy Jones **Date of Birth: 1/1/1980**
Medications: Flovent **BID**; Albuterol **prn**; Singulair **QDay**
Allergies: **NKDA**

Subjective:

Mrs. Jones presents to the office today with a 5-day history of wheezing. She has been using her albuterol at home, but she noticed an **acute** increase in her coughing and wheezing 2 days ago. She also reports **progressively** worse congestion, sneezing, and a runny nose. These **symptoms** have also increased in the past 2 days. She has been **afebrile**. She denies chest pain or difficulty breathing.

Objective:

Vital Signs: **T**: 98.8 **HR**: 72 **RR**: 24 **BP**: 118/72 **Pulse Ox**: 92% on room air

Physical Exam:

Gen: **WDWN.**
HEENT: PERRLA, lips slightly dry.
CV: RRR, no murmurs.
Resp: Wheezing heard **bilaterally** on **auscultation.**
Abd: Soft, nontender.
Skin: Good capillary refill.
Imaging: Chest x-ray: Mild hyperinflation. No opacities.

Assessment:

1. Asthma **exacerbation**
2. Allergies

Plan:

1. Steroids **PO** x 3 days.
2. Continue albuterol **Q4-6 hours prn wheezing.**
3. **Supportive care** for the allergies, including over-the-counter antihistamines.
4. **F/u** 3 weeks in my office.

—Signed electronically by: **Elaine Frank, MD**

Learning Outcome 2.5 Exercises

EXERCISE 1 *Match the term on the left with its definition on the right.*

______	1. symptom		a. well developed, well nourished
______	2. progressive		b. pupils are equal, round, and reactive to light and accommodation
______	3. acute		c. to listen
______	4. auscultation		d. symptoms just started
______	5. afebrile		e. more and more each day
______	6. exacerbation		f. something the patient feels
______	7. PERRLA		g. to not have a fever
______	8. WDWN		h. the symptoms are getting worse

EXERCISE 2 *Fill in the blanks.*

1. The name of the patient is: ______________________________
2. The author of this health record is: ______________________________
3. The patient's temperature is: ______________________________
4. The patient's heart rate is: ______________________________
5. The patient's respiratory rate is: ______________________________
6. The patient's blood pressure is: ______________________________

EXERCISE 3 *True or false questions. Indicate true answers with a T and false answers with an F.*

1. The patient has had a fever. __________
2. Two days ago the patient's coughing and wheezing suddenly increased. __________
3. The patient has an irregular heart rate and rhythm. __________
4. The patient has wheezing on both sides of her body. __________
5. As part of the patient's plan, she will take steroids by mouth for 3 days. __________

EXERCISE 4 *Multiple-choice questions. Select the correct answer.*

1. The patient takes Flovent:
   a. once a day
   b. twice a day
   c. three times a day
   d. as needed
2. The patient takes albuterol:
   a. once a day
   b. twice a day
   c. three times a day
   d. as needed
3. The patient takes Singulair:
   a. once a day
   b. twice a day
   c. three times a day
   d. as needed
4. The term that means "to treat the symptoms and make the patient feel better" is:
   a. discharge
   b. palliative
   c. reassurance
   d. supportive care

Consult Note

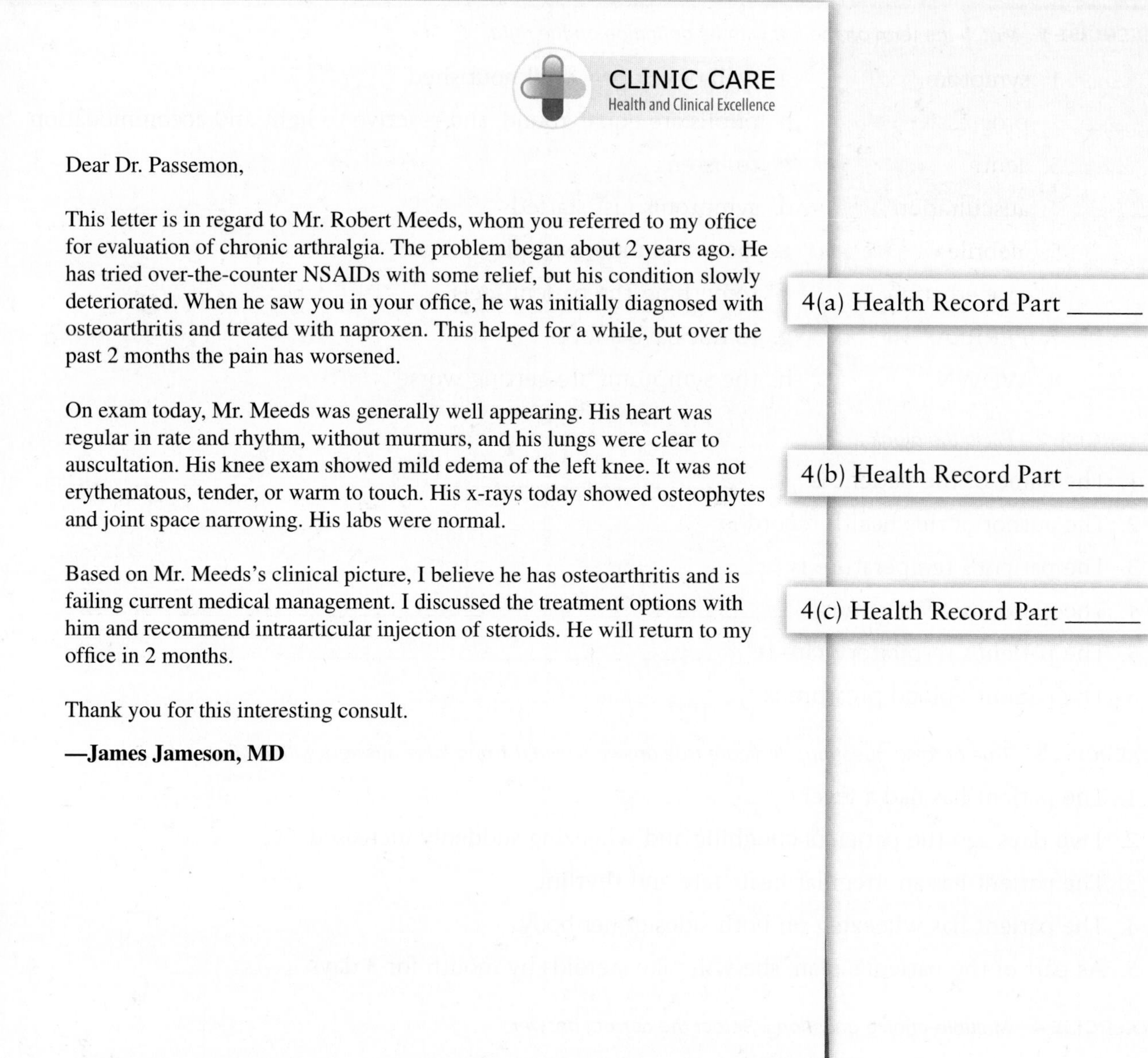

CLINIC CARE
Health and Clinical Excellence

Dear Dr. Passemon,

This letter is in regard to Mr. Robert Meeds, whom you referred to my office for evaluation of chronic arthralgia. The problem began about 2 years ago. He has tried over-the-counter NSAIDs with some relief, but his condition slowly deteriorated. When he saw you in your office, he was initially diagnosed with osteoarthritis and treated with naproxen. This helped for a while, but over the past 2 months the pain has worsened.

4(a) Health Record Part ______

On exam today, Mr. Meeds was generally well appearing. His heart was regular in rate and rhythm, without murmurs, and his lungs were clear to auscultation. His knee exam showed mild edema of the left knee. It was not erythematous, tender, or warm to touch. His x-rays today showed osteophytes and joint space narrowing. His labs were normal.

4(b) Health Record Part ______

Based on Mr. Meeds's clinical picture, I believe he has osteoarthritis and is failing current medical management. I discussed the treatment options with him and recommend intraarticular injection of steroids. He will return to my office in 2 months.

4(c) Health Record Part ______

Thank you for this interesting consult.

—James Jameson, MD

EXERCISE 5 *Based on the sample health record, fill in the blanks and label parts as noted in Question #4 that follows.*

1. The patient's name is: ______________________________
2. The author of the health record is: ______________________________
3. The name of the doctor who referred the patient is: ______________________________
4. In the blanks alongside the sample, label the correct parts of the health record using the letter associated with each section.

   S–Subjective

   O–Objective

   A–Assessment

   P–Plan

Emergency Department Note

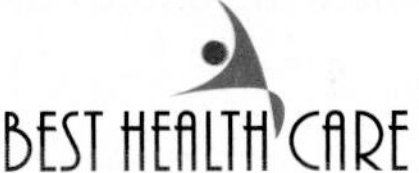

Chief Complaint: Cough

History of Present Illness: Mr. Stephen Dufresne is a 43-year-old male with a 3-day history of cough with wheezing. He has used his inhaler of albuterol but noticed the prescription had expired 3 years ago. The inhaled treatments were mildly effective, but his wheezing returned after 2 hours. He has not been febrile. He does report a runny nose, congestion, and mild headache. He has not had any shortness of breath or chest pain.

PMHx: Asthma.
Past Surgical History: None.
Social History: Lives with his wife and two children. Nonsmoker. Drinks 4 glasses of wine a week.
FHx:
Father: Deceased at 68 years of age from stroke.
Mother: Alive, high blood pressure.

6(a) Health Record Part ______

Medications: Albuterol, prn.

6(b) Health Record Part ______

Allergies: No known drug allergies.

6(c) Health Record Part ______

Physical Exam:

VS: T: 98.8 HR: 80 RR: 28
Gen: WDWN. Mild respiratory distress.
HEENT: TMs normal. Nasal passage patent with clear discharge. mucous membranes moist and pink.
CV: RRR without murmur.
Resp: Wheezing throughout. Fair air entry. Minimal nasal flaring. Mild retractions.
Abdomen: Soft, nontender.
Skin: Pink, good cap refill.

6(d) Health Record Part ______

Emergency Department Course:

Mr. Dufresne arrived to the ER in no apparent distress. A chest x-ray showed mild hyperinflation of his lungs and peribronchial cuffing. No focal infiltrates were noted. We treated him with oxygen and bronchodilators via nebulizer. He also recieved IV steroids. After two treatments of albuterol, he improved. He was no longer in distress. His lungs were clear. He was diagnosed with acute asthma exacerbation and treated wtih oral steroids and a new inhaler of asthma.

6(e) Health Record Part ______

Disposition:

Discharged to home, with follow-up in three days with his PCP.

6(f) Health Record Part ______

—Christine Christenson, MD

Learning Outcome 2.5 Exercises

EXERCISE 6 *Match the abbreviation on the left with its definition on the right.*

_____	1. IV	a. past medical history
_____	2. ER	b. chief complaint
_____	3. PCP	c. well developed, well nourished
_____	4. CC	d. family history
_____	5. FHx	e. respiratory rate
_____	6. PMHx	f. regular rate and rhythm
_____	7. WDWN	g. emergency room
_____	8. RR	h. intravenous
_____	9. RRR	i. primary care physician

EXERCISE 7 *Based on the sample health record, fill in the blanks and label parts as noted in Question #6 that follows.*

1. The patient's name is: ______________________________
2. The patient's temperature is: ______________________________
3. The patient's heart rate is: ______________________________
4. The patient's respiratory rate is: ______________________________
5. The author of this health record is: ______________________________
6. In the blanks alongside the sample, label the correct parts of the health record using the letter associated with each section.

   S–Subjective

   O–Objective

   A–Assessment

   P–Plan

EXERCISE 8 *True or false questions. Indicate true answers with a T and false answers with an F.*

1. The patient has not had a fever. __________
2. Along with wheezing and a mild headache, the patient has had SOB. __________
3. Mr. Dufresne was diagnosed with asthma that just started recently and was getting worse. __________
4. The patient was sent home. __________

Admission Note

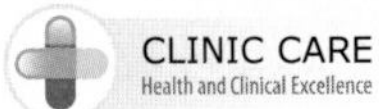

Chief Complaint: Chest pain

5(a) Health Record Part ______

HPI: Mr. William Burns is a 45-year-old male with a 2 day h/o chest pain. The pain is worse when lying **supine**, begins **medially,** and travels down the **lateral** part of his left arm. He has also had mild **SOB.** He took over-the-counter pain medicine, which helped some at first, but now he has **recurrent** pain.
ROS: Positive for **malaise** for 3 days prior to admission. He has not had any coughing, fever, or fainting.
Medications: None.
Allergies: No known drug allergies.
PMHx: Malignant lung mass 5 years ago removed surgically and treated with chemotherapy. His cancer is now in **remission.**
Past Surgical Hx: Tonsillectomy/adenoidectomy at 3 years of age. Tumor removal as above.
Social Hx: 1-pack-per-day smoker. Social alcohol intake. Divorced. Denies sexually risky behavior.
FHx: Father passed away at 40 y/o from unknown **etiology.**

5(b) Health Record Part ______

Vital Signs: Temp: 99.0 HR: 80 RR: 20 BP: 140/92

5(c) Health Record Part ______

Physical Exam

General: NAD. Alert.
HEENT: WNL. Normal fundoscopic exam.
CV: RRR with no murmurs. No carotid bruits.
Resp: Clear to auscultation.
Abd: **WNL.**

5(d) Health Record Part ______

Labs: Elevated glucose: 180. Cardiac enzymes **pending.**

5(e) Health Record Part ______

Imaging: Chest x-ray: normal

5(f) Health Record Part ______

Assessment/Plan

1. Chest pain: The **differential diagnosis** includes heart attack, pneumonia, recurrent lung cancer, and muscular soreness. We will admit him for **observation** while his labs are pending. We will treat him with **supportive care,** including pain relievers.
2. Elevated blood sugar: He did have a large meal prior to coming to the emergency department. We will check his blood sugars **QAC, QPC,** and **QHS.**

5(g) Health Record Part ______

—Madison Ginger, MD

Learning Outcome 2.5 Exercises

EXERCISE 9 *Match the term on the left with its definition on the right.*

	Term		Definition
_______	1. remission	a.	to have again
_______	2. observation	b.	not feeling well
_______	3. pending	c.	dangerous; a problem
_______	4. recurrent	d.	most often used to refer to cancer when it gets better; not the same as a cure
_______	5. malignant	e.	cause
_______	6. malaise	f.	waiting on
_______	7. etiology	g.	to keep an eye on

EXERCISE 10 *Based on the sample health record, fill in the blanks and label parts as noted in Question #5 that follows.*

1. The health record type is: ______________________________
2. The patient's name is: ______________________________
3. The author of this medical note is: ______________________________
4. This health record was written at a(n): ______________________________
5. In the blanks alongside the sample, label the correct parts of the health record using the letter associated with each section.

   S–Subjective

   O–Objective

   A–Assessment

   P–Plan
6. Using the data recorded at the patient's discharge physical examination, fill in the following blanks.
   a. The patient's temperature is: ______________________________
   b. The patient's heart rate is: ______________________________
   c. The patient's respiratory rate is: ______________________________
   d. The patient's blood pressure is: ______________________________

EXERCISE 11 *Translate the following abbreviations.*

1. Hx ______________________________
2. PMHx ______________________________
3. FHx ______________________________
4. y/o ______________________________
5. h/o ______________________________
6. CC ______________________________
7. SOB ______________________________
8. HPI ______________________________
9. ROS ______________________________
10. NAD ______________________________
11. WNL ______________________________
12. RRR ______________________________

Learning Outcome 2.5 Exercises

EXERCISE 12 *Multiple-choice questions. Select the correct answer.*

1. Mr. Burns's pain:
   a. begins in the middle of his chest and travels out to the side
   b. begins in the middle of his chest and travels toward the middle of his left arm
   c. begins on the side of his chest and moves toward the middle
   d. begins on the side of his chest and moves down his left arm
2. Based on the patient's symptoms and exams, the chest pain may be caused by:
   a. heart attack or recurrent lung cancer
   b. pneumonia
   c. muscular soreness
   d. all of these
   e. none of these
3. Supportive care is intended to:
   a. treat the symptoms, but not get rid of the cause
   b. help the patient feel better
   c. prevent the patient from getting sick
   d. monitor the patient to make sure the symptoms do not get worse

EXERCISE 13 *True or false questions. Indicate true answers with a T and false answers with an F.*

1. The patient's father died from lung cancer. __________
2. The patient was admitted to monitor his chest pain while waiting for the lab results. __________
3. The patient had been feeling well prior to admission to the hospital. __________
4. The patient's chest pain is worse when he is lying on his back. __________
5. The patent's lung cancer has been cured. __________
6. The patient looked very ill when he was admitted to the hospital. __________

Discharge Summary

CLINIC CORNER

Patient Name: Regina Klebs

DATE OF ADMISSION: 01/18/2015
DATE OF DISCHARGE: 01/30/2015

4(a) Health Record Part ______

ADMISSION DIAGNOSIS:

1. Pneumonia
2. Respiratory distress

4(b) Health Record Part ______

DISCHARGE DIAGNOSIS:

1. Pneumonia—resolved
2. Cellulitis—resolved

4(c) Health Record Part ______

DISCHARGE CONDITION:

Stable

4(d) Health Record Part ______

CONSULTATIONS:

Pulmonology

4(e) Health Record Part ______

PROCEDURES:

None

LABS:

Blood culture: 1/20/2015 positive for *Staph aureus*
1/24/2015 negative

4(f) Health Record Part ______

Imaging:

Chest x-ray: 1/18/2015: right upper lobe pneumonia
1/24/2015: improving pneumonia
1/30/2015: normal

4(g) Health Record Part ______

HPI:

Ms. Regina Klebs is a 28-year-old woman admitted to hospital from the emergency department with pneumonia. She initially presented with coughing, fever, and shortness of breath. In the **ER,** she had mildly low oxygen levels and was in **acute distress.** A chest x-ray showed pneumonia in the right upper lobe. She was admitted for oxygen and **IV** antibiotics.

4(h) Health Record Part ______

HOSPITAL COURSE:

Ms. Klebs was admitted to the hospital and placed on oxygen and IV antibiotics. Her status improved until day 3 of her hospitalization, when her conditions **abruptly degenerated.** She was noted as **febrile** and **lethargic.** She had a **marked** increased in pain at her IV site and it was red and tender to **palpation.** A culture was sent and came back positive. She was transferred to the **ICU.**

-1-

CLINIC CORNER

A **PICC** line was placed and she was given IV antibiotics. Her condition quickly improved and she was transferred back to the hospital floor. After completing her course of antibiotics, she was discharged to home. Given the risk of significant **morbidity** with her type of infection, we sent her home with **prophylactic topical** antibiotics to put in the nostrils of all her family members.

4(i) Health Record Part ______

DISCHARGE PHYSICAL EXAMINATION:

VS: T: 98.6 **HR:** 64 **RR:** 20 **BP:** 112/74 **Pulse Ox:** 94% on room air

4(j) Health Record Part ______

PE:

Gen: **Alert and oriented. NAD.**
HEENT: PERRLA. Mucous membranes moist.
CV: **RRR,** no murmurs.
Resp: **CTA.**
Abd: Soft, nontender.
Skin: Mild redness to the **proximal** third of the **ventral** side of the right forearm, where the IV site had been. Improving from previous exams.

4(k) Health Record Part ______

ACTIVITY:

No restrictions.

DIET:

Normal.

MEDS:

Topical antibiotic ointment to the nostrils of family members **TID** x 5 days.

FOLLOW-UP:

Appointment—**PCP** (Dr. Primo) in 1 week.

4(l) Health Record Part ______

—Francis Jerome, MD

-2-

Learning Outcome 2.5 Exercises

EXERCISE 14 *Based on the sample health record, fill in the blanks and label parts as noted in Question #4 that follows.*

1. The health record type is: ______________________________
2. The patient's name is: ______________________________
3. This health record was written at a(n): ______________________________
4. In the blanks alongside the sample, label the correct parts of the health record using the letter associated with each section.

   S–Subjective

   O–Objective

   A–Assessment

   P–Plan
5. Using the data recorded at the patient's discharge physical examination, fill in the following blanks.
   a. The patient's temperature is: ______________________________
   b. The patient's heart rate is: ______________________________
   c. The patient's respiratory rate is: ______________________________
   d. The patient's blood pressure is: ______________________________
6. The patient's primary care physician is: ______________________________
7. The patient was transferred to the ICU, which stands for ______________________________.
8. The patient's heart had RRR, which means ________ and ______________________________.
9. The patient's respiratory exam was CTA, or ______________________________ to auscultation.

EXERCISE 15 *Match the term on the left with its definition on the right.*

	Term		Definition
______	1. discharge	a.	what the patient has
______	2. diagnosis	b.	to have a fever
______	3. marked	c.	a decrease in level of consciousness
______	4. lethargic	d.	something that really stands out
______	5. febrile	e.	to feel
______	6. auscultation	f.	peripherally inserted central catheter
______	7. palpation	g.	literally, *to unload*; to send home
______	8. morbidity	h.	the risk for being sick
______	9. PICC	i.	pupils are equal, round, and reactive to light and accommodation
______	10. PERRLA	j.	to listen

EXERCISE 16 *True or false questions. Indicate true answers with a T and false answers with an F.*

1. The patient was admitted to the hospital from the ER. ____________
2. The patient was admitted for oxygen and oral antibiotics. ____________
3. The patient was A&O upon discharge, without any acute distress. ____________
4. The patient's family will be given medication three times a day for 5 days. ____________

Learning Outcome 2.5 Exercises

EXERCISE 17 *Multiple-choice questions. Select the correct answer.*

1. The record indicates that Ms. Klebs was in *acute distress* in the emergency department. This means that her distress:

   a. was getting worse
   b. had been going on for a while
   c. started recently
   d. was unrelated to her chief complaint

2. The record indicates that Ms. Klebs's condition *abruptly degenerated*, which means it:

   a. suddenly got better
   b. suddenly got worse
   c. got better over time
   d. got worse over time

3. The record indicates that the hospital discharged the patient with *prophylactic topical antibiotics* to put in the nostrils of all her family members. These topical antibiotics are intended to:

   a. treat the symptoms but not the actual cause of the illness
   b. prevent an illness
   c. treat the symptoms of an illness to make a patient feel better
   d. create a clean, germ-free environment

4. The record indicates the patient has "mild redness to the *proximal* third of the *ventral* side of the right forearm where the IV site had been." The redness is located on which part of her forearm?

   a. the front, closer to the center
   b. the front, farther away from the center
   c. the back, closer to the center
   d. the back, farther away from the center

Operative Report

CLINIC CORNER

Preoperative Diagnosis: Appendicitis
Postoperative Diagnosis: Appendicitis

Procedure: Appendectomy
Anesthesia: General

Indication: The patient, Wallace Simpson, is a 25-year-old man with acute onset of abdominal pain and fever.
Operative Findings: The patient had a grossly inflamed appendix and local peritonitis.

Description of Procedure: Mr. Simpson was brought to the operating room for suspected appendicitis. He was intubated and placed under general anesthesia. He was prepped and wrapped in sterile technique. A transverse incision was made in right lower quadrant over McBurney's point. Further incision was made through the underlying fascia and the abdominal muscles were separated. The appendix was located and noted to be grossly abnormal. The appendix was dissected, ligated, and sutured. The area was irrigated with normal saline. The cecum was inspected. The peritoneum and fascia were sutured, as well as the skin incision. The wound was cleaned and bandaged with benzoin and steristrips. All gauze and instruments were accounted for.

Disposition: Mr. Simpson was sent to the PACU in stable condition.

—James Cutter, MD

3(a) Health Record Part ______

3(b) Health Record Part ______

3(c) Health Record Part ______

3(d) Health Record Part ______

EXERCISE 18 *Based on the sample health record, fill in the blanks and label parts as noted in Question #3 that follows.*

1. The health record type is: ______________________________
2. The author of this health record is: ______________________________
3. In the blanks alongside the sample, label the correct parts of the health record using the letter associated with each section.

   S–Subjective

   O–Objective

   A–Assessment

   P–Plan
4. The patient was transferred to the PACU, which stands for ______________________________ ______________________________.

Daily Hospital Note/Progress Note

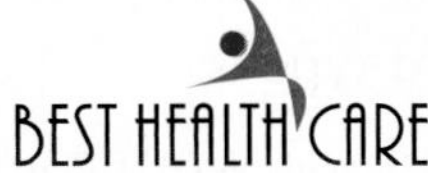

Subjective:

Since yesterday, the patient, Penelope Gates, has vomited 3 times, but she has experienced no vomiting in the past 6 hours. The emesis was not bloody or bilious. She also had 5 episodes of nonbloody, nonmucoid diarrhea in the past 24 hours. She has been afebrile and is without other complaints.

Objective:

Vital Signs: **T**: 99.0 **HR**: 100 **RR**: 24 **Intake:** 1,500 ml **Output**: 1,200 ml

Physical Exam:

General: Tired but responsive and alert.
HEENT: PERRLA, TMs normal, mucous membranes slightly dry and pink.
CV: RRR without murmurs, gallops, or rubs.
Respiratory: CTA without wheezes, rales, or rhonchi.
Abdomen: Soft, nondistended. Minimal generalized tenderness. Normoactive bowel sounds.
Skin: Pink, warm, and dry.
Labs: Na 139. Cl 120 CO_2 14. K 3.8 BUN 15 Cr. 0.4 Glc 100

Assessment/Plan:

1. Acute gastroenteritis: No change. Continue IV fluids. Will give another dose of ondansetron. If patient has no vomiting for 4 hours, then we will advance diet as tolerated. If the patient tolerates it well, will decrease IVF accordingly.
2. Metabolic acidosis: Noticed this AM on lab work. We will begin the patient on sodium bicarbonate.

—Harry Harrison, MD

Learning Outcome 2.5 Exercises

EXERCISE 19 *Fill in the blanks based on the sample health record.*

1. The health record type is: ________________________________
2. This health record was written at a(n): ________________________________
3. The author of this health record is: ________________________________
4. Using the data recorded at the patient's discharge physical examination, fill in the following blanks.
   a. The patient's temperature is: ________________________________
   b. The patient's heart rate is: ________________________________
   c. The patient's respiratory rate is: ________________________________
   d. The patient's I/O is: ________________________________

EXERCISE 20 *Translate the following terms.*

1. T ________________________________
2. HR ________________________________
3. RR ________________________________
4. I/O ________________________________
5. PERRLA ________________________________
6. RRR ________________________________
7. CTA ________________________________
8. IV ________________________________

EXERCISE 21 *True or false questions. Indicate true answers with a T and false answers with an F.*

1. The patient has been without fever. ________
2. The patient vomited three times on the day of the report. ________
3. The physician decided to begin IV fluids. ________
4. Before declaring the patient clear to auscultation, the physician first listened to the lungs to see how they sounded. ________
5. The patient's gastroenteritis is getting worse. ________

Radiology Report

CLINIC CORNER

Reason for Study: Abdominal pain.

Technique: CT of abdomen and pelvis with and without contrast.

Findings: Liver and spleen are normal in size. Appendix measures 9 mm in diameter. Appendicolith noted with thickening of the appendix wall. Kidneys, adrenal glands, pancreas, and gallbladder are unremarkable.

Impression: 1. Appendicitis

—Roxanne Pawlenty, MD

EXERCISE 22 *Multiple-choice questions. Select the correct answer.*

1. Dr. Pawlenty is most likely a:
   a. cardiologist
   b. pathologist
   c. radiologist
   d. surgeon
2. The CT was ordered because the patient had:
   a. abdominal pain
   b. prophylaxis
   c. sequelae
   d. history of appendicitis
3. What technique was used in this study?
   a. CT of abdomen with contrast
   b. CT of abdomen with and without contrast
   c. CT of abdomen and pelvis with contrast
   d. CT of abdomen and pelvis with and without contrast
4. The Findings section of the report would be considered which part of a SOAP note?
   a. S–Subjective
   b. O–Objective
   c. A–Assessment
   d. P–Plan
5. The liver and spleen are:
   a. exacerbated
   b. febrile
   c. marked
   d. unremarkable
6. The kidneys and gallbladder:
   a. are exacerbated
   b. are larger than normal
   c. are normal
   d. require further testing
7. The impression of appendicitis is considered which part of a SOAP note?
   a. S–Subjective
   b. O–Objective
   c. A–Assessment
   d. P–Plan

Pathology Report

BEST HEALTH CARE

Clinical History: Mrs. Linda Genner, a 48-year-old woman, had a suspicious mass seen on a CT scan.

Specimen: Lung, right upper lobe resection.

Gross description: A single specimen measuring 2.3 cm x 4.5 cm x 8.2 cm. The surface of the specimen is smooth, red, and pearly. 1 cm bronchial margin. No invasion of surrounding pleura.

Diagnosis: Right upper lobe: Adenocarcinoma Grade 1.

—Brendan Kellstrom, MD

3(a) Health Record Part ______

3(b) Health Record Part ______

3(c) Health Record Part ______

EXERCISE 23 *Based on the sample health record, fill in the blanks and label parts as noted in Question #3 that follows.*

1. The health record type is: ____________________
2. The author of this health record is: ____________________
3. In the blanks alongside the sample, label the correct parts of the health record using the letter associated with each section.

   S–Subjective

   O–Objective

   A–Assessment

   P–Plan

Prescription

CLINIC CORNER

Albuterol inhaler

Sig: 2-3 puffs inhaled q-4 hours prn wheezing

Disp: 1

Refill: 2

3(a) Health Record Part ______

3(b) Health Record Part ______

3(c) Health Record Part ______

3(d) Health Record Part ______

EXERCISE 24 *Based on the sample health record, fill in the blanks and label parts as noted in Question #3 that follows.*

1. The health record type is: ____

2. Which part of the SOAP note is included in this health record (select one)?

   a. S–Subjective

   b. O–Objective

   c. A–Assessment

   d. P–Plan

3. Label the parts of the health record with:

   a. name and strength of the medicine

   b. patient instructions

   c. how much medicine to give the patient

   d. refill information

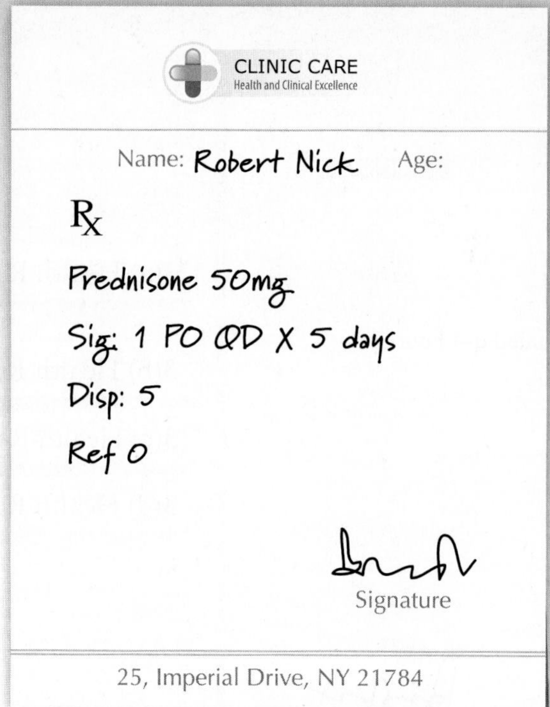
CLINIC CARE
Health and Clinical Excellence

Name: Robert Nick Age:

℞

Prednisone 50mg

Sig: 1 PO QD X 5 days

Disp: 5

Ref 0

Signature

25, Imperial Drive, NY 21784

EXERCISE 25 *Multiple-choice questions. Select the correct answer.*

1. This is a:
   a. prescription
   b. part of the plan for a patient
   c. instructions for the pharmacist
   d. all of these
   e. none of these
2. The first line is the:
   a. name of the medication
   b. strength of the medication
   c. name and strength of the medication
   d. pharmacist instructions
3. The abbreviation *Sig:*
   a. means the instructions for the patient
   b. means the instructions for the pharmacist
   c. is short for *signa,* from Latin for "label"
   d. means the instructions for the patient and is short for *signa,* from Latin for "label"
   e. means the instructions for the pharmacist and is short for *signa,* from Latin for "label"
4. The patient will take the medication:
   a. five pills a day by mouth
   b. four times a day by mouth
   c. daily by mouth for 5 days
   d. four times daily by mouth for 5 days
5. The pharmacist will dispense how many pills?
   a. 1
   b. 5
   c. 20
   d. 25

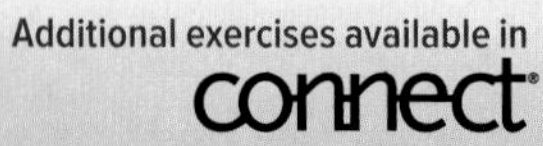

Additional practice items are available in Connect!

The Integumentary System—Dermatology 3

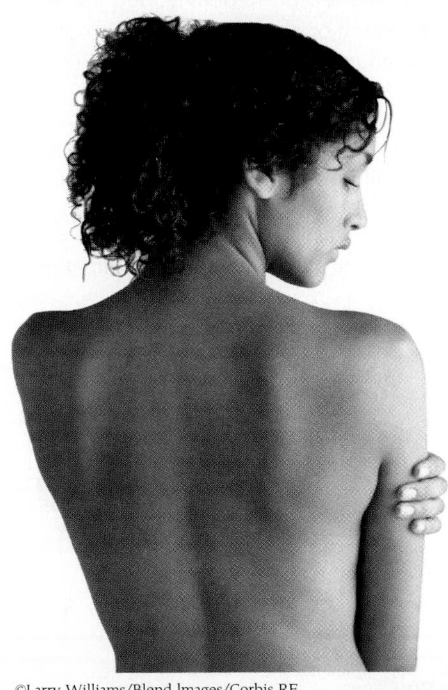

©Larry Williams/Blend Images/Corbis RF

learning outcomes

Upon completion of this chapter, you will be able to:

3.1 Identify the **roots/word parts** associated with the **integumentary system.**

(S) **3.2** Translate the **Subjective** terms associated with the **integumentary system.**

(O) **3.3** Translate the **Objective** terms associated with the **integumentary system.**

(A) **3.4** Translate the **Assessment** terms associated with the **integumentary system.**

(P) **3.5** Translate the **Plan** terms associated with the **integumentary system.**

3.6 Use **abbreviations** associated with the **integumentary system.**

3.7 Distinguish terms associated with the **integumentary system** in the context of **electronic health records.**

Introduction and Overview of Dermatology

For thousands of years, walls of earth, wood, or stone surrounded cities. These outside walls defined the city boundaries. More importantly, they protected the city's inhabitants. By limiting access to the inside of the city and offering a strategic point of attack, walls deterred would-be invaders. In addition, walls provided a convenient vantage point to view the surrounding countryside. In effect, the walls offered protection and surveillance.

Skin serves a similar function as city walls. As an outer protective barrier, skin is the first line of defense from germs and irritants. It also serves as the body's first point of contact with its surroundings.

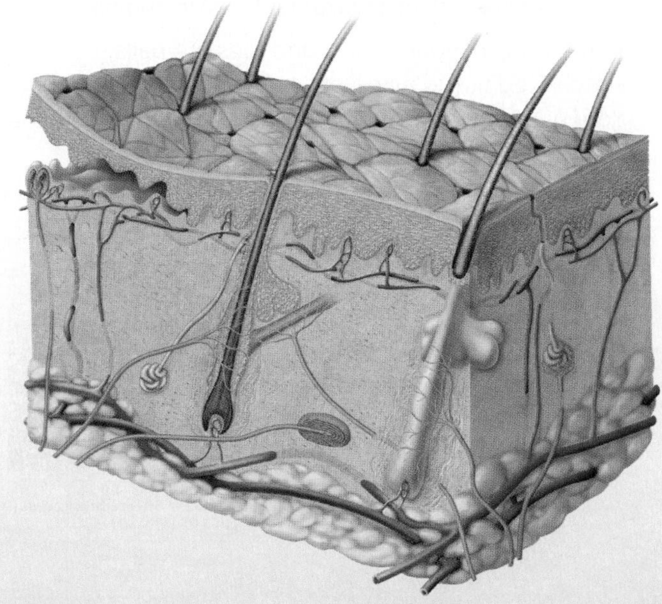

Your skin is your largest organ. It serves as your body's first point of contact with its surroundings.

3.1 Word Parts of the Integumentary System

Word Parts Associated with the Anatomy of the Integumentary System

At first glance, the skin appears to be very simple—just a thin layer of tissue covering our bodies. However, the truth is that the **integumentary system** (the skin) is very complex. Your skin (roots: *cutaneo/dermo*) has many structures, each of which has its own special job.

The outermost layer, the one that is visible, is the **epidermis**. It is made of large cells that look like the scales of a fish under the microscope. The term *squamous cell* refers to this scaly appearance.

Under the epidermis lies a deeper layer known as the **dermis**. This layer, which is much thicker than the epidermis, has fewer cells and more thick fibers to give the skin strength and flexibility. The dermis is also home to hair follicles, nerves, and glands.

- Hair follicles are the roots of your hair (*pilo/tricho*). The follicles anchor the hair to the skin and provide nourishment to it.
- The nerves of the dermis detect fine pressure, deep pressure, temperature, and pain. The vast network of nerves in your skin makes it the largest sensory organ in your body.
- The skin has two types of glands, which are groups of cells that release fluid. Sweat glands (*hidro*) release sweat to rid the body of waste and to cool the body. Sebaceous glands (*sebaceo*) secrete oil as a natural moisturizer for the skin and hair.

At the ends of your fingers and toes are nails, specialized tissue made of a hard substance (keratin). Your nails (*onycho/unguo*) protect your fingers and toes and provide a good base for movement.

fat

ROOTS: ***adip/o, lip/o, steat/o***

EXAMPLES: adipocyte, lipoma, steatosis

NOTES: Next time you are offered a fatty food, you can tell the person who is offering it that you try to avoid *adipogenic* foods.

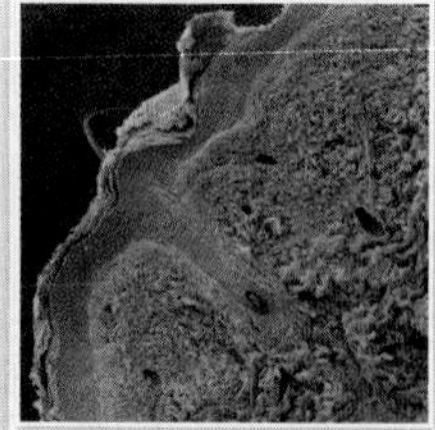

©Eye of Science/Science Source

skin

ROOTS: ***cutane/o, derm/o, dermat/o***

EXAMPLES: subcutaneous, epidermal, dermatology

NOTES: A patient once sought medical treatment for a rash around the mouth. When the health care professional diagnosed her with *perioral dermatitis,* the patient thought to herself, "Duh! You just said the same thing I said—just in a different language." Think about it: What does *perioral dermatitis* mean? You can break it down easily: *peri* = around, *oral* = mouth, *dermat* = skin, and *itis* = inflammation.

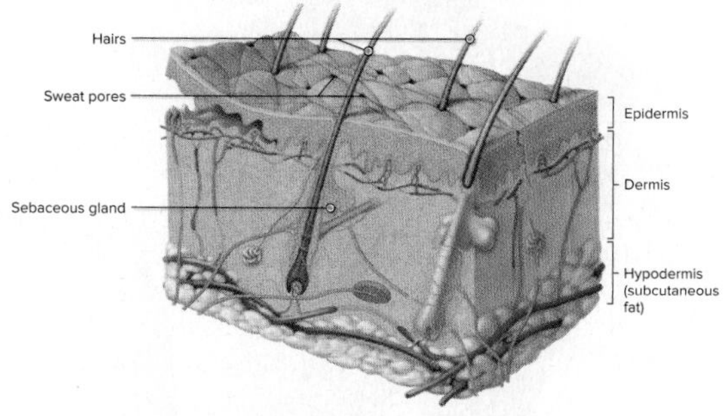

Structure of the Skin.

hair

ROOTS: ***pil/o, trich/o***

EXAMPLES: piloid, atrichosis

NOTES: The word *caterpillar* is believed to come from two Latin words: *catta*, meaning "cat," and *pila*, meaning "hair"; thus, *caterpillar*, meaning "hairy cat." Have you ever had split ends? If you do, you can always ask your hairstylist for a treatment for your *schizotrichia*.

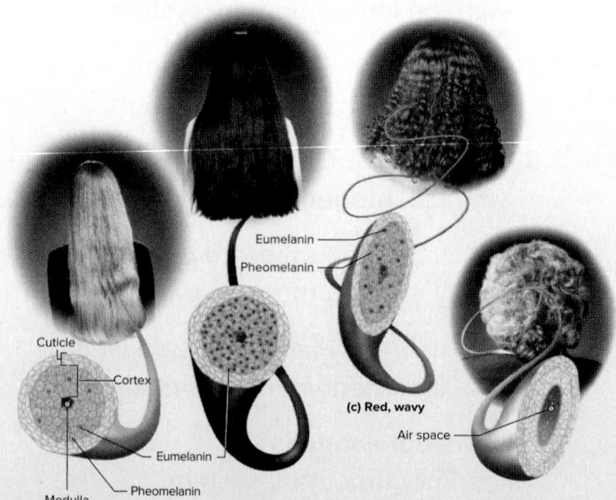

(a): ©McGraw-Hill Education/Joe DeGrandis, photographer; (b): ©McGraw-Hill Education/Joe DeGrandis, photographer; (c): ©McGraw-Hill Education/Joe DeGrandis, photographer; (d): ©McGraw-Hill Education/Joe DeGrandis, photographer

sweat

ROOT: ***hidr/o***

EXAMPLES: hyperhidrosis, hypohidrosis

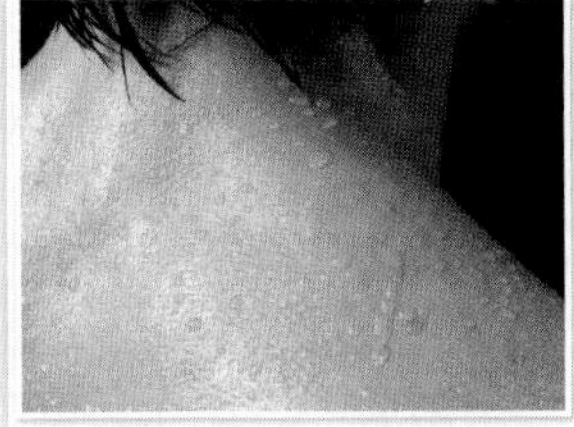

©Scott Kleinman/The Image Bank/Getty Images

NOTES: Humans have gone to great lengths to keep the environment cool—inventing air conditioning and fans, for example—which suggests that humans do not like to get sweaty. But if you didn't have the ability to sweat, your body would have a very hard time regulating its temperature. In fact, *hypohidrosis*, which means "a lack of sweat," can be a sign that something is wrong.

Unlike humans, dogs cannot sweat. Instead, they pant—their bodies are cooled by the air passing over their moist tongues.

scale

ROOT: ***squam/o***

EXAMPLE: squamous layer

NOTES: Have you ever gotten a sunburn that led to peeling skin? Have you ever removed the scales from a fresh fish before cooking it? Either process can be referred to as *desquamation*, a Latin word meaning "to remove the scales from a fish."

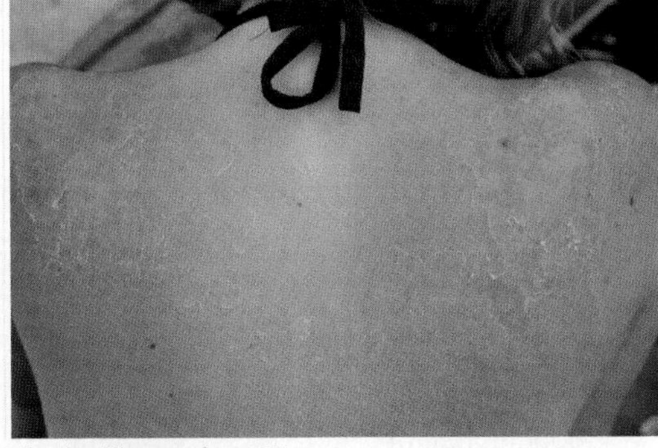

©Alonafoto/Shutterstock.com RF

nail

ROOTS: ***onych/o, ungu/o***

EXAMPLES: onychalgia, subungual

NOTES: Have you noticed that it is time to trim your nails? Excuse yourself to take care of that task by telling your friends you need to step outside to *exungulate*. If the situation is more complicated, and there is a broken nail, you can mention that you have diagnosed yourself with *onychoclasis*.

oil

ROOTS: ***seb/o, sebace/o***

EXAMPLES: sebolith, pilosebaceous

NOTES: Later, when you learn more about the ears, you will learn the root *cerumen*, which refers to ear wax. Actually, *cerumen* is just sebum that is produced in the ears.

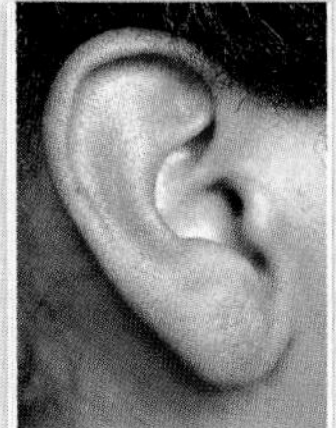

©McGraw-Hill Education/Joe DeGrandis, photographer

Word Parts Associated with Pathology—Change

Skin abnormalities are generally categorized into two groups: unusual skin texture and unusual skin color. Problems with skin texture include hardness or horniness (*kerato-*) and dryness (*xero-*). Of course, skin tones differ from person to person and ethnicity to ethnicity, but certain prefixes are used to describe abnormal skin conditions: whiteness (*leuko-*), redness (*erythro-*), yellowness (*xantho-*), and blackness (*melano-*).

hidden

ROOT: ***crypt/o***

EXAMPLE: onychocryptosis

NOTES: A person who specializes in breaking codes and deciphering secret messages is called a *cryptolinguist. Onychocryptosis* is an ingrown, or hidden, toenail.

The word *crypt* used by itself can refer to a room or vault hidden beneath the floor. It is usually associated with a chamber in which corpses are placed, whether it is located in a church (generally beneath the floor) or a mausoleum (generally above ground).

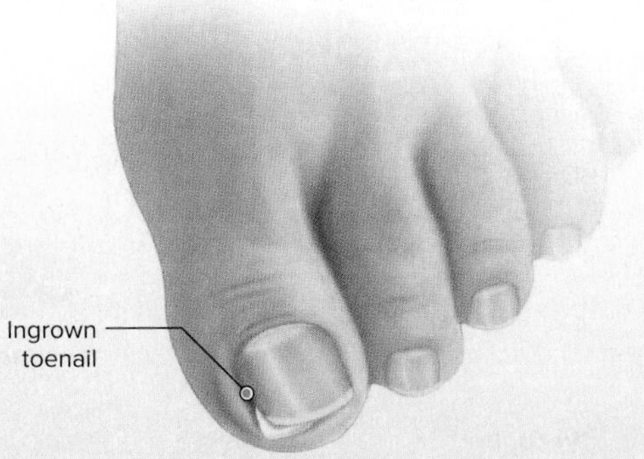

hard, horny

ROOT: ***kerat/o***

EXAMPLES: keratosis, keratoderma

NOTES: The *rhinoceros* is so named because it has a *horn* on its *nose*. The dinosaur *Triceratops* was so named because of the three (*tri*) horns (*kerat*) on its head.

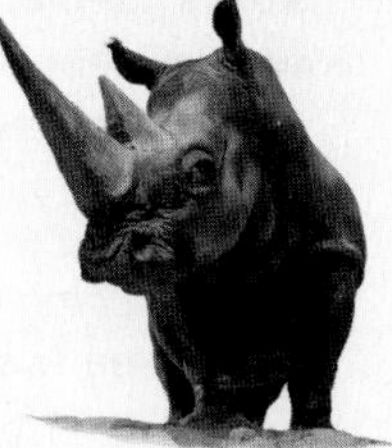

©Valerie Shaff/Stone/Getty Images

dry

ROOT: ***xer/o***

EXAMPLE: xeroderma

NOTES: People who live in dry or desert regions often forgo lawns and instead use *xeriscaping*, which means “landscaping using plants that require little water.” Because grounds that are xeriscaped are typically rocky and brown, some think this type of landscaping is spelled *zeroscaping*—and the fact that the *x* is pronounced like a *z* probably does not help.

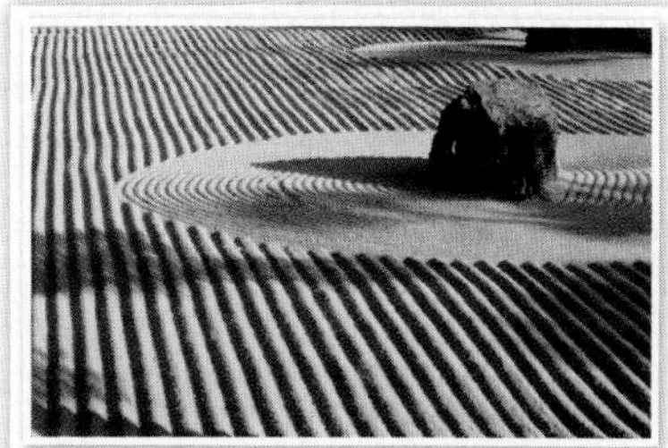

©Akira Kaede/Photodisc/Getty Images RF

Word Parts Associated with Pathology—Skin Conditions Involving Color

One important aspect of diagnosing skin conditions is noting changes. This section gives the roots that refer to the most commonly occurring changes in skin color.

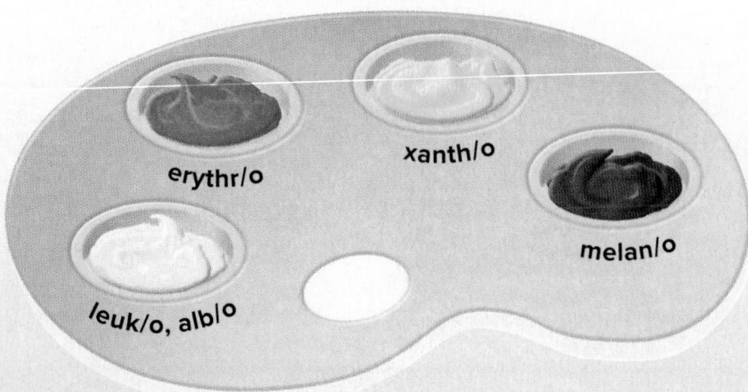

yellow

ROOT: ***xanth/o***

EXAMPLE: xanthoderma

NOTES: If you are unable to see the color yellow, you may have *axanthopsia*.

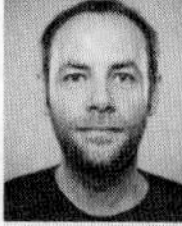

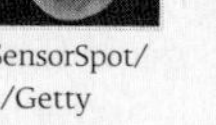

©SensorSpot/E+/Getty Images RF

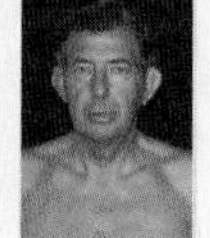

©Dr P. Marazzi/Science Source

red

ROOT: ***erythr/o***

EXAMPLE: erythroderma

NOTES: *Erythroderma* is a redness of the skin. The Red Sea, a sea that separates Africa from Egypt, was originally called the Erythraen (or Red) Sea. The country Eritrea, which lies on the Red Sea between the Sudan and Ethiopia, gets its name from this ancient moniker for the sea.

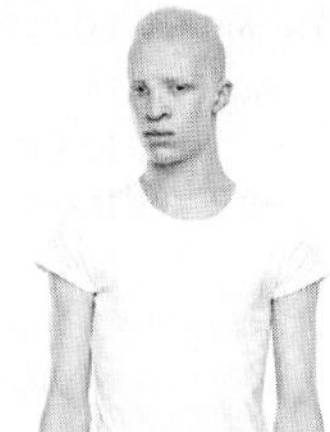

Source: Centers for Disease Control and Prevention/Public Health Image Library

white

ROOTS: ***leuk/o, alb/o***

EXAMPLES: leukoderma, albinism

NOTES: A person with white hair has *leukotrichia*. A complete lack of skin pigment is known as *albinism*.

The *albatross* is a white seabird. Its name is derived in part from a need to distinguish it from a common seabird called the frigate bird, which looks very similar except that it has black feathers.

©ImageSource/Digital Vision/Getty Images RF

black

ROOT: ***melan/o***

EXAMPLE: melanoma

NOTES: Ancient Greeks thought that the human body was filled with four substances they called *humors:* bile (*chole*), black bile (*melan chole*), phlegm (*phlegma*), and blood (*sanguis*). According to this system, a healthy person must have all four humors in perfect balance. If a person was sick, an imbalance of the humors was to blame, and a physician’s goal was to figure out which humor was too plentiful and which was insufficient. *Bloodletting* was developed to help rid the body of excess blood. The word *melancholy* also comes from belief in a balance of the humors, because it was believed that a person who was sad or depressed had too much black bile.

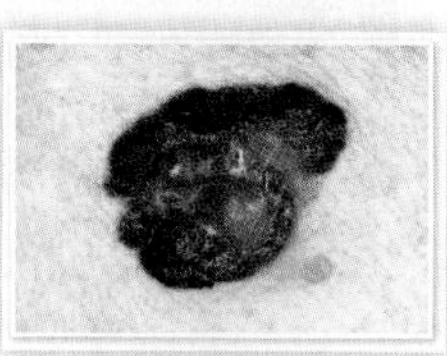

©James Stevenson/SPL/Science Source

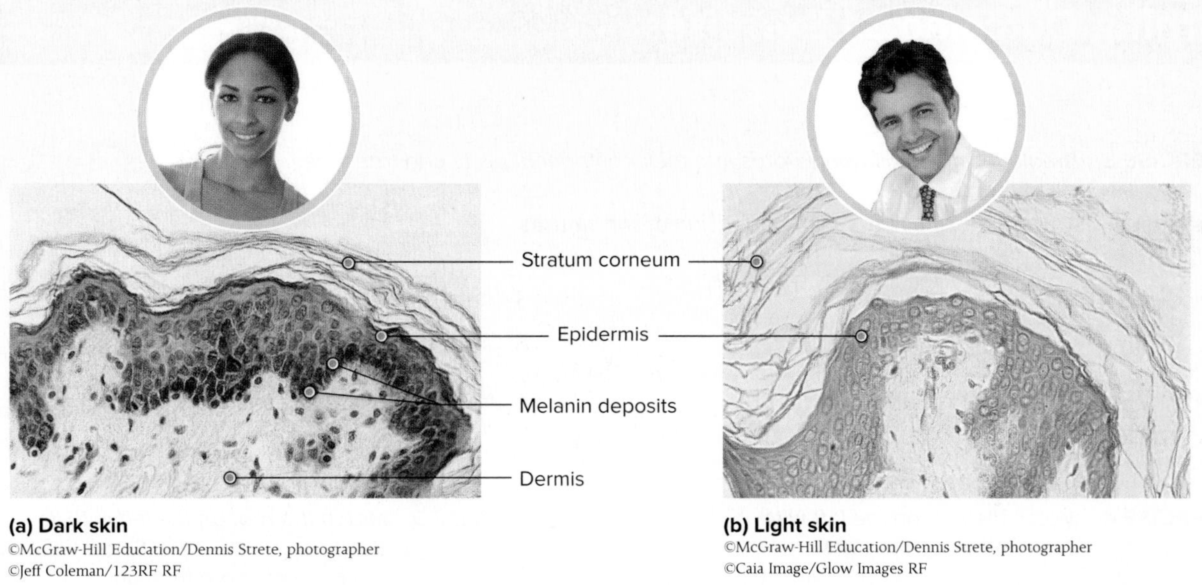

(a) Dark skin
©McGraw-Hill Education/Dennis Strete, photographer
©Jeff Coleman/123RF RF

(b) Light skin
©McGraw-Hill Education/Dennis Strete, photographer
©Caia Image/Glow Images RF

The differences in skin color are caused by the varying levels of melanin deposited in the basal layer. Picture (a) has heavy deposits while picture (b) contains little visible melanin in the basal layer.

Learning Outcome 3.1 Exercises

Additional exercises available in connect®

TRANSLATION

EXERCISE 1 *Match the root on the left with its definition on the right. Some definitions will be used more than once.*

______	1. lip/o	a.	fat
______	2. derm/o	b.	skin
______	3. dermat/o	c.	hair
______	4. hidr/o	d.	sweat
______	5. ungu/o	e.	nail
______	6. adip/o	f.	oil
______	7. cutane/o		
______	8. seb/o		
______	9. pil/o		
______	10. steat/o		
______	11. sebace/o		
______	12. trich/o		
______	13. onych/o		

EXERCISE 2 *Translate the following roots.*

1. derm/o ______________________
2. lip/o ______________________
3. cutane/o ______________________
4. onych/o ______________________
5. adip/o ______________________
6. dermat/o ______________________
7. seb/o ______________________
8. pil/o ______________________
9. hidr/o ______________________
10. ungu/o ______________________
11. steat/o ______________________
12. sebace/o ______________________
13. trich/o ______________________

Learning Outcome 3.1 Exercises

EXERCISE 3 *Break down the following words into their component parts and translate.*

EXAMPLE: sinusitis *sinus | itis* *inflammation of the sinuses*

1. dermatology ______
2. lipoma ______
3. steatosis ______
4. epidermal ______
5. subungual ______
6. subcutaneous ______
7. onychalgia ______

EXERCISE 4 *Match the root on the left with its definition on the right.*

______	1. crypt/o	a. hidden
______	2. xer/o	b. dry
______	3. kerat/o	c. hard, horny

EXERCISE 5 *Provide the roots for the following definitions.*

1. hard, horny ______
2. dry ______
3. hidden ______

EXERCISE 6 *Break down the following words into their component parts and translate.*

EXAMPLE: sinusitis *sinus | itis*
inflammation of the sinuses

1. xeroderma ______
______
2. keratosis ______
______
3. onychocryptosis ______
______

EXERCISE 7 *Identify the roots for the following definitions.*

1. dry ______
2. hard, horny ______
3. hidden ______

EXERCISE 8 *Build a medical term from the information provided.*

1. hard/horny skin ______
2. dry skin ______
3. dry conditions ______

EXERCISE 9 *Match the root on the left with its definition on the right. Some definitions will be used more than once.*

______	1. alb/o	a. black
______	2. melan/o	b. red
______	3. leuk/o	c. white
______	4. erythr/o	d. yellow
______	5. xanth/o	

EXERCISE 10 *Translate the following roots.*

1. melan/o ______
2. leuk/o ______
3. alb/o ______
4. xanth/o ______
5. erythr/o ______

EXERCISE 11 *Break down the following words into their component parts and translate.*

EXAMPLE: sinusitis *sinus | itis*
inflammation of the sinuses

1. leukoderma ______
2. xanthoderma ______
3. erythroderma ______
4. melanoma ______

Learning Outcome 3.1 Exercises

GENERATION

EXERCISE 12 *Identify the roots for the following definitions.*

1. skin (3 roots) ______________________
2. fat (3 roots) ______________________
3. sweat (1 root) ______________________
4. scale (1 root) ______________________
5. oil (2 roots) ______________________
6. hair (2 roots) ______________________
7. nail (2 roots) ______________________

EXERCISE 13 *Build a medical term from the information provided.*

1. inflammation of the skin ______________________
2. inflammation of fat tissue ______________________
3. nail disease ______________________
4. pertaining to the skin ______________________

EXERCISE 14 *Identify the roots for the following definitions.*

1. white (2 roots) ______________________
2. black (1 root) ______________________
3. red (1 root) ______________________
4. yellow (1 root) ______________________

EXERCISE 15 *Build a medical term from the information provided.*

1. red skin ______________________
2. white skin ______________________
3. yellow skin ______________________

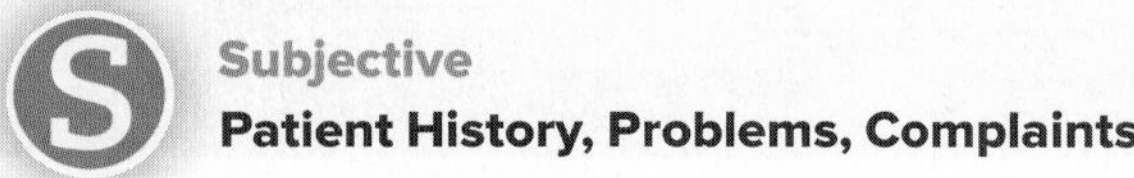

Subjective
Patient History, Problems, Complaints

Objective
Observation and Discovery

Assessment
Diagnosis and Pathology

Plan
Treatments and Therapies

This section contains medical terms built from the roots presented in the previous section. The purpose of this section is to expose you to words used in dermatology that are built from the word roots you learned earlier in the chapter.

The focus of this book is to teach you the process of learning roots and translating them in context. Each term is presented with the correct pronunciation followed by a word analysis that breaks down the word into its component parts, a definition that provides a literal translation of the word, and supplemental information (if the literal translation deviates from its medical use).

The terms are organized using a health care professional's SOAP note (see Chapter 2) as a model.

SUBJECTIVE

3.2 Patient History, Problems, Complaints

The most common reason a person seeks medical care in relation to his or her skin is a new rash. The rash may be painful (*dermatalgia/dermatodynia*) or itchy (*pruritus*). The rash may appear as hives (*urticaria*) or as an oily secretion (*seborrhea*). The rash may be very dry (*xerosis*) or very wet (*macerate*). Patients may also notice that they are producing too much sweat (*hyperhidrosis*) or not enough sweat (*anhidrosis*).

Sometimes the patient's concern is change in normal skin color. These color changes may involve a loss of pigment (*depigmentation*) or darkening of the skin (*hypermelanosis*). Some people lack pigment altogether, as in *albinism*.

Another reason a patient might consult a dermatologist is problems with the hair. Hair falls under the responsibility of a dermatologist because the hair follicles are embedded in the skin. The most common hair complaint for men is hair loss (*alopecia*), but it occurs in women as well. Another hair problem is too much hair (*hypertrichosis*).

dermatological terms

Term	Word Analysis
abrasion uh-BRAY-zhun **Definition** scraping away of skin	**ab / rasion** away / scrape
albinism AL-bin-ism **Definition** lack of pigment in skin causing patient to look white	**albin / ism** white / condition
albino al-BAI-noh **Definition** a person afflicted with albinism	**albino**

3.2 Patient History, Problems, Complaints

dermatological terms *continued*

Term	Word Analysis
alopecia a-loh-PEE-sha **Definition** baldness	**from Greek, for** *fox* ©Africa Studio/Shutterstock.com RF
anhidrosis an-ih-DROH-sis **Definition** lack of sweating	**an / hidr / osis** no / sweat / condition
comedo koh-MEE-doh **Definition** a hair follicle that is plugged with sebum (black head, white head)	**from Latin, for** *to eat up* Closed comedo Open comedo
cyanidrosis sai-yan-ih-DROH-sis **Definition** blue sweat	**cyan / idr / osis** blue / sweat / condition
depigmentation DE-pig-men-TAY-shun **Definition** loss of pigmentation	**de / pigment / ation** away / pigment / condition
dermatalgia der-mah-TAL-jah **Definition** skin pain	**dermat / algia** skin / pain
dermatodynia der-MA-toh-DIH-nee-ah **Definition** skin pain	**dermato / dynia** skin / pain
dermatolysis der-mah-TAWL-ih-sis **Definition** loose skin	**dermato / lysis** skin / loose
erythema eh-rih-THEE-ma **Definition** redness	**from Greek, for** *redness*
erythroderma eh-RIH-throh-DER-ma **Definition** red skin	**erythro / derma** red / skin

3.2 Patient History, Problems, Complaints

dermatological terms *continued*

Term	Word Analysis
hemathidrosis heh-mat-ih-DROH-sis **Definition** sweating blood	**hemat / hidr / osis** blood / sweat / condition
NOTE: This word doesn't use a combining vowel. It just mushes the *t* and the *h* together and pronounces just the *t*. Because of this, the word is also spelled without the *h*: *hematidrosis*. We spell it with the *h* so you can see the root. But you should recognize both.	
hidropoiesis hih-droh-poh-EE-sis **Definition** the formation of sweat	**hidro / poiesis** sweat / formation
hyperhidrosis hai-per-hih-DROH-sis **Definition** excessive sweating	**hyper / hidr / osis** over / sweat / condition
hyperkerotosis hai-per-ker-ah-TOH-sis **Definition** excessive growth of horny skin	**hyper / kerat / osis** over / horny / condition
hypermelanosis hai-per-mel-an-OH-sis **Definition** excessive melanin in the skin	**hyper / melan / osis** over / black / condition
hyperpigmentation hai-per-pig-men-TAY-shun **Definition** excessive pigment in the skin	**hyper / pigment / ation** over / pigment / condition
hypohidrosis hai-poh-hih-DROH-sis **Definition** diminished sweating	**hypo / hidr / osis** under / sweat / condition
hypomelanosis hai-poh-mel-an-OH-sis **Definition** diminished melanin in the skin	**hypo / melan / osis** under / black / condition
hypopigmentation hai-poh-pig-men-TAY-shun **Definition** diminished pigment in the skin	**hypo / pigment / ation** under / pigment / condition
leukoderma loo-koh-DER-mah **Definition** white skin	**leuko / derma** white / skin ©ImageSource/Digital Vision/Getty Images RF
macerate MAS-ir-ayt **Definition** to soften the skin	**from Latin, for to make soft**

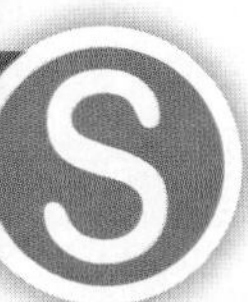

3.2 Patient History, Problems, Complaints

dermatological terms *continued*

Term	Word Analysis
onychophagia aw-nih-koh-FAY-jah **Definition** eating or biting the nails	**onycho / phagia** nail / eat ©James Darell/Getty Images RF
pruritus prur-AI-tis **Definition** an itch **NOTE:** The ending on this word is easily confused with *-itis.*	**from Latin, for** *itching*
rhytidermia rih-tih-DER-mee-ah **Definition** wrinkled skin **NOTE:** The root is actually rhytid/o but because *rhytid-* ends with a *d* and *-dermia* starts with one, the *d* from the root is eliminated.	**rhyti / dermia** wrinkle / skin
sebopoiesis see-boh-poh-EE-sis **Definition** formation of oil (sebum)	**sebo / poiesis** oil / formation
seborrhea seh-boh-REE-ah **Definition** discharge of oil (sebum)	**sebo / rrhea** oil / discharge
trichomegaly tri-koh-MEG-ah-lee **Definition** abnormally thick hair	**tricho / megaly** hair / enlargement
urticaria ur-tih-KAR-ee-ah **Definition** swollen raised itchy areas of the skin	**from Latin, for** *burning nettle*
xanthoderma zan-thoh-DER-mah **Definition** yellow skin	**xantho / derma** yellow / skin
xeroderma zeh-roh-DER-mah **Definition** dry skin	**xero / derma** dry / skin
xerosis ze-ROH-sis **Definition** condition of dryness	**xer / osis** dry / condition

Learning Outcome 3.2 Exercises

PRONUNCIATION

EXERCISE 1 *Indicate which syllable receives emphasis when pronounced.*

EXAMPLE: bronchitis bron**chi**tis

1. albinism ______
2. anhidrosis ______
3. dermatolysis ______
4. dermatalgia ______
5. erythema ______
6. hyperhidrosis ______
7. hyperpigmentation ______
8. macerate ______
9. pruritus ______
10. hyperkerotosis ______
11. rhytidermia ______
12. trichomegaly ______
13. urticaria ______
14. xerosis ______

TRANSLATION

EXERCISE 2 *Break down the following words into their component parts.*

EXAMPLE: nasopharyngoscope *naso | pharyngo | scope*

1. leukoderma ______
2. rhytidermia ______
3. hidropoiesis ______
4. anhidrosis ______
5. dermatolysis ______
6. hyperkeratosis ______
7. hypohidrosis ______
8. hypopigmentation ______
9. hyperpigmentation ______
10. sebopoiesis ______
11. xeroderma ______
12. depigmentation ______

Learning Outcome 3.2 Exercises

EXERCISE 3 *Underline and define the word parts from this chapter in the following terms.*

1. dermatalgia ______
2. albinism ______
3. onychophagia ______
4. seborrhea ______
5. trichomegaly ______
6. xerosis ______
7. hyperhidrosis ______
8. hypomelanosis ______
9. xanthoderma (2 roots) ______
10. erythroderma (2 roots) ______
11. hypermelanosis ______
12. hemathidrosis ______
13. cyanidrosis ______

EXERCISE 4 *Match the term on the left with its definition on the right.*

______	1. albino	a.	scraping away of skin
______	2. erythema	b.	a person with a lack of skin pigment, causing the person to look completely white
______	3. alopecia	c.	baldness
______	4. abrasion	d.	redness
______	5. macerate	e.	to soften the skin
______	6. comedo	f.	an itch
______	7. pruritus	g.	swollen, raised, itchy areas of the skin
______	8. urticaria	h.	a follicle plugged with sebum (black head, white head)

EXERCISE 5 *Translate the following terms as literally as possible.*

EXAMPLE: nasopharyngoscope *an instrument for looking at the nose and throat*

1. albinism ______
2. xerosis ______
3. leukoderma ______
4. rhytidermia ______
5. seborrhea ______
6. depigmentation ______
7. hypomelanosis ______
8. hypopigmentation ______
9. trichomegaly ______
10. erythema ______
11. erythroderma ______
12. hyperhidrosis ______
13. hyperkeratosis ______

S Learning Outcome 3.2 Exercises

GENERATION

EXERCISE 6 *Build a medical term from the information provided.*

EXAMPLE: inflammation of the sinuses *sinusitis*

1. yellow skin ______
2. dry skin ______
3. loose skin ______
4. skin pain ______
5. no sweat condition ______
6. nail eating ______
7. oil formation ______
8. sweat formation ______
9. under sweat condition ______
10. over black condition ______
11. over pigment condition ______
12. blue sweat condition ______
13. blood sweat condition ______

EXERCISE 7 *Multiple-choice questions. Select the correct answer.*

1. From the Latin, meaning "to eat up," which term describes a hair follicle plugged with sebum (black head, white head)?
   a. abrasion
   b. comedo
   c. macerate
   d. pruritus
2. A person with albinism has what color skin?
   a. black
   b. red
   c. yellow
   d. white
3. Which term means "to soften the skin"?
   a. abrasion
   b. comedo
   c. macerate
   d. pruritus
4. *Pruritus* describes
   a. an itch
   b. soft skin
   c. scraped skin
   d. dry skin
5. Which term comes from the Latin, meaning "burning nettle," and describes swollen, raised, itchy areas of the skin?
   a. pruritus
   b. urticaria
   c. albinism
   d. comedo
6. Select all terms below that have roots that mean "skin."
   a. anhidrosis
   b. albinism
   c. cyanidrosis
   d. dermatolysis
   e. erythema
   f. hemathidrosis
   g. hypohidrosis
   h. leukoderma
   i. rhytidermia
   j. xanthoderma
   k. xeroderma
   l. xerosis
7. Select all terms below that have roots meaning "sweat."
   a. anhidrosis
   b. albinism
   c. cyanidrosis
   d. dermatolysis
   e. erythema
   f. hemathidrosis
   g. hypohidrosis
   h. leukoderma
   i. rhytidermia
   j. xanthoderma
   k. xeroderma
   l. xerosis
8. Select all terms below that have roots meaning "white."
   a. anhidrosis
   b. albinism
   c. cyanidrosis
   d. dermatolysis
   e. erythema
   f. hemathidrosis
   g. hypohidrosis
   h. leukoderma
   i. rhytidermia
   j. xanthoderma
   k. xeroderma
   l. xerosis

OBJECTIVE

3.3 Observation and Discovery

A very specific language applies to rashes. This allows medical professionals to tell one another about rashes even when the patient is not present or no photo is available. These descriptions relate to the location, size, color, texture, and filling of the rash or its pustules, and they also describe whether the rash is flat or raised.

Usually, skin conditions are first described by their location. If the rash is limited to a specific area, it is *localized*. If the rash is all over the body, it is called a *generalized* rash. Some rashes begin in one area and spread to another. Rashes that start from the middle and work their way outward are *centrifugal*. Rashes that spread from the outside inward are *centripetal*.

Small bumps (under 1 cm) are called *papules*. When they become larger—specifically over 1 cm—they are called *nodules*. If they are large and flat like a plateau, they are known as *plaques*.

What is inside the rash is important as well. Small bumps (less than 1 cm) filled with clear fluid are called *vesicles*. If the bumps are filled with pus, they are known as *pustules*. A larger vesicle, such as a blister, is called a *bulla*, and larger pustules are called *abscesses*. Small, flat spots, such as freckles, are known as *macules*. Larger macules are *patches*.

Some skin findings are actually caused by blood vessels of the skin or just below the skin. Too many blood vessels formed in one area can cause a mass called a *cherry angioma*. A heavy concentration of blood vessels that is flat but still visible is called a *telangiectasia*. Small bruises under the skin are *petechiae*. Larger bruises are known as *ecchymosis*.

One specific type of injury to the skin is a burn. A burn is an injury to skin cells that is caused by exposure to harmful agent. It can be caused by heat, radiation, chemicals, electricity, or friction. When the skin is burned, three very important skin functions are impaired: the ability to regulate heat, the ability to regulate hydration, and the ability to fight infection. Burns can range in severity from minor injuries to medical emergencies based on how much of the body has been burned and how deep the burn is. Categorizing a burn depends on how deep the trauma goes. A first-degree burn only affects the superficial layer of the skin, or epidermis. A sunburn is the most common example. A deeper burn involving the dermis is known as a second-degree burn. A third-degree burn injures the subcutaneous layer, and a fourth-degree burn involves the underlying tissues like the bone, muscle, or fascia.

Diagnostic procedures in dermatology are limited. If the skin is being *cultured* for infection, it is being sampled to see if it harbors bacteria (culture and sensitivity), a virus, or a fungus. The most common diagnostic procedure is a *skin biopsy*. Many skin conditions can only be clearly distinguished from one another when examined under a microscope. Thus, the skin biopsy is a mainstay of dermatology. A skin biopsy can involve removal of the entire lesion. It can also be *excisional*, which means removal of a part of the lesion. It can be removed with a slice of the blade (a *shave biopsy*), or it can be punched out using a device similar to the hole punches used for paper.

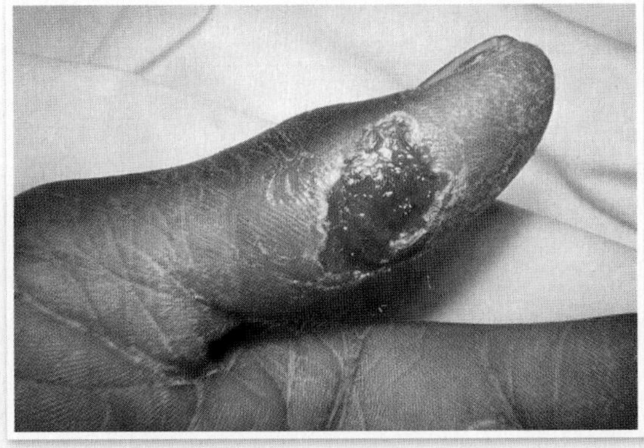

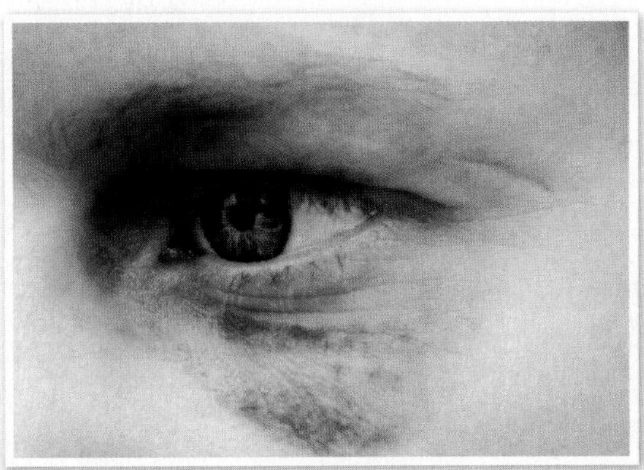

Common skin conditions observed by doctors include abscesses and black eyes.

Sources: (left): Centers for Disease Control and Prevention/Public Health Image Library; (right): ©Ingram Publishing RF

3.3 Observation and Discovery

primary lesions

Term	Word Analysis
Flat, Nonpalpable	
macule, macula (freckle) MA-kyool, MAW-koo-lah **Definition** small, flat, discolored area	**from Latin, for** "spot" **or** "stain" ©Digital Vision/Getty Images RF
patch (vitiligo) pach (vih-tih-LAI-goh) **Definition** larger, flat, discolored area	
Elevated, Palpable, Solid Mass	
papule PA-pyool **Definition** a small solid mass	**from Latin, for** "pimple"
plaque PLAK **Definition** a solid mass on the surface of the skin	
nodule NAWD-jyool **Definition** a solid mass that extends deeper into the skin	
tumor TOO-mur **Definition** a larger solid mass	
Elevated, Fluid-Filled	
vesicle VEH-sih-kul **Definition** a smaller blister	**ves / icle** **bladder / little**
bulla BUL-lah	**from Latin, for** "bubble"

primary lesions *continued*

Term	Word Analysis
pustule PUS-tyool **Definition** a pus-filled blister	**from Latin, for** "little blister" ©McGraw-Hill Education
abscess AB-ses **Definition** a localized collection of pus in the body **NOTE:** The reason this word means *going away* is because in ancient times, it was believed that the harmful humors of the body would "go away" from the body via pus leaking from an abscess.	**ab / scess** away / go Source: Centers for Disease Control and Prevention

secondary lesions

Term	Word Analysis
Loss of Skin Surface	
erosion ee-ROH-zhun **Definition** loss of skin **NOTE:** The root *ros* is where we get the word *rodent* because they gnaw on everything	**e / rosion** away / gnaw/eat
ulcer UL-sir **Definition** a sore	**from Latin, for** "sore" Source: Centers for Disease Control and Prevention/Public Health Image Library
excoriation eks-kor-ee-A-shun **Definition** a scratch	**ex / cori / ation** out / skin / condition
fissure FIH-zhur **Definition** a crack in the skin	**from Latin, for a** "split" **or** "divide"
scale SKAYL **Definition** skin flaking off	

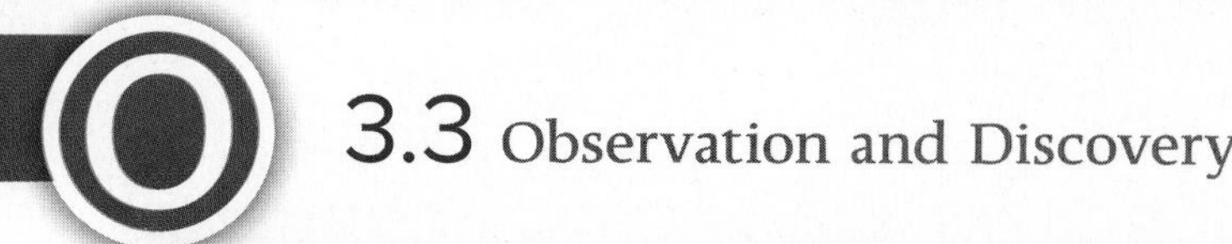

3.3 Observation and Discovery

secondary lesions *continued*

Term	Word Analysis
Material on Skin Surface	
crust KRUST **Definition** a dried substance (i.e., blood, pus) on the skin	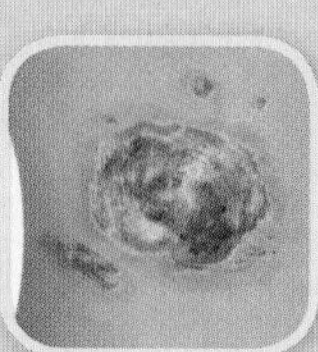

vascular lesions

Term	Word Analysis
vascular lesion VAS-kyoo-lar LEE-zhun **Definition** wounds related to blood vessels	**vascular lesion** **blood vessel wound**
cherry angioma CHEH-ree an-gee-OH-mah **Definition** a small blood vessel tumor	**angi / oma** blood vessel / tumor
telangiectasia (spider angioma) tel-an-jee-ek-TAY-zhuh **Definition** the overexpansion of the end of a blood vessel; sometimes called a *spider angioma* because of how it looks on the skin	**tel / angi / ectasia** end / blood vessel / expansion
petechia puh-TEE-kee-yah **Definition** a small bruise	**from Latin, for** "freckle" **or** "spot" 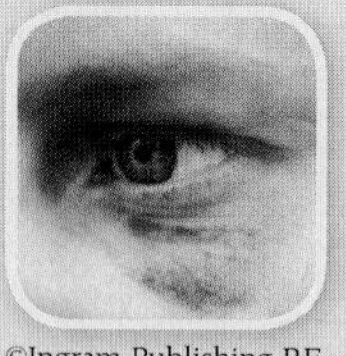 ©Ingram Publishing RF
ecchymosis eh-kih-MOH-sis **Definition** a larger bruise	**from Greek, for** "to pour out"
cicatrix (plural: cicatrices) SIK-ah-triks **Definition** scar	**from Latin, for** "scar"
keloid KEE-loid **Definition** overgrowth of scar tissue	**kel / oid** tumor / resembling

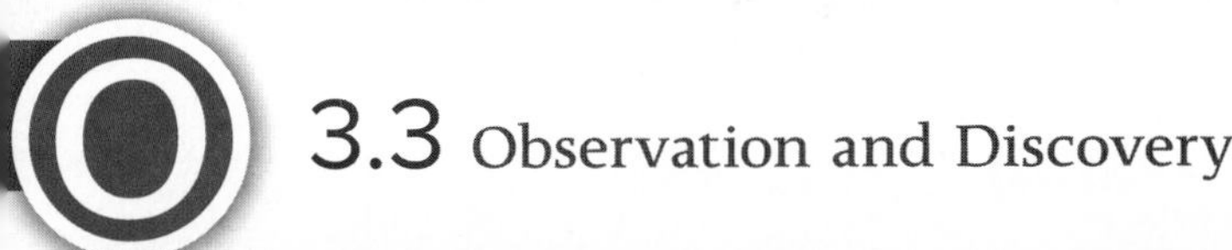

3.3 Observation and Discovery

epidermal tumors

Term	Word Analysis
epidermal tumors eh-pi-DER-mal TOO-murs **Definition** tumors on the skin	**epi / derm / al tumor** upon / skin / pertaining to tumor
nevus NEE-vus **Definition** mole	**from Latin, for** "birthmark" **or** "mole" 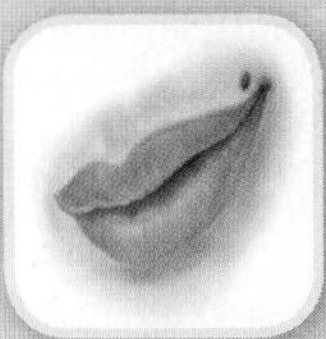
dysplastic nevus dis-PLAS-tic NEE-vus **Definition** a mole with bad changes/formations (often precancerous)	**dys / plastic nevus** bad / formation mole
verruca vah-ROO-kah **Definition** wart	**from Latin, for** "wart"

diagnostic procedures

Term	Word Analysis
culture and sensitivity (C&S) KUL-chur and sin-sih-TIV-ih-tee **Definition** growing microorganisms in isolation in order to determine which drugs they might respond to	
biopsy (Bx) BAI-op-see **Definition** removal of tissue in order to examine it (with your own two eyes)	**bi / ops / y** two / eye / procedure
excisional biopsy ek-SIH-zhun-al **Definition** removal of an entire lesion for examination (to cut it out)	**ex / cision / al** out / cut / pertaining to
incisional biopsy in-SIH-zhun-al **Definition** removal of a portion of a lesion for examination (to cut into it)	**in / cision / al** in / cut / pertaining to 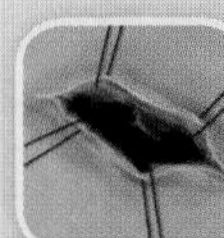
dermatoscope dir-MA-toh-SKOHP **Definition** instrument used to look at the skin	**dermato / scope** skin / instrument to look

diagnostic procedures *continued*

Term	Word Analysis
dermoscopy der-MAW-skoh-pee **Definition** procedure for looking at the skin **NOTE:** The root changes from *dermato to derm* when the suffix changes from *-scope* to *-scopy*. This is unusual, but whoever came up with these terms decided that different roots sounded better—and we agree.	**dermo / scopy** skin / looking procedure 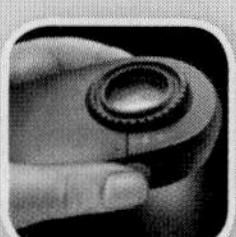

pathology

Term	Word Analysis
adipocele a-dih-poh-SEEL **Definition** a hernia filled with fatty tissue **NOTE:** *cele* originally means "tumor" or "swelling" but is frequently used to refer to types of hernia.	**adipo / cele** fat / tumor (hermia)
dermatofibroma der-MA-toh-fai-BROH-mah **Definition** a fibrous skin tumor	**dermato / fibr / oma** skin / fiber / tumor
erythrocyanosis eh-RITH-roh-sai-an-OH-sis **Definition** a red and/or blue discoloration of the skin	**erytho / cyan / osis** red / blue / condition
keratogenic keh-RAH-toh-jen-ik **Definition** causing horny tissue development	**kerato / gen / ic** horny / creation / pertaining to
keratosis KEH-rah-TOH-sis **Definition** horny tissue condition	**kerat / osis** horny / condition 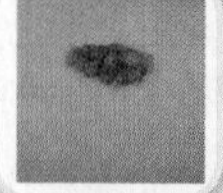
necrosis neh-KROH-sis **Definition** tissue death	**necr / osis** death / condition
onychia oh-NIK-ee-ah **Definition** a nail condition	**onych / ia** nail / condition

pathology *continued*

Term	Word Analysis
onychocryptosis AW-nih-koh-krip-TOH-sis **Definition** an ingrown nail	**onycho / crypt / osis** nail / hidden / condition
onycholysis AW-nih-KAWL-ih-sis **Definition** the loss of a nail	**onycho / lysis** nail / loose
onychomalacia AW-nih-koh-mah-LAY-shah **Definition** abnormal softening of a nail	**onycho / malacia** nail / softening
onychopathy aw-nik-AW-pah-thee **Definition** nail disease	**onycho / pathy** nail / disease
onychophagia aw-nih-koh-FAY-jah **Definition** eating (biting) the nail	**onycho / phagia** nail / eat
pachyderma pa-kih-DER-mah **Definition** tough skin	**pachy / derma** thick / skin
paronychia par-aw-NIH-kee-ah **Definition** a condition of the tissue around a nail **NOTE:** The prefix *para-* has been modified here to *par-* because the root that follows it begins with a vowel.	**par / onych / ia** around / nail / condition
steatoma STAY-ah-TOH-ma **Definition** a fatty tumor	**steat / oma** fat / tumor
xanthoma zan-THOH-mah **Definition** a yellow tumor	**xanth / oma** yellow / tumor

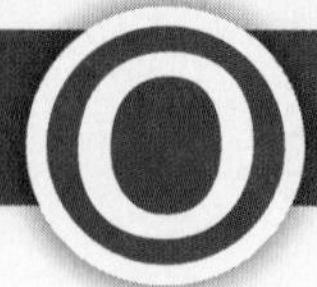

Learning Outcome 3.3 Exercises

PRONUNCIATION

EXERCISE 1 *Indicate which syllable receives emphasis when pronounced.*

EXAMPLE: bronchitis bron**chi**tis

1. vitiligo ________
2. papule ________
3. nodule ________
4. vesicle ________
5. pustule ________
6. excoriation ________
7. angioma ________
8. telangiectasia ________
9. petechia ________
10. ecchymosis ________
11. dysplastic nevus ________
12. verruca ________
13. excisional ________
14. dermatofibroma ________
15. keratogenic ________
16. keratosis ________
17. onychia ________
18. onycholysis ________
19. onychopathy ________
20. pachyderma ________

TRANSLATION

EXERCISE 2 *Break down the following words into their component parts.*

EXAMPLE: nasopharyngoscope *naso | pharyngo | scope*

1. excisional biopsy ________
2. incisional biopsy ________
3. dysplastic nevus ________
4. telangiectasia ________
5. biopsy ________
6. keratosis ________
7. necrosis ________
8. onychocryptosis ________
9. onychopathy ________
10. pachyderma ________
11. dermatoscope ________

EXERCISE 3 *Underline and define the word parts from this chapter in the following terms.*

1. epidermal tumor ________
2. adipocele ________
3. dermatofibroma ________
4. erythocyanosis ________
5. keratogenic ________
6. onychia ________
7. onycholysis ________
8. onychomalacia ________
9. onychophagia ________
10. paronychia ________
11. steatoma ________
12. xanthoma ________

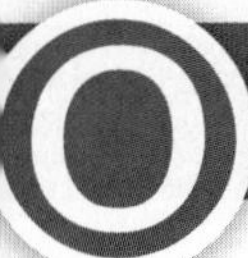

Learning Outcome 3.3 Exercises

EXERCISE 4 *Match the term on the left with its definition on the right.*

______	1. tumor	a.	freckle; small, flat, discolored area
______	2. abscess	b.	larger, flat, discolored area
______	3. pustule	c.	from Latin, for "pimple," a small solid mass
______	4. culture and sensitivity	d.	a solid mass on the surface of the skin
______	5. nodule	e.	a solid mass that extends deeper into the skin
______	6. patch (vitiligo)	f.	a larger solid mass
______	7. plaque	g.	a small blister
______	8. vesicle	h.	a large blister
______	9. macule	i.	a pus-filled blister
______	10. papule	j.	a localized collection of pus in the body
______	11. bulla	k.	diagnostic procedure in dermatology

EXERCISE 5 *Match the term on the left with its definition on the right.*

______	1. ulcer	a.	a small bruise
______	2. erosion	b.	a large bruise
______	3. petechia	c.	a small blood vessel tumor
______	4. scale	d.	a crack in the skin
______	5. crust	e.	loss of skin
______	6. cherry angioma	f.	skin flaking off
______	7. fissure	g.	a sore
______	8. keloid	h.	dried substance (i.e., blood, pus) on the skin
______	9. verruca	i.	a scratch
______	10. nevus	j.	scar
______	11. cicatrix	k.	overgrowth of scar tissue
______	12. ecchymosis	l.	mole
______	13. excoriation	m.	wart

EXERCISE 6 *Translate the following terms as literally as possible.*

EXAMPLE: nasopharyngoscope *an instrument for looking at the nose and throat*

1. vesicle ______________________
2. abscess ______________________
3. erosion ______________________
4. keloid ______________________
5. epidermal tumor ______________________
6. dysplastic nevus ______________________
7. biopsy ______________________
8. incisional biopsy ______________________
9. dermatofibroma ______________________
10. erythocyanosis ______________________
11. keratosis ______________________
12. necrosis ______________________
13. onychocryptosis ______________________
14. onycholysis ______________________
15. pachyderma ______________________

Learning Outcome 3.3 Exercises

GENERATION

EXERCISE 7 *Build a medical term from the information provided.*

EXAMPLE: inflammation of the sinuses *sinusitis*

1. nail condition ____________
2. nail disease ____________
3. fat tumor (2 terms) ____________
4. to cut it out ____________
5. pertaining to horny tissue creation ____________
6. nail softness condition ____________
7. yellow tumor ____________
8. eating the nail ____________
9. procedure to look at the skin ____________
10. (over) expansion of the end of a blood vessel ____________
11. a condition of the tissue around the nail ____________
12. blood vessel tumor ____________

EXERCISE 8 *Multiple-choice questions. Select the correct answer(s).*

1. Select all terms below that refer to flat, nonpalpable lesions.
   - a. abscess
   - b. bulla
   - c. macule
   - d. nodule
   - e. papule
   - f. patch
   - g. plaque
   - h. pustule
   - i. tumor
   - j. vesicle
   - k. vitiligo
2. Select all terms below that refer to elevated, palpable, solid-mass lesions.
   - a. abscess
   - b. bulla
   - c. macule
   - d. nodule
   - e. papule
   - f. patch
   - g. plaque
   - h. pustule
   - i. tumor
   - j. vesicle
   - k. vitiligo
3. Select all terms below that refer to elevated, fluid-filled lesions.
   - a. abscess
   - b. bulla
   - c. macule
   - d. nodule
   - e. papule
   - f. patch
   - g. plaque
   - h. pustule
   - i. tumor
   - j. vesicle
   - k. vitiligo
4. Which flat, nonpalpable lesion is the smallest?
   - a. macule
   - b. papule
   - c. patch
   - d. vitiligo
5. Which elevated, palpable, solid-mass lesion is the largest?
   - a. papule
   - b. plaque
   - c. nodule
   - d. tumor
6. Which elevated, fluid-filled lesion is pus-filled?
   - a. bulla
   - b. plaque
   - c. pustule
   - d. vesicle
7. Select all terms below that refer to lesions involving the loss of skin surface.
   - a. crust
   - b. erosion
   - c. excoriation
   - d. fissure
   - e. scale
   - f. ulcer
8. Select all terms below that refer to lesions involving material on the skin surface.
   - a. crust
   - b. erosion
   - c. excoriation
   - d. fissure
   - e. scale
   - f. ulcer
9. Select all terms below that refer to vascular lesions.
   - a. cherry angioma
   - b. cicatrix
   - c. dysplastic nevus
   - d. ecchymosis
   - e. keloid
   - f. nevus
   - g. petechia
   - h. telangiectasia
   - i. verruca

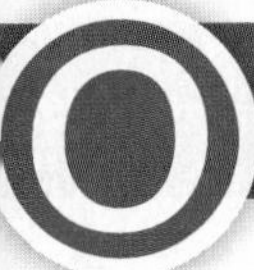

Learning Outcome 3.3 Exercises

10. Select all terms below that refer to scar formation.
    a. cherry angioma
    b. cicatrix
    c. dysplastic nevus
    d. ecchymosis
    e. keloid
    f. nevus
    g. petechia
    h. telangiectasia
    i. verruca

11. Select all terms below that refer to epidermal tumors.
    a. cherry angioma
    b. cicatrix
    c. dysplastic nevus
    d. ecchymosis
    e. keloid
    f. nevus
    g. petechia
    h. telangiectasia
    i. verruca

12. Which diagnostic procedure involves growing microorganisms in order to determine what drugs it might respond to best?
    a. biopsy
    b. culture and sensitivity
    c. excisional biopsy
    d. incisional biopsy

13. Rashes that start from the middle and work their way outward are ______________.
    a. centrifugal
    b. centripetal
    c. generalized
    d. localized

14. Rashes that spread from the outside inward are ______________.
    a. centrifugal
    b. centripetal
    c. generalized
    d. localized

15. If the rash is limited to a specific area, it is a ______________ rash.
    a. centrifugal
    b. centripetal
    c. generalized
    d. localized

16. If the rash is all over the body, it is a ______________ rash.
    a. centrifugal
    b. centripetal
    c. generalized
    d. localized

EXERCISE 9 *Define the following terms.*

1. macule ______________
2. vitiligo ______________
3. patch ______________
4. papule ______________
5. plaque ______________
6. nodule ______________
7. tumor ______________
8. bulla ______________
9. pustule ______________
10. ulcer ______________
11. excoriation ______________
12. fissure ______________
13. scale ______________
14. crust ______________
15. petechia ______________
16. ecchymosis ______________
17. cicatrix ______________
18. verruca ______________
19. nevus ______________

3.4 Diagnosis and Pathology

Skin problems are fairly limited in variety. For the most part, skin problems are infections, inflammations, tumors, or changes in the skin. Bacterial infections of the skin can be a small yellow crust, like *impetigo*, or a more extensive one, like *cellulitis*, which invades deeper layers of skin.

Other skin structures may be infected by bacteria as well: *Hidradenitis* is an infection of the sweat glands in the skin. *Acne* is similar. It is an infection of the *sebaceous* glands that commonly occurs in puberty because of the increase in hormones. Skin can be infected with a fungus (*mycosis*), and fingernails and toenails can also be infected with a fungus (*onychomycosis*). Nail infections typically require a long course of treatment.

Skin may be inflamed without being infected. *Dermatitis* is a general term for skin inflammation that does not indicate its cause. *Actinic dermatitis* is a skin condition related to sun exposure. *Seborrheic dermatitis* is a scaly red rash common in infants and elderly people. General skin problems, such as atopic dermatitis, can affect large areas of the body. *Atopic dermatitis* is very sensitive skin that is common in people with allergies and asthma. The skin is very dry and itchy. *Ichthyosis* is a condition that involves the skin becoming very thick and scaly.

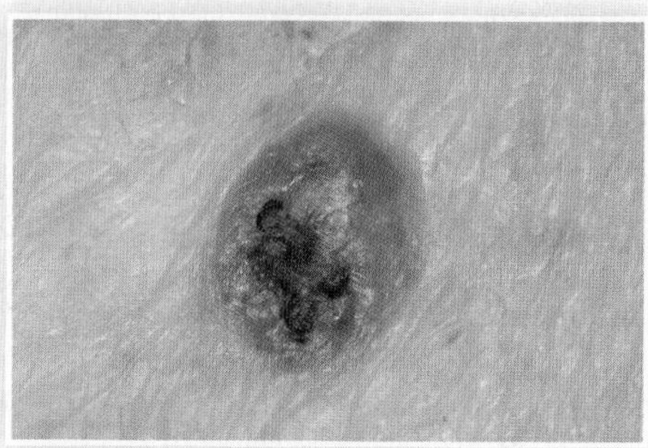

Basal cell carcinoma

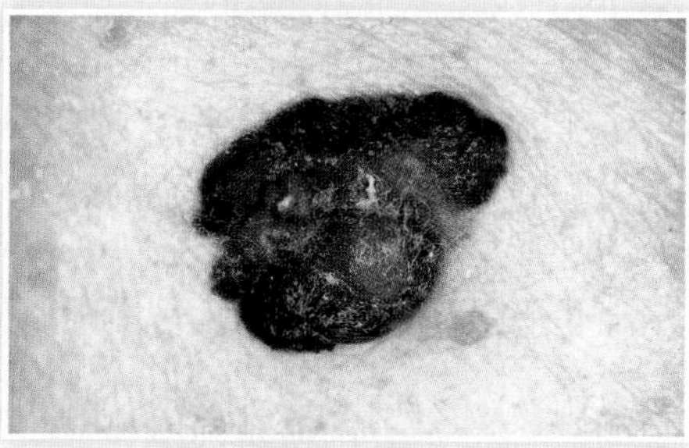

Malignant melanoma

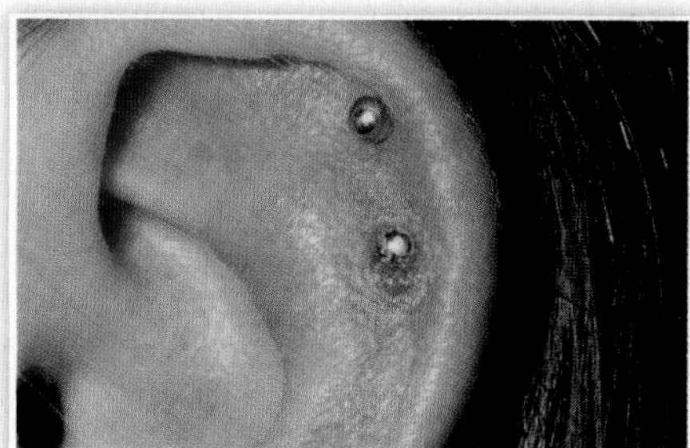

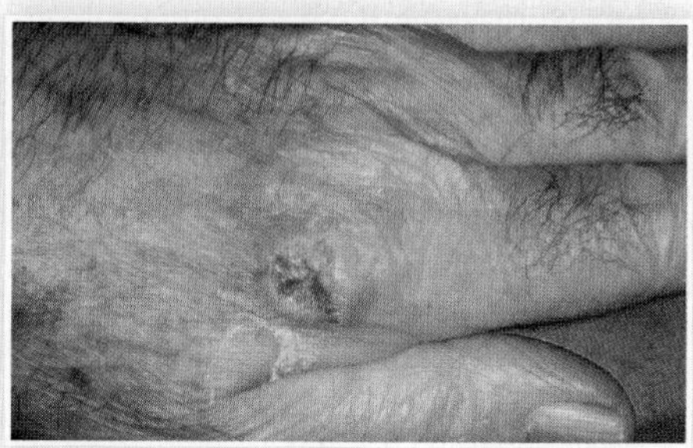

Squamous cell carcinoma

Most tumors of the skin are related to ultraviolet (UV) exposure from the sun. As a result, dermatologists often spend at least part of their visits with their patients explaining how to avoid sun exposure. Basal cell carcinomas, melanomas, and squamous cell carcinomas are all tumors associated with sun exposure.

- *Basal cell carcinoma*, the most common cancer of the skin, often presents as a round, flesh-colored, and pearly nodule.
- While *melanoma*, a cancer of the pigment-producing cells in the skin, is not the most common form of skin cancer, it is responsible for the most deaths. Melanomas are brown in color.
- *Squamous cell carcinoma* can occur anywhere in the skin where squamous cells are found. Squamous cell carcinoma of the skin begins as a small papule but eventually leads to an ulcer.
- *Actinic keratosis* is a precancerous condition also associated with sun exposure.

A decubitus ulcer is a large erosion of skin often seen in bedridden people. When the skin is under constant pressure, it can break down and cause an ulcer.

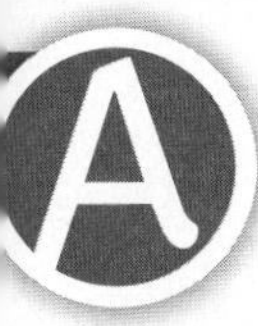

3.4 Diagnosis and Pathology

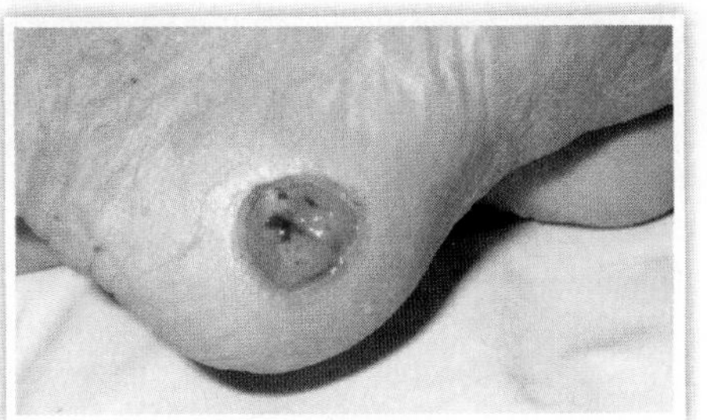

©Medical-on-line/Alamy Stock Photo

general skin changes

Term	Word Analysis
decubitus ulcer deh-KYOO-bih-tus UL-sir **Definition** bed sore	**de / cubitus ulcer** down / lie sore ©Medical-on-line/Alamy Stock Photo
dermatosis der-mah-TOH-sis **Definition** skin condition	**dermat / osis** skin / condition
dermopathy der-MAW-pa-thee **Definition** skin disease	**dermo / pathy** skin / disease
atopic dermatitis AY-taw-pik der-mah-TAI-tis **Definition** a chronic dry inflammatory disease characterized by itching **Note:** *Atopic* literally means *not in the right place and thus unusual.* Eczema is another word for atopic dermatitis.	**a / top / ic dermat / itis** not / place / pertaining to skin / inflammation
hypertrichosis HAI-per-trih-KOH-sis **Definition** excessive growth of hair	**hyper / trich / osis** over / hair / condition
ichthyosis ik-thee-OH-sis **Definition** a condition in the skin is dry and scaly resembling fish scales	**ichthy / osis** fish scale / condiion
postpartum alopecia post-PAR-tum al-oh-PEE-shah **Definition** baldness experienced by women after a pregnancy	**post / partum alopecia** after / birth baldness
psoriasis tor-AI-ah-sis **Definition** a skin condition characterized by patches of itchy, red, scaly skin	**psor / iasis** itch / presence of

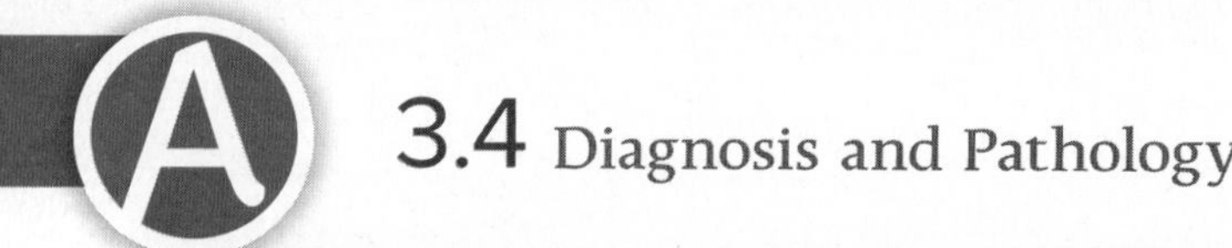

3.4 Diagnosis and Pathology

general skin changes *continued*

Term	Word Analysis
sclerodermatitis skleh-roh-der-mah-TAI-tis **Definition** inflammation of the skin accompanied by thickening and hardening	**sclero / dermat / itis** hard / skin / inflammation
scleronychia skleh-raw-NIH-kee-ah **Definition** thickening and hardening of the nails	**scler / onych / ia** hard / nail / condition
xanthosis zan-THOH-sis **Definition** yellowing of the skin	**xanth / osis** yellow / condition

oncology

Term	Word Analysis
actinic keratosis ak-TIN-ik keh-rah-TOH-sis **Definition** horny skin condition caused by sun exposure **NOTE:** This condition is not cancerous, but it is listed here because it is precancerous and frequently does develop into cancer.	**actin / ic kerat / osis** sun ray / pertaining to horny / condition
basal cell carcinoma BAY-zul sell kar-sih-NOH-mah **Definition** cancerous tumor of basal skin cells	**basal cell carcin / oma** base cell cancer / tumor
hidradenoma hih-drad-eh-NOH-mah **Definition** tumor of the sweat gland	**hidr / aden / oma** sweat / gland / tumor
malignant cutaneous neoplasm mah-LIG-nant kuh-TAY-nee-us NEE-oh-plaz-um **Definition** a harmful new formation of skin tissue (i.e., skin cancer)	**malignant cutane / ous neo / plasm** harmful skin / pertaining to new / formation
malignant melanoma ma-LIG-nant meh-lah-NOH-mah **Definition** a harmful tumor of melanin cells	**malignant melan / oma** bad black / tumor ©James Stevenson/Science Source
squamous cell carcinoma SKWAY-mus sell kar-sih-NO-mah **Definition** cancerous tumor of squamous skin cells	**squam / ous cell carcin / oma** scale / pertaining to cell cancer / tumor 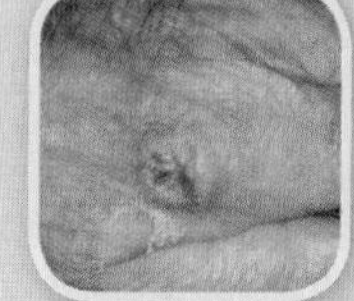 ©Biophoto Assoc./Science Source

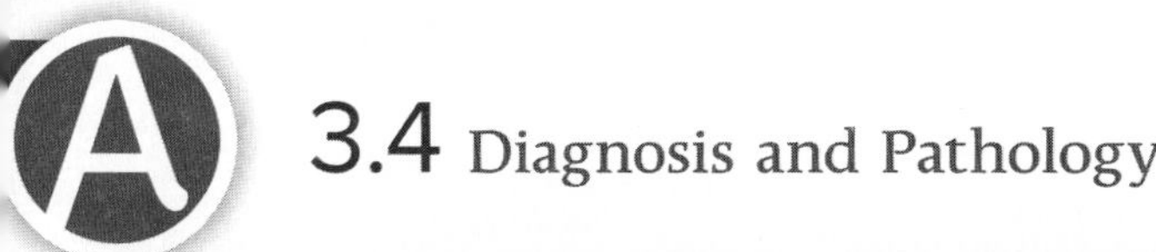

3.4 Diagnosis and Pathology

infections

Term	Word Analysis
acne vulgaris AK-nee vul-GAR-is **Definition** inflammation of the skin follicles	**acne vulgaris** acne common
dermatomycosis der-mah-toh-mai-KOH-sis **Definition** a fungal skin condition	**dermato / myc / osis** skin / fungus / condition Source: Centers for Disease Control and Prevention
hidradenitis hih-dra-deh-NAI-tis **Definition** inflammation of the sweat glands	**hidr / aden / itis** sweat / gland / inflammation
impetigo im-peh-TAI-goh **Definition** a highly contagious bacterial infection of the skin	**from Latin, for** *to attack*
mycodermatitis mai-koh-der-mah-TAI-tis **Definition** inflammation of the skin caused by fungus	**myco / dermat / itis** fungus / skin / inflammation
mycosis mai-KOH-sis **Definition** a fungal condition	**myc / osis** fungus / condition
onychodystrophy AW-ni-koh-DIS-troh-fee **Definition** poor nourishment (and development) of the nail	**onycho / dys / trophy** nail / bad / nourishment
onychomycosis AW-nih-koh-mai-KOH-sis **Definition** a fungal condition of the nail	**onycho / myc / osis** nail / fungus / condition
tinea TIH-nee-ah **Definition** a fungal condition often called "ringworm" due to its circular appearance **NOTE:** Despite its name, it is a fungus and not a bug. It can also have adjectives added onto it to describe where on the body it occurs: *tinea pedis* (foot, sometimes called "athlete's foot"); *tinea cruris* (groin, sometimes called "jock itch"), *tinea capitis* (scalp), *tinea unguium* (nails)	**from the Latin word** "tinea" **means** "worm"
trichomycosis trik-koh-mai-KOH-sis **Definition** a fungal condition of the hair	**tricho / myc / osis** hair / fungus / condition

3.4 Diagnosis and Pathology

inflammations

Term	Word Analysis
actinic dermatitis ak-TIN-ik der-mah-TAI-tis **Definition** inflammation of the skin caused by sun exposure	**actin / ic dermat / itis** sun ray / pertaining to skin / inflammation
dermatitis der-mah-TAI-tis **Definition** inflammation of the skin	**dermat / itis** skin / inflammation
seborrheic dermatitis se-boh-RAY-ik der-mah-TAI-tis **Definition** inflammation of the skin caused by the discharge of oil (sebum)	**sebo / rrhe / ic dermat / itis** oil / discharge / pertaining to skin / inflammation
steatitis stay-ah-TAI-tis **Definition** inflammation of fat tissue	**steat / itis** fat / inflammation

burns

Term	Word Analysis
first-degree burn first deh-GREE birn **Definition** burn affecting only the epidermis or superficial layer of the skin	**first-degree burn** 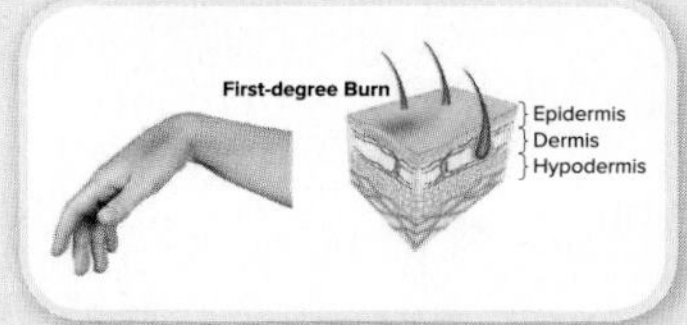
second-degree burn SEH-kund deh-GREE birn **Definition** deeper burn affecting both the epidermis and dermis	**second-degree burn** 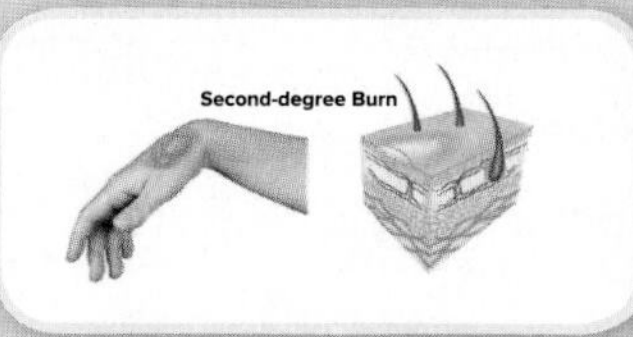
third-degree burn third deh-GREE birn **Definition** deep burn affecting the epidermis, dermis, and subcutaneous layer	**third-degree burn** 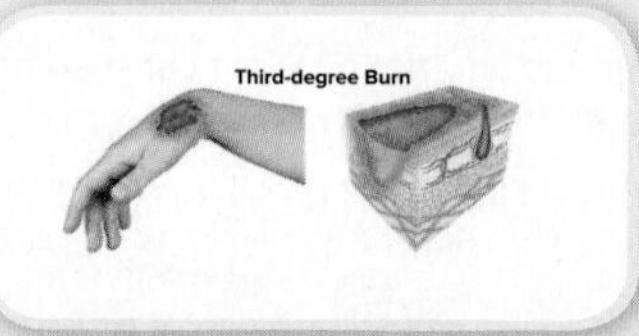
fourth-degree burn forth deh-GREE birn **Definition** deep burn affecting not just all layers of the skin (epidermis, dermis, and subcutaneous layer) but also underlying tissues like muscle, fascia, or bone	**fourth-degree burn**

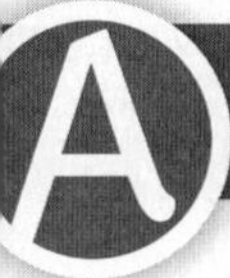

Learning Outcome 3.4 Exercises

PRONUNCIATION

EXERCISE 1 *Indicate which syllable receives emphasis when pronounced.*

EXAMPLE: bronchitis bron**chi**tis

1. actinic ______
2. xanthosis ______
3. dermatomycosis ______
4. onychomycosis ______
5. hidradenitis ______
6. mycodermatitis ______
7. mycosis ______
8. hidradenoma ______
9. dermopathy ______
10. eczema ______
11. sclerodermatitis ______

TRANSLATION

EXERCISE 2 *Break down the following words into their component parts.*

EXAMPLE: nasopharyngoscope *naso | pharyngo | scope*

1. dermopathy ______
2. mycodermatitis ______
3. mycosis ______
4. onychomycosis ______
5. dermatitis ______
6. sclerodermatitis ______
7. hidradenoma ______
8. malignant melanoma ______
9. dermatosis ______
10. atopic dermatitis ______
11. psoriasis ______

EXERCISE 3 *Underline and define the word parts from this chapter in the following terms.*

1. hidradenitis ______
2. dermatomycosis ______
3. onychodystrophy ______
4. trichomycosis ______
5. actinic dermatitis ______
6. seborrhetic ______
7. steatitis ______
8. keratosis ______
9. squamous cell carcinoma ______
10. scleronychia (2 roots) ______
11. xanthosis ______

EXERCISE 4 *Match the term on the left with its definition on the right.*

______ 1. impetigo
______ 2. acne vulgaris
______ 3. decubitus ulcer
______ 4. eczema
______ 5. postpartum alopecia
______ 6. malignant cutaneous neoplasm

a. a highly contagious bacterial infection of the skin
b. horny skin condition caused by sun exposure
c. a harmful new formation of skin tissue
d. a deep burn affecting not just all layers of the skin (epidermis, dermis, and subcutaneous layer) but also underlying tissues like muscle, fascia, or bone
e. a burn affecting only the epidermis or superficial layer of the skin
f. fungal infection sometimes called "ringworm"

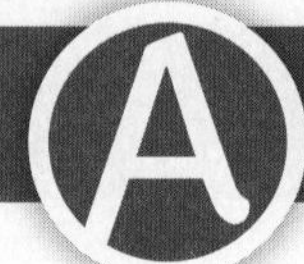

Learning Outcome 3.4 Exercises

_____	7. ichthyosis	g.	a deeper burn affecting both the epidermis and dermis
_____	8. actinic keratosis	h.	a deep burn affecting the epidermis, dermis, and subcutaneous layer
_____	9. tinea	i.	a red, itchy rash that may weep or ooze and then become crusted and scaly
_____	10. first-degree burn	j.	a skin condition that is dry and scaly
_____	11. second-degree burn	k.	bed sore
_____	12. third-degree burn	l.	baldness experienced by women after a pregnancy
_____	13. fourth-degree burn	m.	common acne

EXERCISE 5 *Translate the following terms as literally as possible.*

EXAMPLE: nasopharyngoscope *an instrument for looking at the nose and throat*

1. dermatosis _____
2. mycosis _____
3. steatitis _____
4. mycodermatitis _____
5. sclerodermatitis _____
6. scleronychia _____
7. basal cell carcinoma _____
8. hidradenoma _____
9. ichthyosis _____
10. malignant melanoma _____

GENERATION

EXERCISE 6 *Build a medical term from the information provided.*

EXAMPLE: inflammation of the sinuses *sinusitis*

1. skin disease _____
2. skin inflammation _____
3. sweat gland inflammation _____
4. a fungal condition of the nail _____
5. a fungal condition of the hair _____
6. a fungal condition of the skin _____
7. yellowing of the skin _____
8. an unusual inflammation of the skin _____
9. cancerous tumor of squamous skin cells _____
10. baldness experienced by women after a pregnancy _____

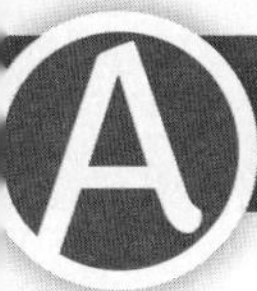

Learning Outcome 3.4 Exercises

EXERCISE 7 *Multiple-choice questions. Select the correct answer.*

1. *Acne vulgaris* means:
   a. common acne
   b. inflammation of the skin follicles
   c. both common acne and inflammation of the skin follicles
   d. neither common acne nor inflammation of the skin follicles
2. Impetigo is a:
   a. bacterial infection
   b. fungal infection
   c. viral infection
   d. none of these
3. *Onychodysptrophy* is:
   a. poor nourishment (and development) of the nail
   b. a fungal condition of the nail
   c. a bad infection of the nail
   d. inflammation of the nail
4. Inflammation of the skin caused by sun exposure is:
   a. dermatoconiosis
   b. seborrheic dermatitis
   c. actinic dermatitis
   d. actinic keratosis
5. Eczema is:
   a. from Greek, for *to boil over*
   b. from Latin, for *to attack*
   c. from Greek, for *to boil over*; and from Latin, for *to attack*
   d. neither from Greek, for *to boil over*; nor from Latin, for *to attack*
6. A skin condition caused by the discharge of oil is:
   a. dermatoconiosis
   b. seborrheic dermatitis
   c. actinic dermatitis
   d. actinic keratosis
7. A horny skin condition caused by sun exposure is:
   a. dermatoconiosis
   b. seborrheic dermatitis
   c. actinic dermatitis
   d. actinic keratosis
8. A *malignant cutaneous neoplasm* is:
   a. a harmful new formation of the skin tissue (i.e., skin cancer)
   b. a harmful tumor of melanin cells
   c. a cancerous tumor of squamous skin cells
   d. a tumor of the sweat gland
9. A bed sore is a(n):
   a. ichthyosis
   b. decubitus ulcer
   c. steatitis
   d. scleronychia

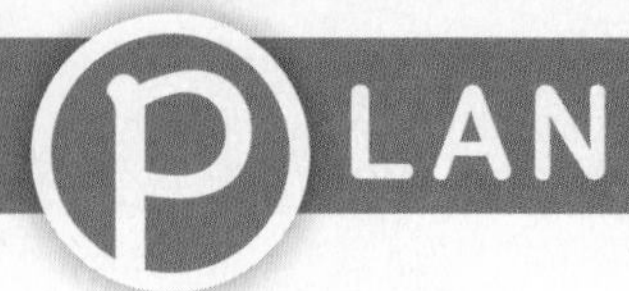

3.5 Treatments and Therapies

There is an old joke in the health community that treatment options in dermatology are very simple: If it's wet, dry it; if it's dry, wet it; and if nothing else works, use steroids. The medicines available in skin care have increased significantly, but they mostly fall in one of a few categories: anti-infection or cleansing (*antibiotics, antiseptics*), anti-immune (*steroids* or related), and anti-itch or allergy (*antihistamines*). In contrast to the limited number of medicines, the field of dermatology employs a variety of types of procedures in eradicating disease. They use chemicals (*chemosurgery* and *chemotherapy*), vacuums (*liposuction*), cold (*cryosurgery*), lasers (*dermabrasion*), and even electricity (*electrosurgery, electrodesiccation*). Of the many different surgical techniques to treat cancer, one of the oldest is Mohs micrographic surgery. The procedure involves removing very thin layers of tissue, examining them under the microscope for cancer, and continuing to remove skin layers until the cancer can no longer be detected. Originally, this technique involved the use of a chemical to "fix" the tissue in place; hence, the original term was *chemosurgery.* Chemicals are no longer used to fix the skin. The newer term, *micrography*, reflects the use of "mapping" out the skin for cancer under the microscope. This procedure and many others still rely on cold, hard steel for cutting, incision and drainage of an abscess and removing all or part of a nail (*onychectomy*); and biopsies still generally rely on the use of a scalpel.

One very challenging and important area of skin surgery is transplanting or grafting new skin in place of old skin. This is needed in areas where skin has been burned, scraped off, or killed. The transplanted skin can come from the patient (*autograft*), another person (*homograft*), or even another species (*heterograft*). While not all health care workers perform such in-depth procedures, most do perform skin-related procedures many times a day—specifically, injections. Inserting a needle into the skin to give medicine is a very routine part of many medical fields.

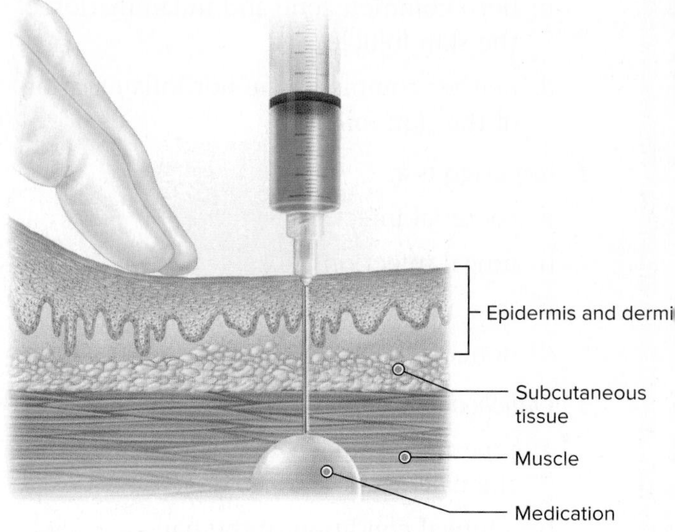

A wide variety of medications are administered via hypodermic needle. As the name suggests, it injects the medicine beneath (*hypo-*) the skin (*dermic*).

pharmacology

Term	Word Analysis
anesthetic an-es-THET-ik **Definition** a drug that temporarily blocks sensation	**an / esthetic** no / sensation
antibiotic an-tai-bai-OH-tk **Definition** a drug that destroys or opposes growth of microorganisms **NOTE:** The life that the drug is fighting is not the life of the patient but the life of microorganisms; similarly, a drug that encourages the growth of microorganisms (especially in the digestive system) is called a probiotic. Antibiotics don't work on viruses because viruses are not living organisms.	**anti / biotic** against / life ©McGraw-Hill Education/Christopher Kerrigan, photographer

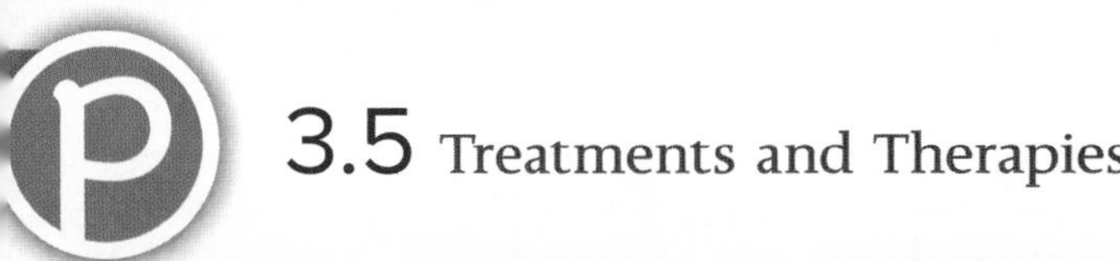

pharmacology *continued*

Term	Word Analysis
antihistamine an-tee-HIS-tah-meen **Definition** a drug that opposes the effects of histamine	**anti / histamine** against / histamine ©McGraw-Hill Education/Christopher Kerrigan, photographer
antipruritic an-tee-pruh-RIH-tik **Definition** a drug that prevents or relieves itching	**anti / pruritic** against / itching
antiseptic an-tee-SEP-tik **Definition** a drug that prevents sepsis (rotting of flesh) by killing microorganisms	**anti / septic** against / rotting

general terms

Term	Word Analysis
epidermal eh-pih-DER-mal **Definition** pertaining to the skin	**epi / derm / al** upon / skin / pertaining to
hypodermic hai-poh-DER-mik **Definition** pertaining to beneath the skin	**hypo / derm / ic** beneath / skin / pertaining to
intradermal in-tra-DER-mal **Definition** pertaining to inside the skin	**intra / derm / al** inside / skin / pertaining to
percutaneous per-kyoo-TAY-nee-us **Definition** pertaining to through the skin	**per / cutane / ous** through / skin / pertaining to
subcutaneous sub-kyoo-TAY-nee-us **Definition** pertaining to beneath the skin	**sub / cutane / ous** beneath / skin / pertaining to

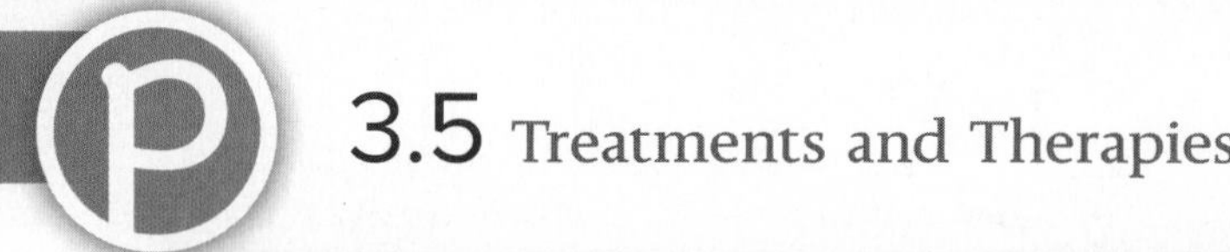

3.5 Treatments and Therapies

general terms *continued*

Term	Word Analysis
topical TAW-pih-cal	**topic / al** place / pertaining to

Definition applied directly to the skin

NOTE: *Topic/o* and *Top/o* mean "place." You might have seen the term *topographical* used with maps. In dermatology, it refers to medicine applied to the skin as opposed to taken by mouth.

Term	Word Analysis
transdermal trans-DER-mal	**trans / derm / al** through / skin / pertaining to

Definition pertaining to through the skin

procedures

Term	Word Analysis
chemosurgery KEE-moh-SIR-juh-ree	**chemo / surgery** chemical / surgery

Definition removal of tissue that has been destroyed using chemicals

Term	Word Analysis
chemotherapy KEE-moh-THEH-rah-pee	**chemo / therapy** chemical / treatment

Definition treatment using chemicals

Term	Word Analysis
cryosurgery KRAI-oh-SIR-juh-ree	**cryo / surgery** cold / surgery

Definition destruction of tissue through freezing

NOTE: Also known as *cryotherapy*

Term	Word Analysis
dermabrasion der-mah-BRAY-zhun	**derm / ab / rasion** skin / away / rub

Definition rubbing or scraping away the outer surface of skin

Term	Word Analysis
electrocauterization e-LEK-troh-KAW-ter-ai-ZAY-shun	**electro / cauteriz / ation** electricity / burn / process

Definition using electricity to destroy tissue by burning it

Term	Word Analysis
electrodesiccation e-LEK-troh-deh-sih-KAY-shun	**electro / desicc / ation** electricity / drying / process

Definition using electricity to destroy tissue by drying it

NOTE: That little packet labeled "Do Not Eat" that you sometimes find in packages is called a *desiccant* because it absorbs moisture and keeps the product dry.

Term	Word Analysis
incision and drainage (I&D) in-SIH-zhun and DRAY-nij	**in / cision** in / cut

Definition to cut into a wound to allow trapped infected liquid to drain

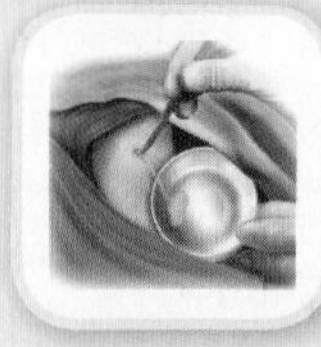

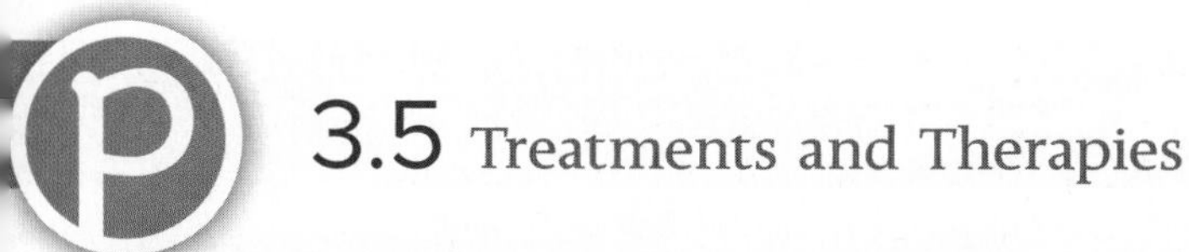

3.5 Treatments and Therapies

procedures *continued*

Term	Word Analysis
lipectomy lih-PEK-toh-mee **Definition** removal of fatty tissue	**lip / ectomy** fat / removal
liposuction LAI-poh-SUK-shun **Definition** removal of fatty tissue using a vacuum	**lipo / suction** fat / vacuum
onychectomy aw-nik-EK-toh-mee **Definition** remove of a nail	**onych / ectomy** nail / removal
onychotomy aw-ni-KAW-toh-mee **Definition** incision into a nail	**onycho / tomy** nail / incision
rhytidoplasty rih-tih-doh-PLAS-tee **Definition** reconstruction of wrinkled skin	**rhytido / plasty** wrinkle / reconstruction

skin grafting

Term	Word Analysis
autograft AW-toh-GRAFT **Definition** skin transplant taken from a different place on the patient's body	**auto / graft** self / transplant
homograft (allograft) HOH-moh-GRAFT (A-loh-GRAFT) **Definition** skin transplant taken from another member of the patient's species (*homo*, because it is from a similar species, and *allo*, because it is from another person)	**homo / graft (allo / graft)** similar / transplant (other / transplant)
heterograft HEH-ter-oh-GRAFT **Definition** skin transplant taken from a species other than the patient's	**hetero / graft** different / transplant
xenograft ZEE-noh-graft **Definition** skin transplant taken from a species other than the patient's	**xeno / graft** foreign / transplant

NOTE: The terms *heterograft* and *xenograft* are interchangeable and mean basically the same thing: *hetero* because it is a different species, and *xeno* because it is a foreign species.

Learning Outcome 3.5 Exercises

PRONUNCIATION

EXERCISE 1 *Indicate which syllable receives emphasis when pronounced.*

EXAMPLE: bronchitis bron**chi**tis

1. dermabrasion ____________
2. lipectomy ____________
3. onychectomy ____________
4. onychotomy ____________
5. xenograft ____________
6. epidermal ____________
7. transdermal ____________
8. percutaneous ____________
9. hypodermic ____________
10. intradermal ____________
11. antihistamine ____________
12. antipruritic ____________
13. topical ____________

TRANSLATION

EXERCISE 2 *Break down the following words into their component parts.*

EXAMPLE: nasopharyngoscope *naso | pharyngo | scope*

1. incision ____________
2. autograft ____________
3. homograft ____________
4. allograft ____________
5. heterograft ____________
6. xenograft ____________
7. intradermal ____________
8. transdermal ____________
9. chemosurgery ____________
10. chemotherapy ____________
11. cryosurgery ____________
12. liposuction ____________
13. onychotomy ____________

EXERCISE 3 *Underline and define the word parts from this chapter in the following terms.*

1. dermabrasion ____________
2. lipectomy ____________
3. hypodermic ____________
4. onychectomy ____________
5. rhytidoplasty ____________
6. epidermal ____________
7. percutaneous ____________
8. subcutaneous ____________

EXERCISE 4 *Match the term on the left with its definition on the right.*

_____ 1. anesthetic
_____ 2. antibiotic
_____ 3. antihistamine
_____ 4. antipruritic
_____ 5. antiseptic
_____ 6. electrocauterization
_____ 7. electrodesiccation

a. using electricity to destroy tissue by burning it
b. a drug that destroys or opposes growth of microorganisms
c. to cut into a wound to allow infected liquid to drain
d. a drug that opposes the effects of histamine
e. a drug that prevents sepsis (rotting of flesh) by killing microorganisms
f. a drug that prevents or relieves itching
g. using electricity to destroy tissue by drying it

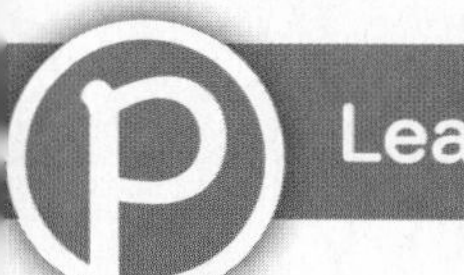

Learning Outcome 3.5 Exercises

______	8. incision and drainage (I&D)	h.	a drug that temporarily blocks sensation
______	9. topical	i.	applied directly to the skin

EXERCISE 5 *Translate the following terms as literally as possible.*

EXAMPLE: nasopharyngoscope *an instrument for looking at the nose and throat*

1. chemosurgery ______
2. cryosurgery ______
3. dermabrasion ______
4. electrocauterization ______
5. incision ______
6. liposuction ______
7. onychotomy ______
8. rhytidoplasty ______
9. homograft ______
10. allograft ______
11. heterograft ______
12. xenograft ______

GENERATION

EXERCISE 6 *Build a medical term from the information provided.*

EXAMPLE: inflammation of the sinuses *sinusitis*

1. pertaining to upon the skin ______
2. pertaining to beneath the skin (use *cutaneo*) ______
3. pertaining to inside the skin ______
4. pertaining to through the skin (2 terms) ______
5. pertaining to beneath the skin (use *dermo*) ______
6. chemical treatment ______
7. removing fatty tissue ______
8. removing a nail ______
9. using electricity to destroy tissue by drying it ______
10. skin transplant taken from a different place on the patient's body ______

EXERCISE 7 *Describe the purpose of the following drugs.*

1. anesthetic ______
2. antibiotic ______
3. antihistamine ______
4. antipruritic ______
5. antiseptic ______

3.6 Abbreviations of the Integumentry System

Abbreviations provide medical professionals with a shorthand for writing words that commonly occur in their field. In dermatology, these abbreviations can refer to things ranging from procedures (C&S), to common diagnoses (AK), or even to mnemonic devices for remembering steps in analysis (ABCDE).

integumentary system abbreviations

Abbreviation	Definition
ABCDE	asymmetry, border, color, diameter, evolving
AK	actinic keratosis
Bx	biopsy
C&S	culture and sensitivity
derm	dermatology
ID	intradermal
SC	subcutaneous
SQ	subcutaneous

Learning Outcome 3.6 Exercises

TRANSLATION

EXERCISE 1 *Define the following abbreviations.*

1. derm ______
2. C&S ______
4. SC ______
6. ID ______
5. ABCDE ______

EXERCISE 2 *Give the abbreviations for the following terms.*

1. biopsy ______
2. dermatology ______
3. asymmetry, border, color, diameter, evolving ______
4. culture and sensitivity ______
5. actinic keratosis ______

Learning Outcome 3.6 Exercises

EXERCISE 3 *Match the abbreviation on the left with its definition on the right.*

______	1. ID	a. horny skin condition caused by sun exposure
______	2. C&S	b. intradermal; within the skin
______	3. Bx	c. subcutaneous; below the skin
______	4. SQ	d. growing microorganisms in isolation in order to determine which drugs they might respond best to
______	5. AK	e. removal of tissue in order to examine it

3.7 Electronic Health Records

Consult Note

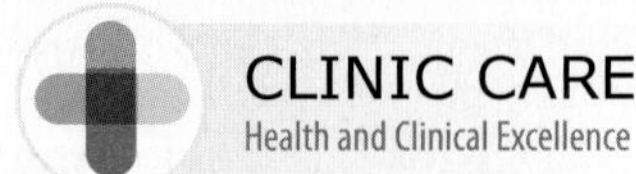

Reason for Consult: Rash

I had the pleasure of seeing your patient in my clinic. As you know, Mr. Skein is a 39-year-old male with a chronic history of **atopic dermatitis.** His atopic dermatitis was well controlled with **topical corticosteroids** until 3 weeks ago, when he developed a new rash consisting of **vesicles** overlying the areas of xerosis on his extremities. He was initially diagnosed with **impetigo** and treated with topical antibiotic therapy. He returned in 1 week without any improvement and was put on **oral** antibiotics at that time. He has now come to my office for a second opinion.

Mr. Skein reports mild pain and **pruritus,** but denies fever/chills, wheezing, or **edema** of his extremities. He had a recent cold sore prior to the new rash. Except for a case of **tinea pedis** and **tinea corporis,** Mr. Skein's dermatological history is unremarkable.

The physical exam showed **erythematous, xerotic patches** in the flexural creases of his elbows and knees as well as the extensor surface of his legs. He has numerous red crusts and **vesicles,** along with scattered excoriations and erosions. The rest of the exam was unremarkable except mild scalp **alopecia.**

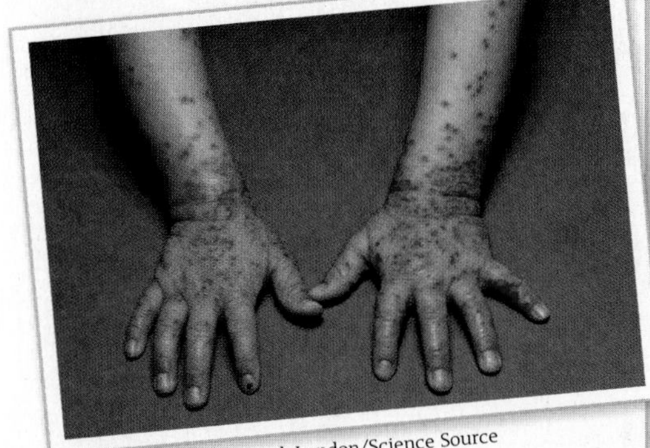

©St Bartholomew's Hospital, London/Science Source

Laboratory testing with viral culture confirmed the diagnosis of **eczema herpeticum.** I treated him with oral antiviral medicine and he will follow up in my office in 2 weeks.

Thank you for this interesting consult.

Sincerely,
Robertra Mandel, MD

Learning Outcome 3.7 Exercises

EXERCISE 1 *Match the term on the left with its definition on the right.*

_____	1. atopic dermatitis	a.	an itch
_____	2. vesicle	b.	loss of skin
_____	3. xerosis	c.	a small blister
_____	4. impetigo	d.	larger, flat, discolored areas
_____	5. antibiotic	e.	a drug that destroys or opposes the growth of microorganisms
_____	6. pruritus	f.	condition of dryness
_____	7. patch	g.	a scratch
_____	8. crust	h.	baldness
_____	9. excoriation	i.	an unusual inflammation of the skin
_____	10. erosion	j.	a highly contagious bacterial infection of the skin
_____	11. alopecia	k.	a red, itchy rash that may weep or ooze, then become crusted and scaly
_____	12. eczema	l.	dried substance (i.e., blood, pus) on the skin

EXERCISE 2 *Fill in the blanks.*

1. The patient has a history of ______________________________ (an unusual inflammation of the skin).
2. The new rash consisted of vesicles overlying the areas of *xerosis* (give definition: ____________________ ____).
3. Mr. Skein reports mild pain and ______________________________ (an itch).
4. The physical exam shows *xerotic* ______________________________ (larger, flat, discolored areas).
5. The patient had mild scalp *alopecia* (give definition: ______________________________).

EXERCISE 3 *True or false questions. Indicate true answers with a T and false answers with an F.*

1. The patient did respond to topical antibiotic therapy. _____
2. The physical exam showed dry red patches in the creases of his elbows and knees. _____
3. The patient was given an antiviral medication by a shot in the arm. _____

Learning Outcome 3.7 Exercises

EXERCISE 4 *Multiple-choice questions. Select the correct answer.*

1. The patient's new rash consisted of:
   a. small blisters
   b. large blisters
   c. warts
   d. moles
2. The initial diagnosis was a highly contagious bacterial infection of the skin called:
   a. dermatomycosis
   b. eczema
   c. hyperkeratosis
   d. impetigo
3. The patient's impetigo was treated with a drug that:
   a. temporarily blocks sensation
   b. destroys or opposes growth of microorganisms
   c. opposes the effects of histamine
   d. prevents or relieves itching
4. "Physical exam showed erythematous, xerotic patches in his flexural creases of his elbows and knees as well as the extensor surface of his legs." The root of *erythematous* means:
   a. black
   b. red
   c. white
   d. yellow

Use the health professional's note "He has numerous hemorrhagic crusts and vesicles along with scattered excoriations and erosions" to answer the following questions:

5. Which symptom is NOT described by the health professional?
   a. localized collection of pus in the body
   b. dried substance (i.e., pus, blood) on the skin
   c. scratches
   d. skin loss
   e. small blisters
6. The patient was diagnosed with *eczema herpticum.* Which of the following symptoms is NOT characteristic of eczema?
   a. erythroderma
   b. pruritus
   c. crusts
   d. ecchymosis

Dermatology Clinic Note

S Subjective

Mrs. Smith is a 53-year-old woman with a 2-year history of worsening rash on her knees and elbows. She has had mild **pruritus,** but otherwise minimal discomfort. She came to my office today because the rash is worsening, and she also has problems with her toenails. She has tried topical moisturizer, which has not helped at all.

Social Hx: 1-pack-per-day smoker. Social drinker; 3–4 glasses of wine a week.

Family Hx: Positive for **psoriasis** in mother.

PMHx: **Dermatofibromas** x 3 on legs removed via **cryotherapy** 3 years ago.

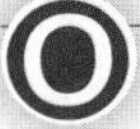

Objective

Temp: 98.7; HR: 74; RR: 16; BP: 115/73

Gen: Woman with healthy appearance, alert and oriented.

HEENT: ears normal. **Xanthochromic**/stained teeth. Mucous membranes moist and pink.

CV: RRR no murmurs.

Resp: CTA.

Skin: **Erythematous papules** and **plaques** with a silver **scale** on the extensor surface of knees, elbows, and back; **onycholysis** of toe nails.

Skin Bx: **Epidermal hyperplasia.**

Assessment

DDx:

1. Rash: **Plaque psoriasis, seborrheic dermatitis, atopic dermatitis.**
2. Onycholysis: Psoriatic vs. **onychomycosis.**

Given that the rash is found on the extensor surface and not the flexural creases, in addition to the presence of a silver scale, I suspected psoriasis. My diagnosis was confirmed with **histologic** appearance on the biopsy.

Plan

I will begin her on topical corticosteroids and have her follow up in 2–4 months. For any unresponsive areas I will try **photochemotherapy.** For the patient's onycholysis, I have referred her to a podiatrist **onychectomy.**

–Electronically signed by
Joaquin Hernandez, MD

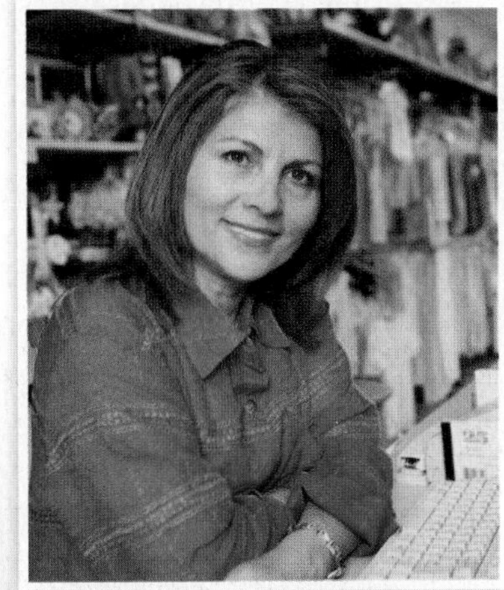

Learning Outcome 3.7 Exercises

EXERCISE 5 *Match the term on the left with its definition on the right.*

_____	1. pruritus	a. skin flaking off
_____	2. dermatofibroma	b. a solid mass on the surface of the skin
_____	3. onychectomy	c. a fibrous skin tumor
_____	4. papule	d. inflammation of the skin caused by the discharge of oil
_____	5. plaque	e. a fungal condition of the nail
_____	6. scale	f. to remove a nail
_____	7. onycholysis	g. the loss of a nail
_____	8. seborrheic dermatitis	h. a small, solid mass
_____	9. atopic dermatitis	i. an itch
_____	10. onychomycosis	j. an unusual inflammation of the skin

EXERCISE 6 *Fill in the blanks.*

1. Mrs. Smith has mild ______________________________ (an itch).
2. Mrs. Smith had three *dermatofibromas* (define: ______________________________) removed with ______________________________ (treatment using cold).
3. The dermatology assessment showed erythematous *papules* (define: ______________________________) and plaques (define: ______________________________) with a silver ______________________________ (skin flaking off).
4. The health care professional referred Mrs. Smith to a podiatrist *onychectomy* (define: ______________________________).

EXERCISE 7 *True or false questions. Indicate true answers with a T and false answers with an F.*

1. Topical moisturizers have helped Mrs. Smith's worsening pruritus. _____
2. Mrs. Smith is losing her toenails. _____
3. The health professional performed a biopsy. _____
4. Seborrheic dermatitis is inflammation of the nail caused by oil. _____
5. *Atopic dermatitis* is a term to describe routine skin inflammation and is quite common. _____
6. Mrs. Smith has psoriasis. _____

Learning Outcome 3.7 Exercises

EXERCISE 8 *Multiple-choice questions. Select the correct answer.*

1. Mrs. Smith has teeth that are stained:
   a. white
   b. black
   c. brown
   d. yellow
2. The papules on Mrs. Smith's skin are *erythematous,* which means they are:
   a. red
   b. itchy
   c. raised
   d. blistered
3. *Bx* is an abbreviation for:
   a. biopsy
   b. bulla
   c. basal cell
   d. cicatrix
4. Mrs. Smith's biopsy revealed hyperplasia that pertained to:
   a. the nail
   b. the skin
   c. the teeth
   d. the rash
5. The root words in *onychomycosis* are *onycho,* meaning "nail," and *myco,* meaning:
   a. fungus
   b. bacteria
   c. virus
   d. tumor

Dermatology Consult Note

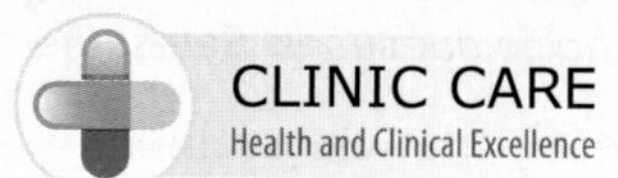

Dermatology Consult

I had the pleasure of seeing your patient John Johnson in my clinic on February 14. Your office referred him to me regarding a rash on sun-exposed areas of his body. He is a 45-year-old landscape architect who spends a large part of his days outdoors. He had noticed several spots on his arms, but did not seek medical care at that time. At his routine physical, his care provider noticed the rash on his arms.

Physical exam revealed a well-developed, well-nourished, fair-skinned male. His heart was regular in rate and rhythm. His lungs were clear. His mucous membranes were moist and pink. His skin exam was significant for papules of **hyperkeratosis** with surrounding **erythema.** A few of the lesions are **hyperpigmented.** He has larger patches on his scalp.

A skin biospy performed in my office confirmed the diagnosis of **actinic keratosis (AK).** After explaining the results to Mr. Johnson, I recommended **cryosurgery** for the smaller lesions on his arms and **dermabrasion** for his scalp lesions. I explained to Mr. Johnson that **AK** can lead to **squamous cell carcinoma** and taught him about the risks of sun exposure, including further AKs and **melanoma.**

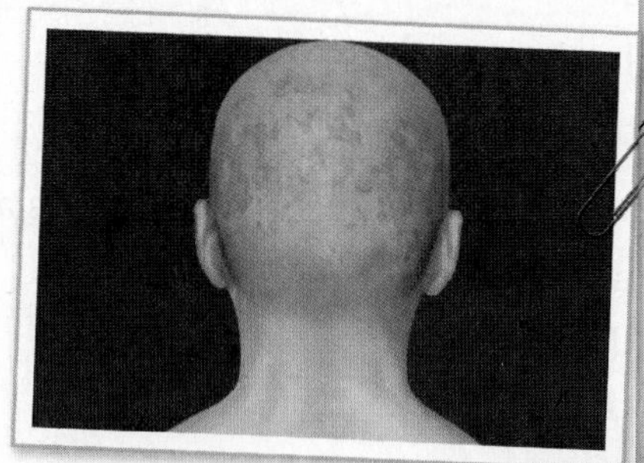

Thank you for this interesting consult.

— James Skinner, MD

EXERCISE 9 *Match the term on the left with its definition on the right.*

_____ 1. papule — a. horny skin condition caused by sun exposure

_____ 2. hyperkeratosis — b. redness

_____ 3. erythema — c. removal of tissue in order to examine it

_____ 4. hyperpigmented — d. excessive growth of horny skin

_____ 5. patch — e. treatment of the skin using cold

_____ 6. biopsy — f. actinic keratosis

_____ 7. actinic keratosis — g. a small, solid mass

_____ 8. cryosurgery — h. larger, flat, discolored area

_____ 9. dermabrasion — i. tumor of melanin cells

_____ 10. AK — j. excessive pigment in the skin

_____ 11. squamous cell carcinoma — k. cancerous tumor of squamous skin cells

_____ 12. melanoma — l. rubbing or scraping away the outer surface of skin

Learning Outcome 3.7 Exercises

EXERCISE 10 *Fill in the blanks.*

1. The patient's skin exam was significant for ______________________________ (small, solid masses) of *hyperkeratosis* (excessive growth of ______________________________ skin) with surrounding *erythema* (define: ______________________________).

2. He has larger ______________________________ (larger, flat, discolored areas) on his scalp.

3. *Actinic* ______________________________ is a horny skin condition caused by ______________________________.

EXERCISE 11 *Multiple-choice questions. Select the correct answer.*

1. A few of Mr. Johnson's lesions are *hyperpigmented,* which means:
   - a. excessive pigmentation
   - b. underpigmentation
   - c. loss of pigmentation
   - d. creation of pigmentation
2. *Actinic keratosis* is:
   - a. inflammation of the skin caused by sun exposure
   - b. horny skin condition caused by sun exposure
   - c. a harmful new formation of the skin tissue (i.e., skin cancer)
   - d. common acne
3. The diagnosis of actinic keratosis was confirmed by performing:
   - a. biopsy
   - b. cryosurgery
   - c. dermabrasion
   - d. C&S
4. Which treatment option was NOT recommended for the patient?
   - a. biopsy
   - b. treatment using cold
   - c. rubbing or scraping away the outer surface of skin
   - d. corticosteroids
5. The root word in *squamous* means:
   - a. scaly
   - b. dry
   - c. oily
   - d. yellow
6. The root word in *melanoma* means:
   - a. white
   - b. black
   - c. yellow
   - d. red

Quick Reference

quick reference glossary of roots

Root	Definition	Root	Definition	Root	Definition
adip/o	fat	**kerat/o**	hard, horny	**seb/o**	oil
alb/o	white	**leuk/o**	white	**squam/o**	scale
crypt/o	hidden	**lip/o**	fat	**steat/o**	fat
cutane/o	skin	**melan/o**	black	**trich/o**	hair
dermat/o	skin	**onych/o**	nail	**ungu/o**	nail
derm/o	skin	**pachy/o**	thick	**xanth/o**	yellow
erythr/o	red	**pil/o**	hair	**xer/o**	dry
hidr/o	sweat	**sebace/o**	oil		

quick reference glossary of terms

Term	Definition
abrasion	a scraping away of skin
abscess	a localized collection of pus in the body
acne vulgaris	common acne; an inflammation of the skin follicles
actinic dermatitis	inflammation of the skin caused by sun exposure
actinic keratosis	horny skin condition caused by sun exposure
adipocele	a hernia filled with fatty tissue
albinism	lack of pigment in skin causing patient to look white
albino	a person afflicted with albinism
allograft	*see* homograft
alopecia	baldness
anesthetic	a drug that temporarily blocks sensation
anhidrosis	lack of sweating
antibiotic	a drug that destroys or opposes the growth of microorganisms
antihistamine	a drug that opposes the effects of histamine
antipruritic	a drug that prevents or relieves itching
antiseptic	a drug that prevents sepsis (rotting of flesh) by killing microorganisms

quick reference glossary of terms *continued*

Term	Definition
atopic dermatitis	an unusual inflammation of the skin (*atopic* usually means "not in the right place")
autograft	skin transplant taken from a different place on the patient's body
basal cell carcinoma	cancerous tumor of basal skin cells
biopsy	removal of tissue in order to examine it
bulla	from Latin, for "bubble"; a larger blister
chemosurgery	removal of tissue that has been destroyed using chemicals
chemotherapy	treatment using chemicals
cherry angioma	a small blood vessel tumor
cicatrix (plural cicatrices)	from Latin, for "scar"; a scar
comedo	from Latin, for "to eat up"; a hair follicle plugged with sebum (black head, white head)
crust	dried substance (i.e., blood, pus) on the skin
cryosurgery	destruction of tissue through freezing
culture & sensitivity	growing microorganisms in isolation in order to determine which drugs they might respond to
cyanidrosis	blue sweat
decubitus ulcer	bed sore
depigmentation	loss of skin pigmentation
dermabrasion	rubbing or scraping away the outer surface of skin
dermatitis	inflammation of the skin
dermatofibroma	a fibrous skin tumor
dermatolysis	loss of skin
dermatomycosis	a fungal skin condition
dermatoscope	instrument used to look at the skin
dermatosis	skin condition
dermopathy	skin disease
dermoscopy	procedure for looking at the skin
dysplastic nevus	a mole with bad changes/formations (often precancerous)
ecchymosis	from Greek, for "to pour out"; a larger bruise
eczema	from Greek, for "to boil over"; a red, itchy rash that may weep or ooze, then become crusted and scaly
electrocauterization	using electricity to destroy tissue by burning it

quick reference glossary of terms *continued*

Term	Definition
electrodesiccation	using electricity to destroy tissue by drying it
epidermal	pertaining to the skin
epidermal tumor	tumors on the skin
erosion	loss of skin
erythema	from Greek, for "redness"; redness
erythrocyanosis	a red and/or blue discoloration of the skin
erythroderma	red skin
excisional biopsy	removal of an entire lesion for examination (to cut it out)
excoriation	a scratch
first-degree burn	a burn affecting only the epidermis or superficial layer of the skin
fissure	from Latin, for a "split" or "divide"; a crack in the skin
fourth-degree burn	a deep burn affecting not just all layers of the skin (epidermis, dermis, and subcutaneous layer) but also underlying tissues like muscle, fascia, or bone
hemathidrosis	sweating blood
heterograft (xenograft)	skin transplant taken from a species other than the patient's (*hetero* because it is a different species; *xeno* because it is a foreign species)
hidradenitis	inflammation of the sweat glands
hidradenoma	tumor of the sweat gland
hidropoiesis	the formation of sweat
homograft (allograft)	skin transplant taken from another member of the patient's species (*homo* because it is from a similar species; *allo* because it is from another person)
hyperhidrosis	excessive sweating
hyperkeratosis	excessive growth of horny skin
hypermelanosis	excessive melanin in the skin
hyperpigmentation	excessive pigment in the skin
hypodermia	pertaining to beneath the skin
hypohidrosis	diminished sweating
hypomelanosis	diminished melanin in the skin
hypopigmentation	diminished pigment in the skin
ichthyosis	a condition in the skin that is dry and scaly resembling fish scales
impetigo	from Latin, for "to attack"; a highly contagious bacterial infection of the skin
incision and drainage (I&D)	to cut into a wound to allow trapped infected liquid to drain

quick reference glossary of terms *continued*

Term	Definition
incisional biopsy	removal of a portion of a lesion for examination (to cut into)
intradermal	pertaining to inside the skin
keloid	overgrowth of scar tissue
keratogenic	causing horny tissue development
keratosis	horny tissue condition
leukoderma	white skin
lipectomy	removal of fatty tissue
liposuction	removal of fatty tissue using a vacuum
macerate	from Latin, for "to make soft"; to soften the skin
macule	from Latin, for "spot" or "stain"; small, flat, discolored area (freckle)
malignant cutaneous neoplasm	a harmful new formation of the skin tissue (i.e., skin cancer)
malignant melanoma	a harmful tumor of melanin cell
mycodermatitis	inflammation of the skin caused by fungus
mycosis	fungus condition
necrosis	tissue death
nevus	from Latin, for "birthmark" or "mole"; a mole
nodule	a solid mass that extends deeper into the skin
onychectomy	remove a nail
onychia	a nail condition
onychocryptosis	an ingrown nail
onychodystrophy	poor nourishment (and development) of the nail
onycholysis	the loss of a nail
onychomalacia	abnormal softening of a nail
onychomycosis	a fungal condition of the nail
onychopathy	nail disease
onychophagia	eating (biting) the nail
onychotomy	incision into a nail
pachyderma	tough skin
papule	from Latin, for "pimple"; a small, solid mass
paronychia	a condition of the tissue around a nail
patch (vitiligo)	larger, flat, discolored area

quick reference glossary of terms *continued*

Term	Definition
percutaneous	pertaining to through the skin
petechia	from Latin, for "freckle" or "spot"; a small bruise
plaque	a solid mass on the surface of the skin
postpartum alopecia	baldness experienced by women after a pregnancy
pruritus	from Latin, for "burning nettle"; swollen, raised, itchy areas of the skin
psoriasis	a skin condition characterized by patches of itchy, red, scaly skin
pustule	from Latin, for "little blister"; a pus-filled blister
rhytidoplasty	reconstruction of wrinkled skin
scale	skin flaking off
sclerodermatitis	inflammation of the skin accompanied by thickening and hardening
scleronychia	thickening and hardening of the nails
seborrheic dermatitis	inflammation of the skin caused by the discharge of oil (sebum)
second-degree burn	a deeper burn affecting both the epidermis and dermis
spider angioma	*see* telangiectasia
squamous cell carcinoma	cancerous tumor of squamous skin cells
steatitis	inflammation of fat tissue
steatoma	a fatty tumor
subcutaneous	pertaining to beneath the skin
telangiectasia (spider angioma)	the overexpansion of the blood vessel, sometimes called a spider angioma because of how it looks on the skin
third-degree burn	a deep burn affecting the epidermis, dermis, and subcutaneous layer
tinea	a fungal condition often called "ringworm" due to its circular appearance
transdermal	pertaining to through the skin
trichomycosis	a fungal condition of the hair
tumor	a larger solid mass
ulcer	from Latin, for "sore"; a sore
vascular lesion	wounds related to blood vessels
verruca	from Latin, for "wart"; a wart
vesicle	from Latin, for "little bladder"; a small blister
vitiligo	*see* patch
xanthoderma	yellow skin

quick reference glossary of terms *continued*

Term	Definition
xanthoma	a yellow tumor
xanthosis	yellowing of the skin
xenograft	*see* heterograft
xeroderma	dry skin
xerosis	condition of dryness

review of terms by roots

Root	Term(s)	
adip/o	adipocele	
alb/o	albinism albino	
crypt/o	onychocryptosis	
cutane/o	malignant cutaneous neoplasm percutaneous subcutaneous	
derm/o, dermat/o	actinic dermatitis atopic dermatitis dermabrasion dermatitis dermatofibroma dermatolysis dermatomycosis dermatoscope dermatosis dermopathy dermoscopy epidermal	epidermal erythroderma hypodermia intradermal leukoderma mycodermatitis pachyderma sclerodermatitis seborrheic dermatitis transdermal xeroderma
erythr/o	erythema erythrocyanosis erythroderma	
hidr/o	anhidrosis cyanidrosis hemathidrosis hidradenitis	hidradenoma hidropoiesis hyperhidrosis hypohidrosis

review of terms by roots *continued*

Root	Term(s)	
kerat/o	actinic keratosis hyperkeratosis keratogenic keratosis	
leuk/o	leukoderma	
lip/o	lipectomy liposuction	
melan/o	hypermelanosis hypomelanosis malignant melanoma	
onych/o	onychomalacia onychectomy onychia onychocryptosis onychodystrophy onycholysis	onychomycosis onychopathy onychophagia onychotomy paronychia scleronychia
seb/o	seborrheic dermatitis	
squam/o	squamous cell carcinoma	
steat/o	steatitis steatoma	
trich/o	trichomycosis	
xanth/o	xanthoderma xanthoma xanthosis	
xer/o	xeroderma xerosis	

other terms

abrasion	fissure
abscess	fourth-degree burn
acne vulgaris	heterograft
allograft	homograft hyperpigmentation
alopecia	hypopigmentation
anesthetic	impetigo

other terms *continued*

antibiotic	incision and drainage
antihistamine	incisional biopsy
antipruritic	keloid
antiseptic	macerate
autograft	macule
basal cell carcinoma	mycosis
biopsy	necrosis
bulla	nevus
chemosurgery	nodule
chemotherapy	papule
cherry angioma	patch
cicatrix	petechia
comedo	plaque
crust	postpartum alopecia
cryosurgery	pruritus
culture & sensitivity	pustule
decubitus ulcer	scale
depigmentation	second-degree burn spider angioma
dysplastic nevus	telangiectasia
ecchymosis	third-degree burn topical
eczema	tumor
electrocauterization	ulcer
electrodesiccation	vascular lesion
erosion	verruca
excisional biopsy	vesicle
excoriation	vitiligo
first-degree burn	xenograft

The Musculoskeletal System—Orthopedics 4

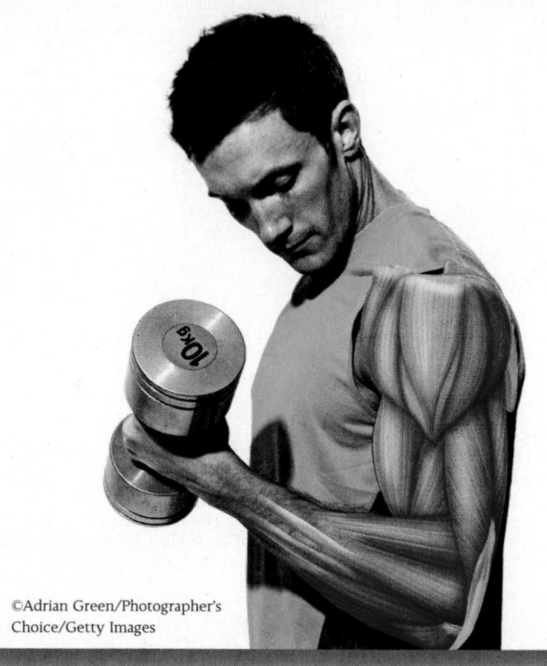

©Adrian Green/Photographer's Choice/Getty Images

learning outcomes

Upon completion of this chapter, you will be able to:

4.1 Identify the **roots/word parts** associated with the **musculoskeletal system.**

S **4.2** Translate the **Subjective** terms associated with the **musculoskeletal system.**

O **4.3** Translate the **Objective** terms associated with the **musculoskeletal system.**

A **4.4** Translate the **Assessment** terms associated with the **musculoskeletal system.**

P **4.5** Translate the **Plan** terms associated with the **musculoskeletal system.**

4.6 Use **abbreviations** associated with the **musculoskeletal system.**

4.7 Distinguish terms associated with the **musculoskeletal system** in the context of **electronic health records.**

Introduction and Overview of the Musculoskeletal System

Think of a crane at a construction site. It's an impressive piece of machinery. All the parts work together to move some very heavy objects.

Your body, specifically your musculoskeletal system, is also an amazing machine. All the parts work just right to allow you to make big movements, like lifting a heavy box, and fine movements, like writing a note on the box.

Continuing the crane analogy, your bones are like the metal fused together to make the framework of the crane. Like the metal, your bones are strong and sturdy. They make the framework of your body. This framework supports your body and protects your internal organs. Your bones are lighter than the steel of a crane, but like steel, they are incredibly strong.

Unlike steel, however, your bones are living organs. They can grow, maintain themselves, and even self-repair.

If you look at a crane up close, you'll notice that the framework is not one solid piece. Instead, it is made up of many smaller pieces that are welded, bolted, or hinged together. Some connection points are immobile, while others allow movement. Your joints are the connection points in your body. They keep the parts together and allow for movement so the crane can actually move things.

The crane couldn't move anything without any power, though. Your muscles are the workhorses of your musculoskeletal system. They act as powerful movers and stabilizers. Some muscles, like those in your thighs, are thick and strong, while others, like those in your hands, are smaller and are made for delicate movements. In fact, the muscles of your eyes are at work even now as you read these words. Together, your bones, joints, and muscles move you, protect you, and give your body support.

4.1 Word Parts of the Musculoskeletal System

Bones

Bones start as cartilage. Blood vessels penetrate the cartilage and bone cells (*osteocytes*) begin the process of replacing the cartilage model with actual bone. This process begins well before you are born and does not finish until puberty ends. Many bones harden from the center outward. Some bones, however, grow at special growth centers called the epiphyseal plate (also known as the growth plate). This growth center lies in the *metaphysis,* the area between the end of the bone (*epiphysis*) and the long shaft of the bone (*diaphysis*).

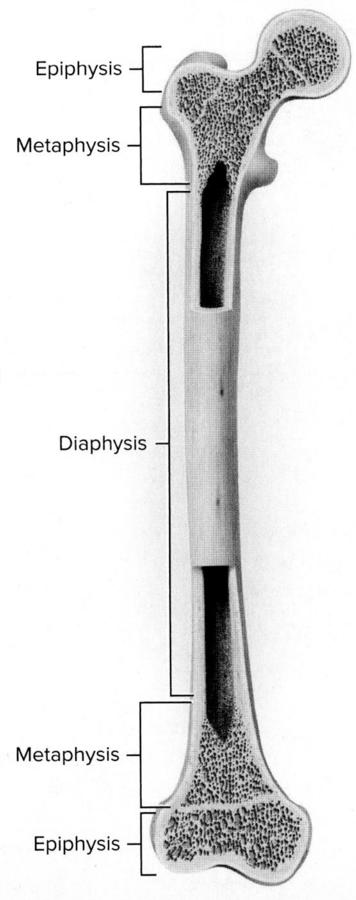

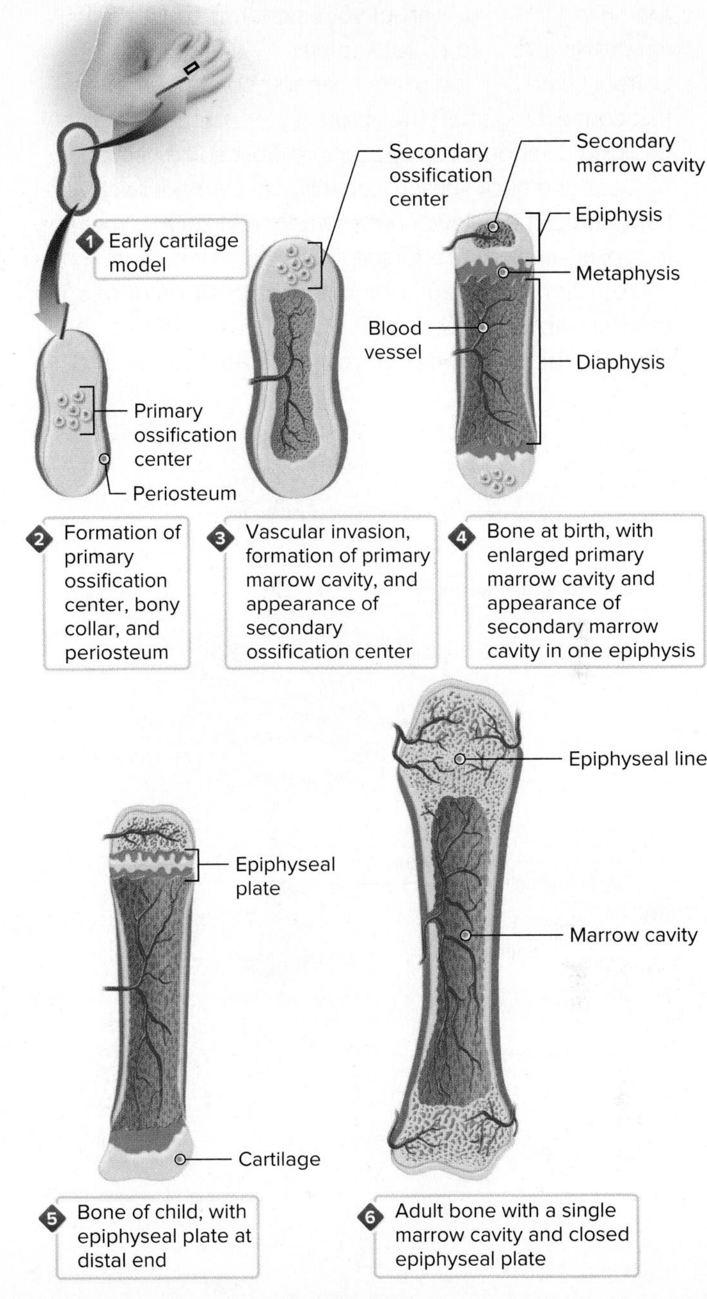

growth

SUFFIX: -***physis***

EXAMPLES: epiphysis, diaphysis, metaphysis

NOTES: *Physics* is the study of matter, energy, and motion. You might think that a subject like quantum physics is completely disconnected from health care, but physics comes from a Greek word meaning "growth" and once referred to the study of nature and living things. The Greek term is also the root of the terms *physical* and *physician.*

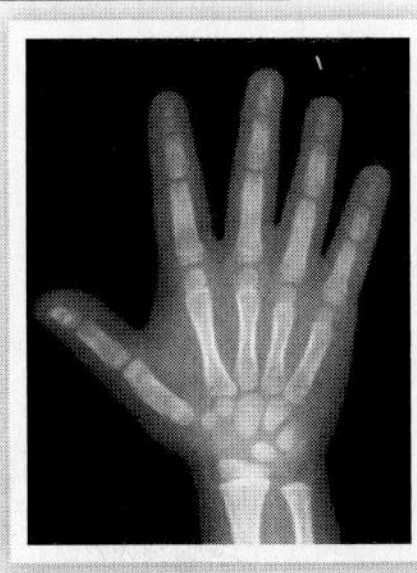

The Skeleton

Your bones make up the framework of your body—your skeleton. Like any good design, your skeleton has a specific layout. The bones in the middle of the skeleton are called the *axial* part of your skeleton. Your skull (*cranio*) is attached to your spine.

Your spine is made of many smaller bones (*vertebrae*) that connect together. They protect your spinal cord, a very fragile and important body structure. Your spine has four sections: the neck section (*cervical*), chest/upper back section (*thoracic*), and lower back (*lumbar* and *sacral*). Your ribs (*costo*) attach to the vertebrae of the thoracic section.

Your arms and legs branch off both sides of this central part of the skeleton. Your upper arm (*brachio*) leads to the two bones of your forearm (*radius* and *ulna*), then to your wrist (*carpe*), and finally to your fingers (*phalanges*). Your legs begin with your thigh bone (*femur*), work down to the two shin bones (*tibia* and *fibula*), move on to your ankle (*tarsal*), and ultimately reach your toes (*phalanges* again, just like the fingers).

bone

ROOT: ***oste/o***

EXAMPLES: osteopathy, periosteum

NOTES: At birth, you had over 300 bones, but no kneecaps. As a full-grown adult, you now have 206 bones including two kneecaps—a net loss of at least 96 bones. A human's neck also contains the same number of bones as a giraffe's.

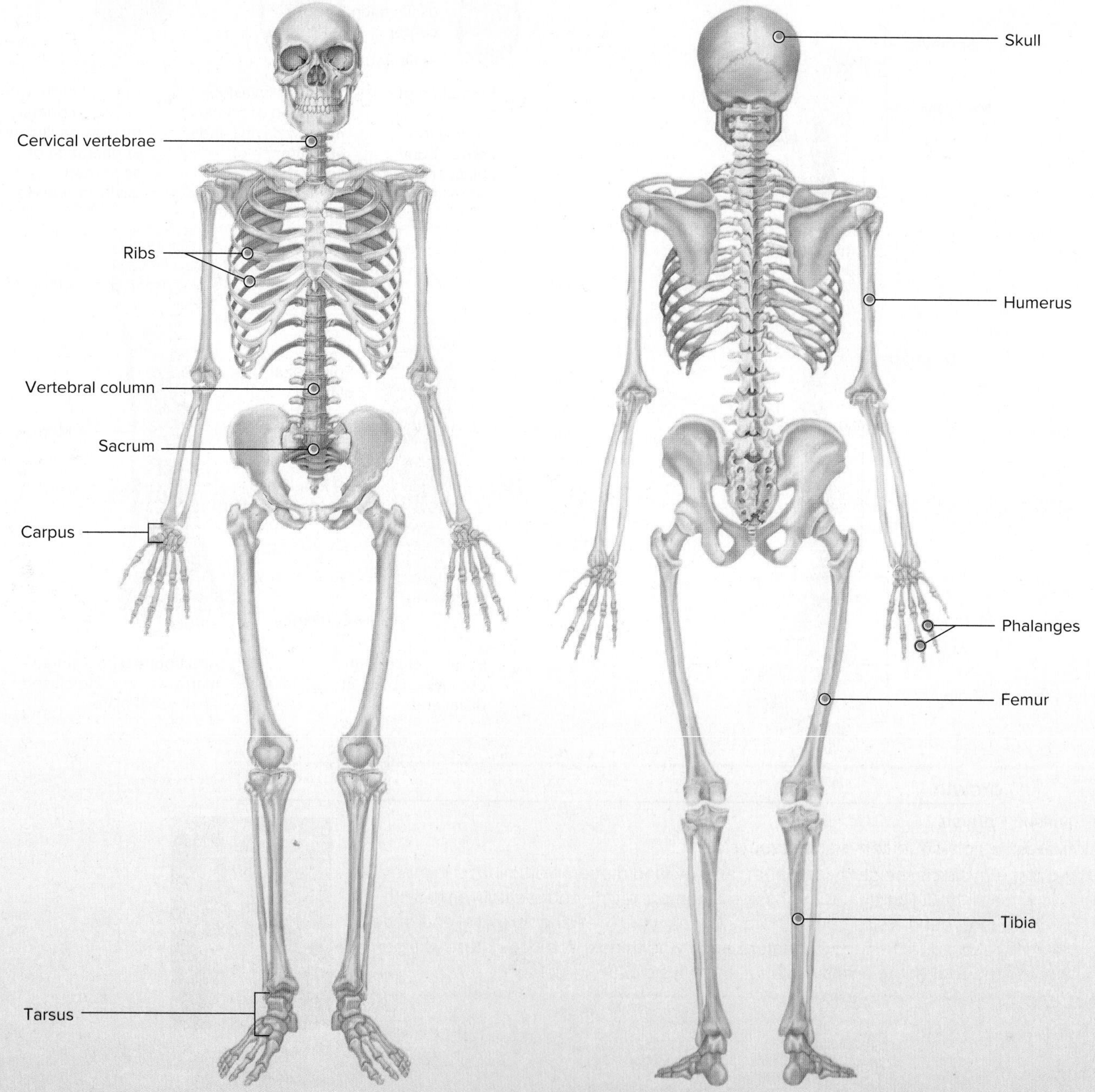

head, skull

ROOT: ***crani/o***

EXAMPLES: craniometer, craniomalacia

NOTES: The term *migraine* comes from the word *hemicrania,* meaning "half the head." The term reflects the fact that most migraines are localized in half the patient's head.

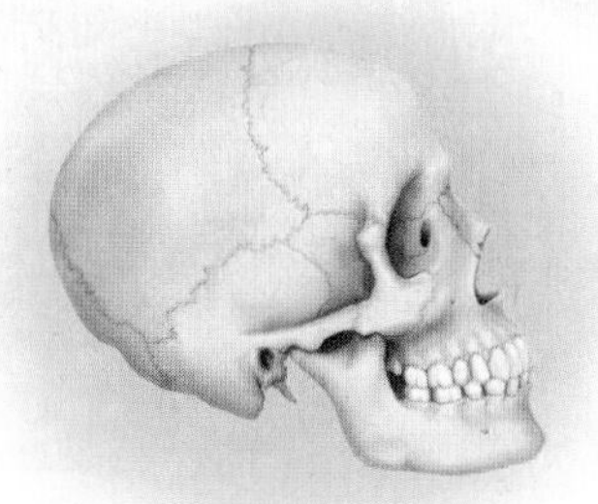

neck

ROOT: ***cervic/o***

EXAMPLES: cervical spine, cervicitis

NOTES: Remember: When a *c* is followed by *a, o,* or *u,* it is pronounced hard like a *k.* When followed by *e* or *i,* it is pronounced soft like an *s.* Therefore, the two example words above are pronounced SIR-vih-kal and SIR-vih-SAI-tis.

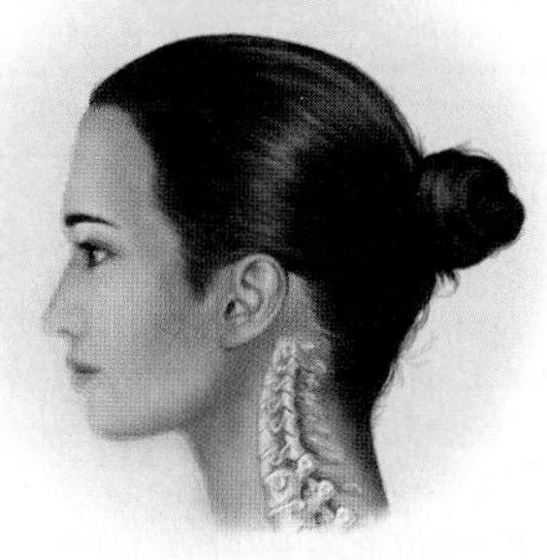

vertebra

ROOT: ***spondyl/o***

EXAMPLES: invertebrate, spondylitis

NOTES: *Vertebra* comes from Latin, for *to* "turn." It is called this because the spine was once thought of as the hinge or center around which all other bones turned.

loin, lower back

ROOT: ***lumb/o***

EXAMPLES: lumbar, lumbodynia

NOTES: The root *lumbo* comes from the Latin *lumbo,* for "loin." It refers to the region between the rib cage and the pelvis, but, frankly, it makes us think about steak.

arm

ROOT: ***brachi/o***

EXAMPLES: brachiocephalic, brachialgia

NOTES: The term *brace,* which comes from this word, originally referred to armor used to cover a knight's upper arm. This root can also be seen in the word *embrace,* which literally means "to put someone in your arms."

finger

ROOT: ***dactyl/o***

EXAMPLES: adactyly, dactylalgia

NOTES: The flying dinosaur called the pterodactyl gets its name from *ptero* (winged) + *dactly* (fingers), which obviously literally means "winged fingers."

wrist

ROOT: ***carp/o***

EXAMPLES: carpectomy, metacarpal

NOTES: The *carpal tunnel* is the area in the wrist where the nerves enter the hand. Repetitive motions using the wrist can cause the nerve to swell, press against the walls of the carpal tunnel, and result in numbness in the hand; this condition is called *carpal tunnel syndrome.*

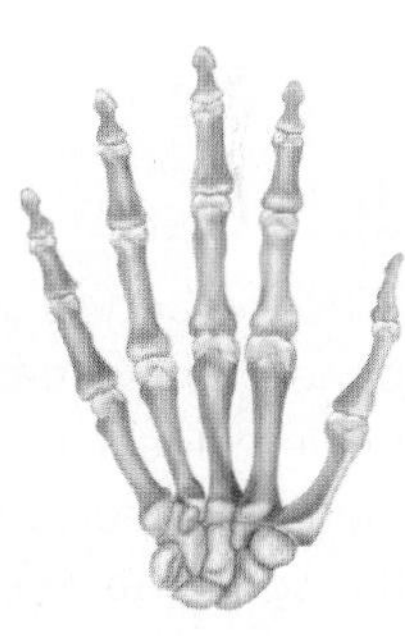

rib

ROOT: ***cost/o***

EXAMPLES: costectomy, intercostal

NOTES: The English word *coast* comes from this word. Think of a country's coasts as its ribs or sides. Also, the word *accost,* which means "to come alongside someone," comes from this word.

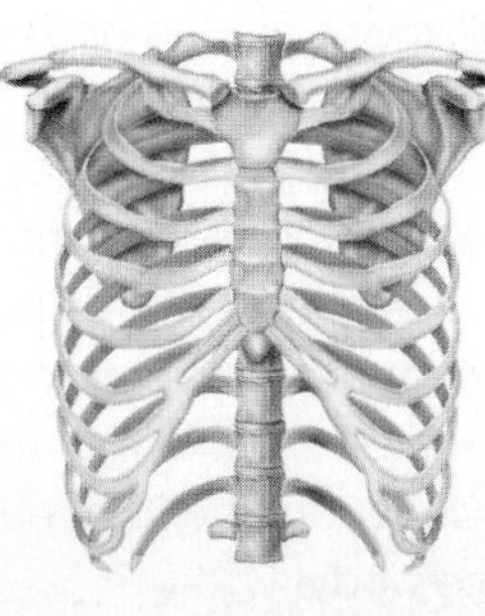

femur (thighbone)

ROOT: ***femor/o***

EXAMPLES: femoral artery

NOTES: The femur is the strongest bone in the human body (nonetheless, a hyena can bite right through it—*ouch*). The femur makes up about a fourth of a person's overall height.

tibia (shinbone)

ROOT: ***tibi/o***

EXAMPLES: tibiaglia

NOTES: The term *tibia* originally meant "pipe" or "flute." Evidently, the person who named this bone thought the shinbone bore a resemblance to this instrument.

ankle

ROOT: ***tars/o***

EXAMPLES: tarsitis, tarsalgia

NOTES: The root *tarso* comes from the Latin word *tarsus,* which can refer to the ankle or in general to the entire foot. But what makes this truly intriguing is that the word *tarsus* in Latin was derived from the Latin word *terra,* which means "earth." The foot was called the *tarsus* because it is the body part that touches the *terra* most.

Joints

"The toe bone's connected to the heel bone. The heel bone's connected to the foot bone . . ." and so it goes. While it doesn't exactly reflect the way anatomy is taught in medical school, the old children's song has the right idea. Every bone in the body except the hyoid bone is connected to another, and these connection points are known as *joints.*

Not all joints allow movement. For example, the bones in your skull are bound together tightly. Usually when we think of joints, we picture the moving ones, because, after all, these are the ones that we hurt when participating in sports or that cause problems in older age.

Moving joints allow motions like bending and rotating. When a joint bends, it's called *flexion.* When it straightens, it's called *extension. Abduction* is the widening of a joint to move parts away from the body. The term *adduction* means just the opposite—during adduction, the joint narrows to bring parts back toward the body.

Moving joints often have surrounding support tissues to absorb shock, keep the bones aligned, and keep the bones moving smoothly. *Tendons* hold muscle to bone. *Ligaments* hold bone to bone. *Cartilage* surrounds bones at the joints and allows smooth movement among them. Under many tendons lie sacs of fluid, known as *bursae,* which help keep muscles and bones moving smoothly as well.

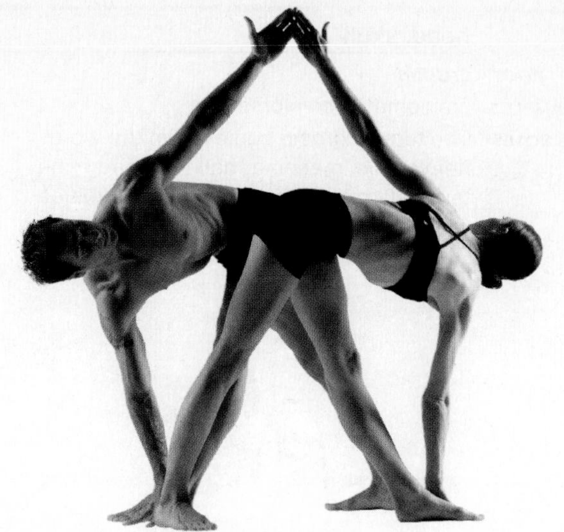

cartilage

ROOT: ***chondr/o***

EXAMPLES: chondritis, chondrodynia

NOTES: People who always think they are sick are called *hypochondriacs.* This term comes from *hypo* (beneath) + *chondro* (cartilage—here specifically referring to the ribs) and reflects an ancient belief that such thoughts came from deep within the rib cage.

joint

ROOT: ***arthr/o***

EXAMPLES: arthritis, arthroscopic surgery

NOTES: Insects, spiders, scorpions, and shellfish belong to the animal family known as *arthropods.* This term comes from *arthro* (joint) + *pod* (feet) and refers to their segmented limbs. If you have ever eaten crab legs, you know exactly what I mean.

bursa

ROOT: ***burs/o***

EXAMPLES: bursitis, bursectomy

NOTES: A *bursa* is a small fluid-filled sac found near the body's joints. Bursae reduce friction and act as cushions. The word comes from the Greek word meaning "purse" or "bag." In some places, the treasurer of an organization is called a *bursar* because he handles the purse. Also, to be *reim**burs**ed* means to have money "put back in your purse."

Muscles

Think of a thick rope. Unlike a piece of string, it is not one strand but numerous strands bundled together. This design makes the rope much stronger. Your skeletal muscles are similar, as they are a collection of thousands of muscle fibers bundled together. The bundles are grouped together to form a muscle. The bundles appear as lines under a microscope, called striations. For this reason, skeletal muscle is also known as striated muscle. While cardiac muscle also has striations, it is slightly different in its packaging and only found in the heart. Both cardiac and skeletal muscle differ from smooth muscle, which has no specific bundles. It lines hollow organs like blood vessels and airways. Cardiac and smooth muscle move involuntarily and are not actually part of the musculoskeletal system.

Skeletal muscle is encased in a thick membrane called *fascia*. The fascia helps keep the muscle together. Skeletal muscles attach to bones. If they didn't, they wouldn't be very useful. Their job is to move the bones, after all. The muscles attach to bones via *tendons*, which are thick bands of connective tissue.

tendon (connective tissue connecting muscle to bone)

ROOTS: ***ten/o, tend/o, tendin/o***

EXAMPLES: tenodynia, tendolysis, tendinitis

NOTES: From Latin, for to stretch. This root is also found in the English word *attend,* which means "to stretch toward."

muscle

ROOTS: ***muscul/o, my/o, myos/o***

EXAMPLES: musculoskeletal, myopathy, myositis

NOTES: The term *muscle* comes from Latin, for "little mouse." It was once thought that the movement of certain muscles looked like mice running underneath the skin. Personally, we don't see the connection, but linking muscle and mouse must have been commonplace, as Greek, German, and Arabic all have similar words for *muscle* and *mouse.*

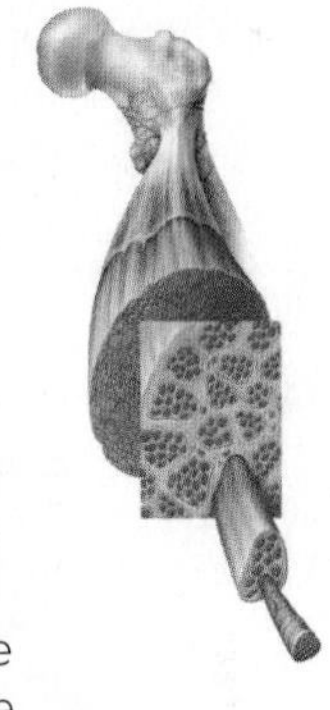

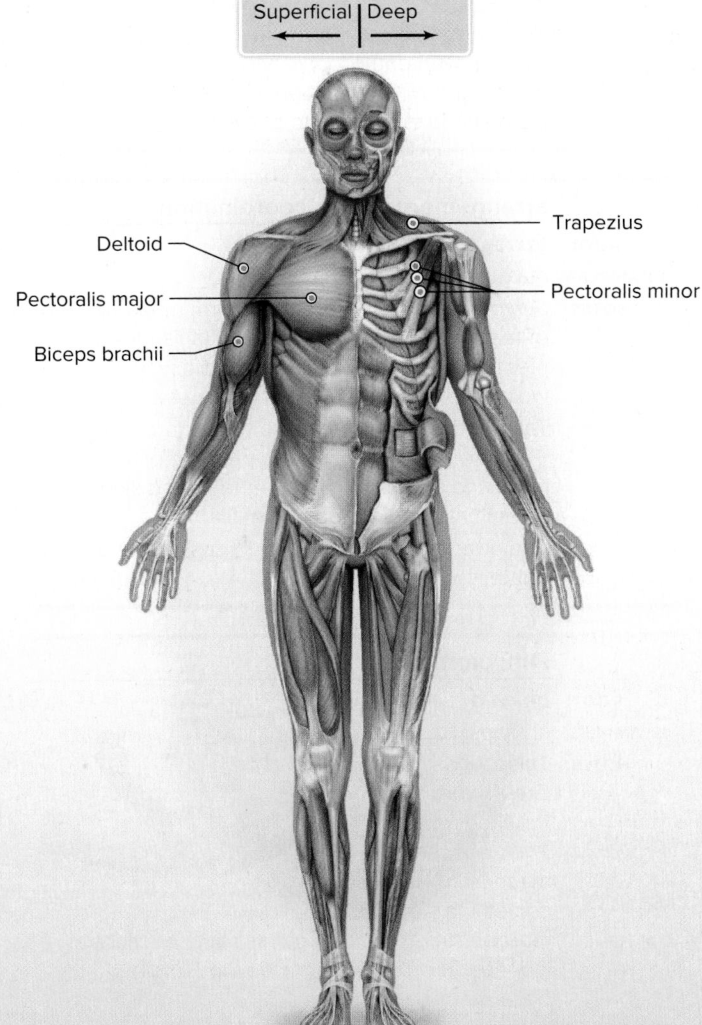

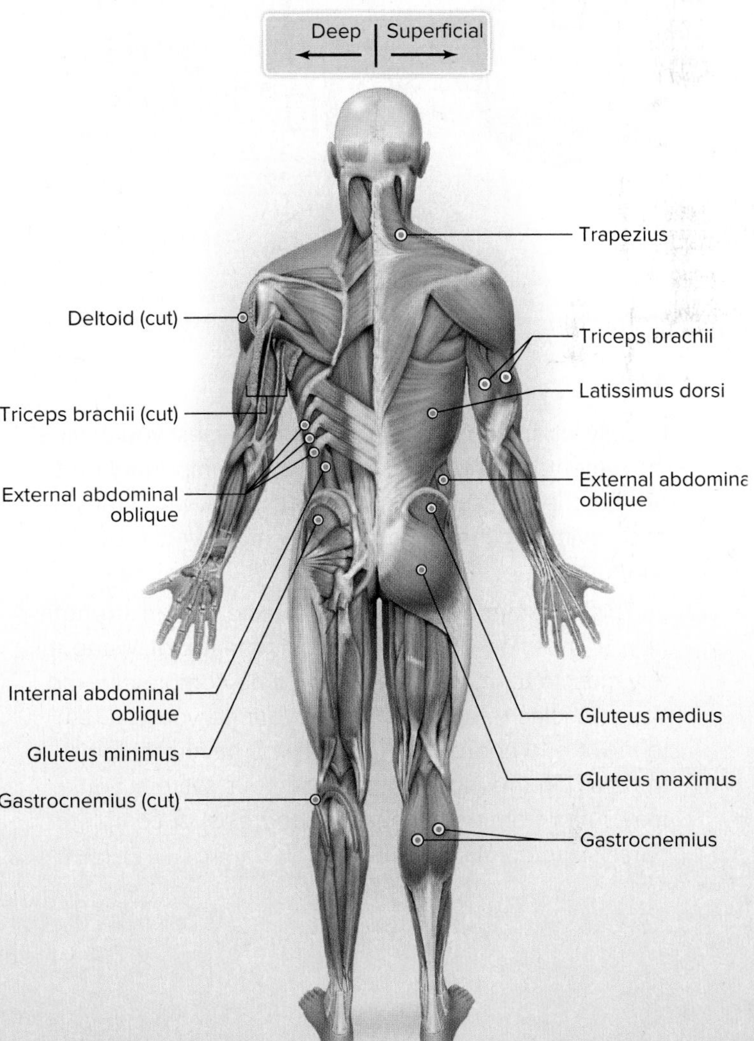

fascia (fibrous connective tissue binding muscles together)

ROOT: ***fasci/o***

EXAMPLES: fasciotomy, fasciitis

NOTES: *Fasciae* are fibrous connective tissues that bind muscles together. The name comes from the Latin word *fasces,* which means "bundle of sticks." In ancient Rome, these bundles of sticks also included axes protruding from the center, and political leaders carried fasces with them wherever they went as symbols of their power and authority. In the early twentieth century, when the leader Benito Mussolini came to power in Italy, his form of government was dubbed *fascism* because it relied heavily on strength in order to maintain control.

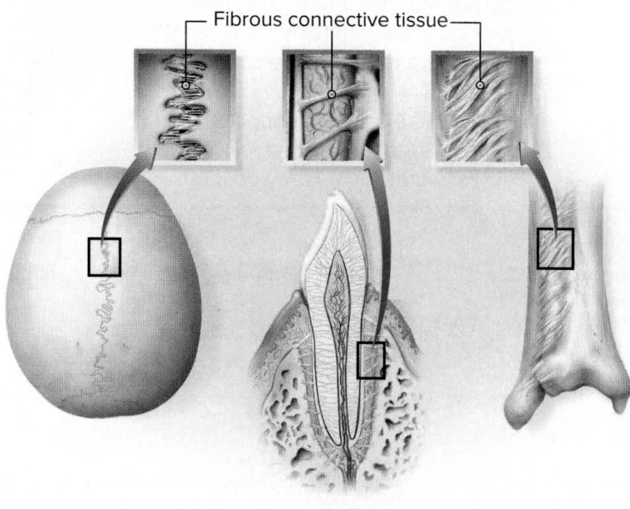

Motion

Usually when you think about your muscles, you think of movement (*kinesio*). While this is a very important part of what they do, they're also hard at work when they're not moving. Your muscles not only move you, they also support you.

This constant holding together—the built-in strength of your muscles—is your muscles' tone (*tono*). Without any muscle tone, your body would be completely limp. Your muscles require input from your nervous system to move and coordinate (*taxo*). If you have problems transferring this input from the nervous system, you may suffer from partial paralysis (*paresis*) or complete paralysis (*plegia*).

tone, tension

ROOT: ***ton/o***

EXAMPLES: dystonia, tonograph

NOTES: *Tonic* is a word for a medicinal drink. This term was used because medicinal drinks were once thought to restore a person's good muscle tone.

Today, tonic water still has medicinal value. Although some people think tonic water is simply another name for carbonated soda water, tonic is actually a form of carbonated soda water in which quinine, a drug used to treat malaria, has been dissolved. Tonic water was developed to treat people who lived in tropical areas, where malaria is often prevalent.

movement, motion

ROOTS: ***kinesi/o*** **(also sometimes *kinet/o*)**

EXAMPLES: kinesiology, hyperkinesia, kinetic energy

NOTES: *Akinetopsia* (pronounce ah-KEE-no-TOP-see-ah) comes from the roots *a* (no) + *kinet* (movement) + *opsia* (vision) and refers to a condition where a patient can see an object if it is still, but is unable to see it if it is moving.

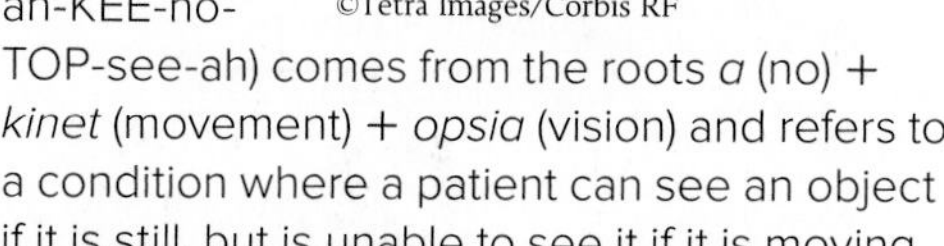

©Tetra Images/Corbis RF

arrangement, order, coordination

ROOT: ***tax/o***

EXAMPLES: ataxia, hypotaxia

NOTES: *Syntax* is an English grammar term made up of the roots *syn* (together) + *tax* (arrangement) and refers to the study of the way words are arranged in a sentence.

Taxidermy, which comes from *taxo* (arrange) + *dermy* (skin), refers to the practice of removing and displaying the head and skin of an animal killed during a hunt.

The arrangement of military forces before a battle is called *tactics.*

stiff, bent

ROOT: ***ankyl/o***

EXAMPLES: ankylosis, ankylodactyly

NOTES: This root comes from a Greek word meaning "hooked" or "bent." The word came to mean "stiff" because if something stays bent, it must be stiff. Your ankle got its name because it bends. People who fish are called *anglers* because they use hooks.

©McGraw-Hill Education/JW Ramsay, photographer

Learning Outcome 4.1 Exercises

Additional exercises available in connect®

TRANSLATION

EXERCISE 1 *Match the word part on the left with its definition on the right.*

_____	1. crani/o	a. ankle
_____	2. oste/o	b. arm
_____	3. lumb/o	c. bone
_____	4. femor/o	d. finger
_____	5. cervic/o	e. growth
_____	6. dactyl/o	f. head, skull
_____	7. cost/o	g. loin, lower back
_____	8. carp/o	h. neck
_____	9. tars/o	i. rib
_____	10. brachi/o	j. thighbone
_____	11. spondyl/o	k. vertebra
_____	12. -physis	l. wrist

EXERCISE 2 *Translate the following word parts.*

1. femor/o _______________
2. crani/o _______________
3. oste/o _______________
4. cervic/o _______________
5. lumb/o _______________
6. dactyl/o _______________
7. -physis _______________
8. brachi/o _______________
9. tars/o _______________
10. carp/o _______________
11. spondyl/o _______________

EXERCISE 3 *Break down the following words into their component parts and translate.*

EXAMPLE: sinusitis *sinus | itis* *inflammation of the sinuses*

1. costalgia _______________
2. tibialgia _______________
3. cervicodynia _______________
4. osteodynia _______________
5. carpectomy _______________
6. tarsectomy _______________
7. spondylomalacia _______________
8. craniomalacia _______________

Learning Outcome 4.1 Exercises

EXERCISE 4 *Match the word part on the left with its definition on the right. Some definitions will be used more than once.*

______	1. burs/o	a.	arrangement, order, coordination
______	2. muscul/o	b.	bursa
______	3. arthr/o	c.	cartilage
______	4. ten/o, tend/o, tendin/o	d.	fibrous connective tissue binding muscles together
______	5. ton/o	e.	joint
______	6. my/o, myos/o	f.	movement, motion
______	7. kinesi/o	g.	muscle
______	8. -plegia	h.	paralysis
______	9. chondr/o	i.	stiff, bent
______	10. ankyl/o	j.	tendon
______	11. tax/o	k.	tone, tension
______	12. fasci/o		

EXERCISE 5 *Translate the following word parts.*

1. ankyl/o ______________________
2. arthr/o ______________________
3. burs/o ______________________
4. chondr/o ______________________
5. fasci/o ______________________
6. kinesi/o ______________________
7. muscul/o ______________________
8. my/o, myos/o ______________________
9. -plegia ______________________
10. tax/o ______________________
11. ten/o, tend/o, tendin/o ______________________
12. ton/o ______________________

EXERCISE 6 *Break down the following words into their component parts and translate.*

EXAMPLE: sinusitis *sinus | itis* *inflammation of the sinuses*

1. fasciitis ______________________
2. tenalgia ______________________
3. arthralgia ______________________
4. myodynia ______________________
5. chondroma ______________________
6. hypertonia ______________________
7. hyperkinesia ______________________
8. bursotomy ______________________
9. ankylosis ______________________

Learning Outcome 4.1 Exercises

GENERATION

EXERCISE 7 *Identify the word parts for the following definitions.*

1. tibia __________
2. growth __________
3. thighbone __________
4. arm __________
5. head, skull __________
6. loin, lower back __________
7. ankle __________
8. neck __________
9. finger __________
10. rib __________

EXERCISE 8 *Build a medical term from the information provided.*

1. bone inflammation __________
2. wrist inflammation __________
3. finger inflammation __________
4. inflammation of the vertebra __________
5. removal of a rib __________

EXERCISE 9 *Identify the word parts for the following definitions.*

1. tendon (3 roots) __________
2. bursa __________
3. tone, tension __________
4. joint __________
5. fascia __________
6. movement, motion __________
7. muscle (3 roots) __________
8. paralysis __________
9. stiff, bent __________
10. arrangement, order, coordination __________
11. cartilage __________

EXERCISE 10 *Build a medical term from the information provided.*

1. inflammation of the tendon __________
2. inflammation of the bursa __________
3. joint inflammation __________
4. incision into fascia __________
5. decrease in muscle tone or tightness __________
6. decrease in muscle movement or activity __________
7. softening of a muscle __________
8. abnormal softening of the cartilage __________

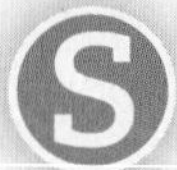

Subjective

Patient History, Problems, Complaints

Bones

Joints

Muscles

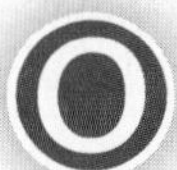

Objective

Observation and Discovery

Diagnostic procedures

Spinal curvatures

Bones

Joints

Muscles

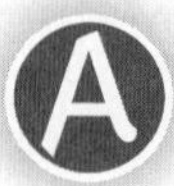

Assessment

Diagnosis and Pathology

Bones

Joints

Muscles

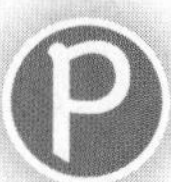

Plan

Treatments and Therapies

Drugs

Bones

Joints

Muscles

This section contains medical terms built from the roots presented in the previous section. The purpose of this section is to expose you to words used in the musculoskeletal system that are built from the word roots presented earlier. The focus of this book is to teach you the process of learning roots and translating them in context. Each term is presented with the correct pronunciation, followed by a word analysis that breaks down the word into its component parts, a definition that provides a literal translation of the word, as well as supplemental information if the literal translation deviates from its medical use.

The terms are organized using a health care professional's SOAP note (first introduced in Chapter 2) as a model.

S UBJECTIVE

4.2 Patient History, Problems, Complaints

Pain is the most common musculoskeletal medical complaint. A patient could have pain in a bone (*ostalgia/ ostealgia*), joint (*arthralgia/arthrodynia*), tendon (*tenalgia*), or a muscle (*myalgia/myodynia*). A patient may also notice a change in a muscle's appearance—a muscle may be wasting away (*atrophy*) or abnormally large (*hypertrophy*). A parent may notice that his or her child is either bow-legged (*genu varum*) or knock-kneed (*genu valgum*). Most of the other problems people experience relate to a change in how their muscles or joints are working. For instance, they may notice that their joints don't work as well as normal. The joint may be stiff/bent (*ankylosis*) or it may make crackling sounds when moved (*crepitus*). Patients may also notice changes in their muscle function. They may experience a decrease in muscle tone (*hypotonia*) or muscle tone that is exaggerated (*hypertonia*). Diseases of the nervous system can lead to problems with coordination (*dystaxia* or *ataxia*), movements (*dykinesia* or *bradykinesia*), or twitches (*myospasms*).

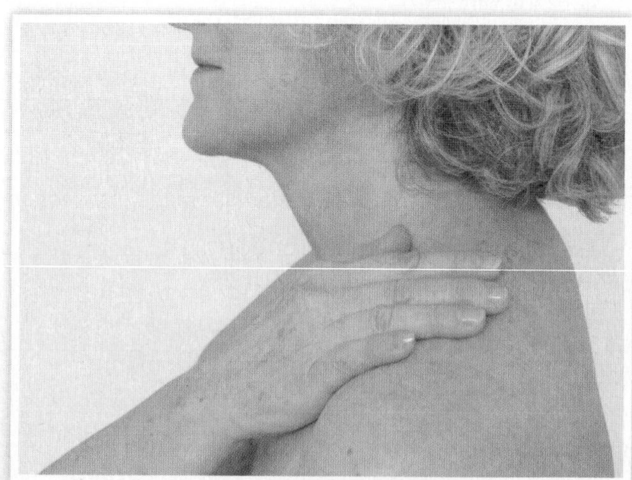

Pain is the most common musculoskeletal medical complaint.

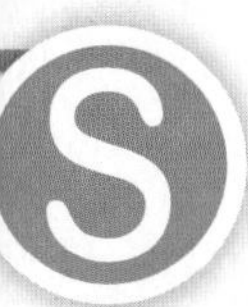

4.2 Patient History, Problems, Complaints

bones

Term	Word Analysis
costalgia kaws-TAL-jah **Definition** rib pain	**cost / algia** rib / pain
metatarsalgia meh-tah-tar-SAL-jah **Definition** pain in the bones of the foot	**meta / tars / algia** after / ankle / pain
ostalgia aws-TAL-jah **Definition** bone pain **NOTE:** An alternate spelling of this term is ostealgia.	**ost / algia** bone / pain
osteodynia aws-tee-oh-DIH-nee-ah **Definition** bone pain	**osteo / dynia** bone / pain
spondylodynia spawn-dih-loh-DIH-nee-ah **Definition** vertebra pain	**spondylo / dynia** vertebra / pain
tibialgia tih-bee-AL-ja **Definition** tibia (shin) pain	**tibi / algia** tibia / pain

joints

Term	Word Analysis
ankylosis an-kih-LOH-sis **Definition** joint stiffness	**ankyl / osis** stiff / condition
arthralgia ar-THRAL-jah **Definition** joint pain	**arthr / algia** joint / pain
arthrodynia ar-throh-DIH-nee-ah **Definition** joint pain	**arthro / dynia** joint / pain

joints *continued*

Term	Word Analysis
cervicodynia sir-vih-koh-DAI-nee-ah **Definition** neck pain	**cervico / dynia** neck / pain
crepitation kreh-pih-TAY-shun **Definition** a crackling sound heard in joints	**from Latin, for "rattle" or "creaking"**
genu valgum JEH-noo VAL-gum **Definition** knock-kneed	**genu valgum** knee pointed in
genu varum JEH-noo VAH-rum **Definition** bowlegged	**genu varum** knee bowed out

muscles

Term	Word Analysis
bradykinesia bray-dih-kih-NEE-zhah **Definition** slow movement	**brady / kinesia** slow / movement
dyskinesia dis-kih-NEE-zhah **Definition** inability to control movement	**dys / kinesia** bad / movement
dystaxia dis-TAK-see-ah **Definition** poor coordination	**dys / taxia** bad / coordination
dystonia dis-TOH-nee-ah **Definition** poor muscle tone	**dys / tonia** bad / muscle tone

4.2 Patient History, Problems, Complaints

muscles *continued*

Term	Word Analysis
graphospasm gra-foh-SPAZM **Definition** writer's cramp	**grapho / spasm** write / involuntary contraction ©Image Source/AGE Fotostock RF
hyperkinesia hai-per-kih-NEE-zhah **Definition** increase in muscle movement or activity	**hyper / kinesia** over / movement
hypertonia hai-per-TOH-nee-yah **Definition** increased muscle tone or tightness	**hyper / tonia** over / muscle tone
hypokinesia hai-poh-kih-NEE-zhah **Definition** decrease in muscle movement or activity	**hypo / kinesia** under / movement
hypotonia hai-poh-TOH-nee-yah **Definition** decrease in muscle tone or tightness	**hypo / tonia** under / muscle tone
myalgia mai-AL-jah **Definition** muscle pain	**my / algia** muscle / pain
myasthenia mai-as-THEH-nee-ah **Definition** muscle weakness	**my / asthenia** muscle / weakness
myodynia mai-oh-DAI-nee-ah **Definition** muscle pain	**myo / dynia** muscle / pain
myospasm mai-oh-SPAZ-um **Definition** muscle spasm	**myo / spasm** muscle / involuntary contraction
tenalgia ten-AL-jah **Definition** tendon pain	**ten / algia** tendon / pain

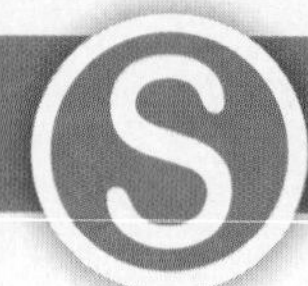

Learning Outcome 4.2 Exercises

PRONUNCIATION

EXERCISE 1 *Indicate which syllable is emphasized when pronounced.*

EXAMPLE: bronchitis bron**chi**tis

1. ostalgia ____________
2. tibialgia ____________
3. costalgia ____________
4. arthralgia ____________
5. myalgia ____________
6. ankylosis ____________
7. myospasm ____________
8. crepitation ____________
9. arthrodynia ____________
10. hyperkinesia ____________

TRANSLATION

EXERCISE 2 *Break down the following words into their component parts.*

EXAMPLE: nasopharyngoscope *naso | pharyngo | scope*

1. ostealgia ____________
2. arthralgia ____________
3. myospasm ____________
4. myasthenia ____________
5. bradykinesia ____________
6. graphospasm ____________

EXERCISE 3 *Underline and define the word parts from this chapter in the following terms.*

1. tenalgia ____________
2. tibialgia ____________
3. ostalgia ____________
4. myalgia ____________
5. costalgia ____________
6. metatarsalgia ____________
7. myodynia ____________
8. osteodynia ____________
9. arthrodynia ____________
10. spondylodynia ____________
11. cervicodynia ____________
12. ankylosis ____________
13. dyskinesia ____________
14. dystaxia ____________
15. dystonia ____________

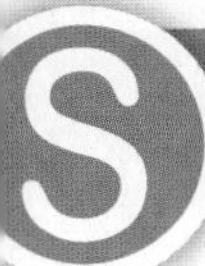

Learning Outcome 4.2 Exercises

EXERCISE 4 *Match the term on the left with its definition on the right.*

_____	1. crepitation	a.	increase in muscle movement or activity
_____	2. genu valgum	b.	increased muscle tone or tightness
_____	3. genu varum	c.	decrease in muscle movement or activity
_____	4. hyperkinesia	d.	decrease in muscle tightness
_____	5. hypertonia	e.	bowlegged
_____	6. hypokinesia	f.	knock-kneed
_____	7. hypotonia	g.	from Latin, for "rattle" or "creaking"; a crackling sound heard in joints

EXERCISE 5 *Translate the following terms as literally as possible.*

EXAMPLE: nasopharyngoscope *an instrument for looking at the nose and throat*

1. dystonia _______________
2. dyskinesia _______________
3. hyperkinesia _______________
4. hypertonia _______________
5. metatarsalgia _______________
6. myasthenia _______________
7. graphospasm _______________
8. ankylosis _______________

GENERATION

EXERCISE 6 *Build a medical term from the information provided.*

EXAMPLE: inflammation of the sinuses *sinusitis*

1. tendon pain _______________
2. tibia (shin) pain _______________
3. rib pain _______________
4. vertebra pain _______________
5. neck pain _______________
6. muscle spasm _______________
7. decrease in muscle movement _______________
8. decrease in muscle tone _______________
9. slow movement _______________
10. poor coordination _______________

Learning Outcome 4.2 Exercises

EXERCISE 7 *Multiple-choice questions. Select the correct answer(s).*

1. Select the terms that mean "bone pain."
   a. arthralgia
   b. myalgia
   c. ostalgia
   d. ostealgia
   e. arthrodynia
   f. myodynia
   g. osteodynia
2. Select the terms that mean "joint pain."
   a. arthralgia
   b. myalgia
   c. ostalgia
   d. ostealgia
   e. arthrodynia
   f. myodynia
   g. osteodynia
3. Select the terms that mean "muscle pain."
   a. arthralgia
   b. myalgia
   c. ostalgia
   d. ostealgia
   e. arthrodynia
   f. myodynia
   g. osteodynia
4. Which of the following terms comes from Latin, for "rattle" or "creaking"?
   a. crepitation
   b. genu varum
   c. genu valgum
   d. kyphosis
5. A person whose knees point inward has which of the following conditions?
   a. crepitation
   b. genu varum
   c. genu valgum
   d. kyphosis
6. A person whose knees are curved outward (bowed) has which of the following conditions?
   a. crepitation
   b. genu varum
   c. genu valgum
   d. kyphosis

OBJECTIVE

4.3 Observation and Discovery

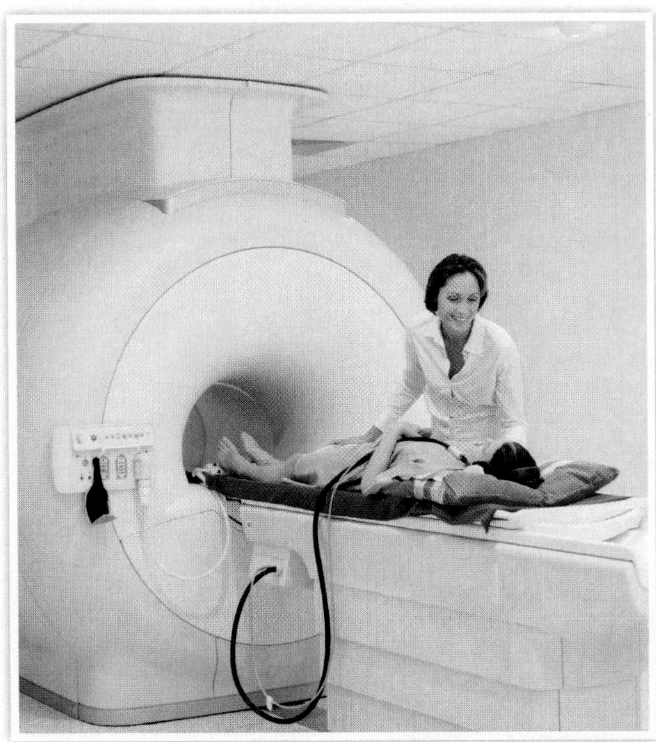

Evaluation of bone issues is commonly performed with imaging, including MRI (magnetic resonance imaging).

When a patient with musculoskeletal problems is evaluated, the physical exam is very important. The exam of the muscles and bones focuses mainly on typical signs of inflammation: redness, swelling, heat, and pain. Any of these symptoms can indicate that an infection or inflammation is present.

There are not many skills that are specific to evaluating bones. Patients with fractured bones may present with a limp or pain upon touching or pressure. A newborn may have extra fingers (*polydactyly*) or fused fingers (*syndactyly*).

Much evaluation of bone issues is performed with imaging. The bread-and-butter imaging method for bones is the simple x-ray. An x-ray can reveal fractures, bone destruction (*osteolysis*), and even extra bone growth (*exostosis*). More involved imaging methods include computed tomography (CT), computed axial tomography (CAT), or magnetic resonance imaging (MRI).

Examining a patient's joint is usually more involved. While the health care provider also checks for the same signs of inflammation, the joint's ability to move also needs to be checked. This is called the joint's range of motion. The provider also checks to make sure the joint is not moving in a direction that it's not supposed to move in. This extra movement is called joint laxity. The provider also checks for fluid around the joint (*effusion*). While the fluid is usually the result of inflammation, it may be pus from an infection (*pyarthrosis*) or blood from an injury (*hemarthrosis*). There are several diagnostic procedures specific to the joints. To get a better view, the health care provider can inject dye into the joint and perform an MRI. This specialized MRI is called an *MR angiogram*. Other means of investigating a joint include injecting a needle and collecting fluid to send to the lab (*arthrocentesis*) or even using a camera-like device to look inside the joint (*arthroscope*).

Examining muscles often means checking how they work. The function of muscles can be evaluated by checking their muscle tone (*myotonia*) or strength. A more involved way to check this is electromyography. In this procedure, two needles are inserted into a muscle to measure the muscle activity.

4.3 Observation and Discovery

diagnostic procedures

Term	Word Analysis
arthrocentesis ar-throh-sin-TEE-sis **Definition** puncture of a joint	**arthro / centesis** joint / puncture 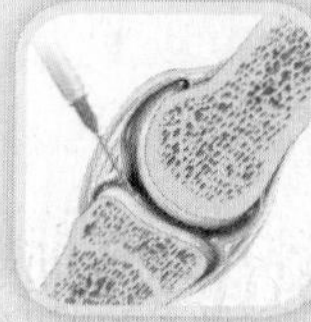
arthroscope AR-throh-skohp **Definition** instrument for looking into a joint	**arthro / scope** joint / instrument to look
arthroscopy ar-THRAW-skoh-pee **Definition** procedure of looking into a joint	**arthro / scopy** joint / procedure to look 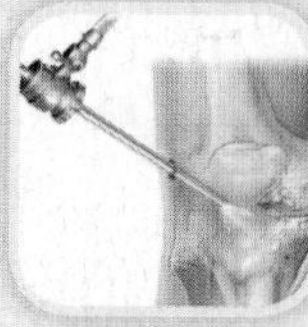
electromyogram eh-lek-troh-MAI-o-gram **Definition** a record of the electrical activity of a muscle	**electro / myo / gram** electricity / muscle / record
electromyography eh-LEK-troh-mai-AW-grah-fee **Definition** procedure for measuring the electrical activity of a muscle	**electro / myo / graphy** electricity / muscle / writing procedure
myography mai-AW-grah-fee **Definition** procedure for studying muscles	**myo / graphy** muscle / writing procedure

radiology

Term	Word Analysis
arthrogram AR-throh-gram **Definition** visual record of a joint	**arthro / gram** joint / record
arthrography ar-THRAW-grah-fee **Definition** procedure used to examine a joint	**arthro / graphy** joint / writing procedure
computed axial tomography (CAT or CT) kom-PYOO-ted AK-see-al taw-MAW-grah-fee **Definition** imaging procedure using a computer to produce cross sections along an axis	**axi / al tomo / graphy** axis / pertaining to cut / writing procedure

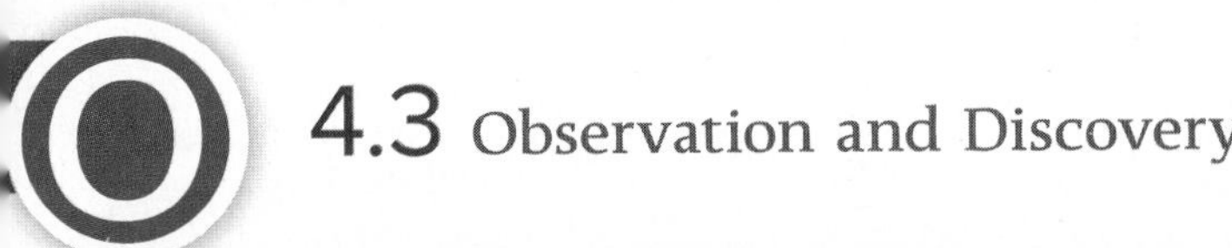

spinal curvatures

Term	Word Analysis
kyphosis kai-FOH-sis **Definition** humped back; abnormal forward curvature of the upper spine	**kyph / osis** bent / condition 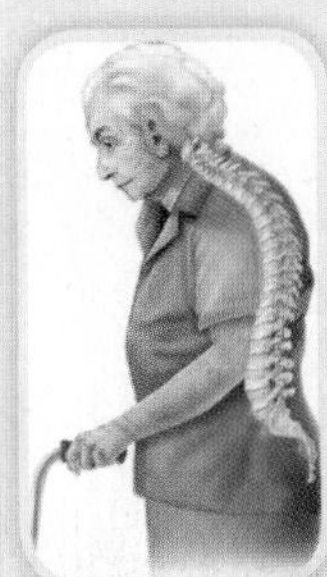
lordosis lor-DOH-sis **Definition** sway back; abnormal forward curvature of the lower spine	**lord / osis** bent backward / condition 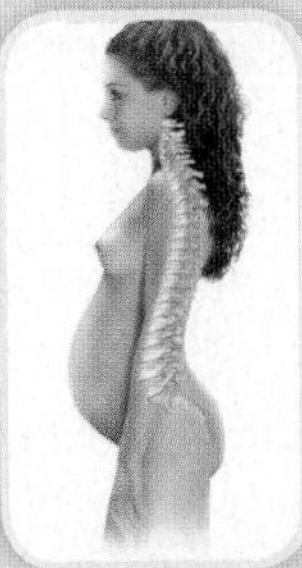
scoliosis SKOH-lee-OH-sis **Definition** crooked back; abnormal lateral curvature of the spine	**scoli / osis** crooked / condition 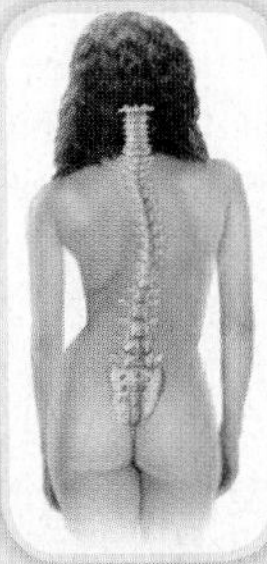

bones

Term	Word Analysis
carpitis kar-PAI-tis **Definition** wrist inflammation	**carp / itis** wrist / inflammation
craniomalacia kray-nee-oh-mah-LAY-shah **Definition** softening of the skull	**cranio / malacia** skull / softening
exostosis eks-aws-TOH-sis **Definition** an abnormal growth of bone out of another bone	**ex / ost / osis** out / bone / condition

bones *continued*

Term	Word Analysis
fracture FRAK-shur **Definition** a bone break	**from Latin, for "break"**
Transverse · Oblique · Spiral · Angulated · Displaced · Angulated & displaced	
osteodystrophy aws-tee-oh-DIH-stroh-fee **Definition** poor bone development	**osteo / dys / trophy** bone / bad / nourishment
osteolysis aw-stee-AW-lih-sis **Definition** bone loss	**osteo / lysis** bone / loss
osteonecrosis aw-stee-oh-nih-KROH-sis **Definition** death of bone	**osteo / necr / osis** bone / death / condition
osteosclerosis aw-stee-oh-skleh-ROH-sis **Definition** abnormal hardening of bone	**osteo / scler / osis** bone / hardening / condition
polydactyly paw-lee-DAK-tih-lee **Definition** having more than the normal number of fingers (or toes)	**poly / dactyl / y** many / finger / condition
spondylitis spawn-dih-LAI-tis **Definition** vertebra inflammation	**spondyl / itis** vertebra / inflammation

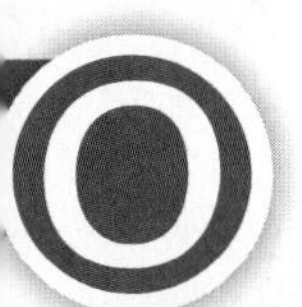

4.3 Observation and Discovery

bones *continued*

Term	Word Analysis
spondylomalacia spawn-dih-loh-mah-LAY-shah **Definition** softening of the vertebra	**spondylo / malacia** vertebra / softening
syndactyly sin-DAK-tih-lee **Definition** fusion (sometimes called webbing) of fingers (or toes)	**syn / dactyl / y** together / finger / condition
tarsoptosis tar-sawp-TOH-sis **Definition** flat feet	**tarso / ptosis** ankle / drooping condition

joints

Term	Word Analysis
bursolith BIR-soh-lith **Definition** a stone in a bursa	**burso / lith** bursa / stone
effusion ee-FYOO-zhun **Definition** fluid buildup	**ef / fusion** out / pour
NOTE: The prefix on *effusion* is actually *ex-;* the *x* turns to an *f* when followed by an *f.* Why? Say *exfusion* 10 times. Most people slur *exfusion* into *effusion* because it is easier to say.	
hemarthrosis hee-mar-THROH-sis **Definition** blood in a joint	**hem / arthr / osis** blood / joint / condition
hydrarthrosis hai-drar-THROH-sis **Definition** water (fluid) in a joint	**hydr / arthr / osis** water / joint / condition
pyarthrosis pai-ar-THROH-sis **Definition** pus in a joint	**py / arthr / osis** pus / joint / condition

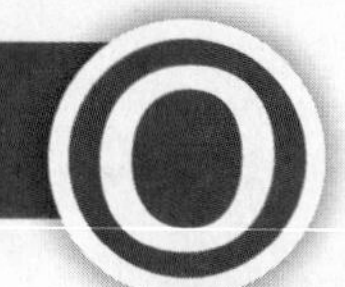

4.3 Observation and Discovery

muscles

Term	Word Analysis
atrophy A-troh-fee **Definition** underdevelopment, decrease, or loss of muscle tissue	**a / trophy** no / nourishment Normal
hypertrophy hai-PER-troh-fee **Definition** overdevelopment of muscle tissue	**hyper / trophy** over / nourishment
myocele MAI-oh-seel **Definition** hernia of muscle tissue	**myo / cele** muscle / hernia
myolysis mai-AW-lih-sis **Definition** loss of muscle tissue	**myo / lysis** muscle / loss
myomalacia mai-oh-mah-LAY-shah **Definition** softening of a muscle	**myo / malacia** muscle / softening
myosclerosis mai-oh-skleh-ROH-sis **Definition** hardening of a muscle	**myo / scler / osis** muscle / hardening / condition
myotasis mai-AW-tah-sis **Definition** stretching of a muscle **Note:** The *-tasis* suffix appears as *-ectasis* in blood vessels (*angiectasis*) and lungs (*bronchiectasis*).	**myo / tasis** muscle / expansion
myotonia mai-oh-TOH-nee-ah **Definition** muscle tone	**myo / tonia** muscle / tone

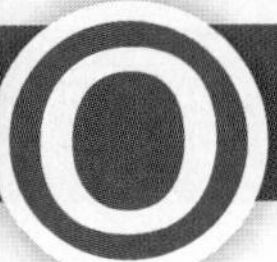

Learning Outcome 4.3 Exercises

PRONUNCIATION

EXERCISE 1 *Indicate which syllable is emphasized when pronounced.*

EXAMPLE: bronchitis bron**chi**tis

1. atrophy ______
2. effusion ______
3. arthroscope ______
4. arthroscopy ______
5. lordosis ______
6. craniomalacia ______
7. osteolysis ______
8. spondylitis ______
9. osteodystrophy ______
10. pyarthrosis ______
11. myotasis ______
12. myomalacia ______
13. electromyography ______

TRANSLATION

EXERCISE 2 *Break down the following words into their component parts.*

EXAMPLE: nasopharyngoscope *naso | pharyngo | scope*

1. arthrogram ______
2. arthroscope ______
3. myocele ______
4. myography ______
5. electromyography ______
6. spondylomalacia ______
7. arthrocentesis ______
8. myolysis ______
9. osteolysis ______
10. osteonecrosis ______
11. osteosclerosis ______
12. myosclerosis ______
13. hydrarthrosis ______
14. polydactyly ______
15. exostosis ______

EXERCISE 3 *Underline and define the word parts from this chapter in the following terms.*

1. carpitis ______
2. spondylitis ______
3. bursolith ______
4. arthroscopy ______
5. arthrography ______
6. myomalacia ______
7. craniomalacia ______
8. myotasis ______
9. syndactyly ______
10. tarsoptosis ______
11. osteodystophy ______
12. electromyogram ______
13. hemarthrosis ______
14. pyarthrosis ______
15. myotonia (2 roots) ______

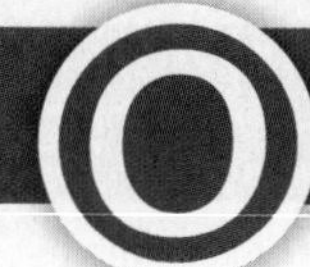

Learning Outcome 4.3 Exercises

EXERCISE 4 *Match the term on the left with its definition on the right.*

_____ 1. fracture

_____ 2. atrophy

_____ 3. scoliosis

_____ 4. computed axial tomography

_____ 5. hypertrophy

_____ 6. effusion

_____ 7. lordosis

_____ 8. kyphosis

a. imaging procedure using a computer to produce cross sections along an axis

b. humped back; abnormal forward curvature of the upper spine

c. sway back; abnormal forward curvature of the lower spine

d. crooked back; abnormal lateral curvature of the spine

e. from Latin, for "break"; a bone break

f. fluid buildup

g. underdevelopment, decrease, or loss of muscle tissue

h. overdevelopment of muscle tissue

EXERCISE 5 *Translate the following terms as literally as possible.*

EXAMPLE: nasopharyngoscope *an instrument for looking at the nose and throat*

1. osteonecrosis _____
2. syndactyly _____
3. bursolith _____
4. myotasis _____
5. hydrarthrosis _____
6. hemarthrosis _____
7. pyarthrosis _____
8. tarsoptosis _____
9. kyphosis _____
10. lordosis _____
11. scoliosis _____

GENERATION

EXERCISE 6 *Build a medical term from the information provided.*

EXAMPLE: inflammation of the sinuses *sinusitis*

1. wrist inflammation _____
2. vertebra inflammation _____
3. softening of the skull _____
4. softening of a muscle _____
5. softening of the vertebra _____
6. muscle tone _____
7. many finger condition _____
8. instrument for looking into a joint _____
9. procedure of looking into a joint _____
10. procedure for measuring bone _____

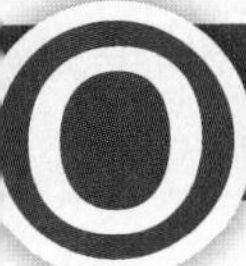

Learning Outcome 4.3 Exercises

EXERCISE 7 *Multiple-choice questions. Select the correct answer(s).*

1. Select the terms that pertain to bone.
   a. fracture
   b. exostosis
   c. arthrocentesis
   d. myography
   e. arthrography
   f. electromyogram
   g. electromyography
   h. atrophy
   i. hypertrophy
   j. osteodystrophy
2. Select the terms that pertain to joints.
   a. fracture
   b. exostosis
   c. arthrocentesis
   d. myography
   e. arthrography
   f. electromyogram
   g. electromyography
   h. atrophy
   i. hypertrophy
   j. osteodystrophy
3. Select the terms that pertain to muscle.
   a. fracture
   b. exostosis
   c. arthrocentesis
   d. myography
   e. arthrography
   f. electromyogram
   g. electromyography
   h. atrophy
   i. hypertrophy
   j. osteodystrophy
4. What does the abbreviation CAT stand for?
   a. chondro-arthrodysplasia tenotomy
   b. computed axial tomography
   c. computed arthrography telectasia
   d. chondro-axial tomography
5. Which of the following terms means "fluid buildup"?
   a. affusion
   b. effusion
   c. effision
   d. exfusure

EXERCISE 8 *Briefly describe the difference between each pair of terms.*

1. osteolysis, myolysis ____________________
2. osteosclerosis, myosclerosis ____________________
3. arthrogram, myogram ____________________
4. arthrocele, myocele ____________________

ASSESSMENT

4.4 Diagnosis and Pathology

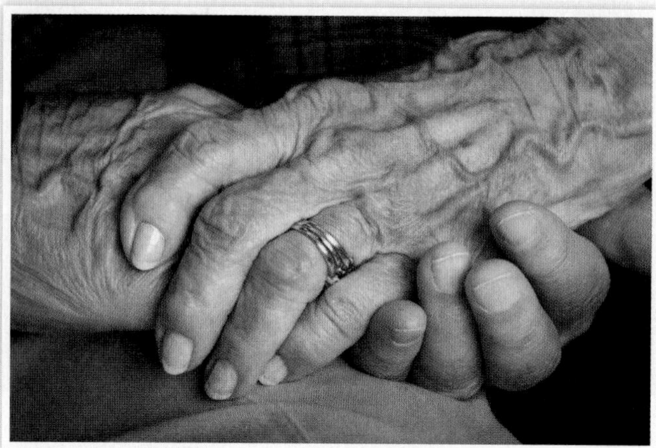
©dszc/iStock/Getty Images RF

As mentioned earlier, fractures are a common reason why patients see health care providers. Fractures are more common in people with weaker bones. Bone loss (*osteopenia*) can be related to age or to a diet that is deficient in calcium. Osteopenia leads to soft bones in children (*osteomalacia*) or weak, frail bones in adults (*osteoporosis*). Some patients suffer from infections of the bone (*osteomyelitis*), a serious illness that often requires hospitalization.

The vertebral column of bones is susceptible to injury. Gymnasts, football players, or weight lifters who bend their backs too far can suffer small stress fractures of their vertebrae (*spondylolysis*). If the fracture is severe, the vertebrae can slip onto one another (*spondylolisthesis*). A very serious version of this condition can advance to problems with a narrowing of the space for the spinal cord (*spinal stenosis*).

You move your joints all the time. They act as shock absorbers for your body, and they take a lot of abuse. It should come as no surprise, then, that joint problems are a very common medical concern. A swollen, painful joint (*arthritis*) can have many causes—the most common being excessive wear and tear. This type is called *osteoarthritis*. As the cartilage between the bones in a joint breaks down, the bones eventually rub together and the joint becomes painful to move. This is a very common reason for a joint replacement surgery.

Other causes for arthritis include infection (*septic arthritis*) and a disease of joint inflammation (*rheumatoid arthritis*). Other parts of the joint area that can cause problems are the bursa (*bursitis*) and tendon (*tendonitis*). These are not usually caused by an injury; instead, they are a result of normal wear and tear over time.

Unusual inflammatory conditions also affect the muscles. Muscles can become inflamed individually (*myositis*) or in groups (*polymyositis*). Sometimes this can involve the skin as well (*dermatomyositis*). General problems with all the muscles are called *myopathies*. *Myasthenia gravis* and *muscular dystrophy* are two of the most common types of myopathy.

Like any system in the body, the musculoskeletal system can develop tumors. Tumors can develop in the bones (*osteosarcoma, osteocarcinoma, osteochondroma*) or they can spread to the bones from other parts of the body. Your muscles can get tumors (*myoma*) as well—one example is an *myosarcoma*.

bones

Term	Word Analysis
ankylosing spondylitis an-kih-LOH-sing spawn-dih-LAI-tis **Definition** a stiffening inflammation of the vertebrae	ankylos / ing spondyl / itis stiffen / causing vertebra / inflammation
chondro-osteodystrophy KAWN-droh-AW-stee-oh-DIH-stroh-fee **Definition** poor development of bones and cartilage	chondro / osteo / dys / trophy cartilage / bone / bad / nourishment

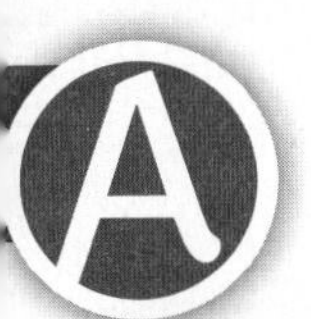

4.4 Diagnosis and Pathology

bones *continued*

Term	Word Analysis
craniosynostosis KRAY-nee-oh-SIN-aw-STOH-sis **Definition** the premature fusing of the skull bones	cranio /syn / ost / osis skull / together / bone / condition Normal
dactylitis DAK-tih-LAI-tis **Definition** finger inflammation	dactyl / itis finger / inflammation
hypertrophic spondylitis HAI-per-TROH-fik spon-dih-LAI-tis **Definition** overdevelopment of the vertebrae causing inflammation	hyper / trophic spondyl / itis over / nourishment vertebra / inflammation
osteitis AW-stee-AI-tis **Definition** bone inflammation	oste / itis bone / inflammation
osteochondritis AW-stee-oh-kon-DRAI-tis **Definition** inflammation of bone and cartilage	osteo / chondr / itis bone / cartilage / inflammation
osteogenesis imperfecta AW-stee-oh-JIN-eh-sis IM-per-FEK-tah **Definition** a disease in which the bones do not develop correctly, also known as *brittle bone disease*	osteo / genesis im / perfecta bone / creation not / complete
osteomalacia AW-stee-oh-mah-LAY-shah **Definition** softening of the bone	osteo / malacia bone / softening
osteomyelitis AW-stee-oh-MAI-eh-LAI-tis **Definition** inflammation of the bone and bone marrow	osteo / myel / itis bone / marrow / inflammation
osteopathy AW-stee-AW-pah-thee **Definition** bone disease	osteo / pathy bone / disease
osteopenia AW-stee-oh-PEE-nee-yah **Definition** reduction in bone volume	osteo / penia bone / deficiency

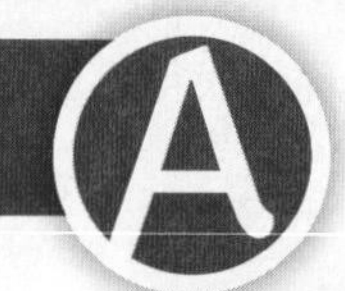

4.4 Diagnosis and Pathology

bones *continued*

Term	Word Analysis
osteoporosis AW-stee-oh-por-OH-sis **Definition** loss of bone density	**osteo / por / osis** bone / pore / condition Normal
spinal stenosis SPAI-nal stih-NOH-sis **Definition** abnormal narrowing of the spine	**spinal sten / osis** spine narrow / condition
spondyloarthropathy SPAWN-dih-loh-ar-THRAW-pah-thee **Definition** joint disease of the vertebrae	**spondylo / arthro / pathy** vertebra / joint / disease
spondylolisthesis SPAWN-dih-loh-lis-THEE-sis **Definition** the slipping or dislocation of a vertebra	**spondylo / listhesis** vertebra / slipping
spondylolysis SPAWN-dih-LO-li-sis **Definition** loss of vertebra structure	**spondylo / lysis** vertebra / loss
spondylosis SPAWN-dih-LOH-sis **Definition** vertebra condition	**spondyl / osis** vertebra / condition

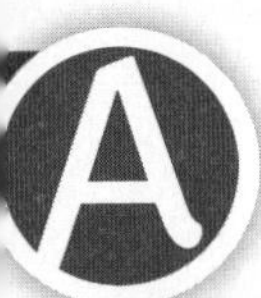

4.4 Diagnosis and Pathology

joints

Term	Word Analysis
arthritis ar-THRAI-tis **Definition** joint inflammation	**arthr / itis** joint / inflammation
rheumatoid arthritis ROO-mah-toyd ar-THRAI-tis **Definition** inflammation of the joints; it is called *rheumatoid* because its symptoms resemble those of rheumatic fever	**rheumat / oid arthr / itis** rheumatic fever / resembling joint / inflammation ©Adam J/Shutterstock.com RF
septic arthritis SEP-tik ar-THRAI-tis **Definition** inflammation of the joint caused by infection	**septic arthr / itis** rotting joint / inflammation
osteoarthritis AW-stee-oh-ar-THRAI-tis **Definition** inflammation of the joints, specifically those that bear weight	**osteo / arthr / itis** bone / joint / inflammation
arthrocele AR-throh-seel **Definition** hernia of a joint	**arthro / cele** joint / hernia
arthrodysplasia AR-throh-dis-PLAY-zhah **Definition** abnormal joint development	**arthro / dys / plasia** joint / bad / formation
arthropathy ar-THRAW-pah-thee **Definition** joint disease	**arthro / pathy** joint / disease
arthrosclerosis AR-throh-skleh-ROH-sis **Definition** hardening of the joints	**arthro / scler / osis** joint / hardening / condition
bursitis bur-SAI-tis **Definition** inflammation of the bursa	**burs / itis** bursa / inflammation
bursopathy bur-SAW-pah-thee **Definition** disease of the bursa	**burso / pathy** bursa / disease

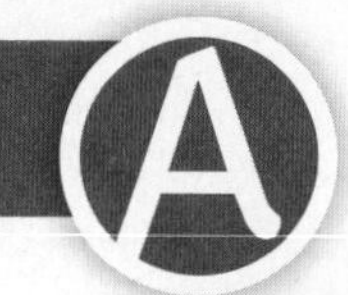

4.4 Diagnosis and Pathology

joints *continued*

Term	Word Analysis
subluxation sub-luk-SAY-shun **Definition** partial dislocation of a joint	**sub / luxation** beneath / dislocation

muscles

Term	Word Analysis
achondroplasia AY-kawn-droh-PLAY-zhah **Definition** a defect in the formation of cartilage	**a / chondro / plasia** no / cartilage / formation
chondromalacia KAWN-droh-mah-LAY-shah **Definition** abnormal softening of the cartilage	**chondro / malacia** cartilage / softening
costochondritis KAW-stoh-kawn-DRAI-tis **Definition** inflammation of the cartilage of the rib	**costo / chondr / itis** rib / cartilage / inflammation
fasciitis FA-shee-AI-tis **Definition** inflammation of the fascia	**fasci / itis** fascia / inflammation
muscular dystrophy MUS-kyoo-lar DIS-troh-fee **Definition** disorder characterized by poor muscle development	**muscul / ar dys / trophy** muscle / pertaining to bad / nourishment
myoclonus MAI-oh-KLAWN-us **Definition** violent muscle contraction	**myo / clonus** muscle / turmoil

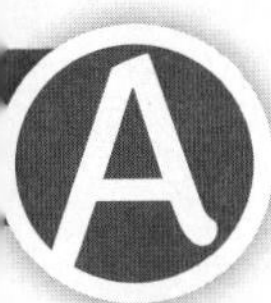

4.4 Diagnosis and Pathology

muscles *continued*

Term	Word Analysis
myopathy mai-AW-pah-thee **Definition** muscle disease	**myo / pathy** muscle / disease
myasthenia MAI-as-THEE-nee-ah **Definition** muscle weakness	**my / asthenia** muscle / weakness
myofasciitis MAI-oh- FA-shee-AI-tis **Definition** inflammation of muscle and fascia	**myo / fasci / itis** muscle / fascia / inflammation
myositis MAI-oh-SAI-tis **Definition** muscle inflammation	**myos / itis** muscle / inflammation
necrotizing fasciitis NEH-kroh-TAI-zing FA-shee-AI-tis **Definition** inflammation of the fascia, causing the death of tissue	**necrot / izing fasci / itis** death / causing fascia / inflammation
polymyositis PAW-lee-MAI-oh-SAI-tis **Definition** inflammation of multiple muscles	**poly / myos / itis** many / muscle / inflammation
tardive dyskinesia TAR-div DIS-kin-EE-zhah **Definition** condition characterized by the loss of muscle control	**tardive dys / kinesia** slow bad / movement
tendinitis TEN-dih-NAI-tis	**tendin / itis** tendon / inflammation
tendonitis TEN-dah-NAI-tis **Definition** tendon inflammation **NOTE:** These words are both accepted spellings for the same condition.	**tendon / itis** tendon / inflammation

oncology

Term	Word Analysis
chondroma kawn-DROH-mah **Definition** a tumorlike growth of cartilage tissue	**chondr / oma** cartilage / tumor
myoma mai-OH-mah **Definition** a muscle tumor	**my / oma** muscle / tumor
myosarcoma MAI-oh-sar-KOH-mah **Definition** a cancerous muscle tumor	**myo / sarc / oma** muscle / flesh / tumor

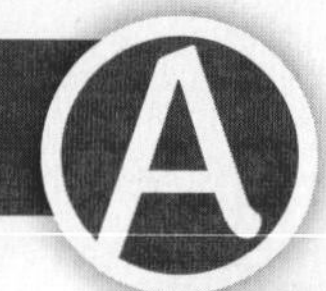

4.4 Diagnosis and Pathology

oncology *continued*

Term	Word Analysis
osteocarcinoma AW-stee-oh-KAR-sih-NOH-mah **Definition** bone cancer tumor **NOTE:** You will notice that certain tumors (-*oma*) have additional designations such as *carcino* or *sarco*. The designation identifies the source from which the cancer develops. Carcinomas develop from surface or epithelial cells. Sarcomas develop from interior or mesenchymal stem cells.	**osteo / carcin / oma** bone / cancer / tumor 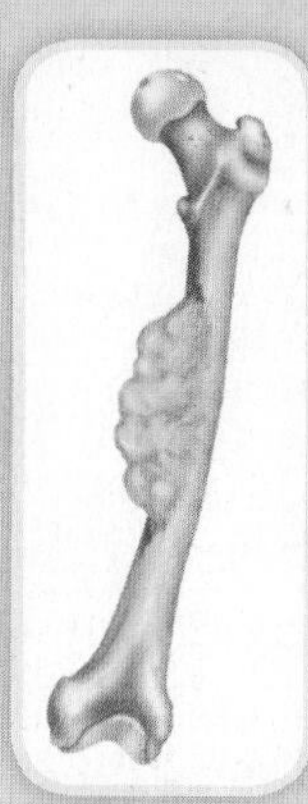
osteochondroma AW-stee-oh-kon-DROH-mah **Definition** a tumor made up of bone and cartilage, also known as an exostosis made up of cartilage	**osteo / chondr / oma** bone / cartilage / tumor
osteosarcoma AW-stee-oh-sar-KOH-mah **Definition** cancerous tumor arising out of bone cells	**osteo / sarc / oma** bone / flesh / tumor

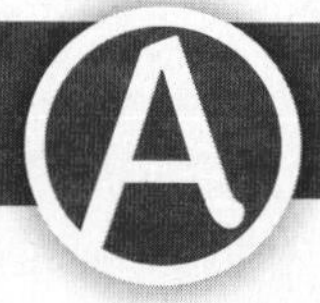

Learning Outcome 4.4 Exercises

PRONUNCIATION

EXERCISE 1 *Indicate which syllable is emphasized when pronounced.*

EXAMPLE: bronchitis bron**chi**tis

1. arthritis ______________
2. osteitis ______________
3. bursitis ______________
4. myoma ______________
5. chondroma ______________
6. arthropathy ______________
7. bursopathy ______________
8. myopathy ______________
9. subluxation ______________

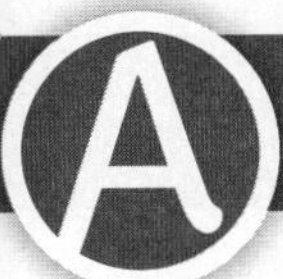

Learning Outcome 4.4 Exercises

TRANSLATION

EXERCISE 2 *Break down the following words into their component parts.*

EXAMPLE: nasopharyngoscope *naso | pharyngo | scope*

1. myopathy ____________
2. myoclonus ____________
3. polymyositis ____________
4. myofasciitis ____________
5. arthrocele ____________
6. arthropathy ____________
7. arthritis ____________
8. bursitis ____________
9. hypertrophic spondylitis ____________
10. chondroma ____________
11. osteoarthritis ____________
12. osteochondritis ____________
13. osteomyelitis ____________
14. osteosarcoma ____________
15. osteocarcinoma ____________
16. chondroosteodystrophy ____________

EXERCISE 3 *Underline and define the word parts from this chapter in the following terms.*

1. bursopathy ____________
2. fasciitis ____________
3. dactylitis ____________
4. osteitis ____________
5. tendinitis ____________
6. tendonitis ____________
7. myositis ____________
8. rheumatoid arthritis ____________
9. myoma ____________
10. muscular dystrophy ____________
11. osteomalacia ____________
12. osteopenia ____________
13. osteogenesis imperfecta ____________
14. osteochondroma (2 roots) ____________
15. chondromalacia ____________
16. myasthenia ____________
17. spondylolisthesis ____________
18. spondylolysis ____________
19. tardive dyskinesia ____________
20. costochondritis (2 roots) ____________
21. craniosynostosis (2 roots) ____________
22. ankylosing spondylitis (2 roots) ____________

EXERCISE 4 *Match the term on the left with its definition on the right.*

______	1. achondroplasia	a.	bone disease
______	2. arthrodysplasia	b.	loss of bone density
______	3. arthrosclerosis	c.	abnormal narrowing of the spine
______	4. myosarcoma	d.	joint disease of the vertebrae
______	5. necrotizing fasciitis	e.	vertebrate condition
______	6. osteopathy	f.	inflammation of the joints, caused by infection
______	7. osteoporosis	g.	abnormal joint development
______	8. septic arthritis	h.	hardening of the joints
______	9. spinal stenosis	i.	a defect in the formation of cartilage
______	10. spondylosis	j.	inflammation of the fascia, causing the death of tissue
______	11. spondyloarthropathy	k.	partial dislocation of a joint
______	12. subluxation	l.	a cancerous muscle tumor

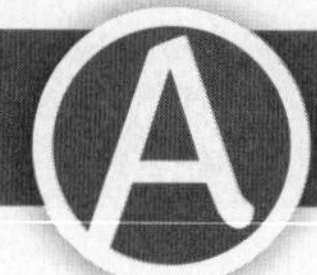

Learning Outcome 4.4 Exercises

EXERCISE 5 *Translate the following terms as literally as possible.*

EXAMPLE: nasopharyngoscope *an instrument for looking at the nose and throat*

1. tendinitis ____________
2. tendonitis ____________
3. arthropathy ____________
4. bursopathy ____________
5. spinal stenosis ____________
6. polymyositis ____________
7. craniosynostosis ____________
8. tardive dyskinesia ____________
9. osteogenesis imperfecta ____________
10. osteomyelitis ____________
11. osteoporosis ____________
12. spondylolisthesis ____________
13. arthrodysplasia ____________
14. subluxation ____________
15. achondroplasia ____________

GENERATION

EXERCISE 6 *Build a medical term from the information provided.*

EXAMPLE: inflammation of the sinuses *sinusitis*

1. inflammation of the bursa ____________
2. inflammation of the fascia ____________
3. finger inflammation ____________
4. inflammation of the cartilage and rib ____________
5. a stiffening inflammation of the vertebrae ____________
6. overdevelopment (*trophic*) vertebrae inflammation ____________
7. joint hardening condition ____________
8. bone disease ____________
9. bone deficiency ____________
10. muscle weakness ____________

EXERCISE 7 *Multiple-choice questions. Select the correct answer(s).*

1. Select the terms that have the root meaning "muscle."
   a. osteitis
   b. arthritis
   c. myositis
   d. myofasciitis
   e. osteoarthritis
   f. osteochondritis

2. Select the terms that have the root meaning "joint."
   a. osteitis
   b. arthritis
   c. myositis
   d. myofasciitis
   e. osteoarthritis
   f. osteochondritis

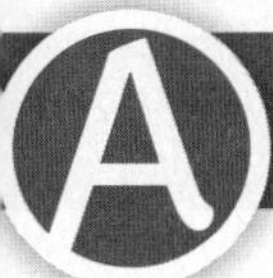

Learning Outcome 4.4 Exercises

3. Select the terms that have the root meaning "cartilage."
   a. osteitis
   b. arthritis
   c. myositis
   d. myofasciitis
   e. osteoarthritis
   f. osteochondritis

4. Select the terms that have the root meaning "bone."
   a. osteitis
   b. arthritis
   c. myositis
   d. myofasciitis
   e. osteoarthritis
   f. osteochondritis

5. *Necrotizing fasciitis* is:
   a. inflammation of the fascia, causing the regeneration of muscle
   b. inflammation of muscle, causing the death of tissue
   c. a disease of the fascia, causing abnormal tissue growth
   d. inflammation of the fascia, causing the death of tissue

6. A violent muscle contraction is called:
   a. myotonic
   b. myoclonus
   c. myodysplasia
   d. muscular dystrophy

7. A disorder characterized by poor muscle development is known as:
   a. myotonic
   b. myoclonus
   c. myodysplasia
   d. muscular dystrophy

EXERCISE 8 *Match the term on the left with its definition on the right*

______	1. rheumatoid arthritis	a.	bone cancer tumor
______	2. arthrocele	b.	a tumor made up of bone and cartilage
______	3. septic arthritis	c.	a cancerous muscle tumor
______	4. myoma	d.	cancerous tumor arising out of bone cells
______	5. myosarcoma	e.	inflammation of the joints, the symptoms of which resemble rheumatic fever
______	6. osteosarcoma	f.	inflammation of the joint, caused by infection
______	7. osteocarcinoma	g.	poor development of bones and cartilage
______	8. chondroma	h.	muscle tumor
______	9. osteochondroma	i.	hernia of a joint
______	10. chondroosteodystrophy	j.	a tumorlike growth of cartilage tissue

EXERCISE 9 *Briefly describe the difference between each pair of terms.*

1. osteomalacia, chondromalacia ______________________________
2. spondyloarthropathy, myopathy ______________________________
3. spondylolysis, spondylosis ______________________________

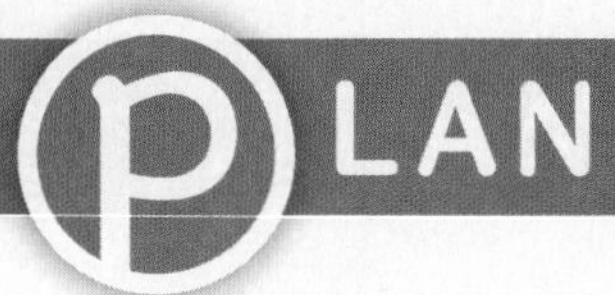

4.5 Treatments and Therapies

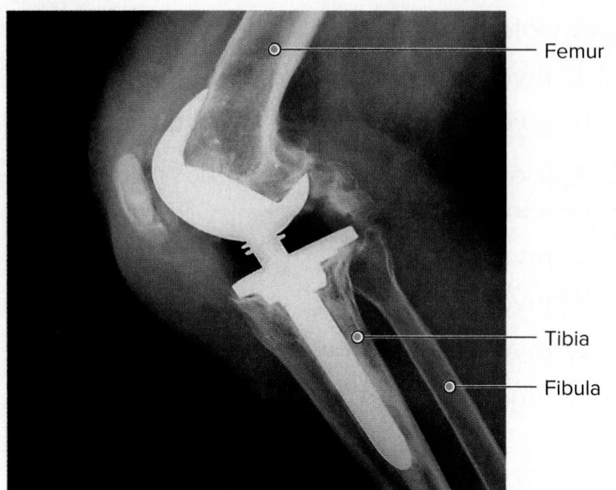

Common procedures for the musculoskeletal system include knee and hip replacements.

©Zephyr/Science Source

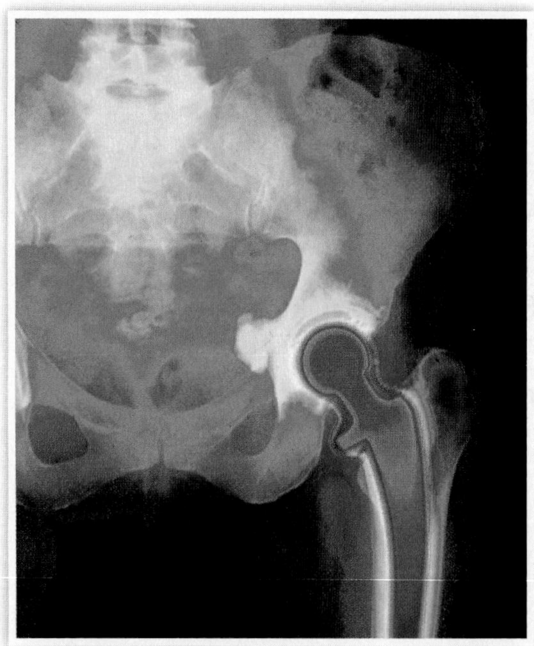

©Mehau Kulyk/Science Source

The medicines used to treat musculoskeletal problems are designed to decrease pain (*analgesic*) or inflammation (*anti-inflammatory*). The most commonly used medicines for both are known as nonsteroidal anti-inflammatory drugs (NSAIDs). Ibuprofen is a common example of this type of medicine. Other nonsurgical treatments include doing *physical therapy,* in which patients exercise and stretch in order to heal injuries, or wearing a device used to relieve tension on a joint (*orthotics*). Shoe inserts are a very common type of orthotic.

When nonsurgical treatment fails, surgery may be necessary. *Orthopedic* surgery deals with joints and bones. Many of the tools used in orthopedic surgery look like they came from a home improvement store—including drills, saws, and hammers. These tools are used to cut into bone (*osteotomy*), joints (*arthrotomy*), or muscle (*myotomy*). Sometimes they remove part or all of these structures (*osteectomy, arthrectomy, myectomy*).

When defective areas or cancer are present in a bone, the diseased area of bone must be removed before new bone (*graft*) or artificial hardware (*prosthesis*) can be installed. This reconstruction of bone procedure is called *osteoplasty.*

Similar procedures exist for joints. Sometimes, removal of a diseased joint (*arthrectomy*) is necessary, followed by a reconstruction of the joint with a prosthesis (*arthroplasty*). These are common treatments for diseased knees and hips. A less aggressive surgery for fixing diseased joints, *chondroplasty,* involves fixing the bad cartilage of a joint. It is very common in athletes and older patients with chronic osteoarthritis.

Not all orthopedic surgery involves complete reconstruction of a bone or joint. Sometimes something that has snapped must be repaired, as in a tendon repair (*tenorrhaphy*) or a muscle repair (*myorrhaphy*). Other times, new attachments must be made. This can involve attaching leftover muscle to bone (*myodesis*) after an amputation or fixing two bones surrounding a joint (*arthrodesis*). While the latter procedure results in immobility of the joint, it may be necessary to relieve pain.

Correcting fractures are among the most common problems encountered when working with bones. Sometimes, the fractured bones end up out of place. Putting them back in place is known as *reduction.* Often, a fracture can be reduced without surgery (*closed reduction*), but sometimes the problem must be corrected surgically (*open reduction*). Once a fracture is corrected, it may need to be held in place with hardware (*fixation*). When hardware is installed inside the body, the procedure is referred to as *internal fixation.* Often, this involves drilling a metal plate into bones and affixing it to the bones with screws. When hardware is installed outside the body, the procedure is referred to as *external fixation.*

4.5 Treatments and Therapies

pharmacology

Term	Word Analysis
analgesic A-nal-JEE-zik **Definition** a drug that relieves pain	**an / alge / sic** no / pain / agent ©Burazin/Photographer's Choice/Getty Images RF
antiarthritic AN-tee-ar-THRIH-tik **Definition** a drug that opposes joint inflammation	**anti / arthri / tic** against / joint (pain) / agent
anti-inflammatory AN-tee-in-FLA-mah-TOR-ee **Definition** a drug that opposes inflammation	**anti / inflammatory** against / inflammation
antipyretic AN-tee-pir-ih-tik **Definition** a drug that opposes fever	**anti / pyre / tic** against / fever / agent

procedures for bones

Term	Word Analysis
carpectomy kar-PEK-toh-mee **Definition** removal of all or part of the wrist	**carp / ectomy** wrist / removal
costectomy kaws-TEK-toh-mee **Definition** removal of a rib	**cost / ectomy** rib / removal
craniectomy KRAY-nee-EK-toh-mee **Definition** removal of a portion of the skull	**crani / ectomy** skull / removal
craniotomy KRAY-nee-AW-toh-mee **Definition** removal of a portion of the skull	**cranio / tomy** skull / incision

NOTE: The difference between a craniectomy and a craniotomy is whether or not the piece of bone is replaced. After a craniotomy, the piece of bone that was removed to allow surgical access to the brain is replaced. In a craniectomy, the piece of bone is not replaced.

procedures for bones *continued*

Term	Word Analysis
external fixation EKS-tir-nal fik-SAY-shun **Definition** the fixation of a fractured bone from the outside (i.e., using casts, splints, stabilizers) **NOTE:** Though external fixation refers to things attached outside the body, things like stabilizers often require surgery to attach.	**external fix / ation** outside fix / procedure 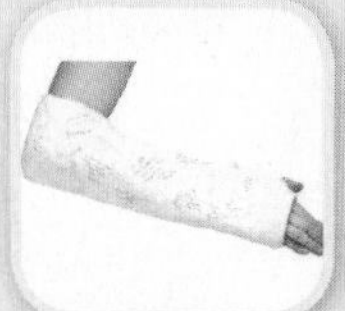 ©Comstock/Alamy Stock Photo RF
internal fixation IN-tir-nal fik-SAY-shun **Definition** the fixation of a fractured bone from the inside (i.e., using screws, pins, plates)	**internal fix / ation** inside fix / procedure
closed reduction klohzd ree-DUK-shun **Definition** returning bones to their proper position without the use of surgery	**closed re / duc / tion** closed back / lead / procedure
open reduction OH-pen ree-DUK-shun **Definition** returning bones to their proper position through the use of surgery	**open re / duc / tion** open back / lead / procedure
metacarpectomy MEH-tah-kar-PEK-toh-mee **Definition** removal of a bone in the hand	**meta / carp / ectomy** after / wrist / removal
orthotics or-THAW-tiks **Definition** a device that aids in the straightening or stabilizing of a part of the body	**ortho / tics** straight / agent 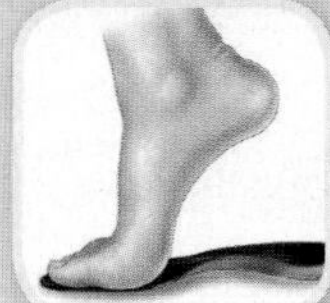
ostectomy aws-TEK-toh-mee **Definition** removal of a bone	**ost / ectomy** bone / removal
osteectomy aws-tee-EK-toh-mee **Definition** removal of a bone	**oste / ectomy** bone / removal
osteoclasia AWS-tee-oh-KLAY-zhah **Definition** the surgical breaking of a bone (often done to remedy a deformity)	**osteo / clasia** bone / breaking
osteoplasty AWS-tee-oh-PLAS-tee **Definition** reconstruction of a bone	**osteo / plasty** bone / reconstruction
osteotomy AWS-tee-AW-toh-mee **Definition** incision into a bone	**osteo / tomy** bone / incision

procedures for bones *continued*

Term	Word Analysis
prosthesis praws-THEE-sis **Definition** a device that is added to a body to replace a missing part or lost function	**pros / thesis** toward / place ©Vereshchagin Dmitry/123RF RF
spondylosyndesis SPAWN-dih-loh-sin-DEE-sis **Definition** fusing together of multiple vertebrae	**spondylo / syn / desis** vertebra / together / binding
sternotomy stir-NAW-toh-mee **Definition** incision into the sternum	**sterno / tomy** sternum / incision
tarsectomy tar-SEK-toh-mee **Definition** removal of all or a portion of the ankle	**tars / ectomy** ankle / removal
tarsoclasia TAR-soh-KLAY-zhah **Definition** surgical fracture of the ankle (i.e., to treat clubfoot)	**tarso / clasia** ankle / breaking

procedures for joints

Term	Word Analysis
arthrectomy ar-THREK-toh-mee **Definition** removal of a joint	**arthr / ectomy** joint / removal
arthroclasia AR-throh-KLAY-zhah **Definition** the therapeutic breaking of a joint to allow for increased mobility	**arthro / clasia** joint / breaking
arthrodesis AR-throh-DEE-sis **Definition** surgical fixation of a joint	**arthro / desis** joining / binding

procedures for joints *continued*

Term	Word Analysis
arthrolysis ar-THRAW-lih-sis **Definition** loosening a stiff joint	**arthro / lysis** joint / loose
arthroplasty AR-throh-PLAS-tee **Definition** reconstruction of a joint	**arthro / plasty** joint / reconstruction
arthrotomy ar-THRAW-toh-mee **Definition** incision into a joint	**arthro / tomy** joint / incision
bursectomy bir-SEK-toh-mee **Definition** removal of a bursa	**burs / ectomy** bursa / removal
bursotomy bir-SAW-toh-mee **Definition** incision into a bursa	**burso / tomy** bursa / incision
chondrectomy kawn-DREK-toh-mee **Definition** removal of cartilage	**chondr / ectomy** cartilage / removal
chondroplasty KAWN-droh-PLAS-tee **Definition** reconstruction of cartilage	**chondro / plasty** cartilage / reconstruction

procedures for muscles

Term	Word Analysis
fasciectomy FA-shee-EK-toh-mee **Definition** removal of fascia	**fasci / ectomy** fascia / removal
fasciodesis FA-shoh-DEE-sis **Definition** binding of fascia	**fascio / desis** fascia / binding
fascioplasty FA-shoh-PLAS-tee **Definition** reconstruction of fascia	**fascio / plasty** fascia / reconstruction
fasciorrhaphy fah-SHOR-ah-fee **Definition** suturing of fascia	**fascio / rrhaphy** fascia / suture

procedures for muscles *continued*

Term	Word Analysis
fasciotomy FA-shee-AW-toh-mee **Definition** incision into fascia	**fascio / tomy** fascia / incision
myectomy mai-EK-toh-mee **Definition** removal of muscle	**my / ectomy** muscle / removal
myodesis MAI-oh-DEE-sis **Definition** binding of a muscle	**myo / desis** muscle / binding
myomectomy MAI-oh-MEK-toh-mee **Definition** removal of a muscle tumor **Note:** It is easy to miss the *oma* root in this word because the *o* looks like it belongs with *myo* and the *a* gets swallowed up by *ectomy.* The *m* is your clue. Don't just read over it—it needs to be explained.	**my / om / ectomy** muscle / tumor / removal
myoplasty MAI-oh-PLAS-tee **Definition** muscle reconstruction	**myo / plasty** muscle / reconstruction
myorrhaphy mai-OR-ah-fee **Definition** muscle suture	**myo / rrhaphy** muscle / suture
myotomy mai-AW-toh-mee **Definition** incision into muscle	**myo / tomy** muscle / incision
tendectomy ten-DEK-toh-mee **Definition** removal of a tendon	**tend / ectomy** tendon / removal
tendoplasty TEN-doh-PLAS-tee **Definition** reconstruction of a tendon	**tendo / plasty** tendon / reconstruction
tenodesis TEN-oh-DEE-sis **Definition** binding of a tendon	**teno / desis** tendon / binding
tenolysis ten-AW-lih-sis **Definition** freeing/loosening a tendon	**teno / lysis** tendon / loosen
tenonectomy TEN-oh-NEK-toh-mee **Definition** removal of a tendon	**tenon / ectomy** tendon / removal
tenoplasty TEN-oh-PLAS-tee **Definition** reconstruction of a tendon	**teno / plasty** tendon / reconstruction

4.5 Treatments and Therapies

procedures for muscles *continued*

Term	Word Analysis
tenorrhaphy ten-OR-ah-fee **Definition** suture of a tendon	**teno / rrhaphy** tendon / suture
tenotomy ten-AW-toh-mee **Definition** incision into a tendon	**teno / tomy** tendon / incision

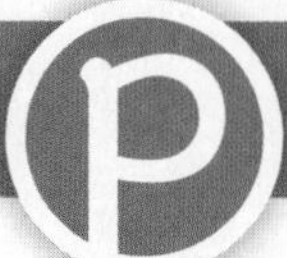

Learning Outcome 4.5 Exercises

PRONUNCIATION

EXERCISE 1 *Indicate which syllable is emphasized when pronounced.*

EXAMPLE: bronchitis bron**chi**tis

1. orthotics ____________
2. prosthesis ____________
3. myotomy ____________
4. tenotomy ____________
5. bursotomy ____________
6. sternotomy ____________
7. arthrotomy ____________
8. carpectomy ____________
9. chondrectomy ____________
10. bursectomy ____________
11. myectomy ____________
12. tendectomy ____________
13. costectomy ____________
14. ostectomy ____________
15. tarsectomy ____________
16. arthrectomy ____________
17. arthrolysis ____________
18. tenolysis ____________
19. fasciorrhaphy ____________

TRANSLATION

EXERCISE 2 *Break down the following words into their component parts.*

EXAMPLE: nasopharyngoscope *naso | pharyngo | scope*

1. analgesic ____________
2. anti-inflammatory ____________
3. osteectomy ____________
4. osteoplasty ____________
5. arthrolysis ____________
6. fascioplasty ____________
7. fasciodesis ____________
8. myoplasty ____________
9. myorrhaphy ____________
10. tenodesis ____________
11. tenoplasty ____________
12. tenorrhaphy ____________
13. carpectomy ____________

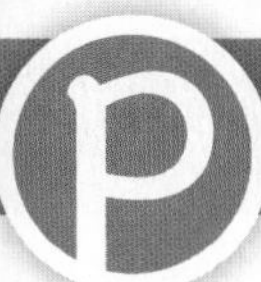

Learning Outcome 4.5 Exercises

EXERCISE 3 *Underline and define the word parts from this chapter in the following terms.*

1. myodesis ______
2. arthrodesis ______
3. arthroplasty ______
4. tendoplasty ______
5. chondroplasty ______
6. bursectomy ______
7. costectomy ______
8. craniectomy ______
9. tenonectomy ______
10. metacarpectomy ______
11. myomectomy ______
12. fasciorrhaphy ______
13. tarsoclasia ______
14. osteoclasia ______
15. tenolysis ______
16. spondylosyndesis ______

EXERCISE 4 *Match the term on the left with its definition on the right.*

______	1. arthrectomy	a.	incision into a bone
______	2. arthrotomy	b.	incision into a bursa
______	3. bursotomy	c.	incision into a joint
______	4. carpectomy	d.	incision into a muscle
______	5. chondrectomy	e.	incision into a tendon
______	6. craniotomy	f.	incision into fascia
______	7. fasciectomy	g.	incision into the skull
______	8. fasciotomy	h.	incision into the sternum
______	9. myectomy	i.	removal of a bone
______	10. myotomy	j.	removal of a joint
______	11. ostectomy	k.	removal of a tendon
______	12. osteotomy	l.	removal of all or a portion of the ankle
______	13. sternotomy	m.	removal of all or part of the wrist
______	14. tarsectomy	n.	removal of cartilage
______	15. tendectomy	o.	removal of fascia
______	16. tenotomy	p.	removal of muscle

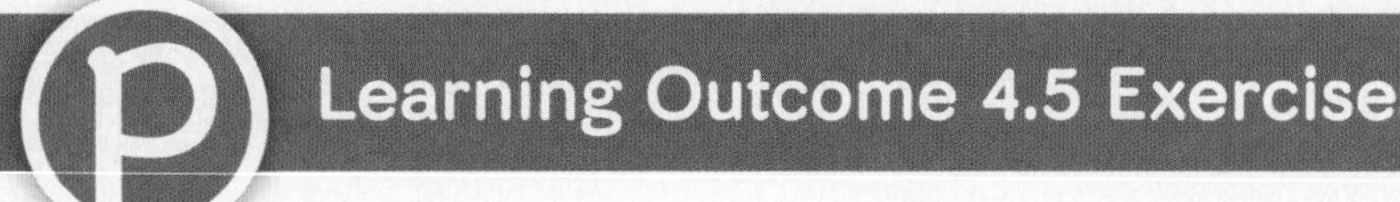

Learning Outcome 4.5 Exercises

EXERCISE 5 *Match the term on the left with its definition on the right.*

______	1. arthroclasia	a. the fixation of a fractured bone from the outside
______	2. closed reduction	b. the fixation of a fractured bone from the inside
______	3. external fixation	c. a device that aids in the straightening or stabilizing of a part of the body
______	4. internal fixation	d. a device that is added to a body to replace a missing part or lost function
______	5. open reduction	e. returning bones to their proper position without the use of surgery
______	6. orthotics	f. returning bones to their proper position through the use of surgery
______	7. prosthesis	g. the therapeutic breaking of a joint to allow for increased mobility

EXERCISE 6 *Translate the following terms as literally as possible.*

EXAMPLE: nasopharyngoscope *an instrument for looking at the nose and throat*

1. bursotomy ______
2. fasciotomy ______
3. myotomy ______
4. tenotomy ______
5. osteotomy ______
6. sternotomy ______
7. ostectomy ______
8. osteectomy ______
9. tendectomy ______
10. tenonectomy ______
11. metacarpectomy ______
12. arthrodesis ______
13. fasciodesis ______
14. myodesis ______
15. tenodesis ______
16. spondylosyndesis ______
17. tenoplasty ______
18. tendoplasty ______
19. analgesic ______
20. antiarthritic ______
21. anti-inflammatory ______
22. antipyretic ______

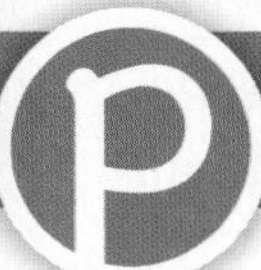

Learning Outcome 4.5 Exercises

GENERATION

EXERCISE 7 *Build a medical term from the information provided.*

EXAMPLE: inflammation of the sinuses *sinusitis*

1. reconstruction of a bone ____________
2. reconstruction of a joint ____________
3. reconstruction of a muscle ____________
4. reconstruction of a tendon ____________
5. reconstruction of fascia ____________
6. reconstruction of cartilage ____________
7. removal of a bursa ____________
8. removal of a tendon ____________
9. removal of fascia ____________
10. removal of a rib ____________
11. removal of all or part of the ankle ____________
12. removal of all or part of the wrist ____________
13. removal of cartilage ____________
14. breaking of a bone ____________
15. breaking of a joint ____________
16. breaking of an ankle ____________
17. suture of a muscle ____________
18. suturing of fascia ____________
19. suture of a tendon ____________

EXERCISE 8 *Briefly describe the difference between each pair of terms.*

1. arthrolysis, tenolysis ____________
2. arthrectomy, arthrotomy ____________
3. myectomy, myomectomy ____________
4. external fixation, internal fixation ____________
5. closed reduction, open reduction ____________
6. craniectomy, craniotomy ____________
7. orthotics, prosthesis ____________

4.6 Abbreviations of the Musculoskeletal System

Abbreviations provide a shorthand way of referring to things that either recur often or are too long to write out. When dealing with bones, joints, and muscles, these abbreviations can refer to everything from observational findings (Hx, ROM), to specific body parts (PCL, MCL), diagnoses (CTS, RA), and treatments (THR, ORIF).

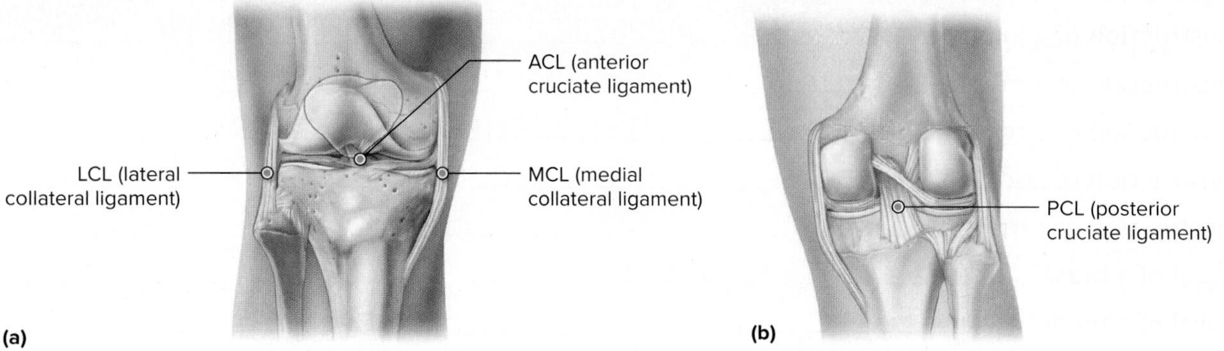

Ligaments of the knee: (a) anterior and lateral ligaments, (b) posterior ligaments

musculoskeletal system abbreviations

Abbreviation	Definition
Hx	history
Fx	fracture
Tx	traction or treatment
ACL	anterior cruciate ligament
MCL	medial collateral ligament
LCL	lateral collateral ligament
PCL	posterior cruciate ligament
C1–C7	cervical (of the neck) vertebrae
T1–T12	thoracic (of the chest) vertebrae
L1–L5	lumbar (of the loin) vertebrae
S1–S5	sacral vertebrae
DTR	deep tendon reflex (this is what doctors are testing when they tap the knee with a reflex hammer)
EMG	electromyogram
FROM	full range of motion
NSAID	nonsteroidal anti-inflammatory drug
OA	osteoarthritis
ORIF	open reduction internal fixation
PT	physical therapy
RA	rheumatoid arthritis

musculoskeletal system abbreviations *continued*

Abbreviation	Definition
RICE	rest, ice, compression, elevation ©McGraw-Hill Education/Rick Brady, photographer
ROM	range of motion
WB	weight bearing
WBAT	weight bearing as tolerated

Learning Outcome 4.6 Exercises

TRANSLATION

EXERCISE 1 *Define the following abbreviations.*

1. Hx ______
2. EMG ______
3. FROM ______
4. ROM ______
5. C1–C7 ______
6. T1–T12 ______
7. L1–L5 ______
8. Fx ______
9. OA ______
10. RA ______
11. NSAID ______
12. PT ______
13. DTR ______

EXERCISE 2 *Give the abbreviations for the following definitions.*

1. anterior cruciate ligament ______
2. lateral collateral ligament ______
3. medial collateral ligament ______
4. posterior cruciate ligament ______
5. open reduction internal fixation ______
6. rest, ice, compression, elevation ______
7. traction ______
8. weight bearing as tolerated ______

Learning Outcome 4.6 Exercises

EXERCISE 3 *Multiple-choice questions. Select the correct answer.*

1. C1–C7 refer to the vertebrae of the:
   a. neck
   b. chest/upper back
   c. lower back
   d. sacrum
2. T1–T12 refer to the vertebrae of the:
   a. neck
   b. chest/upper back
   c. lower back
   d. sacrum
3. L1–L5 refer to the vertebrae of the:
   a. neck
   b. chest/upper back
   c. lower back
   d. sacrum
4. An NSAID is a(n):
   a. anti-inflammatory
   b. steroid
   c. antipyretic
   d. antiarthritic
5. What is the abbreviation for a record of the electrical activity of a muscle?
   a. EAM
   b. EMG
   c. RAM
   d. EEG
6. Select the procedures that would require surgery.
   a. ORIF
   b. PT
   c. RICE
   d. THR
   e. TKR
7. Select the procedures that do NOT require surgery.
   a. ORIF
   b. PT
   c. RICE
   d. THR
   e. TKR
8. RICE means:
   a. rheumatic internal chondrectomy
   b. rest, ice, compression, elevation
   c. range in circular electromyograms
   d. risk for internal fixation and elevation
9. A patient with OA has:
   a. inflammation of the bones
   b. inflammation of the joints
   c. inflammation of the joints, specifically those that bear weight
   d. inflammation of the joints and bones
10. Which of the following acronyms does NOT refer to a part of the body?
    a. ACL
    b. LCL
    c. MCL
    d. C1–C7
    e. T1–T12
    f. L1–L5
    g. M1–M9

4.7 Electronic Health Records

Orthopedic Clinic Note

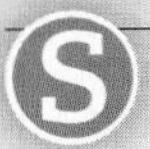

Subjective

History of Present Illness:

Mrs. Maureen Goldman presented to the orthopedic clinic with a chronic history of **arthralgia.** She has been previously diagnosed with **osteoarthritis.** She was initially treated with **NSAIDs** and an **orthotic** that helped for a time; however, Mrs. Goldman's condition worsened and was eventually treated with an intraarticular steroid injection. She reported improved pain and range of motion. The knee pain returned last year, however, and she was treated in our clinic with **arthroscopic** surgery. While it helped some, she reports it didn't completely get rid of her symptoms, and she returns today for evaluation.

PMHx: **Septic arthritis** requiring hospitalization and **IV** antibiotics 4 years ago.

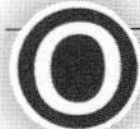

Objective

Physical Exam:

RR: 16; HR: 70; Temp: 98.6; BP: 110/60

Gen: Alert, oriented.

CV: RRR, no murmurs.

Resp: CTA.

Musculoskeletal: **Crepitation** in right knee, decreased **ROM.** Mild **effusion.** Mild muscular **atrophy** of right quadriceps muscle compared to left.

Labs: **ESR** normal, **arthrocentesis:** joint fluid normal.

X-ray: **Subchondral cysts, subchondral sclerosis,** joint space narrowing.

Assessment

DDx: Includes **osteoarthritis, rheumatoid arthritis,** and **bursitis.** Given her history of osteoarthritis on exam and the results of the x-ray and joint aspiration, I believe Mrs. Goldman has **OA** that has failed to respond to previous treatments.

Plan

I have discussed treatment options, and the patient prefers surgery. I have explained the risks and benefits of a **total knee arthroplasty** and she understands. I have scheduled her for surgery next month.

–Electronically signed by
Ricchelle Mitchell, MD
01/26/2015 11:22 AM

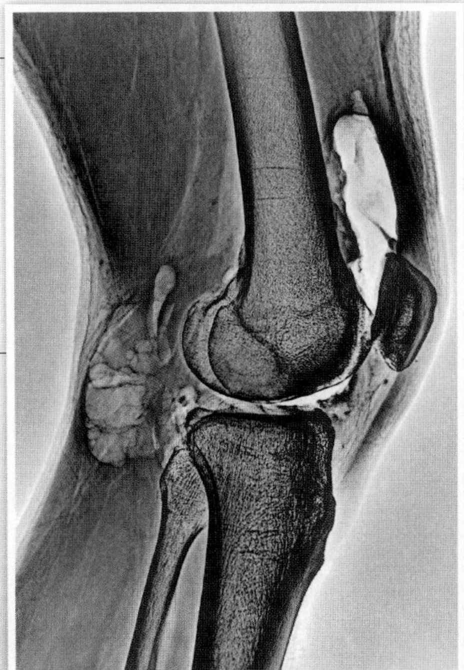

Learning Outcome 4.7 Exercises

EXERCISE 1 *Match the term on the left with its definition on the right.*

______	1. ROM	a. underdevelopment, decrease, or loss of muscle tissue
______	2. atrophy	b. procedure of looking into a joint
______	3. osteoarthritis	c. beneath the cartilage
______	4. arthroplasty	d. reconstruction of a joint
______	5. arthroscopy	e. range of motion
______	6. subchondral	f. inflammation of the joints, specifically those that bear weight

EXERCISE 2 *Fill in the blanks.*

1. Mrs. Goldman was previously diagnosed with ______________ (abbreviation for inflammation of the joints, specifically those that bear weight).
2. Along with ______________ (nonsteroidal anti-inflammatory drugs), she was given an *orthotic* (give definition: ____ ____).
3. Upon evaluation, Mrs. Goldman's right knee had a noticeable creaking sound, or ______________ ______________, as well as mild *effusion* (give definition: ______________________).

EXERCISE 3 *True or false questions. Indicate true answers with a T and false answers with an F.*

1. Mrs. Goldman has a chronic history of bone pain. ______
2. Mrs. Goldman was initially treated with nonsteroidal anti-inflammatory drugs. ______
3. After the intraarticular steroid injection, Mrs. Goldman reported improved arthralgia and ROM. ______
4. Mrs. Goldman was previously hospitalized for joint inflammation caused by infection. ______
5. Mrs. Goldman's right quadriceps muscle had an unusual new growth. ______
6. Mrs. Goldman's x-ray revealed hardening of the cartilage. ______
7. After understanding the risks involved, Mrs. Goldman has agreed to a TKR joint reconstruction. ______

EXERCISE 4 *Multiple-choice questions. Select the correct answer.*

1. *Arthroscopic surgery* is:
   a. closed reduction
   b. external fixation
   c. surgery on a bone
   d. surgery on a joint
2. *Septic arthritis* requires which of the following forms of treatment?
   a. antibiotics
   b. prosthesis
   c. osteectomy
   d. myomectomy
3. The term *subchondral* means:
   a. beneath the cartilage
   b. beneath the knee
   c. beneath the joint
   d. beneath the muscle
4. The term *arthrostenosis* means:
   a. joint narrowing
   b. muscle narrowing
   c. joint hardening
   d. muscle hardening

Discharge Summary

Patient Name: Decker Macmillan

Date of Admission: 1/1/15
Date of Discharge: 1/4/15

Admission Diagnosis
1. **Hypotonia**
2. **Lordosis**

Discharge Diagnosis
1. **Muscular dystrophy**
2. Scoliosis

Discharge Condition: Stable
Consultations: Neurology, cardiology, orthopedic surgery

Procedures
1. **Electromyography**
2. **Muscle biopsy**

Labs: Complete blood count, complete metabolic profile, normal muscle enzyme levels
Imaging: None

HPI
Decker Macmillan is an 8-year-old boy admitted directly to the pediatric floor for workup of chronic progressive **hypotonia.** His parents report they have noticed progressive weakness. Decker has had increasing difficulty running, jumping, and climbing stairs. His parents initially thought his problems were due to his asthma, but they noticed that he also had a waddling gait. They took him to their primary care provider, who referred him for evaluation. On admission, Decker denied any history of **myalgia, arthrodynia,** or **dystaxia.** His problem appeared limited to muscle tone.

Hospital Course
Neuro: On admission exam, Decker was found to have mild **lumbar lordosis, pseudohypertrophy** of his calf muscles, and a waddling gait. He did not have any **genu varum** or **genu valgus.** Reflexes were normal. The initial concern was muscular dystrophy. Given a family history of **polymyositis,** that was considered as well. Decker's labs were consistent with muscular dystrophy. An **electromyography** showed **myopathic** changes. A muscle biopsy was then performed to help distinguish which of the muscular dystrophies the patient has. The results are pending.
CV: Cardiology was consulted, given the strong risk for developing **cardiomyopathy.**
Resp: No problems were seen throughout the hospital stay. Decker was educated in performing breathing exercises and also about the respiratory problems often seen later on in the condition.
Ortho: Orthopedic surgery was consulted for the patient's scoliosis.
Social: Much of the hospital stay focused on patient education.

Discharge Physical Examination
Temp: 98.6; RR: 24; HR: 86; BP: 100/64
Gen: WDWN. Alert.
CV: RRR.
Resp: CTA.
Neuro: Hypotonia of legs. Waddling gait. Using assistance to get up from seated position. Normal reflexes. Marked enlargement of calves.

Activity: No restrictions. Referral to **PT** on discharge. First appointment is next week.
Diet: Calcium/vit. D supplement to prevent **osteoporosis.**
Meds: steroids.

Follow-Up Appointments
- Primary care provider: Dr. Klim in 1 week.
- Neurology: Dr. Willis in 2 weeks.
- Cardiology: Dr. Chatham in 6 months.
- Orthopedic: Dr. Pye in 6 months.

Learning Outcome 4.7 Exercises

EXERCISE 5 *Match the term on the left with its definition on the right.*

______	1. osteoporosis	a.	decrease in muscle tone
______	2. electromyography	b.	crooked back; abnormal lateral curvature of the spine
______	3. scoliosis	c.	disorder characterized by poor muscle development
______	4. myalgia	d.	procedure for measuring the electrical activity of a muscle
______	5. muscular dystrophy	e.	muscle tone
______	6. myotonia	f.	muscle pain
______	7. hypotonia	g.	joint pain
______	8. arthrodynia	h.	poor coordination
______	9. dystaxia	i.	loss of bone density

EXERCISE 6 *Fill in the blanks.*

1. Decker's discharge diagnosis included ______________ (abbreviation for *muscular dystrophy*).
2. Decker did not have any *genu valgum* (give definition: ______________) or *genu varum* (give definition: ______________).
3. Due to Decker's family history, ______________ (inflammation of multiple muscles) was considered in the diagnosis.
4. A(n) ______________ (abbreviation for *electromyography*) showed *myopathic* (pertaining to ______________) changes.
5. The patient will be referred to PT (give definition: ______________).

EXERCISE 7 *True or false questions. Indicate true answers with a T and false answers with an F.*

1. The patient's muscle tone suddenly began to decrease, which is why he is being referred for an evaluation. ______________
2. The patient's problems appear limited to myotonia. ______________
3. The patient denies any joint or muscle pain. ______________
4. The patient has a family history of muscular dystrophy. ______________
5. Calcium and vitamin D supplements were recommended to boost muscle development. ______________

EXERCISE 8 *Multiple-choice questions. Select the correct answer.*

1. Decker's admission diagnosis included:
   a. decrease in muscle tone and abnormal forward curvature of the lower spine
   b. decrease in muscle tone and abnormal forward curvature of the upper spine
   c. increase in muscle tone and abnormal forward curvature of the lower spine
   d. increase in muscle tone and abnormal forward curvature of the upper spine
2. Procedures performed on the patient included:
   a. EAG and muscle Fx
   b. EEG and muscle Bx
   c. EKG and muscle Fx
   d. EMG and muscle Bx

3. The patient does NOT have a history of:
   a. poor coordination
   b. muscle pain
   c. joint pain
   d. all of these
   e. none of these
4. The term *lumbar lordosis* means:
   a. abnormal forward curvature of the lower spine
   b. abnormal forward curvature of the upper spine
   c. abnormal lateral curvature of the lower spine
   d. abnormal lateral curvature of the upper spine
5. *Pseudohypertrophia* is a medical term derived from the combining form *pseudo,* meaning "false," and *hypertrophia,* meaning:
   a. underdevelopment of muscle
   b. overdevelopment of muscle
   c. poor muscle coordination
   d. decrease in muscle movement or activity
6. *Cardiomyopathy* is a disease of:
   a. the muscles of the heart
   b. the growth of the heart
   c. the bursa of the heart
   d. the joints of the heart

Orthopedic Consult Note

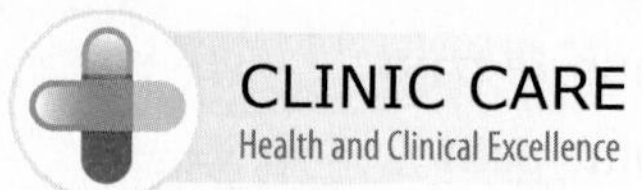

Re: Sam Samuels

Dear Dr. Childs,

Thank you for referring Mr. Samuels to my office. I saw him on March 3, 2015. Mr. Samuels has a 4-month history of increasing pain in his right **distal femur.** He first noticed pain after being kicked in the leg at a soccer game and was evaluated in your office 3 weeks later for persistent pain. There was a soft tissue mass in his distal femur that was tender to touch. An x-ray was performed to rule out a **fracture** or **chronic osteomyelitis.** The x-ray showed both **osteolysis** of the **metaphysis** and **periosteal** new bone formation. Labs were drawn including CBC, CPK, and ESR. He was referred to my office for further evaluation of the x-ray findings.

On exam, Mr. Samuels was a pleasant young man, well developed and well nourished, and in no acute distress. His lungs were clear and heart was regular in rate and rhythm. No murmurs were heard. Examination of his right leg revealed a significant soft tissue mass over his distal femur on the right. The mass was tender. He did not have any knee **effusion.** I reviewed the labs and x-ray. His findings were consistent with **osteosarcoma.**

I discussed the next steps with Mr. Samuels and his family, including staging the tumor and scheduling a biopsy to confirm the diagnosis. I discussed the surgery with Mr. Samuels and his family in the office. His tumor will likely require tumor resection with partial **ostectomy** of the femur with **osteoplasty.** I discussed the benefits of a metal **endoprosthesis** versus an **allograft** for the osteoplasty. Mr. Samuels is scheduled to return to my office 1 week following his biopsy to discuss the results.

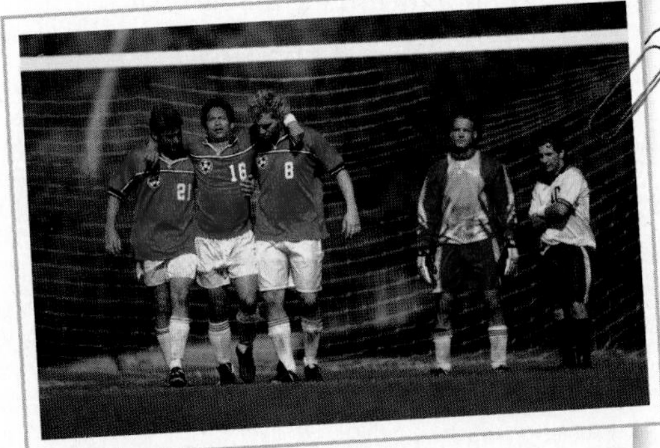

Thank you for this interesting consult.

—Phyllis Sanchez, MD, FAAOS

Learning Outcome 4.7 Exercises

EXERCISE 9 *Match the term on the left with its definition on the right.*

	Term	Definition
______	1. effusion	a. bone pain
______	2. ostalgia	b. a device that is added to a body to replace a missing part or lost function
______	3. ostectomy	c. inflammation of the bone and bone marrow
______	4. osteoplasty	d. bone loss
______	5. osteomyelitis	e. fluid buildup
______	6. osteosarcoma	f. cancerous tumor arising out of bone cells
______	7. osteolysis	g. removal of a bone
______	8. prosthesis	h. reconstruction of a bone

EXERCISE 10 *Fill in the blanks.*

1. An x-ray was performed to rule out ______________ (bone break) or chronic *osteomyelitis* (give definition: ______________________________).
2. Mr. Samuels did not have any fluid buildup in his knee, which is also known as ______________.
3. The labs and x-ray findings were consistent with an *osteosarcoma* (give definition: ______________________________).
4. The patient's tumor will likely require tumor resection with partial *ostectomy* (give definition: ______________) and ______________ (reconstruction of the bone).

EXERCISE 11 *Multiple-choice questions. Select the correct answer.*

1. Mr. Samuels has a 4-month history of:
   a. progressive ostealgia in his femur
   b. acute ostealgia in his femur
   c. progressive myalgia in his femur
   d. acute myalgia in his femur
2. *Osteomyelitis* is:
   a. inflammation of the bone and muscle
   b. inflammation of the bone and bone marrow
   c. disease of the bone and muscle
   d. disease of the bone and bone marrow
3. The root word of *periosteal* means:
   a. bone
   c. cartilage
   b. muscle
   d. joints
4. An *osteosarcoma* is:
   a. a tumor made up of bone and cartilage
   b. a tumor arising from the cartilage of the vertebrae
   c. a tumor arising from bone cells
   d. a benign mass
5. The patient's tumor will likely require:
   a. partial removal of the bone
   b. complete removal of the bone
   c. an incision into the bone
   d. closed reduction
6. The term *endoprosthesis* is created by combining the prefix *endo-*, meaning "within," and *prosthesis,* which is a device that:
   a. is added to a body to replace a missing part or lost function
   b. aids in the straightening or stabilizing of a part of the body
   c. is used to internally fix a broken bone (i.e., screw, pin, plate)
   d. is used to externally immobilize a fractured bone (i.e., cast or splint)

Additional exercises available in connect®

Chapter Review exercises, along with additional practice items, are available in Connect!

Quick Reference

quick reference glossary of roots

Root	Definition	Root	Definition
ankyl/o	stiff, bent	**kinesi/o**	movement, motion
arthr/o	joint	**lumb/o**	loin, lower back
brachi/o	arm	**muscul/o**	muscle
burs/o	bursa (a small fluid-filled sac found near the body's joint)	**my/o, myos/o**	muscle
carp/o	wrist	**oste/o**	bone
cervic/o	neck	**-physis**	growth
chondr/o	cartilage	**spondyl/o**	vertebra
cost/o	rib	**tars/o**	ankle
crani/o	head, skull	**tax/o**	arrangement, order, coordination
dactyl/o	finger	**ten/o, tend/o, tendin/o**	tendon
fasci/o	fascia (fibrous connective tissue binding muscles together)	**tibi/o**	tibia (shinbone)
femor/o	femur (thighbone)	**ton/o**	tone, tension

quick reference glossary of terms

Term	Definition
achondroplasia	a defect in the formation of cartilage
analgesic	a drug that relieves pain
ankylosing spondylitis	a stiffening inflammation of the vertebrae
ankylosis	joint stiffness
antiarthritic	a drug that opposes joint inflammation
anti-inflammatory	a drug that opposes inflammation
antipyretic	a drug that opposes fever
arthrodysplasia	abnormal joint development
arthralgia	joint pain

quick reference glossary of terms *continued*

Term	Definition
arthritis	joint inflammation
arthrocele	hernia of a joint
arthrocentesis	puncture of a joint
arthroclasia	the therapeutic breaking of a joint to allow for increased mobility
arthrodesis	the surgical fixation of a joint
arthrodynia	joint pain
arthrectomy	removal of a joint
arthrogram	visual record of a joint
arthrography	procedure used to examine a joint
arthrolysis	loosening a stiff joint
arthropathy	joint disease
arthroplasty	reconstruction of a joint
arthrosclerosis	hardening of the joints
arthroscope	instrument for looking into a joint
arthroscopy	procedure of looking into a joint
arthrotomy	incision into a joint
atrophy	underdevelopment, decrease, or loss of muscle tissue
bradykinesia	slow movement
bursectomy	removal of a bursa
bursitis	inflammation of the bursa
bursolith	a stone in a bursa
bursopathy	disease of the bursa
bursotomy	incision into a bursa
carpectomy	removal of all or part of the wrist
carpitis	wrist inflammation
cervicodynia	neck pain
chondrectomy	removal of cartilage
chondroma	a tumorlike growth of cartilage tissue
chondromalacia	abnormal softening of the cartilage
chrondro-osteodystrophy	poor development of bones and cartilage

quick reference glossary of terms *continued*

Term	Definition
chondroplasty	reconstruction of cartilage
closed reduction	returning bones to their proper position without the use of surgery
computed axial tomography (CAT or CT)	imaging procedure using a computer to produce cross sections along an axis
costalgia	rib pain
costectomy	removal of a rib
costochondritis	inflammation of the cartilage of the rib
craniectomy	removal of a portion of the skull (bone is not replaced)
craniomalacia	softening of the skull
craniosynostosis	the premature fusing of the skull bones
craniotomy	removal of a portion of the skull (bone is later replaced)
crepitation	from Latin, for "rattle" or "creaking"; a crackling sound heard in joints
dactylitis	finger inflammation
dyskinesia	inability to control movement
dystaxia	poor coordination
dystonia	poor muscle tone
effusion	fluid buildup
electromyogram	record of the electrical activity of a muscle
electromyography	procedure for measuring the electrical activity of a muscle
exostosis	an abnormal growth of bone out of another bone
external fixation	a fixation of a fractured bone from the outside (i.e., using a cast or splint)
fasciectomy	removal of fascia
fasciitis	inflammation of the fascia
fasciodesis	binding of fascia
fascioplasty	reconstruction of fascia
fasciorrhaphy	suturing of fascia
fasciotomy	incision into fascia
fracture	from Latin, for "break"; a bone break
genu valgum	knock-kneed

quick reference glossary of terms *continued*

Term	Definition
genu varum	bowlegged
graphospasm	writer's cramp
hemarthrosis	blood in a joint
hydrarthrosis	water (fluid) in a joint
hyperkinesia	increase in muscle movement or activity
hypertonia	increased muscle tone or tightness
hypertrophic spondylitis	overdevelopment of the vertebrae, causing inflammation
hypertrophy	overdevelopment of muscle tissue
hypokinesia	decrease in muscle movement or activity
hypotonia	decrease in muscle tone or tightness
internal fixation	the fixation of a fractured bone from the inside (i.e., using screws, pins, plates)
kyphosis	humped back—abnormal forward curvature of the upper spine
lordosis	sway back—abnormal forward curvature of the lower spine
metacarpectomy	removal of a bone of the hand
metatarsalgia	pain in the bones of the foot
muscular dystrophy	disorder characterized by poor muscle development
myalgia	muscle pain
myasthenia	muscle weakness
myectomy	removal of muscle
myocele	hernia of muscle tissue
myoclonus	violent muscle contraction
myodesis	binding of muscle
myodynia	muscle pain
myofasciitis	inflammation of the muscle and fascia
myography	procedure for studying muscles
myolysis	loss of muscle tissue
myoma	a muscle tumor

quick reference glossary of terms *continued*

Term	Definition
myomalacia	softening of a muscle
myomectomy	removal of a muscle tumor
myopathy	muscle disease
myoplasty	muscle reconstruction
myorrhaphy	muscle suture
myosarcoma	a cancerous muscle tumor
myosclerosis	hardening of a muscle
myositis	muscle inflammation
myospasm	muscle spasm
myotasis	stretching of a muscle
myotomy	incision into muscle
myotonia	muscle tone
necrotizing fasciitis	inflammation of the fascia, causing the death of tissue
open reduction	returning bones to their proper position through the use of surgery
orthotics	a device that aids in the straightening or stabilizing of a part of the body
ostalgia **ostealgia (alt)**	bone pain
ostectomy	removal of a bone
osteectomy	removal of a bone
osteitis	bone inflammation
osteoarthritis	inflammation of the joints, specifically those that bear weight
osteocarcinoma	bone cancer tumor
osteochondritis	inflammation of bone and cartilage
osteochondroma	a tumor made up of bone and cartilage
osteodynia	bone pain
osteodystrophy	poor bone development
osteogenesis imperfecta	a disease in which the bones do not develop correctly; also known as *brittle bone disease*
osteolysis	bone loss
osteomalacia	softening of the bone
osteomyelitis	inflammation of the bone and bone marrow
osteonecrosis	death of bone
osteopathy	bone disease

quick reference glossary of terms *continued*

Term	Definition
osteopenia	reduction in bone volume
osteoplasty	reconstruction of a bone
osteoporosis	loss of bone density
osteosarcoma	cancerous tumor arising out of bone cells
osteosclerosis	abnormal hardening of bone
osteotomy	incision into a bone
polydactyly	having more than the normal number of fingers (or toes)
polymyositis	inflammation of multiple muscles
prosthesis	a device that is added to a body to replace a missing part or lost function
pyarthrosis	pus in a joint
rheumatoid arthritis	inflammation of the joint is called rheumatoid because its symptoms resemble those of rheumatic fever
scoliosis	crooked back, or abnormal lateral curvature of the spine
septic arthritis	inflammation of the joint caused by infection
spinal stenosis	abnormal narrowing of the spine
spondylitis	inflammation of the vertebra
spondyloarthropathy	joint disease of the vertebrae
spondylolisthesis	the slipping or dislocation of a vertebra
spondylolysis	loss of vertebra structure
spondylomalacia	softening of the vertebra
spondylonia	vertebra pain
spondylosis	vertebra condition
spondylosyndesis	fusing together of multiple vertebrae
sternotomy	incision into the sternum
subluxation	partial dislocation of a joint
syndactyly	fusion (sometimes called webbing) of fingers or toes
tardive dyskinesia	condition characterized by the loss of muscle control
tarsectomy	removal of all or a portion of the ankle
tarsoclasia	the surgical fracture of the ankle (i.e., to treat clubfoot)
tarsoptosis	flat feet
tenalgia	tendon pain
tendectomy	removal of a tendon

quick reference glossary of terms *continued*

Term	Definition
tendonitis **tendinitis (alt)**	tendon inflammation
tendoplasty	reconstruction of a tendon
tenodesis	binding of a tendon
tenolysis	freeing/loosening a tendon
tenonectomy	removal of a tendon
tenoplasty	reconstruction of a tendon
tenorrhaphy	suture of a tendon
tenotomy	incision into a tendon
tibialgia	tibia (shin) pain

review of terms by roots

Root	Term(s)	
ankyl/o	ankylosing spondylitis ankylosis	
arthr/o	antiarthritic arthrectomy arthralgia arthritis arthrocele arthrocentesis arthroclasia arthrodesis arthrodynia arthrodysplasia arthrogram arthrography arthrolysis	arthropathy arthroplasty arthrosclerosis arthroscope arthroscopy arthrotomy hemarthrosis hydrarthrosis osteoarthritis pyarthrosis rheumatoid arthritis septic arthritis spondyloarthropathy
burs/o	bursectomy bursitis bursolith	bursopathy bursotomy
carp/o	carpectomy carpitis	metacarpectomy
cervic/o	cervicodynia	
chondr/o	achondroplasia costochondritis chondrectomy chondroma chondromalacia	chondroosteodystrophy chondroplasty osteochondritis osteochondroma

review of terms by roots *continued*

Root	Term(s)	
cost/o	costalgia costectomy	costochondritis
crani/o	craniectomy craniomalacia	craniosynostosis craniotomy
dactyl/o	dactylitis polydactyly	syndactyly
fasci/o	fasciectomy fasciitis fasciodesis fascioplasty	fasciorrhaphy fasciotomy myofasciitis necrotizing fasciitis
kinesi/o	bradykinesia dyskinesia hyperkinesias	hypokinesia tardive dyskinesia
muscul/o	muscular dystrophy	
my/o	electromyogram	
myos/o	electromyography myalgia myasthenia myectomy myocele myoclonus myodesis myodynia myofasciitis myography myospasm myotasis myotomy	myolysis myoma myomalacia myomectomy myopathy myoplasty myorrhaphy myosarcoma myosclerosis myositis myotonia polymyositis
oste/o	chondroosteodystrophy craniosynostosis exostosis ostalgia ostealgia ostectomy osteectomy osteitis osteoarthritis osteocarcinoma osteochondritis osteochondroma osteodynia osteodystrophy	osteogenesis imperfecta osteolysis osteomalacia osteomyelitis osteonecrosis osteopathy osteopenia osteoplasty osteoporosis osteosarcoma osteosclerosis osteotomy

review of terms by roots *continued*

Root	Term(s)	
spondyl/o	ankylosing spondylitis hypertrophic spondylitis spondylitis spondyloarthropathy spondylodynia	spondylolisthesis spondylolysis spondylomalacia spondylosis spondylosyndesis
tars/o	metatarsalgia tarsectomy	tarsoclasia tarsoptosis
tax/o	dystaxia	
ten/o **tend/o** **tendin/o**	tenalgia tendectomy tendinitis tendonitis tendoplasty tenodesis tenolysis	tenonectomy tenoplasty tenorrhaphy tenotomy
tibi/o	tibialgia	
ton/o	dystonia hypertonia	hypotonia myotonia

other terms

analgesic	genu varum
anti-inflammatory	graphospasm
antipyretic	hypertrophy
atrophy	internal fixation
closed reduction	open reduction
computed axial tomography (CAT or CT)	orthotics
crepitation	prosthesis
effusion	spinal stenosis
external fixation	sternotomy
fracture	subluxation
genu valgum	

The Nervous System—Neurology and Psychiatry

5

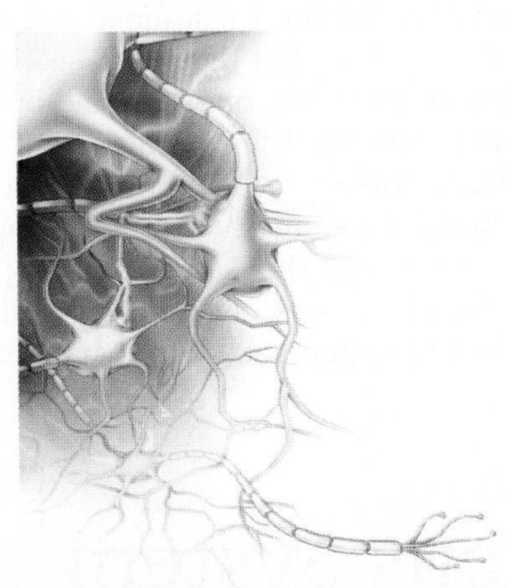

learning outcomes

Upon completion of this chapter, you will be able to:

5.1 Identify the **roots/word parts** associated with the **nervous system**.

S **5.2** Translate the **Subjective** terms associated with the **nervous system**.

O **5.3** Translate the **Objective** terms associated with the **nervous system**.

A **5.4** Translate the **Assessment** terms associated with the **nervous system**.

P **5.5** Translate the **Plan** terms associated with the **nervous system**.

5.6 Use **abbreviations** associated with the **nervous system**.

5.7 Distinguish terms associated with the **nervous system** in the context of **electronic health records**.

Introduction and Overview of the Nervous System

One of our defining characteristics is our ability to think. Aristotle distinguished humans as "rational animals." French philosopher René Descartes famously remarked, "I think, therefore I am." Thinking is one of the most important parts of what makes us who we are. Our knowledge, perception, and response to the world around us are due to the center of thought in our body: the nervous system. More than just the center of conscious thought, the nervous system is always at work gathering information from the world around us, deciding what to do about it, and telling the rest of the body how to respond. It functions as the body's command center for data processing, thought, and action for the conglomerate of many cells, organs, and systems that make up the human body. Thanks to the nervous system, the body acts as a coordinated team reacting to its surroundings with alacrity and precision. The nervous system serves as the body's communications network, coordinating data reception with appropriate reaction.

This network is composed of two parts: the peripheral nervous system and central nervous system. The peripheral nervous system collects data. It receives information such as temperature, pain, light, and pressure from its surroundings. As quickly as it receives input, it transmits it to an analytic center via special conduits known as nerves. The unified collection of cells in the brain and spine are known as the central nervous system. The central nervous system processes the details and formulates a response. Commands are directed back to the appropriate body parts via nerves. This constant progression of receiving, reasoning, and reacting repeats itself continuously as we go about our daily lives.

The nervous system handles both voluntary and involuntary action of the body. In addition, we associate the brain and nervous system with conscious thought and actions. The voluntary command of the body's actions is known as the somatic nervous system. Most often, this voluntary system involves the relationship of the nervous system with the musculoskeletal system. Nerves detect input from the surroundings and send this specific information to the central nervous system for processing. These incoming nerves are called afferent neurons or nerves. The person chooses how to respond and the central nervous system directs the body how to respond through signals sent by efferent neurons. Often these are commands sent to muscles. The signal travels down the nerve through an electric current and connects to the muscle at a special connection point (the neuromuscular junction). This voluntary observation and response represents a small part of the work of the nervous system. The central nervous system also directs the involuntary actions of the body, things that our body does without our conscious choice or awareness. This background control is called the autonomic nervous system and encompasses everything from the beating of our heart, to sweating, to digesting food.

The central nervous system also possesses supporting structures to protect and maintain itself. The skull serves as a dense external layer to protect the brain from common injury. The body also produces cerebrospinal fluid, which surrounds the brain and spinal cord and acts as a shock absorber cushioning them from injury. The brain consumes 20 to 25 percent of the body's oxygen. This huge need for oxygen necessitates a rich blood supply. Nearly 20 percent of the blood pumped from the heart is sent to the brain. This demand is met through an extensive network of blood vessels.

But the brain is more than the neurological controller of the human body's physical processes. What we see, hear, and feel affects our general perception of the world around us. We don't just move and react. We behave. We are more than just digestion, heartbeats, and breathing. We have emotions, opinions, and beliefs. We have more than brains. We have minds we call *psyche* (Greek for "mind"). These more complex functions fit under the umbrella of psychiatry and psychology, both of whose roots come from the Greek word *psyche,* which means "mind" or "soul." These fields deal with problems in our perceptions, emotions, and behavior.

5.1 Word Parts of the Nervous System

Word Parts Associated with the Structure of the Nervous System

Your sensory system—specifically your eyes, ears, nose, and skin—collects data from your surroundings and sends the information to your brain (*encephalo*) by wires known as nerves (*neuro*). Your brain then makes sense of the data and determines the appropriate action. Then it sends out the action plan to the rest of the body via a web of nerves.

Together, your brain and the collecting/acting nerves make up your nervous system. The nerves that send and receive signals from the brain are collectively known as the peripheral nervous system.

Your brain and spinal cord (*myelo*) are called the central nervous system. The brain has several sections (*lobes*) and is divided in two halves (*hemispheres*). The largest portion of your brain is the cerebrum. Under the cerebrum is the *cerebellum,* which controls things like coordination of movements. Your central nervous system is fragile and needs a protective membrane (*meninges*). The tough outer layer is known as the *dura.*

brain

ROOTS: ***cerebr/o, encephal/o***

EXAMPLES: cerebropathy, cerebrospinal, encephalitis, encephalogram

NOTES: The *encephalo* root comes from *en* (inside) and *cephalus* (head) and literally means "the stuff inside your head."

cerebellum

ROOT: ***cerebell/o***

EXAMPLES: cerebellar, cerebellitis

NOTES: This word is just the word *cerebrum* (brain) plus a diminutive suffix. It means the "little brain." It refers to the region of the brain that controls voluntary movements and looks somewhat like a little version of the whole brain.

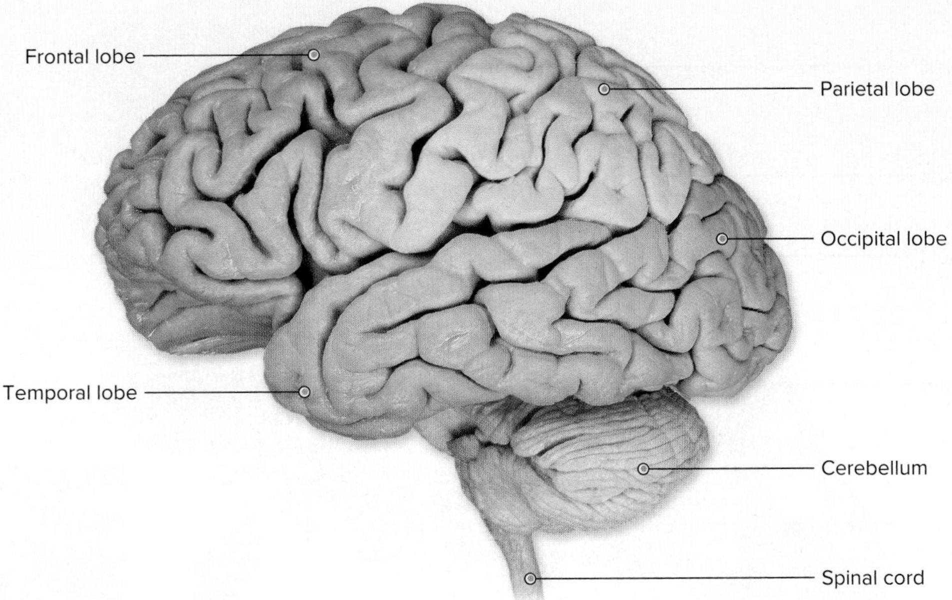

©McGraw-Hill Education/Photo and Dissection by Christine Ecke

lobe

ROOT: ***lob/o***

EXAMPLES: lobotomy, lobectomy

NOTES: The term *lobotomy* is commonly used as a word meaning "a brain operation that changes one's personality." In reality, the term means "incision into a lobe." Lobes are smaller subdivisions of any organ—including the brain, liver, lungs, and, of course, the ears.

The connection between the term *lobotomy* and personality changes probably started with Phineas Gage, a railroad worker in the mid-1800s, who lost a large piece of his brain's frontal lobe in a railroad explosion.

Gage's job was to pack holes full of explosives in order to blast away rock. On one occasion, while Gage was packing a hole, the explosives ignited and sent a rod that was more than 1 inch thick and more than 3 feet long through the front of his skull. Surprisingly, Gage recovered, but he had a much more reserved personality.

This led doctors to understand the role the front lobe of the brain plays in human personality and was the genesis of the use of the term *lobotomy*—which Gage accidentally performed on himself—to describe a brain operation used to make a person more sedate and controlled.

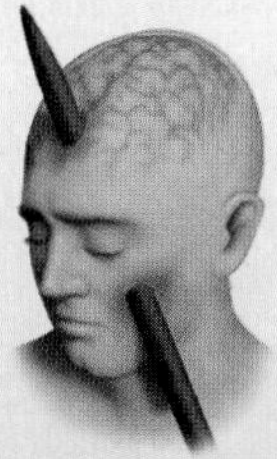

head

ROOT: ***cephal/o***

EXAMPLES: microcephaly, macrocephaly

NOTES: The scientific term for octopus, squid, and other sea creatures that are made up of a head and tentacles is *cephalopod*—literally head (*cephalo*) + feet (*pod*).

head, skull

ROOT: ***crani/o***

EXAMPLES: craniometer, craniomalacia

NOTES: The term *migraine* comes from the word *hemicranias*, meaning "half the head." It reflects the fact most migraines are localized on half the patient's head.

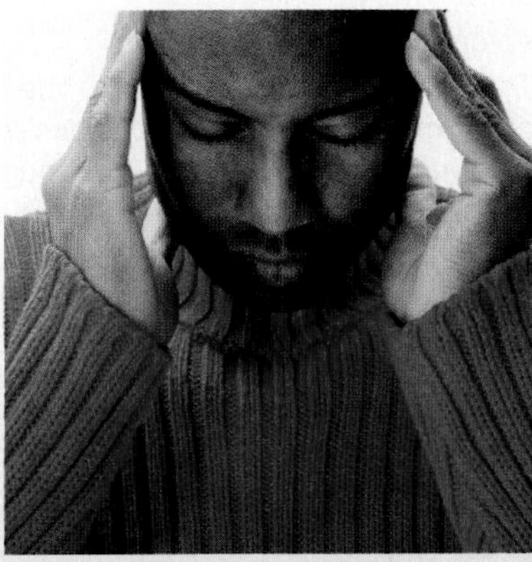

©Ned Frisk/Blend Images/Getty Images RF

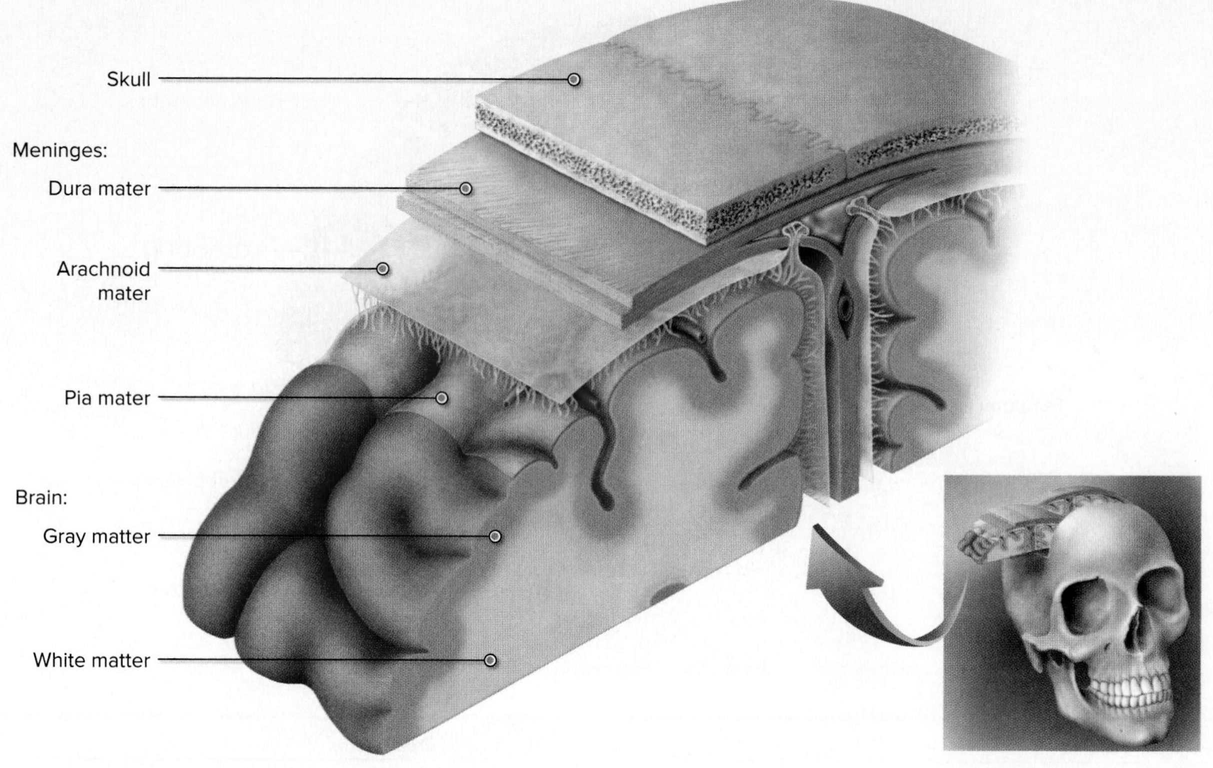

meninges (membrane surrounding the brain and spinal cord)

ROOTS: ***mening/o, meningi/o***

EXAMPLES: meningitis, meningopathy

NOTES: When the letter *g* is followed by an *e* or an *i*, it is pronounced soft (like *j* in *jar*): men-in-JAI-tis. When the letter *g* is followed by an *a, o,* or *u,* it is pronounced hard (like *g* in *gas*): men-in-GOH-pah-thee

dura (tough outer membrane surrounding the brain and spinal cord)

ROOT: ***dur/o***

EXAMPLES: epidural, subdural hematoma

NOTES: This root literally means "hard." The full name of the membrane it refers to is *dura mater cerebri,* which translates to "the tough mother of the brain." Words like *endurance* and *durable* come from the same word.

nerve

ROOT: ***neur/o***

EXAMPLES: neuralgia, neuropathy

NOTES: *Neuron* comes from a Greek word meaning "tendon" or "string." In ancient times, when people first began examining brains, they thought neurons looked like string.

nerve bundle

ROOT: ***gangli/o***

EXAMPLES: ganglion, gangliitis

NOTES: According to Galen, a doctor in ancient Rome, the term *ganglion* means "knot" and could refer to anything gathered up into a ball, which is what Galen thought nerve tissue coming out of the brain looked like.

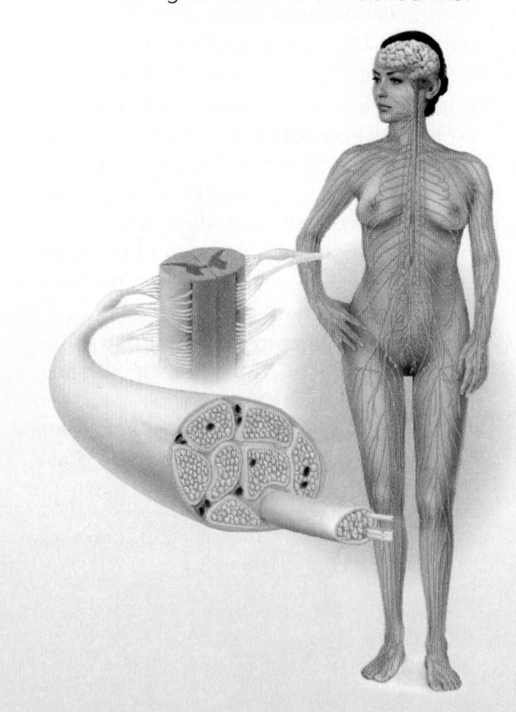

spinal cord, bone marrow

ROOT: ***myel/o***

EXAMPLES: myelitis, myelodysplasia

NOTES: This root comes from a Greek word meaning "the innermost part" and is used in medicine to refer to two different things—bone marrow and the spinal cord. But if you think about it, it makes sense, as both are in the innermost part of something else. Bone marrow is in the center of bones. The spinal cord is in the center of the spine.

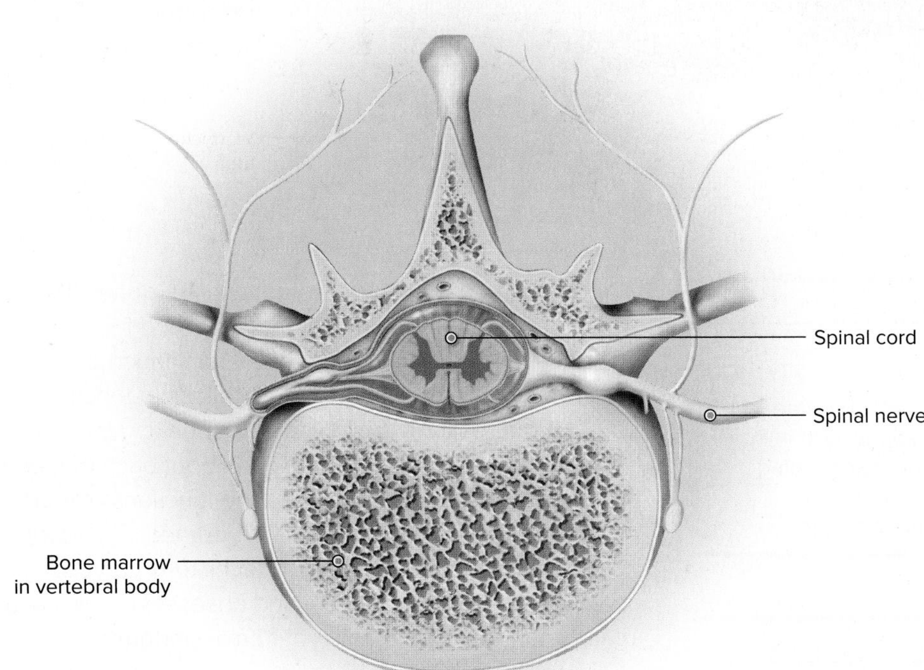

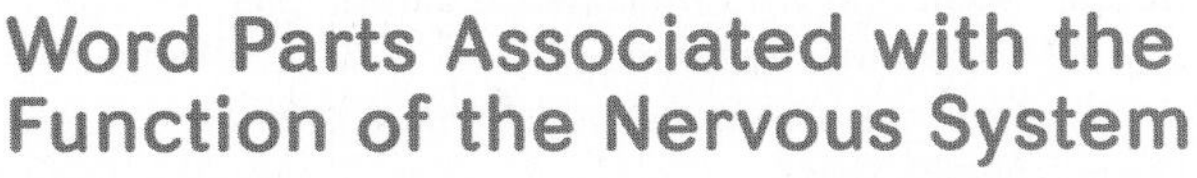

Word Parts Associated with the Function of the Nervous System

While your brain is constantly responding to the world around you, there is more to your mind than just collecting and responding to information. This is where the example of the detective show can go only so far. On those shows, the end result is generally the same—arresting a criminal.

Not all of the data that go to your brain lead to a specific action, though. Much of what you see, hear, and feel affects your general perception of the world around you. It affects your emotions, opinions, or beliefs.

Neurology focuses on actions. The more complex functions often fit under the umbrella of what we call *psyche* (from Greek, for "mind"). We don't just move and react. We *behave*. This is the realm of psychiatry and psychology. These fields of study deal with problems in human perceptions, emotions, and behavior.

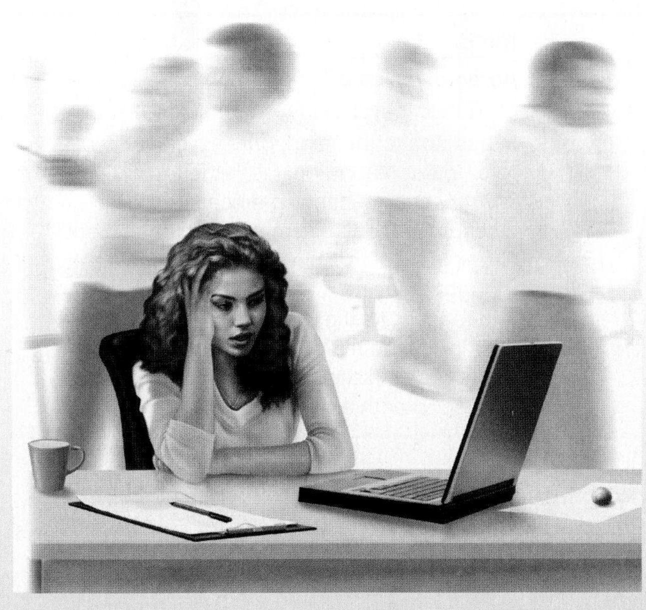

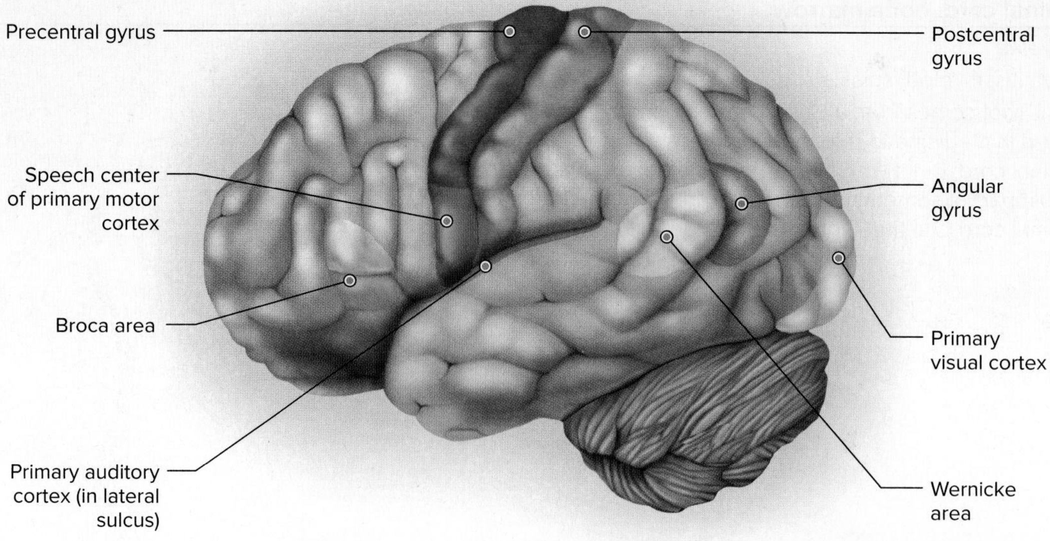

feeling, sensation

ROOT: ***esthesi/o***

EXAMPLES: anesthesia, hyperesthesia

NOTES: *Esthetics* (also sometimes spelled *aesthetics*) is the study of art and philosophy as it pertains to beauty. What makes something beautiful? Can you measure beauty? Is beauty really in the eye of the beholder?

speech

ROOT: ***phas/o***

EXAMPLE: aphasia

NOTES: If a friend is talking too fast, perhaps he or she is stricken with the disease *tachyphasia.*

mind

ROOTS: ***phren/o, psych/o***

EXAMPLES: phrenetic, psychology

NOTES: In addition to the mind, *phren/o* can also refer to the diaphragm (as in the term *phrenospasm,* a fancy medical term for a hiccup). The reason comes from the ancient Greek view of the mind. Early on, the Greeks thought of the chest as the seat of emotion and reason. As that view changed and the location of the mind moved from the chest to the brain, this term for mind began to be applied to both areas of the body.

"You don't know what you've got until it's gone." It's a catchy phrase used in country songs and fortune cookies, and it also applies to the brain. Much of neurology and psychiatry deals with loss of function. A break from reality (*schizo*), a loss of speaking (*phaso*), the inability to feel (*esthesio*)—thinking about each of these conditions helps you appreciate the functions of your brain. When your mind can't keep your fears (*phobia*) or passions (*mania*) at a healthy level, they can cause problems as well. Even fears and obsessions provide a glimpse of the subtler jobs your brain performs.

sleep

ROOTS: ***somn/o, somn/i, hypn/o***

EXAMPLES: somnography, insomnia, hypnosis

NOTES: Someone who walks while sleeping is experiencing *somnambulation,* which comes from the words *somno* (sleep) + *ambulo* (walk).

know

ROOT: ***gnosi/o***

EXAMPLES: agnosia, diagnosis, prognosis

NOTES: Frequently, people who have had a limb amputated report feeling or sensing the missing limb. Such an experience is called *autosomatognosis,* from *auto* (self) + *somato* (body) + *gnosis* (know).

excessive desire

SUFFIX: ***-mania***

EXAMPLES: pyromania, kleptomania

NOTES: Because of the commonly used psychological term *manic-depressive,* some people mistakenly assume that *manic* refers to a type of depression. "He doesn't just have depression, he has *manic* depression." On the contrary—it actually refers to the exact opposite state. Manic-depression is characterized by intense swings of emotion. At times, sufferers are extremely energetic (the *manic* state) and at other times, they are extremely sad (the *depressed* state). Because of these swings in mood, people with this condition are sometimes referred to as being *bipolar,* because their personality is always swinging from one extreme (pole) to the other.

excessive fear or sensitivity

SUFFIX: ***-phobia***

EXAMPLES: photophobia, hydrophobia

NOTES: Phobias can refer to actual symptoms or anxieties. For example, hydrophobia is a main symptom of rabies. Agoraphobia, which is the fear of being outdoors or in public spaces and comes from the Greek word *agora,* meaning "marketplace," is common in people who have experienced major traumatic accidents. Consider these interesting phobias:

- ablutophobia—the fear of taking a bath
- acrophobia—the fear of heights
- alektorophobia—the fear of chickens
- arachnophobia—the fear of spiders
- cynophobia—the fear of dogs
- dendrophobia—the fear of trees
- gynophobia—the fear of women
- ichthyphobia—the fear of fish
- nyctophobia—the fear of night
- phobophobia—the fear of being afraid
- triskaidekaphobia—the fear of the number 13

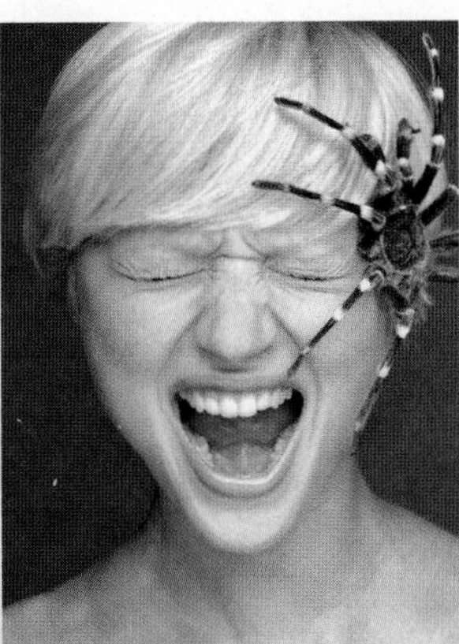

©Serge Krouglikoff/The Image Bank/Getty Images

slight or partial paralysis

SUFFIX: ***-paresis***

EXAMPLE: hemiparesis

NOTES: *Paresis* comes from Greek, for "to let go" or "to slacken"; it is used in health care to refer not to complete loss of sensation or control but instead to a partial or isolated form of paralysis.

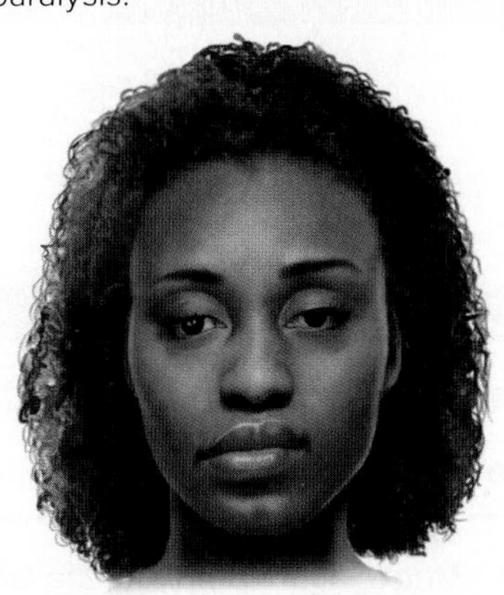

muscle tone, tension, pressure

ROOT: ***ton/o***

EXAMPLES: dystonia, tonograph

NOTES: *Tonic* is used to refer to a medicinal drink. The term was used because these drinks were once thought to restore a person to good muscle *tone.* Today's tonic water still has medicinal value. Though some people think *tonic water* is simply another name for carbonated soda water, tonic is actually a form of carbonated soda water in which quinine, a drug used to treat malaria, has been dissolved. Tonic water was developed for consumption by people living in tropical areas, where malaria is commonplace.

arrangement, order, coordination

ROOT: ***tax/o***

EXAMPLES: ataxia, hypotaxia

NOTES: *Syntax* is an English grammar term made up of the prefix *syn* (together) and the root *tax* (arrangement). It refers to the study of the way words are arranged in a sentence. *Taxidermy,* which comes from *taxo* (arrange) and *dermy* (skin), refers to the practice of removing and displaying the head and skin of an animal killed during a hunt. The arrangement of military forces before a battle is called *tactics.*

paralysis

SUFFIX: ***-plegia***

EXAMPLE: quadriplegia

NOTES: *Plegia* is from Greek, for "to strike." So a word like *thermoplegia* doesn't mean "heat paralysis"; instead, it means "heat stroke."

weakness

SUFFIX: ***-asthenia***

EXAMPLES: myasthenia, phonasthenia

NOTES: Several years back, reports surfaced that a cat in a very rural region of China had spontaneously grown wings. Upon examination by a vet, the cat was diagnosed with a skin condition that causes the skin along the back to become loose and then harden into flat, winglike protrusions. The term for this is *feline* (cat) *cutaneous* (skin) *asthenia* (weakness).

Learning Outcome 5.1 Exercises

Additional exercises available in connect®

TRANSLATION

EXERCISE 1 *Match the word part on the left with its definition on the right. Some definitions will be used more than once.*

_____	1. mening/o	a. head
_____	2. cerebell/o	b. cerebellum
_____	3. neur/o	c. brain
_____	4. crani/o	d. head, skull
_____	5. cerebr/o	e. tough outer membrane surrounding the brain and spinal cord
_____	6. lob/o	f. nerve bundle
_____	7. encephal/o	g. meninges; membrane surrounding the brain and spinal cord
_____	8. cephal/o	h. nerve
_____	9. gangli/o	i. lobe
_____	10. myel/o	j. spinal cord
_____	11. dur/o	

EXERCISE 2 *Translate the following word parts.*

1. crani/o _____
2. cerebr/o _____
3. cerebell/o _____
4. cephal/o _____
5. encephal/o _____
6. mening/o, meningi/o _____
7. neur/o _____
8. dur/o _____
9. myel/o _____
10. gangli/o _____

EXERCISE 3 *Break down the word into its component parts and translate.*

EXAMPLE: sinusitis *sinus | itis* *inflammation of the sinuses*

1. cerebral _____
2. epidural _____

3. meningitis ______________________________
4. myelitis ______________________________
5. cerebellitis ______________________________
6. cephalalgia ______________________________
7. neuralgia ______________________________
8. lobotomy ______________________________
9. craniotomy ______________________________
10. encephalopathy ______________________________

EXERCISE 4 *Match the word part on the left with its definition on the right. Some definitions will be used more than once.*

______	1. psych/o	a.	weakness
______	2. somn/o	b.	feeling, sensation
______	3. -phobia	c.	know
______	4. -mania	d.	sleep
______	5. ton/o	e.	movement, motion
______	6. kinesi/o	f.	excessive desire
______	7. hypn/o	g.	slight or partial paralysis
______	8. -plegia	h.	speech
______	9. -paresis	i.	excessive fear or sensitivity
______	10. esthesi/o	j.	mind
______	11. gnosi/o	k.	arrangement, order, coordination
______	12. phas/o	l.	muscle tone, tension
______	13. tax/o	m.	paralysis
______	14. -asthenia		
______	15. phren/o		

EXERCISE 5 *Translate the following word parts*

1. -phobia ______________________________
2. -mania ______________________________
3. -paresis ______________________________
4. somn/o ______________________________
5. phren/o ______________________________
6. tax/o ______________________________

Learning Outcome 5.1 Exercises

EXERCISE 6 *Break down the following words into their component parts and translate.*

EXAMPLE:	sinusitis	*sinus / itis*	*inflammation of the sinuses*

1. psychology ______________________
2. hypnotic ______________________
3. anesthetic ______________________
4. dystonia ______________________
5. aphasia ______________________
6. neurasthenia ______________________
7. monoplegia ______________________

GENERATION

EXERCISE 7 *Underline and define the word parts from this chapter in the following terms.*

1. cerebral thrombosis ______________________
2. subdural hematoma ______________________
3. lobectomy ______________________
4. craniosclerosis ______________________
5. encephalocele ______________________
6. ganglioma ______________________
7. meningioma ______________________
8. cephalodynia ______________________
9. myelodysplasia ______________________
10. neuropharmacology ______________________

EXERCISE 8 *For the following words, identify and translate the word parts from this chapter.*

1. pyromania ______________________
2. hydrophobia ______________________
3. schizophrenia ______________________
4. psychosomatic ______________________
5. somnambulism ______________________
6. hemiparesis ______________________
7. myasthenia ______________________

Learning Outcome 5.1 Exercises

EXERCISE 9 *Build a medical term from the information provided.*

1. incision into the brain (use *cerebral*) ____________________
2. incision into the skull ____________________
3. incision into a nerve ____________________
4. inflammation of the ganglion ____________________
5. inflammation of the dura ____________________
6. inflammation of the cerebellum ____________________
7. hernia of the meninges ____________________
8. hernia of the spinal cord ____________________
9. hernia of the brain (use *encephalo*) ____________________
10. large head (use *cephalo*) ____________________

EXERCISE 10 *Build a medical term from the information provided.*

1. pertaining to muscle tone ____________________
2. half paralysis (use *-plegia*) ____________________
3. bad feeling (use *dys-*) ____________________
4. bad speaking condition ____________________
5. no coordination condition ____________________
6. sleep agent (use *hypno*) ____________________

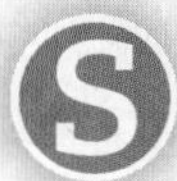

Subjective

Patient History, Problems, Complaints

- Impairments
- Pain
- Paralysis
- Sensation/feeling
- Phobia/mania

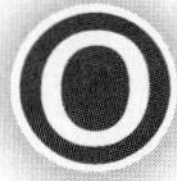

Objective

Observation and Discovery

- Diagnostic procedures
- Structure
- Function
- Professional terms
- Seizure

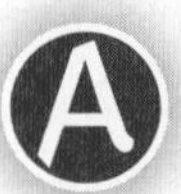

Assessment

Diagnosis and Pathology

- Structure
- Function

Plan

Treatments and Therapies

- Anesthesia
- Drugs
- Surgical procedures

This section contains medical terms built from the roots presented in the previous section. The purpose of this section is to expose you to words used in neurology that are built from the word roots presented earlier. The focus of this book is to teach you the process of learning roots and translating them in context. Each term is presented with the correct pronunciation, followed by a word analysis that breaks down the word into its component parts, a definition that provides a literal translation of the word, as well as supplemental information if the literal translation deviates from its medical use.

The terms are organized using a health care professional's SOAP note (first introduced in Chapter 2) as a model.

SUBJECTIVE

5.2 Patient History, Problems, Complaints

When someone comes to a health care professional with neurological complaints, the complaint will usually fall into problems with either the peripheral or central nervous system. Some patients with peripheral nervous system complaints have problems with the signals being sent to the brain. Their brains may be sending painful signals (*neuralgia, causalgia*) or their brains could have problems receiving sensations (*hyperesthesia, dysesthesia*). Other problems with the peripheral nervous system relate to interruptions in receiving signals from the brain or spinal cord, which could lead to partial or complete paralysis. Central nervous system problems can affect the entire body, as with fainting (*syncope*). Other problems can be more focused, such as problems with speaking (*aphasia, dysphasia*) and reading (*dyslexia*).

The most common psychiatric complaints health care professionals see deal with emotions, such as depression and anxiety. Other common complaints may include concerns over erratic behaviors, abnormal fears (*phobias*), or unhealthy obsessions (*manias*). When a patient enters a sudden state of confusion or abrupt loss of awareness of his or her surroundings, it is *delirium*. When it is a more permanent loss in orientation and thinking ability, it is *dementia*.

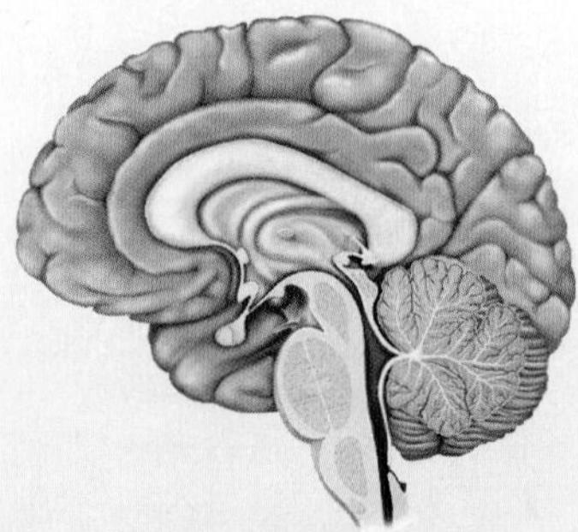

A sagittal cross section of the brain showing the cerebrum, cerebellum, brain stem, and other supporting structures.

5.2 Patient History, Problems, Complaints

impairments

Term	Word Analysis
aphasia ah-FAY-zhah **Definition** inability to speak	a / phas / ia not / speaking / condition
ataxia ah-TAK-see-ah **Definition** lack of coordination	a / taxia no / coordination
catatonia KAT-ah-TOH-nee-ah **Definition** condition characterized by reduced muscle tone	cata / ton / ia down / muscle / tone
delirium deh-LEER-ee-um **Definition** brief loss of mental function	from Latin, for "to plow outside the furrow"; perhaps translates to "go off the tracks"
dementia da-MEN-chah **Definition** loss/decline in mental function	de / ment / ia down / mind / condition
dyskinesia dis-kih-NEE-zhah **Definition** difficulty moving	dys / kinesia bad / movement
dyslexia dis-LEK-see-ah **Definition** difficulty reading	dys / lex / ia bad / reading / condition
dysphasia dis-FAY-zhah **Definition** difficulty speaking	dys / phas / ia bad / speaking / condition
dystonia dis-TOH-nee-ah **Definition** condition characterized by involuntary muscle movements	dys / ton / ia bad / muscle tone / condition
insomnia in-SOM-nee-ah **Definition** inability to sleep	in / somn / ia not / sleeping / condition

5.2 Patient History, Problems, Complaints

impairments *continued*

Term	Word Analysis
myoclonus mai-AWK-loh-nus **Definition** muscle twitching	**myo / clonus** muscle / turmoil
myospasm MAI-oh-spazm **Definition** involuntary muscle contraction	**myo / spasm** muscle / involuntary contraction
neurasthenia NUR-as-THEN-ee-ah **Definition** nerve weakness	**neur / asthenia** nerve / weakness
somnambulism sawm-NAM-byoo-liz-um **Definition** sleep walking	**somn / ambul / ism** sleep / walk / condition
syncope SIN-koh-pee **Definition** fainting; losing consciousness due to temporary loss of blood flow to brain	**from Greek, for** "contraction" **or** "cut off"

pain

Term	Word Analysis
cephalalgia SEH-ful-AL-jah **Definition** head pain	**cephal / algia** head / pain
cephalodynia SEH-fah-loh-DIH-nee-ah **Definition** head pain	**cephalo / dynia** head / pain
encephalalgia in-SE-ful-AL-jah **Definition** brain pain	**encephal / algia** brain / pain
neuralgia nur-AL-jah **Definition** nerve pain	**neur / algia** nerve / pain
neurodynia NUR-oh-DIH-nee-ah **Definition** nerve pain	**neuro / dynia** nerve / pain

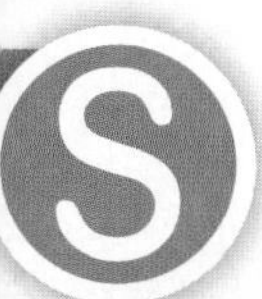

5.2 Patient History, Problems, Complaints

paralysis

Term	Word Analysis
hemiparesis HEH-mee-puh-REE-sis **Definition** partial paralysis on half the body	**hemi / paresis** half / partial paralysis
hemiplegia HEH-mee-PLEE-jah **Definition** paralysis on half the body	**hemi / plegia** half / paralysis
monoparesis MAW-noh-puh-REE-sis **Definition** partial paralysis of one limb	**mono / paresis** one / partial paralysis
monoplegia MAW-noh-PLEE-jah **Definition** paralysis of one limb	**mono / plegia** one / paralysis
paralysis puh-RAH-lu-sis **Definition** complete loss of sensation and motor function	**from Greek, for** "to disable"
paresis puh-REE-sis **Definition** partial paralysis characterized by varying degrees of sensation and motor function	**from Greek, for** "to let go"

sensation/feeling

Term	Word Analysis
causalgia kaw-ZAL-jah **Definition** painful sensation of burning	**caus / algia** burn / pain
dysesthesia DIS-es-THEE-zhah **Definition** bad feeling	**dys / esthesia** bad / sensation
hyperesthesia HAI-per-es-THEE-zhah **Definition** increased sensation	**hyper / esthesia** over / sensation

sensation/feeling *continued*

Term	Word Analysis
paresthesia PAR-es-THEE-zhah **Definition** abnormal sensation (usually numbness or tingling in the skin)	**par / esthesia** beside / sensation
pseudesthesia SOO-des-THEE-zhah **Definition** false sensation	**pseud / esthesia** false / sensation
synesthesia SIN-es-THEE-zhah **Definition** condition where one sensation is experienced as another	**syn / esthesia** together / sensation

phobia/mania

Term	Word Analysis
acrophobia AK-roh-FOH-bee-ah **Definition** fear of heights	**acro / phobia** heights / excessive fear
agoraphobia ah-GOR-ah-FOH-bee-ah **Definition** fear of outdoor spaces **Note:** *Agora* is Greek for "marketplace"; similar to the Roman *forum*.	**agora / phobia** marketplace / excessive fear
hydrophobia HAI-druh-FOH-bee-ah **Definition** fear of water	**hydro / phobia** water / excessive fear
kleptomania KLEP-toh-MAY-nee-ah **Definition** desire to steal	**klepto / mania** theft / excessive desire
photophobia FOH-toh-FOH-bee-ah **Definition** excessive sensitivity to light **Note:** This is an example of *phobia* meaning not just "fear of" but also "sensitivity to" something. Someone with photophobia isn't afraid of light, but rather is extremely sensitive to light.	**photo / phobia** light / excessive sensitivity
pyromania PAI-roh-MAY-nee-ah **Definition** desire to set fire	**pyro / mania** fire / excessive desire

Learning Outcome 5.2 Exercises

PRONUNCIATION

EXERCISE 1 *Indicate which syllable is emphasized when pronounced.*

EXAMPLE: bronchitis bron**chi**tis

1. dystonia ______
2. ataxia ______
3. paresis ______
4. neuralgia ______
5. causalgia ______
6. aphasia ______
7. paralysis ______
8. dysphasia ______
9. somnambulism ______

TRANSLATION

EXERCISE 2 *Break down the following words into their component parts.*

EXAMPLE: nasopharyngoscope *naso | pharyngo | scope*

1. dementia ______
2. pseudesthesia ______
3. synesthesia ______
4. causalgia ______
5. pyromania ______
6. hydrophobia ______
7. dysphasia ______
8. myoclonus ______
9. dyslexia ______
10. neuralgia ______

EXERCISE 3 *Underline and define the word parts from this chapter in the following terms.*

1. neurasthenia ______
2. neurodynia ______
3. cephalalgia ______
4. encephalalgia ______
5. dyskinesia ______
6. dysesthesia ______
7. paresthesia ______
8. kleptomania ______
9. agoraphobia ______
10. photophobia ______
11. monoparesis ______
12. monoplegia ______
13. aphasia ______
14. ataxia ______
15. insomnia ______
16. catatonia ______
17. myospasm ______

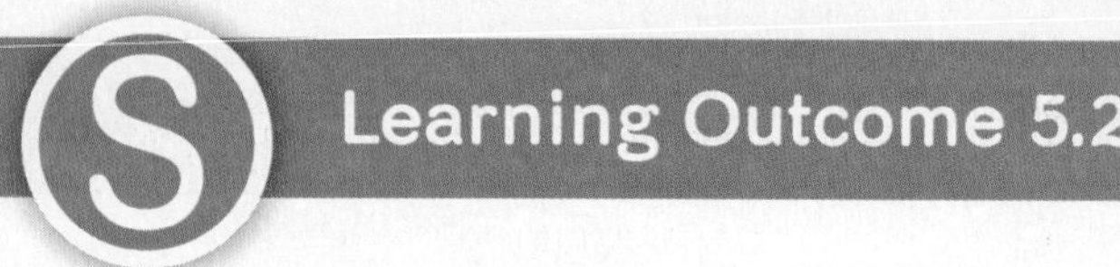

Learning Outcome 5.2 Exercises

EXERCISE 4 *Match the term on the left with its definition on the right.*

______ 1. paralysis
______ 2. delirium
______ 3. insomnia
______ 4. acrophobia
______ 5. cephalodynia
______ 6. hemiparesis
______ 7. syncope
______ 8. hyperesthesia
______ 9. dystonia
______ 10. hemiplegia
______ 11. paresis

a. head pain
b. brief loss of mental function
c. increased sensation
d. fear of heights
e. fainting; losing consciousness due to temporary loss of blood flow to the brain
f. partial paralysis on half the body
g. paralysis on half the body
h. inability to sleep
i. condition characterized by involuntary movements
j. from Greek, for "to disable"; complete loss of sensation and motor function
k. from Greek, for "to let go"; partial paralysis characterized by varying degrees of sensation and motor function

EXERCISE 5 *Translate the following terms as literally as possible.*

EXAMPLE: nasopharyngoscope *an instrument for looking at the nose and throat*

1. aphasia ______
2. catatonia ______
3. somnambulism ______
4. myoclonus ______
5. cephalodynia ______
6. encephalalgia ______
7. monoplegia ______
8. monoparesis ______
9. neurodynia ______
10. pseudesthesia ______
11. synesthesia ______
12. hydrophobia ______
13. pyromania ______

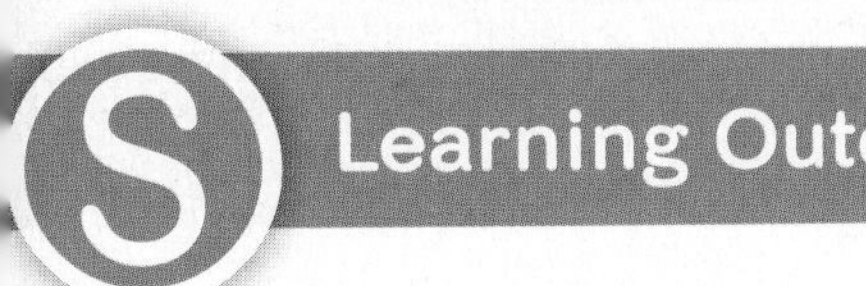

Learning Outcome 5.2 Exercises

GENERATION

EXERCISE 6 *Multiple-choice questions. Select the correct answer(s).*

1. The main categories for nerve complaints are:
   a. peripheral and central nervous system problems
   b. central nervous system and psychiatric problems
   c. peripheral and psychiatric problems
   d. autonomic and pyramidal problems
2. Select the terms that pertain to peripheral nerve problems.
   a. sending painful signals to the brain (*algia*)
   b. problems receiving sensation (*esthesia*)
   c. excessive desire (*mania*)
   d. problems speaking (*phaso*)
   e. abnormal fear (*phobia*)
   f. paralysis (*plegia*)
3. Select the terms that pertain to central nervous system problems.
   a. sending painful signals to the brain (*algia*)
   b. problems receiving sensation (*esthesia*)
   c. excessive desire (*mania*)
   d. problems speaking (*phaso*)
   e. abnormal fear (*phobia*)
   f. paralysis (*plegia*)
4. Select the terms that pertain to psychiatric problems.
   a. sending painful signals to the brain (*algia*)
   b. problems receiving sensation (*esthesia*)
   c. excessive desire (*mania*)
   d. problems speaking (*phaso*)
   e. abnormal fear (*phobia*)
   f. paralysis (*plegia*)

EXERCISE 7 *Build a medical term from the information provided.*

EXAMPLE: inflammation of the sinuses *sinusitis*

1. bad speaking condition __________
2. no coordination condition __________
3. bad muscle tone condition __________
4. bad feeling __________
5. increased sensation __________
6. not sleeping condition __________
7. difficulty moving __________
8. involuntary muscle contraction __________
9. nerve weakness __________
10. partial paralysis on half the body __________
11. paralysis on half the body __________
12. fear of outdoor spaces __________
13. excessive sensitivity to light __________
14. desire to steal __________

Learning Outcome 5.2 Exercises

EXERCISE 8 *Multiple-choice questions. Select the correct answer.*

1. Which of the following means "fear of heights"?
   - a. hydrophobia
   - b. agoraphobia
   - c. acrophobia
   - d. photophobia
2. Which of the following literally means "beside sensation" and normally refers to numbness or tingling in the skin?
   - a. dysesthesia
   - b. hyperesthesia
   - c. paresthesia
   - d. pseudesthesia
   - e. synesthesia
3. Which of the following is a painful sensation of burning?
   - a. causalgia
   - b. cephalalgia
   - c. pyromania
   - d. anosmia
4. A person who lacks a sense of smell has:
   - a. ataxia
   - b. anosmia
   - c. syncope
   - d. dyskinesia

EXERCISE 9 *Briefly describe the difference between each pair of terms.*

1. paralysis, paresis ____________________
2. neuralgia, cephalalgia ____________________
3. dementia, delirium ____________________
4. dyslexia, dyskinesia ____________________

OBJECTIVE

5.3 Observation and Discovery

When a health care professional sees a patient with a neurologic or psychiatric problem, the exam is often quite involved. The neurologic exam involves checking the patient's muscle strength and coordination, sensation, and reflexes. A reflex is a muscle contraction that bypasses the brain. When certain tendons are tapped, an impulse flows directly to the spinal cord, which sends a quick command to the nearby muscle to contract. Checking sensation involves studying afferent nerve paths, which are the paths that lead from the peripheral to the central nervous system. Strength and coordination check efferent pathways, the pathways that lead from the brain to the peripheral nerves. Psychiatric evaluation is very involved, because it depends on extensive questions and history to help discover the root of the patient's problem.

The most common lab work done in the evaluation of the neurologic system focuses on testing a patient's cerebrospinal fluid, which is obtained via lumbar puncture. This is a procedure in which a needle is gently inserted between the vertebrae of the lower spine and a small amount of fluid is drawn and evaluated for signs of infection and other types of inflammation.

Imaging of the brain is commonly performed to evaluate for bleeding after an injury, to determine the presence of diseased brain tissue, and to look for brain tumors. The most common imaging technique is the computed tomography (CT) scan, which is a complex type of x-ray. The benefit of a CT is its speed. When a more detailed view is needed, or when the cerebellum is of special importance, a magnetic resonance image (MRI) is beneficial. Ultrasounds can be used to assess blood circulation to the brain and monitor the speed of the blood passing through the vessels, helpful in detecting both blockages and bleeding. For a more involved view of the vessels, dye can be injected into the bloodstream and an MRI performed. This special image is known as magnetic resonance angiography (MRA). Another type of image utilizing dye is a myelogram, in which an x-ray of the spine is completed after dye is injected into the vertebrae. Another very common procedure for analyzing the electric function of the brain is an electroencephalogram (EEG). An EEG is not exactly an image of the brain; electrodes are placed around the skull and the brain's electric currents are monitored. This is the most effective means to detect seizure activity in the brain.

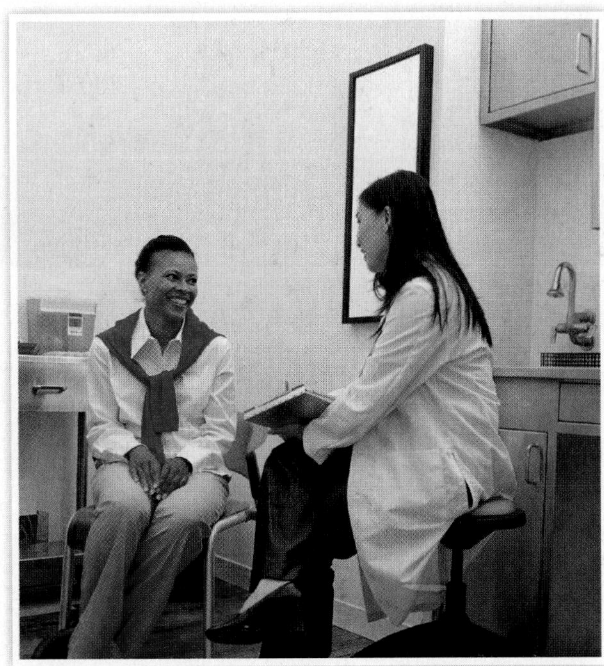

Two of the most common ways of obtaining data to be used in diagnosing neurological or psychiatric disorders involve patient interview and imaging.

©Photomondo/Digital Vision/Getty Images RF

diagnostic procedures

Term	Word Analysis
echoencephalography EH-koh-in-SEH-fah-LAW-grah-fee	**echo / encephalo / graphy** echo / brain / writing procedure

Definition procedure used to examine the brain using sound waves

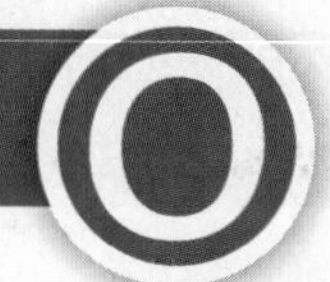

5.3 Observation and Discovery

diagnostic procedures *continued*

Term	Word Analysis
electroencephalography (EEG) eh-LEK-troh-in-SEH-fah-LAW-grah-fee **Definition** procedure used to examine the electrical activity of the brain	**electro / encephalo / graphy** electricity / brain / writing procedure 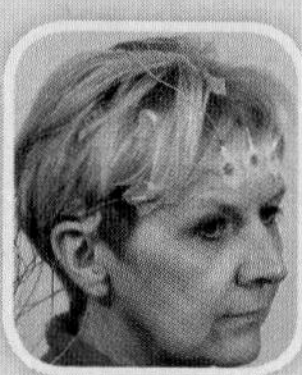 ©McGraw-Hill Education/Bob Coyle, photographer
lumbar puncture (LP) LUM-bar PUNK-chir **Definition** inserting a needle into the lumbar region of the spine in order to collect spinal fluid, commonly called a *spinal tap*	**lumb / ar puncture** lower back / pertaining to 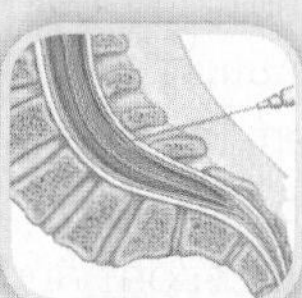

radiology

Term	Word Analysis
cerebral angiography seh-REE-bral AN-gee-AW-grah-fee **Definition** procedure used to examine blood vessels in the brain	**cerebr / al angio / graphy** brain / pertaining to vessel / writing procedure
magnetic resonance angiography (MRA) mag-NET-ik REH-zawn-ants AN-gee-AW-grah-fee **Definition** procedure used to examine blood vessels	**angio / graphy** vessel / writing procedure 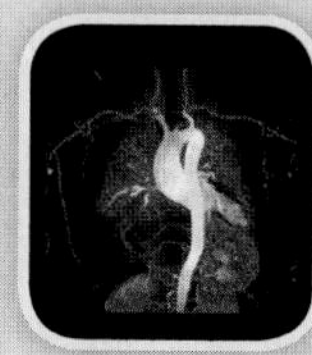 ©Living Art Enterprises/Photo Researchers/Getty Images
myelogram MAI-el-oh-gram **Definition** image of the spinal cord, usually done using x-ray	**myelo / gram** spinal cord / record
positron emission tomography (PET) scan PAWZ-ih-trawn ee-MISH-un taw-MAW-gra-fee **Definition** an imaging procedure that uses radiation (positrons) to produce cross sections of the brain	**e / mission tomo / graphy** out / send cut / writing procedure
transcranial Doppler sonography tranz-KRAY-nee-al DAW-plir saw-NAW-gra-fee **Definition** an imaging technique that produces an image of the brain using sound waves sent through the skull	**trans / cranial Doppler sono / graphy** through / skull Doppler sound / writing procedure

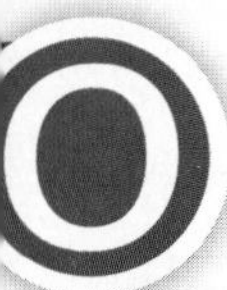

5.3 Observation and Discovery

structure

Term	Word Analysis
cerebellitis ser-eh-bell-AI-tis **Definition** inflammation of the cerebellum	**cerebell / itis** cerebellum / inflammation
cerebral atrophy seh-REE-bral A-troh-fee **Definition** wasting away of brain tissue	**cerebr / al** **a / trophy** brain / pertaining to no / nourishment
duritis dur-AI-tis **Definition** inflammation of the dura	**dur / itis** dura / inflammation
encephalocele en-SEF-ah-loh-SEEL **Definition** hernia of the brain (normally through a defect in the skull)	**encephalo / cele** brain / hernia
hematoma HEE-mah-TOH-mah **Definition** a tumorlike mass made up of blood	**hemat / oma** blood / tumor
cranial hematoma KRAY-nee-al HEE-mah-TOH-mah **Definition** a hematoma beneath the skull	**crani / al** **hemat / oma** skull / pertaining to blood / tumor
epidural hematoma EH-pi-DIR-al HEE-mah-TOH-mah **Definition** a hematoma located on top of the dura	**epi / dur / al** **hemat / oma** upon / dura / pertaining to blood / tumor
intracerebral hematoma IN-trah-se-REE-bral HEE-mah-TOH-mah **Definition** a hematoma located inside the brain	**intra / cerebr / al** **hemat / oma** inside / brain / pertaining to blood / tumor
subdural hematoma sub-DIR-al HEE-mah-TOH-mah **Definition** a hematoma located beneath the dura	**sub / dur / al** **hemat / oma** beneath / dura / pertaining to blood / tumor ©Medical Body Scans/Photo Researchers/Getty Images
macrocephaly MA-kroh-SEH-fah-lee **Definition** abnormally large head	**macro / cephal / y** large / head / condition
microcephaly MAI-kroh-SEH-fah-lee **Definition** abnormally small head	**micro / cephal / y** small / head / condition

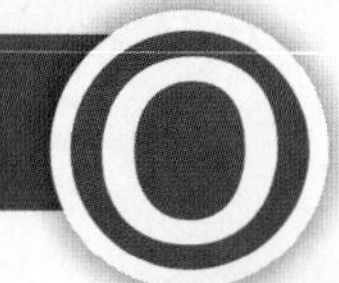

5.3 Observation and Discovery

structure *continued*

Term	Word Analysis
meningocele meh-NIN-goh-seel **Definition** a hernia of the meninges	**meningo / cele** meninges / hernia
myelocele MAI-eh-loh-SEEL **Definition** a hernia of the spinal cord	**myelo / cele** spinal cord / hernia
myelomalacia MAI-eh-loh-mah-LAY-shah **Definition** abnormal softening of the spinal cord	**myelo / malacia** spinal cord / softening
myelomeningocele MAI-eh-loh-meh-NIN-goh-seel **Definition** a hernia of the spinal cord and meninges	**myelo / meningo / cele** spinal cord / meninges / hernia
neuritis nir-AI-tis **Definition** nerve inflammation	**neur / itis** nerve / inflammation
neuroma nir-OH-mah **Definition** a nerve tumor	**neur / oma** nerve / tumor
neurosclerosis NIR-oh-skleh-ROH-sis **Definition** hardening of nerves	**neuro / scler / osis** nerve / hardening / condition
polyneuritis PAW-lee-nir-AI-tis **Definition** inflammation of multiple nerves	**poly / neur / itis** many / nerve / inflammation

function

Term	Word Analysis
agnosia AG-noh-zhah **Definition** inability to comprehend	**a / gnos / ia** not / knowledge / condition
apathy A-pah-thee **Definition** lack of emotion	**a / path / y** no / suffering / condition

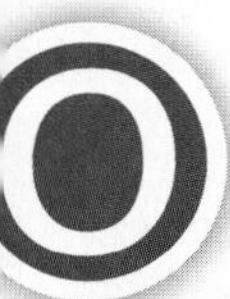

function *continued*

Term	Word Analysis
hyperkinesia HAI-per-kih-NEE-shah **Definition** increase in muscle movement or activity	**hyper / kinesia** over / movement
neurasthenia NIR-as-THEN-ee-ah **Definition** nerve weakness	**neur / asthenia** nerve / weakness
neuroglycopenia NIR-oh-GLAI-koh-PEE-nee-ah **Definition** deficiency of sugar that interferes with normal brain activity	**neuro / glyco / penia** nerve / sugar / deficiency
nystagmus nih-STAG-mus **Definition** involuntary back and forth eye movements	**from Greek, for "to nod"**
prosopagnosia PRAW-soh-pag-NOH-zhah **Definition** inability to recognize faces	**prosop / a / gnos / ia** face / no / knowledge / condition

professional terms

Term	Word Analysis
anesthesiologist A-neh-STHEE-zee-AW-loh-jist **Definition** doctor who specializes in anesthesiology	**an / esthesio / logist** no / sensation / specialist ©Fuse/Getty Images RF
afferent nerve A-fir-ent nirv **Definition** a nerve that carries impulses toward the central nervous system **Note:** The prefix *af-* is actually *ad-* (toward), like in *admit* or *address*. When *ad-* is added to *-ferent*, the word *adferent* changes to *afferent*—it's just easier to say.	**af / ferent nerve** toward / carry
efferent nerve EH-fir-ent nirv **Definition** a nerve that carries impulses away from the central nervous system **Note:** The prefix *ef-* is actually *ex-* (out or away), like in *exit*. When added to *-ferent*, it changes for the same reasons as described for *afferent*.	**ef / ferent nerve** away / carry
neurogenic NIR-oh-JIN-ik **Definition** originating from/created by nerves	**neuro / gen / ic** nerve / creation / pertaining to

professional terms *continued*

Term	Word Analysis
psychiatrist sai-KAI-ah-trist **Definition** doctor who specializes in the treatment of the mind	**psych / iatrist** mind / specialist 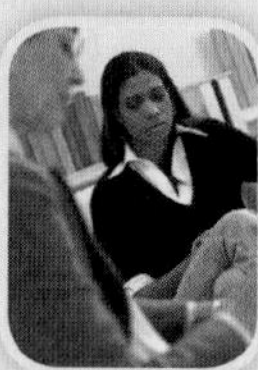 ©Andrea Morini/Getty Images RF
psychiatry sai-KAI-ah-tree **Definition** branch of medicine that focuses on the treatment of the mind	**psych / iatry** mind / specialty
psychogenic SAI-koh-JIN-ik **Definition** originating in/created by the mind	**psycho / gen / ic** mind / creation / pertaining to
psychologist sai-KAW-loh-jist **Definition** doctor who specializes in the study of the mind	**psycho / logist** mind / specialist
psychology sai-KAW-loh-jee **Definition** branch of medicine that focuses on the study of the mind **NOTE:** The chief differences between a psychologist and a psychiatrist are their training and approach; a psychologist has a PhD and normally uses psychotherapy, and a psychiatrist has an MD or a DO and can prescribe medication.	**psycho / logy** mind / study
psychosomatic SAI-koh-soh-MA-tik **Definition** pertaining to the relationship between the body and the mind	**psycho / somat / ic** mind / body / pertaining to

seizure

Term	Word Analysis
idiopathic IH-dee-oh-PAH-thik **Definition** having no known cause or origin **NOTE:** *idio-* means "private" and comes from the Greek word *idiotes*, meaning "private person." Greeks were such social people that anybody who kept to themselves was called an *idiot*.	**idio / path / ic** private / disease / pertaining to
interictal IN-ter-IK-tal **Definition** time between seizures	**inter / ictal** between / seizure
postictal post-IK-tal **Definition** time after a seizure	**post / ictal** after / seizure

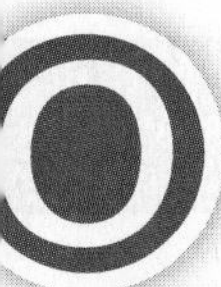

seizure *continued*

Term	Word Analysis
preictal pree-IK-tal **Definition** time before a seizure	**pre / ictal** before / seizure
tonic TAW-nik **Definition** pertaining to muscle tone (normally weak or unresponsive)	**ton / ic** muscle / pertaining to
clonus CLAH-nis **Definition** muscle spasm or twitching	**from Greek,** for "violent"
tonic-clonic seizure TAW-nik CLAH-nik SEE-zhir **Definition** a seizure characterized by both a tonic and a clonic phase	**ton / ic** **clon / ic** muscle / pertaining to spasm / pertaining to

PRONUNCIATION

EXERCISE 1 *Indicate which syllable is emphasized when pronounced.*

EXAMPLE: bronchitis bron**chi**tis

1. tonic ______________________
2. clonus ______________________
3. psychiatrist ______________________
4. psychologist ______________________
5. neuritis ______________________
6. myelogram ______________________
7. agnosia ______________________

TRANSLATION

EXERCISE 2 *Break down the following words into their component parts.*

EXAMPLE: nasopharyngoscope *naso | pharyngo | scope*

1. neuroma ______________________
2. tonic ______________________
3. duritis ______________________
4. neuritis ______________________

Learning Outcome 5.3 Exercises

5. polyneuritis ______
6. myelomalacia ______
7. microcephaly ______
8. psychiatry ______
9. psychology ______
10. psychosomatic ______
11. cerebral atrophy ______
12. myelomeningocele ______
13. neuroglycopenia ______
14. cranial hematoma ______
15. intracerebral hematoma ______
16. subdural hematoma ______
17. electroencephalography ______
18. echoencephalography ______

EXERCISE 3 *Underline and define the word parts from this chapter in the following terms.*

1. hyperkinesia ______
2. cerebellitis ______
3. neurogenic ______
4. psychogenic ______
5. psychologist ______
6. myelocele ______
7. meningocele ______
8. encephalocele ______
9. macrocephaly ______
10. neurosclerosis ______
11. agnosia ______
12. prosopagnosia ______
13. myelogram ______
14. cerebral angiography ______
15. transcranial Doppler sonography ______
16. neurasthenia (2 word parts) ______
17. epidural hematoma ______
18. tonic-clonic seizure ______
19. anesthesiologist ______
20. electroencephalography ______

EXERCISE 4 *Match the term on the left with its definition on the right.*

______ 1. apathy

______ 2. hematoma

______ 3. idiopathic

______ 4. lumbar puncture (LP)

______ 5. postictal

a. inserting a needle into the lumbar (lower back) region of the spine in order to collect spinal fluid

b. procedure used to examine blood vessels

c. an imaging procedure that uses radiation (positrons) to produce cross sections of the brain

d. lack of emotion

e. involuntary back and forth eye movements

Learning Outcome 5.3 Exercises

_____	6. preictal	f.	a nerve that carries impulses toward the CNS
_____	7. interictal	g.	a nerve that carries impulses away from the CNS
_____	8. magnetic resonance angiography (MRA)	h.	time between seizures
_____	9. positron emission tomography (PET) scan	i.	time after a seizure
_____	10. nystagmus	j.	time before a seizure
_____	11. clonus	k.	from Greek, for "violent"; muscle spasm or twitching
_____	12. afferent nerve	l.	having no known cause or origin
_____	13. efferent nerve	m.	a tumorlike mass made up of blood

EXERCISE 5 *Translate the following terms as literally as possible.*

EXAMPLE: nasopharyngoscope *an instrument for looking at the nose and throat*

1. neuroma _______________
2. encephalocele _______________
3. myelocele _______________
4. myelomalacia _______________
5. polyneuritis _______________
6. psychosomatic _______________
7. anesthesiologist _______________
8. afferent nerve _______________
9. efferent nerve _______________

GENERATION

EXERCISE 6 *Build a medical term from the information provided.*

EXAMPLE: inflammation of the sinuses *sinusitis*

1. inflammation of the nerves _______________
2. inflammation of the cerebellum _______________
3. inflammation of the dura _______________
4. no knowledge condition _______________
5. over movement condition _______________
6. pertaining to muscle tone _______________
7. a hernia of the meninges _______________

Learning Outcome 5.3 Exercises

8. a hernia of the spinal cord and meninges ____________
9. brain writing procedure (use *encephalo*) ____________
10. spinal cord record ____________
11. nerve weakness ____________
12. branch of medicine that focuses on the treatment of the mind ____________
13. branch of medicine that focuses on the study of the mind ____________

EXERCISE 7 *Multiple-choice questions. Select the correct answer(s).*

1. Select the terms that pertain to seizures.
   a. afferent
   b. agnostic
   c. apathetic
   d. clonus
   e. efferent
   f. idiopathic
   g. interictal
   h. tonic-clonic
2. Which diagnostic procedure is used to examine blood vessels in the brain?
   a. cerebral angiography
   b. lumbar puncture
   c. positron emission tomography
   d. transcranial Doppler sonography
3. During a lumbar puncture (LP), the needle is inserted into what part of the body?
   a. arm
   b. brain
   c. heart
   d. spine
4. A person with *apathy* lacks:
   a. knowledge/comprehension
   b. emotion
   c. sensation
   d. sleep
5. A person with *prosopagnosia* cannot:
   a. comprehend
   b. feel emotion
   c. locate a sensation
   d. recognize faces
6. Which term means "hardening of nerves"?
   a. neuroglycopenia
   b. neurosclerosis
   c. neurasthenia
   d. polyneuritis
7. Which term means "deficiency of sugar that interferes with normal brain activity"?
   a. neuroglycopenia
   b. neurosclerosis
   c. neurasthenia
   d. polyneuritis
8. Which term means "a tumorlike mass made up of blood located beneath the skull"?
   a. cranial hematoma
   b. intracerebral hematoma
   c. subdural hematoma
   d. encephaloma
9. Which term means "a tumorlike mass made up of blood located inside the brain"?
   a. cranial hematoma
   b. intracerebral hematoma
   c. subdural hematoma
   d. encephaloma
10. *Nystagmus* comes from the Greek word meaning:
    a. back and forth
    b. repetition
    c. to nod
    d. to jump

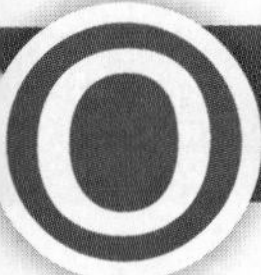

Learning Outcome 5.3 Exercises

EXERCISE 8 *Briefly describe the difference between each pair of terms.*

1. macrocephaly, microcephaly ______
2. neurogenic, psychogenic ______
3. psychiatrist, psychologist ______
4. preictal, postictal ______
5. afferent nerve, efferent nerve ______
6. epidural hematoma, subdural hematoma ______
7. echoencephalography, electroencephalography ______

ASSESSMENT

5.4 Diagnosis and Pathology

When assessing a patient with neuropsychiatric problems, it's helpful to determine whether the problem originates from the nervous system (*neurogenic*) or mind (*psychogenic*).

Neurogenic problems may arise from conditions involving the supporting structures, like the skull or blood supply. Disorders of the skull, like premature closure of the bones (*craniosynostosis*), can limit brain growth and lead to pressure on the brain. Increased pressure can also arise from too much fluid around the brain, as seen in hydrocephalus. Pressure in the brain (*intracranial hypertension*) from these conditions can present as headache and vomiting. Disruption of critical blood supply to the brain presents with sudden changes in neurologic function, like slurring of speech. It can happen from a rupture in the blood vessel (*hemorrhagic stroke*) or a blockage cutting off blood supply (*ischemic stroke*). These vascular events constitute a medical emergency.

Problems of the central nervous system may also arise from direct injury or irritation to nerves or brain cells. The symptoms depend on which part of the nervous system is affected. For example, problems involving only the spinal cord, like myelitis or spinal injury, do not cause problems with thought but can lead to muscle weakness or even paralysis. Infections of the tissue surrounding the brain and spinal cord (*meningitis*) cause headache and a stiff neck, while infections of the brain matter (*encephalitis*) lead to generalized dysfunction of the brain, characterized by an altered mental state (*encephalopathy*). Other causes of encephalopathy include prolonged deprivation of oxygen, exposure to toxins, increased pressure in the brain, or chronic injuries. Not all conditions of the brain matter lead to changes in general mental state. Abnormal firing of nerves leads to involuntary changes in muscle tone (*seizure*), and a dysfunction in higher functions like personal interaction and communication is seen in autism.

Nerves can be affected directly by injury or compression, or indirectly through diseases or toxins. Typically, injury or compression will cause a decrease or total loss of function of a single nerve or a group of nerves that exits the spinal cord in the same place. This may lead to pain (*neuralgia*) and/or loss of function (*paresis* or *paralysis*). Diseases such as diabetes and medicines like chemotherapy drugs can be toxic to nerves. Often, this has a greater effect on the nerves that are farther from the brain and spinal cord (*peripheral neuropathy*).

Tumors of the nervous system happen much more often in the central nervous system. Commonly known as brain tumors, central nervous system tumors are named after the type of cells from which they are made. These include *astrocytomas*, *glioblastomas*, and *medulloblastomas*. Common symptoms include headaches, seizures, sensory changes, and changes in emotions or thinking.

Common psychogenic problems include depression and anxiety. Some people have an inability to control their urges for periods of time, which is known as mania. Most often, these manic phases alternate with bouts of depression, producing a condition known as bipolar disorder or manic-depressive disorder. Some patients have an altered perception of reality known as a psychosis. One of the more common psychotic conditions is schizophrenia. Patients often struggle with distorted perceptions of reality (*delusions*) and may even hear or see things that are not there (*hallucinations*). Furthermore, their thinking patterns are disorganized and emotions are erratic. Another condition characterized by a patient's distorted view of reality occurs in eating disorders. Rather than misunderstanding the world around them, patients with eating disorders such as anorexia and bulimia suffer from an altered perception of their own body.

structure

Term	Word Analysis
Cerebrovascular Accident	
cerebrovascular accident (CVA) seh-REE-broh-VAS-kyoo-lar AK-sih-dent	**cerebro / vascul / ar** brain / blood vessel / pertaining to

Definition an accident involving the blood vessels of the brain

5.4 Diagnosis and Pathology

structure *continued*

Term	Word Analysis
stroke STROHK **Definition** loss of brain function caused by interruption of blood flow/supply to the brain	**stroke** 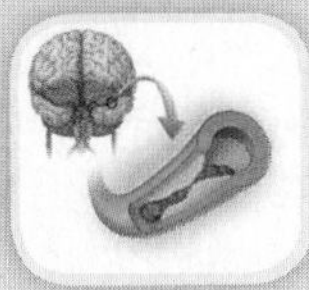
hemorrhagic stroke HEM-oh-RA-jik STROHK **Definition** a stroke where the blood loss is caused by the rupture of a blood vessel	**hemo / rrhag / ic** blood / excessive bleeding / pertaining to
ischemic stroke ihs-KEE-mik STROHK **Definition** a stroke where the blood loss is caused by a blockage	**isch / em / ic** hold back / blood / pertaining to
transient ischemic attack (TIA) TRAN-zee-ent ih-SKEE-mik ah-TAK **Definition** a "mini-stroke" caused by the blockage of a blood vessel, which resolves (goes away) within 24 hours	**trans / ient isch / em / ic** across / go hold back / blood / pertaining to
Cerebrovascular Disease	
cerebrovascular disease seh-REE-broh-VAS-kyoo-lar dih-ZEEZ **Definition** a disease of the blood vessels of the brain	**cerebro / vascul / ar** brain / blood vessel / pertaining to
cerebral aneurysm seh-REE-bral AN-yir-IZ-um **Definition** the widening or abnormal dilation of a blood vessel in the brain **Note:** In *aneurysm*, the *an-* prefix doesn't come from *a* (not) but from *ana* (meaning "up" or "out"). Another word you can see this in is *analysis*, *ana* (up) + *lysis* (loose). So to *analyze* something means "to break something up and look at the parts."	**cerebr / al an / eury / sm** brain / pertaining to out / wide / condition 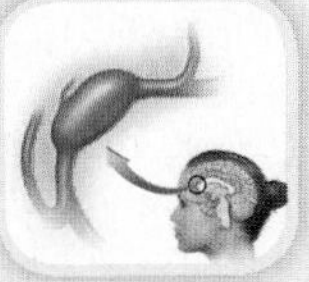
cerebral arteriosclerosis seh-REE-bral ar-TIH-ree-oh-skleh-ROH-sis **Definition** the hardening of an artery in the brain	**cerebr / al arterio / scler / osis** brain / pertaining to artery / hardening / condition
cerebral atherosclerosis seh-REE-bral ATH-er-oh-skleh-ROH-sis **Definition** the hardening of an artery in the brain caused by the buildup of fatty plaque	**cerebr / al athero / scler / osis** brain / pertaining to fatty / hardening / condition 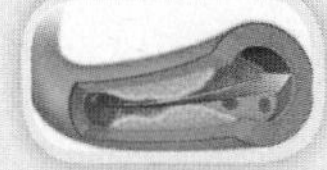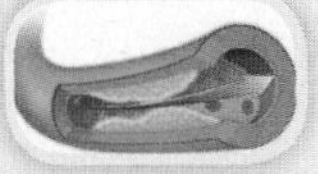
cerebral embolism seh-REE-bral EM-boh-lih-zum **Definition** the blockage of a blood vessel in the brain caused by a foreign object (*embolus*) such as fat or bacteria **Note:** *Embolus* is a Greek word meaning "stopper" or "plug."	**cerebr / al embol / ism** brain / pertaining to stopper / condition 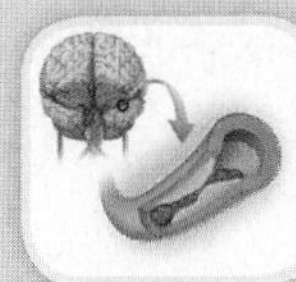

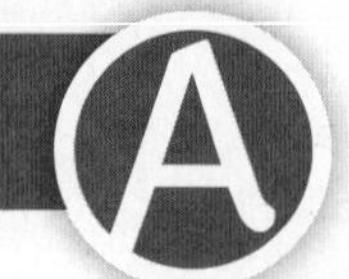

5.4 Diagnosis and Pathology

structure *continued*

Term	Word Analysis
cerebral thrombosis seh-REE-bral throm-BOH-sis **Definition** the blockage of a blood vessel in the brain caused by a blood clot	**cerebr / al** — brain / pertaining to **thromb / osis** — clot / condition
Skull	
craniomalacia KRAY-nee-oh-mah-LAY-shah **Definition** abnormal softening of the skull	**cranio / malacia** skull / softening
craniosclerosis KRAY-nee-oh-skleh-ROH-sis **Definition** abnormal hardening of the skull	**cranio / scler / osis** skull / hardening / condition
craniostenosis KRAY-nee-oh-steh-NOH-sis **Definition** abnormal narrowing of the skull	**cranio / sten / osis** skull / narrow / condition
craniosynostosis KRAY-nee-oh-SIN-aw-STOH-sis **Definition** premature fusing of the skull bones	**cranio / syn / ost / osis** skull / together / bone / condition
hydrocephaly HAI-droh-SEH-fah-lee **Definition** abnormal accumulation of spinal fluid in the brain	**hydro / cephal / y** water / head / condition 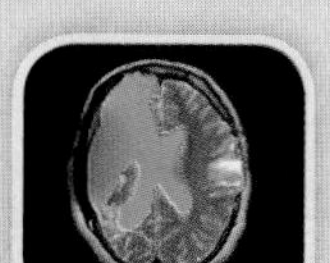 ©Medical Body Scans/Photo Researchers/Getty Images
Oncology	
astrocytoma ASS-troh-sai-TOH-mah **Definition** a tumor of arising from astrocyte glial cells **Note:** Astrocytes are a star-shaped type of glial cell (see note on gliobastoma) found in the brain.	**astro / cyt / oma** star / cell / tumor
ganglioma GAN-glee-OH-mah **Definition** ganglion tumor	**gangli / oma** ganglion / tumor
glioblastoma GLEE-oh-blas-TOH-mah **Definition** a brain tumor arising from glioblast cells **Note:** *Glio* means "glue" and refers to cells in the brain that serve as support structures for neurons.	**glio / blast / oma** glue / sprout / tumor **Note:** *Blast* means "sprout" or "seed" and refers to a type of early formative cell that grows or develops into a mature cell later on.

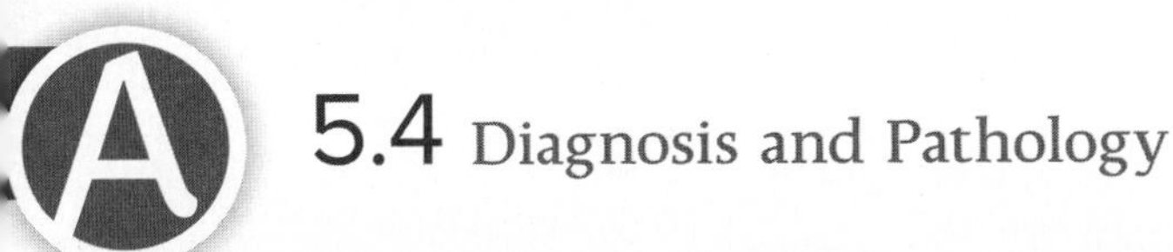

5.4 Diagnosis and Pathology

structure *continued*

Term	Word Analysis
meningioma meh-NIN-jee-OH-mah **Definition** tumor of the meninges	**meningi / oma** meninges / tumor
Other	
cerebellitis SEH-rah-bell-AI-tis **Definition** inflammation of the cerebellum	**cerebell / itis** cerebellum / inflammation
cerebromeningitis seh-REE-broh-MEN-in-JAI-tis **Definition** inflammation of the brain and meninges	**cerebro / mening / itis** brain / meninges / inflammation
encephalitis in-SEF-ah-LAI-tis **Definition** inflammation of the brain	**encephal / itis** brain / inflammation
encephalomyelitis in-SEF-ah-loh-MAI-eh-LAI-tis **Definition** inflammation of the brain and spinal cord	**encephalo / myel / itis** brain / spinal cord / inflammation
encephalomyeloneuropathy in-SEF-ah-loh-MAI-el-oh-nir-AW-pah-thee **Definition** disease of the brain, spinal cord, and nerves	**encephalo / myelo / neuro / pathy** brain / spinal cord / nerve / disease
encephalopathy in-SEF-ah-LAW-pah-thee **Definition** disease of the brain	**encephalo / pathy** brain / disease
encephalopyosis in-SEF-ah-loh-pai-OH-sis **Definition** a pus-filled abscess in the brain	**encephalo / py / osis** brain / pus / condition ©McGraw-Hill Education
gangliitis GAN-glee-AI-tis **Definition** inflammation of a ganglion	**gangli / itis** ganglion / inflammation
intracerebral hemorrhage IN-trah-sih-REE-bral HIH-moh-rij **Definition** excessive bleeding inside the brain	**intra / cerebr / al** inside / brain / pertaining to **hemo / rrhage** blood / excessive bleeding ©McGraw-Hill Education

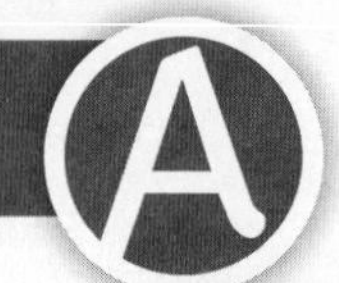

5.4 Diagnosis and Pathology

structure *continued*

Term	Word Analysis
meningopathy MEH-nin-GAW-pah-thee **Definition** disease of the meninges	**meningo / pathy** meninges / disease
meningitis MEH-nin-JAI-tus **Definition** inflammation of the meninges	**mening / itis** meninges / inflammation
meningoencephalitis meh-NIN-goh-in-SEF-ah-LAI-tis **Definition** inflammation of the meninges and brain	**meningo / encephal / itis** meninges / brain / inflammation
myelitis MAI-eh-LAI-tis **Definition** inflammation of the spinal cord	**myel / itis** spinal cord / inflammation
myelodysplasia MAI-eh-loh-dis-PLAY-zhah **Definition** defective formation of the spinal cord **NOTE:** Since the root *myelo* can be used for both spinal cord and bone marrow, this term is also used to mean "bad bone marrow formation"; you can tell them apart by considering the context they occur in.	**myelo / dys / plas / ia** spinal cord / bad / formation / condition
myelopathy MAI-el-AW-pah-thee **Definition** disease of the spinal cord	**myelo / pathy** spinal cord / disease
neuroarthropathy NIR-oh-ar-THRAW-pah-thee **Definition** disease of the joint associated with nerves	**neuro / arthro / pathy** nerve / joint / disease
neuroencephalomyelopathy NIR-oh-in-SEF-ah-loh-MAI-el-AW-pah-thee **Definition** disease of the nerves, brain, and spinal cord	**neuro / encephalo / myelo / pathy** nerve / brain / spinal cord / disease
neuropathy nir-AW-pah-thee **Definition** disease of the nervous system	**neuro / pathy** nerve / disease
poliomyelitis POH-lee-oh-MAI-el-AI-tis **Definition** inflammation of the gray matter of the spinal cord **NOTE:** This is the full name of the disease known as polio.	**polio / myel / itis** gray / spinal cord / inflammation
polyneuropathy PAW-lee-nir-AW-pah-thee **Definition** disease affecting multiple nerves	**poly / neuro / pathy** many / nerve / disease

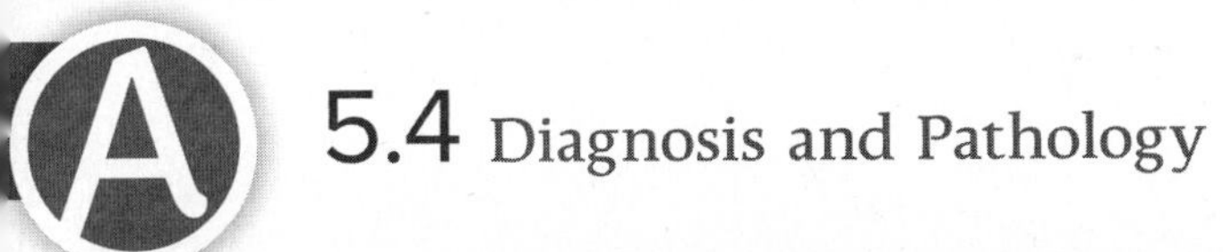

5.4 Diagnosis and Pathology

function

Term	Word Analysis
amyotrophic lateral sclerosis (ALS) a-MAI-aw-TROH-fik LAT-tih-ral skleh-ROH-sis	a / myo / troph / ic lateral scler / osis not / muscle / nourishment / pertaining to side hardening / condition
Definition a degenerative disease of the central nervous system causing loss of muscle control. Literally, the hardening (*sclerosis*) of the nerve cells on the sides (*lateral*) of the spine leading to the loss of muscle tissue from disuse. **NOTE:** This disease is more commonly known as Lou Gehrig's disease, after the famous baseball player was diagnosed with it in 1939.	
anorexia a-noh-REK-see-ah	an / orex / ia no / appetite / condition
Definition an eating disorder characterized by the patient's refusal to eat	
autism AH-tiz-um	aut / ism self / condition
Definition a psychiatric disorder characterized by withdrawal from communication with others; the patient is focused only on the self	
bulimia boo-LEE-mee-ah	bu / lim / ia ox / hunger / condition
Definition an eating disorder characterized by overeating and usually followed by forced vomiting	
cerebral palsy seh-REE-bral PAL-zee	cerebr / al palsy brain / pertaining to paralysis
Definition paralysis caused by damage to the area of the brain responsible for movement **NOTE:** *Palsy* is a less common word for paralysis.	
dysphoria dis-FOR-ee-ah	dys / phor / ia bad / carry / condition
Definition a negative emotional state	
epilepsy eh-pih-LEP-see	epi / lepsy upon / seize
Definition a disease marked by seizures	
euphoria yoo-FOR-ee-ah	eu / phor / ia good / carry / condition
Definition a positive emotional state	
hypomania HAI-poh-MAY-nee-ah	hypo / mania under / excessive anger
Definition a mental state just below mania	
manic depression (bipolar) MAN-ik de-PREH-shun	manic depression excitement depression
Definition a psychiatric disorder characterized by alternating bouts of excitement and depression **NOTE:** This disease is referred to by the name *bipolar* because the patient fluctuates between two extremes.	
myasthenia mai-as-THEH-nee-ah	my / asthenia muscle / weakness
Definition muscle weakness	
narcolepsy NAR-coh-LEP-see	narco / lepsy sleep / seize
Definition a disease characterized by sudden, uncontrolled sleepiness	
neurosis neh-ROH-sis	neur / osis nerve / condition
Definition a nerve condition	

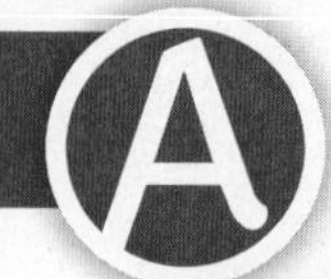

5.4 Diagnosis and Pathology

function *continued*

Term	Word Analysis
psychosis sai-KOH-sis **Definition** a mind condition	**psych / osis** mind / condition
NOTE: Both *neurosis* and *psychosis* are general terms of psychiatric conditions, but a neurosis doesn't interfere with rational thought or daily functioning; a psychosis involves some sort of break with reality.	
psychopathy sai-KAW-pah-thee **Definition** a mental illness	**psycho / pathy** mind / disease
schizophrenia SKIT-zoh-FREH-nee-ah **Definition** a mental illness characterized by delusions, hallucinations, and disordered speech	**schizo / phren / ia** divide / mind / condition
NOTE: *Schizo* refers to the division in the mind between the mind itself and reality, not the division of the mind into multiple personalities.	

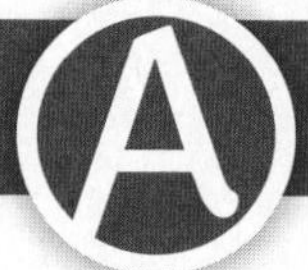

Learning Outcome 5.4 Exercises

PRONUNCIATION

EXERCISE 1 *Indicate which syllable is emphasized when pronounced.*

EXAMPLE: bronchitis bron**chi**tis

1. neuropathy ______
2. anorexia ______
3. autism ______
4. bulimia ______
5. dysphoria ______
6. euphoria ______
7. epilepsy ______
8. neurosis ______
9. psychosis ______
10. psychopathy ______
11. myelodysplasia ______
12. ganglioma ______
13. craniosclerosis ______
14. meningitis ______

TRANSLATION

EXERCISE 2 *Break down the following words into their component parts.*

EXAMPLE: nasopharyngoscope *naso | pharyngo | scope*

1. hypomania ______
2. dysphoria ______
3. euphoria ______
4. psychopathy ______
5. intracerebral ______
6. cerebrovascular ______
7. craniosclerosis ______
8. craniostenosis ______

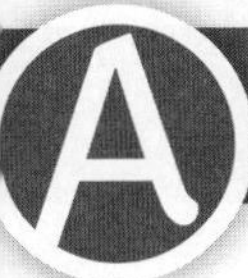

Learning Outcome 5.4 Exercises

9. gangliitis ______
10. meningitis ______
11. cerebromeningitis ______
12. encephalitis ______
13. encephalomyelitis ______
14. poliomyelitis ______
15. encephalopathy ______
16. encephalomyeloneuropathy ______
17. neuroarthropathy ______
18. myelodysplasia ______

EXERCISE 3 *Underline and define the word parts from this chapter in the following terms.*

1. encephalopyosis ______
2. cerebral aneurysm ______
3. cerebral embolism ______
4. craniomalacia ______
5. craniosynostosis ______
6. hydrocephaly ______
7. cerebellitis ______
8. ganglioma ______
9. meningopathy ______
10. meningioma ______
11. meningoencephalitis (2 roots) ______
12. myelitis ______
13. myelopathy ______
14. neuropathy ______
15. polyneuropathy ______
16. amyotrophic lateral sclerosis ______
17. cerebral palsy ______
18. manic depression ______
19. myasthenia ______
20. neurosis ______
21. psychosis ______
22. schizophrenia ______

EXERCISE 4 *Match the term on the left with its definition on the right.*

Term	Definition
______ 1. autism	a. an accident involving the blood vessels of the brain
______ 2. bulimia	b. loss of brain function caused by interruption of blood flow/supply to the brain
______ 3. anorexia	c. a stroke where the blood loss is caused by the rupture of a blood vessel
______ 4. epilepsy	d. a stroke where the blood loss is caused by blockage
______ 5. stroke	e. a mini-stroke caused by the blockage of a blood vessel that resolves (goes away) within 24 hours
______ 6. transient ischemic attack (TIA)	f. the hardening of an artery in the brain
______ 7. hemorrhagic stroke	g. the hardening of an artery in the brain caused by the buildup of fatty plaque
______ 8. narcolepsy	h. the blockage of a blood vessel in the brain caused by a blood clot
______ 9. cerebral atherosclerosis	i. an eating disorder characterized by overeating and usually followed by forced vomiting
______ 10. cerebral thrombosis	j. an eating disorder characterized by the patient's refusal to eat
______ 11. cerebral arteriosclerosis	k. a psychiatric disorder characterized by the withdrawal from communication with others; the patient is focused only on the self
______ 12. cerebrovascular accident (CVA)	l. a disease marked by seizures
______ 13. ischemic stroke	m. a disease characterized by sudden, uncontrolled sleepiness

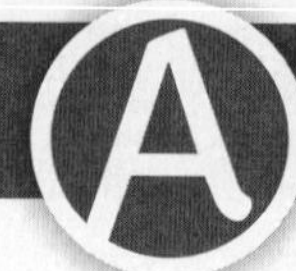

Learning Outcome 5.4 Exercises

EXERCISE 5 *Translate the following terms as literally as possible.*

EXAMPLE: nasopharyngoscope *an instrument for looking at the nose and throat*

1. hypomania ______
2. gangliitis ______
3. meningitis ______
4. meningoencephalitis ______
5. meningopathy ______
6. psychopathy ______
7. encephalopathy ______
8. encephalomyeloneuropathy ______
9. encephalopyosis ______
10. myelodysplasia ______
11. myelopathy ______
12. neuropathy ______
13. polyneuropathy ______
14. poliomyelitis ______
15. dysphoria ______
16. euphoria ______
17. bulimia ______
18. cerebrovascular accident ______
19. craniosynostosis ______

GENERATION

EXERCISE 6 *Build a medical term from the information provided.*

EXAMPLE: inflammation of the sinuses *sinusitis*

1. ganglion tumor ______
2. meninges tumor ______
3. inflammation of the spinal cord ______
4. inflammation of the cerebellum ______
5. inflammation of the brain (*cerebro*) and meninges ______
6. inflammation of the brain (use *encephalo*) ______
7. inflammation of the brain (*encephalo*) and spinal cord ______
8. abnormal narrowing of the skull ______

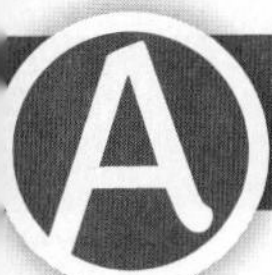

Learning Outcome 5.4 Exercises

9. literally, *water head condition* ________________
10. a disease of the blood vessels of the brain ________________
11. disease of the joint associated with nerves ________________
12. muscle weakness condition ________________

EXERCISE 7 *Multiple-choice questions. Select the correct answer.*

1. Anorexia is:
   a. a disease marked by seizures
   b. an eating disorder characterized by the patient's refusal to eat
   c. an eating disorder characterized by overeating and usually followed by forced vomiting
   d. a psychiatric disorder characterized by the withdrawal from communication with others
2. Autism is:
   a. a disease marked by seizures
   b. an eating disorder characterized by the patient's refusal to eat
   c. an eating disorder characterized by overeating and usually followed by forced vomiting
   d. a psychiatric disorder characterized by the withdrawal from communication with others
3. Epilepsy is:
   a. a disease marked by seizures
   b. an eating disorder characterized by the patient's refusal to eat
   c. an eating disorder characterized by overeating and usually followed by forced vomiting
   d. a psychiatric disorder characterized by the withdrawal from communication with others
4. A person who is *narcoleptic* has a disease characterized by sudden, uncontrolled:
   a. desire for food
   b. sleepiness
   c. desire for medication
   d. withdrawal into self
5. A person with *cerebral palsy* has paralysis caused by damage to the area of the brain responsible for:
   a. emotion
   b. hunger
   c. movement
   d. feeling/sensation
6. A loss of brain function caused by interruption of blood flow/supply to the brain is:
   a. stroke
   b. hemorrhagia
   c. cerebral aneurysm
   d. cerebrovascular disease
   e. intracerebral hemorrhage
7. The widening or abnormal dilation of a blood vessel in the brain is a(n):
   a. stroke
   b. hemorrhagia
   c. cerebral aneurysm
   d. cerebrovascular disease
   e. intracerebral hemorrhage
8. Excessive bleeding inside the brain is a(n):
   a. stroke
   b. hemorrhagia
   c. cerebral aneurysm
   d. cerebrovascular disease
   e. intracerebral hemorrhage
9. The common name for this disease is Lou Gehrig's disease.
   a. poliomyelitis
   b. cerebral palsy
   c. encephalomyelitis
   d. amyotrophic lateral sclerosis (ALS)

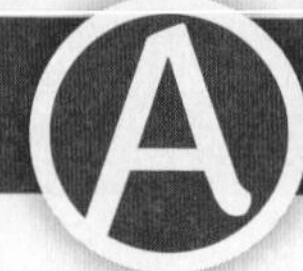

Learning Outcome 5.4 Exercises

10. An alternate term for someone who has *manic depression* is:
    a. bipolar
    b. autistic
    c. phrenetic
    d. schizophrenic

11. Which of the following characteristics is *not* displayed by a schizophrenic?
    a. delusions
    b. disordered speech
    c. hallucinations
    d. multiple personalities

EXERCISE 8 *Briefly describe the difference between each pair of terms.*

1. craniomalacia, craniosclerosis ____________________
2. neurosis, psychosis ____________________
3. hemorrhagic stroke, ischemic stroke ____________________
4. ischemic stroke, transient ischemic attack (TIA) ____________________
5. cerebral arteriosclerosis, cerebral atherosclerosis ____________________
6. cerebral embolism, cerebral thrombosis ____________________

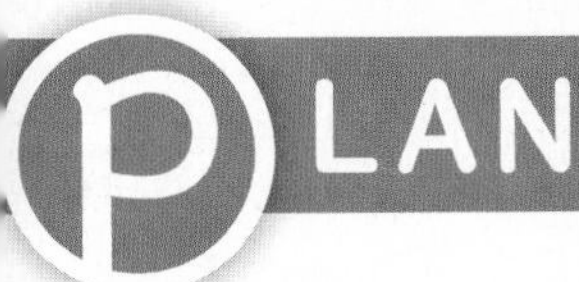

5.5 Treatments and Therapies

There are few medicines that work directly on the neurologic system. The largest class of neurologic medicine works to dull the pain reception from nerves (*anesthetics*). Anesthetics have revolutionized medicine. They may be injected into a small area (*local*), injected into a group of nerves (*epidural*), or even affect the entire body (*general*). In fact, this type of medicine is so critical, there is an entire medical specialty devoted to its use (*anesthesiology*). Another large class of neurologic medicine treats seizures (*anticonvulsants*).

Perhaps one of the fastest-growing areas in drug development has been the field of psychiatry. There are numerous medicines to treat problems of the mind. Whether they treat depression (*antidepressants*), anxiety (*anxiolytics*), or psychosis (*antipsychotics*), these medicines all work in a similar fashion—by altering the response or availability of the chemicals that allow communication between nerves (*neurotransmitters*). Psychiatric medicines work by increasing or decreasing the activity of specific neurotransmitters that lead to an increase or decrease in activity of certain areas of the brain.

Surgical interventions to treat neurologic disorders can involve direct cutting and cleaning of a partially blocked artery, as in *endarterectomy*. Treating diseased blood vessels in the brain may also be carried out by less-invasive techniques such as radiology guided therapy. In endovascular neurology, medicines are injected into specific areas to cause or destroy clots, depending on the need. Neurosurgery can also be used to treat problems of the nervous system's support structures. These procedures can help remedy skull problems (*cranioplasty*), or to remove part of the vertebral bone (*laminectomy*) or an intervertebral disc (*discectomy*). In cases of hydrocephalus, a special drain can be inserted leading from the brain into another part of the body. Most commonly, the drain is placed in the open area surrounding the inside of the abdomen. This type of shunt is called a ventriculoperitoneal (VP) shunt. Invasive brain surgery may be necessary to remove a tumor, to place a device to monitor the pressure in the brain, to insert a device to treat seizures, or to remove part of a lobe of the brain (*lobectomy*). Nerves have traditionally posed a challenge to repair surgically, but advances are being made that allow for nerves to be reconnected (*neurorrhaphy*).

anesthesiology

Term	Word Analysis
anesthetic an-es-THET-ik **Definition** a drug that causes loss of sensation	**an / esthetic** not / sensation
general anesthetic JEH-nir-al an-es-THET-ik **Definition** anesthetic that causes complete loss of consciousness	**general anesthetic**
local anesthetic LOH-kal an-es-THET-ik **Definition** anesthetic that does not affect consciousness	**local anesthetic**
regional anesthetic REE-jih-nal an-es-THET-ik **Definition** anesthetic that is injected into a nerve causing loss of sensation over a particular area	**regional anesthetic**
topical anesthetic TAW-pih-kal an-es-THET-ik **Definition** local anesthesia applied to the surface of the area to be anesthetized	**topical anesthetic**

anesthesiology *continued*

Term	Word Analysis
epidural anesthetic eh-pih-DUH-ral an-es-THET-ik **Definition** anesthetic applied in the dural region of the spinal cord	**epi / dur / al** upon / dura

pharmacology

Term	Word Analysis
analgesic an-al-JEE-zik **Definition** a drug that relieves pain	**an / alge / sic** not / pain / agent
anticonvulsant AN-tee-kon-VUL-sant **Definition** a drug that opposes convulsions	**anti / convuls / ant** against / convulsion / agent
antidepressant AN-tee-deh-PREH-sant **Definition** a drug that opposes depression	**anti / depress / ant** against / depression / agent
antipsychotic AN-tee-sai-KAW-tik **Definition** a drug that opposes psychoses	**anti / psycho / tic** against / psychosis / agent
anxiolytic ANG-zee-oh-LIH-tik **Definition** a drug that lessens anxiety	**anxio / lytic** anxiety / breakdown agent
hypnotic hip-NAWT-ik **Definition** a drug that aids sleep	**hypno / tic** sleep / agent
neuropharmacology nir-oh-FAR-mah-KAW-loh-jee **Definition** the study of the effects of drugs on the nervous system	**neuro / pharmaco / logy** nerve / drug / study ©Image Source/Image Source/Getty Images RF
psychopharmacology SAI-koh-FAR- mah-KAW-loh-jee **Definition** the study of the effects of drugs on mental processes	**psycho / pharmaco / logy** mind / drug / study

pharmacology *continued*

Term	Word Analysis
pyschotropic SAI-koh-TROH-pik **Definition** drugs that are able to turn the mind	**psycho / trop / ic** mind / turn / agent
thrombolytic THRAWM-boh-LIT-ik **Definition** a drug that dissolves clots	**thrombo / lytic** clot / breakdown agent

surgical procedures and treatments

Term	Word Analysis
cerebrotomy seh-ree-BRAW-toh-mee **Definition** incision into the brain	**cerebro / tomy** brain / incision
chemotherapy KEE-moh-THER-ah-pee **Definition** treatment using chemicals	**chemo / therapy** chemical / treatment 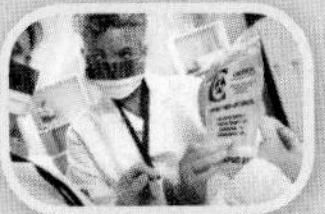 ©fstop123/E+/Getty Images RF
craniectomy KRAY-nee-EK-toh-mee **Definition** removal of a piece of the skull	**crani / ectomy** skull / removal
craniotomy KRAY-nee-AW-toh-mee **Definition** incision into the skull	**cranio / tomy** skull / incision
endarterectomy EN-dar-tir-EK-toh-mee **Definition** removal of the inside of an artery	**end / arter / ectomy** inside / artery / removal
endovascular neurosurgery EN-doh-VAS-kyoo-lar NIR-oh-SIR-jir-ee **Definition** surgery on the nervous system performed by entering the body through blood vessels	**endo / vascul / ar neuro / surgery** inside / vessel / pertaining to nerve / surgery
lobectomy loh-BEK-toh-mee **Definition** removal of a lobe	**lob / ectomy** lobe / removal
lobotomy loh-BAW-toh-mee **Definition** incision into a lobe	**lobo / tomy** lobe / incision
neurectomy nir-EK-toh-mee **Definition** removal of a nerve	**neur / ectomy** nerve / removal

surgical procedures and treatments *continued*

Term	Word Analysis
neurolysis nir-AW-lih-sis **Definition** destruction of nerve tissue **NOTE:** You may wonder why this term is under treatment and not disease; the reason is because one common treatment for chronic nerve pain is to destroy the nerve causing it.	**neuro / lysis** nerve / loose
neuroplasty NIR-oh-PLAS-tee **Definition** reconstruction of a nerve	**neuro / plasty** nerve / reconstruction
neurorrhaphy nir-OR-ah-fee **Definition** suturing of a nerve (often the severed ends of a nerve)	**neuro / rrhaphy** nerve / suture
neurotomy nir-AW-toh-mee **Definition** incision into a nerve	**neuro / tomy** nerve / incision

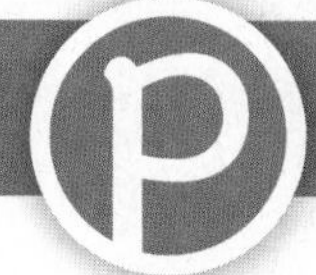

Learning Outcome 5.5 Exercises

PRONUNCIATION

EXERCISE 1 *Indicate which syllable is emphasized when pronounced.*

EXAMPLE: bronchitis bron**chi**tis

1. anesthetic ____________
2. antidepressant ____________
3. craniectomy ____________
4. craniotomy ____________
5. endarterectomy ____________
6. neuroplasty ____________
7. epidural anesthetic ____________
8. thrombolytic ____________
9. anticonvulsant ____________
10. chemotherapy ____________
11. hypnotic ____________
12. lobotomy ____________
13. neurotomy ____________
14. cerebrotomy ____________
15. lobectomy ____________
16. neurectomy ____________
17. anxiolytic ____________
18. neurolysis ____________

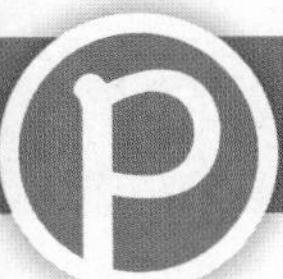

Learning Outcome 5.5 Exercises

TRANSLATION

EXERCISE 2 *Break down the following words into their component parts.*

EXAMPLE: nasopharyngoscope *naso | pharyngo | scope*

1. craniotomy ______
2. lobotomy ______
3. neurotomy ______
4. neurolysis ______
5. neuroplasty ______
6. antipsychotic ______
7. neuropharmacology ______
8. psychopharmacology ______

EXERCISE 3 *Underline and define the word parts from this chapter in the following terms.*

1. anesthetic ______
2. epidural ______
3. hypnotic ______
4. psychotropic ______
5. cerebrotomy ______
6. lobectomy ______
7. neurectomy ______
8. craniectomy ______
9. neurorrhaphy ______
10. endovascular neurosurgery ______

EXERCISE 4 *Match the term on the left with its definition on the right.*

______	1. analgesic	a.	anesthetic that causes complete loss of consciousness
______	2. anticonvulsant	b.	anesthetic that does not affect consciousness
______	3. antidepressant	c.	anesthetic that is injected into a nerve, causing loss of sensation over a particular area
______	4. anxiolytic	d.	local anesthesia applied to the surface of the treatment area using chemicals
______	5. chemotherapy	e.	a drug that relieves pain
______	6. endarterectomy	f.	a drug that opposes convulsions
______	7. general anesthetic	g.	a drug that opposes depression
______	8. local anesthetic	h.	a drug that lessens anxiety

_____ 9. regional anesthetic — i. a drug that dissolves clots

_____ 10. thrombolytic — j. treatment using chemicals

_____ 11. topical anesthetic — k. removal of the inside of an artery

EXERCISE 5 *Translate the following terms as literally as possible.*

EXAMPLE: nasopharyngoscope *an instrument for looking at the nose and throat*

1. anesthetic ______________________
2. craniectomy ______________________
3. lobotomy ______________________
4. neurotomy ______________________
5. neurolysis ______________________
6. neurorrhaphy ______________________
7. neuropharmacology ______________________
8. psychopharmacology ______________________

GENERATION

EXERCISE 6 *Build a medical term from the information provided.*

EXAMPLE: inflammation of the sinuses *sinusitis*

1. sleep agent ______________________
2. brain incision ______________________
3. skull incision ______________________
4. lobe removal ______________________
5. nerve removal ______________________
6. nerve reconstruction ______________________
7. chemical treatment ______________________
8. anesthetic applied in the dural region of the spinal cord ______________________
9. a drug (literally, agent) that opposes psychosis ______________________

EXERCISE 7 *Multiple-choice questions. Select the correct answer.*

1. *Endovascular neurosurgery* is surgery on the nervous system performed by entering the body through:

   a. the heart
   b. the spine
   c. nerve tissue
   d. blood vessels

2. A medical professional may recommend which drug to relieve pain?

   a. analgesic
   b. anxiolytic
   c. general anesthetic
   d. thrombolytic

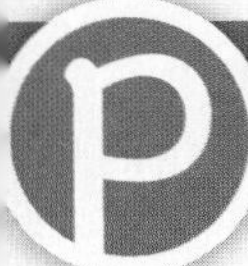

Learning Outcome 5.5 Exercises

3. The root *trope* in the term *psychotropic* means
   - a. to turn
   - b. to lessen
   - c. to oppose
   - d. to remove

4. Which term means "the removal of the inside of an artery"?
   - a. endarterectomy
   - b. subarterectomy
   - c. endarterotomy
   - d. subarterotomy

EXERCISE 8 *Briefly describe the difference between each pair of terms.*

1. anticonvulsant, antidepressant ________________
2. anxiolytic, thrombolytic ________________
3. general anesthetic, local anesthetic ________________
4. regional anesthetic, topical anesthetic ________________

5.6 Abbreviations

Abbreviations provide medical professionals with a shorthand for writing words that commonly occur in their field. In neurology and psychiatry, these abbreviations can refer to things ranging from procedures (EEG), to common diagnoses (MS), to parts of the system itself (CNS).

nervous system abbreviations

Abbreviation	Definition
ADHD	attention-deficit hyperactivity disorder
ALS	amyotrophic lateral sclerosis (Lou Gehrig's disease)
CNS	central nervous system
CP	cerebral palsy
CSF	cerebrospinal fluid
CVA	cerebrovascular accident
EEG	electroencephalogram
EMG	electromyogram
ICP	intracranial pressure
LOC	level of consciousness
LP	lumbar puncture
MRA	magnetic resonance angiography
MS	multiple sclerosis
OCD	obsessive compulsive disorder
PET	positron emission tomography
PNS	peripheral nervous system
TIA	transient ischemic attack

Learning Outcome 5.6 Exercises

EXERCISE 1 *Define the following abbreviations.*

1. ADHD ______
2. MS ______
3. TIA ______
4. ALS ______
5. CSF ______
6. PET ______
7. LOC ______
8. ICP ______
9. PNS ______
10. CP ______

EXERCISE 2 *Give the abbreviations for the following definitions.*

1. lumbar puncture ______
2. central nervous system ______
3. obsessive compulsive disorder ______
4. magnetic resonance angiography ______
5. cerebrovascular accident ______
6. electromyogram ______
7. electroencephalogram ______
8. stereotactic radiosurgery ______
9. amyotrophic lateral sclerosis ______

Learning Outcome 5.6 Exercises

EXERCISE 3 *Multiple-choice questions. Select the correct answer.*

1. Problems with which part of the body can result in a person having problems sending or receiving signals to the brain?
   a. CNS
   b. CSF
   c. PET
   d. PNS
2. Problems with which part of the body can affect the entire body?
   a. CNS
   b. CSF
   c. PET
   d. PNS
3. Which of the following is NOT a medical procedure?
   a. EEG
   b. LP
   c. MRA
   d. CSF
4. A person who has an accident involving the blood vessels of the brain has a(n):
   a. CVA
   b. CNS
   c. MS
   d. PNS
5. A mini-stroke caused by the blockage of a blood vessel that resolves within 24 hours is a(n):
   a. ICP
   b. LOC
   c. ADHD
   d. TIA
6. A procedure used to examine the electrical activity of the brain is a(n):
   a. CSF
   b. CVA
   c. EEG
   d. EMG

5.7 Electronic Health Records

Subjective

Mrs. Voxenhead is here for follow-up for her **schizophrenia**. At her last visit, she complained of **dystonia** on her haloperidol. I changed her to a newer **antipsychotic**, and she is here today to follow up the results. Overall, her condition is improved, and she has not had any new hallucinations. Her only concern today is recent **insomnia** (the past week). She noticed the insomnia started when she began a new job. She says that learning her new job has been stressful. She has been anxious at night, and that has made it hard for her to sleep.

Objective

General: She does not appear agitated. Her affect is flat. Her mood is not **dysphoric**. She is alert, oriented.

HEENT: Pupils equal, round, and reactive to light. Tonsils normal size.

Resp: Clear breath sounds.

CV: RRR without murmur, gallop, rubs.

Neuro: Normal movement. No **dyskinesia**. Normal muscle tone.

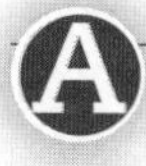

Assessment

1. Schizophrenia: Stable on new medical regimen.
2. Insomnia. Likely related to new job stress.

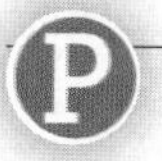

Plan

1. I will begin her short term on an **anxiolytic**.
2. Continue antipsychotic.
3. Follow-up visit in 2 months.
4. Continue following up with **psychologist**.

–Electronically signed by
Dale Kelly, MD
03/04/2015 9:30 AM

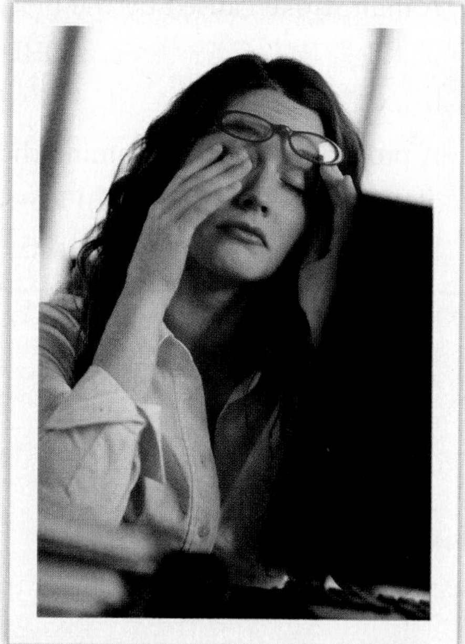

Learning Outcome 5.7 Exercises

EXERCISE 1 *Match the term on the left with its definition on the right.*

______	1. schizophrenia	a. a drug that opposes psychosis
______	2. dystonia	b. a condition characterized by involuntary muscle movements
______	3. antipsychotic	c. a mental illness characterized by delusions, hallucinations, and disordered speech
______	4. insomnia	d. inability to sleep
______	5. dysphoric	e. a negative emotional state
______	6. dyskinesia	f. difficulty moving
______	7. anxiolytic	g. a drug that lessens anxiety
______	8. psychologist	h. a doctor who specializes in the study of the mind

EXERCISE 2 *Refer to the document on the previous page and fill in the blanks.*

1. Mrs. Voxenhead is following up on her *schizophrenia* (give definition: ______________________).
2. Her mood is not characterized as ______________________ (negative emotional state).
3. Learning her new job has made Mrs. Voxenhead stressed; this is likely related to her *insomnia* (give definition: ______________________).
4. Mrs. Voxenhead will continue to follow up with a(n) ______________________ (doctor who specializes in the study of the mind).

EXERCISE 3 *True or false questions. Refer to the document on the previous page and indicate true answers with a T and false answers with an F.*

1. The patient suffers from a mental illness characterized by hallucinations. ________
2. Mrs. Voxenhead complained of involuntary muscle movements during her last visit. ________
3. The antipsychotic has helped her sleep much better. ________
4. Mrs. Voxenhead will continue to follow up with a psychopharmacologist. ________

EXERCISE 4 *Multiple-choice questions. Refer to the document on the previous page and select the correct answer.*

1. An *anxiolytic* and *antipsychotic* are both:
   a. drugs that lessen and/or oppose
   b. drugs that increase and/or heighten
   c. drugs that remove sensation
2. The plan for treating Mrs. Voxenhead is to:
   a. discontinue her antipsychotic and begin an anxiolytic
   b. continue her antipsychotic and begin an anxiolytic
   c. discontinue her anxiolytic and begin an antipsychotic
   d. continue her anxiolytic and begin an antipsychotic
3. The medical professional who wrote the health record for Mrs. Voxenhead is Dale Kelly, MD. Dr. Kelly is a:
   a. psychologist
   b. psychiatrist
   c. psychogenist
   d. neuropharmacologist

Emergency Department Visit

Patient Name: Manuel Skayken

Chief Complaint: Confusion, fever.

History of Present Illness:

Manuel Skayken is a 15-year-old boy who presents with a 2-day history of fever to 104°F. He has been more lethargic today and his headache has worsened. He has **photophobia** and his parents are concerned that he is acting abnormally. He is not using his right arm and legs as much as his left. He appears **ataxic** in his gait and has been **hypersomnolent** at home. His parents are concerned that he is not responding to questions normally.

Past Medical History: **Somnambulation,** otherwise noncontributory.

Medications: None.

Allergies: NKDA.

Social History: Lives at home with his parents.

Sophomore in high school. A/B student. Nonsmoker.

Surgical History: None.

Physical Exam:

RR: 30; HR: 98; Temp: 104.2; BP: 88/60

Gen: WDWN. Lethargic.

Confused and disoriented.

HEENT: PERRLA, mild **nystagmus.**

Neck: Stiff.

CV: Mildly fast heart rate. No murmurs.

Resp: Clear.

GI: Normal.

Neuro: CN II-XII grossly intact; DTRs normal.

Hemiparesis: Strength in right arm and leg.

Failed mini-mental status exam.

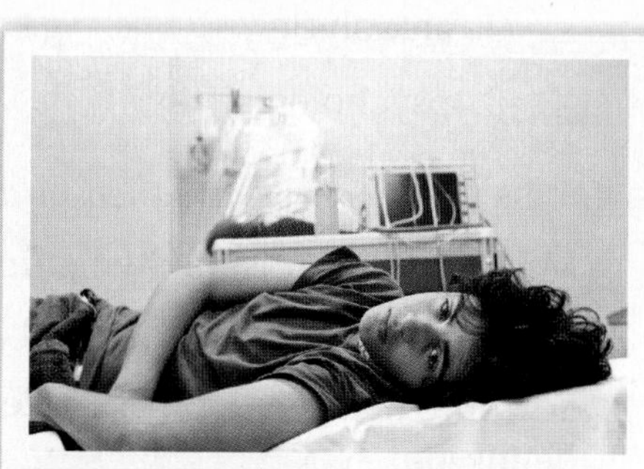

Emergency Department Course:

Manuel was driven to the emergency room by his parents. On arrival, he appeared very confused, though not agitated. With his **encephalopathic** picture, we were most worried about **psychotropic** drug abuse or infection. A normal urine drug screen and an elevated white blood cell count were suspicious for infection. Because **encephalitis** and **meningitis** were the main concerns, we performed a **lumbar puncture**. The opening pressure was consistent with elevated **intracranial pressure**. The **CSF** showed an elevated white blood cell count. The spinal fluid culture is pending. Shortly after his lumbar puncture, Manuel had a **seizure**. We treated him with an **anticonvulsant** and the seizure stopped. The **electroencephalogram** findings were characteristic of herpes encephalitis. The pediatric team was called, and they admitted him to the PICU.

Learning Outcome 5.7 Exercises

EXERCISE 5 *Match the term on the left with its definition on the right.*

_____	1. anticonvulsant	a.	excessive sensitivity to light
_____	2. encephalitis	b.	lack of coordination
_____	3. meningitis	c.	drugs that are able to turn the mind
_____	4. EEG	d.	inflammation of the brain
_____	5. psychotropic	e.	inflammation of the meninges
_____	6. ICP	f.	intracranial pressure
_____	7. photophobia	g.	electroencephalography
_____	8. ataxia	h.	a drug that opposes convulsions

EXERCISE 6 *Refer to the document on the previous page and fill in the blanks.*

1. The patient's gait has been ______________________________ (lacking coordination).
2. The root word in *hypersomnolent* is ______________________________ (sleep).
3. Manuel has mild ______________________________ (involuntary back and forth eye movements).
4. The root word in *encephalopathic* is *encephalo,* which means ______________________________.
5. The term *intracranial* comes from combining __________ (inside) and *cranio,* which means __________.

EXERCISE 7 *True or false questions. Refer to the document on the previous page and indicate true answers with a T and false answers with an F.*

1. Manuel has not been sleeping as much as usual at home. __________
2. The medical professionals worried that Manuel was abusing drugs. __________
3. Because of their concern about encephalitis and meningitis, the health professionals performed an LP. __________
4. In response to his seizure, Manuel was given a thrombolytic. __________

EXERCISE 8 *Multiple-choice questions. Select the correct answer.*

1. *Photophobia* is defined as:
   a. fear of fire
   b. excessive sensitivity to light
   c. fear of pictures
   d. fear of outdoor spaces
2. A seizure characterized by alternating bouts of muscle spasms and weak or unresponsive muscles is:
   a. tonic
   b. clonic
   c. tonic-clonic
   d. ischemic
3. *Hemiparesis* is defined as:
   a. partial paralysis on half of the body
   b. complete paralysis on half of the body
   c. partial paralysis of one limb
   d. complete paralysis of one limb

Learning Outcome 5.7 Exercises

4. The health professionals were concerned about the possibility of which two conditions?
   a. inflammation of the brain and the membrane surrounding the brain and spinal cord
   b. inflammation of the brain and spinal cord
   c. inflammation of the spinal cord and the tough outer membrane surrounding the brain and spinal cord
   d. inflammation of the spinal cord and the membrane surrounding the brain and spinal cord
5. Which procedures were used to assist in the diagnosis and treatment of the patient?
   a. LP, EEG
   b. CSF, EEG
   c. LP, CSF
   d. EEG, LP, ICP
   e. ICP, LP, CSF

Brief Admission Summary Letter

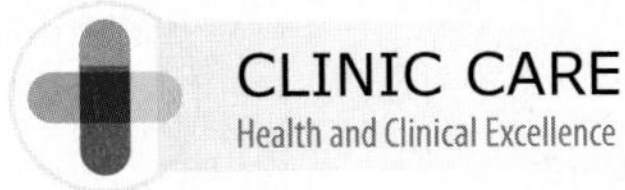

Dear Dr. Dowling,

This letter is to inform you that your patient Sally Chia has been admitted to Bed 4 of the ICU for observation and treatment of recent CVA. As you know, I have been following Mrs. Chia for cerebrovascular disease. She has had two transient ischemic attacks in the past 2 years and underwent a carotid endarterectomy last February. She presented to the ED last night with a sudden onset of left-sided hemiparesis and hyperesthesia. She was also noted to have mild agnosia and aphasia. She was brought to the ED by her husband, who is not sure when the symptoms began. A cerebral CT and CT angiogram showed middle cerebral artery occlusion and ruled out intracranial hemorrhage or hematoma. She was treated with a thrombolytic. Her symptoms have improved.

—I. C. Hilliard, MD

Learning Outcome 5.7 Exercises

EXERCISE 9 *Match the term on the left with its definition on the right.*

______	1. hemiparesis	a. inability to comprehend
______	2. agnosia	b. partial paralysis on half of the body
______	3. hyperesthesia	c. cerebrovascular accident
______	4. aphasia	d. increased sensation
______	5. CVA	e. inability to speak
______	6. transient ischemic attack	f. a mini-stroke caused by the blockage of a blood vessel that resolves (goes away) within 24 hours

EXERCISE 10 *Fill in the blanks.*

1. Last February, Mrs. Chia underwent a carotid ______________________ (removal of the inside of an artery).
2. She was treated with a *thrombolytic* (give definition: ______________________________________).
3. Mrs. Chia's CT scans ruled out *intracranial* (inside the ______________) hemorrhage or ______________ (a tumorlike mass made up of blood).

EXERCISE 11 *True or false questions. Indicate true answers with a T and false answers with an F.*

1. The patient suffered a recent CVA. ________
2. Mrs. Chia has had two TIAs in the past 2 years. ________
3. Dr. Hilliard is writing to Dr. Dowling to inform him that his patient, Mrs. Chia, may have a brain tumor. ________

EXERCISE 12 *Multiple-choice questions. Select the correct answer.*

1. The medical professionals took a CT of her:
   a. brain
   c. nerves
   b. spine
   d. meninges
2. Which symptom was *not* displayed by the patient?
   a. inability to comprehend
   c. increased sensation
   b. inability to speak
   d. complete paralysis on half of the body
3. A transient ischemic attack is caused by:
   a. blockage of a blood vessel
   c. inflammation of the brain
   b. inflammation of the blood vessels
   d. tumor in the brain
4. Dr. Hilliard has been following the patient for a disease of the blood vessels of the brain, which is called:
   a. cerebrovascular accident
   b. cerebrovascular disease
   c. cerebral arteriosclerosis
   d. cerebral atherosclerosis

Additional exercises available in connect

Chapter Review exercises, along with additional practice items, are available in Connect!

Quick Reference

quick reference glossary of roots and suffixes

Term	Definition	Term	Definition
-asthenia	weakness	**-mania**	excessive desire
cephal/o	head	**mening/o, meningi/o**	meninges; membrane surrounding the brain and spinal cord
cerebell/o	cerebellum	**myel/o**	spinal cord, bone marrow
cerebr/o	brain	**neur/o**	nerve
crani/o	head, skull	**-paresis**	slight or partial paralysis
dur/o	tough outer membrane surrounding the brain and spinal cord	**phas/o**	speech
encephal/o	brain	**-phobia**	excessive fear
esthesi/o	feeling, sensation	**phren/o**	mind
gangli/o	nerve bundle	**-plegia**	paralysis
gnosi/o	know	**psych/o**	mind
hypn/o	sleep	**somn/o, somn/i**	sleep
lob/o	lobe	**tax/o**	arrangement, order, coordination
		ton/o	muscle tone, tension

quick reference glossary of terms

Term	Definition
acrophobia	fear of heights
afferent nerve	a nerve that carries impulses toward the central nervous system
agnosia	inability to comprehend
agoraphobia	fear of outdoor spaces
amyotrophic lateral sclerosis (ALS)	a degenerative disease of the central nervous system, causing loss of muscle control; also known as Lou Gehrig's disease
analgesic	a drug that relieves pain
anesthesiologist	doctor who specializes in anesthesiology
anesthetic	a drug that causes loss of sensation
anorexia	an eating disorder characterized by the patient's refusal to eat
anticonvulsant	a drug that opposes convulsions
antidepressant	a drug that opposes depression

quick reference glossary of terms *continued*

Term	Definition
antipsychotic	a drug that opposes psychosis
anxiolytic	a drug that lessens anxiety
apathy	lack of emotion
aphasia	inability to speak
astrocytoma	a tumor arising from astrocyte glial cell
ataxia	lack of coordination
autism	a psychiatric disorder characterized by the withdrawal from communication with others; the patient is focused only on the self.
bulimia	an eating disorder characterized by overeating and usually followed by forced vomiting
catatonia	condition characterized by reduced muscle tone
causalgia	painful sensation of burning
cephalalgia	head pain
cephalodynia	head pain
cerebellitis	inflammation of the cerebellum
cerebral aneurysm	the widening or abnormal dilation of a blood vessel in the brain
cerebral angiography	procedure used to examine blood vessels in the brain
cerebral arteriosclerosis	the hardening of an artery in the brain
cerebral atherosclerosis	the hardening of an artery in the brain caused by the buildup of fatty plaque
cerebral atrophy	wasting away of brain tissue
cerebral embolism	the blockage of a blood vessel in the brain caused by a foreign object (embolus) such as fat or bacteria
cerebral palsy	paralysis caused by damage to the area of the brain responsible for movement
cerebral thrombosis	the blockage of a blood vessel in the brain caused by a clot
cerebromeningitis	inflammation of the brain and meninges
cerebrotomy	incision into the brain
cerebrovascular accident (CVA)	an accident involving the blood vessels of the brain
cerebrovascular disease	a disease of the blood vessels of the brain
chemotherapy	treatment using chemicals
clonus	muscle spasm or twitching
cranial hematoma	a hematoma beneath the skull
craniectomy	removal of a piece of the skull
craniomalacia	abnormal softening of the skull

quick reference glossary of terms *continued*

Term	Definition
craniosclerosis	abnormal hardening of the skull
craniostenosis	abnormal narrowing of the skull
craniosynostosis	the premature fusing of the skull bones
craniotomy	incision into the skull
delirium	brief loss of mental function
dementia	loss/decline in mental function
duritis	inflammation of the dura
dysesthesia	bad feeling
dyskinesia	difficulty moving
dyslexia	difficulty reading
dysphasia	difficulty speaking
dysphoria	a negative emotional state
dystonia	condition characterized by involuntary muscle movements
echoencephalography	procedure used to examine the brain using sound waves
efferent nerve	a nerve that carries impulses away from the central nervous system
electroencephalography (EEG)	procedure used to examine the electrical activity of the brain
encephalalgia	brain pain
encephalitis	inflammation of the brain
encephalocele	hernia of the brain (normally through a defect in the skull)
encephalography	procedure for studying the brain
encephalomyelitis	inflammation of the brain and spinal cord
encephalomyeloneuropathy	disease of the brain, spinal cord, and nerves
encephalopathy	disease of the brain
encephalopyosis	a pus-filled abscess in the brain
endarterectomy	removal of the inside of an artery
endovascular neurosurgery	surgery on the nervous system performed by entering the body through blood vessels
epidural anesthetic	anesthetic applied in the dural region of the spinal cord
epidural hematoma	a hematoma located on top of the dura
epilepsy	a disease marked by seizures
euphoria	a positive emotional state
gangliitis	inflammation of the ganglion
ganglioma	ganglion tumor

quick reference glossary of terms *continued*

Term	Definition
general anesthetic	anesthetic that causes complete loss of consciousness
glioblastoma	a brain tumor arising from glioblast cells
hematoma	a tumorlike mass made up of blood
hemiparesis	partial paralysis on half of the body
hemiplegia	paralysis on half the body
hemorrhagic stroke	a stroke where blood loss is caused by the rupture of a blood vessel
hydrocephaly	abnormal accumulation of spinal fluid in the brain
hydrophobia	fear of water
hyperesthesia	increased sensation
hyperkinesia	increase in muscle movement or activity
hypnotic	a drug that aids sleep
hypomania	a mental state just below mania
idiopathic	having no known cause or origin
insomnia	inability to sleep
interictal	time between seizures
intracerebral hematoma	a hematoma located inside the brain
intracerebral hemorrhage	excessive bleeding inside the brain
ischemic stroke	a stroke where blood loss is caused by a blockage
kleptomania	desire to steal
lobectomy	removal of a lobe
lobotomy	incision into a lobe
local anesthetic	any anesthetic that does not affect consciousness
lumbar puncture (LP)	inserting a needle into the lumbar region of the spine in order to collect spinal fluid
macrocephaly	abnormally large head
magnetic resonance angiography (MRA)	procedure used to examine blood vessels
manic depression (bipolar)	a psychiatric disorder characterized by alternating bouts of excitement and depression
meningioma	tumor of the meninges
meningitis	inflammation of the meninges
meningocele	a hernia of the meninges
meningoencephalitis	inflammation of the meninges and brain
meningopathy	disease of the meninges

quick reference glossary of terms *continued*

Term	Definition
microcephaly	abnormally small head
monoparesis	partial paralysis of one limb
monoplegia	paralysis of one limb
myasthenia	condition characterized by muscle weakness
myelitis	inflammation of the spinal cord
myelocele	a hernia of the spinal cord
myelodysplasia	defective formation of the spinal cord
myelogram	image of the spinal cord, usually done using x-ray
myelomalacia	abnormal softening of the spinal cord
myelomeningocele	a hernia of the spinal cord and meninges
myelopathy	disease of the spinal cord
myoclonus	muscle twitching
myospasm	involuntary muscle contraction
narcolepsy	a disease characterized by sudden, uncontrolled sleepiness
neuralgia	nerve pain
neurasthenia	nerve weakness
neurectomy	removal of a nerve
neuritis	nerve inflammation
neuroarthropathy	disease of the joint associated with nerves
neurodynia	nerve pain
neuroencephalomyelopathy	disease of the nerves, brain, and spinal cord
neurogenic	originating from/created by nerves
neuroglycopenia	deficiency of sugar that interferes with normal brain activity
neurolysis	destruction of nerve tissue
neuroma	a nerve tumor
neuropathy	disease of the nervous system
neuropharmacology	the study of the effects of drugs on the nervous system
neuroplasty	reconstruction of a nerve
neurorrhaphy	suturing of a nerve (often the severed ends of a nerve)
neurosclerosis	hardening of nerves
neurosis	a nerve condition
neurotomy	incision into a nerve
nystagmus	involuntary back and forth eye movements

quick reference glossary of terms *continued*

Term	Definition
paralysis	complete loss of sensation and motor function
paresis	partial paralysis characterized by varying degrees of sensation and motor function
paresthesia	abnormal sensation (usually numbness or tingling in the skin)
photophobia	excessive sensitivity to light
poliomyelitis	inflammation of the gray matter of the spinal cord
polyneuritis	inflammation of multiple nerves
polyneuropathy	disease affecting multiple nerves
positron emission tomography (PET) scan	an imaging procedure that uses radiation (positrons) to produce cross sections of the brain
postictal	time after a seizure
preictal	time before a seizure
prosopagnosia	inability to recognize faces
pseudoesthesia	false sensation
psychiatrist	doctor who specializes in treatment of the mind
psychiatry	branch of medicine that focuses on the treatment of the mind
psychogenic	originating in/created by the mind
psychologist	doctor who specializes in the study of the mind
psychology	branch of medicine that focuses on the study of the mind
psychopathy	a mental illness
psychopharmacology	the study of the effects of drugs on mental processes
psychosis	a mind condition (involves some sort of break with reality interfering with rational thought or daily functioning)
psychosomatic	pertaining to the relationship between the body and the mind
psychotropic	drugs that are able to turn the mind
pyromania	desire to set fires
regional anesthesia	anesthetic that is injected into a nerve, causing loss of sensation over a particular area
schizophrenia	a mental illness characterized by delusions, hallucinations, and disordered speech
somnambulism	sleep walking
stroke	loss of brain function caused by interruption of blood flow/supply to the brain
subdural hematoma	a hematoma located beneath the dura

quick reference glossary of terms *continued*

Term	Definition
syncope	fainting; losing consciousness due to temporary loss of blood flow to the brain
synesthesia	condition where one sensation is experienced as another
thrombolytic	a drug that dissolves clots
tonic	pertaining to muscle tone (normally weak or unresponsive)
tonic-clonic seizure	a seizure characterized by both a tonic and a clonic phase
topical anesthetic	local anesthesia applied to the surface of the area to be anesthetized
transcranial Doppler sonography	an imaging technique that produces an image of the brain using sound waves sent through the skull
transient ischemic attack (TIA)	a mini-stroke caused by the blockage of a blood vessel that resolves (goes away) within 24 hours

review of terms by roots

Root	Term(s)	
-asthenia	myasthenia neurasthenia	
cephal/o	cephalalgia cephalodynia hydrocephaly	macrocephaly microcephaly
cerebell/o	cerebellitis	
cerebr/o	cerebral aneurysm cerebral angiography cerebral arteriosclerosis cerebral atherosclerosis cerebral embolism cerebral palsy cerebral thrombosis	cerebromeningitis cerebrotomy cerebrovascular accident cerebrovascular disease intracerebral hematoma intracerebral hemorrhage
crani/o	cranial hematoma craniectomy craniomalacia craniosclerosis	craniostenosis craniosynostosis craniotomy transcranial Doppler sonography
dur/o	duritis epidural anesthetic	epidural hematoma subdural hematoma
encephal/o	echoencephalography electroencephalography encephalalgia encephalitis encephalocele encephalography	encephalomyelitis pencephalomyeloneuropathy encephalopathy encephalopyosis meningoencephalitis neuroencephalomyelopathy

review of terms by roots *continued*

Root	Term(s)	
esthesi/o	anesthesiologist anesthetic dysesthesia epidural anesthetic general anesthetic hyperesthesia	local anesthetic parasthesia pseudesthesia regional anesthetic synesthesia topical anesthetic
gangli/o	gangliitis ganglioma	
gnosi/o	agnosia atopognosis prosopagnosia	
hypn/o	hypnotic	
kinesi/o	hyperkinesia dyskinesia	
lob/o	lobectomy lobotomy	
-mania	hypomania kleptomania	manic depression (bipolar) pyromania
mening/o, meningi/o	cerebromeningitis meningioma meningitis meningocele	meningoencephalitis meningopathy myelomeningocele
myel/o	encephalomyelitis encephalomyeloneuropathy myelitis myelocele myelodysplasia myelogram	myelomalacia myelomeningocele myelopathy neuroencephalomyelopathy poliomyelitis
neur/o	encephalomyeloneuropathy endovascular neurosurgery neuralgia neurasthenia neurectomy neuritis neuroarthropathy neurodynia neuroencephalomyelopathy neurogenic neuroglypenia	neurolysis neuroma neuropathy neuropharmacology neuroplasty neurorrhaphy neurosclerosis neurosis neurotomy polyneuritis polyneuropathy
-paresis	hemiparesis monoparesis	
phas/o	aphasia dysphasia	

review of terms by roots *continued*

Root	Term(s)	
-phobia	acrophobia agoraphobia	hydrophobia photophobia
phren/o	schizophrenia	
-plegia	hemiplegia monoplegia	
psych/o	antipsychotic psychiatrist psychiatry psychogenic psychologist psychology	psychopathy psychopharmacology psychosis psychosomatic psychotropic
somn/o	insomnia somnambulism	
tax/o	ataxia	
ton/o	catatonia dystonia	tonic tonic-clonic seizure

other terms

afferent nerve	hematoma
amyotrophic lateral sclerosis (ALS)	hemorrhagic stroke
analgesic	idiopathic
anorexia	interictal
anosmia	ischemic stroke
anticonvulsant	lumbar puncture (LP)
antidepressant	magnetic resonance angiography (MRA)
anxiolytic	myoclonus
apathy	myospasm
autism	narcolepsy
bulimia	nystagmus
causalgia	paralysis
clonus	paresis
delirium	positron emission tomography (PET) scan
dementia	postictal
dyslexia	preictal
dysphoria	stroke
efferent nerve	syncope
endarterectomy	thrombolytic
epilepsy	transient ischemic attack (TIA)
euphoria	

The Sensory System—Ophthalmology and Otolaryngology

6

Introduction and Overview of Sensory Organs

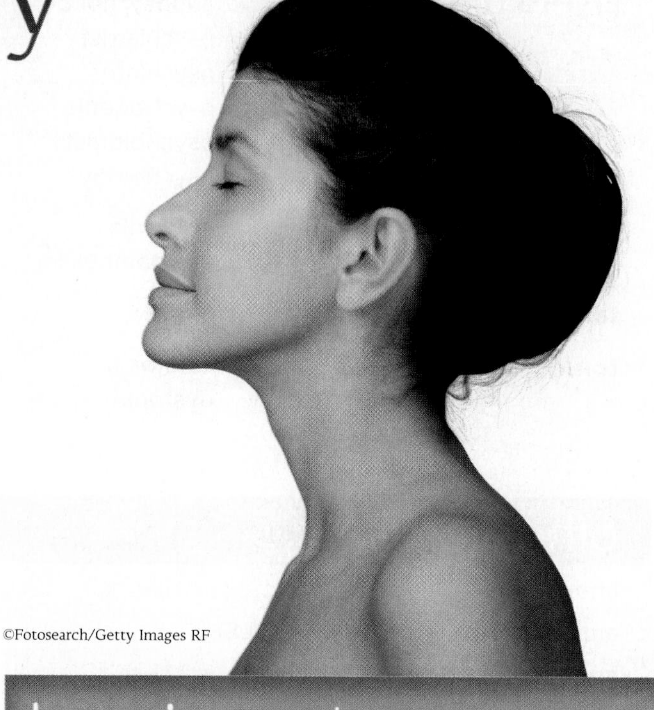
©Fotosearch/Getty Images RF

You are standing at a music festival listening to live music. The feeling is electric and the experience is unforgettable. What makes it so memorable? The sound is fantastic, but you could download the music. The sights are great. The band is in top form and everyone around you is excited. However, you could watch and hear it all online. There are distinct smells. Many of them are unpleasant, but for some reason, as part of a whole, they are acceptable. You feel the bass. You sweat as you dance. Overall, the experience is far greater than the parts. Why is that the case? Your brain processes each component of these things and integrates them into a whole. Yet each sense is important in defining the experience. The function of the sensory system is collecting specific details about the surroundings and sending the information on to the central nervous system.

Sensory organs and cells are found throughout your entire body. As mentioned before, your skin is your largest sensory organ. It contains thousands upon thousands of cells sending information to your brain, including information about pain, pressure, and temperature. Your most complex sensory organs, however, are your eyes and ears. They provide you with a wealth of information about the world around you.

learning outcomes

Upon completion of this chapter, you will be able to:

6.1 Identify the **roots/word parts** associated with the **sensory system**.

(S) **6.2** Translate the **Subjective** terms associated with the **sensory system**.

(O) **6.3** Translate the **Objective** terms associated with the **sensory system**.

(A) **6.4** Translate the **Assessment** terms associated with the **sensory system**.

(P) **6.5** Translate the **Plan** terms associated with the **sensory system**.

6.6 Use **abbreviations** associated with the **sensory system**.

6.7 Distinguish terms associated with the **sensory system** in the context of **electronic health records**.

6.1 Word Parts of the Sensory System

Word Roots Associated with the Eye

OUTER STRUCTURES AND VISION

The eye (*oculo*) is a very valuable but vulnerable organ. There are many protective structures around the eye that help keep it safe and wet. The eye rests in a socket made of seven connecting bones in the skull. This socket is also known as the orbit. Just outside the eye is a set of eyelids (*blepharo*) that protect the eyes from dust and other floating particles in the air. In addition, eyelids aid in keeping the eye moist. It is extremely important for the eye to remain wet. For this reason, there are additional structures that help keep the eye moist. The lacrimal gland is a small gland that sits just above and to the side of the eye. It produces tears that stream across the eye and keep it wet. Finally, the eyes and eyelids are lined with a thin invisible membrane known as the conjunctiva.

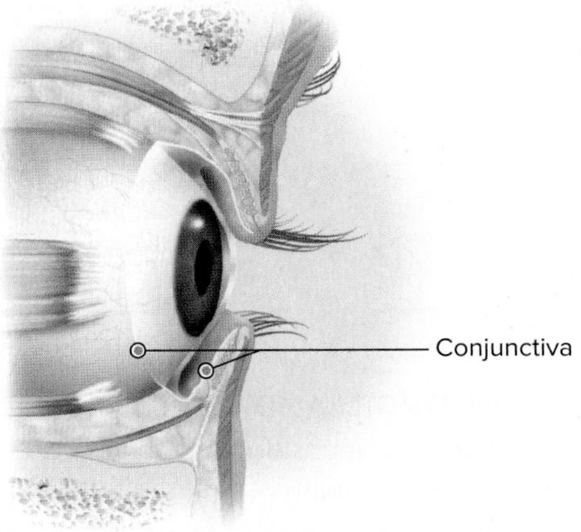

tear

ROOTS: ***lacrim/o, dacry/o***

EXAMPLES: lacrimation, dacryorrhea

NOTES: Often the term *lacrimal* is used interchangeably for the word *tear.* Keep in mind that the lacrimal gland and the tear gland refer to the same thing.

Although it isn't the origin of the term, you may find it easy to remember that *dacryo* means "tear" because it has the word *cry* in the middle of it—daCRYo.

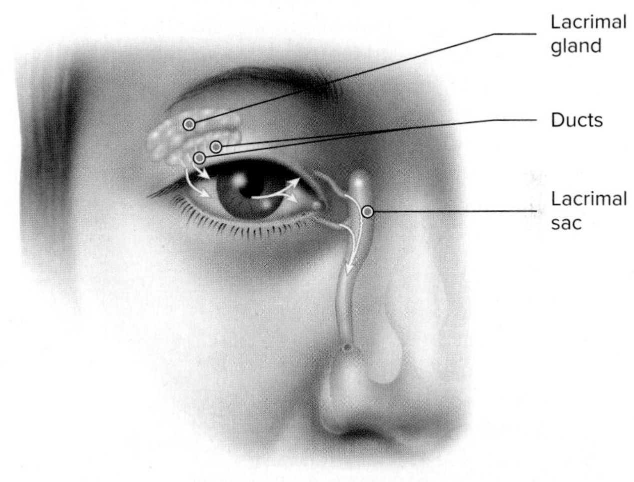

eye

ROOTS: ***ocul/o, ophthalm/o, opt/o***

EXAMPLES: oculopathy, ophthalmologists, optometrist

NOTES: It might sound nitpicky, but *ophthalmo* has two *h*s, not one. Many people think the root is *OPthalmo* but it is actually *OPHthalmo.*

Some people think the word *antler* comes from the Latin phrase *ante ocular,* which means "in front of the eye," because that is where the horns grow on deer and cows.

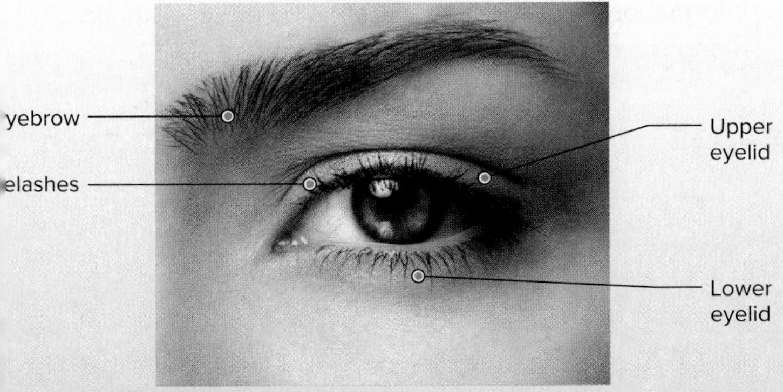

nk P Wartenberg/Picture Press/Getty Images

vision condition

SUFFIXES: ***-opia, -opsia***

EXAMPLES: hyperopia, akinetopsia

NOTES: Akinetopsia = *a* + *kinet* + *-opsia* = no movement vision condition. It refers to a condition where patients are unable to see objects in motion.

eyelid

ROOT: ***blephar/o***

EXAMPLES: blepharedema, blepharoplasty

NOTES: Blepharoplasty = *blepharo* + *plasty* = surgical reconstruction of the eyelid.

Also, remember that the *ph* is pronounced *f.* The word is ble*ph*aroplasty, *not* ble*p*aroplasty.

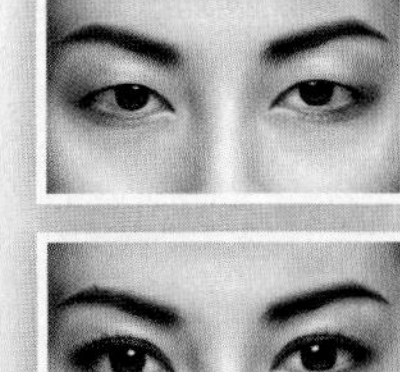

SCLERA AND CORNEA

An eye is like a video camera with three layers. The outermost layer includes the *sclera* and the *cornea.* The *sclera* is the white part of the eye—a dense, protective layer, like the hard shell on the outside of the video camera. The *cornea* is a clear surface in the middle of the eye. Like the glass on a video camera, the cornea protects the lens and begins the work of focusing light to the back of the eye.

cornea

ROOTS: ***corne/o, kerat/o***

EXAMPLES: corneal transplant, keratitis

NOTES: *Kerato* is a tricky root because it has multiple meanings. In the context of the eye, *kerato* means "cornea." In the context of the skin, *kerato* refers to a horny texture to the skin. What's the connection? *Kerato* comes from a Greek word meaning "horn" (think of a rhinoCEROS) and *corneo* comes from a Latin word meaning "horn" (think of a CORNUcopia, a horn of plenty). Apparently someone thought the cornea of the eye looked like a horn.

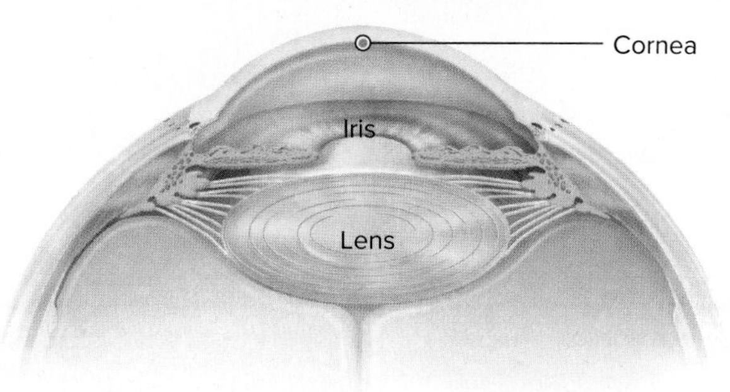

conjunctiva

ROOT: ***conjunctiv/o***

EXAMPLE: conjunctivitis

NOTES: The *conjunctiva* is a clear membrane that covers the sclera and lines the eyelids. The root comes from two Latin words, *con* (with/together) and *junct* (join). Evidently, someone thought it joined the eye to the rest of body.

sclera (the white of the eye)

ROOT: ***scler/o***

EXAMPLE: scleritis

NOTES: Just like *kerato,* sclera has multiple meanings. In other contexts, *sclero* means "hard" and can refer to the abnormal hardening of any tissue or organ. In the eye, it refers to the white, tough, and fibrous protective covering of the eye. Words having to do with the eye use *sclero* in both ways:

phacosclerosis = *phaco* + *scler* + *osis* = an abnormal hardening of the lens

scleromalacia = *sclero* + *malacia* = an abnormal softening of the sclera

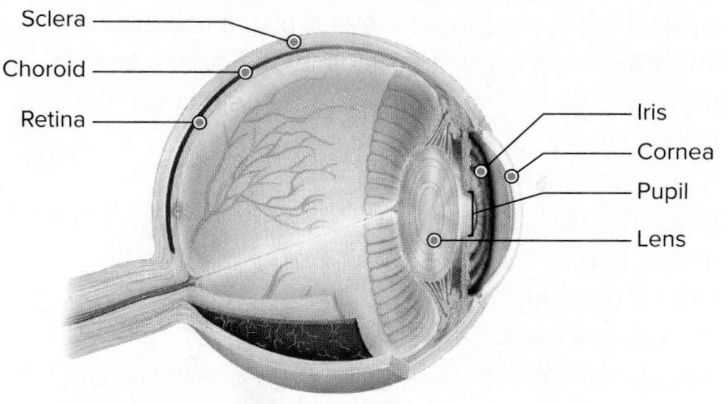

CHOROID AND RETINA

The next layer down is the *choroid.* It includes the *lens,* which gathers light and focuses on images in the same way a lens on a camera does. The choroid also includes the *iris* and the *ciliary muscles.*

The iris is what gives eyes their color. By expanding (*dilating*) or shrinking (*constricting*) the pupils, the irises control how much light hits the back of the eye.

The ciliary muscles adjust the shape of the eye and lens to focus on near or far objects. As light passes through the lens, it passes through liquid in the eye (*vitreous*) that bends the light and aims it to the back of the eyeball—all the way to the deepest layer, the *retina,* which is the eye's image processor. The retina helps turn visual stimuli into electric signals. The collected information is then sent to the brain by electric signals along the optic nerve.

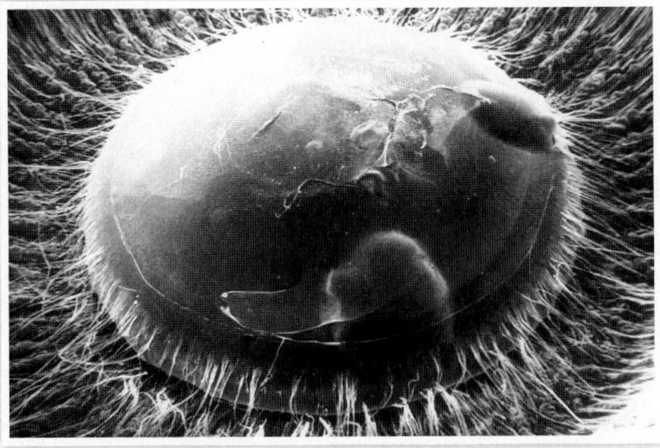

An up-close picture of the eye's lens.

vitreous liquid (also called vitreous humor)

ROOT: ***vitre/o***

EXAMPLES: vitreous liquid, vitrectomy

NOTES: The root *vitreo* means "glass" and refers to the liquid in the eye that helps focus light on the back of the retina. You're probably more familiar with the root *vitreo* in the term *in vitro fertilization*. This is the scientific word for a test-tube baby, an embryo that is fertilized not in the body but *in vitro*, which means "in a glass tube."

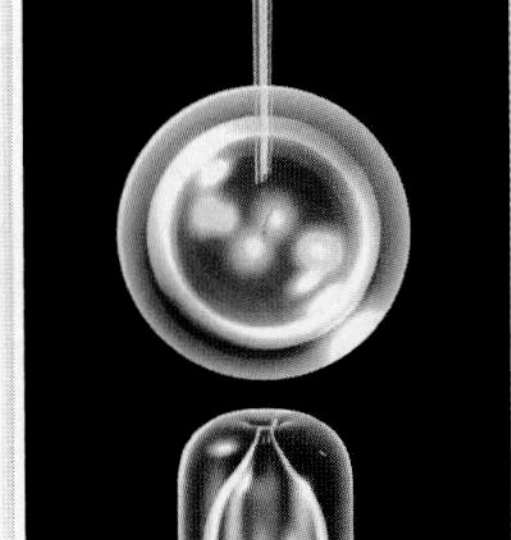

ciliary body

ROOT: ***cycl/o***

EXAMPLE: cycloplegia

NOTES: The *ciliary body* is a circle of tissue surrounding the lens. One of its primary jobs is to change the shape of the lens of the eye in order to allow the eye to maintain focus, a process called accommodation. Someone who can't read things close up without the help of glasses has ciliary bodies that are unable to sufficiently focus their lenses. When this happens in old age, it is called *presbyopia*.

retina

ROOT: ***retin/o***

EXAMPLES: retinitis, retinoscope

NOTES: *Retina* comes from a word that means "net"; it refers to the netlike pattern of light-sensitive tissue on the inside surface of the eye.

iris

ROOTS: ***ir/o, irid/o***

EXAMPLES: iritis, iridalgia

NOTES: The iris is the colored part of the eye. It is responsible for adjusting the size of the pupil to control the amount of light that enters the eye. In Greek mythology, Iris was a female messenger of the gods. She was the personification of the rainbow, which is why her name was given to the colored part of the eye.

lens

ROOTS: ***phac/o, phak/o***

EXAMPLES: phacoscope, phakitis

NOTES: *Phaco* is a Greek word meaning "lentil," a type of bean, which is where we get the word *lens*. Notice that *phaco* can be spelled with a *c* (*phaco*) or a *k* (*phako*). Because *c* sounds like *s* before *i* and e, the *k* sound is used sometimes to be sure the syllable is pronounced hard. For example, *phacitis* could be pronounced fah-SAI-tis. To avoid confusion, the word is sometimes spelled *phakitis* so it is pronounced fah-KAI-tis.

Word Roots Associated with the Ear

THE EAR AND HEARING

Ears work like stereo speakers in reverse. While stereo speakers turn electrical signals into sounds (*acouso, audio*), ears (*auro, oto*) turn sounds into electrical signals. First, they collect sounds. Next, they turn the energy from the sound into movement, and then they convert it again into electrical signals. Last, they send the signals to the brain, where it all gets sorted out into meaning.

ear

ROOTS: ***aur/o, ot/o***

EXAMPLES: aural, otoscope

NOTES: If you learn better by hearing something than by reading it, then you are an *aural learner.* It's easy to confuse *aural* with *oral.* But since *oral* means "mouth," we guess an oral learner would be someone who learns by eating. Also, the root *oto* is pronounced OH- toh, not AW-toh. An instrument a doctor uses to look in the ear is called an *otoscope,* which is pronounced OH-toh-skohp, not AW-toh-skohp.

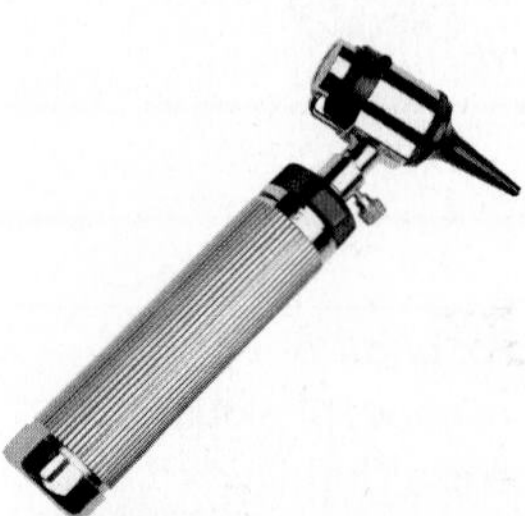

©Photodisc Collection/Getty Images RF

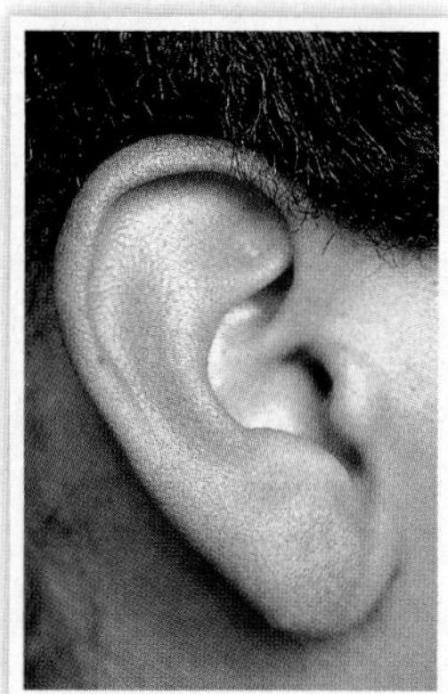

©McGraw-Hill Education/Joe DeGrandis, photographer

sound, hearing

ROOTS: ***acous/o, audi/o***

EXAMPLES: acoustic, audiogram

NOTES: Sound travels at 768 miles per hour. That's about 12 miles per minute, or about 1 mile every 5 seconds. Light, however, travels a lot faster—186,282 miles per second, which is about 5.6 million miles per minute, or more than 335 million miles per hour. That's why you see a flash of lightning before you hear the thunder.

©Hill Street Studios/Photolibray/Getty Images

hearing condition

SUFFIX: ***-acusis***

EXAMPLES: hyperacusis, osteoacusis

NOTES: Have you ever wondered why your voice sounds different to you than it does to other people, or why you seem to sound different when you hear a recording of yourself? That's because of *osteoacusis* (*osteo* + *-acusis* = bone hearing condition). When you speak, your voice passes through the air and hits other people's eardrums. But it reaches your own ear in two very different ways—through the air, as it does for others, but also through the bones of your head, which is why you can hear yourself talk even if you plug your ears. Sound waves travel differently through bone than through air, so your voice sounds different to you than it does to other people.

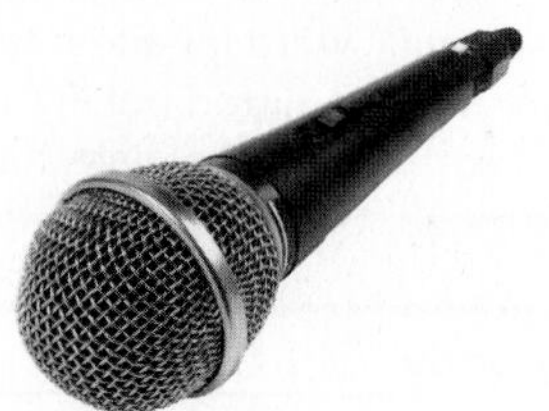

©Stockbyte/Punchstock RF

OUTER/MIDDLE EAR

There are three main divisions of the ear: the outer ear, the middle ear, and the inner ear.

The outer ear includes the *pinna* and the *ear canal.* The pinna is what we first think of when we think about the ear—it's the fleshy part we pierce, tug on, and cover up in the winter. The pinna sits on the mastoid bone of the skull. Its funnel shape helps collect sound from the air and send it down the ear canal toward the eardrum (*tympanic membrane*).

The eardrum is part of the middle ear and is a very important structure. It turns sound waves into physical energy. To keep the eardrum free from interference, the body protects it from both sides. From the outside, the ear canal produces ear wax (*cerumen*). Despite its gross appearance, ear wax is very helpful—it is a natural antibiotic and also a lubricant that keeps the ear canal moist. On the other side of the eardrum is a drainage system. The middle ear is connected to the nose and throat through a tube (*salpinx*). This tube helps drain the ear of any fluid and keeps the pressure inside the middle ear the same as outside the ear. Your eardrum is attached to three bones that make up the rest of the middle ear. These bones are the *incus, stapes,* and *malleus* (anvil, stirrup, and hammer). When the eardrum moves, these tiny bones move too. They transfer their movement to the inner ear.

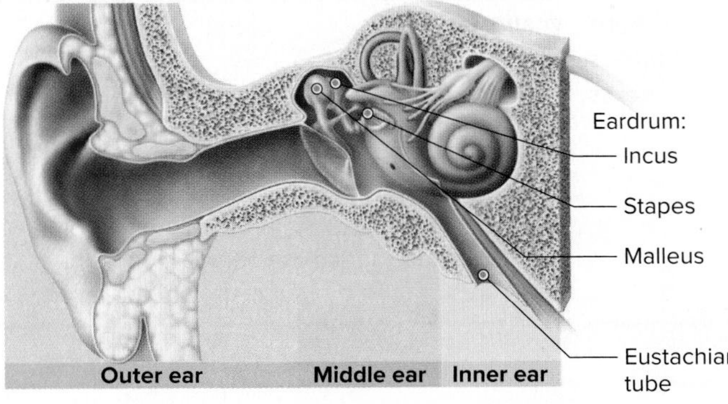

ear wax

ROOT: ***cerumin/o***

EXAMPLE: ceruminolysis

NOTES: Remember: *C* is pronounced like an *s* before *e* and *i* and like a *k* before *a, o,* and *u.* So *cerumen* is pronounced SEH-roo-men.

eustachian tube

ROOT: ***salping/o***

EXAMPLE: rhinosalpingitis

NOTES: *Salpingo* is derived from the Latin word *salpinx,* which means "trumpet." It refers to the long, straight kind used by Roman legions in battle, not the curvy kind with keys that is used today. This is important because *salpingo* is used in two body systems: in the ear, referring to the eustachian tubes, and in the female reproductive system, referring to the fallopian tubes. Both have long, tubelike shapes.

And what are eustachian tubes? They connect the middle ear to the throat. Hold your nose, close your mouth, and blow. You'll make your eardrum pop by forcing air into your middle ear through the eustachian tubes. Ear infections occur when the eustachian tubes are prevented from draining fluid out of the middle ear.

eardrum

ROOTS: ***tympan/o, myring/o***

EXAMPLES: tympanostomy, myringotomy

NOTES: The root *tympano* comes from a Greek word meaning "drum." Orchestras' big kettledrums are called *tympany,* so "eardrum" is not a bad translation. If you take a peek inside someone's ear sometime, you'll probably agree that it does resemble a drum.

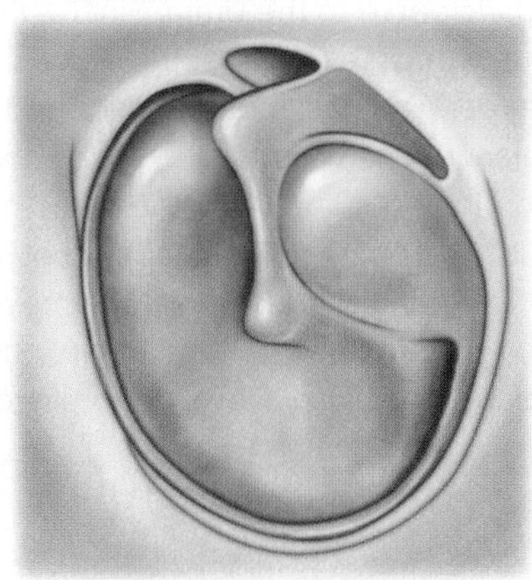

mastoid process

ROOT: ***mastoid/o***

EXAMPLE: mastoiditis

NOTES: Put your hand on the protruding part of your skull behind your ear—that's the mastoid process. It sticks out from the side rear portion of the skull. Its name comes from *mast* (breast) + *oid* (resembling) = resembling a breast.

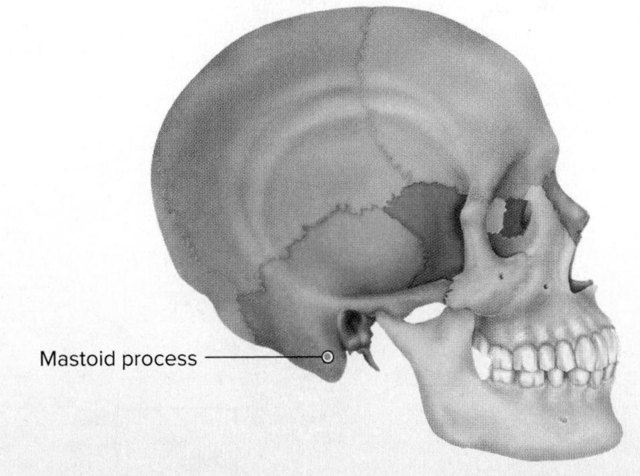

INNER EAR

The bones of the middle ear are connected to the *cochlea,* a shell-shaped organ in your inner ear (*labyrinth*) filled with fluid and hair. When the *stapes* (pronounced STAY-peez) moves, it presses on the cochlea and causes the fluid to move. Just as the ocean waters move through seaweed, when the fluid moves, the hairs bend. The hairs, which are connected to the nervous system, create an electric signal carried by the *acoustic nerve* to the brain. Finally, the brain receives and processes the electric signals.

The inner ear also has another critical job: helping maintain balance. The *vestibular system* sends information to the brain about the tilt, rotation, and motion of the head. Like the cochlea, it is made up of small canals filled with fluid and hair. These hairs are moved not by sound but by movement and head angle. This helps maintain balance and also allows the brain to coordinate movement with the eyes.

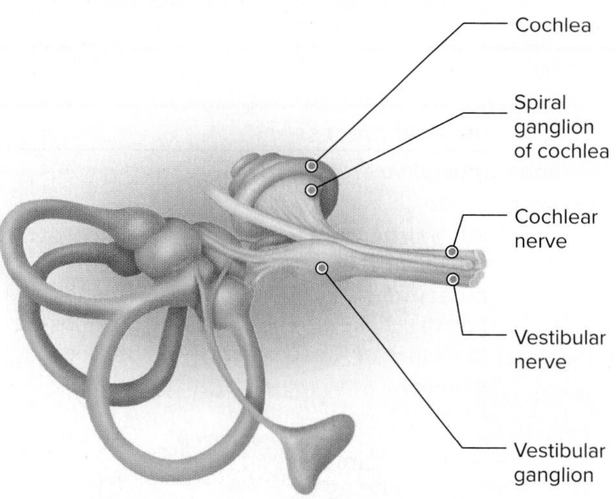

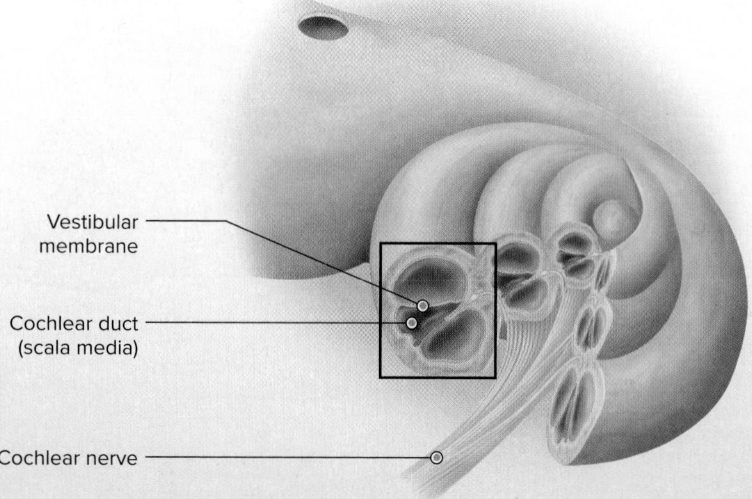

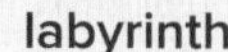

labyrinth

ROOT: ***labyrinth/o***

EXAMPLE: labyrinthitis

NOTES: The *labyrinth* is the innermost part of the ear. It contains two structures: the *cochlea,* which controls hearing, and the *vestibular system,* which controls balance. The term *labyrinth* comes from Greek mythology. It is the name of an elaborate maze built by King Minos to imprison the Minotaur, a half-man, half-bull creature.

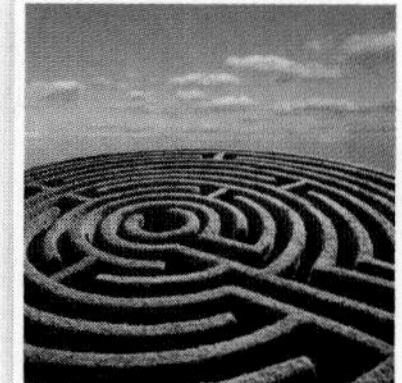

vestibule

ROOT: ***vestibul/o***

EXAMPLE: vestibulitis

NOTES: The term *vestibule* literally means "the lobby of a building." Sometimes church lobbies are called vestibules. In medicine, *vestibule* refers to a small space at the beginning of a canal. In the ear, it refers to the area in front of semicircular canals (hence the name); it contains structures that help regulate balance.

cochlea

ROOT: ***cochle/o***

EXAMPLE: cochleitis

NOTES: From Greek, for "snail shell," the *cochlea* (pronounced KOH-klee-ah) is a spiral, snail shell–shaped tube in the inner ear that contains hearing receptors.

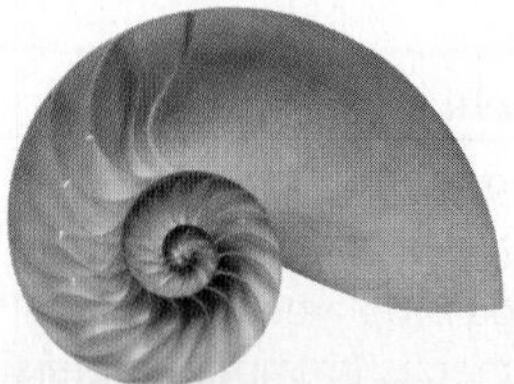

Learning Outcome 6.1 Exercises

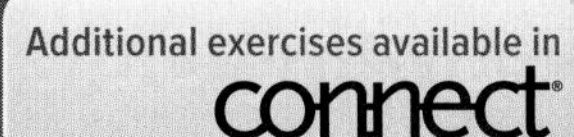

TRANSLATION

EXERCISE 1 *Match the word part on the left with its definition on the right.*

_____	1. ophthalm/o	a. eye
_____	2. dacry/o	b. eye condition
_____	3. -opia	c. eyelid
_____	4. blephar/o	d. tear

EXERCISE 2 *Translate the following word parts.*

1. opt/o ______________________
2. ocul/o ______________________
3. -opsia ______________________
4. opthalm/o ______________________
5. blephar/o ______________________
6. dacry/o ______________________
7. lacrim/o ______________________

EXERCISE 3 *Break down the following words into their component parts and translate.*

EXAMPLE: sinusitis *sinus | itis* *inflammation of the sinuses*

1. optic ______________________
2. oculopathy ______________________
3. ophthalmitis ______________________
4. blepharitis ______________________
5. hyperopia ______________________
6. dacryorrhea ______________________

EXERCISE 4 *Match the word part on the left with its definition on the right.*

_____	1. retin/o	a. ciliary body
_____	2. corne/o	b. conjunctiva
_____	3. conjunctiv/o	c. cornea
_____	4. scler/o	d. iris
_____	5. ir/o	e. lens
_____	6. vitre/o	f. retina
_____	7. phac/o	g. sclera
_____	8. cycl/o	h. vitreous liquid

EXERCISE 5 *Translate the following roots.*

1. corne/o ______________________
2. retin/o ______________________
3. irid/o ______________________
4. conjunctiv/o ______________________
5. ir/o ______________________
6. phac/o ______________________
7. cycl/o ______________________
8. kerat/o ______________________
9. phak/o ______________________

Learning Outcome 6.1 Exercises

EXERCISE 6 *Break down the following words into their component parts and translate.*

EXAMPLE: sinusitis *sinus | itis* *inflammation of the sinuses*

1. corneal transplant ____________________
2. conjunctivitis ____________________
3. iritis ____________________
4. scleromalacia ____________________
5. retinopathy ____________________
6. keratopathy ____________________
7. cyclotomy ____________________
8. phacoscope ____________________
9. iridalgia ____________________
10. vitrectomy ____________________
11. sclerokeratitis ____________________

EXERCISE 7 *Match the word part on the left with its definition on the right. Some definitions will be used more than once.*

______	1. audi/o	a. ear
______	2. -acusis	b. hearing condition
______	3. acous/o	c. sound
______	4. aur/o	
______	5. ot/o	

EXERCISE 8 *Translate the following word parts.*

1. -acusis ____________________
2. acous/o ____________________
3. aur/o ____________________
4. audi/o ____________________
5. ot/o ____________________

EXERCISE 9 *Break down the following words into their component parts and translate.*

EXAMPLE: sinusitis *sinus | itis* *inflammation of the sinuses*

1. audiologist ____________________
2. hyperacusis ____________________
3. hypoacusis ____________________
4. otalgia ____________________
5. otoscope ____________________
6. acoustic neuroma ____________________

Learning Outcome 6.1 Exercises

EXERCISE 10 *Match the word part on the left with its definition on the right.*

_____	1. cochle/o	a. cochlea
_____	2. vestibul/o	b. eardrum
_____	3. labyrinth/o	c. ear wax
_____	4. mastoid/o	d. eustachian tube
_____	5. myring/o	e. labyrinth
_____	6. cerumin/o	f. mastoid process
_____	7. salping/o	g. vestibule

EXERCISE 11 *Translate the following word parts.*

1. cochle/o _______________
2. mastoid/o _______________
3. vestibul/o _______________
4. labyrinth/o _______________
5. tympan/o _______________
6. cerumin/o _______________
7. myring/o _______________
8. salping/o _______________

EXERCISE 12 *Break down the following words into their component parts and translate.*

EXAMPLE: sinusitis *sinus | itis* *inflammation of the sinuses*

1. cochleitis _______________
2. labyrinthitis _______________
3. vestibulitis _______________
4. myringitis _______________
5. mastoidalgia _______________
6. salpingoscope _______________
7. ceruminoma _______________
8. tympanometry _______________
9. labyrinthectomy _______________
10. myringodermatitis _______________

GENERATION

EXERCISE 13 *Identify the word parts from this chapter for the following terms.*

1. amblyopia _______________
2. ophthalmologist _______________
3. blepharospasm _______________
4. lacrimation _______________
5. oculomycosis _______________
6. optomyometer _______________
7. hemianopsia _______________
8. dacryohemorrhea _______________
9. optokinetic _______________

EXERCISE 14 *Build a medical term from the information provided.*

1. surgical reconstruction of the eye (use *ocul/o*) _______________
2. surgical reconstruction of the eyelid _______________
3. disease of the eye (use *ophthalm/o*) _______________
4. specialist in measuring the eye (use *opt/o*) _______________
5. weak vision condition (use *-opia*) _______________
6. tear stone (use *dacry/o*) _______________
7. inflammation of the optic nerve _______________

Learning Outcome 6.1 Exercises

EXERCISE 15 *Identify the word parts from this chapter for the following terms.*

1. corneal xerosis ______
2. keratomalacia ______
3. retinopexy ______
4. cycloplegia ______
5. iridemia ______
6. phacoemulsification ______
7. aphakia ______
8. blepharoconjunctivitis ______
9. sclerokeratoiritis ______

EXERCISE 16 *Build a medical term from the information provided.*

1. inflammation of the lens (use *phak/o*) ______
2. inflammation of the conjunctiva ______
3. inflammation of the cornea (use *kerat/o*) ______
4. inflammation of the ciliary body and cornea (use *kerat/o*) ______
5. inflammation of the iris and ciliary body (use *irid/o*) ______
6. inflammation of the sclera and iris (use *ir/o*) ______
7. lens softening (use *phac/o*) ______
8. incision into the retina ______
9. incision into the sclera ______

EXERCISE 17 *Identify the word parts from this chapter for the following terms.*

1. otitis media ______
2. aural ______
3. audiogram ______
4. auditory prosthesis ______
5. pneumatic otoscopy ______
6. osteoacusis ______
7. otoneurology ______

EXERCISE 18 *Build a medical term from the information provided.*

1. pertaining to the ear (use *aur/o*) ______
2. pertaining to sound/hearing (use *acous/o*) ______
3. surgical reconstruction of the ear (use *ot/o*) ______
4. ear hardening condition (use *ot/o*) ______
5. procedure for looking in the ear (use *ot/o*) ______
6. procedure for measuring hearing (use *audi/o*) ______
7. instrument for measuring hearing (use *audi/o*) ______

Learning Outcome 6.1 Exercises

EXERCISE 19 *Identify the word parts from this chapter for the following terms.*

1. tympanic perforation ______
2. cochlear implant ______
3. mastoidectomy ______
4. ceruminolysis ______
5. vestibular neuritis ______
6. myringomycosis ______
7. salpingopharyngeal ______

EXERCISE 20 *Build a medical term from the information provided.*

1. inflammation of the mastoid ______
2. inflammation of the cochlea ______
3. ear wax condition ______
4. surgical reconstruction of the eardrum (use *myring/o*) ______
5. surgical reconstruction of the eardrum (use *tympan/o*) ______
6. incision into the vestibule ______
7. incision into the labyrinth ______
8. instrument for looking at the eustachian tubes ______

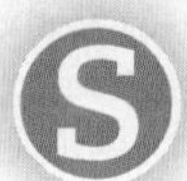

Subjective

Patient History, Problems, Complaints

Eye
- Vision conditions
- Outer structures and vision
- Sclera
- Choroid/retina

Ear
- Hearing conditions
- Outer/middle ear
- Inner ear

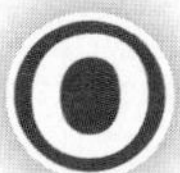

Objective

Observation and Discovery

Eye
- Diagnostic procedures
- Professional terms
- Outer structures and vision
- Sclera
- Choroid/retina

Ear
- Diagnostic procedures
- Professional terms
- Outer ear
- Middle ear

Assessment

Diagnosis and Pathology

Eye
- Outer structures and vision
- Sclera
- Choroid/retina

Ear
- Outer ear
- Middle ear
- Inner ear

Plan

Treatments and Therapies

Eye
- Outer structures and vision
- Sclera
- Choroid/retina

Ear
- Outer ear
- Middle ear
- Inner ear

This section contains medical terms built from the roots presented in the previous section. The purpose of this section is to expose you to words used in ophthalmology and otolaryngology that are built from the word roots presented earlier. The focus of this book is to teach you the process of learning roots and translating them in context. Each term is presented with the correct pronunciation, followed by a word analysis that breaks down the word into its component parts, a definition that provides a literal translation of the word, as well as supplemental information if the literal translation deviates from its medical use.

The terms are organized using a health care professional's SOAP note (first introduced in Chapter 2) as a model.

SUBJECTIVE

6.2 Patient History, Problems, Complaints

The Eye

When a patient goes to a health clinic for an eye problem, often the problem deals with a change in vision. While many people think of vision problems only in terms of either nearsightedeness (*myopia*) or farsightedness (*hyperopia*), vision problems can also be much more specific in nature. For example, a patient could have blindness in half of her field of vision (*hemianopsia*).

Complaints relating to the tear glands are very common as well. Excessive tearing (*dacryorrhea*) or excessive dryness (*xerophthalmia*) can both cause a patient discomfort.

Patients may also experience problems with their eyelids. An eyelid twitch (*blepharospasm*) is not serious, but it can be very uncomfortable and distracting.

6.2 Patient History, Problems, Complaints

As with any part of the body, patients can experience pain in their eyes. The pain may be generalized (*ophthmalgia*) or specific to a part of the eye (*iridalgia* or *keratalgia*). Finally, patients may notice that their pupils are either large (*mydriasis*) or small (*miosis*).

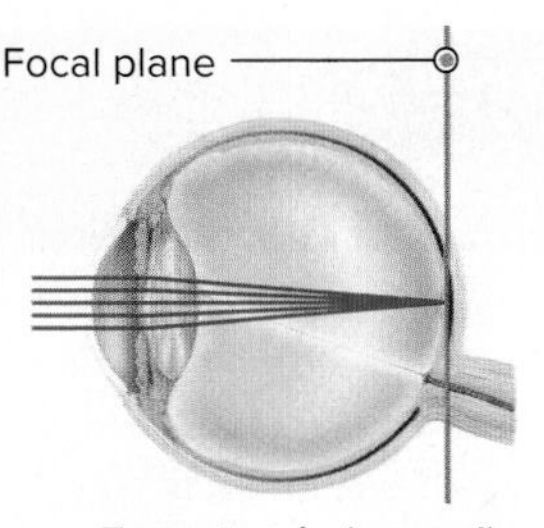

Emmetropia (normal)

The Ear

A change in hearing, like a change in vision, is a common ear complaint. A patient may complain of decreased (*hypoacusis*) or increased (*hyperacusis*) sensitivity to sound. Patients might also complain of ringing in the ears (*tinnitus*). Ear pain (*otalgia/ otodynia*) and discharge (*otorrhea*) are especially common in children with ear infections. Pain in the mastoid (*mastoidalgia*) may indicate a dangerous spread of the ear infection into the mastoid bone. *Vertigo* is a severe form of dizziness that often indicates problems with the patient's inner ear.

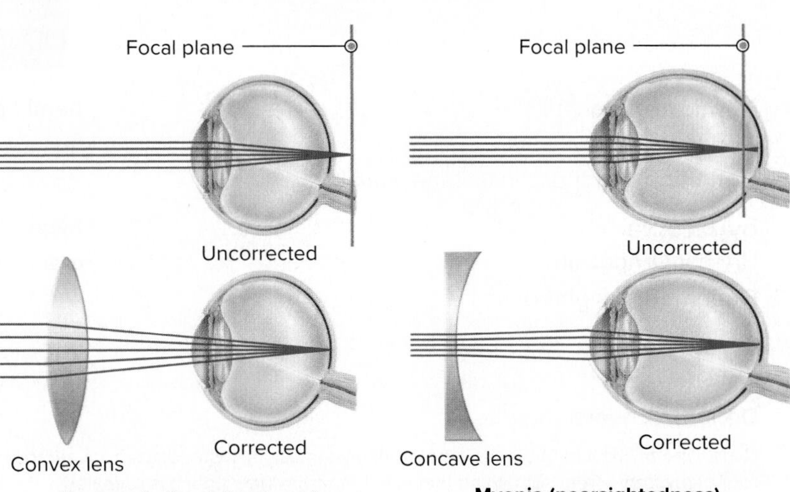

Hyperopia (farsightedness) — Myopia (nearsightedness)

eye

Term	Word Analysis
Vision Conditions—Opias	
akinetopsia uh-KEE-nah-TOP-see-ah **Definition** inability to see objects in motion	**a / kinet / opsia** no / movement / vision condition
ambiopia AM-bee-OH-pee-ah **Definition** double vision	**ambi / opia** both / vision condition
amblyopia AM-blih-OH-pee-ah **Definition** decreased vision; when it occurs in one eye, it is referred to as *lazy eye*	**ambly / opia** dull / vision condition
asthenopia AS-then-OH-pee-ah **Definition** weak vision (i.e., eye strain)	**asthen / opia** weak / vision condition

eye *continued*

Term	Word Analysis
diplopia dih-PLOH-pee-ah **Definition** double vision	**dipl / opia** double / vision condition
hemianopsia HEH-mee-an-OP-see-ah **Definition** blindness in half the visual field	**hemi / an / opsia** half / no / vision condition
hyperopia HAI-per-OH-pee-ah **Definition** farsightedness	**hyper / opia** over / vision condition
myopia mai-OH-pee-ah **Definition** nearsightedness **NOTE:** The *my* root in this word is not from *myo* (muscle); instead, it's from another word that means "to shut" that is related to the word at the root of *mystery*—from something that is hidden from view until it is revealed.	**my / opia** shut / vision condition
presbyopia PREZ-bee-OH-pee-ah **Definition** decreased vision caused by old age	**presby / opia** old age / vision condition
scotopia skaw-TOH-pee-ah **Definition** adjustment of the eye to seeing in darkness	**scot / opia** darkness / vision condition
Eye—Outer Structures and Vision	
blepharoplegia BLEF-ah-roh-PLEE-jah **Definition** paralysis of the eyelid	**blepharo / plegia** eyelid / paralysis ©Dr. P. Marazzi/Science Source
blepharospasm BLEF-ah-roh-SPAZ-um **Definition** involuntary contraction of an eyelid	**blepharo / spasm** eyelid / involuntary contraction

6.2 Patient History, Problems, Complaints

eye *continued*

Term	Word Analysis
dacryoadenalgia DAK-ree-oh-AD-en-AL-jah **Definition** pain in the tear gland	**dacryo / aden / algia** tear / gland / pain
dacryocystalgia DAK-ree-oh-sis-TAL-jah **Definition** pain in the tear sac	**dacryo / cyst / algia** tear / sac / pain
dacryohemorrhea DAK-ree-oh-HIM-oh-REE-ah **Definition** blood in the tears	**dacryo / hemo / rrhea** tear / blood / excessive discharge
dacryorrhea DAK-ree-oh-REE-ah **Definition** excessive tearing	**dacryo / rrhea** tear / excessive discharge
ophthalmalgia awf-thal-MAL-jah **Definition** eye pain	**ophthalm / algia** eye / pain
ophthalmoplegia awf-THAL-moh-PLEE-jah **Definition** eye paralysis	**ophthalmo / plegia** eye / paralysis
xerophthalmia ZER-off-THAL-mee-ah **Definition** dry eyes	**xer / ophthalm / ia** dry / eye / condition
Eye—Sclera	
astigmatism ah-STIG-mah-TIZ-um **Definition** vision problem caused by the fact that light rays entering the eye aren't focused on a single point in the back of the eye	**a / stigmat / ism** no / point / condition
corneal xerosis KOR-nee-al ZER-oh-sis **Definition** dryness of the cornea	**corne / al** **xer / osis** cornea / pertaining to dry / condition
keratalgia KEH-rah-TAL-jah **Definition** pain in the cornea	**kerat / algia** cornea / pain

6.2 Patient History, Problems, Complaints

eye *continued*

Term	Word Analysis
Eye—Choroid/Retina	
cycloplegia SAI-kloh-PLEE-jah **Definition** paralysis of the ciliary body	**cyclo / plegia** ciliary body / paralysis
iridalgia IH-rid-AL-jah **Definition** pain in the iris	**irid / algia** iris / pain
miosis mai-OH-sis **Definition** abnormal contraction of the pupil	**from Greek, for** "to lessen"
mydriasis mi-DRAI-ah-sis **Definition** abnormal dilation of pupil **NOTE:** We don't really see the connection—do you?	**from Greek, for** "red-hot metal"
scotoma skaw-TOH-mah **Definition** dark spot in the visual field	**scot / oma** darkness / tumor ©Design Pics/Ben Welsh RF

ear

Term	Word Analysis
Hearing Conditions—Acuses	
hyperacusis HAI-per-ah-KOO-sis **Definition** excessively sensitive hearing	**hyper / acusis** over / hearing condition
hypoacusis HAI-poh-ah-KOO-sis **Definition** excessively insensitive hearing	**hypo / acusis** under / hearing condition

6.2 Patient History, Problems, Complaints

ear *continued*

Term	Word Analysis
osteoacusis AW-stee-oh-ah-KOO-sis **Definition** hearing through bone	**osteo / acusis** bone / hearing condition
presbycusis PREZ-bih-KOO-sis **Definition** loss of hearing in old age **NOTE:** The *a* in *acusis* was swallowed up by the *y* at the end of *presby*. The word is sometimes written as *presbyacusis*, but that's a lot harder to pronounce.	**presby / cusis** old age / hearing condition
Outer/Middle Ear	
mastoidalgia MAS-toid-AL-jah **Definition** pain in the mastoid	**mastoid / algia** mastoid / pain
otalgia oh-TAL-jah **Definition** ear pain	**ot / algia** ear / pain
otodynia OH-toh-DAI-nee-ah **Definition** ear pain	**oto / dynia** ear / pain
otorrhea OH-toh-REE-ah **Definition** discharge from the ear	**oto / rrhea** ear / excessive discharge
Inner Ear	
tinnitus tih-NAI-tis **Definition** ringing in the ears	**from Latin, for "to ring or jingle"** ©Peter Dazeley/Photographer's Choice/Getty Images
vertigo VER-tih-goh **Definition** sensation of moving through space (while stationary)	**from Latin, for "to whirl around"**

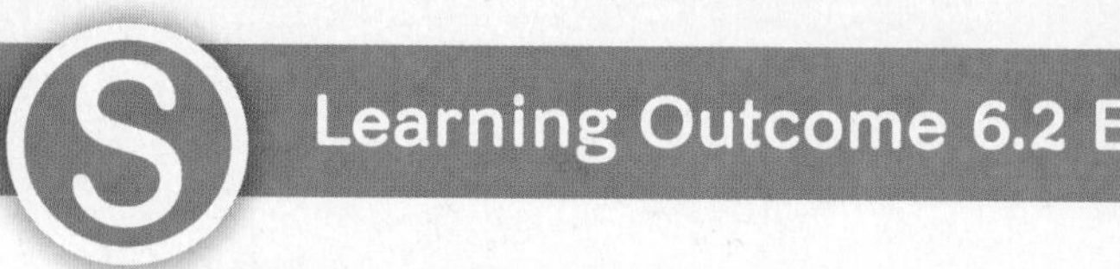

Learning Outcome 6.2 Exercises

PRONUNCIATION

EXERCISE 1 *Indicate which syllable is emphasized when pronounced.*

EXAMPLE: bronchitis bron**chi**tis

1. diplopia ______
2. myopia ______
3. miosis ______
4. otalgia ______
5. mydriasis ______
6. scotoma ______
7. tinnitus ______

TRANSLATION

EXERCISE 2 *Break down the following words into their component parts.*

EXAMPLE: nasopharyngoscope *naso | pharyngo | scope*

1. otalgia ______
2. otorrhea ______
3. asthenopia ______
4. hyperopia ______
5. hyperacusis ______
6. osteoacusis ______
7. hemianopsia ______
8. akinetopsia ______
9. blepharospasm ______
10. ophthalmoplegia ______
11. dacryoadenalgia ______
12. dacryocystalgia ______
13. dacryohemorrhea ______
14. xerophthalmia ______

EXERCISE 3 *Underline and define the word parts from this chapter in the following terms.*

1. dacryorrhea ______
2. iridalgia ______
3. keratalgia ______
4. mastoidalgia ______
5. ophthalmalgia ______
6. otodynia ______
7. cycloplegia ______
8. scotopia ______
9. diplopia ______
10. myopia ______
11. hypoacusis ______
12. corneal xerosis ______

Learning Outcome 6.2 Exercises

EXERCISE 4 *Match the term on the left with its definition on the right.*

______	1. vertigo	a.	vision problem caused by the fact that light rays entering the eye aren't focused on a single point in the back of the eye
______	2. astigmatism	b.	abnormal contraction of the pupil
______	3. ambiopia	c.	abnormal dilation of the pupil
______	4. amblyopia	d.	dark spot in the visual field
______	5. presbyopia	e.	decreased vision (when it occurs in one eye, it is referred to as *lazy eye*)
______	6. presbycusis	f.	decreased vision caused by old age
______	7. tinnitus	g.	double vision
______	8. scotoma	h.	loss of hearing in old age
______	9. mydriasis	i.	ringing in the ears
______	10. miosis	j.	the sensation of moving through space (while stationary)

EXERCISE 5 *Translate the following terms as literally as possible.*

EXAMPLE: nasopharyngoscope *an instrument for looking at the nose and throat*

1. otalgia ______________________
2. otodynia ______________________
3. ophthalmalgia ______________________
4. ambiopia ______________________
5. diplopia ______________________
6. hemianopsia ______________________
7. osteoacusis ______________________
8. presbycusis ______________________
9. akinetopsia ______________________
10. corneal xerosis ______________________
11. xerophthalmia ______________________
12. dacryoadenalgia ______________________
13. dacryocystalgia ______________________
14. dacryohemorrhea ______________________
15. astigmatism ______________________

Learning Outcome 6.2 Exercises

GENERATION

EXERCISE 6 *Build a medical term from the information provided.*

EXAMPLE: inflammation of the sinuses *sinusitis*

1. eye paralysis (use *ophthalm/o*) ______
2. paralysis of the ciliary body ______
3. paralysis of the eyelid ______
4. involuntary contraction of an eyelid ______
5. pain in the cornea (use *kerat/o*) ______
6. pain in the mastoid ______
7. pain in the iris ______
8. discharge from the ear (use *ot/o*) ______
9. excessive tearing (use *dacry/o*) ______
10. over vision condition (farsightedness) ______
11. decreased vision caused by old age ______

EXERCISE 7 *Multiple-choice questions. Select the correct answer.*

1. The medical term for nearsightedness is:
   a. amblyopia c. myopia
   b. asthenopia d. tinnitus
2. When this condition occurs in one eye, it is known as *lazy eye.*
   a. amblyopia c. myopia
   b. asthenopia d. tinnitus
3. The medical term for "eye strain" is:
   a. amblyopia c. myopia
   b. asthenopia d. tinnitus
4. The medical term used to describe "ringing in the ears" is:
   a. amblyopia c. myopia
   b. asthenopia d. tinnitus
5. *Vertigo* is a condition of the:
   a. inner ear c. inner eye
   b. outer/middle ear d. outer eye

EXERCISE 8 *Briefly describe the difference between each pair of terms.*

1. hyperacusis, hypoacusis ______
2. myopia, hyperopia ______
3. dacryohemorrhea, dacryorrhea ______
4. scotopia, scotoma ______
5. miosis, mydriasis ______

OBJECTIVE

6.3 Observation and Discovery

The Eye

As you might imagine, the physical exam of the eye is mainly limited to visual inspection. Often an eye exam begins with looking at the parts that surround it. An examiner might observe swelling (*blepharedema*) or drooping (*blepharoptosis*) around the eyelids. If pus is draining from the eyelids (*blepharopyorrhea*), that's a strong sign of infection.

After checking the eyelids, a health care professional might examine the position of the eye. An eye bulging from the orbit is known as *exophthalmos,* a condition commonly seen in hyperthyroidism.

The main areas of emphasis when inspecting the eye during a routine exam are the color of the sclera, the size of the pupils, and the movement of the eyes. The sclera of the eye is normally white. The blood vessels of the conjunctiva are normally so small that they are invisible. If the conjunctiva becomes inflamed, the vessels increase in size and the sclera may appear red. If one of the vessels in the conjunctiva ruptures, a small collection of blood may remain. Using a penlight or specialized light for examining eyes (*ophthalmoscope*), an examiner can check the size of a patient's pupils and determine how they react to light. They should constrict when exposed to light (*miosis*) and dilate when the light is dimmed.

Both eyes should work together. Shining a light in one eye should cause both pupils to constrict. The pupils should appear symmetric when looking straight ahead. One eye angled inward (*esotropia*) or outward (*exotropia*) is known as *strabismus.* A jittery, abnormal movement of the eye is called *nystagmus.* This may be a sign of an eye problem or a problem with the nervous system.

Further inspection of the eye may require specialized tools. An ophthalmoscope may be used to examine the back of a patient's eyes. It may show swelling of the optic nerve (*papilledema*). Other tools look at specific parts of the eye (*retinoscope, phacoscope*) or check for the pressure inside the eye (*tonometer*).

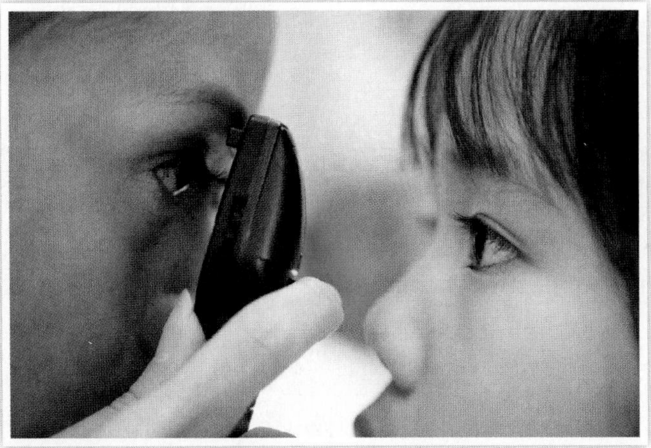

The doctor's primary instruments for observation of the eye and ear are the ophthalmoscope and the otoscope.

The Ear

When a patient presents with an ear problem, a health care professional is likely to first examine the outer part of the ear, including its size (*macrotia/microtia*) and signs of inflammation, like redness and swelling. To inspect the ear canal and eardrum, a special light known as an *otoscope* is needed.

One common finding is an excessive amount of ear wax in the ear (*ceruminosis/cerminoma*) that makes it difficult to see the eardrum. Upon visualizing the eardrum, the examiner looks for signs of fluid behind the ear. If the eardrum is red or bulging outward, an ear infection may be present. If the ear infection is bad enough, the eardrum may burst (*tympanic perforation*). Once the burst eardrum heals, the perforation may leave small, visible scars (*tympanosclerosis*).

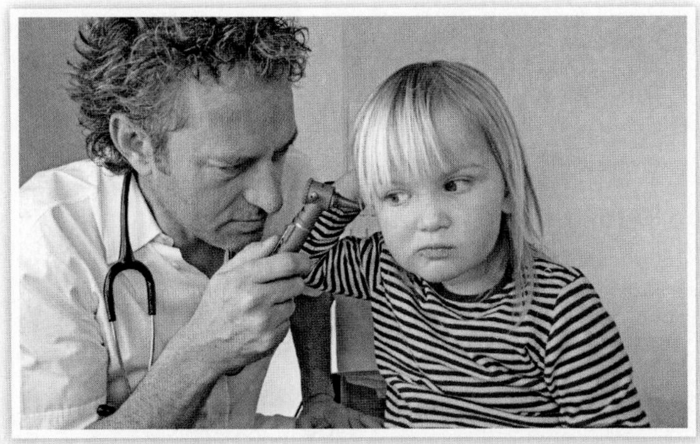

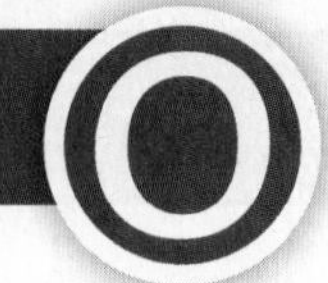

6.3 Observation and Discovery

The visualization of the ear canal and eardrum with an otoscope is called *otoscopy.* While very important, it can be difficult to determine the presence of an ear infection just by looking. If otoscopy alone does not reveal the presence of an ear infection, forcing air into the ear canal to see if it moves the eardrum (*pneumatic otoscopy*) may work.

Other tools to evaluate the ear include the *audiometer,* an instrument commonly used to check a patient's hearing, and the *salpingoscope,* a specialized instrument for examining the tubes that connect the middle ear to the nose and throat.

eye

Term	Word Analysis
Diagnostic Procedures	
ophthalmoscope awf-THAL-mah-SKOHP **Definition** instrument for looking at the eye	**ophthalmo / scope** eye / instrument for looking ©Keith Brofsky/Getty Images RF
optomyometer AWP-toh-MAI-oh-MEE-tir **Definition** device used to determine the strength of eye muscles	**opto / myo / meter** eye / muscle / instrument for measuring
phacoscope FAY-koh-SKOHP **Definition** instrument for looking at the lens	**phaco / scope** lens / instrument for looking
retinoscope RET-in-aw-SKOP **Definition** instrument for looking at the retina	**retino / scope** retina / instrument for looking
retinoscopy RET-in-AWS-koh-pee **Definition** procedure for looking at the retina	**retino / scopy** retina / looking procedure
tonometer TOH-naw-MEE-tir **Definition** instrument for measuring tension or pressure in the eye (intraocular pressure)	**tono / meter** tension / instrument for measuring
Professional Terms	
binocular bai-NAW-kyoo-lar **Definition** pertaining to both eyes	**bin / ocul / ar** two / eye / pertaining to
iridokinesis IR-ih-doh-kin-EE-sis **Definition** the movement of the iris	**irido / kinesis** iris / movement

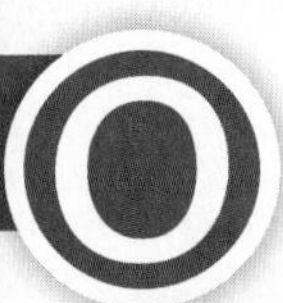

eye *continued*

Term	Word Analysis
lacrimation LAH-krih-MAY-shun **Definition** formation of tears (i.e., crying)	**lacrim / ation** tear / condition
nasolacrimal NAY-zoh-LAH-krih-mal **Definition** pertaining to the nose and tear system	**naso / lacrim / al** nose / tear / pertaining to
ophthalmic awf-THAL-mik **Definition** pertaining to the eye	**ophthalm / ic** eye / pertaining to
ophthalmologist AWF-thal-MAW-loh-jist **Definition** eye specialist	**ophthalmo / logist** eye / specialist ©Sean Justice/Corbis RF
optic AWP-tik **Definition** pertaining to the eye	**opt / ic** eye / pertaining to
optokinetic AWP-toh-kih-NEH-tik **Definition** pertaining to eye movement	**opto / kinet / ic** eye / movement / pertaining to
optometrist awp-TAW-meh-trist **Definition** specialist in measuring the eye	**opto / metr / ist** eye / measure / specialist
retinal REH-tih-nal **Definition** pertaining to the retina	**retin / al** retina / pertaining to
Outer Structures and Vision	
blepharedema BLEF-ar-eh-DEE-mah **Definition** eyelid swelling	**blephar / edema** eyelid / swelling
blepharoptosis BLEF-ar-awp-TOH-sis **Definition** drooping eyelid	**blepharo / ptosis** eyelid / drooping condition

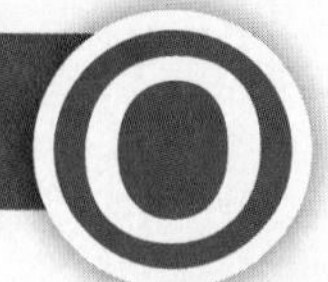

6.3 Observation and Discovery

eye *continued*

Term	Word Analysis
blepharopyorrhea BLEF-ah-roh-PAI-oh-REE-ah **Definition** discharge of pus from the eyelid	**blepharo / pyo / rrhea** eyelid / pus / discharge
dacryolith DAK-ree-oh-lith **Definition** hard formation (stone) in the tear system	**dacryo / lith** tear / stone
dacryopyorrhea DAK-ree-oh-pai-REE-ah **Definition** discharge of pus in tears	**dacryo / pyo / rrhea** tear / pus / discharge
ectropion ek-TROH-pee-on **Definition** outward turning of the eyelid, away from the eye	**ec / tropion** out / turn
entropion en-TROH-pee-on **Definition** inward turning of the eyelid, toward the eye	**en / tropion** in / turn
exophthalmus EKS-of-THAL-mus **Definition** protrusion of the eyes out of the eye socket	**ex / ophthalmus** out / eye
nystagmus nih-STAG-mus **Definition** involuntary back-and-forth movement of the eyes	**from Greek, for** "to nod"
strabismus stuh-BIZ-mus **Definition** condition where the eyes deviate when looking at the same object	**from Latin, for** "to squint"
esotropia AY-soh-TROH-pee-ah **Definition** inward turning of the eye, toward the nose	**eso / trop / ia** inward / turn / condition

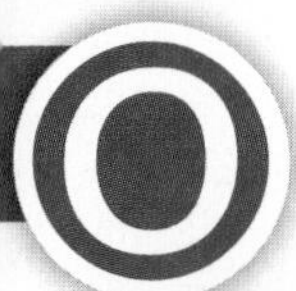

6.3 Observation and Discovery

eye *continued*

Term	Word Analysis
exotropia EK-soh-TROH-pee-ah **Definition** outward turning of the eye, away from the nose	**exo / trop / ia** outward / turn / condition
Sclera	
keratomalacia ker-AH-toh-mah-LAY-shah **Definition** abnormal softening of the cornea	**kerato / malacia** cornea / softening
pterygium ter-IH-jee-um **Definition** winglike growth of conjunctival tissue extending to the cornea **Note:** Think of the pterodactyl, a flying dinosaur whose name means "winged fingers."	**from Greek, for "wing"** 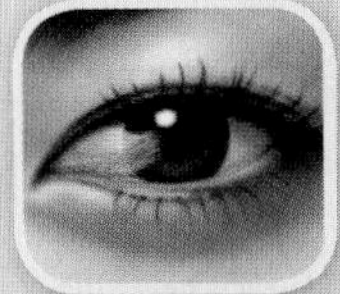
scleromalacia SKLEH-roh-mah-LAY-shah **Definition** abnormal softening of the sclera	**sclero / malacia** sclera / softening
Choroid/Retina	
papilledema PAH-pil-ah-DEE-mah **Definition** swelling of the optic nerve where it enters the retina **Note:** *Papilla* is the term for the place in the back of the eye where the optic nerve enters the retina. It looks like a nipple, so that is what they named it.	**papill / edema** nipple / swelling 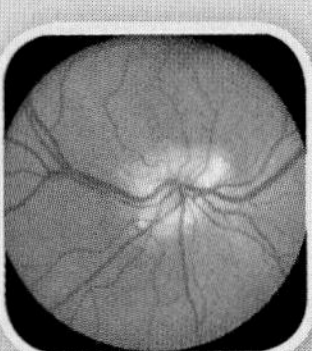 ©Biophoto Associates/Science Source
phacomalacia FAH-koh-mah-LAY-shah **Definition** abnormal softening of the lens	**phaco / malacia** lens / softening
phacosclerosis FAH-koh-skleh-ROH-sis **Definition** abnormal hardening of the lens	**phaco / scler / osis** lens / hardening / condition

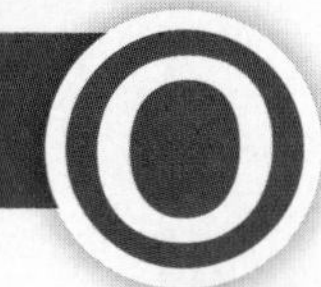

6.3 Observation and Discovery

ear

Term	Word Analysis
Diagnostic Procedures	
audiogram AW-dee-oh-GRAM **Definition** record produced by an audiometer	**audio / gram** hearing / record
audiometer aw-dee-AW-meh-ter **Definition** instrument for measuring hearing	**audio / meter** hearing / instrument for measuring
audiometry aw-dee-AW-meh-tree **Definition** procedure for measuring hearing	**audio / metry** hearing / measuring procedure
otoscope OH-toh-SKOHP **Definition** instrument for looking in the ear	**oto / scope** ear / instrument for looking
otoscopy oh-TAW-skoh-pee **Definition** procedure for examining the ear	**oto / scopy** ear / looking procedure ©Creatas/PunchStock RF
pneumatic otoscopy noo-MA-tik oh-TAW-skoh-pee **Definition** procedure for examining the ear using air **NOTE:** Air is pushed against the eardrum to see how much it moves. Less movement indicates that fluid has built up—an indicator of otitis media.	**pneumat / ic** **oto / scopy** air / pertaining to ear / looking procedure
salpingoscope sal-PING-goh-skohp **Definition** instrument for examining the eustachian tubes	**salpingo / scope** eustachian tube / instrument for looking
tympanometry tim-pan-AW-meh-tree **Definition** procedure for measuring the eardrum **NOTE:** In this context, *measurement* is not about size of the eardrum, but about how much it moves.	**tympano / metry** eardrum / measuring process

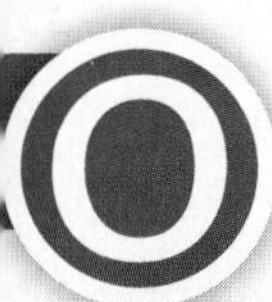

6.3 Observation and Discovery

ear *continued*

Term	Word Analysis
Professional Terms	
audiologist aw-dee-AW-loh-jist **Definition** hearing specialist	**audio / logist** hearing / specialist
aural AW-ral **Definition** pertaining to the ear **NOTE:** This word is easily confused with *oral*.	**aur / al** ear / pertaining to
otolaryngologist OH-toh-LAH-rin-GAW-loh-jist **Definition** specialist in the ear and throat	**oto / laryngo / logist** ear / throat / specialist
otoneurologist OH-toh-nih-RAW-loh-jist **Definition** specialist in the nerve connections between the ear and brain	**oto / neuro / logist** ear / nerve / specialist
otorhinolaryngologist OH-toh-RAI-noh-LAH-rin-GAW-loh-jist **Definition** specialist in the ear, nose, and throat	**oto / rhino / laryngo / logist** ear / nose / throat / specialist
otosteal oh-TAWS-tee-all **Definition** pertaining to the bones of the ear	**ot / oste / al** ear / bone / pertaining to
salpingopharyngeal sal-PING-goh-fah-RIN-jee-al **Definition** pertaining to the eustachian tubes and the throat	**salpingo / pharyng / eal** eustachian tube / throat / pertaining to
Outer Ear	
ceruminoma seh-ROO-min-OH-mah **Definition** benign tumor of the cerumen-secreting glands of the ear	**cerumin / oma** ear wax / tumor
ceruminosis seh-ROO-min-OH-sis **Definition** excessive formation of ear wax	**cerumin / osis** ear wax / condition
macrotia mah-KROH-shee-ah **Definition** abnormally large ears	**macr / ot / ia** big / ear / condition
microtia mai-KROH-shee-ah **Definition** abnormally small ears	**micr / ot / ia** small / ear / condition

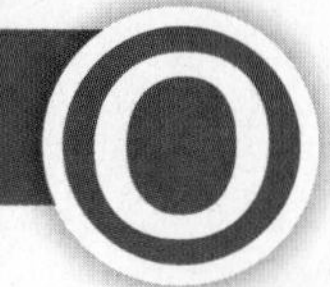

6.3 Observation and Discovery

ear *continued*

Term	Word Analysis
otopyorrhea OH-toh-PAI-oh-REE-ah **Definition** discharge of pus from the ears	**oto / pyo / rrhea** ear / pus / discharge
Middle Ear	
otosclerosis OH-toh-skleh-ROH-sis **Definition** hearing loss caused by the hardening of the bones of the middle ear	**oto / scler / osis** ear / hardening / condition
tympanic perforation tim-PAN-ik per-fer-AY-shun **Definition** tear or hole in the eardrum	**tympan / ic** **per / for / ation** eardrum / pertaining to through / pierce / condition 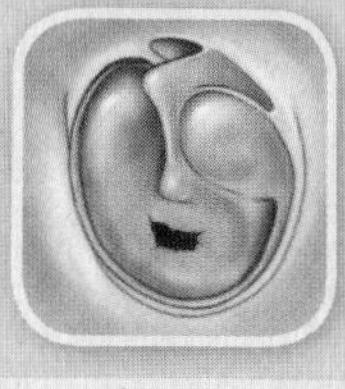
tympanosclerosis tim-PAN-oh-skleh-ROH-sis **Definition** hardening of the eardrum	**tympano / scler / osis** eardrum / hardening / condition

PRONUNCIATION

EXERCISE 1 *Indicate which syllable is emphasized when pronounced.*

EXAMPLE: bronchitis bron**chi**tis

1. retinal ______
2. otoscopy ______
3. dacryolith ______
4. ophthalmic ______
5. audiometer ______
6. audiometry ______
7. audiologist ______
8. ectropion ______
9. entropion ______
10. strabismus ______
11. nystagmus ______
12. macrotia ______
13. microtia ______
14. tympanometry ______

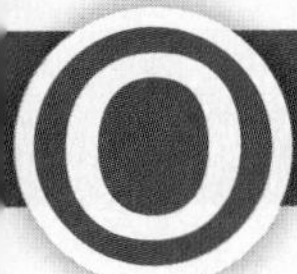

Learning Outcome 6.3 Exercises

TRANSLATION

EXERCISE 2 *Break down the following words into their component parts.*

EXAMPLE: nasopharyngoscope *naso | pharyngo | scope*

1. audiogram ______
2. audiometer ______
3. aural ______
4. microtia ______
5. optometrist ______
6. optokinetic ______
7. otosclerosis ______
8. phacosclerosis ______
9. tympanosclerosis ______
10. ceruminosis ______
11. nasolacrimal ______
12. blepharoptosis ______
13. blepharopyorrhea ______
14. dacryopyorrhea ______
15. exophthalmus ______
16. otoneurology ______
17. otolaryngologist ______
18. otorhinolaryngologist ______
19. salpingopharyngeal ______

EXERCISE 3 *Underline and define the word parts from this chapter in the following terms.*

1. optic ______
2. retinal ______
3. otoscopy ______
4. otosteal ______
5. audiometry ______
6. tympanometry ______
7. ophthalmic ______
8. audiologist ______
9. ophthalmologist ______
10. dacryolith ______
11. retinoscopy ______
12. keratomalacia ______
13. phacomalacia ______
14. scleromalacia ______
15. tonometer ______
16. binocular ______
17. otopyorrhea ______
18. optomyometer ______
19. iridokinesis ______
20. lacrimation ______

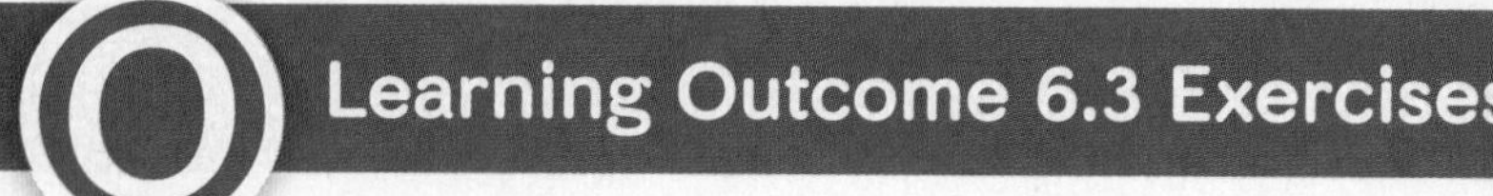

21. blepharedema ______________________
22. ceruminoma ______________________
23. pneumatic otoscopy ______________________
24. macrotia ______________________

EXERCISE 4 *Match the term on the left with its definition on the right.*

____	1. tympanic perforation	a.	condition where the eyes deviate when looking at the same object
____	2. papilledema	b.	tear or hole in the eardrum
____	3. pterygium	c.	winglike growth of conjunctival tissue extending to the cornea
____	4. exotropia	d.	involuntary back-and-forth movement of the eyes
____	5. esotropia	e.	swelling of the optic nerve where it enters the retina
____	6. ectropion	f.	inward turning of the eye, toward the nose
____	7. entropion	g.	outward turning of the eye, away from the nose
____	8. nystagmus	h.	inward turning of the eyelid, toward the eye
____	9. strabismus	i.	outward turning of the eyelid, away from the eye

EXERCISE 5 *Match the term on the left with its definition on the right.*

____	1. retinoscope	a.	instrument for looking at the eustachian tubes
____	2. otoscope	b.	instrument for looking at the eye
____	3. ophthalmoscope	c.	instrument for looking at the lens
____	4. salpingoscope	d.	instrument for looking at the retina
____	5. phacoscope	e.	instrument for looking in the ear

EXERCISE 6 *Translate the following terms as literally as possible.*

EXAMPLE: nasopharyngoscope *an instrument for looking at the nose and throat*

1. optomyometer ______________________
2. retinoscopy ______________________
3. tonometer ______________________
4. binocular ______________________
5. nasolacrimal ______________________
6. retinal ______________________
7. blepharopyrorrhea ______________________
8. dacryolith ______________________
9. dacryopyorrhea ______________________
10. exophthalmus ______________________
11. audiometer ______________________

Learning Outcome 6.3 Exercises

12. audiometry ______
13. tympanometry ______
14. aural ______
15. otolaryngologist ______
16. otorhinolaryngologist ______
17. salpingopharyngeal ______
18. ceruminosis ______
19. macrotia ______
20. otopyorrhea ______
21. tympanic perforation ______

GENERATION

EXERCISE 7 *Build a medical term from the information provided.*

EXAMPLE: inflammation of the sinuses *sinusitis*

1. instrument for looking at the eye (use *ophthalm/o*) ______
2. instrument for looking in the ear (use *ot/o*) ______
3. instrument for looking at the lens ______
4. instrument for looking at the retina ______
5. instrument for looking at the eustachian tubes ______
6. abnormal softening of the cornea (use *kerat/o*) ______
7. ear wax tumor ______
8. procedure for looking in the ear (use *ot/o*) ______
9. procedure for looking in the ear using air ______
10. hearing record (use *audi/o*) ______
11. hearing specialist (use *audi/o*) ______
12. ear nerve specialist (use *ot/o*) ______
13. pertaining to the eye (use *ophthalm/o*) ______
14. pertaining to the eye (use *opt/o*) ______
15. pertaining to eye movement (use *opt/o*) ______
16. pertaining to the bones of the ear (use *ot/o*) ______
17. the movement of the iris (use *irid/o*) ______

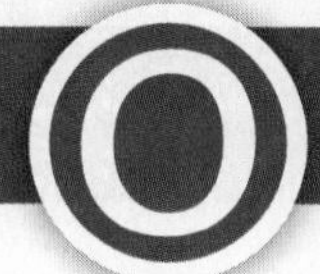

Learning Outcome 6.3 Exercises

EXERCISE 8 *Multiple-choice questions. Select the correct answer.*

1. The swelling of the optic nerve where it enters is retina is known as:
   a. nystagmus
   b. papilledema
   c. pterygium
   d. strabismus
2. This term comes from Greek, for "wing," and describes a winglike growth of conjunctival tissue extending to the cornea.
   a. lacrimation
   b. papilledema
   c. pterygium
   d. strabismus
3. The medical term for tear formation, or "crying," is:
   a. lacrimation
   b. nystagmus
   c. pterygium
   d. strabismus
4. A condition where the eyes deviate when looking at the same object is:
   a. lacrimation
   b. nystagmus
   c. papilledema
   d. strabismus
5. Involuntary back-and-forth movement of the eyes is called:
   a. lacrimation
   b. nystagmus
   c. papilledema
   d. pterygium

EXERCISE 9 *Briefly describe the difference between each pair of terms.*

1. microtia, macrotia ____________________
2. tympanosclerosis, otosclerosis ____________________
3. phacomalacia, scleromalacia ____________________
4. phacomalacia, phacosclerosis ____________________
5. optometrist, ophthalmologist ____________________
6. blepharedema, blepharoptosis ____________________
7. ectropion, entropion ____________________
8. esotropia, exotropia ____________________

6.4 Diagnosis and Pathology

The Eye

OUTER STRUCTURES

Structures around the eye often get inflamed. *Blepharitis* is usually caused by a mild bacterial skin infection. *Dacryoadenitis* is inflammation of the tear gland. The cause is not well understood, but it's thought to be an extension of inflammation of the conjunctiva.

More common is inflammation of the tear duct that drains the eye. In infants, this drainage system can be blocked (*dacryostenosis*) and can lead to a mild infection (*dacryocystitis*). Probably the most common eye complaint seen in most doctors' offices is inflammation of the conjunctiva (*conjunctivitis*). This can result from allergies, irritants in the eye, or infection. Infections of the conjunctiva (commonly known as *pink eye*) are usually caused by a virus or bacteria.

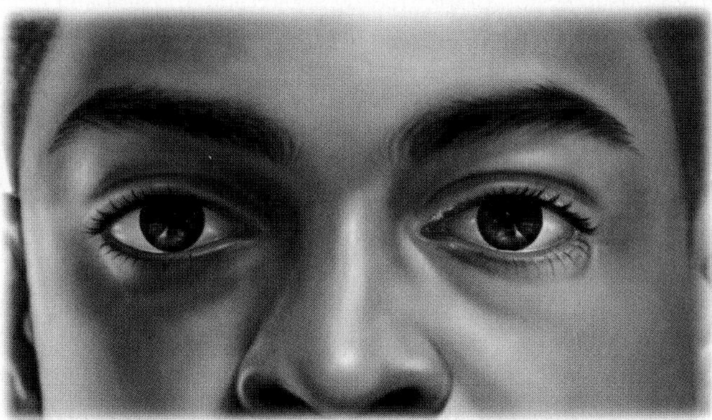

Infections of the conjunctiva are commonly known as pink eye.

OUTER LAYER

The sclera has few general problems—the main one being *scleritis*. This painful, chronic illness is often due to general inflammatory disorders like *rheumatoid arthritis*. Problems with the cornea (*keratopathy*) include scratching from a foreign object (*corneal abrasion*) and inflammation (*keratitis*). Often caused by infection, keratitis is generally a very serious condition.

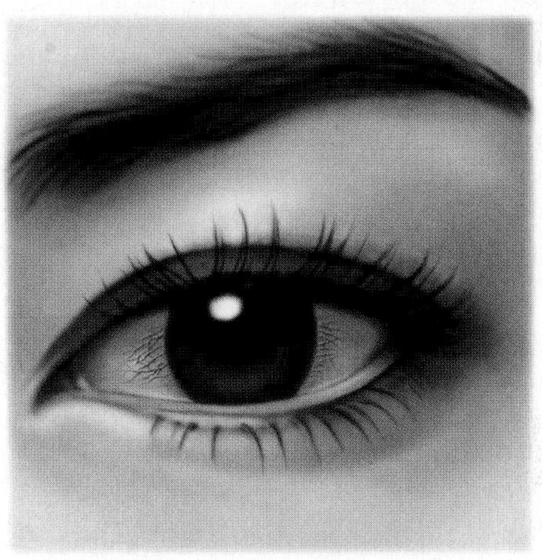

Inflamed blood vessels in the sclera

MIDDLE LAYER

The most common concern of the lens is clouding (*cataract*). The lens may also be undeveloped/absent (*aphakia*). Often aphakia is a result of surgical removal. Iridopathies, or disorders of the iris, include bleeding (*iridemia*). Inflammation of the iris (*iritis*) and iris with extension to the ciliary muscle (*iridocyclitis*) are unusual and painful.

INNER LAYER

The optic nerve is vulnerable to pressure from inside the eye (*glaucoma*) or from the brain; pressure from the brain can lead to swelling of the optic disc (*papilledema*). Like the other parts of the eye, the optic nerve can become inflamed (*optic neuritis*).

The retina can become detached from the blood supply. This emergency situation requires immediate reattachment, or blindness will occur. General retinal damage (*retinopathy*) can result from diabetes or blood disorders. Premature infants sometimes develop retinopathy after receiving oxygen as treatment for a lung disease.

The Ear

Many problems of the outer and middle ear involve infection. Infection of the outer ear (*otitis externa*) is a very common problem in summer, as swimmers often get water trapped in the ear canal. The common term for this illness is *swimmer's ear.* Otitis externa can also result from using a cotton swab to clean out the ears, which can push ear wax down into the ear until it forms a hard mass known as *cerumen impaction.*

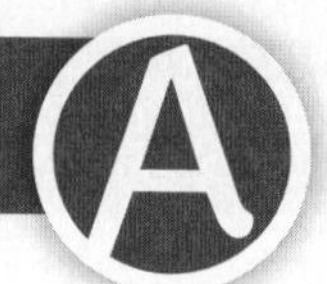

6.4 Diagnosis and Pathology

Infection of the middle ear (*otitis media*) is one of the most common complaints seen in pediatric offices. Occasionally, the eardrum can be so inflamed that it blisters (*bullous myrigitis*). Less commonly, an ear infection can lead to a serious infection of the nearby skull bone (*mastoiditis*).

Inner ear problems manifest as either a loss of hearing (*sensorineural hearing loss*) or *vertigo*. Vertigo arises from inflammation of the inner ear structures (*labyrinthitis*) or the nerve that connects it to the brain (*vestibular neuritis*).

eye

Term	Word Analysis
Outer Structures and Vision	
blepharitis BLEF-ah-RAI-tis **Definition** eyelid inflammation	**blephar / itis** eyelid / inflammation
blepharoconjunctivitis BLEF-ah-roh-con-JUNK-tih-VAI-tis **Definition** inflammation of the eyelid and conjunctiva	**blepharo / conjunctiv / itis** eyelid / conjunctiva / inflammation
dacryocystitis DAK-ree-oh-sis-TAI-tis **Definition** inflammation of the tear sac	**dacryo / cyst / itis** tear / sac / inflammation
dacryoadenitis DAK-ree-oh-AD-en-AI-tis **Definition** inflammation of the tear gland	**dacryo / aden / itis** tear / gland / inflammation
dacryohemorrhea DAK-ree-oh-HEH-moh-REE-ah **Definition** discharge of blood in tears	**dacryo / hemo / rrhea** tear / blood / discharge
dacryolithiasis DAK-ree-oh-lih-THAI-ah-sis **Definition** presence of hard formations (stones) in the tear system	**dacryo / lith / iasis** tear / stone / presence
dacryostenosis DAK-ree-oh-steh-NOH-sis **Definition** narrowing of the tear duct	**dacryo / sten / osis** tear / narrowing / condition
glaucoma glaw-KOH-mah **Definition** eye disease that causes vision loss by damaging the optic nerve	**glaucoma** **from a Greek word meaning** "gray-eyed"

NOTE: Although you might think that this word has an *-oma* suffix and refers to a tumor, it is actually a Greek word that means "gray-eyed" and refers to the fact that until the 1700s doctors didn't distinguish between cataracts and glaucoma.

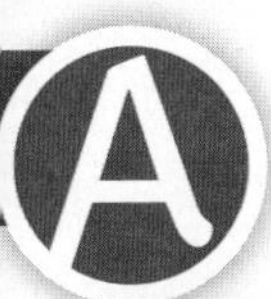

6.4 Diagnosis and Pathology

eye *continued*

Term	Word Analysis
oculomycosis AW-kyoo-loh-mai-KOH-sis **Definition** fungal eye condition	**oculo / myc / osis** eye / fungus / condition
oculopathy AW-kyoo-LAW-pah-thee **Definition** eye disease	**oculo / pathy** eye / disease
ophthalmatrophy AWF-thal-MAW-troh-fee **Definition** atrophy (wasting away) of the eye	**ophthalm / a / trophy** eye / no / nourishment
ophthalmitis AWF-thal-MAI-tis **Definition** inflammation of the eye	**ophthalm / itis** eye / inflammation
ophthalmomycosis awf-THAL-moh-mai-KOH-sis **Definition** fungal eye condition	**ophthalmo / myc / osis** eye / fungus / condition
ophthalmomyitis awf-THAL-moh-mai-AI-tis **Definition** inflammation of the eye muscles	**ophthalmo / my / itis** eye / muscle / inflammation
ophthalmopathy AWF-thal-MOH-pah-thee **Definition** eye disease	**ophthalmo / pathy** eye / disease
trichiasis trih-KAI-ah-sis **Definition** condition caused by eyelashes growing backward and coming in contact with the eye	**trich / iasis** hair / presence
Sclera	
conjunctivitis con-JUNK-tih-VAI-tis **Definition** inflammation of the conjunctiva (also known as *pink eye*)	**conjunctiv / itis** conjunctiva / inflammation Source: Centers for Disease Control and Prevention
keratitis KEH-rah-TAI-tis **Definition** inflammation of the cornea	**kerat / itis** cornea / inflammation

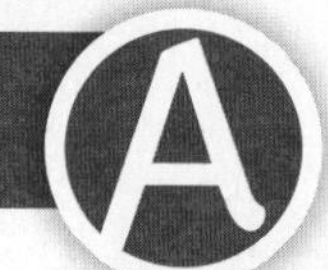

6.4 Diagnosis and Pathology

eye *continued*

Term	Word Analysis
keratopathy KEH-rah-TOP-ah-thee **Definition** disease of the cornea	**kerato / pathy** cornea / disease
sclerectasia SKLER-ek-TAY-zhah **Definition** overexpansion of the sclera	**scler / ectas / ia** sclera / expansion / condition
scleroiritis SKLER-oh-ai-RAI-tis **Definition** inflammation of the sclera and iris	**sclero / ir / itis** sclera / iris / inflammation
sclerokeratitis SKLER-oh-KEH-rah-TAI-tis **Definition** inflammation of the sclera and cornea	**sclero / kerat / itis** sclera / cornea / inflammation
sclerokeratoiritis SKLER-oh-KEH-ra-toh-ai-RAI-tis **Definition** inflammation of the sclera, cornea, and iris	**sclero / kerato / ir / itis** sclera / cornea / iris / inflammation
Choroid/Retina	
aniridia AN-ih-RIH-dee-ah **Definition** absence of an iris	**an / irid / ia** no / iris / condition 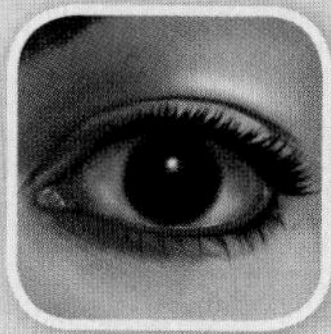
aphakia ah-FAY-kee-ia **Definition** absence of a lens **NOTE:** *Phak* is written with a *k* instead of a *c*. Although both are acceptable spellings, some people use a *k* to make sure the word is pronounced ah-FAY-kee-ia instead of ah-FAY-see-ia, which could be confused with other terms.	**a / phak / ia** no / lens / condition 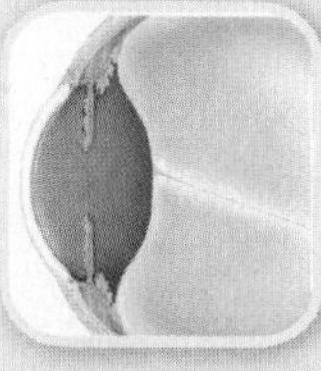
cataract KAT-ah-RAKT **Definition** opacity (cloudiness) of the lens of the eye	**from Latin, for** "waterfall" 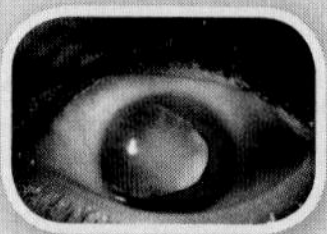 ©Paul Whitten/Science Source

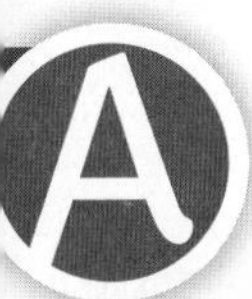

6.4 Diagnosis and Pathology

eye *continued*

Term	Word Analysis
corneal abrasion KOR-nee-al a-BRAY-zhun **Definition** scratch on the cornea	**corne / al ab / rasion** cornea / pertaining to away / rubbing ©Dr. P. Marazzi/Science Source
cyclokeratitis SAI-cloh-keh-rah-TAI-tis **Definition** inflammation of the ciliary body and cornea	**cyclo / kerat / itis** ciliary body / cornea / inflammation
endophthalmitis EN-dof-thal-MAI-tis **Definition** inflammation of the inside of the eye (often a complication from intraocular surgery)	**end / ophthalm / itis** inside / eye / inflammation
iridemia EAR-ih-DEE-mee-ah **Definition** bleeding from the iris	**irid / emia** iris / blood condition
iridocyclitis EAR-ih-doh-sai-KLAI-tis **Definition** inflammation of the iris and ciliary body	**irido / cycl / itis** iris / ciliary body / inflammation
iridokeratitis EAR-ih-doh-keh-rah-TAI-tis **Definition** inflammation of the iris and cornea	**irido / kerat / itis** iris / cornea / inflammation
iridopathy EAR-ih-DOP-ah-thee **Definition** disease of the iris	**irido / pathy** iris / disease
iritis ai-RAI-tis **Definition** inflammation of the iris	**ir / itis** iris / inflammation
optic neuritis OP-tik nir-AI-tis **Definition** inflammation of the optic nerve	**opt / ic neur / itis** eye / pertaining to nerve / inflammation
phakitis fah-KAI-tis **Definition** inflammation of the lens **Note:** *Phak* is written with a *k* instead of a *c*. Although both are acceptable spellings, some people use a *k* to make sure the word is pronounced fah-KAI-tis instead of fah-SAI-tis, which could be confused with other terms.	**phak / itis** lens / inflammation
retinitis REH-tih-NAI-tis **Definition** inflammation of the retina	**retin / itis** retina / inflammation ©Sue Ford/Science Source

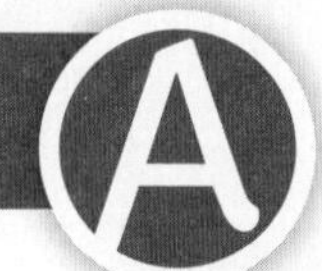

6.4 Diagnosis and Pathology

eye *continued*

Term	Word Analysis
retinopathy REH-tih-NOP-ah-thee **Definition** disease of the retina	**retino / pathy** retina / disease
retinosis REH-tih-NOH-sis **Definition** retinal condition	**retin / osis** retina / condition

ear

Term	Word Analysis
Outer Ear	
cerumen impaction SEH-roo-men im-PAK-shun **Definition** buildup of ear wax blocking ear canal	**cerumen im / pac / tion** ear wax in / drive / condition
mastoiditis MAS-toi-DAI-tis **Definition** inflammation of the mastoid	**mastoid / itis** mastoid / inflammation
otitis externa oh-TAI-tis eks-TERN-nah **Definition** inflammation of the outer ear	**ot / itis externa** ear / inflammation outside
otomycosis oh-toh-mai-KOH-sis **Definition** fungal ear condition	**oto / myc / osis** ear / fungus / condition
Middle Ear	
aerotitis AIR-oh-TAI-tis **Definition** inflammation of the ear caused by air **NOTE:** This one is tricky because, unless you are careful, you will be tempted to miss the *ot* root in the middle. Most people want to divide the word *aero* + *itis*. The problem is the *t* in the middle. That is your clue that a root is hiding in the middle.	**aer / ot / itis** air / ear / inflammation
conductive hearing loss con-DUK-tiv **Definition** hearing loss caused by sound not getting to the middle/inner ear (due to blockages)	**con / duct / ive** together / lead / pertaining to
myringitis MIR-in-JAI-tis **Definition** inflammation of the eardrum	**myring / itis** eardrum / inflammation ©BSIP/Science Source
myringodermatitis mir-IN-goh-DER-mah-TAI-tis **Definition** inflammation of the eardrum and surrounding skin	**myringo / dermat / itis** eardrum / skin / inflammation

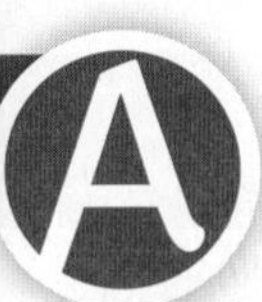

6.4 Diagnosis and Pathology

ear *continued*

Term	Word Analysis
myringomycosis mir-IN-goh-mai-KOH-sis **Definition** fungal condition of the eardrum	**myringo / myc / osis** eardrum / fungus / condition
otitis media oh-TAI-tis MEH-dee-ah **Definition** inflammation of the middle ear	**ot / itis media** ear / inflammation middle
otosclerosis oh-toh-skleh-ROH-sis **Definition** hearing loss caused by the hardening of the bones of the middle ear	**oto / scler / osis** ear / hardening / condition
rhinosalpingitis RAI-noh-SAL-pin-JAI-tis **Definition** inflammation of the nose and eustachian tubes	**rhino / salping / itis** nose / eustachian / tube inflammation
Inner Ear	
acoustic neuroma ah-KOO-stik nir-OH-mah **Definition** tumor on the acoustic nerve	**acous / tic neur / oma** hearing / pertaining to nerve / tumor
cochleitis KOH-klee-AI-tis **Definition** inflammation of the cochlea	**cochle / itis** cochlea / inflammation
labyrinthitis LAB-uh-rinth-AI-tis **Definition** inflammation of the labyrinth	**labyrinth / itis** labyrinth / inflammation
sensorineural hearing loss SEN-sor-ee-NIR-al **Definition** hearing loss caused by sound not being transmitted from the inner ear to the brain (due to problems with the sensory organs or nerves)	**sensori / neur / al** sense / nerve / pertaining to
vestibular neuritis ves-TIH-byoo-lar nir-AI-tis **Definition** inflammation of the vestibular nerve	**vestibul / ar neur / itis** vestibule / pertaining to nerve / inflammation
vestibulitis ves-TIH-byoo-LAI-tis **Definition** inflammation of the vestibule	**vestibul / itis** vestibule / inflammation

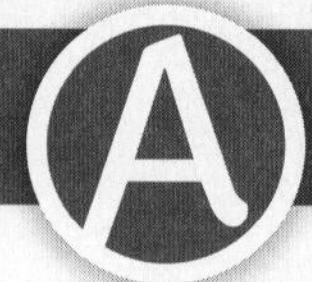

Learning Outcome 6.4 Exercises

PRONUNCIATION

EXERCISE 1 *Indicate which syllable is emphasized when pronounced.*

EXAMPLE: bronchitis bron**chi**tis

1. acoustic ______
2. neuroma ______
3. vestibular ______
4. neuritis ______
5. iritis ______
6. aphakia ______
7. trichiasis ______
8. otomycosis ______

TRANSLATION

EXERCISE 2 *Break down the following words into their component parts.*

EXAMPLE: nasopharyngoscope *naso | pharyngo | scope*

1. iridemia ______
2. retinopathy ______
3. ophthalmopathy ______
4. dacryostenosis ______
5. dacryocystitis ______
6. dacryoadenitis ______
7. otomycosis ______
8. myringomycosis ______
9. ophthalmomycosis ______
10. blepharoconjunctivitis ______
11. sclerokeratoiritis ______

EXERCISE 3 *Underline and define the word parts from this chapter in the following terms.*

1. corneal abrasion ______
2. conjunctivitis ______
3. mastoiditis ______
4. cochleitis ______
5. labyrinthitis ______
6. vestibulitis ______
7. myringitis ______
8. blepharitis ______
9. retinosis ______
10. otosclerosis ______
11. oculopathy ______
12. keratopathy ______
13. iridopathy ______
14. cerumen impaction ______
15. sclerectasia ______
16. aniridia ______
17. aphakia ______
18. ophthalmomyitis ______

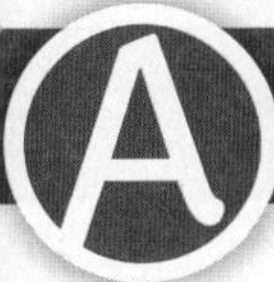

Learning Outcome 6.4 Exercises

EXERCISE 4 *Match the term on the left with its definition on the right.*

	Term		Definition
______	1. cataract	a.	fungal eye condition
______	2. oculomycosis	b.	atrophy (wasting away) of the eye
______	3. ophthalmatrophy	c.	condition caused by eyelashes growing backward and coming in contact with the eye
______	4. dacryolithiasis	d.	discharge of blood in the tears
______	5. dacryohemorrhea	e.	opacity (cloudiness) of the lens of the eye
______	6. trichiasis	f.	presence of hard formations (stones) in the tear system

EXERCISE 5 *Match the term on the left with its definition on the right.*

	Term		Definition
______	1. retinitis	a.	inflammation of the ciliary body and cornea
______	2. keratitis	b.	inflammation of the cornea
______	3. iritis	c.	inflammation of the eye
______	4. ophthalmitis	d.	inflammation of the iris
______	5. phakitis	e.	inflammation of the iris and ciliary body
______	6. optic neuritis	f.	inflammation of the iris and cornea
______	7. iridokeratitis	g.	inflammation of the lens
______	8. iridocyclitis	h.	inflammation of the optic nerve
______	9. scleroiritis	i.	inflammation of the retina
______	10. sclerokeratitis	j.	inflammation of the sclera and cornea
______	11. cyclokeratitis	k.	inflammation of the sclera and iris

EXERCISE 6 *Match the term on the left with its definition on the right.*

	Term		Definition
______	1. otitis media	a.	inflammation of the outer ear
______	2. otitis externa	b.	inflammation of the ear caused by air
______	3. aerotitis	c.	hearing loss caused by sound not getting to the middle/inner ear (due to blockages)
______	4. conductive hearing loss	d.	inflammation of the eardrum and surrounding skin
______	5. sensorineural hearing loss	e.	inflammation of the middle ear
______	6. vestibular neuritis	f.	inflammation of the nose and eustachian tubes
______	7. acoustic neuroma	g.	tumor on the acoustic nerve
______	8. myringodermatitis	h.	hearing loss caused by sound not being transmitted from the inner ear to the brain (due to problems with the sense organs or nerves)
______	9. rhinosalpingitis	i.	inflammation of the vestibular nerve

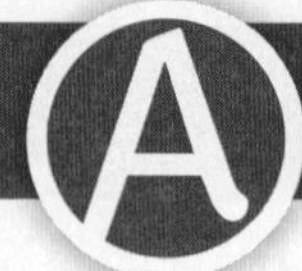

Learning Outcome 6.4 Exercises

EXERCISE 7 *Translate the following terms as literally as possible.*

EXAMPLE: nasopharyngoscope *an instrument for looking at the nose and throat*

1. oculopathy ______
2. ophthalmopathy ______
3. iridemia ______
4. iridokeratitis ______
5. cyclokeratitis ______
6. sclerectasia ______
7. scleroiritis ______
8. sclerokeratoiritis ______
9. blepharoconjunctivitis ______
10. dacryohemorrhea ______
11. dacryolithiasis ______
12. ophthalmomycosis ______
13. myringomycosis ______
14. trichiasis ______
15. optic neuritis ______
16. acoustic neuroma ______
17. vestibular neuritis ______
18. rhinosalpingitis ______

GENERATION

EXERCISE 8 *Build a medical term from the information provided.*

EXAMPLE: inflammation of the sinuses *sinusitis*

1. inflammation of the retina ______
2. inflammation of the mastoid ______
3. inflammation of the cochlea ______
4. inflammation of the labyrinth ______
5. inflammation of the vestibule ______
6. inflammation of the lens ______
7. inflammation of the iris ______
8. inflammation of the iris and ciliary body ______
9. inflammation of the cornea (use *kerat/o*) ______
10. inflammation of the sclera and cornea ______

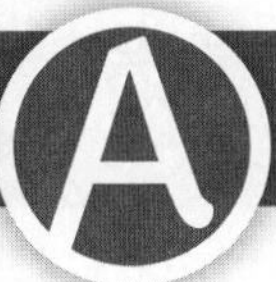

Learning Outcome 6.4 Exercises

11. inflammation of the eardum (use *myring/o*) ______________________
12. inflammation of the eardrum and surrounding skin ______________________
13. inflammation of the eye (use *ophthalm/o*) ______________________
14. inflammation of the eye muscles ______________________
15. Inflammation of the eyelid ______________________
16. Inflammation of the eyelid and conjunctiva ______________________

EXERCISE 9 *Multiple-choice questions. Select the correct answer(s).*

1. Select the terms that pertain to the eye.
   a. aerotitis
   b. aphakia
   c. cataract
   d. cerumen impaction
   e. corneal abrasion
   f. ophthalmatrophy
   g. otitis media

2. Select the terms that pertain to the ear.
   a. aerotitis
   b. aphakia
   c. cataract
   d. cerumen impaction
   e. corneal abrasion
   f. ophthalmatrophy
   g. otitis media

3. The medical term that refers to the atrophy of the eye is:
   a. oculosclerosis
   b. ophthalmatrophy
   c. otomatrophy
   d. otosclerosis

4. A cataract affects what part of the eye?
   a. cornea
   b. lens
   c. optic nerve
   d. retina

5. A scratch on the cornea is called a(n):
   a. aphakia
   b. cataract
   c. corneal abrasion
   d. oculitis externa

6. Cerumen impaction is a:
   a. buildup of ear wax, blocking the ear canal
   b. buildup of ear wax, hindering the function of the eardrum
   c. buildup of fluid, causing pain in the ear canal
   d. buildup of fluid, causing pain in the eardrum

7. Inflammation of the ear caused by air is:
   a. aerotitis
   b. otitis externa
   c. otitis media
   d. pneumatic acoustitis

EXERCISE 10 *Briefly describe the difference between each pair of terms.*

1. iridopathy, keratopathy ______________________
2. retinopathy, retinosis ______________________
3. otitis externa, otitis media ______________________
4. dacryocystitis, dacryoadenitis ______________________
5. oculomycosis, otomycosis ______________________
6. dacryostenosis, otosclerosis ______________________
7. aniridia, aphakia ______________________
8. conductive hearing loss, sensorineural hearing loss ______________________

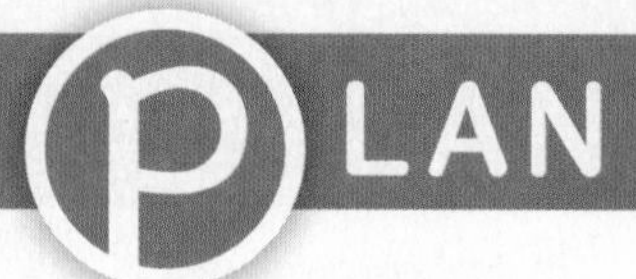

6.5 Treatments and Therapies

The Eye

Many advances have been made in eye surgery in recent years. A skilled surgeon can treat many disorders that could lead to blindness. In the outer layer, the sclera is a common site for making a cut (*sclerotomy*) in order to perform surgery in other parts of the eye.

The cornea is another common site for eye surgery. In a *corneal transplant,* a diseased cornea is removed and replaced with a donor cornea. Another type of corneal surgery, which involves making cuts in the cornea like spokes in a wheel (*radial keratotomy*), corrects myopia.

Many surgeries involve the next layer of the eye. The most common eye surgery is *cataract extraction.* The modern approach involves breaking the original lens up into small pieces, aspirating the pieces out of the eye through a needle (*phacoemulsification*), and then installing a new lens (*intraocular lens implantation*). *Iridotomy* and *iridectomy* are procedures used to treat glaucoma. Retinal detachment requires immediate reattachment (*retinopexy*) in order to prevent blindness.

In the most dire situations, such as aggressive cancer, an eye may need complete removal (*enucleation*). Cosmetic surgeries of the eye usually involve the eyelid (*blepharoplasty*) to remove wrinkles.

There are limited medicines specific to ophthalmology. *Cycloplegics* are used prior to surgery to temporarily paralyze the pupil. *Mydriatics* are used prior to a thorough eye exam to dilate the eyes. *Miotics* were commonly used to treat glaucoma before more effective treatments were discovered.

The Ear

Many treatments of the outer ear first involve a thorough cleaning of the ear canal. This can be done with washing (*ear lavage*) or inserting medicine to clear out the wax (*ceruminolytic*). One outer ear surgery (*otoplasty*) can make a deformed ear appear more normal. Another outer ear intervention is putting in a hearing aid (*auditory prosthesis*). This very common device is used to help people with hearing loss.

Middle ear procedures usually involve just the eardrum. Perhaps the most common surgery children undergo involves making a cut in the eardrum (*myringotomy*) and putting in a *tympanostomy* tube to drain fluid from the ear. Occasionally, when the tube falls out over time, it may leave a hole. In that case, the eardrum will need patching (*tympanoplasty*). In the inner ear, a more advanced electronic device can be placed in the cochlea (*cochlear implant*). Another inner ear surgery, *labryinthectomy,* can be used to treat severe vertigo.

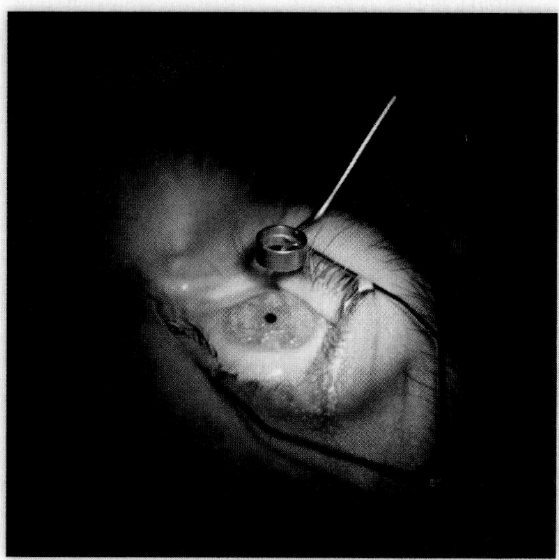

Surgery may be performed to treat a variety of eye disorders.

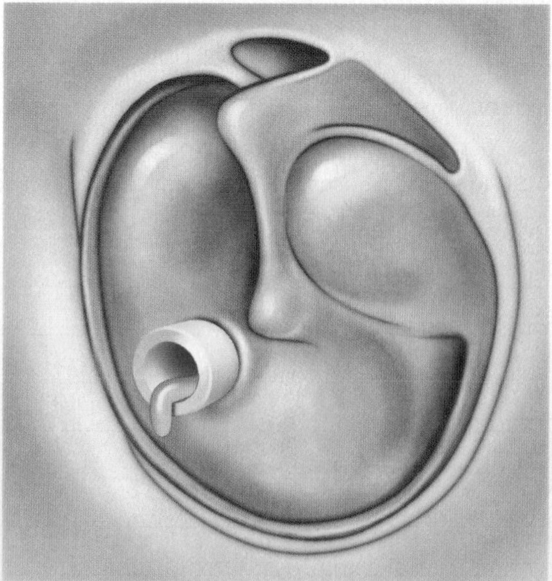

Tubes may be surgically installed in the eardrum to drain fluid from the ear.

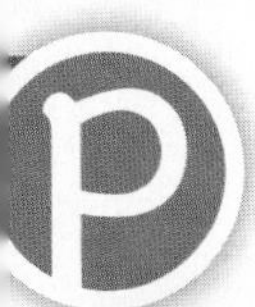

6.5 Treatments and Therapies

pharmacology

Term	Word Analysis
Eye	
miotic mai-AW-tik	**miot / ic** constriction / pertaining to
Definition drug that causes the abnormal contraction of the pupil	
mydriatic MID-ree-AT-ik	**mydriat / ic** dilation / pertaining to
Definition drug that causes the abnormal dilation of the pupil	
cycloplegic SAI-kloh-PLEE-jik	**cyclo / pleg / ic** ciliary body / paralysis / pertaining to
Definition drug that paralyzes the ciliary body	
intravitreal antibiotics IN-trah-VEE-tree-al AN-tai-bai-AW-tiks	**intra / vitre / al anti / biot / ics** inside / vitreous / pertaining to against / life / agent
Definition antibiotics administered directly into the vitreous gel liquid	
Ear	
ceruminolytic seh-ROO-min-oh-LIH-tik	**cerumino / lytic** ear wax / breakdown agent
Definition drug that aids in the breakdown of ear wax	
ototoxic OH-toh-TOK-sik	**oto / tox / ic** ear / poision / pertaining to
Definition drug that is damaging to the ear/hearing	

eye procedures

Term	Word Analysis
Outer Structures and Vision	
blepharoplasty BLEF-ah-roh-PLAS-tee **Definition** surgical reconstruction of the eyelid	**blepharo / plasty** eyelid / reconstruction
blepharotomy BLEF-ah-RAW-toh-mee **Definition** incision into the eyelid	**blepharo / tomy** eyelid / incision
dacryoadenectomy DAK-ree-oh-AD-en-EK-toh-mee **Definition** removal of the tear gland	**dacryo / aden / ectomy** tear / gland / removal

6.5 Treatments and Therapies

eye procedures *continued*

Term	Word Analysis
dacryocystectomy DAK-ree-oh-sis-TEK-toh-mee **Definition** removal of the tear sac	**dacryo / cyst / ectomy** tear / sac / removal
dacryocystorhinostomy DAK-ree-oh-SIS-toh-rai-NAWS-toh-mee **Definition** creation of an opening between the tear sac and the nose	**dacryo / cysto / rhino / stomy** tear / sac / nose / opening
dacryocystotomy DAK-ree-oh-sis-TAWT-oh-mee **Definition** incision into the tear sac	**dacryo / cysto / tomy** tear / sac / incision
enucleation eh-NOO-clee-AY-shun **Definition** removal of an eye	**e / nucle / ation** out / nucleus / procedure
oculoplasty AW-kyoo-loh-PLAS-tee **Definition** surgical reconstruction of the eye	**oculo / plasty** eye / reconstruction
ophthalmectomy AWF-thal-MEK-toh-mee **Definition** removal of the eye	**ophthalm / ectomy** eye / removal
Sclera	
corneal transplant KOR-nee-al TRANZ-plant **Definition** replacement of damaged cornea with donated tissue	**corne / al** **trans / plant** cornea / pertaining to across / place
keratoplasty ker-A-toh-PLAS-tee **Definition** surgical reconstruction of the cornea	**kerato / plasty** cornea / reconstruction
keratotomy KER-ah-TAW-toh-mee **Definition** incision into the cornea	**kerato / tomy** cornea / incision
sclerotomy skler-AW-toh-mee **Definition** incision into the sclera	**sclero / tomy** sclera / incision

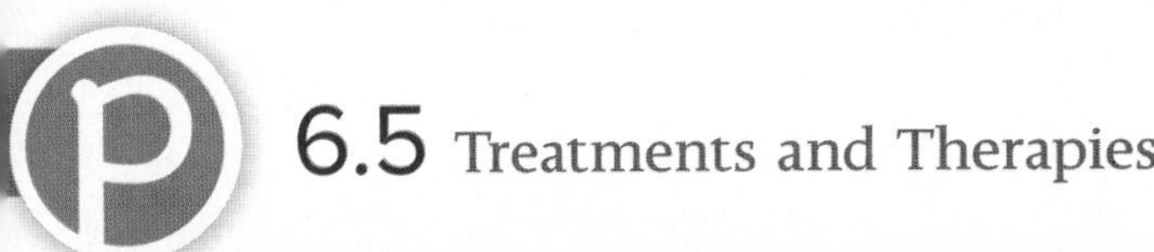

6.5 Treatments and Therapies

eye procedures *continued*

Term	Word Analysis
Choroid/Retina	
cyclotomy sai-KLAW-toh-mee **Definition** incision into the ciliary body	**cyclo / tomy** ciliary body / incision
intraocular lens implant IN-trah-AW-kyoo-lar lenz IM-plant **Definition** insertion of a new lens inside the eye	**intra / ocul / ar lens im / plant** inside / eye / pertaining to lens in / place
iridectomy EAR-id-EK-toh-mee **Definition** removal of the iris	**irid / ec / tomy** iris / out / incision
iridocyclectomy EAR-ih-doh-sai-KLEK-toh-mee **Definition** removal of the iris and ciliary body	**irido / cycl / ectomy** iris / ciliary body / removal
iridotomy EAR-id-AW-toh-mee **Definition** incision into the iris	**irido / tomy** iris / incision
phacoemulsification FAY-koh-ee-MUL-sih-fih-KAY-shun **Definition** fragmentation of an existing lens in order to remove and replace it	**phaco / emulsific / ation** lens / mix up / condition
retinopexy reh-TIH-noh-PEK-see **Definition** surgical fixation (reattachment) of a retina	**retino / pexy** retina / surgical fixation
retinotomy REH-tih-NAW-toh-mee **Definition** incision into the retina	**retino / tomy** retina / cut incision
vitrectomy vih-TREK-toh-mee **Definition** removal of the vitreous liquid from the eye	**vitr / ectomy** vitreous / removal

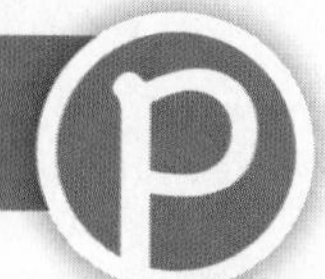

6.5 Treatments and Therapies

ear procedures and treatments

Term	Word Analysis
Outer Ear	
auditory prosthesis AW-dih-TOR-ee praws-THEE-sis **Definition** hearing aid	**auditory pros / thesis** hearing toward / place ©2009Jupiterimages Corporation RF
ceruminolysis seh-ROO-min-AW-lih-sis **Definition** breakdown of ear wax	**cerumino / lysis** ear wax / loose
ear lavage ee-ir lah-VAJ **Definition** rinsing/washing the external ear canal (usually to remove ear wax) **Note:** It's the origin of the English word *lavatory.*	**from Latin, for** "to wash, bathe"
mastoidectomy MAS-toy-DEK-toh-mee **Definition** removal of the mastoid	**mastoid / ectomy** mastoid / removal
mastoidocentesis mas-TOY-doh-sin-TEE-sis **Definition** puncture of the mastoid	**mastoido / centesis** mastoid / puncture
otoplasty OH-toh-PLAS-tee **Definition** surgical reconstruction of the ear	**oto / plasty** ear / reconstruction
Middle Ear	
myringectomy MIR-in-JEK-toh-mee **Definition** removal of the eardrum	**myring / ectomy** eardrum / removal
myringoplasty mir-IN-goh-PLAS-tee **Definition** surgical reconstruction of the eardrum	**myringo / plasty** eardrum / reconstruction
myringotomy mir-in-GAW-toh-mee **Definition** incision into the eardrum	**myringo / tomy** eardrum / incision
tympanocentesis tim-PAN-oh-sin-TEE-sis **Definition** puncture of the eardrum	**tympano / centesis** eardrum / puncture

ear procedures and treatments *continued*

Term	Word Analysis
tympanolabyrinthopexy tim-PAN-oh-lah-buh-RINTH-oh-PEK-see **Definition** surgical fixation of the eardrum to the labyrinth	**tympano / labyrintho / pexy** eardrum / labyrinth / surgical fixation
tympanoplasty tim-PAN-oh-PLAS-tee **Definition** surgical reconstruction of the eardrum	**tympano / plasty** eardrum / reconstruction
tympanostomy TIM-pan-AW-stoh-mee **Definition** creation of an opening in the eardrum	**tympano / stomy** eardrum / opening 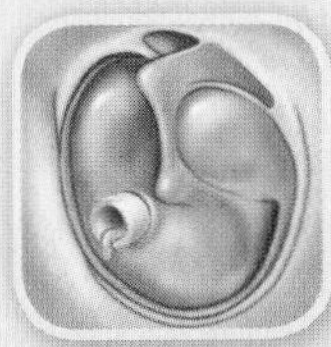
Inner Ear	
cochlear implant KOH-klee-ar IM-plant **Definition** electronic device that stimulates the cochlea; it can give a sense of sound to those who are profoundly deaf	**cochle / ar** **im / plant** cochlea / pertaining to in / place 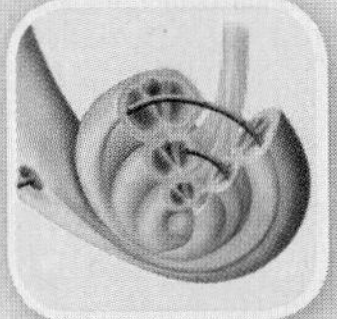
labyrinthectomy LAB-uh-rinth-EK-toh-mee **Definition** removal of the labyrinth	**labyrinth / ectomy** labyrinth / removal
labyrinthotomy LAB-uh-rinth-AW-toh-mee **Definition** incision into the labyrinth	**labyrintho / tomy** labyrinth / incision
vestibulotomy ves-TIH-byoo-LAW-toh-mee **Definition** incision into the vestibule	**vestibulo / tomy** vestibule / incision

Learning Outcome 6.5 Exercises

PRONUNCIATION

EXERCISE 1 *Indicate which syllable is emphasized when pronounced.*

EXAMPLE: bronchitis bron**chi**tis

1. cochlear ____
2. lavage ____
3. miotic ____
4. vitrectomy ____
5. myringotomy ____
6. enucleation ____
7. ototoxic ____
8. blepharotomy ____
9. tympanocentesis ____
10. iridectomy ____

TRANSLATION

EXERCISE 2 *Break down the following words into their component parts.*

EXAMPLE: nasopharyngoscope *naso | pharyngo | scope*

1. keratotomy ____
2. labyrinthotomy ____
3. myringotomy ____
4. cyclotomy ____
5. blepharotomy ____
6. tympanostomy ____
7. labyrinthectomy ____
8. vitrectomy ____
9. myringectomy ____
10. mastoidectomy ____
11. ophthalmectomy ____
12. iridocyclectomy ____
13. dacryoadenectomy ____
14. dacryocystectomy ____
15. dacryocystotomy ____
16. tympanolabyrinthopexy ____

Learning Outcome 6.5 Exercises

EXERCISE 3 *Underline and define the word parts from this chapter in the following terms.*

1. iridectomy ______
2. iridotomy ______
3. retinotomy ______
4. vestibulotomy ______
5. sclerotomy ______
6. oculoplasty ______
7. blepharoplasty ______
8. cycloplegic ______
9. otoplasty ______
10. keratoplasty ______
11. tympanoplasty ______
12. myringoplasty ______
13. ceruminolysis ______
14. mastoidocentesis ______
15. tympanocentesis ______
16. intravitreal antibiotics ______
17. intraocular lens implant ______
18. dacryocystorhinostomy ______

EXERCISE 4 *Match the term on the left with its definition on the right.*

______	1. corneal transplant	a.	drug that is damaging to the ear/hearing
______	2. cochlear implant	b.	hearing aid
______	3. ototoxic	c.	electronic device that stimulates the cochlea
______	4. auditory prosthesis	d.	drug that causes the abnormal contraction of the pupil
______	5. phacoemulsification	e.	drug that causes the abnormal dilation of the pupil
______	6. ear lavage	f.	breakdown of ear wax
______	7. ceruminolytic	g.	fragmentation of an existing lens in order to remove and replace it
______	8. retinopexy	h.	removal of an eye
______	9. mydriatic	i.	replacement of damaged cornea with donated tissue
______	10. miotic	j.	rinsing/washing the external ear canal (usually to remove ear wax)
______	11. enucleation	k.	surgical fixation (reattachment) of a retina

Learning Outcome 6.5 Exercises

EXERCISE 5 *Translate the following terms as literally as possible.*

EXAMPLE: nasopharyngoscope *an instrument for looking at the nose and throat*

1. ototoxic ____________
2. cycloplegic ____________
3. tympanostomy ____________
4. iridectomy ____________
5. vitrectomy ____________
6. mastoidectomy ____________
7. labyrinthectomy ____________
8. myringectomy ____________
9. ophthalmectomy ____________
10. iridocyclectomy ____________
11. phacoemulsification ____________
12. dacryocystorhinostomy ____________

GENERATION

EXERCISE 6 *Build a medical term from the information provided.*

EXAMPLE: inflammation of the sinuses *sinusitis*

1. incision into the eardrum (use *myringo*) ____________
2. incision into the cornea ____________
3. incision into the retina ____________
4. incision into the iris ____________
5. incision into the sclera ____________
6. incision into the labyrinth ____________
7. incision into the vestibule ____________
8. incision into the eyelid ____________
9. incision into the ciliary body ____________
10. incision into the tear sac ____________

Learning Outcome 6.5 Exercises

EXERCISE 7 *Multiple-choice questions. Select the correct answer(s).*

1. Select the terms that pertain to the ear.
   a. blepharoplasty
   b. keratoplasty
   c. myringoplasty
   d. oculoplasty
   e. otoplasty
   f. tympanoplasty
2. Select the terms that pertain to the eye.
   a. blepharoplasty
   b. keratoplasty
   c. myringoplasty
   d. oculoplasty
   e. otoplasty
   f. tympanoplasty
3. Select the terms that mean "removal of an eye."
   a. corneal transplant
   b. enucleation
   c. intraocular lens implant
   d. ophthalmectomy
4. Select the terms than involve surgery of the choroid/retina layer of the eye.
   a. corneal transplant
   b. enucleation
   c. intraocular lens implant
   d. ophthalmectomy
5. Intravitreal antibiotics are administered to which part of the body?
   a. blood vessels in the outer eye
   b. vein
   c. vitreous liquid of the eye
   d. vitreous liquid of the inner ear

EXERCISE 8 *Briefly describe the difference between each pair of terms.*

1. mastoidocentesis, tympanocentesis ______
2. dacryoadenectomy, dacryocystectomy ______
3. retinopexy, tympanolabyrinthopexy ______
4. ceruminolysis, ceruminolytic ______
5. auditory prosthesis, cochlear implant ______
6. mydriatic, miotic ______

6.6 Abbreviations

Abbreviations provide a shorthand way of referring to things that either recur often or are too long to write out. When dealing with the eyes and ears, these abbreviations can refer to everything from body parts (OD, OS, AD, AS, TM) to common observations (PERRLA), common diagnoses (ARMD, OM), and common procedures (LASIK).

eye

Abbreviation	Definition
ARMD	age-related macular degeneration
HEENT	head, eyes, ears, nose, and throat
IOL	intraocular lens
IOP	intraocular pressure
LASIK	laser-assisted in situ keratomileusis
OD	right eye (from Latin—*oculus dexter*)
OS	left eye (from Latin—*oculus sinister*)
OU	both eyes (from Latin—*oculus uterque*)
PERRLA	pupils are equal, round, and reactive to light and accommodation
VA	visual acuity
VF	visual field

ear

Abbreviation	Definition
AD	right ear (from Latin—*auris dextra*)
AOM	acute otitis media
AS	left ear (from Latin—*auris sinistra*)
AU	both ears (from Latin—*auris utraque*)
EENT	eye, ear, nose, and throat
ENT	ear, nose, and throat
OM	otitis media
TM	tympanic membrane

Learning Outcome 6.6 Exercises

EXERCISE 1 *Match the abbreviation on the left with its definition on the right.*

_____	1. AD	a. both ears
_____	2. AS	b. both eyes
_____	3. AU	c. left ear
_____	4. OD	d. left eye
_____	5. OS	e. right ear
_____	6. OU	f. right eye

EXERCISE 2 *Define the following abbreviations.*

1. ARMD _____
2. HEENT _____
3. IOL _____
4. OD _____
5. OS _____
6. OU _____
7. PERRLA _____
8. ENT _____
9. AOM _____
10. OM _____
11. TM _____
12. EENT _____

EXERCISE 3 *Give the abbreviations for the following definitions.*

1. intraocular pressure _____
2. laser-assisted in situ keratomileusis _____
3. right eye _____
4. left eye _____
5. both eyes _____
6. visual acuity _____
7. visual field _____
8. right ear _____
9. left ear _____
10. both ears _____

Learning Outcome 6.6 Exercises

EXERCISE 4 *Multiple-choice questions. Select the correct answer(s).*

1. The TM refers to:
   a. the mastoid process
   b. the membrane of the eardrum
   c. the tear duct
   d. the tear sac

2. An IOL implant is:
   a. a hearing aid
   b. an electronic device that stimulates the cochlea
   c. the insertion of a new lens inside the eye
   d. the replacement of a damaged cornea with donated tissue

3. AOM is:
   a. the progressive inflammation of the middle ear
   b. the progressive inflammation of the outer ear
   c. the rapid onset of inflammation in the middle ear
   d. the rapid onset of inflammation of the outer ear

4. Select the abbreviations that pertain to the eye.
   a. ENT
   b. HEENT
   c. IOP
   d. OM
   e. PERRLA
   f. VA
   g. VF

5. Select the abbreviations that pertain to the ear.
   a. ENT
   b. HEENT
   c. IOP
   d. OM
   e. PERRLA
   f. VA
   g. VF

6. The root word in *keratomileusis* in the term *laser-assisted in situ keratomileusis* (LASIK) means:
   a. ciliary body
   b. cochlea
   c. conjunctiva
   d. cornea

6.7 Electronic Health Records

Discharge Summary

Patient Name: Ms. Susan Cloud
Date of Admission: 6/23/15
Date of Discharge: 6/28/15

Admission Diagnosis
1. **Cataract** extraction

Discharge Diagnosis
1. Post-cataract extraction
2. **Endophthalmitis**

Discharge Condition
Stable

Consultations
Infectious disease

Procedures
1. **Cataract** extraction with **phacoemulsification** and implantation of a posterior chamber **intraocular lens,** right eye.

Labs
CBC: WBC 22.4 on 6/24; 18.5 6/25; 15.1 on 6/27; BCx. negative; **vitreous** culture: *Staphylococcus epidermidis*

Imaging
Ocular u/s: **vitreous** inflammation. No **retinal** detachment.

HPI
Ms. Cloud is a 58-year-old woman who first presented to her **ophthalmologist** with a complaint of cloudy vision. She was also noted to have **nystagmus** and **strabismus.** She was diagnosed with a **cataract.** She was treated surgically with **cataract** extraction and **lens** implantation. She was admitted to the hospital on 6/23/2015 for postoperative observation.

Hospital Course
On postop day 2, Ms. Cloud began complaining of increasing right **ophthalmalgia.** She was noted to be febrile to 102.2. Exam revealed **conjunctival** infection and edema. She was presumed to have postoperative endophthalmitis. **Vitrectomy** was performed under sterile conditions, and samples were sent to lab for culture. She was given **intravitreal** antibiotics. Over the next couple of days, her fever curve trended down and her WBC count improved. Cultures came back positive for *S. epidermidis.* Infectious disease was consulted; they recommended 2 weeks of IV therapy. A PICC line was placed and she was discharged with care instructions.

Activity
Eye rest

Diet
No restrictions

Meds
IV vancomycin via PICC

Follow-Up Appointments
Ophthalmology outpatient clinic in 2 days
Infectious disease clinic in 1 week

–Lynn Holmes, MD

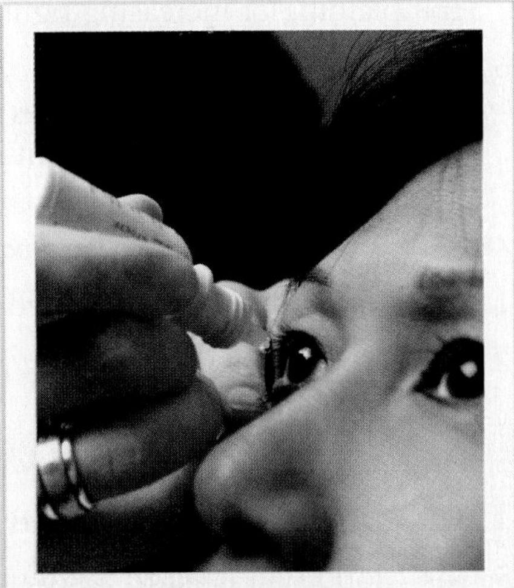

Learning Outcome 6.7 Exercises

EXERCISE 1 *Match the term on the left with its definition on the right.*

	Term		Definition
______	1. conjunctival	a.	condition where the eyes deviate when looking at the same object
______	2. retinal	b.	eye specialist
______	3. ocular	c.	fragmentation of an existing lens in order to remove and replace it
______	4. ophthalmologist	d.	inflammation of the eye
______	5. ophthalmitis	e.	involuntary back-and-forth movement of the eyes
______	6. ophthalmalgia	f.	opacity (cloudiness) of the lens of the eye
______	7. cataract	g.	pain in the eye
______	8. nystagmus	h.	pertaining to the conjunctiva
______	9. strabismus	i.	pertaining to the eye
______	10. phacoemulsification	j.	pertaining to the retina

EXERCISE 2 *Fill in the blanks.*

1. According to the admission diagnosis, Ms. Cloud was admitted for a(n) ____________________.
2. The images performed on Ms. Cloud revealed that she had no *retinal detachment,* or that her ____________________ was still properly attached.
3. Ms. Cloud was first presented to her ____________________ (eye specialist) with cloudy vision, and was noted to have *nystagmus* (give definition: ____________________) and *strabismus* (give definition: ____________________).
4. During her surgery, her ____________________ was removed and a(n) ____________________ was implanted.
5. On *postop* (give definition: ____________________) day 2, Ms. Cloud began complaining of increasing right eye pain, or ____________________.
6. A *vitrectomy* (give definition: ____________________) was performed under sterile conditions, and samples were sent to the lab for culture. She was then begun on ____________________ (antibiotics administered directly inside the vitreous gel liquid).

EXERCISE 3 *True or false questions. Indicate true answers with a T and false answers with an F.*

1. This health record was created at an ophthalmology clinic. ________
2. Ms. Cloud began complaining that her eye felt inflamed the second day after her operation. ________
3. During her second postop day, Ms. Cloud was noted to have a fever. ________
4. The cultures came back negative for an infection. ________
5. Ms. Cloud will need to follow up with an optometrist in 2 days. ________

Learning Outcome 6.7 Exercises

EXERCISE 4 *Multiple-choice questions. Select the correct answer(s).*

1. The patient was admitted to the hospital for:
   a. a cataract extraction
   b. a lens implantation
   c. ophthalmalgia and a fever
   d. postoperative observation

2. The health record indicates that the patient "was presumed to have postoperative endophthalmitis." The term *endophthalmitis* is created by combining the prefix *endo-* with the term *ophthalmitis,* which means:
   a. discharge from the cornea
   b. discharge from the eye
   c. inflammation in the cornea
   d. inflammation in the eye

3. The patient will receive antibiotics via a PICC line, which is a:
   a. peripherally inserted central catheter
   b. peripherally inserted corneal control
   c. phacoemulsification inserted corneal control
   d. phacoemulsification iridocyclectal catheter

4. The abbreviation for the term *intraocular lens* is:
   a. IL
   b. IOL
   c. ICL
   d. OL

5. *S. epidermidis* is a bacteria that gets its name from the *epidermis* (where it is often found). Epidermis is the:
   a. eye
   b. lens
   c. nerves
   d. skin

Eye Consult

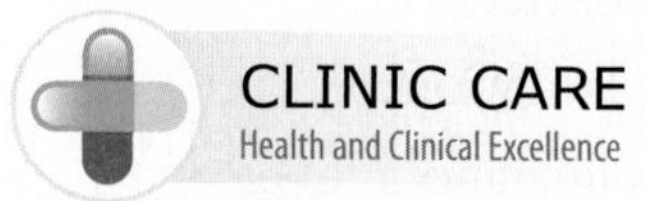

Dr. Strauss,

I saw Mrs. Kelly Robison in my office on 5/7/2015 for routine follow-up. As you know, Mrs. Robison initially presented with nystagmus, strabismus, and noted photophobia. She was diagnosed at the time with aniridia. I have been treating her medically with miotics.

Her resultant visual problems have been corrected with glasses, and she had strabismus surgery in 2013 to help improve her binocular vision. Last year, she was noted to have significant corneal clouding that was successfully treated with keratoplasty.

As is common with this condition, the medicine alone was not enough to prevent glaucoma. I have been routinely monitoring her IOP, and it has risen in the recent past. It is my recommendation to relieve the pressure surgically. I discussed the risks and benefits from the surgery with Mrs. Robison, and she is interested in proceeding. She will contact my staff for scheduling.

If you have any questions, please call me.

Sincerely,

Theodora McIntosh, MD

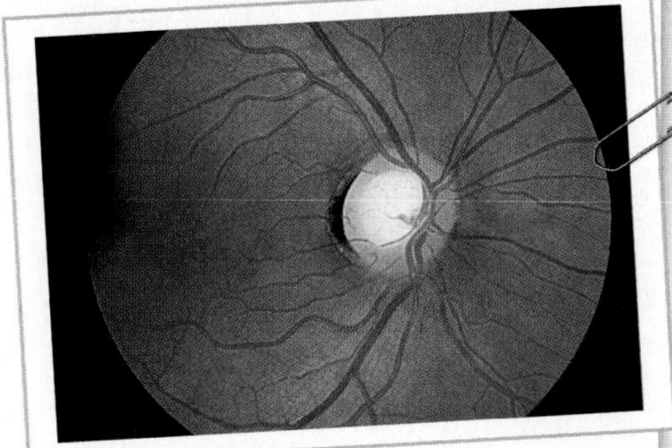

©Jean-Luc Kokel/Science Source

Learning Outcome 6.7 Exercises

EXERCISE 5 *Match the term on the left with its definition on the right.*

_____	1. binocular	a. condition where the eyes deviate when looking at the same object
_____	2. aniridia	b. absence of an iris
_____	3. keratoplasty	c. drug that causes the abnormal contraction of the pupil
_____	4. strabismus	d. involuntary back-and-forth movement of the eyes
_____	5. nystagmus	e. pertaining to both eyes
_____	6. miotic	f. surgical reconstruction of the cornea

EXERCISE 6 *Fill in the blanks.*

1. Mrs. Robison initially presented with ____________________ (involuntary back-and-forth movement of the eyes), ____________________ (a condition where the eyes deviate when looking at the same object), and ____________________ (extreme sensitivity to light).
2. Mrs. Robison was diagnosed with *aniridia* (give definition: ____________________) and treated with *miotics* (give definition: ____________________).
3. Mrs. Robison's corneal clouding was successfully treated with ____________________ (surgical reconstruction of the ____________________).

EXERCISE 7 *True or false questions. Indicate true answers with a T and false answers with an F.*

1. Mrs. Robison is having difficulty hearing. ________
2. Mrs. Robison's initial diagnosis included the absence of a lens in her eye. ________
3. A miotic causes the abnormal contraction of the pupil. ________
4. Keratoplasty was successful in treating the clouding that occurred in the patient's cornea. ________
5. Mrs. Robison has developed glaucoma. ________
6. Dr. McIntosh has been monitoring the pressure in the patient's eye. ________

EXERCISE 8 *Multiple-choice questions. Select the correct answer(s).*

1. The abbreviation IOP stands for
   a. internal ophthalmopathy
   b. intraocular phacoscopy
   c. intraocular pressure
   d. iridopathy
2. Although not mentioned in the note, the type of surgery used to relieve the eye pressure from glaucoma is *trabeculotomy,* a medical term formed by combining *trabecula* (part of the anatomy of the eye) and *-otomy,* which means:
   a. creation of an opening
   b. incision
   c. removal
   d. surgical reconstruction
3. A drug that causes the abnormal contraction of the pupil is called a(n):
   a. ectropion
   b. miotic
   c. mydriatic
   d. ototoxic

Ear Consult

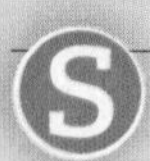

Subjective

Johnny Masur is a 4-year-old boy referred to my clinic for evaluation of **chronic otitis media**. He began with a 1-week history of nasal congestion, runny nose, and cough. He has had a low-grade temperature up to 100.2. He went to his PCP last week for **otopyorrhea** on the left side and **otalgia** on the right side. He was diagnosed with bilateral **acute otitis media** and treated with oral antibiotics. He has failed three separate courses of oral antibiotics.

PMHx

Johnny's history is significant for **tympanostomy** tubes placed bilaterally when he was 2 years old. One tube left a persistent perforation in the **tympanic membrane**, so he had **tympanoplasty** at 3 years of age. He has not had any episodes of otitis media in the past 2 years.

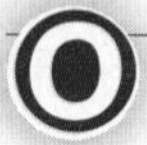

Objective

Physical Exam

RR: 24; HR: 88; Temp: 99.9; BP: 98/68.

Gen: Well-developed 4y/o in no acute distress.

HEENT: Normocephalic. PERRLA. No conjunctival erythema; mild clear nasal discharge; right canal blocked with **cerumen**–after **ceruminolytic** placed and canal clear, the tympanic membrane was seen. It was **erythematous** and full. Some mild **tympanosclerosis** of **TM** noted; the left ear was erythematous and full. Mild **mastoidalgia** on the left, but the ear is not displaced forward.

CV: RRR without murmur.

Resp: CTA.

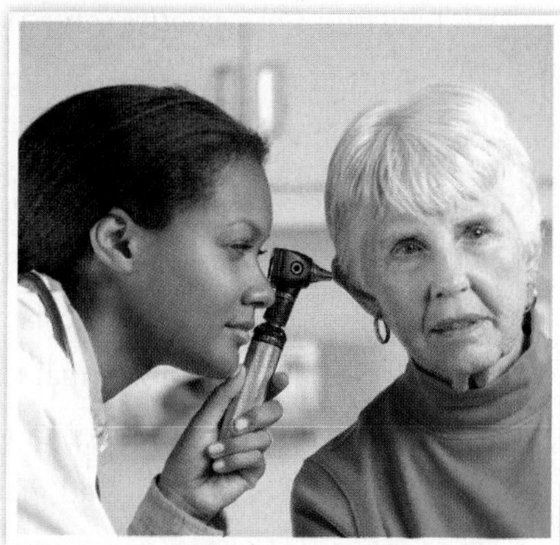

©Monkey Business Images/Shutterstock.com RF

Assessment

Johnny has chronic otitis media failing three courses of oral antibiotics.

Plan

I have performed **tympanocentesis** in the office and sent the fluid for culture. While awaiting the result, we will treat him with an IM antibiotic. I will also send a fungal culture to rule out **otomycosis**. While Johnny has mild mastoidalgia, he is afebrile today and in no distress, and his ear is not displaced. Thus, I do not think he has acute **mastoiditis,** but I told Johnny's parents what to look for.

Given how long Johnny has had this infection, he will need to see audiology for **audiometry** when he is better.

–Johanna Long, MD

Learning Outcome 6.7 Exercises

EXERCISE 9 *Match the term on the left with its definition on the right.*

	Term		Definition
______	1. otitis media	a.	drug that aids in the breakdown of ear wax
______	2. audiometry	b.	fungal ear condition
______	3. tympanoplasty	c.	creation of an opening in the eardrum
______	4. otalgia	d.	discharge of pus from the ear
______	5. mastoidalgia	e.	ear pain
______	6. mastoiditis	f.	hardening of the eardrum
______	7. tympanostomy	g.	inflammation of the mastoid
______	8. ceruminolytic	h.	inflammation of the middle ear
______	9. tympanocentesis	i.	pain in the mastoid
______	10. otopyorrhea	j.	procedure for measuring hearing
______	11. otomycosis	k.	puncture of the eardrum
______	12. tympanosclerosis	l.	surgical reconstruction of the eardrum

EXERCISE 10 *Match the abbreviation on the left with its definition on the right.*

______	1. TM	a.	clear to auscultation
______	2. PCP	b.	head, eyes, ears, nose, and throat
______	3. RRR	c.	primary care provider
______	4. CTA	d.	pupils are equal, round, and reactive to light and accommodation
______	5. HEENT	e.	regular rate and rhythm
______	6. PERRLA	f.	tympanic membrane

EXERCISE 11 *Fill in the blanks.*

1. The patient went to his PCP (give definition: ______________________________) for *otopyorrhea* (discharge of ____________________ from the ear) and *otalgia* (give definition: ______________________________).
2. Johnny had a(n) ____________________ (surgical reconstruction of the eardrum) at 3 years of age.
3. Patient's heart rate: ____________________; respiratory rate: ____________________; blood pressure: ______________________________.
4. Johnny's right ear canal was blocked with *cerumen* (give definition: ______________________________), and was given a(n) ____________________ (a drug that aids in the breakdown of ear wax).

EXERCISE 12 *True or false questions. Indicate true answers with a T and false answers with an F.*

1. The patient was diagnosed by his primary care physician with AOM in both ears. ________
2. Oral antibiotics were an effective treatment for the patient's symptoms in the past. ________
3. Johnny had tubes placed in both of his eardrums when he was 2 years old. ________
4. One tube left a hole in his TM. ________
5. Upon exam, the patient's eardrums were red on both sides. ________
6. Upon exam, the patient had pain in his left ear. ________
7. Part of the physician's plan for care included the puncturing of Johnny's eardrum. ________
8. The patient was diagnosed with otomycosis. ________

Learning Outcome 6.7 Exercises

EXERCISE 13 *Multiple-choice questions. Select the correct answer(s).*

1. The patient visited his physician for *otalgia,* or ear pain. Another medical term for *ear pain* is:
   a. mastoidalgia
   b. myringodynia
   c. ophthalmalgia
   d. otodynia
2. *Otitis media* is an inflammation of the middle ear. An inflammation of the outer ear is called:
   a. macrotia
   b. osteoacusis
   c. otitis externa
   d. otomycosis
3. The patient was referred to this clinic for *chronic otitis media,* which is:
   a. inflammation of the middle ear that has been going on for a while
   b. inflammation of the middle ear that just started recently
   c. inflammation of the outer ear that has been going on for a while
   d. inflammation of the outer ear that just started recently
4. The abbreviation PCP stands for:
   a. past care provider
   b. patient care provider
   c. primary care patient
   d. primary care provider
5. The abbreviation for *acute otitis media* is:
   a. AO
   b. AOM
   c. AOTM
   d. OM
6. Johnny's history is significant for tubes placed in his:
   a. cerumen
   b. cochlea
   c. eardrum
   d. mastoid
7. After clearing the ear canal from ear wax, the tympanic membrane was "erythematous and full." The root *erythro* means:
   a. black
   b. red
   c. white
   d. yellow
8. Because Johnny's ear infection persisted for so long, Dr. Long recommended that the patient visit with audiology for a(n) ______________ when he is better.
   a. antibiotic screening
   b. auditory prosthesis
   c. hearing test
   d. tympanocentesis

Additional exercises available in connect

Chapter Review exercises, along with additional practice items, are available in Connect!

Quick Reference

quick reference glossary of roots

Root	Definition	Root	Definition
acous/o	sound	**mastoid/o**	mastoid process
-acusis	hearing condition	**myring/o**	eardrum
audi/o	sound	**ocul/o**	eye
aur/o	ear	**ophthalm/o**	eye
blephar/o	eyelid	**-opia**	vision condition
cerumin/o	ear wax	**-opsia**	vision condition
cochle/o	cochlea	**opt/o**	eye
conjunctiv/o	conjunctiva	**ot/o**	ear
corne/o	cornea	**phac/o**	lens
cycl/o	ciliary body	**phak/o**	lens
dacry/o	tear	**retin/o**	retina
ir/o	iris	**salping/o**	eustachian tube
irid/o	iris	**scler/o**	sclera (the white of the eye)
kerat/o	cornea	**tympan/o**	eardrum
labyrinth/o	labyrinth	**vestibul/o**	vestibule
lacrim/o	tear		

quick reference glossary of terms

Term	Definition
acoustic neuroma	a tumor on the acoustic nerve
aerotitis	inflammation of the ear caused by air
akinetopsia	the inability to see objects in motion
ambiopia	double vision
amblyopia	decreased vision (when it occurs in one eye, it is referred to as *lazy eye*)
aniridia	absence of an iris
aphakia	absence of a lens
asthenopia	weak vision (i.e., *eye strain*)
astigmatism	vision problem caused by the fact that light rays entering the eye aren't focused on a single point in the back of the eye

quick reference glossary of terms *continued*

Term	Definition
audiogram	record produced by an audiometer
audiologist	hearing specialist
audiometer	instrument for measuring hearing
audiometry	procedure for measuring hearing
auditory prosthesis	hearing aid
aural	pertaining to the ear
binocular	pertaining to both eyes
blepharedema	eyelid swelling
blepharitis	eyelid inflammation
blepharoconjunctivitis	inflammation of the eyelid and conjunctiva
blepharoplasty	surgical reconstruction of the eyelid
blepharoplegia	paralysis of the eyelid
blepharoptosis	drooping eyelid
blepharopyorrhea	discharge of pus from the eyelid
blepharospasm	involuntary contraction of an eyelid
blepharotomy	incision into the eyelid
cataract	opacity (cloudiness) of the lens of the eye (from Latin, for "waterfall")
cerumen impaction	buildup of ear wax blocking the ear canal
ceruminolysis	breakdown of ear wax
ceruminolytic	drug that aids in the breakdown of ear wax
ceruminoma	benign tumor of the cerumen-secreting glands of the ear
ceruminosis	excessive formation of ear wax
cochlear implant	electronic device that stimulates the cochlea; it can give the sense of sound to those who are profoundly deaf
cochleitis	inflammation of the cochlea
conductive hearing loss	sound does not get to the middle/inner ear (due to blockages)
conjunctivitis	inflammation of the conjunctiva (also known as *pink eye*)
corneal abrasion	scratch on the cornea
corneal transplant	replacement of damaged cornea with donated tissue
corneal xerosis	dryness of the cornea
cyclokeratitis	inflammation of the ciliary body and cornea
cycloplegia	paralysis of the ciliary body

quick reference glossary of terms *continued*

Term	Definition
cycloplegic	drug that paralyzes the ciliary body
cyclotomy	incision into the ciliary body
dacrocystitis	inflammation of the tear sac
dacryadenitis	inflammation of the tear gland
dacryoadenalgia	pain in the tear gland
dacryoadenectomy	removal of the tear gland
dacryocystalgia	pain in the tear sac
dacryocystectomy	removal of the tear sac
dacryocystorhinostomy	creation of an opening between the tear sac and the nose
dacryocystotomy	incision into the tear sac
dacryohemorrhea	discharge of blood in the tears
dacryolith	hard formation (stone) in the tear system
dacryolithiasis	presence of hard formations (stones) in the tear system
dacryopyorrhea	discharge of pus in tears
dacryorrhea	excessive tearing
dacryostenosis	narrowing of the tear duct
diplopia	double vision
ear lavage	rinsing/washing the external ear canal (usually to remove ear wax); from Latin, for “to wash, bathe”
ectropion	outward turning of the eyelid, away from the eye
entropion	inward turning of the eyelid, toward the eye
enucleation	removal of an eye
esotropia	inward turning of the eye, toward the nose
exophthalmus	protrusion of the eye out of the eye socket
exotropia	outward turning of the eye, away from the nose
hemianopsia	blindness in half the visual field
hyperacusis	excessively sensitive hearing
hyperopia	farsightedness
hypoacusis	excessively insensitive hearing
intraocular lens implant	insertion of a new lens inside the eye
iridalgia	pain in the iris

quick reference glossary of terms *continued*

Term	Definition
iridectomy	removal of the iris
iridemia	bleeding from the iris
iridocyclectomy	removal of the iris and ciliary body
iridocyclitis	inflammation of the iris and ciliary body
iridokeratitis	inflammation of the iris and cornea
iridokinesis	movement of the iris
iridopathy	disease of the iris
iridotomy	incision into the iris
iritis	inflammation of the iris
keratalgia	pain in the cornea
keratitis	inflammation of the cornea
keratomalacia	abnormal softening of the cornea
keratopathy	disease of the cornea
keratoplasty	surgical reconstruction of the cornea
keratotomy	incision into the cornea
labyrinthectomy	removal of the labyrinth
labyrinthitis	inflammation of the labyrinth
labyrinthotomy	incision into the labyrinth
lacrimation	formation of tears (i.e., crying)
macrotia	abnormally large ears
mastoidalgia	pain in the mastoid
mastoidectomy	removal of the mastoid
mastoiditis	inflammation of the mastoid
mastoidocentesis	puncture of the mastoid
microtia	abnormally small ears
miosis	abnormal contraction of the pupil (from Greek, for "to lessen")
miotic	drug that causes the abnormal contraction of the pupil
mydriasis	abnormal dilation of the pupil
mydriatic	drug that causes the abnormal dilation of the pupil
myopia	nearsightedness
myringectomy	removal of the eardrum

quick reference glossary of terms *continued*

Term	Definition
myringitis	inflammation of the eardrum
myringodermatitis	inflammation of the eardrum and surrounding skin
myringomycosis	fungal condition of the eardrum
myringoplasty	surgical reconstruction of the eardrum
myringotomy	incision into the eardrum
nasolacrimal	pertaining to the nose and tear system
nystagmus	involuntary back-and-forth movement of the eyes (from Greek, for "to nod")
oculomycosis	a fungal eye condition
oculopathy	disease of the eye
oculoplasty	surgical reconstruction of the eye
ophthalmatrophy	atrophy (wasting away) of the eye
ophthalmectomy	removal of the eye
ophthalmic	pertaining to the eye
ophthalmitis	inflammation of the eye
ophthalmologist	eye specialist
ophthalmomycosis	fungal eye condition
ophthalmomyitis	inflammation of the eye muscles
ophthalmopathy	eye disease
ophthalmoplegia	eye paralysis
ophthalmoscope	instrument for looking at the eye
ophthalmalgia	eye pain
optic	pertaining to the eye
optic neuritis	inflammation of the optic nerve
optokinetic	pertaining to eye movement
optometrist	specialist in measuring the eye
optomyometer	device used to determine the strength of eye muscles
osteoacusis	hearing through bone
otalgia	ear pain
otitis externa	inflammation of the outer ear
otitis media	inflammation of the middle ear
otodynia	ear pain

quick reference glossary of terms *continued*

Term	Definition
otolaryngologist	specialist in the ear and throat
otomycosis	fungal ear condition
otoneurology	specialist in the nerve connections between the ear and brain
otoplasty	surgical reconstruction of the ear
otopyorrhea	discharge of pus from the ears
otorhinolaryngologist	specialist in the ear, nose, and throat
otorrhea	discharge from the ear
otosclerosis	hearing loss caused by the hardening of the bones of the middle ear
otoscope	instrument for looking in the ear
otoscopy	procedure for looking in the ear
otosteal	pertaining to the bones of the ear
ototoxic	drug that is damaging to the ear/hearing
papilledema	swelling of the optic nerve where it enters the retina
phacoemulsification	fragmentation of an existing lens in order to remove and replace it
phacomalacia	abnormal softening of the lens
phacosclerosis	abnormal hardening of the lens
phacoscope	instrument for looking at the lens
phakitis	inflammation of the lens
pneumatic otoscopy	procedure for looking in the ear using air
presbycusis	loss of hearing in old age
presbyopia	decreased vision caused by old age
pterygium	winglike growth of conjunctival tissue extending to the cornea (from Greek, for "wing")
retinal	pertaining to the retina
retinitis	inflammation of the retina
retinopathy	disease of the retina
retinopexy	surgical fixation (reattachment) of a retina
retinoscope	instrument for looking at the retina
retinoscopy	procedure for looking at the retina
retinosis	retinal condition
retinotomy	incision into the retina
rhinosalpingitis	inflammation of the nose and eustachian tubes

quick reference glossary of terms *continued*

Term	Definition
salpingopharyngeal	pertaining to the eustachian tubes and the throat
salpingoscope	instrument for looking at the eustachian tubes
sclerectasia	overexpansion of the sclera
scleroiritis	inflammation of the sclera and iris
sclerokeratitis	inflammation of the sclera and cornea
sclerokeratoiritis	inflammation of the sclera, cornea, and iris
scleromalacia	abnormal softening of the sclera
sclerotomy	incision into the sclera
scotoma	dark spot in the visual field
scotopia	adjustment of the eye to seeing in darkness
sensorineural hearing loss	sound is not transmitted from the inner ear to the brain (due to problems with the sense organs or nerves)
strabismus	condition where the eyes deviate when looking at the same object (from Latin, for "to squint")
tinnitus	ringing in the ears (from Latin, for "to ring" or "jingle")
tonometer	instrument for measuring tension or pressure in the eye (intraocular pressure)
trichiasis	condition caused by eyelashes growing backward and coming in contact with the eye
tympanic perforation	tear or hole in the eardrum
tympanocentesis	puncture of the eardrum
tympanolabyrinthopexy	surgical fixation of the eardrum to the labyrinth
tympanometry	procedure for measuring the eardrum
tympanoplasty	surgical reconstruction of the eardrum
tympanosclerosis	hardening of the eardrum
tympanostomy	creation of an opening in the eardrum
vertigo	sensation of moving through space (while stationary); from Latin, for "to whirl around"
vestibular neuritis	inflammation of the vestibular nerve
vestibulitis	inflammation of the vestibule
vestibulotomy	incision into the vestibule
xerophthalmia	dry eyes

review of terms by roots

Root	Term(s)	
acous/o	acoustic neuroma	
-acusis	hyperacusis hypoacusis	osteoacusis presbycusis
audi/o	audiogram audiologist audiometer	audiometry auditory prosthesis
aur/o	aural	
blephar/o	blepharedema blepharitis blepharoconjunctivitis blepharoplasty blepharoplegia	blepharoptosis blepharopyorrhea blepharospasm blepharotomy
cerumin/o	cerumen impaction ceruminolysis ceruminolytic	ceruminoma ceruminosis
cochle/o	cochlear implant cochleitis	
conjunctiv/o	blepharoconjunctivitis conjunctivitis	
corne/o	corneal abrasion corneal transplant	corneal xerosis
cycl/o	cyclokeratitis cycloplegia cycloplegic	cyclotomy iridocyclectomy iridocyclitis
dacry/o	dacrocystitis dacryadenitis dacryoadenalgia dacryoadenectomy dacryocystalgia dacryocystectomy dacryocystorhinostomy	dacryocystotomy dacryohemorrhea dacryolith dacryolithiasis dacryopyorrhea dacryorrhea dacryostenosis
ir/o	iridalgia iridectomy iridemia iridocyclectomy iridocyclitis iridokeratitis	iridokinesis iridopathy iridotomy iritis scleroiritis sclerokeratoiritis
irid/o	aniridia	
kerat/o	iridokeratitis keratalgia keratitis keratomalacia keratopathy	keratoplasty keratotomy sclerokeratitis sclerokeratoiritis

review of terms by roots *continued*

Root	Term(s)	
labyrinth/o	labyrinthectomy labyrinthitis	labyrinthotomy tympanolabyrinthopexy
lacrim/o	lacrimation nasolacrimal	
mastoid/o	mastoidalgia mastoidectomy	mastoiditis mastoidocentesis
myring/o	myringectomy myringitis myringodermatitis	myringomycosis myringoplasty myringotomy
ocul/o	binocular intraocular lens implant oculomycosis	oculopathy oculoplasty
ophthalm/o	exophthalmus ophthalmalgia ophthalmatrophy ophthalmectomy ophthalmic ophthalmitis ophthalmologist	ophthalmomycosis ophthalmomyitis ophthalmopathy ophthalmoplegia ophthalmoscope xerophthalmia
-opia **-opsia**	akinetopsia ambiopia amblyopia asthenopia diplopia	hemianopsia hyperopia myopia presbyopia scotopia
opt/o	optic optic neuritis optokinetic	optometrist optomyometer
ot/o	aerotitis macrotia microtia otalgia otitis externa otitis media otodynia otolaryngologist otomycosis otoneurology	otoplasty otopyorrhea otorhinolaryngologist otorrhea otosclerosis otoscope otoscopy otosteal ototoxic pneumatic otoscopy
phac/o	phacoemulsification phacomalacia	phacosclerosis phacoscope
phak/o	aphakia	phakitis

review of terms by roots *continued*

Root	Term(s)	
retin/o	retinal retinitis retinopathy retinopexy	retinoscope retinoscopy retinosis retinotomy
salping/o	rhinosalpingitis salpingopharyngeal	salpingoscope
scler/o	sclerectasia scleroiritis sclerokeratitis	sclerokeratoiritis scleromalacia sclerotomy
tympan/o	tympanic perforation tympanocentesis tympanolabyrinthopexy tympanometry	tympanoplasty tympanosclerosis tympanostomy
vestibul/o	vestibular neuritis vestibulitis	vestibulotomy

other terms

astigmatism	mydriatic
cataract	nystagmus
conductive hearing loss	papilledema
ear lavage	pterygium
ectropion	scotoma
entropion	sensorineural hearing loss
enucleation	strabismus
esotropia	tinnitus
exotropia	tonometer
miosis	trichiasis
miotic	vertigo
mydriasis	

The Endocrine System–Endocrinology 7

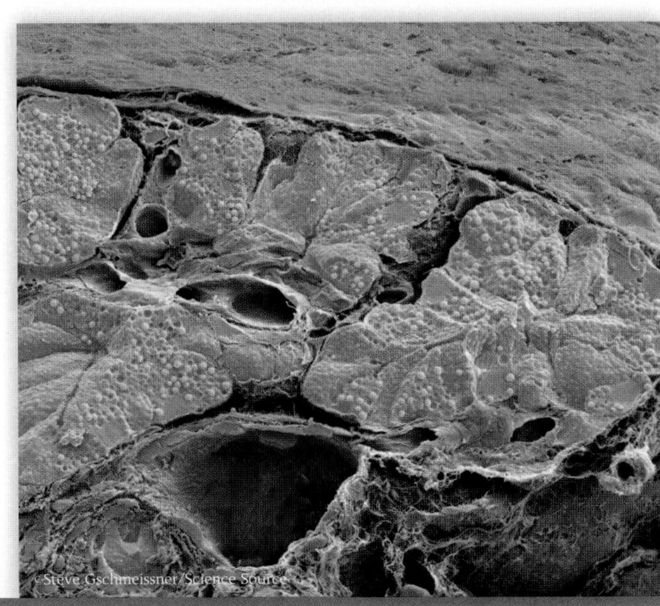
©Steve Gschmeissner/Science Source

learning outcomes

Upon completion of this chapter, you will be able to:

7.1 Identify the **roots/word parts** associated with the **endocrine system.**

S 7.2 Translate the **Subjective** terms associated with the **endocrine system.**

O 7.3 Translate the **Objective** terms associated with the **endocrine system.**

A 7.4 Translate the **Assessment** terms associated with the **endocrine system.**

P 7.5 Translate the **Plan** terms associated with the **endocrine system.**

7.6 Use **abbreviations** associated with the **endocrine system.**

7.7 Distinguish terms associated with the **endocrine system** in the context of **electronic health records.**

Introduction and Overview of the Endocrine System

Any building with heating or air conditioning also has a thermostat. A thermostat watches for changes in the temperature of a space and then responds to keep it in a desired range. When the building is too warm or too cold, the thermostat sends a signal to the heater or air conditioner to turn on or off. For the human body, the endocrine system serves this function of sending signals to keep all the body's many functions in balance.

The endocrine system can be broken down into signal senders, the signals they send, and the signals' outcomes. The main signal senders are the endocrine glands, which include the hypothalamus, pituitary, thyroid, parathyroid, adrenal, pancreas, and gonads (ovaries and testicles). Endocrine glands specifically send chemical signals to different parts of the body. These chemical signals, which are hormones, generally cause slower, subtler changes than the nervous system, which uses electric signals.

The signals travel through the rest of the body via the bloodstream, but only the intended cells in the body respond to these hormonal signals. These cells are keyed with receptors that fit with the hormone–just like two matching puzzle pieces. The hormone then signals the cell to perform a desired job, such as releasing another hormone, releasing or taking in nutrients, or changing the speed at which the body makes certain proteins.

The end result is that the endocrine system can adjust the levels of nutrients in the blood, excrete excess nutrients, help the body respond to its environment, and direct growth and development. For example, the pancreas secretes hormones that help the body control the level of sugar in the blood. The adrenal glands, thyroid gland, and parathyroid gland keep critical minerals like calcium and sodium in balance. The adrenal glands also make hormones for the fight-or-flight response to danger. Growth hormone helps the body grow to adult height and affects metabolism. The gonads make hormones that help drive sexual development. The endocrine system even stimulates milk production in new mothers.

7.1 Word Parts of the Endocrine System

Word Roots for Endocrine Glands

As you recall, the signal makers and senders of the endocrine system are called *glands*. They are located throughout your body, including in your brain, in the area above your kidneys, in your genitals, and in the front part of your neck.

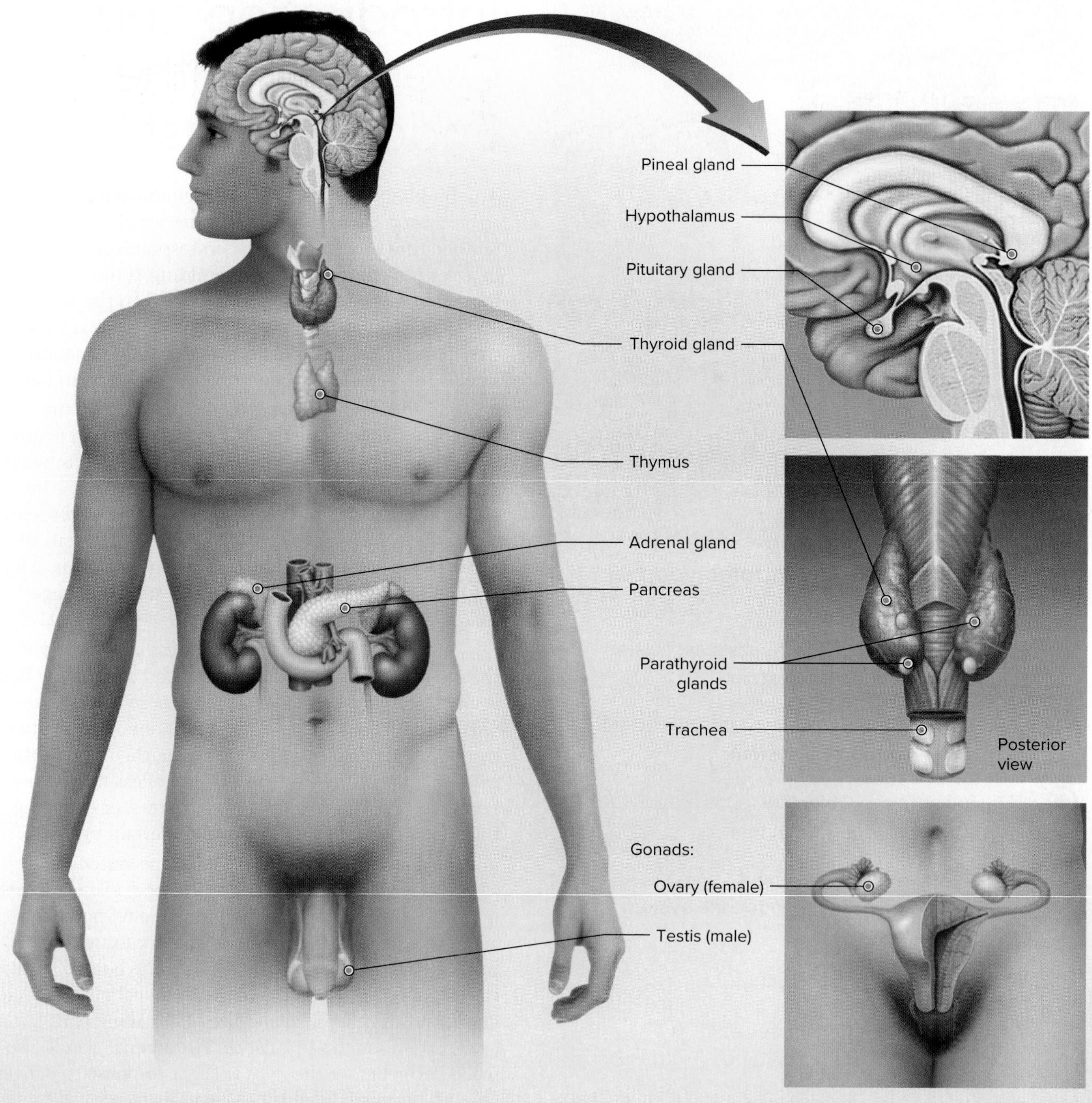

The glands are linked to the nervous system via the *hypothalamus*. It gets its name from its location in the brain, resting just below the thalamus. While part of the brain, the hypothalamus also acts as a gland in that it makes and releases hormones that direct the other glands. The main role of the hypothalamus is to direct the activity of the *pituitary gland*. It can cause the pituitary to make and release its chemical signals via chemicals called *releasing hormones* (example: *gonadotropin-releasing hormone*).

The pituitary gland is made of two parts: the *anterior* (front) and *posterior* (back) pituitary. The anterior pituitary gland is the origin for many very important hormones. These hormones travel by blood and stimulate many other endocrine glands, including your *thyroid* gland, *adrenal* glands, and *gonads*.

Located in the front part of your neck resting just below the Adam's apple is your thyroid gland and just behind it, the *parathyroid* glands. The thyroid gland makes hormones (T3 and T4) that affect the body's metabolism, as well as a hormone that helps control the level of calcium in the blood. The parathyroid glands also make a hormone that works along with the thyroid hormone to control the blood's calcium level.

The *pancreas,* an interesting gland that sits just under your stomach, is both an endocrine gland and a gastrointestinal organ. As an endocrine gland, it sends hormones directly into the bloodstream that help keep the blood sugar level in balance. As a gastrointestinal organ, it secretes enzymes by ducts (*exocrine*) directly into your intestines to help with digestion.

The adrenal gland gets its name from its location in your body, as it lies on top of your kidneys. The adrenal gland has an inner layer that makes the fight-or-flight hormone, *adrenaline*. Its outer layer, or cortex, makes two general types of hormones. One type keeps mineral levels in balance and also maintains the proper volume of water and salt in the blood. The other helps keep blood sugar levels in balance and affects your body's response to inflammation.

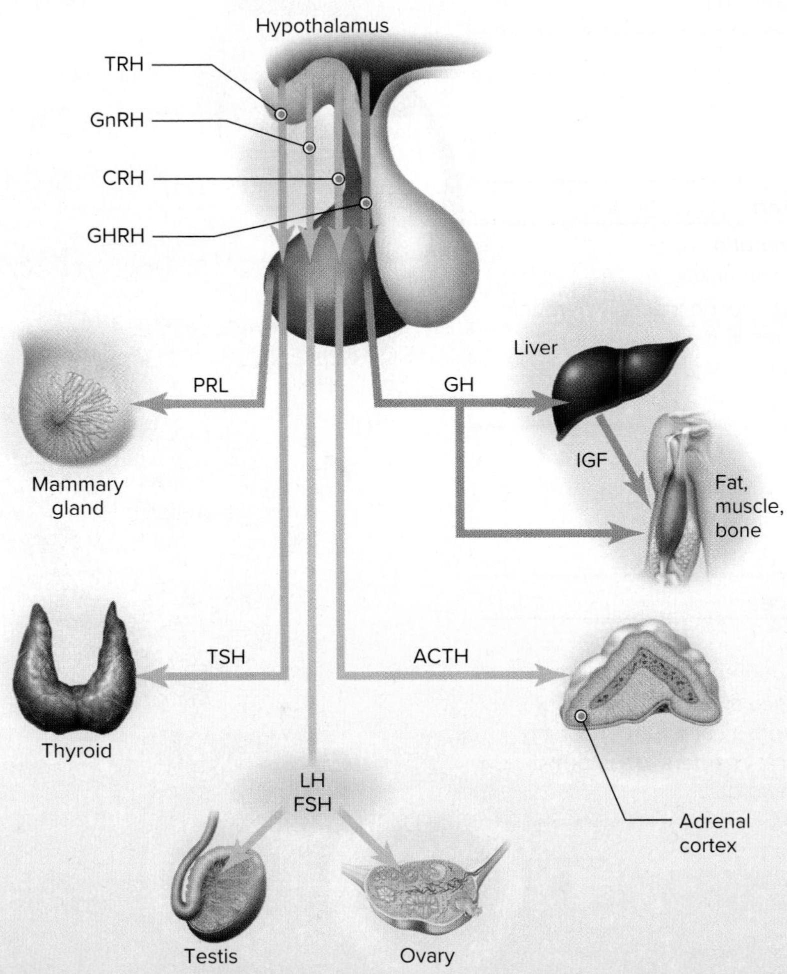

The gonads help with reproduction and with expression of male and female characteristics. The male gonads are the *testes.* They produce the male hormone *testosterone. Ovaries,* the female gonads, secrete *estrogens,* which help the body develop female attributes and help prepare the body for pregnancy.

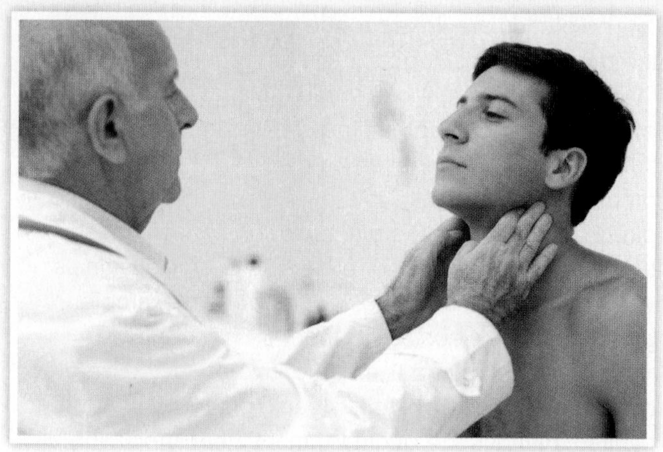

One indicator doctors use in determining health is whether or not the patient has swollen glands.

gland

ROOT: ***aden/o***

EXAMPLES: adenoma, adenopathy

NOTES: This root refers to any gland. Since the endocrine system has a lot of glands, the term comes up often.

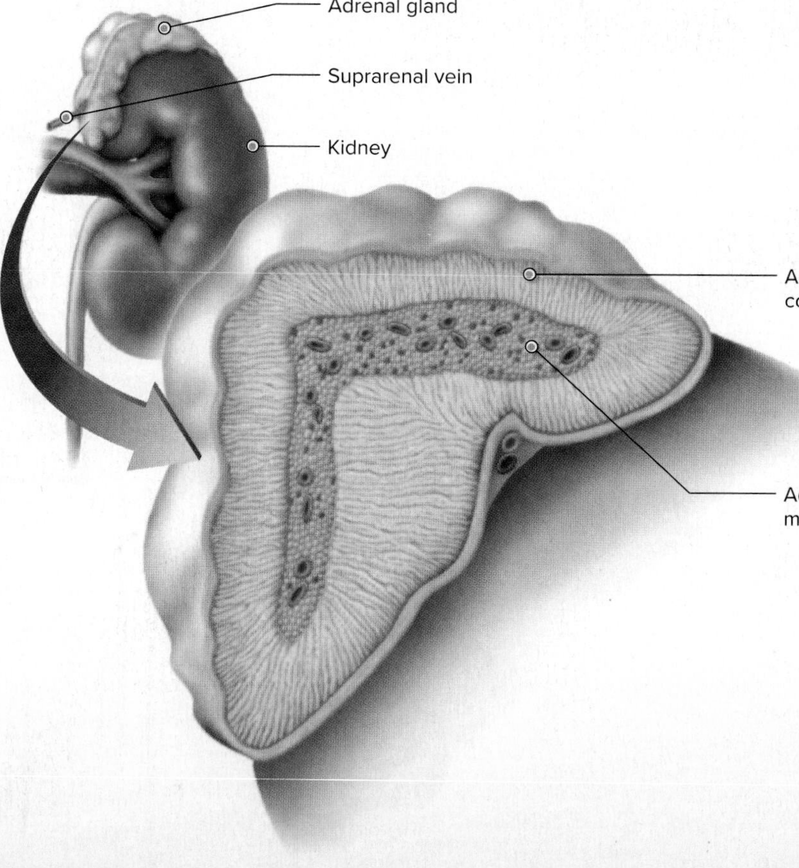

adrenal gland

ROOTS: ***adren/o, adrenal/o***

EXAMPLES: adrenarche, adrenalitis

NOTES: The name *adrenal* describes where this gland is located in the body. It literally means "on the kidney"—*ad* (to, on) + *renal* (kidney).

outer surface

ROOT: ***cortic/o***

EXAMPLES: corticotropic, adrenocorticohyperplasia

NOTES: The root *cortico* and the noun *cortex* both come from a Latin word meaning "bark" or "husk." It refers to the outer surface of any organ.

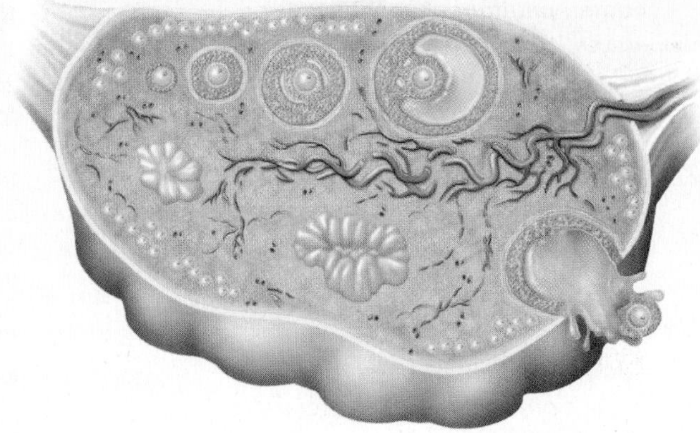

gonads (sex organs)

ROOT: ***gonad/o***

EXAMPLES: gonadopathy, gonadogenesis

NOTES: Although it is sometimes used interchangeably with the term *testicles,* the term *gonad* actually refers to the sex organs of both men and women. In males, of course, the gonads are the testicles, and in females, they are the ovaries.

You can easily recall the term *gonad* by remembering that its first three letters, *gon,* are from the same Greek root that places *gen* in the word *genesis,* which means "to create." That makes sense, because the gonads are the organs that aid in pro*creation*.

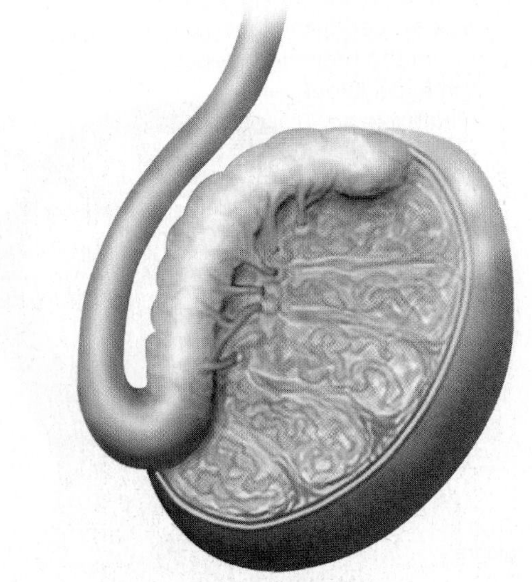

pancreas

ROOT: ***pancreat/o***

EXAMPLES: pancreatitis, pancreatolith

NOTES: The term *pancreas* comes from two Greek words: *pan* (all) and *kreas* (flesh). The reasoning for this has long been debated; some people think the name stuck because of the organ's fleshy consistency.

If you ever find yourself tempted by the word *sweetbreads* on a menu, think carefully before ordering. That's the term used by chefs to mean "cooked pancreas."

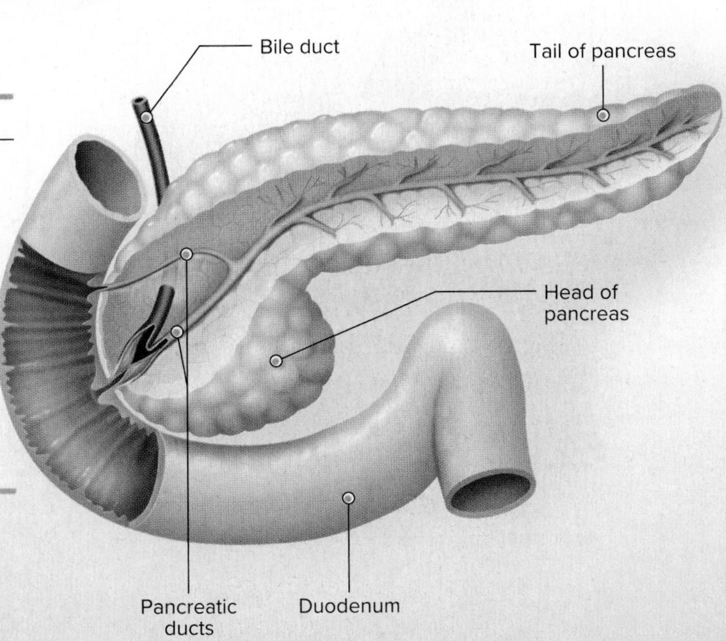

pituitary gland

ROOTS: ***pituitar/o, hypophys/o***

EXAMPLES: hyperpituitarism, hypophysitis

NOTES: The word *pituitary* comes from a Latin word meaning "mucus," because the Romans believed that the pituitary gland channeled mucus from the brain to the nose.

The other root, *hypophyso,* comes from the Greek words *hypo* (under) + *physis* (growth) and refers to the appearance and location of the pituitary gland, a pea-sized gland located under the brain right behind the eyes. It looks a little like an abnormal growth underneath the brain—but it is a critical part of the endocrine system.

thymus

ROOT: ***thym/o***

EXAMPLES: *thymoma, thymectomy*

NOTES: The *thymus* is an organ found in the upper chest, under the sternum and in front of the heart. Its name is derived from the name of the herb *thyme.* To those who first discovered it, the organ looked like a bunch of thyme.

©I. Rozenbaum & F. Cirou/PhotoAlto RF

thyroid

ROOTS: ***thyr/o, thyroid/o***

EXAMPLES: thyrotoxin, thyroidectomy

NOTES: The word *thyroid* comes from the Greek word *thyros,* meaning "shield."

Thyro (shield) + *oid* (resembling) = the gland resembling a shield. It really does look like a shield spread out over the throat, doesn't it?

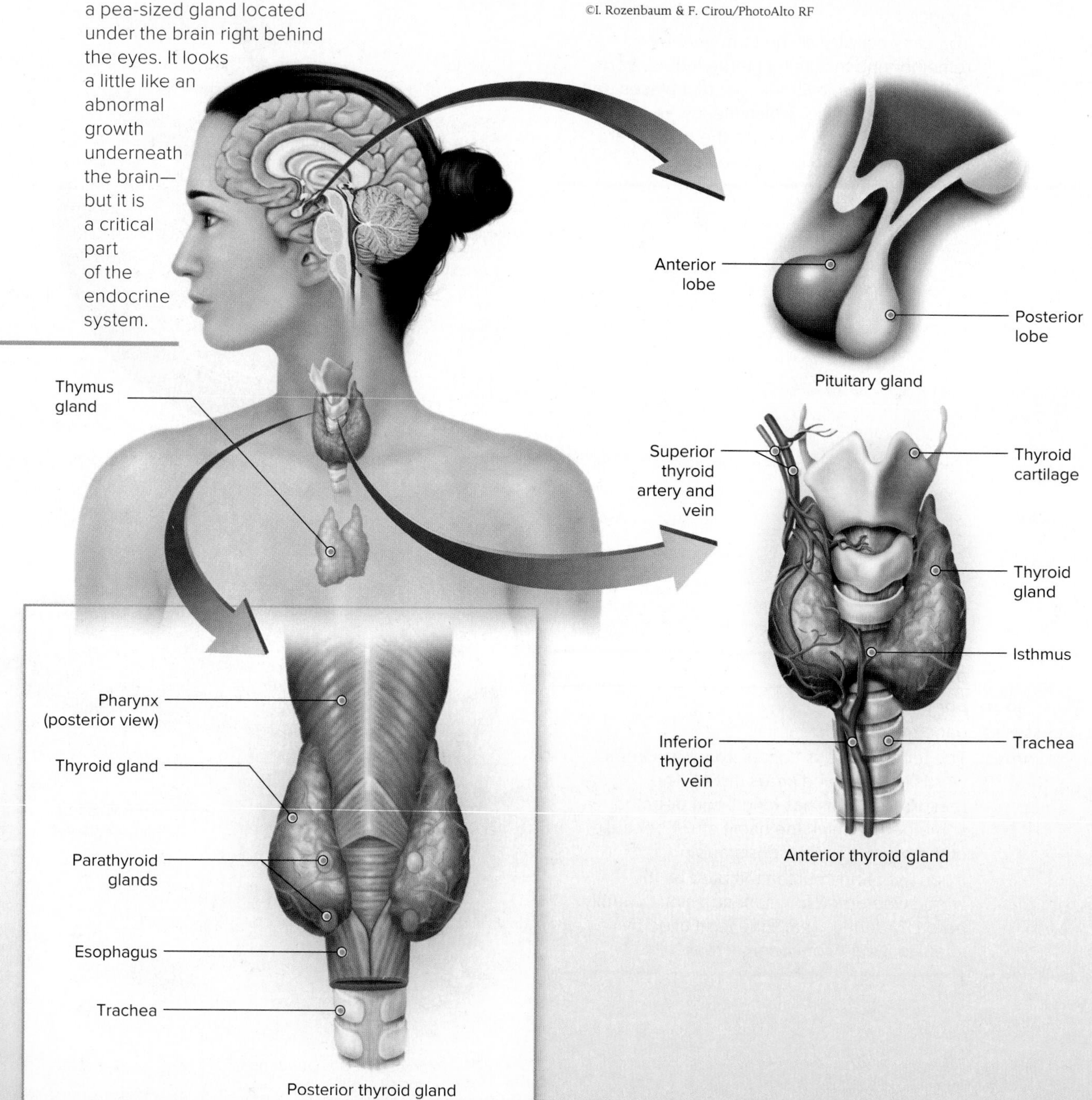

sugar

ROOTS: ***gluc/o, glucos/o, glyc/o***

EXAMPLES: glucocorticoid, glucosuria, hypoglycemia

NOTES: Three common types of sugar are sucrose, glucose, and fructose. *Sucrose* is a complex molecule made up of glucose and fructose. *Glucose* and *fructose* have the same chemical composition but different molecular structures. For some reason, glucose (which requires insulin to break it down) is the universal fuel of all living things and is also used in brain functions. Neurologists often use glucose consumption as an indicator of brain activity. When the brain lacks glucose, certain mental functions, like self-control and decision making, become more difficult.

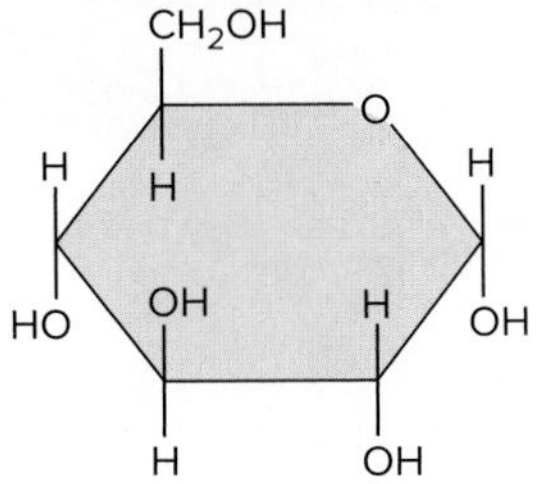

Glucose

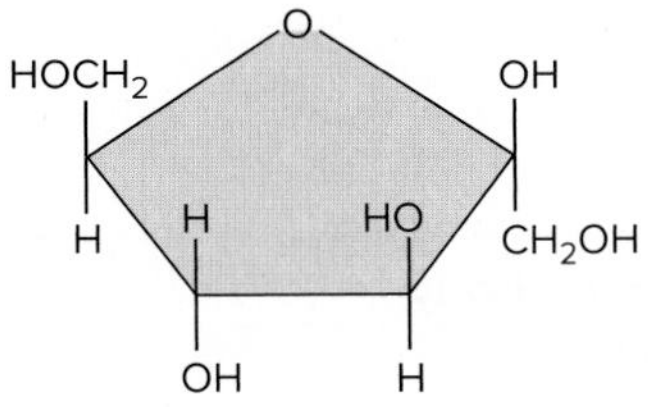

Fructose

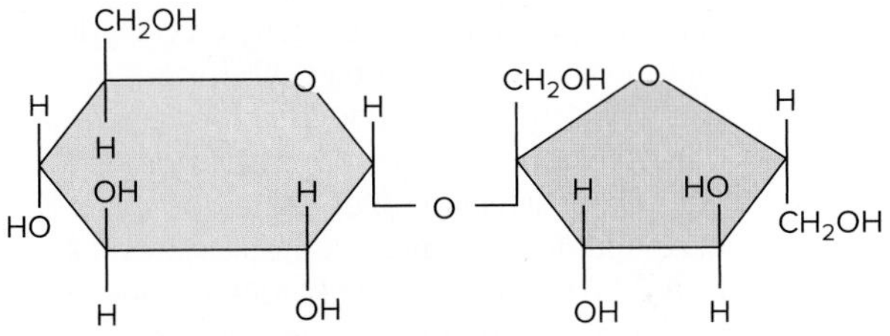

Sucrose

to secrete

ROOT: ***crin/o***

EXAMPLES: endocrine, exocrine

NOTES: *Endocrine* means "to secrete internally"; it refers to chemicals secreted into the bloodstream. The opposite of this is *exocrine,* which means "to secrete externally" and refers to chemicals secreted through ducts to the surface of an organ. Examples of this include sweat glands and salivary glands. Next time you find yourself sweating through a workout or drooling over some food, you can say that you're having an excessive exocrine response.

Word Roots for Secretions, Chemicals, and Blood Work

Once the signals (*hormones*) are made in the endocrine organs, they wait to be secreted (*crino*) to their target body part. Endocrine signals travel via the bloodstream. The *pituitary* gland makes many hormones that encourage other endocrine glands in the body to work. *Adrenocorticotropic hormone (ACTH)* stimulates the outer part of the adrenal gland. *Thyroid-stimulating hormone* (*TSH)* stimulates the thyroid gland. *Luteinizing (LH)* and *follicle-stimulating hormone (FSH)* stimulate the gonads. The pituitary gland also makes growth hormone and prolactin.

The thyroid makes three very important hormones: *T4, T3,* and *calcitonin.* T4 and T3 affect the body's metabolism. An overactive thyroid (*hyperthyroidism*) leads to a higher-than-normal metabolism—everything speeds up. As a result, a person suffering from hyperthyroidism experiences weight loss, increased hunger, diarrhea, and nervousness. On the opposite end, for people with *hypothyroidism,* everything slows down. They typically experience weight gain, decreased energy and appetite, and constipation.

Calcitonin is a hormone that encourages the uptake of calcium in the blood into bone. This keeps the level of calcium in the blood from getting too high. The parathyroid glands make *parathyroid hormone.* This hormone has the opposite effect of calcitonin. It helps keep the level of calcium in the blood from getting too low.

As you recall, the pancreas is both a digestive organ and an endocrine organ. The endocrine part of the pancreas makes two hormones that work together to keep the level of sugar in the blood in balance. *Insulin*

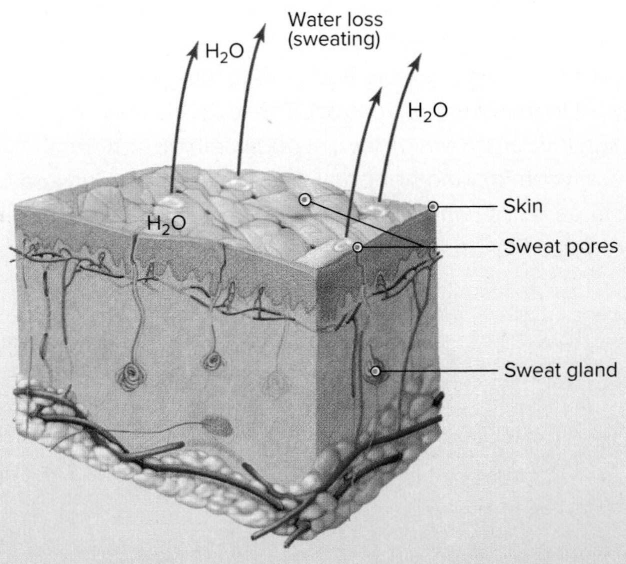

decreases the level of sugar in the blood. It encourages cells to open up to the blood sugar (*glucose*) and take it in. *Glucagon* works against insulin. It tells the liver to make more sugar and thus increases the level of sugar in the blood.

The adrenal gland creates hormones in two parts—the inner part or the outer part. The inner part of the adrenal gland makes *epinephrine,* which was once known as adrenaline. Many people know adrenaline as the chemical that surges in danger and helps mothers lift cars off their babies. While it doesn't truly gift people with superpowers, it does play an important role in the fight-or-flight response by increasing your heart rate and opening your airways to get more oxygen. Norepinephrine, also made in the adrenal gland, causes very similar changes.

The outer part of the adrenal gland (*cortex*) also makes very important hormones. ACTH stimulates the cortex to release *corticosteroids,* which are steroid hormones made in the cortex. The two types of corticosteroids are hormones dealing with mineral balance (*mineralocorticoids*) and hormones dealing with sugar balance (*glucocorticoids*).

Last, the adrenal glands are an extra location for secretion of the sex hormones, testosterone and estrogen. The main source of these hormones, however, is the gonads. The gonads of men and women make different hormones. In men, the testes make testosterone. The testes trigger the production of sperm and the development of masculine body characteristics, like increased muscle and facial hair. Ovaries, the female gonads, secrete estrogens, which cause the development and release of eggs as well as the development of feminine attributes, like breasts and wide hips.

Measuring the level of certain hormones and how they affect the patient's blood is one way of checking the function of the endocrine system. The most common example is checking the glucose level in the blood (*glycemia*). These levels may be high (*hyperglycemia*), low (*hypoglycemia*), or normal (*euglycemia*). Another body fluid that is often measured is a patient's *urine.* Substances like sugar (*glucosuria*) or ketones (*ketonuria*) may be found in the urine.

hormone

ROOT: ***hormon/o***

EXAMPLE: hormonopoesis

NOTES: From the Greek word meaning "to rush" or "push," *hormones* are chemicals secreted by certain glands for the purpose of stimulating an organ or part of the body to do something.

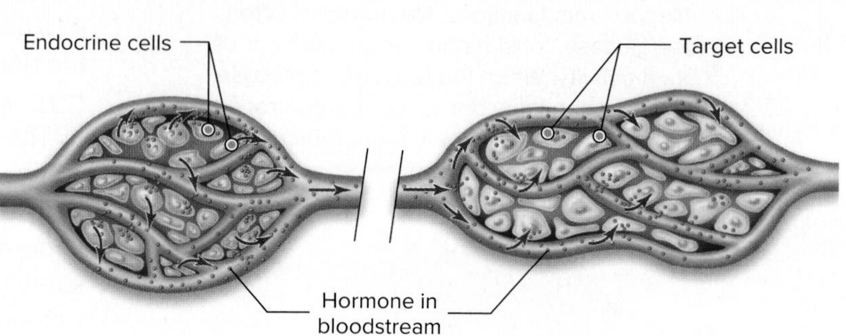

ketone body

ROOT: ***ket/o***

EXAMPLES: ketosis, ketogenic

NOTES: A *ketone body* is a substance that increases in the blood as a result of faulty carbohydrate metabolism. Ketone bodies are toxic chemicals that build up in the blood and are detectable in the urine. When there isn't enough insulin in the blood, the body cannot use sugar for energy, so it breaks down fat instead. The presence of ketone bodies is normally a sign of untreated or poorly controlled diabetes. Oddly enough, although ketones can be secreted in the urine, the primary way the body gets rid of them is through the lungs, giving sufferers fruity-smelling breath.

Suffixes for Secretions, Chemicals, and Blood Work

stimulating hormone

SUFFIX: *-tropin*

EXAMPLES: thyrotropin, gonadotropin

NOTES: If a term has the suffix *-tropin,* it refers to a hormone that has a stimulating effect on a target organ. The suffix comes from a Greek word meaning "to turn"—perhaps because it turns the target organ on and tells it to start working.

-Tropin has the same root as the word *trophy.* In ancient Greece, a *trophy* was a monument built on a battlefield to mark the spot where the battle *turned* in the victor's favor.

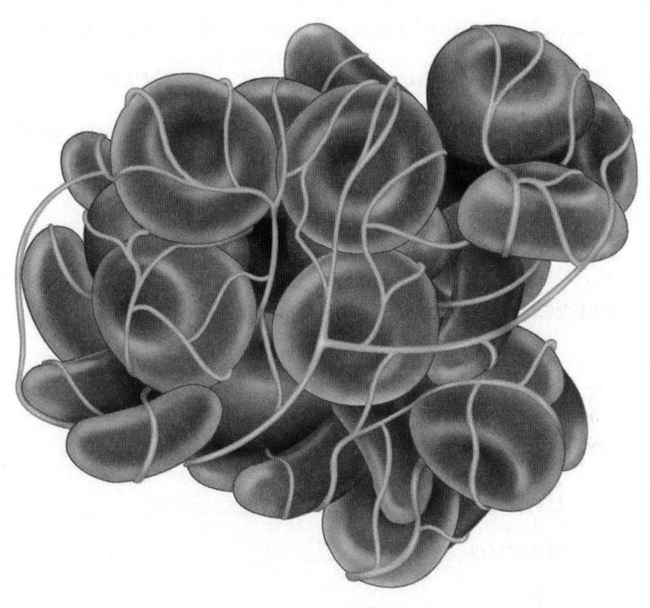

blood condition

SUFFIX: *-emia*

EXAMPLES: glycemia, calcemia

NOTES: Because the endocrine system deals with internal secretions, blood analysis (which is, of course, analysis of a secretion of the body) is usually the best way to detect problems.

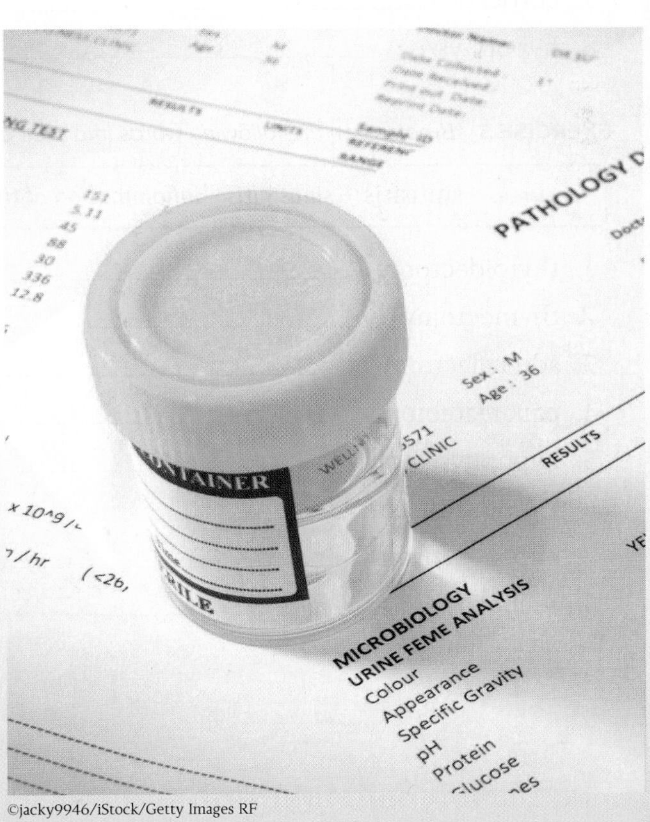

©jacky9946/iStock/Getty Images RF

urine condition

SUFFIX: *-uria*

EXAMPLE: polyuria

NOTES: Substances in the urine can be useful clues in diagnosing endocrine problems.

For example, in 1889, Oscar Minkowski and Joseph von Mering removed the pancreas of a healthy dog. Several days after the dog's pancreas was removed, the researchers noticed that flies were feeding on the dog's urine—something that was not the case prior to the removal of the pancreas. Analysis of the dog's urine revealed the presence of sugar—a discovery that helped established the relationship between the pancreas and diabetes.

Learning Outcome 7.1 Exercises

Additional exercises available in connect

TRANSLATION

EXERCISE 1 *Match the root on the left with its definition on the right.*

_____	1. pancreat/o	a. adrenal gland
_____	2. gonad/o	b. gland
_____	3. pituitar/o	c. gonads (sex organs)
_____	4. adren/o	d. outer surface
_____	5. thym/o	e. pancreas
_____	6. thyr/o	f. pituitary gland
_____	7. aden/o	g. thymus
_____	8. cortic/o	h. thyroid

EXERCISE 2 *Translate the following roots.*

1. adrenal/o ______________________________
2. gonad/o ______________________________
3. pancreat/o ______________________________
4. thyroid/o ______________________________
5. thym/o ______________________________
6. aden/o ______________________________
7. cortic/o ______________________________
8. hypophys/o ______________________________

EXERCISE 3 *Break down the following words into their component parts and translate.*

EXAMPLE: sinusitis *sinus | itis* *inflammation of the sinuses*

1. thyroidectomy ______________________________
2. thymectomy ______________________________
3. adrenalectomy ______________________________
4. pancreatectomy ______________________________
5. hypophysectomy ______________________________
6. hypopituitarism ______________________________
7. hypogonadism ______________________________
8. adenopathy ______________________________

Learning Outcome 7.1 Exercises

EXERCISE 4 *Match the word part on the left with its definition on the right. Some definitions will be used more than once.*

______	1. hormon/o		a. blood condition
______	2. ket/o		b. hormone
______	3. glyc/o		c. ketone body
______	4. gluc/o		d. stimulating hormone
______	5. -emia		e. sugar
______	6. -uria		f. to secrete
______	7. -tropin		g. urine condition
______	8. crin/o		

EXERCISE 5 *Translate the following word parts.*

1. hormon/o ______________________________
2. glucos/o ______________________________
3. ket/o ______________________________
4. crin/o ______________________________
5. glyc/o ______________________________
6. -uria ______________________________
7. -emia ______________________________
8. -tropin ______________________________

EXERCISE 6 *Break down the following words into their component parts and translate.*

EXAMPLE:	sinusitis	*sinus | itis*	*inflammation of the sinuses*

1. hyperglycemia ______________________________
2. euglycemia ______________________________
3. ketonuria ______________________________
4. glucosuria ______________________________
5. gonadotropin ______________________________
6. endocrine ______________________________

Learning Outcome 7.1 Exercises

GENERATION

EXERCISE 7 *Identify the word parts from this chapter for the following terms.*

1. adrenomegaly ____________
2. pancreatalgia ____________
3. corticotropin ____________
4. gonadogenesis ____________
5. hypophysitis ____________
6. thymoma ____________
7. polyadenopathy ____________
8. panhypopituitarism ____________
9. thyrotoxicosis ____________
10. hypothyroidism ____________

EXERCISE 8 *Build a medical term from the information provided.*

1. inflammation of the pancreas ____________
2. inflammation of the thyroid ____________
3. inflammation of a gland ____________
4. good thyroid ____________

EXERCISE 9 *Identify the word parts from this chapter for the following terms.*

1. polyuria ____________
2. exocrine ____________
3. glucogenesis ____________
4. endocrinologist ____________
5. hyperphosphatemia ____________
6. ketogenic diet ____________
7. adrenocortical insufficiency (2 roots) ____________
8. euglycemia (2 roots) ____________
9. adrenocorticotropic hormone (4 roots) ____________

EXERCISE 10 *Build a medical term from the information provided.*

1. sugar urine condition (use *glucoso*) ____________
2. ketone urine condition ____________
3. low blood sugar condition (use *glyco*) ____________
4. thyroid-stimulating hormone (use *thyro*) ____________

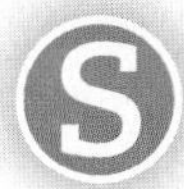

Subjective
Patient History, Problems, Complaints
Adrenal
Gonad
Pancreas
Pituitary
Thyroid

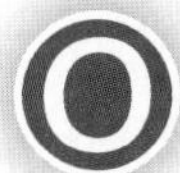

Objective
Observation and Discovery
-emia/-uria
Hormones
Results
Professional terms, diagnostic procedures

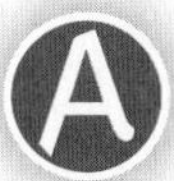

Assessment
Diagnosis and Pathology
General terms
Adrenal
Pancreas
Pituitary
Thyroid

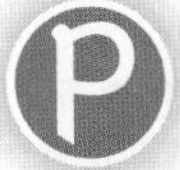

Plan
Treatments and Therapies
General terms
Adrenal
Pancreas
Pituitary
Thyroid

This section contains medical terms built from the roots presented in the previous section. The purpose of this section is to expose you to words used in the endocrine system that are built from the word roots presented earlier. The focus of this book is to teach you the process of learning roots and translating them in context. Each term is presented with the correct pronunciation, followed by a word analysis that breaks down the word into its component parts, a definition that provides a literal translation of the word, as well as supplemental information if the literal translation deviates from its medical use.

The terms are organized using a health care professional's SOAP note (first introduced in Chapter 2) as a model.

SUBJECTIVE

7.2 Patient History, Problems, Complaints

The symptoms a patient experiences from an endocrine problem all depend on which organ is affected. Patients with pituitary problems may present to a health care provider with growth disturbances. This can be on either extreme, from the abnormally large (*pituitary gigantism*) or small (*pituitary dwarfism*). If the extra growth is disproportionate in the face and long bones of the body, it is known as *acromegaly*.

Patients with an overactive thyroid (*hyperthyroidism*) have a higher-than-normal metabolism—everything speeds up. As a result, a person suffering from hyperthyroidism experiences weight loss, increased hunger, diarrhea, and nervousness. Some also have bulging eyes (*exophthalmos*).

On the opposite end, for someone with *hypothyroidism,* everything slows down. Patients with this disease typically experience weight gain, decreased energy, hair loss, decreased appetite, and constipation. They may also experience swelling and puffiness in the hands and face. This grouping of symptoms is called *myxedema*. Both hyperthyroidism and hypothyroidism can present with an enlarged thyroid (*goiter*).

7.2 Patient History, Problems, Complaints

Decreased pancreatic endocrine activity leads to diabetes. Patients with diabetes may complain of excessive thirst (*polydipsia*), excessive urination (*polyuria*), and constant hunger (*polyphagia*), with an unexpected weight loss.

Premature sexual traits may represent a problem with the adrenal gland or the gonads. Males may experience premature puberty from an overactive adrenal gland (*adrenal virilism*). Females with the same problem may report facial hair (*hirsutism*). When a female has a hyperactive gonad (*hypergonadism*) she may present with periods (*menarche*) or breast development (*thelarche*) at a premature age. Females with underfunctioning gonads may complain of lack of menstruation (*amenorrhea*). Males may experience breast development (*gynecomastia*). This is very common in puberty.

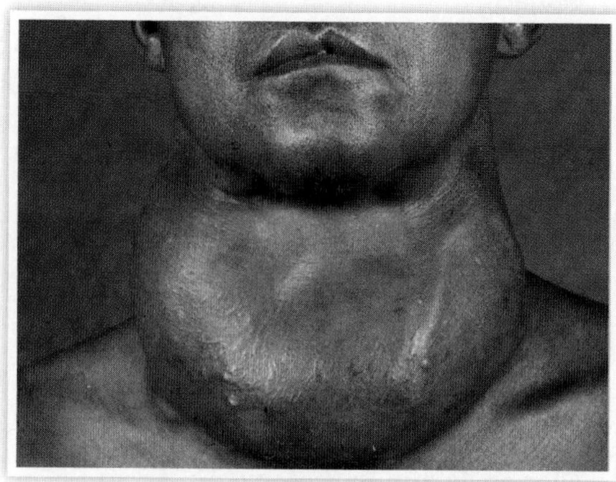

Goiter, or swollen thyroid gland, is most commonly caused by iodine deficiency. The easy solution to this, and to other health problems caused by low iodine, is to add iodine to salt. Check the container of table salt in your home. Chances are good that it's iodized salt.

adrenal

Term	Word Analysis
adenalgia AD-eh-NAL-jah **Definition** pain in a gland	**aden / algia** gland / pain
adrenal virilism ad-REE-nal VIR-il-izm **Definition** development of male secondary sexual characteristics caused by excessive secretion of the adrenal gland	**adrenal viril / ism** adrenal man / condition
adrenarche AD-ren-AR-kay **Definition** beginning of adrenal secretion (at puberty)	**adren / arche** adrenal / beginning
hirsutism HIR-soo-tizm **Definition** excessive growth of facial and body hair in women	**from Latin, for** "shaggy"

gonad

Term	Word Analysis
amenorrhea ah-MEN-oh-REE-ah **Definition** lack of menstrual flow	**a / meno / rrhea** no / menstrual / flow

gonad *continued*

Term	Word Analysis
gynecomastia GAI-neh-koh-MAS-tee-ah **Definition** development of breast tissue in males	**gyneco / mast / ia** woman / breast / condition 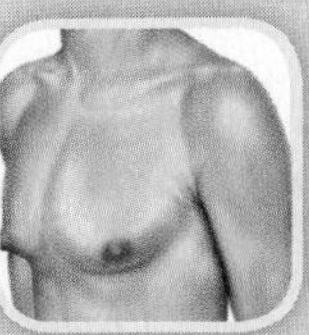
hypergonadism HAI-per-GOH-nad-izm **Definition** condition in which there is excessive secretion of the sex glands	**hyper / gonad / ism** over / gonad / condition
hypogonadism HAI-poh-GOH-nad-izm **Definition** condition in which there is undersecretion of the sex glands	**hypo / gonad / ism** under / gonad / condition
menarche MEN-ar-kee **Definition** beginning or first menstruation	**men / arche** menstrual / beginning
thelarche thee-LAR-kay **Definition** beginning of breast development	**thel / arche** breast / beginning 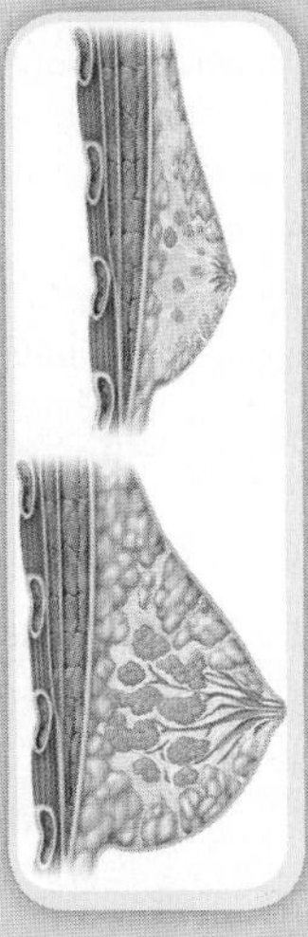

pancreas

Term	Word Analysis
hypoglycemic HAI-poh-glai-SEE-mik **Definition** pertaining to low blood sugar	**hypo / glyc / em / ic** under / sugar / blood / pertaining to
pancreatalgia PAN-kree-ah-TAL-jah **Definition** pain in the pancreas	**pancreat / algia** pancreas / pain

pancreas *continued*

Term	Word Analysis
polydipsia PAW-lee-DIP-see-ah **Definition** excessive thirst	**poly / dips / ia** excessive / thirst / condition
NOTE: You might expect *hyperdipsia*, but the term uses *poly* instead. The reason is because this word is not first a medical word but the ancient Greek term for "excessively thirsty." In Greek, *poly* can mean "*excessive*" as well as "many."	
polyphagia PAW-lee-FAY-jah **Definition** excessive eating	**poly / phag / ia** excessive / eat / condition
polyuria PAW-lee-YOO-ree-ah **Definition** excessive urination	**poly / uria** excessive / urine condition

pituitary

Term	Word Analysis
acromegaly AK-roh-MEH-gah-lee **Definition** abnormal enlargement of the extremities	**acro / megaly** extremities / abnormal enlargement
NOTE: The term *acro* can mean "top" or "high," as in *acrophobia*, the fear of heights, or it can mean "the end" or "extremity," as it does here.	
galactorrhea gah-LAK-toh-REE-ah **Definition** discharge of milk	**galacto / rrhea** milk / discharge
NOTE: The word *galaxy* comes from this root. Our galaxy is called the Milky Way because early stargazers thought it looked like someone sprayed milk in the sky.	
pituitary dwarfism pih-TOO-ih-TER-ee DWAR-fizm **Definition** abnormally short height caused by undersecretion of growth hormone from the pituitary gland	**pituitary dwarfism**
pituitary gigantism pih-TOO-ih-TER-ee jai-GAN-tizm **Definition** abnormally tall height caused by oversecretion of growth hormone from the pituitary gland	**pituitary gigantism**

thyroid

Term	Word Analysis
exophthalmos EKS-of-THAL-mohs **Definition** protrusion of the eyes out of the eye socket	**ex / ophthalmos** out / eye

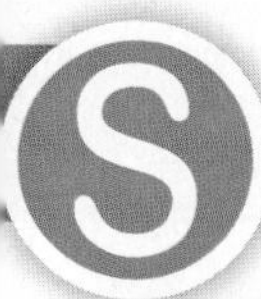

7.2 Patient History, Problems, Complaints

thyroid *continued*

Term	Word Analysis
goiter GOY-ter **Definition** swollen thyroid gland **NOTE:** The most common cause of goiter is iodine deficiency. The easy solution to this, and to other health problems caused by low iodine, is to add iodine to salt.	**from Latin, for** "gutter" (meaning "throat") ©Dr. M.A. Ansary/Science Source
thyrocele THAI-roh-seel **Definition** another name for goiter	**thyro / cele** thyroid / tumor
thyromegaly THAI-roh-MEH-gah-lee **Definition** enlargement of the thyroid	**thyro / megaly** thyroid / enlargement
thyroptosis THAI-rop-TOH-sis **Definition** downward displacement (drooping) of the thryoid	**thyro / ptosis** thyroid / drooping condition

Learning Outcome 7.2 Exercises

PRONUNCIATION

EXERCISE 1 *Indicate which syllable is emphasized when pronounced.*

EXAMPLE: bronchitis bron**chi**tis

1. menarche ____________
2. thelarche ____________
3. polydipsia ____________
4. adenalgia ____________
5. myxedema ____________
6. thyroptosis ____________
7. hypergonadism ____________
8. hypogonadism ____________

Learning Outcome 7.2 Exercises

TRANSLATION

EXERCISE 2 *Underline and define the word parts from this chapter in the following terms.*

1. adenalgia ______
2. thyrocele ______
3. thyromegaly ______
4. polyuria ______
5. adrenal virilism ______
6. hypergonadism ______
7. hypogonadism ______
8. pituitary dwarfism ______
9. pituitary gigantism ______
10. thyroptosis ______
11. exophthalmos ______

EXERCISE 3 *Match the term on the left with its definition on the right.*

______	1. galactorrhea	a.	abnormal enlargement of the extremities
______	2. amenorrhea	b.	discharge of milk
______	3. gynecomastia	c.	excessive eating
______	4. polyuria	d.	excessive growth of facial and body hair in women
______	5. polyphagia	e.	excessive thirst
______	6. polydipsia	f.	excessive urination
______	7. menarche	g.	lack of menstrual flow
______	8. thelarche	h.	swelling of the skin caused by deposits under the skin
______	9. adrenarche	i.	swollen thyroid gland
______	10. goiter	j.	beginning of adrenal secretion
______	11. acromegaly	k.	beginning of breast development
______	12. myxedema	l.	beginning or first menstruation
______	13. hirsutism	m.	development of breast tissue in males

EXERCISE 4 *Translate the following terms as literally as possible.*

EXAMPLE: nasopharyngoscope *an instrument for looking at the nose and throat*

1. thyroptosis ______
2. exophthalmos ______
3. galactorrhea ______
4. amenorrhea ______
5. adrenarche ______
6. gynecomastia ______

S

Learning Outcome 7.2 Exercises

GENERATION

EXERCISE 5 *Build a medical term from the information provided.*

EXAMPLE: inflammation of the sinuses *sinusitis*

1. pain in the pancreas ______________________
2. pain in a gland ______________________
3. thyroid tumor (use *-cele*) ______________________
4. excessive urination ______________________
5. pertaining to low blood sugar ______________________

EXERCISE 6 *Multiple-choice questions. Select the correct answer.*

1. In the condition known as *adrenal virilism,* the adrenal gland secretes excess hormones causing the development of:
   a. a swollen thyroid gland
   b. abnormal enlargement of the extremities
   c. breast tissue in males
   d. male secondary sexual characteristics
   e. all of these

2. The "bearded lady" at the carnival is displaying which condition?
   a. gynecomastia
   b. hirsutism
   c. thyrocele
   d. polydipsia
   e. none of these

3. Another word for *goiter* is:
   a. parathyroid
   b. thyrocele
   c. thyromegaly
   d. thyroptosis
   e. none of these

4. A term that describes excessive thirst is called:
   a. gynecomastia
   b. hirsutism
   c. thyrocele
   d. polydipsia
   e. none of these

5. A person with hyperthyroidism can display which symptoms?
   a. exophthalmos
   b. nervousness
   c. polyphagia
   d. weight loss
   e. all of these

6. Decreased pancreatic endocrine activity leads to diabetes. If a patient has diabetes, he or she may complain of:
   a. polydipsia
   b. polyuria
   c. polyphagia
   d. unexpected weight loss
   e. all of these

7. When a female has a hyperactive gonad (*hypergonadism*), she may present with premature:
   a. periods
   b. menarche
   c. breast development
   d. thelarche
   e. all of these

8. A person who is experiencing weight gain, decreased energy, hair loss, decreased appetite, constipation, or puffy hands and face may be experiencing which of the following conditions?
   a. hyperthyroidism
   b. hypothyroidism
   c. polydipsia
   d. polyphagia
   e. none of these

9. Premature sexual traits may represent a problem with the adrenal gland or the gonads. Males may experience:
   a. adrenal virilism
   b. hirsutism
   c. premature puberty from an overactive adrenal gland
   d. adrenal virilism and hirsutism
   e. adrenal virilism and premature puberty from an overactive adrenal gland

Learning Outcome 7.2 Exercises

10. Premature sexual traits may represent a problem with the adrenal gland or the gonads. Females may come to health care providers complaining of:
    a. facial hair
    b. gynecomastia
    c. hirsutism
    d. facial hair and gynecomastia
    e. facial hair and hirsutism
11. Females with underfunctioning gonads may complain of:
    a. amenorrhea
    b. lack of menstruation
    c. thelarche
    d. amenorrhea and lack of menstruation
    e. lack of menstruation and thelarche
12. Males with underfunctioning gonads may complain of:
    a. breast development
    b. gynecomastia
    c. hirsutism
    d. breast development and gynecomastia
    e. breast development and hirsutism

EXERCISE 7 *Briefly describe the difference between each pair of terms.*

1. hypergonadism, hypogonadism ______________________________
2. pituitary dwarfism, pituitary gigantism ______________________________
3. menarche, thelarche ______________________________
4. polydipsia, polyphagia ______________________________
5. acromegaly, thyromegaly ______________________________

OBJECTIVE

7.3 Observation and Discovery

When a patient is examined for endocrine problems, many of the findings are the same things that the patient noticed and reported. The examiner may notice that the patient is much taller or shorter than average, or that he or she is overweight or underweight. Patients may have incorrect sexual traits, like a male with breast development. Patients may have swelling or fat that is more pronounced in certain parts of their bodies.

Much of what is left for data collection relates to laboratory testing. There are numerous tests in endocrinology. The tests check either the level of hormones in the blood or their effect. Many of the hormones take on similar names to the gland that made them. For example, one of the hormones that the parathyroid glands makes is parathyroid hormone. Adrenal glands make adrenaline (also known as *epinephrine*). They may take on the name from the part of the gland in which they are made. Cortisol is made in the cortex of the adrenal gland. Other hormones are named for the organ they "turn on." These types of hormones are known as *-tropins*. For example, adrenocorticotropic hormone stimulates the cortex of the adrenal gland. Other -tropins include gonadotropins (*LH* and *FSH*) and thyrotopin (*TSH*).

There are two general fluids that can be checked to see the results of hormones: blood and urine. Any lab level that represents a substance in the blood ends in *-emia*. For instance, magnesemia is the level of magnesium in the blood. If the level is higher than normal it has the prefix *hyper-*, and if it is lower than normal it has the prefix *hypo-*. For instance, if a patient has a lower-than-expected level of magnesium in his or her blood, the patient has hypomagnesemia. Any lab level for a substance in the urine ends with *-uria*. If a patient has calcium in his or her urine, the patient has calciuria.

One specific nutrient the endocrine system manages is the sugar level in the blood. It controls how fast sugar is being made (*gluconeogenesis*) and how fast it is broken down (*glycolysis*). If someone has low blood sugar (*hypoglycemia*) then the body releases a hormone to increase the production of sugar and slow the breakdown of sugar. Ketones are a byproduct of this.

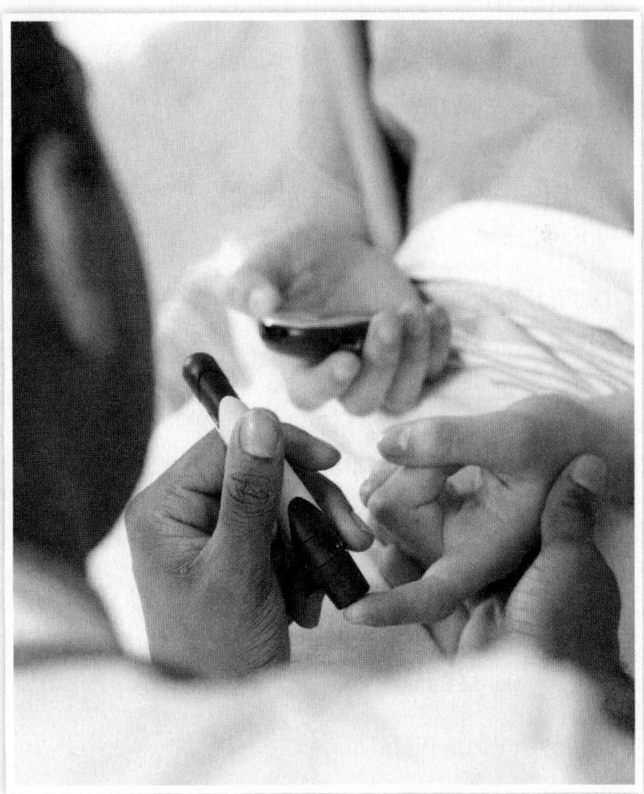

Testing blood is central to gathering data for the endocrine system. A finger prick is the easiest and least invasive path when only a little blood is needed.

blood and urine conditions

Term	Word Analysis
acidemia A-sih-DEE-mee-ah **Definition** abnormal acidity of the blood	**acid / emia** acid / blood condition

blood and urine conditions *continued*

Term	Word Analysis
alkalemia AL-kah-LEE-mee-ah **Definition** abnormal alkalinity (opposite of acidity) of the blood	**alkal / emia** alkali / blood condition
Note: Alkali is a strong base and is the opposite of an acid. The term *alkali* comes from the Arabic, for *al-qaliy*, which means "the ashes" and is the name of a plant that grows well in alkaline soil.	
calciuria CAL-sih-YOO-ree-ah **Definition** calcium in the urine	**calci / uria** calcium / urine condition
chloremia klor-EE-mee-ah **Definition** increased chloride in the blood	**chlor / emia** chloride / blood condition
euglycemia YOO-glai-SEE-mee-ah **Definition** good blood sugar	**eu / glyc / emia** good / sugar / blood condition
glucosuria GLOO-koh-SOO-ree-ah **Definition** sugar in the urine	**glucos / uria** sugar / urine condition
hypercalcemia HAI-per-kal-SEE-mee-ah **Definition** excessive calcium in the blood	**hyper / calc / emia** over / calcium / blood condition
hypercholesterolemia HAI-per-koh-LES-ter-aw-LEE-mee-ah **Definition** excessive cholesterol in the blood	**hyper / cholesterol / emia** excessive / cholesterol / blood condition
Note: The term *cholesterol* breaks down as *chole* (bile) + *stero* (solid) + *ol* (substance) and means "a solid bile substance." It gets the name because it was first discovered in gallstones.	
hyperglycemia HAI-per-glai-SEE-mee-ah **Definition** high blood sugar	**hyper / glyc / emia** excessive / sugar / blood condition
hyperkalemia HAI-per-kah-LEE-mee-ah **Definition** excessive potassium in the blood	**hyper / kal / emia** over / potassium / blood condition
Note: The *kal* root comes from the Latin word *kalium*, which means "potash." The name comes from the fact that potassium is obtained by soaking ashes in water and then evaporating the liquid. This explains why the periodic table's abbreviation for potassium is *K*. The name *potassium* is a Latinization of the words "pot ash." Potassium really does mean "pot-ash-ium."	

blood and urine conditions *continued*

Term	Word Analysis
hyperlipidemia HAI-per-lih-pih-DEE-mee-ah **Definition** excessive fat in the blood	**hyper / lipid / emia** excessive / fat / blood condition 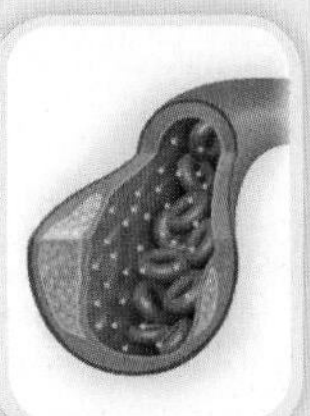
hypernatremia HAI-per-nah-TREE-mee-ah **Definition** excessive sodium in the blood	**hyper / natr / emia** excessive / sodium / blood condition
hyperphosphatemia HAI-per-FAWS-fay-TEE-mee-ah **Definition** excessive phosphate in the blood	**hyper / phosphat / emia** excessive / phosphate / blood condition
hypoglycemia HAI-poh-glai-SEE-mee-ah **Definition** low blood sugar	**hypo / glyc / emia** under / sugar / blood condition 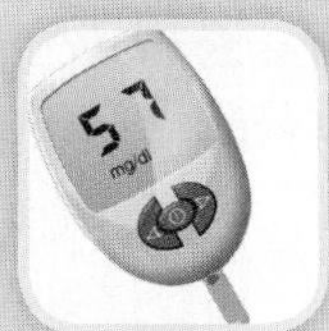
ketonuria KEE-toh-NYOO-ree-ah **Definition** ketone bodies in the urine	**keton / uria** ketone / urine condition
polyuria PAW-lee-YOO-ree-ah **Definition** excessive urination	**poly / uria** excessive / urine condition
uremia yoo-REE-mee-ah **Definition** presence of urinary waste in the blood	**ur / emia** urine / blood condition

hormones

Term	Word Analysis
adrenaline ad-REN-ah-lin **Definition** hormone secreted by the adrenal gland	**ad / renal / ine** on / kidney / chemical
epinephrine EH-pee-NEF-rin **Definition** hormone secreted by the adrenal gland	**epi / nephr / ine** upon / kidney / chemical

NOTE: Both *adrenaline* and *epinephrine* mean the same thing and can be used interchangeably. *Adrenaline comes* from Latin and *epinephrine* from Greek. In America, health care professionals prefer *epinephrine*.

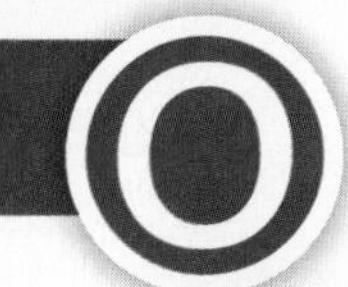

7.3 Observation and Discovery

hormones *continued*

Term	Word Analysis
adrenocorticotropic hormone (ACTH) ah-DREH-noh-KOR-tih-koh-TROH-pik HOR-mohn **Definition** hormone secreted by the pituitary gland that stimulates the cortex of the adrenal gland	**adreno / cortico / trop / ic** adrenal / cortex / stimulating / pertaining to
corticotropin KOR-tih-koh-TROH-pin **Definition** shorter name for adrenocorticotropic hormone	**cortico / tropin** cortex / stimulating
glucagon GLOO-kah-gawn **Definition** hormone secreted by the pancreas that stimulates the liver to increase blood sugar levels	**gluc / agon** sugar / lead
glucocorticoid GLOO-koh-KOR-tih-koyd **Definition** hormone produced by the adrenal cortex with a role in carbohydrate metabolism	**gluco / cortic / oid** sugar / cortex / resembling
gonadotropin goh-NAD-oh-TROH-pin **Definition** hormone that stimulates the gonads	**gonado / tropin** gonad / stimulating
insulin IN-suh-lin **Definition** hormone secreted by the pancreas that controls the metabolism and uptake of sugar and fats **NOTE:** The root used to name this hormone comes from the fact that insulin is secreted by a cluster or *island* of cells in the pancreas called the *islet of Langerhans*.	**insul / in** island / chemical
thyrotropin THAI-roh-TROH-pin **Definition** hormone that stimulates the thyroid	**thyro / tropin** thyroid / stimulating

results

Term	Word Analysis
adenomegaly ah-DEN-oh-MEH-gah-lee **Definition** abnormal enlargement of a gland	**adeno / megaly** gland / enlargement
adrenomegaly ad-REN-oh-MEH-gah-lee **Definition** abnormal enlargement of the adrenal gland	**adreno / megaly** adrenal / enlargement
euthyroid YOO-thai-royd **Definition** normal functioning thyroid	**eu / thyroid** good / thyroid
gluconeogenesis GLOO-koh-NEE-oh-JIN-eh-sis **Definition** formation of glucose from noncarbohydrate sources	**gluco / neo / genesis** sugar / new / formation

results *continued*

Term	Word Analysis
glycolysis glai-KAW-lih-sis **Definition** breakdown of sugar **NOTE:** This is done in cells in order to release energy.	**glyco / lysis** sugar / loosen
glycopenia GLAI-koh-PEE-nee-ah **Definition** deficiency of sugar	**glyco / penia** sugar / deficiency
gonadogenesis goh-NAD-oh-JIN-eh-sis **Definition** creation/development of gonads	**gonado / genesis** gonad / formation
metabolism meh-TAB-oh-LIZM **Definition** breakdown of matter into energy **NOTE:** The root *bol* is the source of the English word *ball*.	**meta / bol / ism** over / throw / condition

professional terms, diagnostic procedures

Term	Word Analysis
endocrine EN-doh-krin **Definition** to secrete internally (i.e., into the bloodstream)	**endo / crine** inside / secretion
endocrinologist EN-doh-krih-NAW-loh-jist **Definition** specialist in internal secretions	**endo / crino / logist** inside / secretion / specialist
exocrine EKS-oh-krin **Definition** to secrete externally (through ducts to the surface of an organ, i.e., sweat glands and salivary glands)	**exo / crine** outside / secretion
glycemic index glai-SEE-mik IN-deks **Definition** ranking of food based on the way it affects sugar levels in the blood	**glyc / em / ic** sugar / blood / pertaining to

Glycemic Index (GI) and Glycemic Load (GL) for Common Foods

Food	GI	Serving Size (g)	Carbs per Serving (g)	GL
Cornflakes	92	1 cup (28 g)	23	21.1
Grape-Nuts	75	1/2 cup (58 g)	42	31.5
Muesli	66	2/3 cup (55 g)	36	23.8
Bran muffin	59	1 med (113 g)	51	30
Soy milk	44	1 cup (245 g)	9	4
Lentils	29	1 cup (198 g)	24	7

7.3 Observation and Discovery

professional terms, diagnostic procedures *continued*

Term	Word Analysis
ketogenesis KEE-toh-JIN-eh-sis **Definition** creation of ketone bodies	**keto / genesis** ketone / creation
thyroid function tests THAI-roid FUNK-shun TESTS **Definition** tests performed to evaluate the function of the thyroid	**thyroid function tests**

radiology

Term	Word Analysis
cholangiopancreatography KOHL-AN-jee-oh-PAN-kree-ah-TAW-grah-fee **Definition** procedure used to examine the bile ducts and pancreas	**chol / angio / pancreato / graphy** bile / vessel / pancreas / writing procedure
endoscopic retrograde cholangiopancreatography EN-doh-SKAW-pik REH-troh-GRAYD KOHL-AN-jee-oh-PAN-kree-ah-TAW-grah-fee **Definition** procedure used to examine the bile ducts and pancreas in which an endoscope is passed backward from the digestive tract into the bile duct	**endo / scop / ic retro / grade** inside / looking / pertaining to backward / step **chol / angio / pancreato / graphy** bile / vessel / pancreas / writing procedure 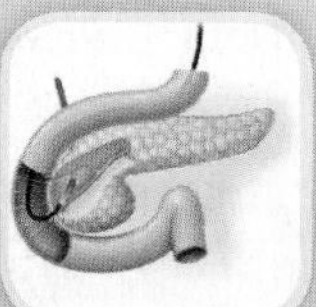

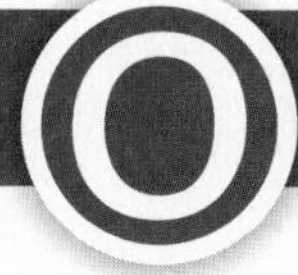

Learning Outcome 7.3 Exercises

PRONUNCIATION

EXERCISE 1 *Indicate which syllable is emphasized when pronounced.*

EXAMPLE: bronchitis bron**chi**tis

1. uremia ______
2. chloremia ______
3. hypernatremia ______
4. insulin ______
5. adrenaline ______
6. endocrine ______
7. exocrine ______
8. glycolysis ______
9. euthyroid ______

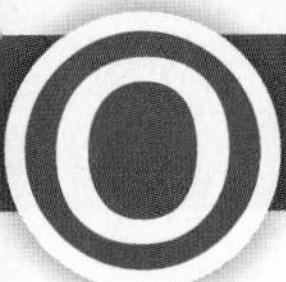

Learning Outcome 7.3 Exercises

TRANSLATION

EXERCISE 2 *Break down the following words into their component parts.*

EXAMPLE: nasopharyngoscope *naso | pharyngo | scope*

1. euthyroid ______
2. adrenomegaly ______
3. gonadogenesis ______
4. gluconeogenesis ______
5. endocrinologist ______
6. hyperlipidemia ______
7. hypercholesterolemia ______
8. adrenocorticotropic hormone ______

EXERCISE 3 *Underline and define the word parts from this chapter in the following terms.*

1. glucagon ______
2. glycolysis ______
3. glycopenia ______
4. ketogenesis ______
5. adenomegaly ______
6. endocrine ______
7. exocrine ______
8. adrenaline ______
9. glycemic index ______
10. hyperkalemia ______
11. glucocorticoid (2 roots) ______
12. gonadotropin (2 roots) ______
13. ketonuria (2 roots) ______
14. corticotropin (2 roots) ______
15. thyrotropin (2 roots) ______

EXERCISE 4 *Match the term on the left with its definition on the right.*

______	1. hypoglycemia	a.	abnormal acidity of the blood
______	2. acidemia	b.	abnormal alkalinity (opposite of acidity) of the blood
______	3. chloremia	c.	calcium in the urine
______	4. polyuria	d.	excessive urination
______	5. euglycemia	e.	good blood sugar
______	6. alkalemia	f.	increased chloride in the blood
______	7. calciuria	g.	ketone bodies in the urine
______	8. ketonuria	h.	low blood sugar
______	9. uremia	i.	presence of urinary waste in the blood
______	10. glucosuria	j.	sugar in the urine

EXERCISE 5 *Fill in the blanks.*

1. hypercholesterolemia = excessive ______ in the blood
2. hypercalcemia = excessive ______ in the blood
3. hyperlipidemia = excessive ______ in the blood
4. hyperglycemia = excessive ______ in the blood

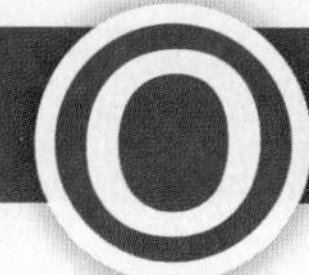

Learning Outcome 7.3 Exercises

5. hyperkalemia = excessive ______________ in the blood
6. hyperphosphatemia = excessive ______________ in the blood
7. hypernatremia = excessive ______________ in the blood

EXERCISE 6 *Translate the following terms as literally as possible.*

EXAMPLE: nasopharyngoscope *an instrument for looking at the nose and throat*

1. euthyroid ______________
2. calciuria ______________
3. glycolysis ______________
4. glycopenia ______________
5. glucocorticoid ______________
6. glucagon ______________
7. endocrinologist ______________
8. hyperlipidemia ______________
9. gluconeogenesis ______________
10. hypernatremia ______________

GENERATION

EXERCISE 7 *Build a medical term from the information provided.*

EXAMPLE: inflammation of the sinuses *sinusitis*

1. sugar in the urine (use *glucos/o*) ______________
2. high blood sugar ______________
3. low blood sugar ______________
4. good blood sugar ______________
5. ketone bodies in the urine ______________
6. presence of urinary waste in the blood ______________
7. a hormone that stimulates the gonads ______________
8. a hormone that stimulates the thyroid ______________
9. abnormal enlargement of a gland ______________
10. abnormal enlargement of the adrenal gland ______________

Learning Outcome 7.3 Exercises

EXERCISE 8 *Multiple-choice questions. Select the correct answer(s).*

1. Select all of the terms below that pertain to blood conditions.
   a. chloremia
   b. glucosuria
   c. hypomagnesemia
   d. hypernatremia
   e. hyperphosphatemia
   f. polyuria
   g. uremia
2. Select all of the terms below that pertain to urine conditions.
   a. chloremia
   b. glucosuria
   c. hypomagnesemia
   d. hypernatremia
   e. hyperphosphatemia
   f. polyuria
   g. uremia
3. The breakdown of matter into energy is called:
   a. adrenaline
   b. epinephrine
   c. glycolysis
   d. metabolism
   e. none of these
4. The *glycemic index* ranks foods based on:
   a. the way they affect sugar levels in the blood
   b. the way they affect sugar levels in the urine
   c. the way the body forms sugar from them
   d. the way the body metabolizes sugar
   e. none of these
5. Select all of the terms below that refer to a hormone secreted by the pituitary gland, which stimulates the cortex of the adrenal gland.
   a. ACTH
   b. adrenaline
   c. adrenocorticotropic hormone
   d. corticotropin
   e. epinephrine
6. Select all of the terms below that refer to a hormone secreted by the adrenal gland.
   a. ACTH
   b. adrenaline
   c. adrenocorticotropic hormone
   d. corticotropin
   e. epinephrine
   f. glucagon
   g. insulin
7. Select all of the terms below that refer to hormones secreted by the pancreas.
   a. ACTH
   b. adrenaline
   c. adrenocorticotropic hormone
   d. corticotropin
   e. epinephrine
   f. glucagon
   g. insulin

EXERCISE 9 *Briefly describe the difference between each pair of terms.*

1. acidemia, alkalemia ______
2. hypercalcemia, calciuria ______
3. adenomegaly, adrenomegaly ______
4. endocrine, exocrine ______
5. gonadogenesis, ketogenesis ______
6. insulin, glucagon ______

ASSESSMENT

7.4 Diagnosis and Pathology

The main types of disorders of the endocrine system result from an organ making either too much of a hormone or not enough of it. When a gland is producing too much hormone, it is labeled with the prefix *hyper-*. An overactive thyroid gland, for example, causes *hyperthyroidism.* A gland that doesn't make enough hormone is labeled with the prefix *hypo-*. When a patient's thyroid gland does not make enough thyroid hormone, the patient develops *hypothyroidism.*

Another way of saying a gland doesn't make enough hormone is to call it *insufficient.* When the cortex of the adrenal gland doesn't make enough cortisol, the condition is called *adrenocortical insufficiency.*

The pancreas is a bit different than many of the other glands in this regard. It produces competing hormones that work against each other: *glucagon* and *insulin.* While problems can occur with either hormone, underproduction of insulin is the most common disorder. This condition leads to *diabetes.*

Many times, overproduction of a hormone is caused by a tumor in the gland that causes it to secrete too much hormone. When a tumor on a gland is benign, it is called an *adenoma;* when a tumor is malignant, it is called an *adenocarcinoma.*

Another cause for the change in the function of a gland is *inflammation.* A patient with *thyroiditis* may initially have high levels of thyroid hormone in his or her blood, followed by hypothyroidism. This initial thyroid hormone is not from overproduction, however. Instead, it originates from the release of already-made hormones. This condition is called *thyrotoxicosis.*

Bleeding into a gland, which causes cells in the gland to die, can also lead to common gland problems. This happens in the case of *pituitary infarctions.* Bleeding into the pituitary decreases the number of gland cells available to make the hormones, thus causing it to function abnormally.

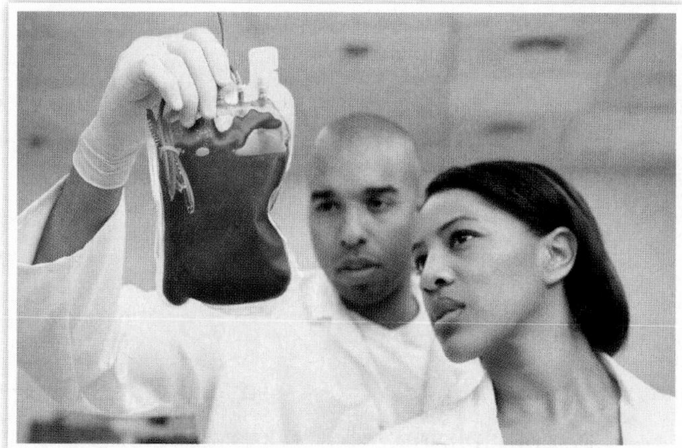

Analyzing blood and urine provides key information about the functioning of the endocrine system.

general terms

Term	Word Analysis
adenitis AD-en-AI-tis **Definition** inflammation of a gland	**aden / itis** gland / inflammation
adenopathy AD-eh-NOP-ah-thee **Definition** gland disease	**adeno / pathy** gland / disease
adenosis AD-en-OH-sis **Definition** gland condition	**aden / osis** gland / condition
dysmetabolic syndrome DIS-meh-tah-BAW-lik SIN-drohm **Definition** combination of medical disorders associated with faulty metabolism	**dys / metabolic syn / drome** bad / metabolism together / running

7.4 Diagnosis and Pathology

general terms *continued*

Term	Word Analysis
ketosis kee-TOH-sis	**ket / osis** ketone body / condition
Definition condition characterized by elevated levels of ketone bodies in the blood	
polyadenopathy PAW-lee-AD-eh-NOP-ah-thee	**poly / adeno / pathy** many / gland / disease
Definition disease involving many glands	

adrenal

Term	Word Analysis
adrenal insufficiency ad-REE-nal IN-suh-FIH-shun-see	**adrenal in / sufficiency** adrenal not / adequate
Definition condition in which the adrenal glands underproduce necessary hormones	
adrenalitis ad-REE-nah-LAI-tis	**adrenal / itis** adrenal / inflammation
Definition inflammation of the adrenal gland	
adrenocortical insufficiency ad-REE-noh-KOR-tih-kal IN-suh-FIH-shun-see	**adreno / cortic / al in / sufficiency** adrenal / cortex / pertaining to not / adequate
Definition condition in which the adrenal cortex underproduces necessary hormones	
adrenocorticohyperplasia ad-REE-noh-KOR-tih-koh-HAI-per-PLAY-zhah	**adreno / cortico / hyper / plasia** adrenal / cortex / over / formation
Definition overdevelopment of the cortex of the adrenal gland	
congenital adrenal hyperplasia kon-JEN-ih-tal ad-REE-nal HAI-per-PLAY-zhah	**con / genit / al adrenal** with / birth / pertaining to adrenal **hyper / plasia** over / formation
Definition genetic disease in which the adrenal gland is overdeveloped, resulting in a deficiency of certain hormones and an overproduction of others	

pancreas

Term	Word Analysis
diabetes mellitus DAI-ah-BEE-teez MEH-lih-tis	**diabetes mellitus** pass through honey
Definition metabolic disease characterized by excessive urination and hyperglycemia **NOTE:** *Diabetes* is an ancient Greek word that refers to any condition that causes excessive urination. *Mellitus* (which means "honey") was added to describe a specific kind of diabetes characterized by excessive sugar in the urine.	
diabetic ketoacidosis DAI-ah-BEH-tik KEE-toh-ASS-ih-DOH-sis	**diabet / ic keto / acid / osis** diabetes / pertaining to ketone / acid / condition
Definition acidity of the blood caused by the presence of ketone bodies produced when the body is unable to burn sugar; thus, it must burn fat for energy	

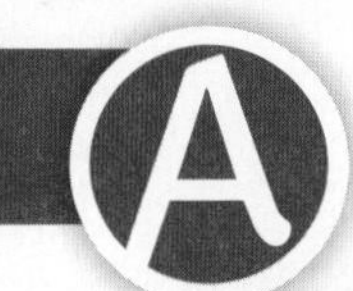

7.4 Diagnosis and Pathology

pancreas *continued*

Term	Word Analysis
pancreatic pseudocyst PAN-kree-at-ik SOO-doh-sist **Definition** abnormally expanded area in the pancreas resembling a cyst	**pancreat / ic** — pancreas / pertaining to **pseudo / cyst** — false / cyst
pancreatitis PAN-kree-ah-TAI-tis **Definition** inflammation of the pancreas	**pancreat / itis** pancreas / inflammation 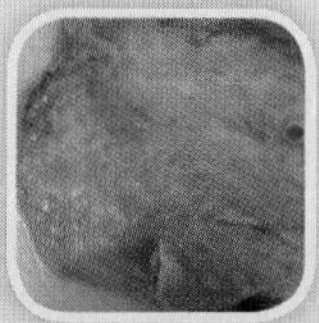 ©McGraw-Hill Education
pancreatolith PAN-kree-AT-oh-lith **Definition** stone in the pancreas	**pancreato / lith** pancreas / stone
pancreatolithiasis PAN-kree-at-oh-lih-THAI-ah-sis **Definition** presence of a stone in the pancreas	**pancreato / lith / iasis** pancreas / stone / presence

pituitary

Term	Word Analysis
hyperpituitarism HAI-per-pih-TOO-ih-tar-IZM **Definition** overfunctioning of the pituitary gland	**hyper / pituitar / ism** over / pituitary / condition 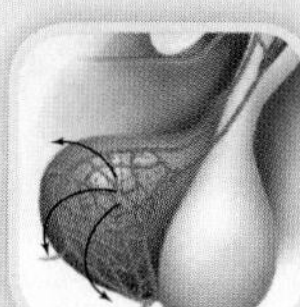
hypophysitis hai-PAWF-ih-SAI-tis **Definition** inflammation of the pituitary gland	**hypophys / itis** pituitary / inflammation
hypopituitarism HAI-poh-pih-TOO-ih-tar-IZM **Definition** condition caused by the undersecretion of the pituitary gland	**hypo / pituitar / ism** under / pituitary / condition
panhypopituitarism PAN-HAI-poh-pih-TOO-ih-tar-IZM **Definition** defective or absent function of the entire pituitary gland	**pan / hypo / pituitar / ism** all / under / pituitary / condition
pituitary infarction pih-TOO-ih-TEH-ree in-FARK-shun **Definition** death of the pituitary gland	**pituitary in / farc / tion** pituitary in / stuff / condition

NOTE: The term *infarction* normally refers to a blocked blood vessel, but it can also refer to the death of tissue resulting from the blockage. In fact, it can refer to the death of any tissue—as is the case here—whether or not a blockage is involved.

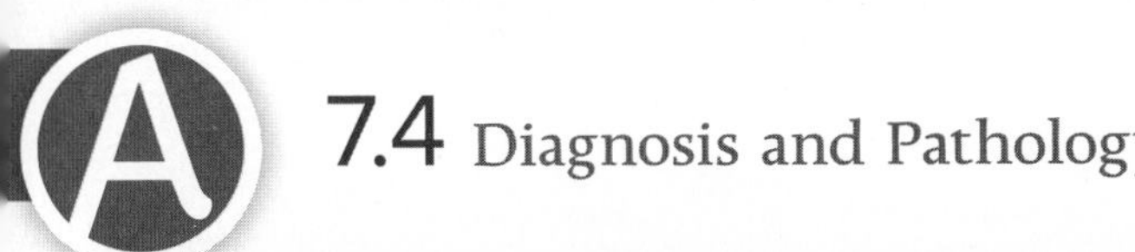

7.4 Diagnosis and Pathology

thyroid

Term	Word Analysis
hyperparathyroidism HAI-per-PAR-ah-THAI-roid-IZM **Definition** overproduction by the parathyroid glands	**hyper / para / thyroid / ism** over / beside / thyroid / condition
hyperthyroidism HAI-per-THAI-roid-IZM **Definition** overproduction by the thyroid	**hyper / thyroid / ism** over / thyroid / condition
hypoparathyroidism HAI-poh-PAR-ah-THAI-roid-IZM **Definition** underproduction by the parathyroid	**hypo / para / thyroid / ism** under / beside / thyroid / condition
hypothyroidism HAI-poh-THAI-roid-IZM **Definition** underproduction by the thyroid	**hypo / thyroid / ism** under / thyroid / condition
thyroiditis THAI-roid-AI-tis **Definition** inflammation of the thyroid	**thyroid / itis** thyroid / inflammation
thyrotoxicosis THAI-roh-TOKS-ih-KOH-sis **Definition** condition caused by the exposure of body tissue to excessive levels of thyroid hormone (an extreme version of this is known as "thyroid storm")	**thyro / toxic / osis** thyroid / poison / condition

oncology

Term	Word Analysis
adenocarcinoma ad-EN-oh-KAR-sih-NOH-mah **Definition** cancerous tumor of a gland	**adeno / carcin / oma** gland / cancer / tumor ©McGraw-Hill Education
adenoma AD-eh-NOH-mah **Definition** glandular tumor	**aden / oma** gland / tumor

oncology *continued*

Term	Word Analysis
adrenal adenoma ad-REE-nal AD-eh-NOH-mah **Definition** tumor of the adrenal gland	**adrenal aden / oma** adrenal gland / tumor
adrenocortical carcinoma ad-REE-noh-KOR-tih-kal KAR-sih-NOH-mah **Definition** cancerous tumor originating in the cortex of the adrenal gland	**adreno / cortic / al carcin / oma** adrenal / cortex / pertaining to cancer / tumor ©McGraw-Hill Education
insulinoma IN-suh-lih-NOH-mah **Definition** tumor that secretes insulin (found in the insulin-producing cells in the pancreas)	**insulin / oma** insulin / tumor
parathyroidoma PAR-ah-THAI-roid-OH-mah **Definition** tumor of the parathyroid	**para / thyroid / oma** beside / thyroid / tumor
pituitary adenoma pih-TOO-ih-TEH-ree AD-eh-NOH-mah **Definition** tumor on the pituitary gland	**pituitary aden / oma** pituitary gland / tumor
thymoma thai-MOH-mah **Definition** tumor of the thymus	**thym / oma** thymus / tumor ©SPL/Science Source

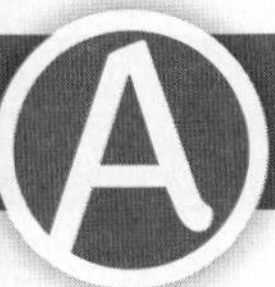

Learning Outcome 7.4 Exercises

PRONUNCIATION

EXERCISE 1 *Indicate which syllable is emphasized when pronounced.*

EXAMPLE: bronchitis bron**chi**tis

1. adenoma ________
2. pituitary adenoma ________
3. diabetes mellitus ________
4. insulinoma ________
5. adenopathy ________
6. polyadenopathy ________
7. thyrotoxicosis ________
8. diabetic ketoacidosis ________
9. pancreatolith ________
10. pancreatolithiasis ________
11. parathyroidoma ________
12. hyperthyroidism ________
13. hypothyroidism ________
14. hyperparathyroidism ________
15. hypoparathyroidism ________
16. adrenocorticohyperplasia ________

TRANSLATION

EXERCISE 2 *Break down the following words into their component parts.*

EXAMPLE: nasopharyngoscope *naso | pharyngo | scope*

1. adenosis ________
2. adrenalitis ________
3. thyroiditis ________
4. pancreatitis ________
5. adenopathy ________
6. adenoma ________
7. insulinoma ________
8. adrenal adenoma ________
9. parathyroidoma ________
10. hypopituitarism ________
11. panhypopituitarism ________
12. pancreatolithiasis ________
13. hyperparathyroidism ________
14. hypoparathyroidism ________
15. adrenocortical carcinoma ________
16. adrenocorticohyperplasia ________

EXERCISE 3 *Underline and define the word parts from this chapter in the following terms.*

1. ketosis ________
2. thymoma ________
3. adenitis ________
4. pancreatolith ________
5. pancreatic pseudocyst ________
6. hyperpituitarism ________
7. hyperthyroidism ________
8. hypothyroidism ________
9. adrenal insufficiency ________
10. congenital adrenal hyperplasia ________
11. adenocarcinoma ________
12. polyadenopathy ________
13. hypophysitis ________
14. thyrotoxicosis ________
15. adrenocortical insufficiency (2 roots) ________
16. pituitary adenoma (2 roots) ________

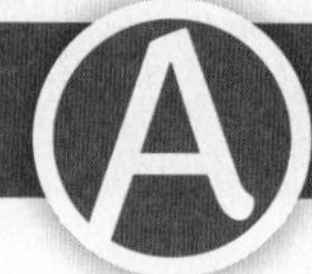

Learning Outcome 7.4 Exercises

EXERCISE 4 *Multiple-choice questions. Select the correct answer.*

1. *Dysmetabolic syndrome* is a combination of medical disorders associated with faulty:
   a. hormone production
   b. metabolism
   c. breakdown of matter into energy
   d. hormone production and metabolism
   e. metabolism and breakdown of matter into energy
2. *Diabetes mellitus* is a metabolic disease characterized by:
   a. excessive urination
   b. hyperglycemia
   c. high blood sugar
   d. polyuria
   e. all of these
3. The name for an acidity of the blood caused by the presence of ketone bodies produced when the body is unable to burn sugar, thus forcing the body to burn fat for energy is:
   a. acidemia
   b. diabetes mellitus
   c. diabetic ketoacidosis
   d. hyperlipidemia
   e. ketonuria
4. The death of the pituitary gland is called:
   a. pituitary adenoma
   b. pituitary infarction
   c. pituitary dwarfism
   d. pituitary gigantism
   e. none of these

EXERCISE 5 *Translate the following terms as literally as possible.*

EXAMPLE: nasopharyngoscope *an instrument for looking at the nose and throat*

1. adenopathy ______
2. polyadenopathy ______
3. adenosis ______
4. ketosis ______
5. pancreatolith ______
6. pancreatolithiasis ______
7. hyperthyroidism ______
8. hypothyroidism ______
9. hyperpituitarism ______
10. hypopituitarism ______
11. panhypopituitarism ______
12. hyperparathyroidism ______
13. hypoparathyroidism ______
14. pancreatic pseudocyst ______
15. thyrotoxicosis ______

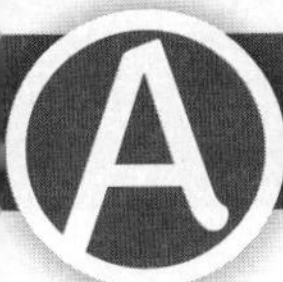

Learning Outcome 7.4 Exercises

GENERATION

EXERCISE 6 *Build a medical term from the information provided.*

EXAMPLE: inflammation of the sinuses *sinusitis*

1. inflammation of the pituitary gland (use *hypophyso*) ______________________
2. inflammation of the thyroid ______________________
3. inflammation of the pancreas ______________________
4. inflammation of the adrenal gland ______________________
5. inflammation of a gland ______________________
6. a tumor of the thymus ______________________
7. a tumor of the adrenal gland (2 words) ______________________
8. a tumor of the parathyroid ______________________
9. a tumor on the pituitary gland (2 words) ______________________
10. a cancerous tumor of a gland ______________________
11. a glandular tumor ______________________
12. a tumor that secretes insulin ______________________

EXERCISE 7 *Match the term on the left with its definition on the right.*

______	1. dysmetabolic syndrome	a.	cancerous tumor originating in the cortex of the adrenal gland
______	2. diabetes mellitus	b.	combination of medical disorders associated with faulty metabolism
______	3. pituitary infarction	c.	condition in which the adrenal cortex underproduces necessary hormones
______	4. adrenocortical insufficiency	d.	condition in which the adrenal glands underproduce necessary hormones
______	5. adrenal insufficiency	e.	genetic disease in which the adrenal gland is overdeveloped
______	6. adrenocortical carcinoma	f.	metabolic disease characterized by excessive urination and hyperglycemia
______	7. congenital adrenal hyperplasia	g.	acidity of the blood caused by the presence of ketone bodies produced when the body is unable to burn sugar, thus it must burn fat for energy
______	8. adrenocorticohyperplasia	h.	death of the pituitary gland
______	9. diabetic ketoacidosis	i.	overdevelopment of the cortex of the adrenal gland

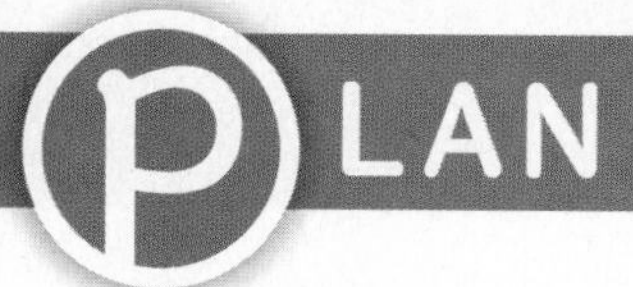

7.5 Treatments and Therapies

Most treatments of endocrine problems involve correcting abnormal hormone levels. If the level of a particular hormone, such as insulin, is too low, the proper treatment involves giving the patient supplemental hormones to bring the levels to normal (*hormone replacement therapy*). There are many routes for delivering the supplemental hormones, including injection, oral, and topical. An even more advanced method is continuous subcutaneous insulin infusion, which is an insulin pump that injects insulin under the skin as needed.

When the hormone level disorder is caused by a tumor or an overactive organ, more aggressive measures may be needed. This can involve taking a medicine that destroys all or part of the problematic gland or undergoing surgery to partially or completely remove the gland (i.e., *adenectomy*).

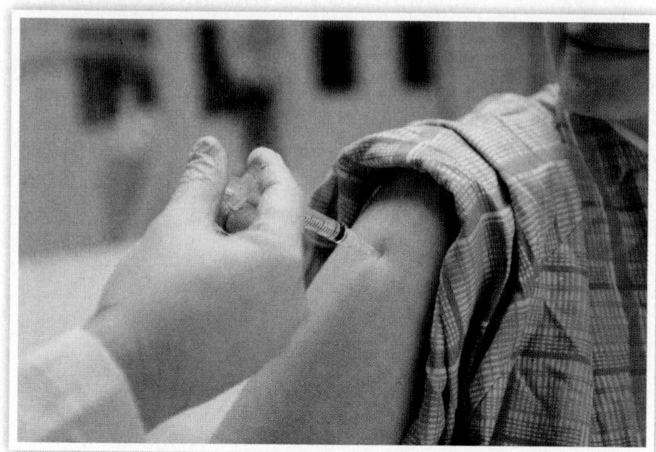

Once an endocrine imbalance has been diagnosed, sometimes the treatment is as easy as supplying the needed hormone.

©M.Constantini/PhotoAlto RF

pharmacology

Term	Word Analysis
continuous subcutaneous insulin infusion kun-TIN-yoo-us SUB-koo-TAY-nee-us IN-suh-lin in-FYOO-zhun **Definition** continuous injection of insulin into the blood from a pump inserted under the skin	**continuous sub / cutaneous** continuous beneath / skin **insulin in / fus / ion** insulin in / pour / process ©Realistic Reflections RF
thyroidotoxin thai-ROID-oh-TOK-sin **Definition** substance poisonous to the thyroid gland	**thyroido / toxin** thyroid / poison

7.5 Treatments and Therapies

general terms

Term	Word Analysis
adenectomy AD-eh-NEK-toh-mee **Definition** removal of a gland	**aden / ectomy** gland / removal
ketogenic diet KEE-toh-JIN-ik DAI-et **Definition** diet that aids in the production of ketones in the body	**keto / genic diet** ketone body / creating
thymectomy thai-MEK-toh-mee **Definition** removal of the thymus	**thym / ectomy** thymus / removal

adrenal

Term	Word Analysis
adrenalectomy ad-REE-nal-EK-toh-mee **Definition** removal of the adrenal gland	**adrenal / ectomy** adrenal / removal
laparoscopic adrenalectomy LAP-ah-roh-SKAW-pik ad-REE-nal-EK-toh-mee **Definition** removal of an adrenal gland by means of a laparascope (instrument inserted into the abdomen for viewing)	**laparo / scop / ic** abdomen / looking / pertaining to **adrenal / ectomy** adrenal / removal

pancreas

Term	Word Analysis
pancreatectomy PAN-kree-ah-TEK-toh-mee **Definition** removal of the pancreas	**pancreat / ectomy** pancreas / removal
pancreatolithectomy PAN-kree-ah-toh-lih-THEK-toh-mee **Definition** removal of a stone in the pancreas	**pancreato / lith / ectomy** pancreas / stone / removal

7.5 Treatments and Therapies

pituitary

Term	Word Analysis
hypophysectomy hai-POF-is-EK-toh-mee **Definition** removal of the pituitary gland	**hypophys / ectomy** pituitary / removal

thyroid

Term	Word Analysis
parathyroidectomy PAR-ah-THAI-roid-EK-toh-mee **Definition** removal of the parathyroid	**para / thyroid / ectomy** beside / thyroid / removal
thyroidectomy THAI-roid-EK-toh-mee **Definition** removal of the thyroid	**thyroid / ectomy** thyroid / removal
thyroidotomy THAI-roid-AW-toh-mee **Definition** incision into the thyroid	**thyroido / tomy** thyroid / incision
thyroparathyroidectomy THAI-roh-PAR-ah-THAI-roid-EK-toh-me **Definition** removal of the thyroid and parathyroid glands	**thyro / para / thyroid / ectomy** thyroid / beside / thyroid / removal

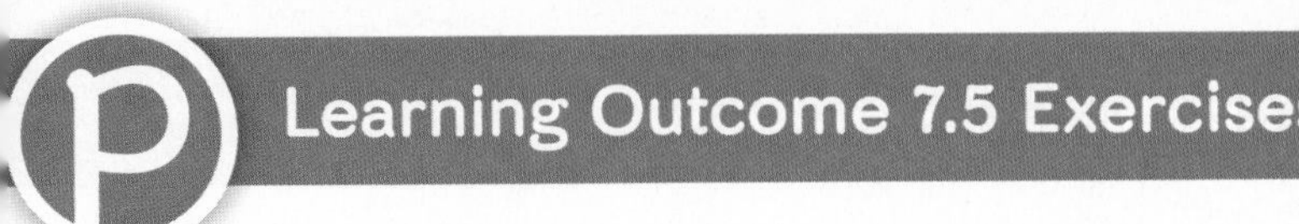

Learning Outcome 7.5 Exercises

PRONUNCIATION

EXERCISE 1 *Indicate which syllable is emphasized when pronounced.*

EXAMPLE: bronchitis bron**chi**tis

1. thyroidectomy ______
2. thyroidotomy ______
3. thyroidotoxin ______
4. adenectomy ______
5. thymectomy ______
6. adrenalectomy ______
7. laparoscopic adrenalectomy ______
8. pancreatectomy ______
9. pancreatolithectomy ______
10. parathyroidectomy ______

TRANSLATION

EXERCISE 2 *Break down the following words into their component parts.*

EXAMPLE: nasopharyngoscope *naso | pharyngo | scope*

1. thymectomy ______
2. adenectomy ______
3. adrenalectomy ______
4. pancreatolithectomy ______
5. thyroidectomy ______
6. parathyroidectomy ______
7. thyroparathyroidectomy ______

EXERCISE 3 *Underline and define the word parts from this chapter in the following terms.*

1. adrenalectomy ______
2. thyroidotomy ______
3. ketogenic diet ______
4. thyroidotoxin ______
5. pancreatectomy ______
6. hypophysectomy ______
7. laparoscopic adrenalectomy ______

Learning Outcome 7.5 Exercises

EXERCISE 4 *Match the term on the left with its definition on the right.*

_____ 1. thymectomy

_____ 2. continuous subcutaneous insulin infusion

_____ 3. laparoscopic adrenalectomy

_____ 4. thyroparathyroidectomy

_____ 5. pancreatolithectomy

a. removal of a stone in the pancreas

b. removal of an adrenal gland by means of a laparascope (an instrument inserted into the abdomen for viewing)

c. removal of thymus

d. continuous injection of insulin into the blood from a pump inserted under the skin

e. removal of the thyroid and parathyroid glands

EXERCISE 5 *Translate the following terms as literally as possible.*

EXAMPLE: nasopharyngoscope *an instrument for looking at the nose and throat*

1. thyroidotomy _____
2. thyroidotoxin _____
3. ketogenic diet _____
4. pancreatolithectomy _____
5. laparoscopic adrenalectomy _____

GENERATION

EXERCISE 6 *Build a medical term from the information provided.*

EXAMPLE: inflammation of the sinuses *sinusitis*

1. removal of the pituitary gland (use *hypophys/o*) _____
2. removal of the pancreas _____
3. removal of the thymus _____
4. removal of the adrenal gland _____
5. removal of a gland _____
6. removal of the thyroid _____
7. removal of the parathyroid _____
8. removal of the thyroid and parathyroid glands _____

7.6 Abbreviations

Abbreviations provide a shorthand way of referring to things that either recur often or are too long to write out. When dealing with the endocrine system, these can refer to common tests (TFT), hormones (GH), diagnoses (DM), or treatments (CSII).

endocrine system abbreviations

Abbreviation	Definition
ACTH	adrenocorticotropic hormone
BS	blood sugar
CGM	continuous glucose monitor
DI	diabetes insipidus
DM	diabetes mellitus
ERCP	endoscopic retrograde cholangiopancreatography
FBS	fasting blood sugar
GDM	gestational diabetes mellitus
GH	growth hormone
GTT	glucose tolerance test
HgA1C	hemoglobin A1C test (used by diabetes patients to monitor blood sugar levels)
HRT	hormone replacement therapy
TFT	thyroid function test
TSH	thyroid-stimulating hormone (also known as thyrotropin)
T3	triiodothyronine (one of two primary hormones produced by the thyroid)
T4	thyroxine (one of two primary hormones produced by the thyroid)

Learning Outcome 7.6 Exercises

EXERCISE 1 *Define the following abbreviations.*

1. BS ______
2. FBS ______
3. TFT ______
4. DM ______
5. DI ______
6. IDDM ______
7. NIDDM ______
8. T4 ______
9. GH ______
10. GTT ______
11. CGM ______
12. HRT ______

13. ERCP ______________________
14. GDM ______________________

EXERCISE 2 *Give the abbreviations for the following definitions.*

1. blood sugar ______________________
2. thyroid function test ______________________
3. diabetes insipidus ______________________
4. diabetes mellitus ______________________
5. fasting blood sugar ______________________
6. growth hormone ______________________
7. glucose tolerance test ______________________
8. continuous glucose monitor ______________________
9. hormone replacement therapy ______________________
10. insulin-dependent diabetes mellitus ______________________
11. non-insulin-dependent diabetes mellitus ______________________
12. endoscopic retrograde cholangiopancreatography ______________________
13. thyroxin levels ______________________
14. thyroid-stimulating hormone ______________________

EXERCISE 3 *Multiple-choice questions. Select the correct answer(s).*

1. Select all the abbreviations below that pertain to diabetes.
   a. BS
   b. CGM
   c. DI
   d. DM
   e. FBS
   f. GH
   g. HRT
   h. IDDM
2. Select all the abbreviations below that pertain to hormones.
   a. BS
   b. CGM
   c. DI
   d. DM
   e. FBS
   f. GH
   g. HRT
   h. IDDM
3. Select all the abbreviations below that pertain to blood sugar.
   a. BS
   b. CGM
   c. DI
   d. DM
   e. FBS
   f. GH
   g. HRT
   h. IDDM
4. Which of the following types of diabetes is dependent on insulin?
   a. CSII
   b. ERCP
   c. IDDM
   d. NIDDM
5. GTT is a test that determines how a patient's body tolerates:
   a. calcium
   b. excess water
   c. fat
   d. sugar
6. A test to evaluate the function of the thyroid is a(n):
   a. CGM
   b. GTT
   c. HRT
   d. TFT

7.7 Electronic Health Records

Endocrinology Clinic Note

S Subjective

Mrs. Moon returned to the clinic today to discuss her blood tests. She first came to the office with a chief complaint of **amenorrhea**. She had also noticed a hump developing on the back of her neck, recent weight gain, and **hirsutism**.

O Objective

Temp: 98.6; HR: 70; RR: 16; BP: 150/94.

Gen: WDWN, NAD. AOx3.

HEENT: NCAT. PERRLA. White sclera. No conjunctival injection. Mucous membranes moist and pink. Normal dentition.

Neck: Supple. Enlarged fat pad over extensor surface of neck.

Resp: CTA without wheezes, rales, or rhonchi.

CV: RRR without murmurs, gallops, or rubs; radial pulses normal.

Abd: Soft, nontender, nondistended. No masses. Striae (*stretch marks*) over abdomen.

Neuro: CN II-XII grossly intact. No focal neurologic deficit.

Ext: Feet pink and warm. No cyanosis, clubbing, or edema.

Skin: Mild increase in hair growth over the lip and chin.

Tests revealed low **ACTH,** increased cortisol, **hyperlipidemia,** and **hyperglycemia.**

A Assessment

Mrs. Moon has **glucocorticoid** excess (specifically cortisol). The differential diagnosis at this point includes adrenal cortical nodular hyperplasia and an **adrenal adenoma**.

P Plan

We will schedule Mrs. Moon for abdominal CT to help clarify the diagnosis. I discussed the case with Dr. Glenz, who is in agreement.

–Mary Masterson, NP

Learning Outcome 7.7 Exercises

EXERCISE 1 *Match the term on the left with its definition on the right.*

______	1. hyperlipidemia	a.	hormone produced by the adrenal cortex with a role in carbohydrate metabolism
______	2. amenorrhea	b.	hormone secreted by the pituitary gland, which stimulates the cortex of the adrenal gland
______	3. hyperlipidemia	c.	tumor of the adrenal gland
______	4. glucocorticoid	d.	excessive fat in the blood
______	5. adrenal adenoma	e.	excessive growth of facial and body hair in women
______	6. hirsutism	f.	high blood sugar
______	7. ACTH	g.	lack of menstrual flow

EXERCISE 2 *Fill in the blanks.*

1. Using the data recorded at the patient's discharge physical examination, fill in the following blanks.
   a. The patient's temperature: ______________________________
   b. The patient's heart rate: ______________________________
   c. The patient's respiratory rate: ______________________________
   d. The patient's blood pressure: ______________________________
   e. HEENT (______________________________):
   NCAT ______________________________
   (pupils equal, round, and reactive to light and accommodation).
2. Her tests revealed low ACTH (give definition: ______________________________), increased cortisol, ______________________________ (excessive fat in the blood), and *hyperglycemia* (give definition: ______________________________).
3. The patient will be scheduled for an abdominal ______________________________ (computed axial tomography) to help clarify the diagnosis.

EXERCISE 3 *True or false questions. Indicate true answers with a T and false answers with an F.*

1. The patient's tests showed too much fat in the blood and high blood sugar. ________
2. One possible diagnosis is an adrenal tumor. ________
3. The patient has a mild increase in hair growth over the lip and chin, which could indicate she has hirsutism. ________

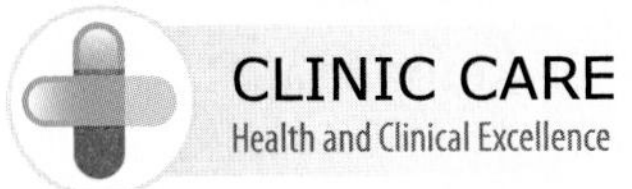

Patient Name: Olivia Sweet
Chief Complaint: Vomiting, lethargy.
History of Present Illness:

Miss Sweet is a 13-year-old female who presented to the ER with a several-hour history of vomiting. She awoke this morning with abdominal pain, which progressed to vomiting. She has not had any fever. She has not been able to keep any food or liquid down, and when she began to look tired, Miss Sweet's parents brought her to the Emergency Department.
Per Miss Sweet's parents, she has had a 2-month history of **polydipsia**, **polyuria**, and **polyphagia**. Despite a recent increase in appetite, they have noticed that she has lost weight.

Past Medical History: Normal. She has not had **menarche**.
Medications: None.
Allergies: NKDA.
Social History: Lives with her parents and two siblings. A/B student on the honor roll.
Surgical History: None.
Family History: Mother: Rheumatoid arthritis; maternal aunt: **Type 2 diabetes**.

Physical Exam:

Temperature: 98.6; Heart Rate: 100; Respiratory Rate: 32; BP: 84/60.
General: Thin. Lethargic.
Head: Normocephalic atraumatic, very dry mucous membranes. **Ketotic** breath (*sweet smelling breath associates with ketosis*). Pupils equal, round, and reactive to light. TMs normal.
Neck: Supple.
Cardiovascular: Mild tachycardia. No murmur, gallop, or rub.
Respiratory: Deep, rapid breathing. Clear to auscultation. No retractions.
Abdomen: Soft, nontender, nondistended. Spleen and liver edge not palpable.
Neurologic: DTRs: patellar and brachial present and equal.
Skin: Dry. Capillary refill > 3 seconds.
Extremities: No cyanosis, clubbing, or edema.

Emergency Department Course:

Miss Sweet arrived in the ED lethargic, but responsive. Given her history and vomiting, we were concerned about **diabetic ketoacidosis**. The patient's finger stick blood sugar test result of 320 confirmed **hyperglycemia**, and a urinalysis revealed both **glucosuria** and **ketonuria**. An IV was started and labs were sent. Chemistry profile showed **hypernatremia**, **hyperkalemia**, and **acidemia**. The pediatric intensive care team was contacted for transfer to the PICU.

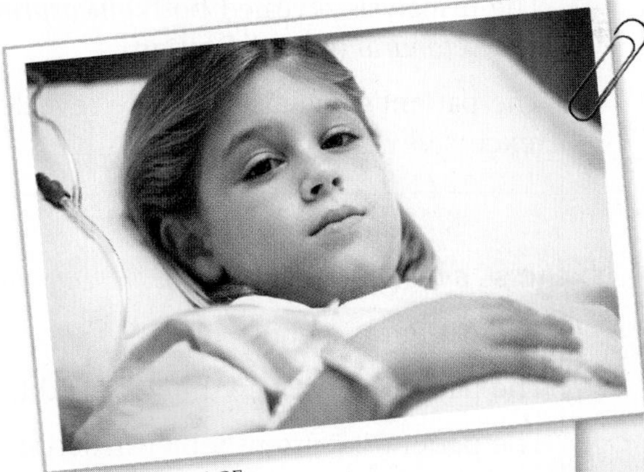
©Creatas/PunchStock RF

Disposition: Transfer to PICU.

—Ed Rhume, MD

Learning Outcome 7.7 Exercises

EXERCISE 4 *Match the term on the left with its definition on the right.*

______	1. hyperglycemia		a. abnormal acidity of the blood
______	2. ketonuria		b. acidity of the blood caused by the presence of ketone bodies produced when the body is unable to burn sugar; thus, it must burn fat for energy
______	3. acidemia		c. excessive eating
______	4. polyuria		d. excessive sodium in the blood
______	5. glucosuria		e. excessive thirst
______	6. menarche		f. excessive urination
______	7. diabetic ketoacidosis		g. high blood sugar
______	8. polydipsia		h. ketone bodies in the urine
______	9. polyphagia		i. sugar in the urine
______	10. hypernatremia		j. beginning or first menstruation

EXERCISE 5 *Fill in the blanks.*

1. Using the data recorded at the patient's discharge physical examination, fill in the following blanks.
   a. T: ______________________________
   b. HR: ______________________________
   c. RR: ______________________________
   d. BP: ______________________________
   e. The patient has a 2-month history of ______________ (excessive thirst), ______________ (excessive hunger), and ______________________ (excessive urination).
2. The urinalysis revealed both *glucosuria* (give definition: ______________________) and *ketonuria* (give definition: ______________________).
3. The patient's chemistry profile revealed *hypernatremia* (excessive sodium in the blood), *hypokalemia* (excessive ______________________ in the blood), and *acidemia* (abnormal acidity of the ______________________).

EXERCISE 6 *True or false questions. Indicate true answers with a T and false answers with an F.*

1. The patient is afebrile. ______
2. The patient is not very hungry or thirsty. ______
3. The patient is currently menstruating. ______
4. The patient has high blood sugar. ______
5. The patient has sugar and ketone bodies in her urine. ______

Learning Outcome 7.7 Exercises

EXERCISE 7 *Multiple-choice questions. Select the correct answer.*

1. *Hypernatremia* is a condition of the:
   a. adrenal gland
   b. blood
   c. thyroid
   d. urine
2. A person with excessive potassium in the blood has:
   a. acidemia
   b. glucosuria
   c. hyperkalemia
   d. hypernatremia
3. PICU stands for:
   a. pediatric intensive care unit
   b. postoperative intensive care unit
   c. preoperative intensive care unit
   d. none of these
4. When a person has faulty carbohydrate metabolism, the result is increased ketone bodies. The body gets rid of them through the lungs, giving sufferers fruity-smelling breath.
   a. Miss Sweet has ketotic breath.
   b. Miss Sweet is experiencing normal carbohydrate metabolism.
   c. Miss Sweet is suffering from faulty carbohydrate metabolism.
   d. Miss Sweet has ketotic breath and is experiencing normal carbohydrate metabolism.
   e. Miss Sweet has ketotic breath and is suffering from faulty carbohydrate metabolism.

Surgery Follow-Up Note

Subjective

Mr. Shield presented to our office today for follow up from his **thyroidectomy**. He initially presented to his primary care physician with concerns over a **goiter**. His PCP noticed mild **exophthalmos** and an enlarged thyroid with palpable nodules. He had **thyroid scintigraphy** and **TFTs** that both revealed active nodules. After discussion with Dr. Sharp during a consultation, Mr. Shield elected for surgical correction. Dr. Sharp performed a thyroidectomy 2 weeks ago. Mr. Shield had postoperative **hypocalcemia** but otherwise had an unremarkable hospital stay. Since discharge, Mr. Shield has done very well.

Objective

Temp: 98.6; HR 60; RR: 16; BP 102/62; Wt: 176.
General: No acute distress. Alert and oriented.
HEENT: PERRLA. No conjunctival injection. Mucous membranes moist and pink. TMs normal.
Neck: Postop incision site is clean, dry, and intact. No erythema, induration, or discharge. No goiter.
Resp: CTA. w/o wheezes, rales, or rhonchi.
CV: RRR without murmur.
Gen: Soft, nontender, nondistended.
Ext: No cyanosis or edema.
Labs: Mildly elevated **TSH** and low T4.
Calcium—normal.

Impression/Plan

Mr. Shield's thyroid labs are still not where I want them to be. We will increase his medicine to help get him **euthyroid**.
No lasting **hypoparathyroidism** from the surgery.
Return for follow-up visit including labs in 1 month.

—Sue Stenson, NP

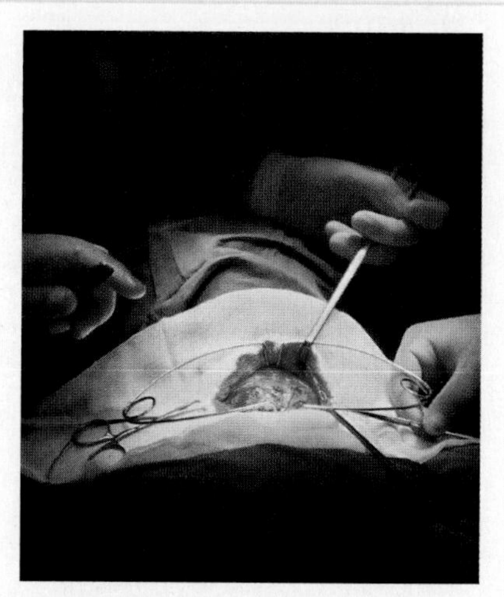

Learning Outcome 7.7 Exercises

EXERCISE 8 *Match the term on the left with its definition on the right.*

______	1. hypocalcemia	1. "good thyroid"
______	2. thyroidectomy	2. swollen thyroid gland
______	3. euthyroid	3. low calcium levels in the blood
______	4. exophthalmos	4. removal of the thyroid
______	5. hypoparathyroidism	5. protrusion of the eyes out of the eye socket
______	6. goiter	6. underproduction by the parathyroid

Learning Outcome 7.7 Exercises

EXERCISE 9 *Fill in the blanks.*

1. Mr. Shield is at the office today to follow up from his *thyroidectomy* (give definition: ____).

2. Using the data recorded at the patient's discharge physical examination, fill in the following blanks.
   a. The patient's temperature: ____________________
   b. The patient's heart rate: ____________________
   c. The patient's respiratory rate: ____________________
   d. The patient's blood pressure: ____________________
   e. HEENT (____________________): ____________________ (pupils equal, round, and reactive to light and accommodation).
   f. Resp: CTA (________________ to ________________).
   g. CV: ____________________ (regular rate and rhythm).

EXERCISE 10 *True or false questions. Indicate true answers with a T and false answers with an F.*

1. The patient recently had his thyroid removed. ________
2. He initially presented to his PCP with concerns over a swollen thyroid gland. ________
3. His thyroid function tests revealed active nodules. ________
4. After Mr. Shield's operation, he had normal blood sugar. ________
5. According to the patient's labs, he has low thyroxin levels. ________

EXERCISE 11 *Multiple-choice questions. Select the correct answer.*

1. The patient suffered from postoperative *hypocalcemia.* Which of the following is a correct breakdown of the term?
   a. *hypo* (over) + *calc* (calcium) + *-emia* (blood condition)
   b. *hypo* (over) + *calc* (calcium) + *-emia* (urine condition)
   c. *hypo* (under) + *calc* (calcium) + *-emia* (blood condition)
   d. *hypo* (under) + *calc* (calcium) + *-emia* (urine condition)

2. The patient has no lasting *hypoparathyroidism.* Which of the following is a correct breakdown of the term?
   a. *hypo* (over) + *para* (in addition to) + *thyroid* (the thyroid gland) + *-ism* (condition)
   b. *hypo* (over) + *parathyroid* (the parathyroid gland) + *-ism* (condition)
   c. *hypo* (under) + *parathyroid* (the parathyroid gland) + *-ism* (condition)
   d. *hypo* (under) + *para* (in addition to) + *thyroid* (the thyroid gland) + *-ism* (condition)

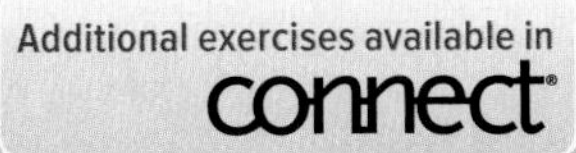

Chapter Review exercises, along with additional practice items, are available in Connect!

Quick Reference

quick reference glossary of roots

Root	Definition	Root	Definition
aden/o	gland	**hypophys/o**	pituitary gland
adren/o, adrenal/o	adrenal gland	**ket/o**	ketone body
cortic/o	outer surface	**pancreat/o**	pancreas
crin/o	secrete	**pituitar/o**	pituitary gland
-emia	blood condition	**thym/o**	thymus
gluc/o, glucos/o, glyc/o	sugar	**thyr/o, thyroid/o**	thyroid
gonad/o	gonads (sex organs)	**-tropin**	stimulating hormone
hormon/o	hormone	**-uria**	urine condition

quick reference glossary of terms

Term	Definition
acidemia	abnormal acidity of the blood
acromegaly	abnormal enlargement of the extremities
adenalgia	pain in a gland
adenectomy	removal of a gland
adenitis	inflammation of a gland
adenocarcinoma	cancerous tumor of a gland
adenoma	glandular tumor
adenomegaly	abnormal enlargement of a gland
adenopathy	gland disease
adenosis	gland condition
adrenal adenoma	tumor of the adrenal gland
adrenal insufficiency	condition in which the adrenal glands underproduce necessary hormones
adrenal virilism	development of male secondary sexual characteristics caused by excessive secretion of the adrenal gland
adrenalectomy	removal of the adrenal gland
adrenaline	hormone secreted by the adrenal gland (from Latin; see also *epinephrine*)
adrenalitis	inflammation of the adrenal gland
adrenarche	beginning of adrenal secretion (at puberty)
adrenocortical carcinoma	cancerous tumor originating in the cortex of the adrenal gland
adrenocortical insufficiency	condition in which the adrenal cortex underproduces necessary hormones
adrenocorticohyperplasia	overdevelopment of the cortex of the adrenal gland

quick reference glossary of terms *continued*

Term	Definition
adrenocorticotropic hormone (ACTH)	hormone secreted by the pituitary gland, which stimulates the cortex of the adrenal gland
adrenomegaly	abnormal enlargement of the adrenal gland
alkalemia	abnormal alkalinity (opposite of acidity) of the blood
amenorrhea	lack of menstrual flow
calciuria	calcium in the urine
chloremia	increased chloride in the blood
cholangiopancreatography	procedure used to examine the bile ducts and pancreas
congenital adrenal hyperplasia	genetic disease in which the adrenal gland is overdeveloped, resulting in a deficiency of certain hormones and an overproduction of others
continuous subcutaneous insulin infusion	continuous injection of insulin into the blood from a pump inserted under the skin
corticotropin	shorter name for adrenocorticotropic hormone
diabetes mellitus	metabolic disease characterized by excessive urination and hyperglycemia
diabetic ketoacidosis	acidity of the blood caused by the presence of ketone bodies produced when the body is unable to burn sugar; thus, it must burn fat for energy
dysmetabolic syndrome	combination of medical disorders associated with faulty metabolism
endocrine	secrete internally (i.e., into the bloodstream)
endocrinologist	specialist in internal secretions
endoscopic retrograde cholangiopancreatography	procedure used to examine the bile ducts and pancreas in which an endoscope is passed backward from the digestive tract into the bile duct
epinephrine	hormone secreted by the adrenal gland (from Greek; see also *adrenaline*)
euglycemia	good blood sugar
euthyroid	a normal functioning thyroid
exocrine	secrete externally through ducts to the surface of an organ (i.e., sweat glands and salivary glands)
exophthalmos	protrusion of the eyes out of the eye sockets
galactorrhea	discharge of milk
glucagon	hormone secreted by the pancreas that stimulates the liver to increase blood sugar levels
glucocorticoid	a hormone produced by the adrenal cortex with a role in carbohydrate metabolism
gluconeogenesis	the formation of glucose from noncarbohydrate sources
glucosuria	sugar in the urine
glycemic index	ranking of food based on the way it affects sugar levels in the blood
glycolysis	breakdown of sugar
glycopenia	deficiency of sugar

quick reference glossary of terms *continued*

Term	Definition
goiter	swollen thyroid gland
gonadogenesis	creation/development of gonads
gonadotropin	hormone that stimulates the gonads
gynecomastia	development of breast tissue in males
hirsutism	excessive growth of facial and body hair in women
hypercalcemia	excessive calcium in the blood
hypercholesterolemia	excessive cholesterol in the blood
hyperglycemia	high blood sugar
hypergonadism	excessive secretion of the sex glands
hyperkalemia	excessive potassium in the blood
hyperlipidemia	excessive fat in the blood
hyperparathyroidism	overproduction by the parathyroid glands
hyperpituitarism	overfunctioning of the pituitary gland
hyperthyroidism	overproduction by the thyroid
hypoglycemia	low blood sugar
hypoglycemic	pertaining to low blood sugar
hypogonadism	undersecretion of the sex glands
hypomagnesemia	deficient magnesium in the blood
hypernatremia	excessive salt in the blood
hypoparathyroidism	underproduction by the parathyroid
hyperphosphatemia	excessive phosphate in the blood
hypophysectomy	removal of the pituitary gland
hypophysitis	inflammation of the pituitary gland
hypopituitarism	condition caused by the undersecretion of the pituitary gland
hypothyroidism	underproduction by the thyroid
insulin	hormone secreted by the pancreas that controls the metabolism and uptake of sugar and fats
insulinoma	tumor that secretes insulin (found in the insulin-producing cells in the pancreas)
ketogenesis	creation of ketone bodies
ketogenic diet	diet that aids in the production of ketones in the body
ketonuria	ketone bodies in the urine
ketosis	condition characterized by elevated levels of ketone bodies in the blood
laparoscopic adrenalectomy	removal of an adrenal gland by means of a laparoscope (an instrument inserted into the abdomen for viewing)

quick reference glossary of terms *continued*

Term	Definition
menarche	beginning or first menstruation
metabolism	breakdown of matter into energy
pancreatalgia	pain in the pancreas
pancreatectomy	removal of the pancreas
pancreatic pseudocyst	abnormally expanded area in the pancreas resembling a cyst
pancreatitis	inflammation of the pancreas
pancreatolith	stone in the pancreas
pancreatolithectomy	removal of a stone in the pancreas
pancreatolithiasis	presence of a stone in the pancreas
panhypopituitarism	defective or absent function of the entire pituitary gland
parathyroid	removal of the parathyroid
parathyroidoma	tumor of the parathyroid
pituitary adenoma	tumor on the pituitary gland
pituitary dwarfism	abnormally short height caused by undersecretions of growth hormone from the pituitary gland
pituitary gigantism	abnormally tall height caused by oversecretion of growth hormone from the pituitary gland
pituitary infarction	death of the pituitary gland
polyadenopathy	disease involving many glands
polydipsia	excessive thirst
polyphagia	excessive eating
polyuria	excessive urination
thelarche	beginning of breast development
thymectomy	removal of the thymus
thymoma	tumor of the thymus
thyrocele	*see* goiter
thyroid function tests	tests performed to evaluate the function of the thyroid
thyroidectomy	removal of the thyroid
thyroiditis	inflammation of the thyroid
thyroidotomy	incision into the thyroid
thyroidotoxin	substance poisonous to the thyroid gland
thyromegaly	enlargement of the thyroid
thyroparathyroidectomy	removal of the thyroid and parathyroid glands
thyroptosis	downward displacement (drooping) of the thyroid

quick reference glossary of terms *continued*

Term	Definition
thyrotoxicosis	condition caused by the exposure of body tissue to excessive levels of thyroid hormone
thyrotropin	hormone that stimulates the thyroid
uremia	presence of urinary waste in the blood

review of terms by roots

Root	Term(s)	
aden/o	adenalgia adenectomy adenitis adenocarcinoma adenoma adenomegaly	adenopathy adenosis adrenal adenoma pituitary adenoma polyadenopathy
adren/o	adrenal adenoma adrenal insufficiency adrenal virilism adrenalectomy adrenaline adrenalitis adrenarche	adrenocortical carcinoma adrenocortical insufficiency adrenocorticohyperplasia adrenocorticotropic hormone (ACTH) adrenomegaly congenital adrenal hyperplasia laparoscopic adrenalectomy
cortic/o	adrenocortical carcinoma adrenocortical insufficiency	adrenocorticohyperplasia adrenocorticotropic hormone (ACTH) corticotropin glucocorticoid
crin/o	endocrine endocrinologist	exocrine
-emia	acidemia alkalemia chloremia euglycemia hypercalcemia hypercholesterolemia hyperglycemia hyperkalemia	hyperlipidemia hypernatremia hyperphosphatemia hypoglycemia hypoglycemic hypomagnesemia uremia
gluc/o	glucagon	
glucos/o	glucocorticoid glucogenesis glucosuria	
glyc/o	euglycemia glycemic index glycolysis glycopenia	hyperglycemia hypoglycemia hypoglycemic
gonad/o	gonadogenesis gonadotropin	hypergonadism hypogonadism
hormon/o	adrenocorticotropic hormone (ACTH)	

review of terms by roots *continued*

Root	Term(s)	
hypophys/o	hypophysectomy hypophysitis	
ket/o	diabetic ketoacidosis ketogenesis ketogenic diet	ketonuria ketosis
pancreat/o	cholangiopancreatography endoscopic retrograde pancreatalgia pancreatectomy pancreatic pseudocyst	pancreatitis pancreatolith pancreatolithectomy pancreatolithiasis
pituitar/o	hyperpituitarism hypopituitarism panhypopituitarism pituitary adenoma	pituitary dwarfism pituitary gigantism pituitary infarction
thym/o	thymectomy thymoma	
thyr/o	euthyroid	
thyroid/o	hyperparathyroidism hyperthyroidism hypoparathyroidism hypothyroidism parathyroidectomy parathyroidoma thyrocele thyroid function tests thyroidectomy	thyroiditis thyroidotomy thyroidotoxin thyromegaly thyroparathyroidectomy thyroptosis thyrotoxicosis thyrotropin
-tropin	adrenocorticotropic hormone (ACTH) corticotropin gonadotropin	thyrotropin
-uria	calciuria glucosuria ketonuria	polyuria uremia

other terms

acromegaly	gynecomastia
amenorrhea	hirsutism
continuous subcutaneous insulin infusion	insulin
diabetes mellitus	insulinoma
dysmetabolic syndrome	menarche
epinephrine	metabolism
exophthalmos	polydipsia
galactorrhea	polyphagia
goiter	thelarche

The Blood and Lymphatic Systems–Hematology and Immunology

8

Introduction and Overview of Hematology and Immunology

People who live together in a community, like an apartment complex or neighborhood, all need certain services. A community needs energy, such as electricity, to provide power for all its lights and appliances. A community needs ways to communicate, like phones or mail service. A community needs recycling and garbage removal systems. Finally, a community needs protection, such as the services rendered by police officers and firefighters.

In many ways, the body is a collection of many communities. The blood and lymphatic systems provide many of these valuable services and resources to the body's communities. These services are absolutely critical to life. If blood flow stops even for a few minutes, hazardous waste will accumulate, and cells will starve. For example, the blood provides energy by delivering sugar and oxygen. The blood carries signals from other parts of the body, allowing for communication. The blood also takes away the waste made by the body's cells.

The lymphatic system provides constant protection by repairing injuries and fighting infections.

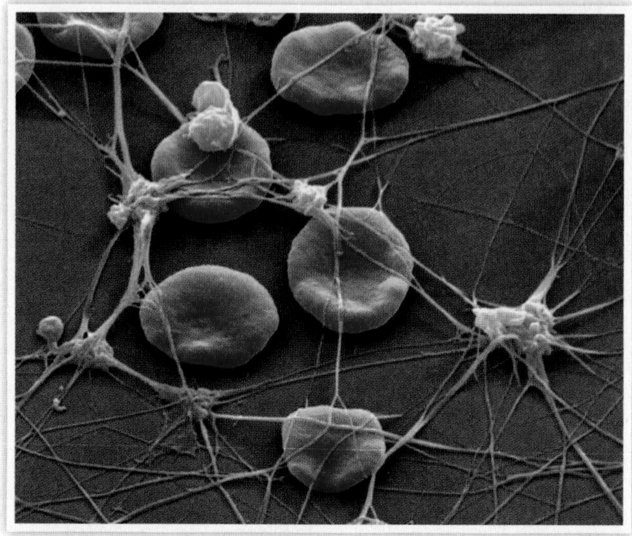

©Eye of Science/Science Source

learning outcomes

Upon completion of this chapter, you will be able to:

8.1 Identify the **roots/word parts** associated with the **hematological/immunological systems**.

(S) **8.2** Translate the **Subjective** terms associated with the **hematological/immunological systems**.

(O) **8.3** Translate the **Objective** terms associated with the **hematological/immunological systems**.

(A) **8.4** Translate the **Assessment** terms associated with the **hematological/immunological systems**.

(P) **8.5** Translate the **Plan** terms associated with the **hematological/immunological systems**.

8.6 Use **abbreviations** associated with the **hematological/immunological systems**.

8.7 Distinguish terms associated with the **hematological/immunological systems** in the context of **electronic health records**.

8.1 Word Parts Associated with the Hematological/Immunological Systems

Word Roots of the Hematological System

Blood has three main types of cells (*cytes*). Red blood cells (*erythrocytes*) are the transport trucks that bring oxygen to all the cells of the body and take away the waste. White blood cells (*leukocytes*) fight infection. Platelets (*thrombocytes*) are the small scab-makers of the body. They patch things up.

Red blood cells are the most common cells in the blood (*hemo/hemato*). They contain a substance called *hemoglobin*. Hemoglobin grabs on to oxygen when the surrounding oxygen levels are high and releases it when the ambient oxygen levels are low. In this way, it helps carry fresh oxygen from the lungs to all the parts of the body that need it.

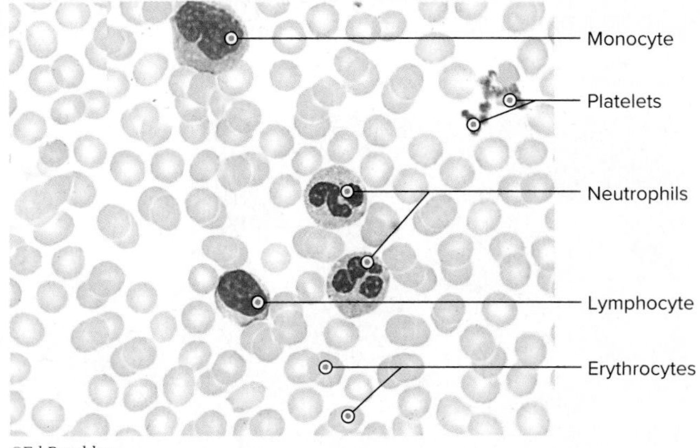

©Ed Reschke

White blood cells protect the body from invasion. The blood contains different types of white blood cells that fight different types of infections (*neutrophils, lymphocytes, basophils,* and *eosinophils*). Each carries out a different job.

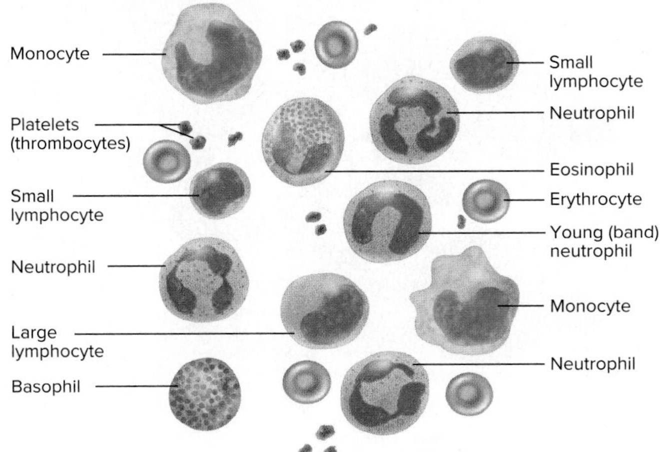

These white blood cells aren't the body's only defense, though. The body also makes special protective proteins as well. These proteins are called *immunoglobulins*. Just like the white blood cells, different types of immunoglobulins are designed for specific tasks. In fact, immunizations are means of forcing the body to make immunoglobulins against dangerous illnesses.

Platelets are the smallest of the cells in the blood. Their job is to patch up any broken blood vessels. Blood vessels constantly develop small leaks. They need a patch system to keep them functioning properly. When a vessel is injured, it attracts platelets that clump together to form a sticky patch. They also send signals that help further form a permanent clot.

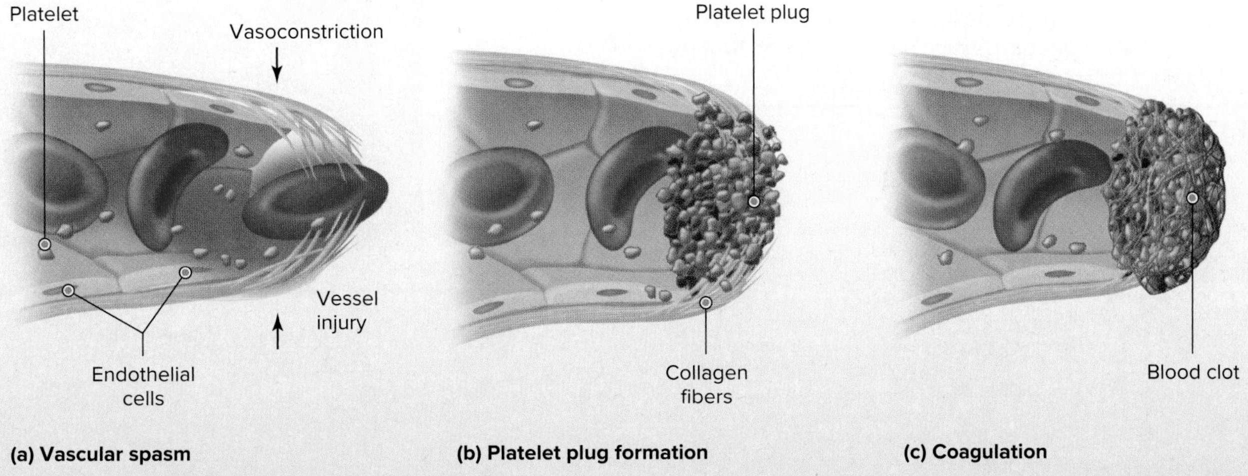

This shows the process of coagulation and the formation of a clot.

coagulation

ROOT: ***coagul/o***

EXAMPLES: anticoagulant, coagulopathy

NOTES: *Coagulo* refers to the blood's ability to form clots. It comes from a Latin word, *coagulum,* which comes from the world of cheese making. *Coagulum* is added to milk to make it curdle and begin the process of turning milk into cheese.

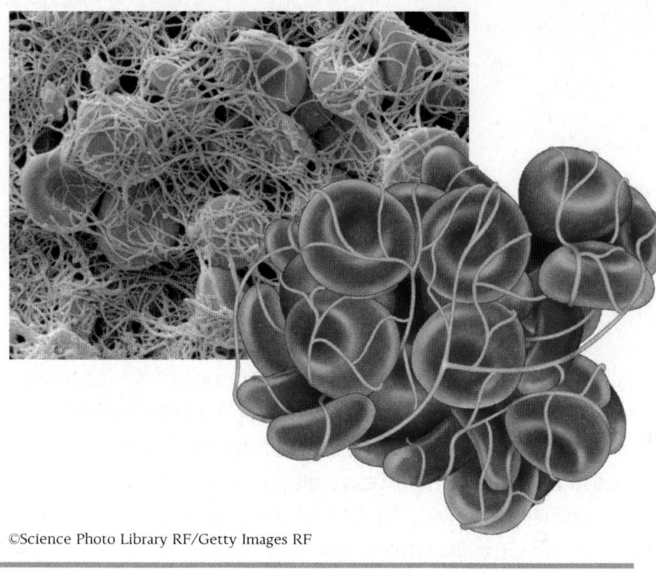

clot

ROOT: ***thromb/o***

EXAMPLES: thrombocyte, thrombosis

NOTES: The blood's ability to clot can be both life saving and life threatening. When the body is wounded, clotting enables the body to stop the bleeding and begin the healing process. *Hemophilia* is a disease in which the blood doesn't clot well, potentially causing minor cuts to become life-threatening injuries. Clots become life threatening when they form in the bloodstream in places where they aren't needed, which can block blood flow to vital organs.

blood

ROOTS: ***hem/o, hemat/o***

EXAMPLES: hemolysis, hematology

NOTES: The average-sized man has almost 6 quarts of blood in his body. The average-sized woman has almost 4 quarts.

cell

ROOT: ***cyt/o***

EXAMPLES: erythrocyte, thrombocytosis

NOTES: *Cyto* comes from a Greek word meaning "jar" or "basket." The word in Greek can also refer to the individual units of a beehive, which is probably where the connection with human cells comes from.

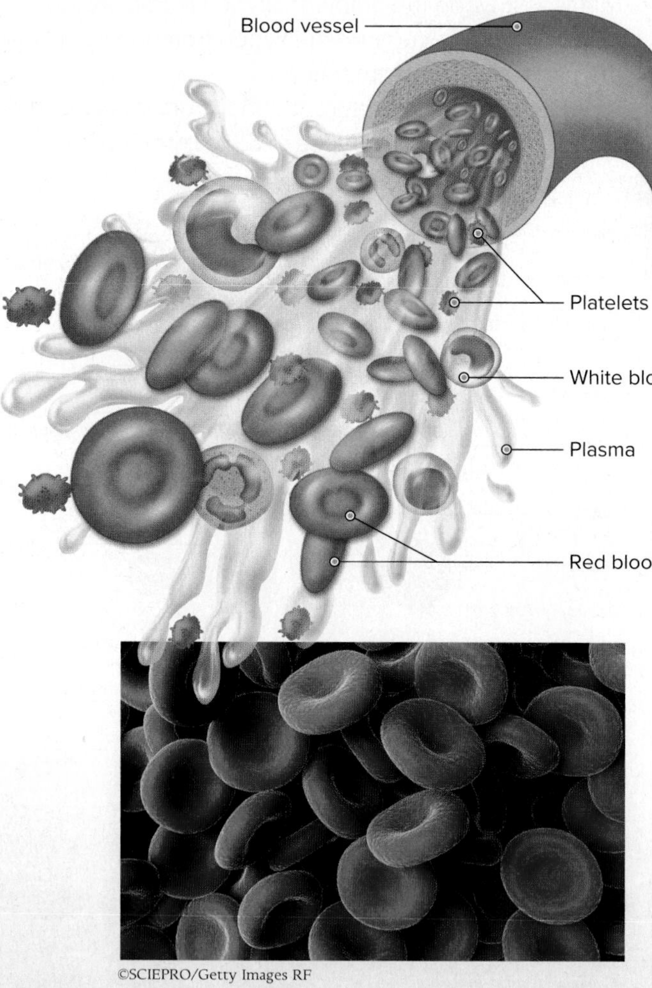

white

ROOT: ***leuk/o***

EXAMPLES: leukocytes, leukemia

NOTES: Leukocytes, which are white blood cells, act as the bloodstream's police force and garbage collectors. They are the primary responders to infection and tissue damage. They also remove debris from the bloodstream through a process called *phagocytosis* (remember: *phago* means "to eat") and begin the process of cell repair.

vein

ROOTS: ***phleb/o, ven/o***

EXAMPLES: phlebotomy, venospasm

NOTES: The term *phlebotomy* comes from *phlebo* (vein) and *tomy* (incision). It is the term used for drawing blood. But make sure you pronounce the word carefully: You don't want to get some blood drawn (*phlebotomy*) and end up having a portion of your brain removed (*lobotomy*).

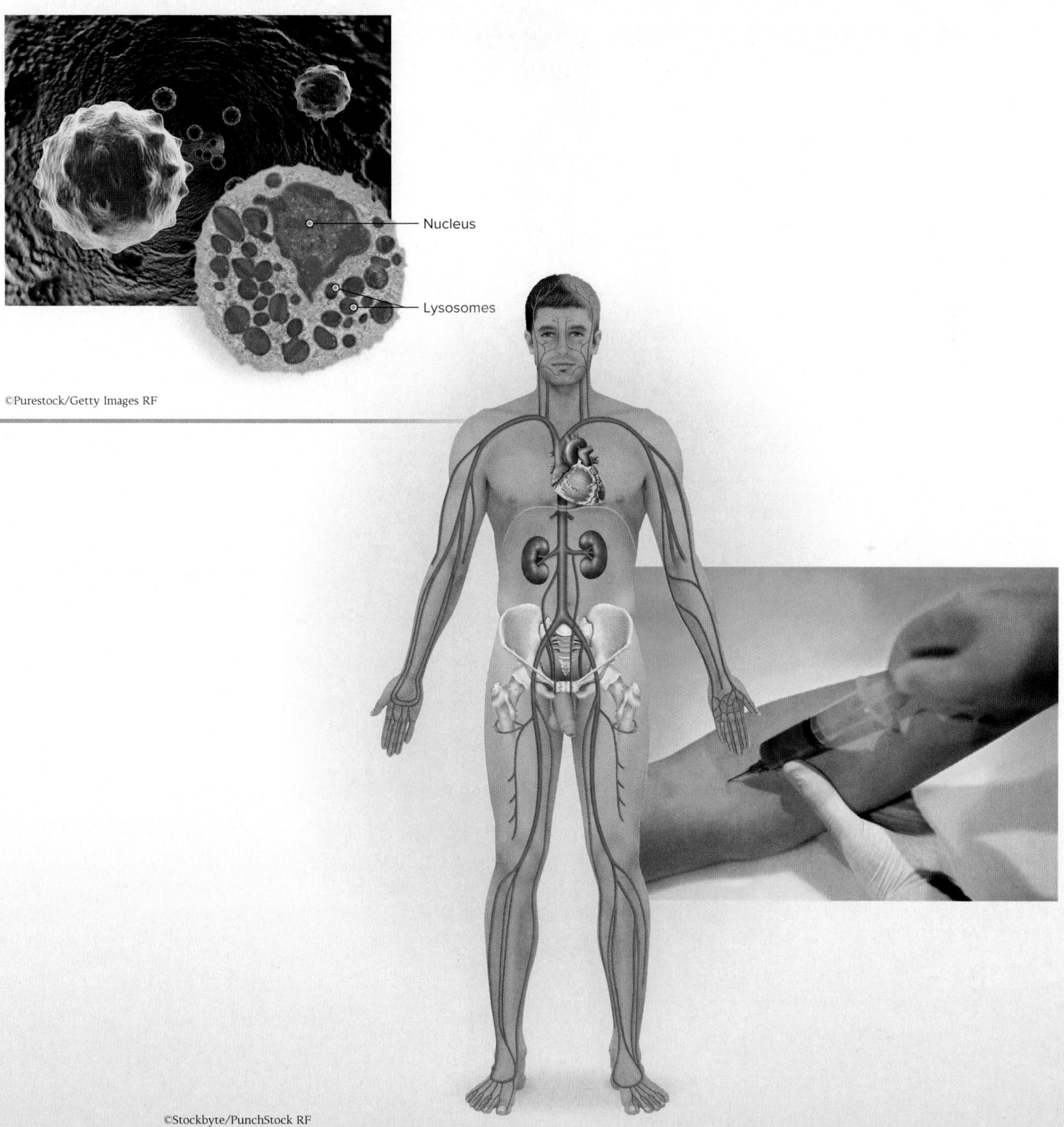

Word Roots of the Immunological System

LYMPHATIC SYSTEM

Runoff water from mountains collects into small tributaries that collect into larger streams, then into rivers, and eventually into the ocean.

The lymphatic system works in a similar way. Excess fluid from body tissues collects into lymph vessels that pour into larger vessels. This fluid then eventually pours back into the "ocean" of the body's blood supply. Along with lymphatic vessels, the lymph system includes lymph nodes, tonsils, a spleen, and a thymus.

Together, the lymphatic system plays a large role in the body's immune system. Lymph vessels carry immune proteins to all parts of the body. Lymph nodes and the spleen act as filters in the body, filtering out dangerous things like infectious agents and cancerous cells.

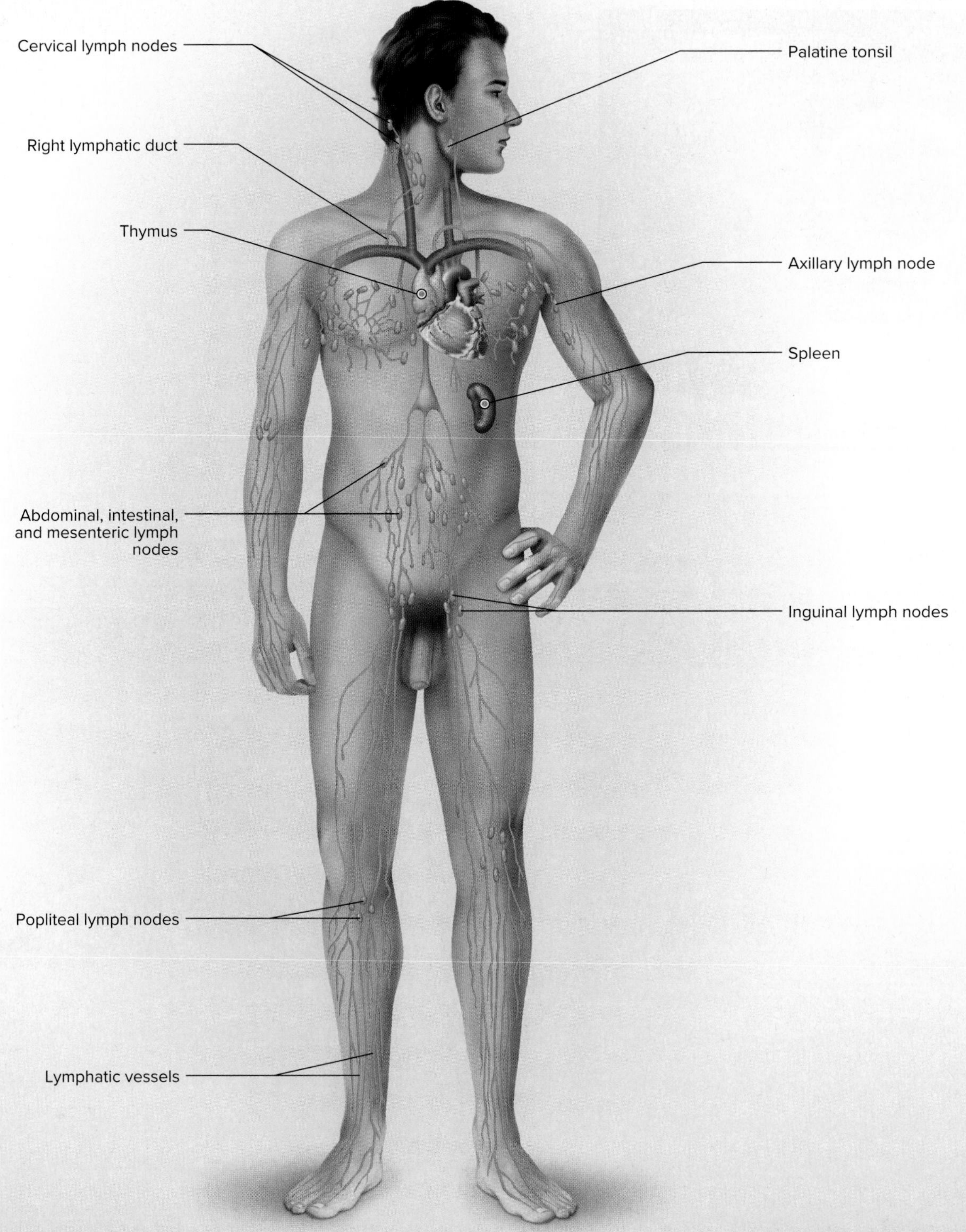

lymph

ROOT: ***lymph/o***

EXAMPLES: lymphadenitis, lymphoma

NOTES: *Lymph* comes from a Latin word meaning "water" or "spring" and refers to a clear liquid that circulates in the body, providing nutrients to cells and removing waste from them.

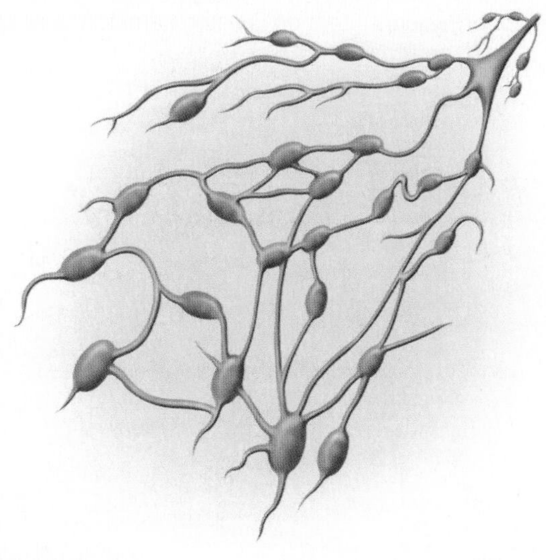

bone marrow, spine

ROOT: ***myel/o***

EXAMPLES: myelitis, myelodysplasia

NOTES: This root comes from a Greek word meaning "the innermost part" and is used in medicine to refer to two different things: bone marrow and the spinal cord. If you think about it, it makes sense: Both are in the innermost part of something else. Bone marrow is in the center of bones. The spinal cord is in the center of the spine.

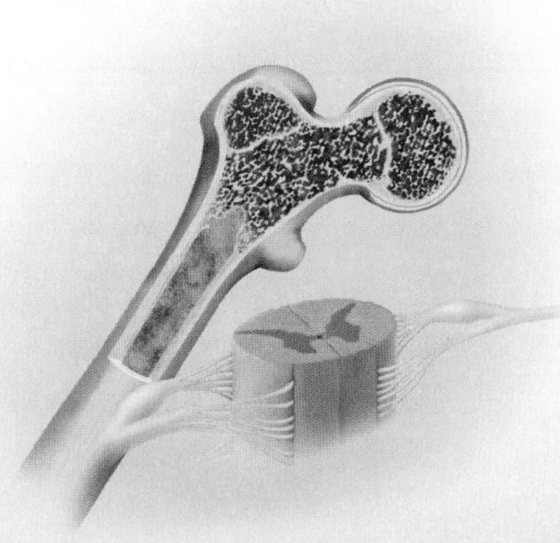

blood condition

SUFFIX: ***-emia***

EXAMPLES: anemia, leukemia

NOTES: *-emia* comes from a combination of *hemo,* meaning "blood," and *-ia,* meaning "condition." The *h* at the beginning of *hemo* got dropped because it is hard to pronounce when added to the end of a word. Think about it. Which is easier to say: *anemia* or *anhemia?*

On occasion, the *h* makes a comeback, in words like *polycythemia.* So watch out.

tonsils

ROOT: ***tonsill/o***

EXAMPLES: tonsillitis, tonsillectomy

NOTES: The *tonsils* are masses of lymphoid tissue located in the back of the mouth at the top of the throat. The word *tonsil* comes from the Latin word meaning "almond," no doubt because of its appearance. The fact that the root has two, and not one, letter *l* is not a spelling mistake. The English word tonsil has one *l*, but its root form has two. That's why the words *tonsillitis* and *tonsillectomy* have two.

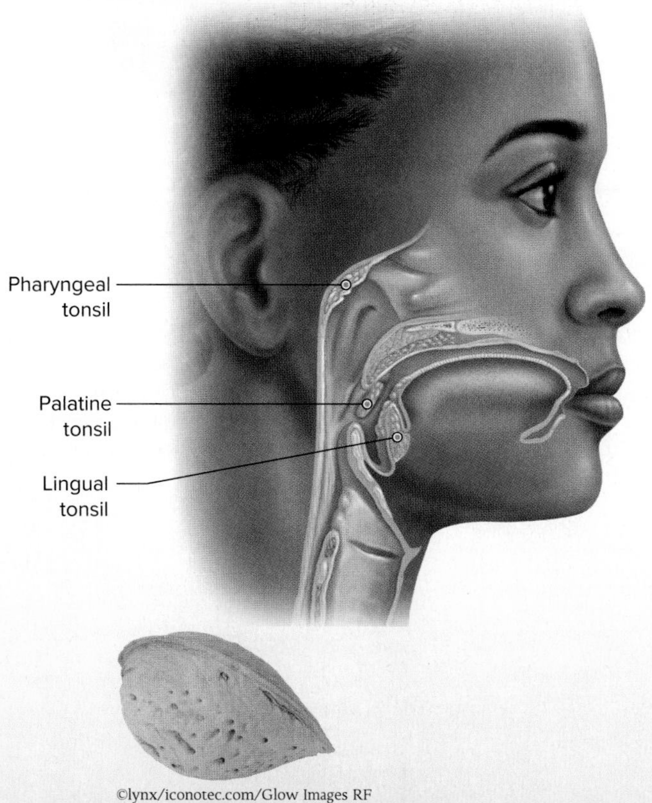

spleen

ROOT: ***splen/o***

EXAMPLES: splenomegaly, splenectomy

NOTES: The spleen is an organ in the upper-left portion of your abdomen. One of its jobs is to filter old red blood cells out of your blood. A human can live without a spleen with no adverse effects, which is good news for motocross and BMX bikers, who have a high rate of spleen injury and removal. Why? Because when they have accidents, their abdomens often crash into the handlebars of their bikes.

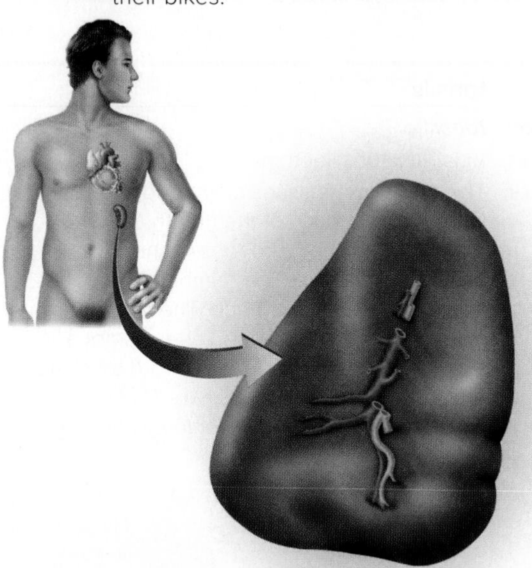

thymus

ROOT: ***thym/o***

EXAMPLES: thymoma, thymectomy

NOTES: The *thymus* is an organ found at the base of the neck. Its name is derived from the herb *thyme*. Evidently, the organ looked like a bunch of thyme to the folks who first discovered it.

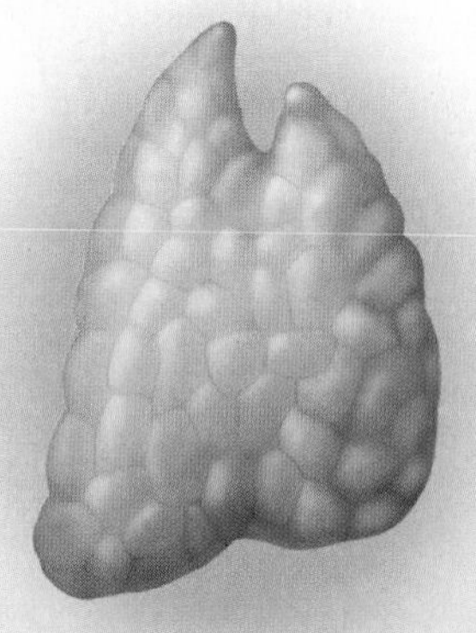

immune system

ROOT: ***immun/o***

EXAMPLES: immunology, immunoglobulin

NOTES: The immune system is the body's defensive system against foreign invaders. Most people don't realize that the skin is a layer of the immune system. It functions as a physical barrier between your vital organs and a world of organisms intent on causing harm to them.

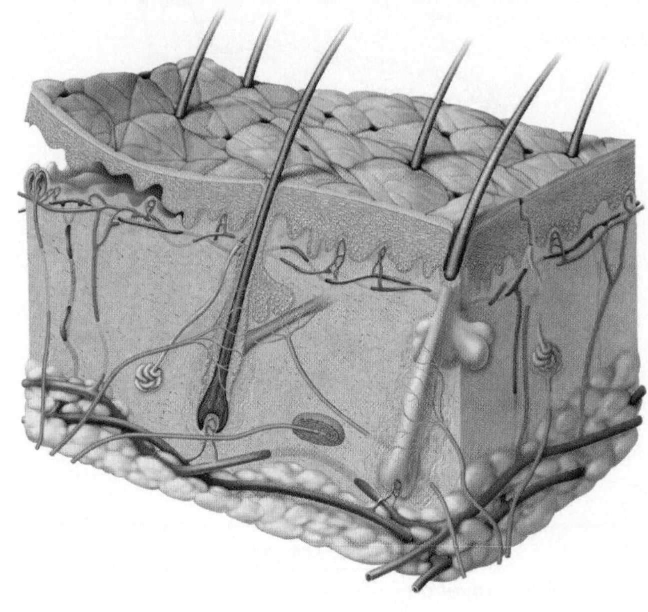

deficiency

SUFFIX: ***-penia***

EXAMPLE: cytopenia

NOTES: *-penia* comes from a Greek word meaning "poverty" or "famine." It is related to the English word *penury,* which means "poverty." But that's a word that doesn't get used much these days.

Learning Outcome 8.1 Exercises

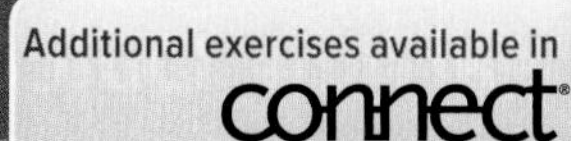

TRANSLATION

EXERCISE 1 *Match the root on the left with its definition on the right. Some definitions will be used more than once.*

_____	1. leuk/o	a. blood
_____	2. cyt/o	b. cell
_____	3. ven/o	c. clot
_____	4. hem/o	d. coagulation
_____	5. hemat/o	e. vein
_____	6. coagul/o	f. white
_____	7. thromb/o	
_____	8. phleb/o	

EXERCISE 2 *Translate the following roots.*

1. leuk/o ____________________
2. cyt/o ____________________
3. ven/o ____________________
4. hem/o ____________________
5. hemat/o ____________________
6. coagul/o ____________________
7. thromb/o ____________________
8. phleb/o ____________________

EXERCISE 3 *Underline and define the word parts from this chapter for the following terms.*

1. leukemia ____________________
2. hematopoiesis ____________________
3. hemoglobinopathy ____________________
4. thromboembolism ____________________
5. hypercoagulability ____________________
6. phlebarteriectasia ____________________
7. phagocytosis ____________________
8. thrombophlebitis (2 roots) ____________________

EXERCISE 4 *Break down the following words into their component parts and translate.*

EXAMPLE: sinusitis *sinus | itis* *inflammation of the sinuses*

1. anticoagulant ____________________
2. leukocyte ____________________
3. thrombocyte ____________________
4. phlebotomy ____________________
5. hematoma ____________________
6. hemolysis ____________________

Learning Outcome 8.1 Exercises

EXERCISE 5 *Match the word part on the left with its definition on the right.*

______	1. tonsill/o	a. blood condition
______	2. immun/o	b. bone marrow
______	3. lymph/o	c. deficiency
______	4. splen/o	d. immune system
______	5. thym/o	e. lymph
______	6. -emia	f. spleen
______	7. myel/o	g. thymus
______	8. -penia	h. tonsil

EXERCISE 6 *Translate the following word parts.*

1. tonsill/o ______________________
2. immun/o ______________________
3. lymph/o ______________________
4. splen/o ______________________
5. thym/o ______________________
6. myel/o ______________________
7. -emia ______________________
8. -penia ______________________

EXERCISE 7 *Underline and define the word parts from this chapter for the following terms.*

1. tonsillectomy ______________________
2. thymic hyperplasia ______________________
3. autoimmune disease ______________________
4. hypervolemia ______________________
5. myelodysplasia ______________________
6. lymphangiectasia ______________________
7. laparosplenectomy ______________________
8. pancytopenia (2 roots) ______________________

EXERCISE 8 *Break down the following words into their component parts and translate.*

EXAMPLE: sinusitis *sinus | itis* *inflammation of the sinuses*

1. tonsillectomy ______________________
2. thymectomy ______________________
3. immunologist ______________________
4. lymphedema ______________________
5. splenalgia ______________________
6. myeloma ______________________
7. lymphocyte ______________________
8. leukopenia ______________________
9. hypercholesterolemia ______________________

Learning Outcome 8.1 Exercises

GENERATION

EXERCISE 9 *Identify the word parts for the following terms.*

1. white ______________________
2. cell ______________________
3. coagulation ______________________
4. clot ______________________
5. blood (2 roots) ______________________
6. vein (2 roots) ______________________

EXERCISE 10 *Build a medical term from the information provided.*

1. normal-sized cell (use the prefix *normo-*) ______________________
2. the study of the blood ______________________
3. the study of veins ______________________
4. coagulation disease ______________________
5. white cell ______________________
6. clot cell ______________________

EXERCISE 11 *Multiple-choice questions. Select the correct answer.*

1. What are the names of the body's three different types of blood cells?
   a. leukocytes, red blood cells, white blood cells
   b. leukocytes, thrombocytes, white blood cells
   c. leukocytes, platelets, thrombocytes
   d. platelets, red blood cells, white blood cells
   e. platelets, red blood cells, thrombocytes
2. The function of a red blood cell is to:
   a. bring oxygen to cells and remove waste
   b. fight infection
   c. patch up broken blood vessels
   d. all of these
   e. none of these
3. The function of a white blood cell is to:
   a. bring oxygen to cells and remove waste
   b. fight infection
   c. patch up broken blood vessels
   d. all of these
   e. none of these
4. The function of a platelet is to:
   a. bring oxygen to cells and remove waste
   b. fight infection
   c. patch up broken blood vessels
   d. all of these
   e. none of these
5. A scab is formed by which type of blood cell?
   a. erythrocyte
   b. leukocyte
   c. platelet
   d. red blood cell
   e. white blood cell
6. Neutrophils, lymphocytes, basophils, and eosinophils are all types of:
   a. erythrocytes
   b. platelets
   c. red blood cells
   d. thrombocytes
   e. white blood cells
7. The type of blood cell that contains *hemoglobin* is a:
   a. leukocyte
   b. platelet
   c. red blood cell
   d. thrombocyte
   e. white blood cell

Learning Outcome 8.1 Exercises

8. Another name for *red blood cell* is:
   a. erythrocyte
   b. leukocyte
   c. platelet
   d. thrombocyte
   e. white blood cell
9. Another name for *white blood cell* is:
   a. erythrocyte
   b. leukocyte
   c. platelet
   d. red blood cell
   e. thrombocyte
10. Another name for *platelet* is:
    a. erythrocyte
    b. leukocyte
    c. red blood cell
    d. thrombocyte
    e. white blood cell
11. Which of the following substances assists a cell in grabbing oxygen where levels are high and then releasing it when the levels are low?
    a. hemoglobin
    b. immunoglobulin
    c. leukocyte
    d. thrombocyte
    e. none of these
12. Which of the following substances is a protein that assists white blood cells in fighting infection?
    a. hemoglobin
    b. immunoglobulin
    c. leukocyte
    d. thrombocyte
    e. none of these

EXERCISE 12 *Identify the word parts for the following terms.*

1. immune system ____________________
2. tonsil ____________________
3. lymph ____________________
4. thymus ____________________
5. spleen ____________________
6. bone marrow ____________________
7. blood condition ____________________
8. deficiency ____________________

EXERCISE 13 *Build a medical term from the information provided.*

1. study of the immune system ____________________
2. inflammation of the tonsil ____________________
3. inflammation of the spleen ____________________
4. disease of the thymus ____________________
5. bone marrow tumor ____________________
6. lymph cell ____________________
7. lymph deficiency ____________________
8. white blood condition ____________________

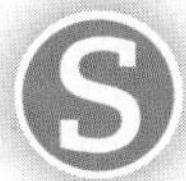

Subjective

Patient History, Problems, Complaints

Blood

Lymph

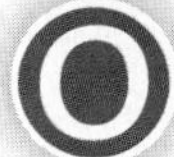

Objective

Observation and Discovery

Blood

Lymph

Professional terms

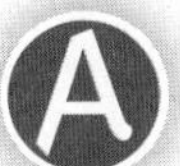

Assessment

Diagnosis and Pathology

Blood

Blood conditions

Lymph

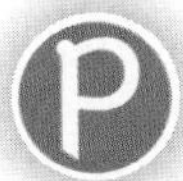

Plan

Treatments and Therapies

Drugs

Surgery

Transfusions

This section contains medical terms built from the roots presented in the previous section. The purpose of this section is to expose you to words used in hematology and immunology that are built from the word roots presented earlier. The focus of this book is to teach you the process of learning roots and translating them in context. Each term is presented with the correct pronunciation, followed by a word analysis that breaks down the word into its component parts, a definition that provides a literal translation of the word, as well as supplemental information if the literal translation deviates from its medical use.

The terms are organized using a health care professional's SOAP note (first introduced in Chapter 2) as a model.

SUBJECTIVE

8.2 Patient History, Problems, Complaints

Patients with blood disorders normally present with the same general symptoms. They usually seek medical care because they suffer from secondary effects of having a low amount of a specific blood cell type.

A patient with anemia may feel weak and run down, and may look paler than normal. If patients' *platelet* levels are too low, they may notice they bruise easily (*ecchymosis*) or that they develop small, flat, red spots on their body (*petechiae*). They may also complain that they tend to bleed (*hemorrhage*) more easily than most people. This can also result from *hemophilia*.

A patient who has a low white blood cell count is more vulnerable to infection; thus, he or she will suffer from more infections than normal. A patient may even present with the chief concern of possible immune deficiency.

Disorders of the lymphatic system also have few symptoms. Most commonly, a patient will present with swollen lymph nodes (*lymphadenopathy*). This can be a sign of many different types of illnesses, which range from mild to serious. Another concern may be swelling in their extremities (*lymphedema*), which can also have serious or harmless causes.

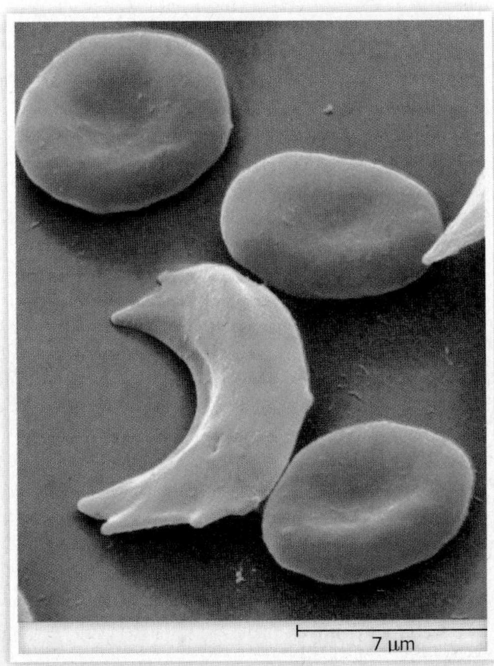

A common type of anemia is sickle-cell anemia, called that because affected red blood cells develop a hard, rigid "sickle" shape that can cause frequent clots in the sufferer.

8.2 Patient History, Problems, Complaints

blood

Term	Word Analysis
anemia ah-NEE-mee-ah	**an / emia** no / blood condition
Definition reduction of red blood cells noticed by the patient as weakness and fatigue	
ecchymosis eh-kih-MOH-sis	**from Greek, for** "to pour out"
Definition large bruise	
hematoma HEE-mah-TOH-mah	**hemat / oma** blood / tumor
Definition mass of blood within an organ, cavity, or tissue	
hemophilia HEE-moh-FEE-lee-ah	**hemo / phil / ia** blood / love / condition
Definition condition in which the blood doesn't clot, thus causing excessive bleeding	
hemorrhage HEM-oh-RIJ	**hemo / rrhage** blood / burst forth
Definition excessive blood loss	
petechia puh-TEE-kee-yah	**from Latin, for** "freckle" **or** "spot"
Definition small bruise	©Dr. P. Marazzi/Science Source
reperfusion injury REE-pir-FYOO-zhun IN-jir-ee	**re / per / fusion injury** again / through / pour
Definition injury to tissue that occurs after blood flow is restored	

lymph

Term	Word Analysis
lymphadenopathy lim-FAD-eh-NAW-pah-thee	**lymph / adeno / pathy** lymph / gland / disease
Definition any disease of a lymph gland (node); used to refer to noticeably swollen lymph nodes, especially in the neck	©McGraw-Hill Education

8.2 Patient History, Problems, Complaints

lymph *continued*

Term	Word Analysis
lymphedema LIMF-ah-DEE-mah	**lymph / edema** lymph / swelling
Definition swelling caused by abnormal accumulation of lymph, usually in the extremities	
splenalgia splee-NAL-jah	**splen / algia** spleen / pain
Definition pain in the spleen	
splenodynia SPLEE-noh-DAI-nee-ah	**spleno / dynia** spleen / pain
Definition pain in the spleen	

Learning Outcome 8.2 Exercises

PRONUNCIATION

EXERCISE 1 *Indicate which syllable is emphasized when pronounced.*

EXAMPLE: bronchitis bron**chi**tis

1. anemia ____________
2. hemophilia ____________
3. hemorrhage ____________
4. hematoma ____________
5. splenodynia ____________
6. splenalgia ____________
7. lymphedema ____________
8. reperfusion injury ____________

TRANSLATION

EXERCISE 2 *Break down the following words into their component parts.*

EXAMPLE: nasopharyngoscope *naso | pharyngo | scope*

1. hematoma ____________
2. hemorrhage ____________
3. splenodynia ____________
4. splenalgia ____________
5. lymphedema ____________
6. hemophilia ____________
7. anemia ____________
8. lymphadenopathy ____________

Learning Outcome 8.2 Exercises

EXERCISE 3 *Underline and define the word parts from this chapter in the following terms.*

1. hemophilia ______________________________
2. hemorrhage ______________________________
3. hematoma ______________________________
4. splenodynia ______________________________
5. splenalgia ______________________________
6. lymphedema ______________________________
7. anemia ______________________________

EXERCISE 4 *Match the term on the left with its definition on the right. Some definitions may be used more than once.*

______	1. anemia	a.	a condition in which the blood doesn't clot, thus causing excessive bleeding
______	2. hemophilia	b.	a mass of blood within an organ, cavity, or tissue
______	3. hemorrhage	c.	excessive blood loss
______	4. hematoma	d.	injury to tissue that occurs after blood flow is restored
______	5. splenalgia	e.	large bruise
______	6. splenodynia	f.	pain in the spleen
______	7. lymphedema	g.	reduction of red blood cells noticed by the patient as weakness and fatigue
______	8. reperfusion injury	h.	small bruise
______	9. ecchymosis	i.	swelling caused by abnormal accumulation of lymph
______	10. petechia		

EXERCISE 5 *Translate the following terms as literally as possible.*

EXAMPLE: nasopharyngoscope *an instrument for looking at the nose and throat*

1. splenodynia ______________________________
2. splenalgia ______________________________
3. hematoma ______________________________
4. hemorrhage ______________________________
5. anemia ______________________________
6. lymphedema ______________________________

Learning Outcome 8.2 Exercises

GENERATION

EXERCISE 6 *Build a medical term from the information provided.*

EXAMPLE: inflammation of the sinuses *sinusitis*

1. spleen pain (use *-dynia*) ____________________
2. spleen pain (use *-algia*) ____________________
3. blood tumor ____________________
4. lymph swelling ____________________
5. no blood condition ____________________
6. any disease of a lymph gland (node) ____________________

OBJECTIVE

8.3 Observation and Discovery

There are two ways of looking at blood cells. The first is to count them. A *complete blood count (CBC)* is one of the most common tests in medicine. A machine counts the number of each type of cell in the blood.

A lower-than-normal number of red blood cells is known as *anemia.* It is the most common blood problem and has a variety of causes. A higher-than-normal number of red blood cells (*erythrocytosis* or *polycythemia*) is much less common. When it is severe, it can be dangerous because the blood becomes too thick to flow well.

A low number of white blood cells (*leukopenia*) can be caused by an infection. If the number is too low, however, it may mean the patient has a weakened immune system (*immunodeficiency*). In general, people are more at risk if they are low in a specific type of white blood cell, neutrophils (*neutropenia*). Having a high number of white blood cells in the blood (*leukocytosis*) is a common marker for infection. Less commonly, it can indicate cancer.

Low platelet numbers (*thrombocytopenia*) can lead to easy bleeding and bruising. Having too many platelets in the blood (*thrombocytosis*) indicates inflammation. If platelet levels are too high, the patient runs the risk of experiencing abnormal blood clotting and forming a floating clot (*thromboembolism*).

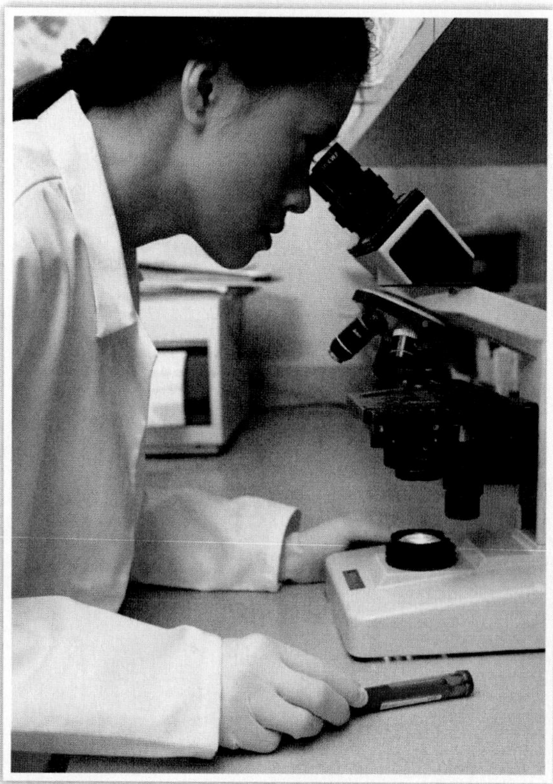

In hematology, a great deal of information is gathered through microscopic analysis of blood samples.

Another way of evaluating blood cells is by looking at their size and shape. The size of red blood cells helps distinguish among different causes for anemia. In fact, it is generally the first step in diagnosing the cause.

Causes for anemia with small red blood cells (*microcytosis*) include iron deficiency and lead poisoning. Anemias with enlarged blood cells (*macrocytosis*) can be a result of folate deficiency or B12 deficiency. Normal-sized blood cell (*normocytic*) anemias include bleeding and anemia from chronic disease. Some problems with the makeup of a red blood cell can cause it to assume abnormal shapes. *Spherocytes* and *elliptocytes* are two types of blood cells with abnormal shapes.

The physical exam of the lymphatic system focuses mainly on the few organs of the system, including the lymph nodes and the spleen. The lymph nodes may be swollen and painful (*lymphadenopathy*). The spleen may also be enlarged (*splenomegaly*). When lymph vessels become swollen, they can cause swelling in arms and legs (*lymphedema*).

There are no lab tests specific to the lymphatic system, but there is a special type of image that examines the lymph vessels (*lymphangiogram*). Most other lymphatic system issues, such as the absence of a spleen (*asplenia*), can be seen on a CT scan.

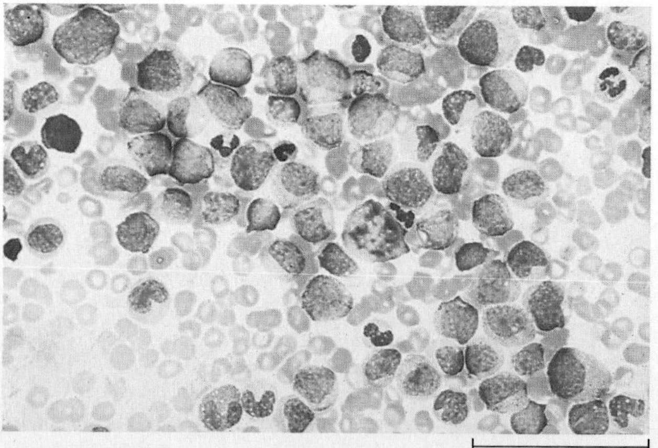

Blood from a patient with acute monocytic leukemia. Note the abnormally high number of white blood cells, especially monocytes.

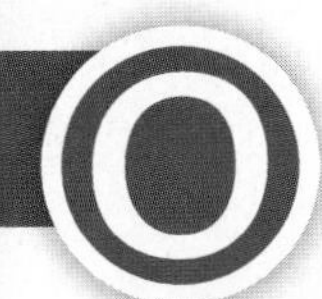

8.3 Observation and Discovery

blood

Term	Word Analysis
anisocytosis AN-ai-soh-SAI-toh-sis	**an / iso / cyt / osis** not / equal / cell / condition
Definition condition characterized by a great inequality in the size of red blood cells	
elliptocyte ee-LIP-toh-SAIT	**ellipto / cyte** oval-shaped / cell
Definition oval red blood cells	
elliptocytosis ee-LIP-toh-SAI-toh-sis	**ellipto / cyt / osis** oval-shaped / cell / condition
Definition condition characterized by an increase in the number of oval-shaped red blood cells	
embolism EM-boh-LIZ-um	**embol / ism** embolus / condition
Definition blockage in a blood vessel caused by an embolus	
embolus EM-boh-lus	**em / bolus** in / throw
Definition mass of matter present in the blood **Note:** In Greek, this word means "stopper," as in a cap for a bottle.	
erythrocyte eh-RIH-throh-SAIT	**erythro / cyte** red / cell
Definition red blood cell	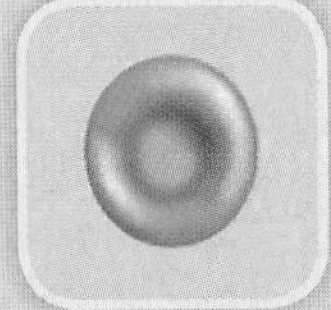
erythrocytosis eh-RIH-throh-sai-TOH-sis	**erythro / cyt / osis** red / cell / condition
Definition abnormal increase in the number of red blood cells	
hematopoiesis heh-MAH-toh-poh-EE-sis	**hemato / poiesis** blood / formation
Definition formation of blood cells	
hemolysis hee-MAW-lih-sis	**hemo / lysis** blood / breakdown
Definition breakdown of blood cells	
leukocyte LOO-koh-sait	**leuko / cyte** white / cell
Definition white blood cell	©MedicalRF.com/Getty Images RF

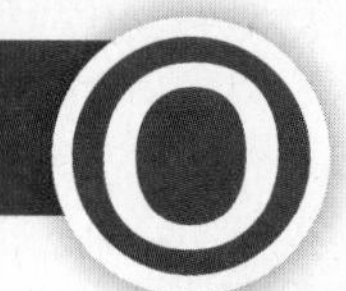

blood *continued*

Term	Word Analysis
leukocytosis LOO-koh-sai-TOH-sis **Definition** increase in the number of white blood cells	**leuko / cyt / osis** white / cell / condition
leukopenia LOO-koh-PEE-nee-ah **Definition** deficiency in white blood cells	**leuko / penia** white / deficiency
macrocytosis MAH-kroh-sai-TOH-sis **Definition** condition characterized by large red blood cells	**macro / cyt / osis** large / cell / condition
microcytosis MAI-kroh-sai-TOH-sis **Definition** condition characterized by small red blood cells	**micro / cyt / osis** small / cell / condition
myelopoiesis MAI-eh-loh-poh-EE-sis **Definition** formation of bone marrow	**myelo / poiesis** bone marrow / formation
neutropenia NOO-troh-PEE-nee-ah **Definition** deficiency in neutrophil **NOTE:** A neutrophil is a type of white blood cell.	**neutro / penia** neutrophil / deficiency
normocyte NOR-moh-sait **Definition** normal-sized red blood cell	**normo / cyte** normal / cell
oligocythemia AW-lih-goh-sih-THEE-mee-ah **Definition** deficiency in the number of red blood cells	**oligo / cyt / hemia** few / cell / blood condition
pancytopenia PAN-SAI-toh-PEE-nee-ah **Definition** deficiency in all cellular components of the blood	**pan / cyto / penia** all / cell / deficiency
phagocytosis FAY-goh-sai-TOH-sis **Definition** process in which phagocytes (a type of white blood cell) destroy (or eat) foreign microorganisms or cell debris	**phago / cyt / osis** eat / cell / condition

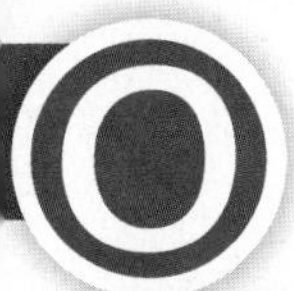

blood *continued*

Term	Word Analysis
poikilocytosis POI-kih-loh-sai-TOH-sis	**poikilo / cyt / osis** various / cell / condition
Definition condition characterized by red blood cells in a variety of shapes	
polycythemia PAW-lee-sih-THEE-mee-ah	**poly / cyt / hemia** many / cell / blood condition
Definition excess of red blood cells	
reticulocyte reh-TIK-yoo-loh-SAIT	**reticulo / cyte** net / cell
Definition immature red blood cell; the root comes from its netlike appearance	
spherocyte SFEE-roh-SAIT	**sphero / cyte** sphere / cell
Definition red blood cell that assumes a spherical shape	
thrombocyte THROM-boh-sait	**thrombo / cyte** clot / cell
Definition cell that helps blood clot; also known as a platelet	
thrombocytopenia THROM-boh-SAI-toh-PEE-nee-ah	**thrombo / cyto / penia** clot / cell / deficiency
Definition deficiency in the number of platelets (clot cells)	
thrombocytosis THROM-boh-sai-TOH-sis	**thrombo / cyt / osis** clot / cell / condition
Definition increase in the number of platelets (clot cells)	
thromboembolism THROM-boh-EM-boh-LIZ-um	**thrombo / embol / ism** clot / embolus / condition
Definition blockage of a vessel (embolism) caused by a clot that has broken off from where it formed	
thrombogenic THROM-boh-JIN-ik	**thrombo / gen / ic** clot / formation / pertaining to
Definition capable of producing a blood clot	
thrombosis throm-BOH-sis	**thromb / osis** clot / condition
Definition the formation of a blood clot	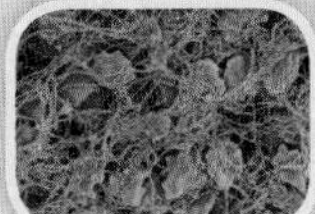 ©Steve Gschmeissner/Science Source

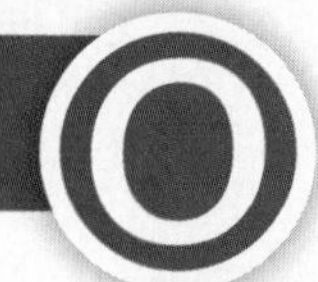

8.3 Observation and Discovery

blood *continued*

Term	Word Analysis
thrombus THROM-bus **Definition** blood clot **Note:** The difference between a thrombus and an embolus is twofold. A thrombus is a clot of blood and is stationary. An embolus is foreign material and is in motion. When a thrombus breaks off, it becomes a *thromboembolus*.	**from Greek, for** "lump, clot," **or even** "curd of milk"

lymph

Term	Word Analysis
asplenia ah-SPLEE-nee-ah **Definition** absence of a spleen or of spleen function	**a / splen / ia** no / spleen / condition
hepatosplenomegaly heh-PAT-oh-SPLEE-noh-MEH-gah-lee **Definition** enlargement of the liver and spleen	**hepato / spleno / megaly** liver / spleen / enlargement ©Dr. M. A. Ansary/Science Source
lymphocyte LIM-foh-SAIT **Definition** lymph cell	**lympho / cyte** lymph / cell
lymphopenia LIM-foh-PEE-nee-ah **Definition** abnormal deficiency in lymph	**lympho / penia** lymph / deficiency
splenectopy splee-NEK-toh-pee **Definition** displacement of the spleen; sometimes called floating spleen	**splen / ec / top / y** spleen / out / place / condition
splenolysis splee-NAW-lih-sis **Definition** breakdown (destruction) of spleen tissue	**spleno / lysis** spleen / breakdown
splenomalacia SPLEE-noh-mah-LAY-shah **Definition** softening of the spleen	**spleno / malacia** spleen / softening
splenomegaly SPLEE-noh-MEH-gah-lee **Definition** enlargement of the spleen	**spleno / megaly** spleen / enlargement ©Bollershot Photo/Science Source

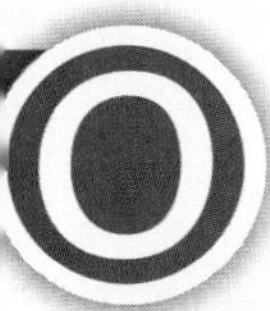

8.3 Observation and Discovery

lymph *continued*

Term	Word Analysis
splenoptosis SPLEE-nawp-TOH-sis	**spleno / ptosis** spleen / drooping condition
Definition downward displacement (drooping) of the spleen	
thymic hyperplasia THAI-mik HAI-per-PLAY-zhah	**thym / ic** **hyper / plasia** thymus / pertaining to over / formation
Definition overdevelopment of the thymus	

professional terms

Term	Word Analysis
antibody AN-tih-BAW-dee	**anti / body** against / body
Definition substance produced by the body in response to an antigen	
NOTE: If you think the word *antibody* seems incomplete and keep asking yourself "an anti-*what* body," you're right. Something *is* missing. This word is a shortened form of *antitoxic body*—that means *against poison*, which makes more sense.	
antigen AN-tih-JIN	**anti / gen** against / creator
Definition substance that causes the body to produce antibodies	
hematocrit hee-MAT-oh-krit	**hemato / crit** blood / judge (separate)
Definition test to judge or separate the blood; it is used to determine the ratio of red blood cells to total blood volume	
NOTE: The root *crit* comes from the Greek word that is the basis of the English word *critic*.	

Withdraw blood
Centrifuge
Plasma (55% of whole blood)
Buffy coat: leukocytes and platelets (< 1% of whole blood)
Erythrocytes (45% of whole blood)
Formed elements

professional terms *continued*

Term	Word Analysis
hematology HEE-mah-TAW-loh-jee **Definition** study of the blood	**hemato / logy** blood / study
hemoglobin HEE-moh-GLOH-bin **Definition** iron-containing pigment in red blood cells that carries oxygen to the cells **NOTE:** *Globin* and *globulin* both come from a Latin word meaning "globe" or "ball." They are used in medical language to refer to proteins.	**hemo / globin** blood / globe
hypoperfusion HAI-poh-per-FYOO-zhun **Definition** inadequate flow of blood	**hypo / per / fusion** under / through / pour
immunoglobulin im-MYOO-noh-GLAW-byoo-lin **Definition** protein that provides protection (immunity) against disease	**immuno / globulin** immune system / sphere
immunology IM-myoo-NAW-loh-jee **Definition** study of the immune system	**immuno / logy** immune system / study
immunologist IM-myoo-NAW-loh-jist **Definition** specialist in the study of the immune system	**immuno / logist** immune system / specialist
lymphangiogram lim-FAN-jee-oh-GRAM **Definition** record of the study of lymph vessels	**lymph / angio / gram** lymph / vessel / record
lymphangiography lim-FAN-jee-AW-grah-fee **Definition** procedure to study the lymph vessels	**lymph / angio / graphy** lymph / vessel / writing procedure
perfusion per-FYOO-zhun **Definition** circulation of blood through tissue	**per / fusion** through / pour
phlebology fleh-BAW-loh-jee **Definition** study of veins	**phlebo / logy** vein / study of
phlebotomist fleh-BAW-toh-mist **Definition** specialist in drawing blood	**phlebo / tom / ist** vein / cut / specialist
phlebotomy fleh-BAW-toh-mee **Definition** incision into a vein; another name for drawing blood	**phlebo / tomy** vein / incision ©liquidlibrary/PictureQuest RF

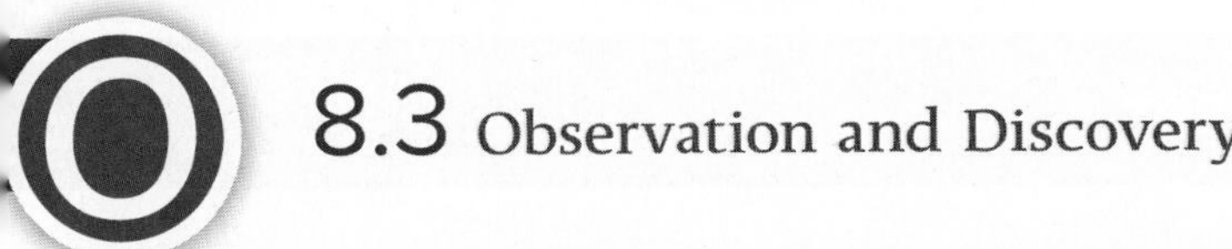

8.3 Observation and Discovery

professional terms *continued*

Term	Word Analysis
sphygmomanometer SFIG-moh-mah-NAW-meh-ter **Definition** fancy name for the device used to measure blood pressure	**sphygmo / mano / meter** strangle / thin / instrument for measuring ©Creatas/PunchStock RF

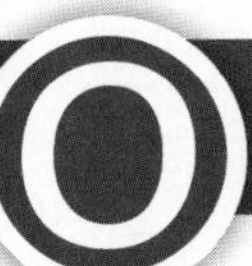

Learning Outcome 8.3 Exercises

PRONUNCIATION

EXERCISE 1 *Indicate which syllable is emphasized when pronounced.*

EXAMPLE: bronchitis bron**chi**tis

1. splenomegaly ______
2. macrocytosis ______
3. microcytosis ______
4. leukocytosis ______
5. thrombocytosis ______
6. elliptocytosis ______
7. erythrocytosis ______
8. poikilocytosis ______
9. splenoptosis ______
10. neutropenia ______
11. pancytopenia ______
12. thrombocytopenia ______
13. myelopoiesis ______
14. lymphangiogram ______
15. hepatosplenomegaly ______
16. sphygmomanometer ______
17. splenectopy ______
18. perfusion ______
19. embolus ______

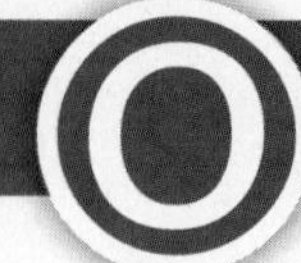

Learning Outcome 8.3 Exercises

20. thrombus ______
21. thrombosis ______
22. leukocyte ______
23. normocyte ______
24. thrombocyte ______
25. phlebotomy ______
26. phlebotomist ______
27. asplenia ______
28. hemolysis ______
29. splenolysis ______

TRANSLATION

EXERCISE 2 *Break down the following words into their component parts.*

EXAMPLE: nasopharyngoscope *naso | pharyngo | scope*

1. hemolysis ______
2. hematocrit ______
3. thrombosis ______
4. immunoglobulin ______
5. hepatosplenomegaly ______
6. splenolysis ______
7. splenomalacia ______
8. splenomegaly ______
9. antibody ______
10. antigen ______
11. hemoglobin ______
12. hypoperfusion ______
13. immunologist ______
14. lymphangiography ______
15. perfusion ______
16. phlebotomist ______
17. sphygmomanometer ______

EXERCISE 3 *Underline and define the word parts from this chapter in the following terms.*

1. immunology ______
2. hematology ______
3. phlebology ______
4. thymic hyperplasia ______
5. splenectopy ______
6. phlebotomy ______
7. splenoptosis ______
8. hematopoiesis ______
9. myelopoiesis ______
10. neutropenia ______

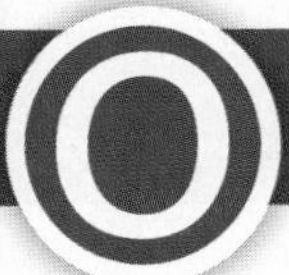

Learning Outcome 8.3 Exercises

11. asplenia ____________________
12. lymphangiography ____________________
13. leukopenia (2 roots) ____________________
14. lymphopenia (2 roots) ____________________
15. pancytopenia (2 roots) ____________________
16. oligocythemia (2 roots) ____________________
17. polycythemia (2 roots) ____________________
18. thrombocytopenia (3 roots) ____________________

EXERCISE 4 *Match the term on the left with its definition on the right.*

_____	1. normocyte	a.	cell that helps blood clot (platelet)
_____	2. lymphocyte	b.	immature red blood cell (netlike appearance)
_____	3. spherocyte	c.	lymph cell
_____	4. leukocyte	d.	normal-sized red blood cell
_____	5. thrombocyte	e.	oval-shaped red blood cell
_____	6. erythrocyte	f.	red blood cell
_____	7. elliptocyte	g.	spherical red blood cell
_____	8. reticulocyte	h.	white blood cell

EXERCISE 5 *Match the term on the left with its definition on the right.*

_____	1. thrombogenic	a.	blockage in a blood vessel caused by an embolus
_____	2. thrombus	b.	blockage of a vessel (embolism) caused by a blood clot (thrombus) that has broken off from where it formed
_____	3. embolism	c.	a mass of matter present in the blood; from the Greek word for "stopper," as in the cap on a bottle
_____	4. embolus	d.	stationary blood clot
_____	5. thromboembolism	e.	capable of producing a blood clot

EXERCISE 6 *Fill in the blanks.*

1. macrocytosis = ____________________ cell condition
2. microcytosis = ____________________ cell condition
3. leukocytosis = ____________________ cell condition
4. thrombocytosis = ____________________ cell condition
5. elliptocytosis = ____________________ cell condition
6. erythrocytosis = ____________________ cell condition
7. phagocytosis = ____________________ cell condition
8. poikilocytosis = ____________________ cell condition
9. anisocytosis = ____________________ cell condition

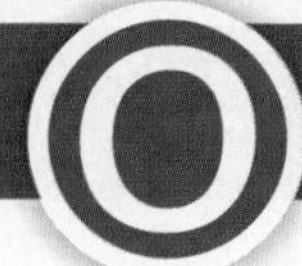

Learning Outcome 8.3 Exercises

EXERCISE 7 *Translate the following terms as literally as possible.*

EXAMPLE: nasopharyngoscope *an instrument for looking at the nose and throat*

1. immunologist ______
2. immunoglobulin ______
3. thrombogenic ______
4. lymphopenia ______
5. neutropenia ______
6. pancytopenia ______
7. splenolysis ______
8. splenoptosis ______
9. hematocrit ______
10. erythrocytosis ______
11. phagocytosis ______
12. anisocytosis ______
13. poikilocytosis ______
14. thymic hyperplasia ______
15. hepatosplenomegaly ______

GENERATION

EXERCISE 8 *Build a medical term from the information provided.*

EXAMPLE: inflammation of the sinuses *sinusitis*

1. study of the immune system ______
2. study of blood ______
3. study of veins ______
4. lymph cell ______
5. white blood cell ______
6. clot cell ______
7. red blood cell ______
8. sphere cell ______
9. normal cell ______
10. softening of the spleen ______
11. enlargement of the spleen ______
12. no spleen condition ______
13. formation of bone marrow ______

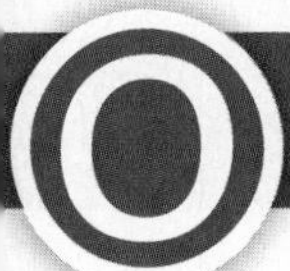

Learning Outcome 8.3 Exercises

EXERCISE 9 *Multiple-choice questions. Select the correct answer(s).*

1. A *sphygmomanometer* measures:
   a. blood pressure
   b. red blood cells
   c. white blood cells
   d. none of these
2. A *floating spleen* is called a:
   a. splenectopy
   b. splenolysis
   c. splenomalacia
   d. splenomegaly
   e. splenoptosis
3. An immature red blood cell that has a netlike appearance is called a(n):
   a. elliptocyte
   b. erythrocyte
   c. reticulocyte
   d. spherocyte
   e. thrombocyte
4. *Hemoglobin:* (select all that apply)
   a. carries oxygen to cells
   b. contains antibodies
   c. contains iron
   d. helps the body fight infection
   e. is found in red blood cells
   f. is found in white blood cells
5. The circulation of blood through tissue is called:
   a. hyperplasia
   b. hypoperfusion
   c. perfusion
   d. none of these
6. An inadequate flow of blood is called:
   a. hyperplasia
   b. hypoperfusion
   c. perfusion
   d. none of these
7. An *embolism* is:
   a. a blockage in a blood vessel caused by a foreign material in motion
   b. a cell capable of producing a blood clot
   c. the formation of a blood clot
   d. none of these
8. A blockage of a vessel caused by a clot that has broken off from where it formed is a(n):
   a. embolism
   b. thromboembolism
   c. thrombosis
   d. thrombus
9. The formation of a blood clot is a(n):
   a. embolism
   b. thromboembolism
   c. thrombosis
   d. thrombus

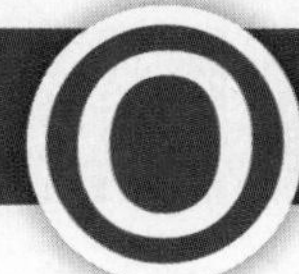

Learning Outcome 8.3 Exercises

EXERCISE 10 *Briefly describe the difference between each pair of terms.*

1. macrocytosis, microcytosis ______
2. elliptocyte, elliptocytosis ______
3. phlebotomist, phlebotomy ______
4. hematopoiesis, hemolysis ______
5. lymphangiogram, lymphangiography ______
6. leukocytosis, leukopenia ______
7. thrombocytopenia, thrombocytosis ______
8. oligocythemia, polycythemia ______
9. antibody, antigen ______
10. embolus, thrombus ______

ASSESSMENT

8.4 Diagnosis and Pathology

Diseases affecting the blood often affect one specific blood cell type. The most common type of red blood cell problem is not having enough of them to do their job (*anemia*), which results from the body not being able to make enough of them. Iron is a necessary mineral for generating blood cells. As a result, a low level of iron can cause a decreased production of red blood cells (*iron deficiency anemia*). The available red blood cells may also be low because they break too easily (*hemolytic anemia*).

Even if there are enough red blood cells, there may be a problem with the blood's *hemoglobin,* the protein that actually carries oxygen. In less common situations, a patient may have too many red blood cells (*polycythemia*). This condition can make the blood thicker, making the flow of blood more difficult.

As with red blood cells, an insufficient number of white blood cells in the body can cause serious problems. A deficiency of white blood cells may cause the patient to be more vulnerable to infections (*immune deficiency*). Sometimes this can be caused by an outside force (*immunosuppression*) like a medication or illness. When the body has a problem with making white blood cells, it may make way too many of them. This is what happens in people who have *leukemia*.

Not having enough platelets in the blood (*thrombocytopenia*) can cause problems with bleeding. It can be mild, causing bruising and bloody noses, or it can be more severe, creating risk for bleeding into major organs like the brain.

On the other hand, if the blood has too many platelets, spontaneous clots (*thrombosis*) may occur. Problems also arise when other parts of the body's clotting team are not working well—whether the blood is not clotting enough (*coagulopathy*) or clotting too easily (*hypercoagulability*).

Finally, blood diseases can be caused by things that are carried in the blood along with blood cells. Infection can spread to the bloodstream (*septicemia*), which can be very dangerous. Fat floats in the blood as well. Too much fat (*hyperlipidemia*) in the blood can eventually lead to heart problems. Another thing that may be seen in the blood is the recycled blood product *bilirubin.* Too much bilirubin in the blood may cause the skin to appear yellow.

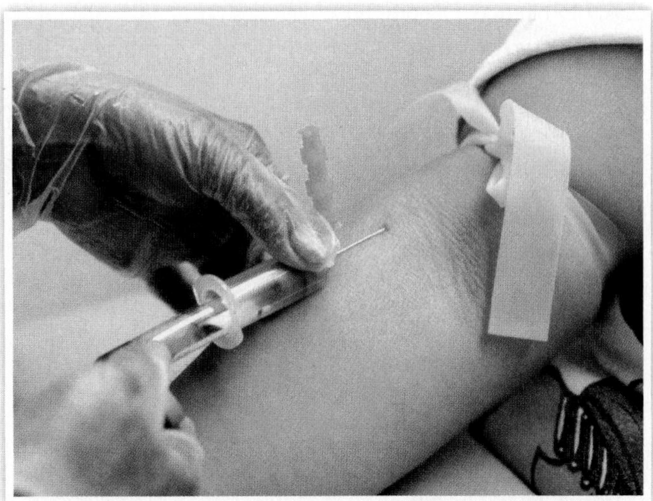

Often, a phlebotomy is the first step in diagnosing blood conditions.

Problems in the lymphatic system are mainly seen in lymph nodes. Lymph nodes can become sore (*lymphadenopathy*) when overworked or infected (*lymphadenitis*). They are also a common site for cancer (*lymphoma*). The main spleen condition patients encounter is an enlarged spleen (*splenomegaly*), which can happen when it is overactive (*hypersplenism*) or, more commonly, as a result of an infection. The most common infection that affects the spleen is *mononucleosis.*

Bone marrow can become infected (*osteomyelitis*) from the bloodstream or from an injury to the bone. These infections are hard to treat and require a long course of antibiotics.

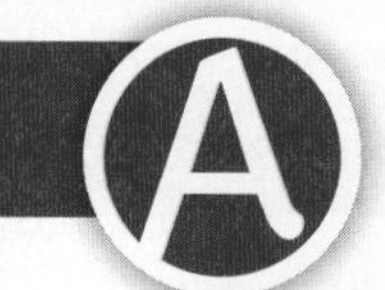

8.4 Diagnosis and Pathology

blood

Term	Word Analysis
autoimmune disease AW-toh-ih-MYOON dih-ZEEZ **Definition** disease caused by the body's immune system attacking the body's own healthy tissue	**auto / immune** self / immune
coagulopathy coh-AG-yoo-LAW-pah-thee **Definition** any disease that deals with problems in blood coagulation	**coagulo / pathy** coagulation / disease
deep vein thrombosis DEEP VAYN throm-BOH-sis **Definition** formation of a blood clot in a vein deep in the body, most commonly the leg	**deep vein thromb / osis** deep vein clot / condition
hemoglobinopathy HEE-maw-GLOH-bin-AW-pah-thee **Definition** disease of the hemoglobin	**hemo / globino / pathy** blood / globe / disease
hypercoagulability HAI-per-koh-AG-yoo-lah-BIL-ih-tee **Definition** increased ability of the blood to coagulate	**hyper / coagul / ability** over / coagulation / ability
immunocompromised ih-MYOO-noh-COM-proh-MAIZD **Definition** having an immune system incapable of responding normally and completely to a pathogen or disease	**immuno / compromised** immune / compromised
immunodeficiency ih-MYOO-noh-deh-FIH-shin-see **Definition** immune system with decreased or compromised response to disease-causing organisms	**immuno / deficiency** immune / deficiency ©Science Source
immunosuppression ih-MYOO-noh-suh-PREH-shun **Definition** reduction in the activity of the body's immune system	**immuno / suppression** immune / suppression
ischemia ih-SKEE-mee-ah **Definition** blockage of blood flow to an organ	**isch / emia** hold back / blood condition

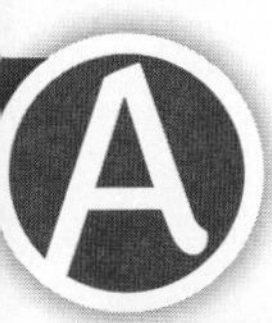

8.4 Diagnosis and Pathology

blood *continued*

Term	Word Analysis
phlebarteriectasia FLEB-ar-TER-ee-ek-TAY-zhah **Definition** dilation of blood vessels	**phleb / arteri / ectasia** vein / artery / dilation 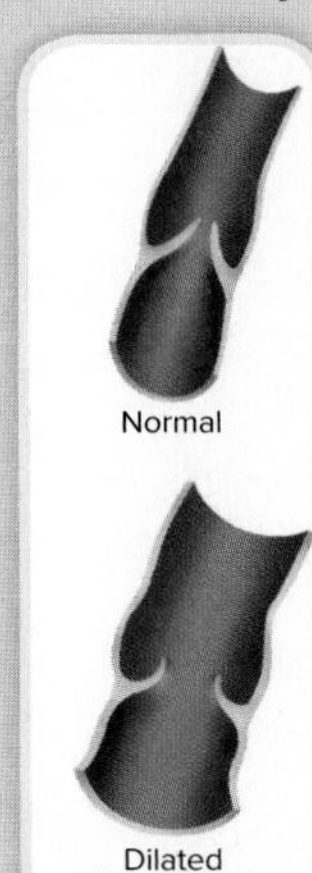
spherocytosis SFEER-oh-sai-TOH-sis **Definition** condition in which red blood cells assume a spherical shape	**sphero / cyt / osis** sphere / cell / condition
thrombophlebitis THROM-boh-fleh-BAI-tis **Definition** inflammation of vein caused by a clot	**thrombo / phleb / itis** clot / vein / inflammation

blood conditions

Term	Word Analysis
anemia ah-NEE-mee-ah **Definition** reduced red blood cells	**an / emia** no / blood condition
aplastic anemia AY-plas-tik ah-NEE-mee-ah **Definition** anemia caused by red blood cells not being formed in sufficient quantities	**a / plas / tic an / emia** no / formation / pertaining to no / blood condition
hemolytic anemia HEE-moh-LIH-tik ah-NEE-mee-ah **Definition** anemia caused by the destruction of red blood cells	**hemo / lytic an / emia** blood / breakdown no / blood condition
iron deficiency anemia AI-ern deh-FIH-shin-see ah-NEE-mee-ah **Definition** anemia caused by inadequate iron intake	**iron deficiency an / emia** iron deficiency no / blood condition
bilirubinemia BIH-lee-ROO-bin-EE-mee-ah **Definition** presence of bilirubin in the blood **NOTE:** *Bilirubin* (red bile) is a substance derived from red blood cells that have completed their life span. Bilirubin is secreted by the liver into the digestive tract.	**bili / rubin / emia** bile / red / blood condition

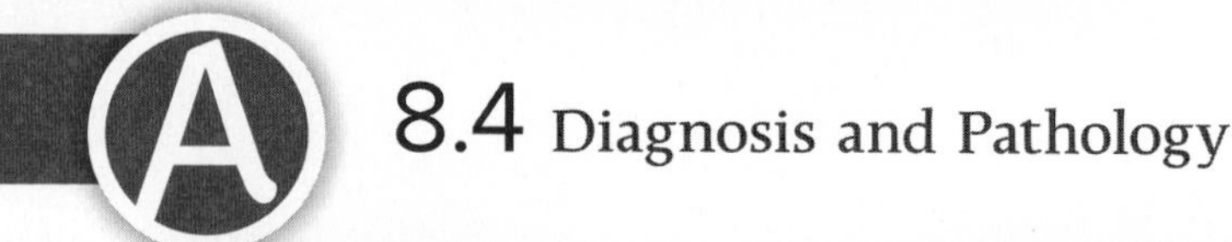

8.4 Diagnosis and Pathology

blood conditions *continued*

Term	Word Analysis
hyperbilirubinemia HAI-per-BIH-lee-ROO-bin-EE-mee-ah **Definition** excessive bilirubin in the blood	**hyper / bili / rubin / emia** over / bile / red / blood condition
hypercholesterolemia HAI-per-koh-LES-ter-ol-EE-mee-ah **Definition** excessive cholesterol in the blood	**hyper / cholesterol / emia** over / cholesterol / blood condition
hyperlipidemia HAI-per-LIH-pid-EE-mee-ah **Definition** excessive fat in the blood	**hyper / lipid / emia** over / fat / blood condition
hypervolemia HAI-per-voh-LEE-mee-ah **Definition** increased blood volume	**hyper / vol / emia** over / volume / blood condition
hypovolemia HAI-poh-voh-LEE-mee-ah **Definition** decreased blood volume	**hypo / vol / emia** under / volume / blood condition
septicemia SEP-tih-SEE-mee-ah **Definition** presence of disease-causing microorganisms in the blood	**septic / emia** rotting / blood condition
uremia yoo-REE-mee-ah **Definition** presence of urine in the blood	**ur / emia** urine / blood condition

lymph

Term	Word Analysis
hepatosplenitis hih-PAT-oh-SPLEEN-ai-tis **Definition** inflammation of the liver and spleen	**hepato / splen / itis** liver / spleen / inflammation
hypersplenism HAI-per-SPLEEN-izm **Definition** increased spleen activity	**hyper / splen / ism** over / spleen / condition

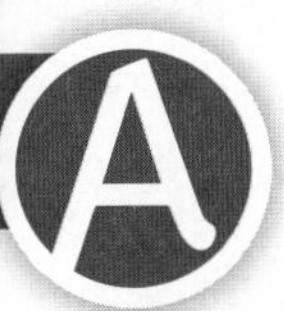

8.4 Diagnosis and Pathology

lymph *continued*

Term	Word Analysis
lymphadenitis LIM-fad-eh-NAI-tis **Definition** inflammation of a lymph gland (node)	**lymph / aden / itis** lymph / gland / inflammation
lymphangiectasia lim-FAN-jee-ek-TAY-zhah **Definition** dilation of a lymph vessel, normally noticed by swelling in the extremities	**lymph / angi / ectasia** lymph / vessel / dilation
lymphangitis LIM-fan-JAI-tis **Definition** inflammation of lymph vessels	**lymph / ang / itis** lymph / vessel / inflammation
mononucleosis MAW-noh-NOO-klee-OH-sis **Definition** condition characterized by an abnormally large number of mononuclear leukocytes	**mono / nucle / osis** one / nucleus / condition
myelodysplasia MAI-el-oh-dis-PLAY-zhah **Definition** disease characterized by poor production of blood cells by the bone marrow	**myelo / dys / plas / ia** bone marrow / bad / formation / condition
osteomyelitis AW-stee-oh-MAI-eh-LAI-tis **Definition** inflammation of bone and bone marrow	**osteo / myel / itis** bone / bone marrow / inflammation
splenitis splee-NAI-tis **Definition** inflammation of the spleen	**splen / itis** spleen / inflammation
splenopathy splee-NAW-pah-thee **Definition** any disease of the spleen	**spleno / pathy** spleen / disease
splenorrhexis SPLEE-noh-REK-sis **Definition** rupture of the spleen	**spleno / rrhexis** spleen / rupture
thymopathy thai-MAW-pah-thee **Definition** disease of the thymus	**thymo / pathy** thymus / disease
tonsillitis TON-sil-AI-tis **Definition** inflammation of a tonsil	**tonsill / itis** tonsil / inflammation Source: Centers for Disease Control and Prevention

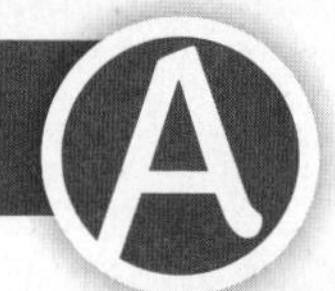

8.4 Diagnosis and Pathology

oncology

Term	Word Analysis
leukemia loo-KEE-mee-ah **Definition** cancer of the blood or bone marrow characterized by the abnormal increase in white blood cells	**leuk / emia** white / blood condition ©Ed Reschke
lymphoma lim-FOH-mah **Definition** tumor originating in lymphocytes	**lymph / oma** lymph / tumor Source: Centers for Disease Control and Prevention
myeloma MAI-eh-LOH-mah **Definition** cancerous tumor of the bone marrow; when the tumors are present in several bones, it is called multiple myeloma	**myel / oma** bone marrow / tumor
thymoma thai-MOH-mah **Definition** tumor of the thymus	**thym / oma** thymus / tumor

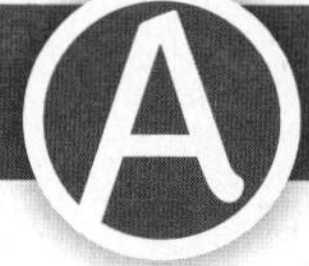

Learning Outcome 8.4 Exercises

PRONUNCIATION

EXERCISE 1 *Indicate which syllable is emphasized when pronounced.*

EXAMPLE: bronchitis bron**chi**tis

1. anemia ______
2. leukemia ______
3. uremia ______
4. lymphoma ______
5. splenitis ______
6. splenopathy ______
7. thymoma ______
8. thymopathy ______
9. coagulopathy ______
10. hemoglobinopathy ______
11. thrombophlebitis ______
12. hyperbilirubinemia ______
13. hypovolemia ______
14. osteomyelitis ______
15. hypersplenism ______

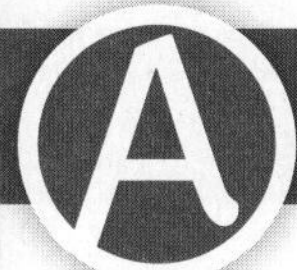

Learning Outcome 8.4 Exercises

TRANSLATION

EXERCISE 2 *Break down the following words into their component parts.*

EXAMPLE: nasopharyngoscope *naso | pharyngo | scope*

1. autoimmune ______
2. splenitis ______
3. splenopathy ______
4. thymopathy ______
5. hemoglobinopathy ______
6. immunocompromised ______
7. immunosuppression ______
8. hypersplenism ______
9. hyperbilirubinemia ______
10. lymphangitis ______
11. osteomyelitis ______
12. hypercoagulability ______

EXERCISE 3 *Underline and define the word parts from this chapter in the following terms.*

1. tonsillitis ______
2. immunodeficiency ______
3. lymphoma ______
4. thymoma ______
5. myeloma ______
6. coagulopathy ______
7. lymphadenitis ______
8. anemia ______
9. deep vein thrombosis ______
10. phlebarteriectasia ______
11. spherocytosis ______
12. lymphangiectasia ______
13. myelodysplasia ______
14. splenorrhexis ______
15. hepatosplenitis ______
16. leukemia (2 roots) ______
17. thrombophlebitis (2 roots) ______

EXERCISE 4 *Match the term on the left with its definition on the right.*

______ 1. hypercholesterolemia
______ 2. iron deficiency anemia
______ 3. bilirubinemia
______ 4. hemolytic anemia
______ 5. aplastic anemia
______ 6. hyperlipidemia
______ 7. hypervolemia
______ 8. hypovolemia
______ 9. septicemia
______ 10. ischemia
______ 11. uremia

a. anemia caused by inadequate iron intake
b. anemia caused by red blood cells not being formed in sufficient quantities
c. anemia caused by the destruction of red blood cells
d. blockage of blood flow to an organ
e. decreased blood volume
f. excessive cholesterol in the blood
g. excessive fat in the blood
h. increased blood volume
i. the presence of bilirubin in the blood
j. the presence of disease-causing microorganisms in the blood
k. the presence of urine in the blood

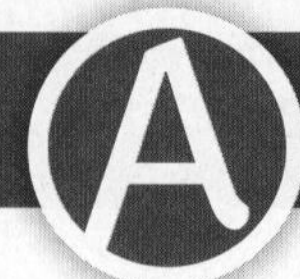

Learning Outcome 8.4 Exercises

EXERCISE 5 *Translate the following terms as literally as possible.*

EXAMPLE: nasopharyngoscope *an instrument for looking at the nose and throat*

1. hypercoagulability ______
2. phlebarteriectasia ______
3. spherocytosis ______
4. thrombophlebitis ______
5. anemia ______
6. hyperbilirubinism ______
7. septicemia ______
8. hepatosplenitis ______
9. hypersplenism ______
10. lymphadenitis ______
11. lymphangiectasia ______
12. lymphangitis ______
13. osteomyelitis ______
14. splenitis ______
15. splenorrhexis ______
16. tonsillitis ______

GENERATION

EXERCISE 6 *Build a medical term from the information provided.*

EXAMPLE: inflammation of the sinuses *sinusitis*

1. lymph tumor ______
2. spleen disease ______
3. thymus disease ______
4. coagulation disease ______
5. a disease of the hemoglobin ______
6. white blood condition ______
7. presence of bilirubin in the blood ______
8. presence of urine in the blood ______
9. excessive cholesterol in the blood ______
10. excessive fat in the blood ______

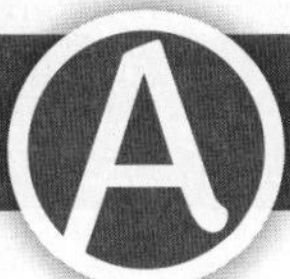

Learning Outcome 8.4 Exercises

EXERCISE 7 *Multiple-choice questions. Select the correct answer.*

1. The root word in *immunocompromised* is:
   a. *compromo*–the lymph system
   b. *compromo*–to protect
   c. *immuno*–the immune system
   d. *immuno*–the platelets and white cells of the body
   e. none of these
2. An immune system with decreased or compromised response to disease-causing organisms is called:
   a. autoimmune
   b. immunodeficiency
   c. immunogenic
   d. immunosuppression
   e. none of these
3. Anemia caused by inadequate iron intake is known as:
   a. aplastic anemia
   b. hematopenia
   c. hemolytic anemia
   d. iron deficiency anemia
   e. none of these
4. The term *ischemia* means:
   a. blockage of blood flow to an organ
   b. decreased blood volume
   c. dilation of blood vessels
   d. inflammation of a vein caused by a clot
   e. none of these
5. The formation of a blood clot deep in the body, most commonly in the leg, is called:
   a. deep vein thrombosis
   b. hyperthrombopathy
   c. phlebarteriectasia
   d. thrombophlebitis
   e. none of these
6. *Bilirubin* is:
   a. red bile
   b. a substance derived from red blood cells
   c. secreted by the liver into the digestive tract
   d. a substance that has completed its life span
   e. all of these
7. A cancer of the blood or bone marrow characterized by the abnormal increase in white blood cells is known as:
   a. leukemia
   b. myeloma
   c. lymphoma
   d. osteomyelitis
   e. none of these
8. A disease characterized by poor production of blood cells by the bone marrow is called:
   a. myelodysplasia
   b. osteomyelitis
   c. myeloma
   d. hematomyelogenopathy
   e. none of these

EXERCISE 8 *Briefly describe the difference between each pair of terms.*

1. myeloma, thymoma ______________________________
2. hypervolemia, hypovolemia ______________________________
3. autoimmune disease, immunosuppression ______________________________
4. aplastic anemia, hemolytic anemia ______________________________

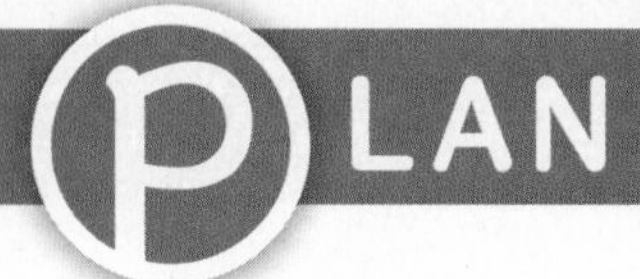

8.5 Treatments and Therapies

Treatment for blood problems generally involves both medicine and transfusions. With red blood cell problems, the treatment often involves blood transfusions (for severe problems), and then fixing the cause. Many times, iron supplements can also be helpful.

White blood cell problems—in particular, severely low white blood cell counts—can be treated with transfusions too. A patient with leukemia is treated with chemotherapy.

When the problem is significant enough, patients with very low platelet levels often are treated with transfusions as well. Other medicines that can help with platelet problems include medicines to break clots (*thrombolytics*) and those that prevent clots (*anticoagulants*).

Treating diseases of the lymphatic system generally involves surgery. Organs of the lymphatic system may be removed, such as the spleen (*splenectomy*) or the thymus (*thymectomy*). Lymph nodes may need removal (*lymphadenectomy*) as well, usually for the purpose of a biopsy.

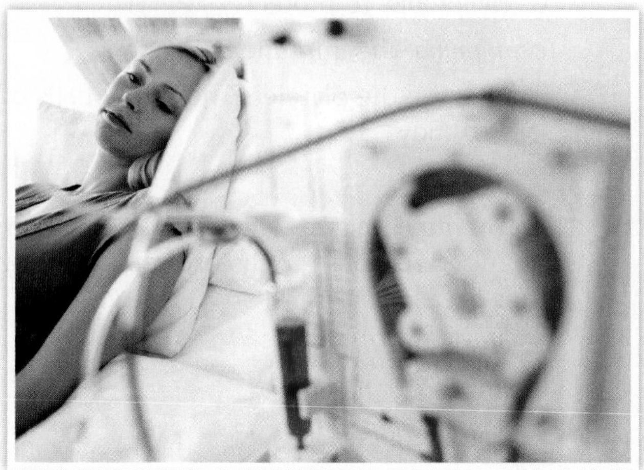

Transfusions and apheresis are important components of treating blood problems.

pharmacology

Term	Word Analysis
anticoagulant AN-tee-coh-AG-yoo-lant **Definition** drug that prevents the coagulation of blood	**anti / coagul / ant** against / coagulation / agent
hemostatic HEE-moh-STAT-ik **Definition** drug that stops the flow of blood	**hemo / static** blood / standing
thrombolytic THROM-boh-LIH-tik **Definition** drug that breaks down blood clots	**thrombo / lytic** clot / breakdown agent

surgical procedures

Term	Word Analysis
laparosplenectomy LAP-ah-roh-splee-NEK-toh-mee **Definition** surgical removal of the spleen through the abdomen	**laparo / splen / ectomy** abdomen / spleen / removal

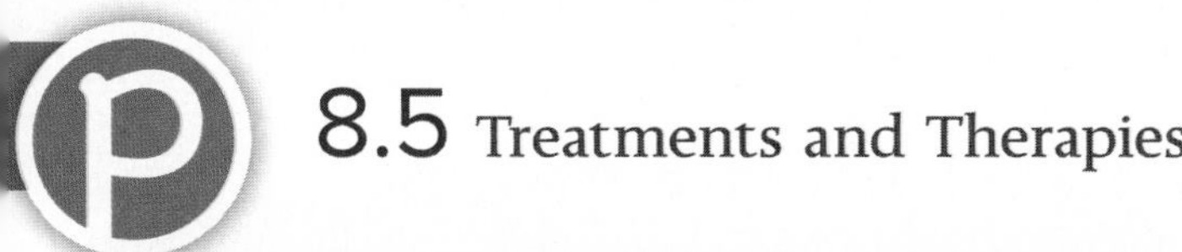

surgical procedures *continued*

Term	Word Analysis
lymphadenectomy lim-FAD-eh-NEK-toh-mee **Definition** surgical removal of a lymph gland (node)	**lymph / aden / ectomy** lymph / gland / removal
lymphadenotomy lim-FAD-eh-NAW-toh-mee **Definition** incision into a lymph gland (node)	**lymph / adeno / tomy** lymph / gland / incision
nephrosplenopexy NEF-roh-SPLEE-noh-PEK-see **Definition** surgical fixation of the spleen and a kidney	**nephro / spleno / pexy** kidney / spleen / fixation
splenectomy spleh-NEK-toh-mee **Definition** surgical removal of the spleen	**splen / ectomy** spleen / removal
thymectomy thai-MEK-toh-mee **Definition** surgical removal of the thymus	**thym / ectomy** thymus / removal
tonsillectomy TON-sil-EK-toh-mee **Definition** surgical removal of a tonsil	**tonsill / ectomy** tonsil / removal

transfusions

Term	Word Analysis
apheresis AH-fer-EE-sis **Definition** general term for a process, similar to dialysis, that draws out a patient's blood, removes something from it, then returns the rest of the blood to the patient's body **Note:** *Apheresis* can also refer to the use of this process to remove unwanted or disease-causing components from the blood.	**from Greek, for** "separation" **Note:** This is the same word that was the origin of the word *heretic*, meaning one who has separated from the traditional teachings of a group. ©Cristina Pedrazzini/Science Source
cytapheresis SAI-tah-fer-EE-sis **Definition** apheresis to remove cellular material	**cyt / apheresis** cell / separation
plasmapheresis PLAZ-mah-feh-REE-sis **Definition** apheresis to remove plasma	**plasm / apheresis** plasma / separation

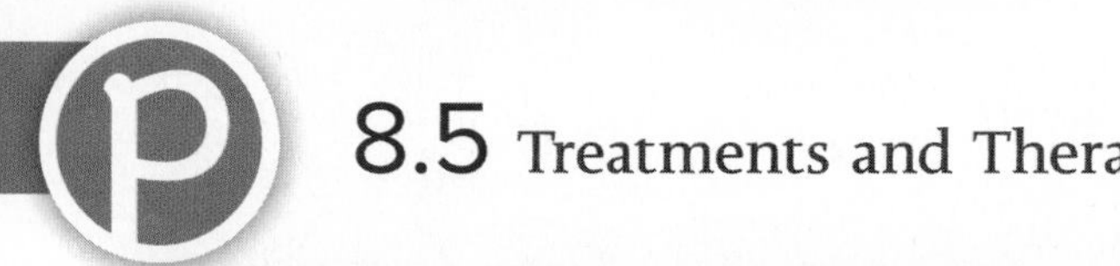

8.5 Treatments and Therapies

transfusions *continued*

Term	Word Analysis
plateletpheresis PLAYT-let-feh-REE-sis	**platelet / pheresis** platelet / separation
Definition apheresis to remove platelets (for the purpose of donating them to patients in need of platelets) **NOTE:** Where did the *a* in *apheresis* go? Probably, this term was developed from the term *plasmapheresis.* But because the first root in that word is *plasma,* someone thought that the *a* in *apheresis* went with it, so when they made this new word, they left the *a* out. Either that, or *platelet-AH-pheresis* didn't sound as good.	
transfusion tranz-FYOO-zhun **Definition** infusion into a patient of blood from another source	**trans / fusion** across / pour ©Martin Barraud/AGE Fotostock RF

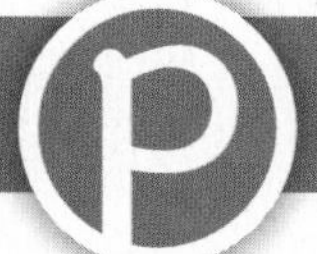

Learning Outcome 8.5 Exercises

PRONUNCIATION

EXERCISE 1 *Indicate which syllable is emphasized when pronounced.*

EXAMPLE: bronchitis bron**chi**tis

1. hemostatic ______________
2. tonsillectomy ______________
3. anticoagulant ______________
4. plasmapheresis ______________
5. plateletpheresis ______________
6. laparosplenectomy ______________
7. transfusion ______________
8. thymectomy ______________
9. splenectomy ______________

Learning Outcome 8.5 Exercises

TRANSLATION

EXERCISE 2 *Break down the following words into their component parts.*

EXAMPLE: nasopharyngoscope *naso | pharyngo | scope*

1. thymectomy ______
2. laparosplenectomy ______
3. transfusion ______
4. plasmapheresis ______
5. plateletpheresis ______
6. lymphadenotomy ______

EXERCISE 3 *Underline and define the word parts from this chapter in the following terms.*

1. tonsillectomy ______
2. thymectomy ______
3. splenectomy ______
4. thrombolytic ______
5. anticoagulant ______
6. hemostatic ______
7. cytapheresis ______
8. lymphadenectomy ______
9. laparosplenectomy ______
10. nephrosplenopexy ______

EXERCISE 4 *Match the term on the left with its definition on the right.*

______ 1. transfusion
______ 2. apheresis
______ 3. plasmapheresis
______ 4. cytapheresis

a. apheresis to remove cellular material
b. apheresis to remove plasma
c. general term for a process, similar to dialysis, that draws blood, removes something from it, then returns the rest of the blood to the patient
d. infusion into a patient of blood from another source

EXERCISE 5 *Translate the following terms as literally as possible.*

EXAMPLE: nasopharyngoscope *an instrument for looking at the nose and throat*

1. thrombolytic ______
2. hemostatic ______
3. cytapheresis ______
4. plateletpheresis ______
5. plasmapheresis ______
6. laparosplenectomy ______
7. nephrosplenopexy ______

Learning Outcome 8.5 Exercises

GENERATION

EXERCISE 6 *Build a medical term from the information provided.*

EXAMPLE: inflammation of the sinuses *sinusitis*

1. surgical removal of the spleen ____________
2. surgical removal of the thymus ____________
3. surgical removal of the tonsil ____________
4. surgical removal of a lymph gland (node) ____________
5. incision into a lymph gland (node) ____________
6. a drug that prevents the coagulation of blood ____________

EXERCISE 7 *Multiple-choice questions. Select the correct answer(s).*

1. A *laparosplenectomy* is:
   a. an incision into the spleen through the abdomen
   b. an incision into the spleen with a laser
   c. the surgical removal of the spleen through the abdomen
   d. the surgical removal of the spleen with a laser
   e. none of these
2. Select all of the below statements that apply to the term *apheresis.*
   a. a process similar to dialysis
   b. can refer to the removal of unwanted or disease-causing components from the blood
   c. from the Greek word meaning "separation"
   d. requires a transfusion
   e. the blood is not returned to the patient once removed
3. After a patient has undergone *plateletpheresis*:
   a. the patient receives a transfusion to replace lost blood
   b. the plasma is cleaned and then returned to the patient
   c. the platelets are often donated to another person in need
   d. the platelets are then returned to the patient
   e. none of these

8.6 Abbreviations

Abbreviations provide a shorthand way of referring to things that either recur often or are too long to write out. When dealing with the the blood and lymph systems, these can refer to common examination findings (NCAT), common lab work (PLT, RBC, WBC), diseases (ALL, AIDS), or treatments (BMT).

blood and lymph abbreviations

Abbreviation	Definition
AIDS	acquired immunodeficiency syndrome ©Science Photo Library RF/Getty Images RF
ALL	acute lymphoblastic leukemia
AML	acute myeloid leukemia
BMT	bone marrow transplant
CBC	complete blood count
CML	chronic myeloid leukemia
DIC	disseminated intravascular coagulopathy
EBV	Epstein-Barr virus
ESR	erythrocyte sedimentation rate
Hct	hematocrit
Hgb	hemoglobin
HIV	human immunodeficiency virus
HSM	hepatosplenomegaly
HUS	hemolytic uremic syndrome
INR	international normalized ratio
ITP	idiopathic thrombocytopenic purpura
IV	intravenous
IVIG	intravenous immunoglobulin
LAD	lymphadenopathy
PLT	platelet count
PT	prothrombin time
PTT	partial thromboplastin time
RBC	red blood count; red blood cell ©Ingram Publishing RF
TTP	thrombotic thrombocytopenic purpura
WBC	white blood count; white blood cell

Learning Outcome 8.6 Exercises

EXERCISE 1 *Define the following abbreviations.*

1. HIV ______
2. AIDS ______
3. CBC ______
4. WBC ______
5. RBC ______
6. Hgb ______
7. PLT ______
8. INR ______
9. AML ______
10. BMT ______
11. CML ______
12. LAD ______
13. IV ______

EXERCISE 2 *Give the abbreviations for the following definitions.*

1. acute lymphoblastic leukemia ______
2. disseminated intravascular coagulopathy ______
3. erythrocyte sedimentation rate ______
4. hemolytic uremic syndrome ______
5. prothrombin time ______
6. partial thromboplastin time ______
7. idiopathic thrombocytopenic purpura ______
8. thrombotic thrombocytopenic purpura ______
9. intravenous immunoglobulin ______
10. hepatosplenomegaly ______
11. hematocrit ______
12. Epstein-Barr virus ______

EXERCISE 3 *Multiple-choice questions. Select the correct answer(s).*

1. Both AIDS and HIV have to do with the:
   a. blood count
   b. bone marrow
   c. immune system
   d. leukemia
   e. none of these
2. BMT is:
   a. blood microcytosis time
   b. blood microcytosis transplant
   c. bone marrow time
   d. bone marrow transplant
   e. none of these
3. PLT is:
   a. partial leukocyte time
   b. platelet count
   c. prothrombin time
   d. thrombocytopenic purpura
   e. none of these
4. HUS, *hemolytic uremic syndrome,* comes from the roots:
   a. *hemo:* blood + *lytic:* breakdown agent + *ur:* urine + *emia:* blood condition
   b. *hemo:* blood + *lytic:* clotting agent + *ur:* urine + *emia:* blood deficiency

Learning Outcome 8.6 Exercises

c. *hemo:* liver + *lytic:* breakdown agent + *ur:* urine + *emia:* blood condition

d. *hemo:* liver + *lytic:* clotting agent + *ur:* urine + *emia:* blood deficiency

e. *hemo:* spleen + *lytic:* clotting agent + *ur:* urine + *emia:* blood deficiency

5. A person with HSM has:
   a. a hardened and enlarged spleen
   b. a hardened liver and spleen
   c. a small and hardened spleen
   d. a small liver and spleen
   e. an enlarged liver and spleen

6. A person with LAD has:
   a. any disease of a lymph gland (node)
   b. lymphadenopathy
   c. noticeably swollen lymph nodes, especially in the neck
   d. all of these
   e. none of these

7. Select the abbreviations below that pertain to leukemia.
   a. ALL
   b. ALT
   c. AML
   d. CML
   e. ITP
   f. PT
   g. PTT
   h. TTP

8. Select the abbreviations below that pertain to blood counts.
   a. BMT
   b. CBC
   c. ESR
   d. Hct
   e. Hgb
   f. RBC
   g. WBC

9. Select the abbreviations below that pertain to red blood cells.
   a. BMT
   b. CBC
   c. ESR
   d. Hct
   e. Hgb
   f. RBC
   g. WBC

8.7 Electronic Health Records

Heme/Onc Clinic

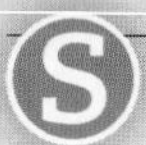

Subjective

Jerry is a 4-year-old male sent to our clinic for evaluation of ostealgia. He has had a 1-month history of intermittent pain in his distal left femur. He also been febrile on and off for the past month and had night sweats. He denies weight loss, weakness, or limping. No other extremities are hurting him.

ROS: No shortness of breath, no chest pain; no headaches; no arthralgias; no new rashes; no gastrointestinal complaints.

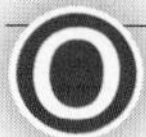

Objective

Physical Exam

RR: 20; HR: 88; Temp: 100; BP: 80/60.

Gen: WDWN, active, playful 4-year-old boy in NAD. AOx3.

HEENT: NCAT. PERRLA. White sclera. No conjunctival injection. Mucous membranes moist and pink. Normal dentition.

Neck: Supple. No **LAD**.

Resp: CTAB without wheezes, rales, or rhonchi; no retractions. Good air exchange.

CV: RRR without murmurs.

Abd: Soft, nontender, nondistended. Mild **hepatosplenomegaly**. No masses.

Neuro: CN II-XII grossly intact. No focal neurologic deficit.

Ext: Distal left femur has mild edema and is tender to palpation. No erythema, warmth, or induration. Multiple palpable inguinal lymph nodes on the left.

Skin: Scattered **petechiae** generalized over body, both above and below the midchest.

Genitalia: SMR I (*a develeopmental staging term*) male testes descended bilaterally.

Laboratory Data: **WBC**: 6,200 (20 neutrophils, 2 bands (*immature neutrophils*), 10 **lymphocytes**, 1 monocyte, 67 lymphoblasts); **hemoglobin** 10.1, hematocrit 30.6, **platelet** count 54,000.

Assessment

4-year-old male with **anemia**, **leukopenia**, and **thrombocytopenia**. The lymphoblasts on the peripheral blood smear indicate an **acute lymphoblastic leukemia.**

Plan

1. We will schedule him for a diagnostic bone marrow aspirate and biopsy.
2. Lumbar puncture to rule out CNS involvement.
3. Abdominal CT to evaluate for nodes.

–Rodger Dodger, PA

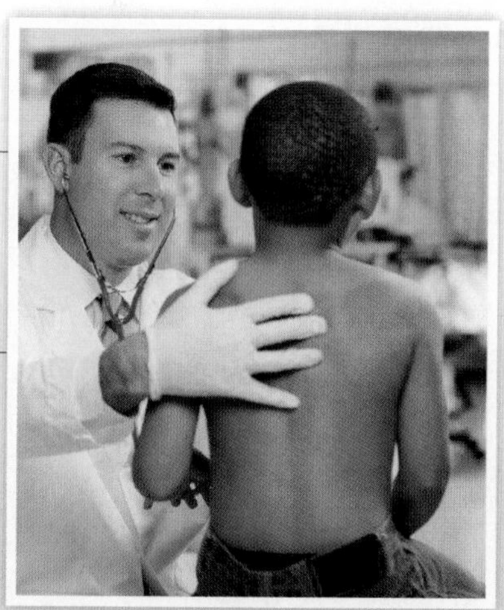

©db2stock/Getty Images RF

Learning Outcome 8.7 Exercises

EXERCISE 1 *Match the term on the left with its definition on the right.*

_____ 1. anemia

_____ 2. hemoglobin

_____ 3. leukopenia

_____ 4. thrombocytopenia

_____ 5. hepatosplenomegaly

a. deficiency in the number of platelets (clot cells)

b. deficiency in white blood cells

c. enlargement of the liver and spleen

d. reduction of red blood cells noticed by the patient by weakness and fatigue

e. the iron-containing pigment in red blood cells that carries oxygen to the cells

EXERCISE 2 *Fill in the blanks.*

1. Using the data recorded at the patient's physical examination, fill in the following blanks.
   a. The patient's temperature: _____
   b. The patient's heart rate: _____
   c. The patient's respiratory rate: _____
   d. The patient's blood pressure: _____
   e. WDWN (_____) active playful 4-year-old boy in NAD (_____).
   f. HEENT: NCAT (_____).
   g. Neck: no LAD (define abbreviation: _____).
   h. CV: _____ (regular rate and rhythm).
2. Using the patient's laboratory data, fill in the following blanks.
   a. WBC (_____): 6,200
   b. 10 *lymphocytes* (give definition: _____)
   c. *hemoglobin* (give definition: _____) 10.1
   d. Hct (define abbreviation: _____) 30.6
   e. Platelet count (give abbreviation: _____) 54,000

EXERCISE 3 *True or false questions. Indicate true answers with a T and false answers with an F.*

1. The patient has had intermittent pain in his *distal* (farther away from the center) left femur. _____
2. The patient has not had a fever. _____
3. The patient has lymphadenopathy in his neck. _____
4. Several of the patient's left lymph nodes are *palpable* (large enough to feel). _____
5. A neutrophil is a type of white blood cell. _____
6. The patient's blood smear indicated an ALL. _____
7. The patient does not need to have a Bx. _____

Learning Outcome 8.7 Exercises

EXERCISE 4 *Multiple-choice questions. Select the correct answer.*

1. The health care professional noticed the patient had *hepatosplenomegaly,* which is a(n):
   a. enlarged spleen and liver
   b. small spleen and liver
   c. displaced spleen and liver
   d. none of these

2. Which of the following is *not* included in the patient's assessment?
   a. reduction of red blood cells
   b. deficiency in white blood cells
   c. deficiency in clotting cells
   d. decreased blood volume

3. The patient's blood smear indicated an *acute lymphoblastic leukemia,* which is:
   a. a cancer of the blood or bone marrow characterized by the abnormal increase in white blood cells, specifically lymphoblasts, that started recently
   b. a cancer of the blood or bone marrow characterized by the abnormal increase in white blood cells, specifically lymphoblasts, that has been going on for a while now
   c. a cancer of the blood or bone marrow characterized by the abnormal increase in red blood cells, specifically lymphoblasts, that started recently
   d. a cancer of the blood or bone marrow characterized by the abnormal increase in red blood cells, specifically lymphoblasts, that has been going on for a while now

4. Which of the following is *not* part of the patient's plan for treatment?
   a. abdominal computer axial tomography
   b. Bx
   c. LP to rule out central nervous system involvement
   d. PTT to determine if there is an additional bleeding disorder

Hospital Progress Note

Subjective

Mrs. Campos was admitted last night for fever and elevated **WBC**. Initial blood culture is coming back positive from gram-positive cocci. She has been on antibiotics for 10 hours now. Last night, the nurses noted hemorrhages. She has noticed **hematuria**, **hemoptysis**, and a bloody nose. In addition, she developed painful swelling in her right calf. She remains febrile, but the fever is improving since admission. She is still very tired. She denies vomiting.

Objective

RR: 18; HR: 70; Temp 101.2; BP: 102/74.

General: Sleeping. Tired but responsive to questions.

HEENT: NCAT, dried bloody crusts in nostrils, mucous membranes moist and pink; PERRLA, EOMI, conjunctivae clear.

Neck: Supple, no **adenopathy,** no JVD.

Resp: No increased effort, clear breath sounds.

CV: Regular, S1, S2, no murmur/rub; pedal pulses 2+ .

Abd: Soft, nontender, nondistended, normoactive bowel sounds, no **HSM.**

Lymph: No enlarged cervical, axillary, or inguinal lymph nodes.

Skin: Scattered **petechiae,** CR 2 seconds.

Ext: Right swelling with tender subcutaneous nodule.

Neuro: Alert and oriented, CN II-XII grossly intact, normal and symmetric strength in UEs and LEs, DTRs 2+ and symmetric.

Labs

Total bilirubin: 6.2

Hgb: 9.2; **WBC:** 20.2; **PLT:** 24.

PT and **PTT** both elevated.

Microangiopathic hemolysis seen on peripheral smear.

Assessment/Plan

1. **Septicemia:** Fever down slightly and WBC decreased from 25.4 to 20.2. Continue current IV antibiotics.
2. **Anemia/Coagulopathy/Thrombocytopenia:** Clinically consistent with **DIC.** We will transfuse a unit of platelets and follow labs in 6 hours.
3. **Calf swelling:** Suspect superficial **thromboembolism.** We will consult hematology/oncology in regard to their opinion on beginning **anticoagulant** medicine.
4. **Hyperbilirubinemia:** I suspect the etiology is liver dysfunction from DIC. Follow labs in the AM.

–Linda Lovegood, MD

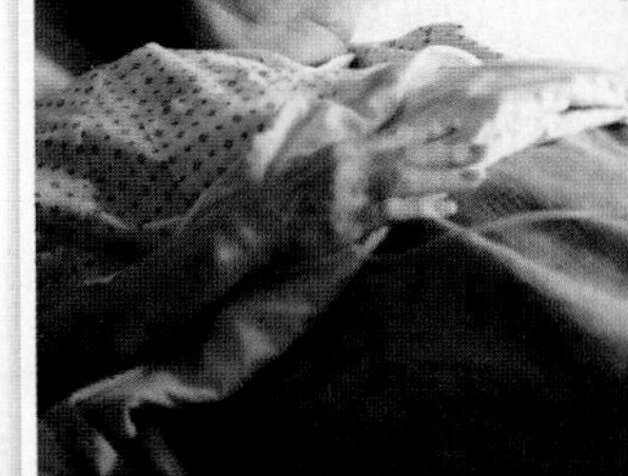

©Rubberball/Nicole Hill/Getty Images RF

Learning Outcome 8.7 Exercises

EXERCISE 5 *Match the term on the left with its definition on the right.*

Term	Definition
_____ 1. anemia	a. a blockage of a vessel (embolism) caused by a clot that has broken off from where it formed
_____ 2. transfusion	b. a drug that prevents the coagulation of blood
_____ 3. hematology	c. any disease that deals with problems in blood coagulation
_____ 4. hemorrhage	d. breakdown of blood cells
_____ 5. hemolysis	e. deficiency in the number of platelets (clot cells)
_____ 6. anticoagulant	f. enlargement of the spleen and liver
_____ 7. coagulopathy	g. excessive bilirubin in the blood
_____ 8. hyperbilirubinemia	h. excessive blood loss
_____ 9. septicemia	i. reduction of red blood cells noticed by the patient by weakness and fatigue
_____ 10. thrombocytopenia	j. the infusion into a patient of blood from another source
_____ 11. hepatosplenomegaly	k. the presence of disease-causing microorganisms in the blood
_____ 12. thromboembolism	l. the study of the blood

EXERCISE 6 *Fill in the blanks.*

1. Using the data recorded at the patient's physical examination, fill in the following blanks.
   a. The patient's temperature: ______________________
   b. The patient's heart rate: ______________________
   c. The patient's respiratory rate: ______________________
   d. The patient's blood pressure: ______________________
   e. HEENT (______________): NCAT. ______________ (pupils equal, round, and reactive to light and accommodation).
   f. Abdomen: no HSM (give definition for abbreviation: ______________________)
2. Using the patient's laboratory data, fill in the following blanks.
   a. Hemoglobin: ______________________
   b. White blood count: ______________________
   c. Platelet count: ______________________
3. According to the physician's assessment/plan:
   a. *septicemia* (give definition: ______________); WBC (give definition for abbreviation: ______________) decreased from 25.4 to 20.2.
   b. ______________ (decreased red blood cells)/ ______________ (any disease that deals with problems in blood coagulation)/ ______________ (deficiency in the number of platelets): clinically consistent with DIC (give definition for abbreviation: ______________).
   c. For suspected ______________ (a blockage of a vessel [embolism] caused by a clot that has broken off from where it formed), the hematology/oncology department will be consulted before beginning *anticoagulants* (give definition: ______________).

Learning Outcome 8.7 Exercises

EXERCISE 7 *True or false questions. Indicate true answers with a T and false answers with an F.*

1. The patient was admitted for an elevated red blood count. ____________
2. Upon admission, the patient was afebrile. ____________
3. The patient's spleen and liver are enlarged. ____________
4. The patient's prothrombin time and partial thromboplastin time are elevated. ____________
5. The patient will receive blood and/or blood components from another source. ____________
6. The patient has increased bilirubin in the blood. ____________

EXERCISE 8 *Multiple-choice questions. Select the correct answer.*

1. The patient has *hematuria,* which is:
   a. blood in the urine
   b. a condition of the liver and blood
   c. decreased blood volume
   d. none of these
2. The patient had *hemoptysis,* which comes from the root *ptysis,* which means "cough," and *hemo,* which means:
   a. blood
   b. bone marrow
   c. liver
   d. lymph system
3. The patient's peripheral blood smear revealed *microangiopathic hemolysis.* The term *microangiopathic* refers to a disease of the small blood vessels. The term *hemolysis* refers to:
   a. breakdown of blood cells
   b. breakdown of clotting cells
   c. creation of blood cells
   d. creation of clotting cells
4. The patient has *hyperbilirubinemia,* which is:
   a. excessive bilirubin in the blood
   b. excessive red bile in the blood
   c. excessive bilirubin in the blood and excessive red bile in the blood
   d. none of these

Hospital Consult

Subjective

Reason for Consult: I was asked to see this 8-year-old boy to evaluate his **anemia.**

History of Present Illness: Billy Caspar presented initially to his primary care provider with decreased energy and **pallor.** He had recently had rash on his hands and a fever, both of which have improved over the past few days. A **hematocrit** was performed in the office and it was critically low. In addition, the patient had a flow murmur and appeared lethargic. He was sent to the hospital for admission. He was **transfused** with two units of **prbcs** and **hematology** was consulted.

Past Medical History: Term delivery. Normal newborn screen. Specifically, no **hemoglobinopathy** on screen. Normal development.

Past Surgical History: None.

Family History: Father with **hereditary spherocytosis.**

Medications: Daily vitamin.

Objective

Exam

Temp: 99.4; Heart Rate: 100; Respiratory Rate: 22; Blood Pressure: 88/64; Pulse Ox 98%.

General: Tired, pale young man in no acute distress.

HEENT: PERRLA. Pale palpebral conjunctiva. Pale, dry mucous membranes. Normal dentition.

Neck: Supple. No **LAD.**

CV: Mild tachycardia and soft systolic flow murmur. No gallop or rub.

Resp: CTA.

Abd: Soft, nontender, nondistended. **Splenomegaly:** spleen tip palpates three finger breadths below ribs. No hepatomegaly.

Ext: Cool to touch. No cyanosis, clubbing (*enlarged finger tips from respiratory disease*), or edema. Delayed capillary refill.

Laboratory Data

CBC: **Normocytic anemia. Reticulocytosis.**

BMP: **Hyperbilirubinemia.**

Smear: **Poikilocytosis.**

Assessment

Billy clearly has a **hemolytic anemia** that is consistent with hereditary spherocytosis. I believe that, given his sudden and severe presentation along with his recent illness, he has **aplastic** crisis. This is likely brought on from infection from the parvo B19 virus. His flow murmur and slow cap refill are concerning for continued **hypovolemia.**

Recommendation

Billy needs another **transfusion** immediately. I have already ordered this. Once his anemia is stabilized, I think he should be seen by surgery to assess for a **splenectomy.** If he does get a splenectomy, he will, of course, need a pneumococcus **vaccine,** as he will be partially **immunocompromised** due to **asplenia.**

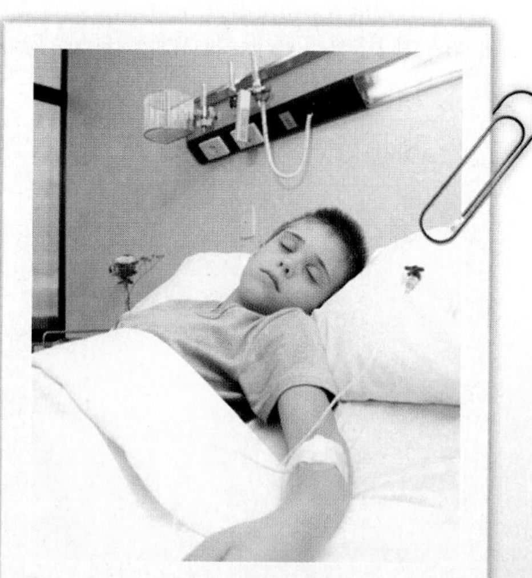

©PhotoAlto Agency RF Collection/Laurence Mouton/Getty Images RF

Thank you for this interesting consult. I will continue to follow up on a daily basis.

–Red Barnes, MD

Learning Outcome 8.7 Exercises

EXERCISE 9 *Match the term on the left with its definition on the right.*

	Term		Definition
______	1. hematology	a.	a condition characterized by red blood cells in a variety of shapes
______	2. anemia	b.	a disease of the hemoglobin
______	3. immunocompromised	c.	a normal-sized red blood cell
______	4. transfusion	d.	condition in which red blood cells assume a spherical shape
______	5. normocyte	e.	absence of a spleen or of spleen function
______	6. hypovolemia	f.	an immature red blood cell (netlike appearance)
______	7. hyperbilirubinemia	g.	anemia caused by the destruction of red blood cells
______	8. hemolytic anemia	h.	decreased blood volume
______	9. splenomegaly	i.	enlargement of the spleen
______	10. splenectomy	j.	excessive bilirubin in the blood
______	11. hemoglobinopathy	k.	having an immune system incapable of responding normally and completely to a pathogen or disease
______	12. spherocytosis	l.	reduction of red blood cells noticed by the patient as weakness and fatigue
______	13. asplenia	m.	study of the blood
______	14. reticulocyte	n.	surgical removal of the spleen
______	15. poikilocytosis	o.	the infusion into a patient of blood from another source

EXERCISE 10 *Fill in the blanks.*

1. The reason for the consult was to evaluate Billy's *anemia* (give definition: ______________________________).
2. According to Billy's past medical history, he did not have ______________________________ (disease of the hemoglobin).
3. Billy's family has a history of *spherocytosis* (give definition: ______________________________).
4. Using the data recorded at Billy's physical examination, fill in the following blanks.
   a. Temp: ______________________________
   b. HR: ______________________________
   c. RR: ______________________________
   d. BP: ______________________________
   e. Neck: no ______________________________ (lymphadenopathy)
   f. Abdomen: ______________________________ (enlarged spleen)
5. Using Billy's laboratory data, fill in the following blanks.
   a. CBC (define abbreviation: ______________________________): *normocytic anemia, reticulocytosis* (condition of the ______________________________ red blood cells).

b. BMP: *hyperbilirubinemia* (give definition: ________________________).

c. Smear: *poikilocytosis* (condition characterized by ________________________ blood cells in a variety of ________________________).

EXERCISE 11 *True or false questions. Indicate true answers with a T and false answers with an F.*

1. An Hct was performed in the office. ________________
2. Billy needs to be given more blood from an outside source. ________________
3. Billy's spleen does not need to be removed. ________________
4. Without a spleen, Billy's immune system will not be compromised. ________________

EXERCISE 12 *Multiple-choice questions. Select the correct answer(s).*

1. Billy has been assessed with *hemolytic anemia,* which is:
   a. anemia caused by red blood cells not being formed in sufficient quantities
   b. anemia caused by the destruction of red blood cells
   c. anemia caused by the destruction of white blood cells
   d. anemia caused by white blood cells not being formed in sufficient quantities
2. The term *normocytic anemia* refers to an anemia of the *normocytes,* which are:
   a. clotting cells
   b. red blood cells
   c. white blood cells
   d. none of these
3. Bilirubin is: (select all that apply)
   a. a substance derived from red blood cells that have completed their life span
   b. a substance derived from white blood cells that have completed their life span
   c. also known as red bile
   d. also known as white bile
   e. normally found in the blood
   f. normally found in the digestive tract
   g. secreted by the liver
   h. secreted by the spleen

Additional exercises available in connect®

Chapter Review exercises, along with additional practice items, are available in Connect!

Quick Reference

quick reference glossary of roots

Root	Definition	Root	Definition
coagul/o	coagulation	**-penia**	deficiency
cyt/o	cell	**phleb/o**	vein
-emia	blood condition	**splen/o**	spleen
hem/o, hemat/o	blood	**thromb/o**	clot
immun/o	immune system	**thym/o**	thymus
leuk/o	white	**tonsill/o**	tonsils
lymph/o	lymph	**ven/o**	vein
myel/o	bone marrow		

quick reference glossary of terms

Term	Definition
anemia	reduction of red blood cells noticed by the patient as weakness and fatigue
anisocytosis	condition characterized by a great inequality in the size of red blood cells
antibody	substance produced by the body in response to an antigen
anticoagulant	drug that prevents the coagulation of blood
antigen	substance that causes the body to produce antibodies
apheresis	general term for a process, similar to dialysis, that draws blood, removes something from it, then returns the rest of the blood to the patient
aplastic anemia	anemia caused by red blood cells not being formed in sufficient quantities
asplenia	absence of a spleen or of spleen function
autoimmune disease	a disease caused by the body's immune system attacking the body's own healthy tissue
bilirubinemia	the presence of bilirubin (red bile; a substance derived from red blood cells that have completed their life span) in the blood
coagulopathy	any disease that deals with problems in blood coagulation
cytapheresis	apheresis to remove cellular material
deep vein thrombosis	the formation of a blood clot in a vein deep in the body, most commonly the leg
ecchymosis	large bruise
elliptocyte	oval-shaped red blood cell
elliptocytosis	condition characterized by an increase in the number of oval-shaped red blood cells
embolism	blockage in a blood vessel caused by an embolus

quick reference glossary of terms *continued*

Term	Definition
embolus	mass of matter present in the blood
erythrocyte	red blood cell
erythrocytosis	abnormal increase in the number of red blood cells
hematocrit	test to judge or separate the blood; used to determine the ratio of red blood cells to total blood volume
hematology	study of the blood
hematoma	mass of blood within an organ, cavity, or tissue
hematopoiesis	formation of blood cells
hemoglobin	iron-containing pigment in red blood cells that carries oxygen to the cells
hemoglobinopathy	disease of the hemoglobin
hemolysis	breakdown of blood cells
hemolytic anemia	anemia caused by the destruction of red blood cells
hemophilia	condition in which the blood doesn't clot, thus causing excessive bleeding
hemorrhage	excessive blood loss
hemostatic	drug that stops the flow of blood
hepatosplenitis	inflammation of the liver and spleen
hepatosplenomegaly	enlargement of the liver and spleen
hyperbilirubinemia	excessive bilirubin in the blood
hypercholesterolemia	excessive cholesterol in the blood
hypercoagulability	increased ability of the blood to coagulate
hyperlipidemia	excessive fat in the blood
hypersplenism	increased spleen activity
hypervolemia	increased blood volume
hypoperfusion	inadequate flow of blood
hypovolemia	decreased blood volume
immunocompromised	having an immune system incapable of responding normally and completely to a pathogen or disease
immunodeficiency	immune system with decreased or compromised response to disease-causing organisms
immunoglobulin	protein that provides protection (immunity) against disease
immunologist	specialist in the immune system
immunology	study of the immune system
immunosuppression	reduction in the activity of the body's immune system
iron deficiency anemia	anemia caused by inadequate iron intake

quick reference glossary of terms *continued*

Term	Definition
ischemia	blockage of blood flow to an organ
laparosplenectomy	surgical removal of the spleen through the abdomen
leukemia	cancer of the blood or bone marrow characterized by the abnormal increase in white blood cells
leukocyte	white blood cell
leukocytosis	increase in the number of white blood cells
leukopenia	deficiency in white blood cells
lymphadenectomy	surgical removal of a lymph gland (node)
lymphadenitis	inflammation of a lymph gland (node)
lymphadenopathy	any disease of a lymph gland (node); used to refer to noticeably swollen lymph nodes, especially in the neck
lymphadenotomy	incision into a lymph gland (node)
lymphangiectasia	dilation of a lymph vessel, normally noticed by swelling in the extremities
lymphangiogram	record of the study of lymph vessels
lymphangiography	procedure to study the lymph vessels
lymphangitis	inflammation of the lymph vessels
lymphedema	swelling caused by abnormal accumulation of lymph
lymphocyte	lymph cell
lymphoma	tumor originating in lymphocytes
lymphopenia	abnormal deficiency in lymph
macrocytosis	condition characterized by large red blood cells
microcytosis	condition characterized by small red blood cells
myelodysplasia	disease characterized by poor production of blood cells by the bone marrow
myeloma	cancerous tumor of the bone marrow
myelopoiesis	formation of bone marrow
nephrosplenopexy	surgical fixation of the spleen and a kidney
neutropenia	deficiency in neutrophil
normocyte	normal-sized red blood cell
oligocythemia	deficiency in the number of red blood cells
osteomyelitis	inflammation of bone and bone marrow
pancytopenia	deficiency in all cellular components of the blood
perfusion	circulation of blood through tissue
petechia	small bruise

quick reference glossary of terms *continued*

Term	Definition
phagocytosis	process in which phagocytes (a type of white blood cell) destroy (or eat) foreign microorganisms or cell debris
phlebarteriectasia	dilation of blood vessels
phlebology	study of veins
phlebotomist	specialist in drawing blood
phlebotomy	incision into a vein (another name for drawing blood)
plasmapheresis	apheresis to remove plasma
plateletpheresis	apheresis to remove platelets (for the purpose of donating them to patients in need of platelets)
poikilocytosis	condition characterized by red blood cells in a variety of shapes
polycythemia	excess of red blood cells
reperfusion injury	injury to tissue that occurs after blood flow is restored
reticulocyte	immature red blood cell
septicemia	presence of disease-causing microorganisms in the blood
spherocyte	red blood cell that assumes a spherical shape
spherocytosis	condition in which red blood cells assume a spherical shape
sphygmomanometer	fancy name for the device used to measure blood pressure
splenalgia	pain in the spleen
splenectomy	surgical removal of the spleen
splenectopy	displacement of the spleen, sometimes called *floating spleen*
splenitis	inflammation of the spleen
splenodynia	pain in the spleen
splenolysis	breakdown (destruction) of spleen tissue
splenomalacia	softening of the spleen
splenomegaly	enlargement of the spleen
splenopathy	any disease of the spleen
splenoptosis	downward displacement (drooping) of the spleen
splenorrhexis	rupture of the spleen
thrombocyte	cell that helps blood clot (also known as a platelet)
thrombocytopenia	deficiency in the number of platelets (clot cells)
thrombocytosis	increase in the number of platelets (clot cells)
thromboembolism	blockage of a vessel (embolism) caused by a clot that has broken off from where it formed
thrombogenic	capable of producing a blood clot

quick reference glossary of terms *continued*

Term	Definition
thrombolytic	drug that breaks down blood clots
thrombophlebitis	inflammation of a vein caused by a clot
thrombosis	formation of a blood clot
thrombus	blood clot
thymectomy	surgical removal of the thymus
thymic hyperplasia	overdevelopment of the thymus
thymoma	tumor of the thymus
thymopathy	disease of the thymus
tonsillectomy	surgical removal of a tonsil
tonsillitis	inflammation of a tonsil
transfusion	infusion into a patient of blood from another source
uremia	presence of urine in the blood

review of terms by roots

Root	Term(s)	
coagul/o	anticoagulant	hypercoagulability
	coagulopathy	
cyt/o	anisocytosis	oligocythemia
	cytapheresis	pancytopenia
	elliptocyte	phagocytosis
	elliptocytosis	poikilocytosis
	erythrocyte	polycythemia
	erythrocytosis	reticulocyte
	leukocyte	spherocyte
	leukocytosis	spherocytosis
	lymphocyte	thrombocyte
	macrocytosis	thrombocytopenia
	microcytosis	thrombocytosis
	normocyte	

review of terms by roots *continued*

Root	Term(s)	
-emia	anemia	hypovolemia
	aplastic anemia	iron deficiency anemia
	bilirubinemia	ischemia
	hemolytic anemia	leukemia
	hyperbilirubinemia	oligocythemia
	hypercholesterolemia	polycythemia
	hyperlipidemia	septicemia
	hypervolemia	uremia
hem/o, hemat/o	hematocrit	hemolysis
	hematology	hemolytic anemia
	hematoma	hemophilia
	hematopoiesis	hemorrhage
	hemoglobin	hemostatic
	hemoglobinopathy	
immun/o	autoimmune disease	immunologist
	immunocompromised	immunology
	immunodeficiency	immunosuppression
	immunoglobulin	
leuk/o	leukemia	leukocytosis
	leukocyte	leukopenia
lymph/o	lymphadenectomy	lymphangiography
	lymphadenitis	lymphangitis
	lymphadenopathy	lymphedema
	lymphadenotomy	lymphocyte
	lymphangiectasia	lymphoma
	lymphangiogram	lymphopenia
myel/o	myelodysplasia	myelopoiesis
	myeloma	osteomyelitis
-penia	leukopenia	pancytopenia
	lymphopenia	thrombocytopenia
	neutropenia	
phleb/o	phlebarteriectasia	phlebotomy
	phlebology	thrombophlebitis
	phlebotomist	

review of terms by roots *continued*

Root	Term(s)	
splen/o	asplenia	splenitis
	hepatosplenitis	splenodynia
	hepatosplenomegaly	splenolysis
	hypersplenism	splenomalacia
	laparosplenectomy	splenomegaly
	nephrosplenopexy	splenopathy
	splenalgia	splenoptosis
	splenectomy	splenorrhexis
	splenectopy	
thromb/o	deep vein thrombosis	thrombogenic
	thrombocyte	thrombolytic
	thrombocytopenia	thrombophlebitis
	thrombocytosis	thrombosis
	thromboembolism	thrombus
thym/o	thymectomy	thymoma
	thymic hyperplasia	thymopathy
tonsill/o	tonsillectomy	
	tonsillitis	

other terms

antibody	perfusion
antigen	petechia
apheresis	plasmapheresis
ecchymosis	plateletpheresis
embolism	reperfusion injury
embolus	sphygmomanometer
hypoperfusion	transfusion

The Cardiovascular System—Cardiology 9

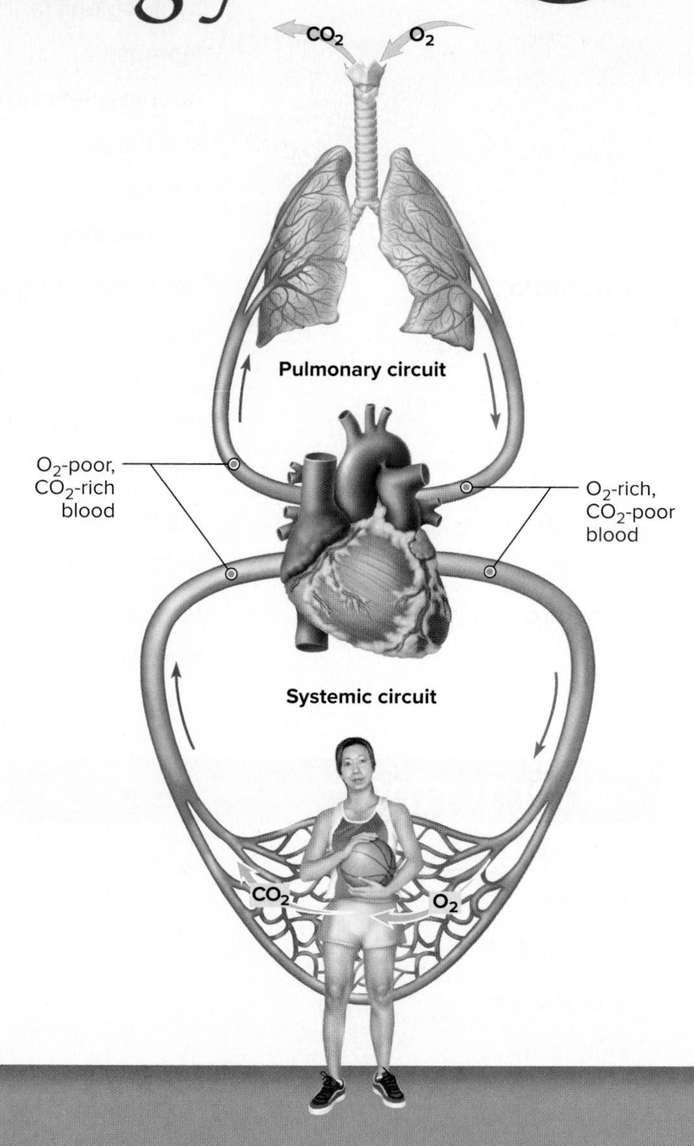

Introduction and Overview of the Cardiovascular System

Imagine a large city without roads or transportation of any type. There would be no way for food to get to stores, no access for emergency services to get to people in need of rescue, and no means for trash to be collected. It wouldn't take long for the city to fall into chaos.

The body is much the same. It needs a system to continually deliver fresh supplies to the cells of the body and remove waste. The body also needs a means to deliver chemical messages from one part of the body to another. The cardiovascular system is the body's transport system that provides nourishment, cleanup services, and communication.

There are two parts to the cardiovascular system: the *cardio* (heart) and the *vascular* (blood vessels). The heart is a big pump that squeezes blood out to the body, and the vessels are the tubes that carry the blood. Together, they transport all manner of essential nutrients, blood cells, and chemical signals. They also work together to help rid the body of waste.

learning outcomes

Upon completion of this chapter, you will be able to:

9.1 Identify the **roots/word parts** associated with the **cardiovascular system.**

S **9.2** Translate the **Subjective** terms associated with the **cardiovascular system.**

O **9.3** Translate the **Objective** terms associated with the **cardiovascular system.**

A **9.4** Translate the **Assessment** terms associated with the **cardiovascular system.**

P **9.5** Translate the **Plan** terms associated with the **cardiovascular system.**

9.6 Use **abbreviations** associated with the **cardiovascular system.**

9.7 Distinguish terms associated with the **cardiovascular system** in the context of **electronic health records.**

9.1 Word Parts of the Cardiovascular System

Heart

The heart is the workhorse of this critical transport system. It constantly pumps, getting blood moving to where it needs to go. The heart is divided into four "rooms," or chambers: the left and right receiving rooms (*atria*) and the left and right sending rooms (*ventricles*).

The left side of the heart handles oxygen-rich blood, and the right side handles the oxygen-poor blood. A thick wall of muscle, the *septum,* divides the left and right sides.

Blood constantly cycles between the body and the heart, and it collects in the atria. Blood that has nourished the body and is ready to go to the lungs for more oxygen collects in the right atrium. After getting a fresh supply of oxygen, blood returns to the heart via the left atrium. From the atria, blood—on both sides—passes through the one-way doors of the valves into the ventricles.

In a normal heart, there is no blood flow between the left and right side. There are connections between the atria and ventricles, and between the ventricles and the blood vessels. The connection between each atrium and ventricle is a valve that allows blood to flow in one direction. On the left side, the *mitral valve* connects the left atrium and ventricle. Then the *aortic valve* connects the left ventricle to the outgoing blood vessel, the *aorta.*

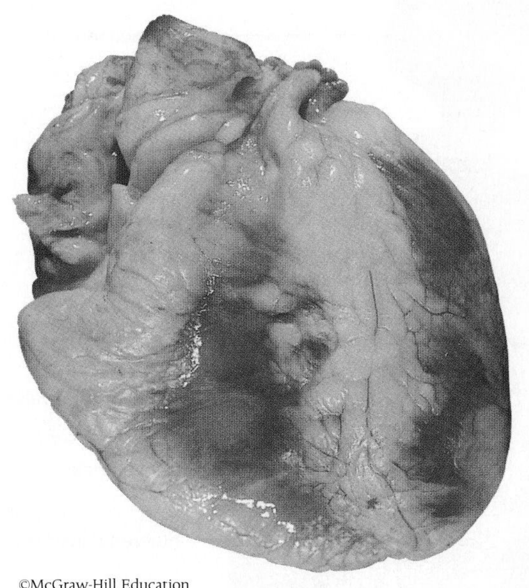

valve

ROOT: ***valvul/o***

EXAMPLES: valvulotomy, valvulitis

NOTES: The heart has four valves: two atrioventricular valves and two valves between the ventricles and arteries. The purpose of heart valves is to prevent blood from flowing backward.

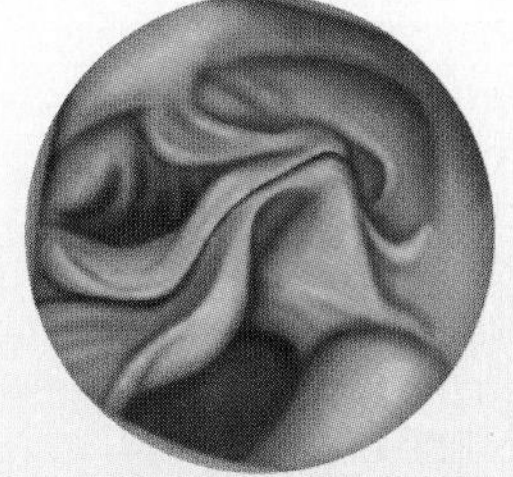

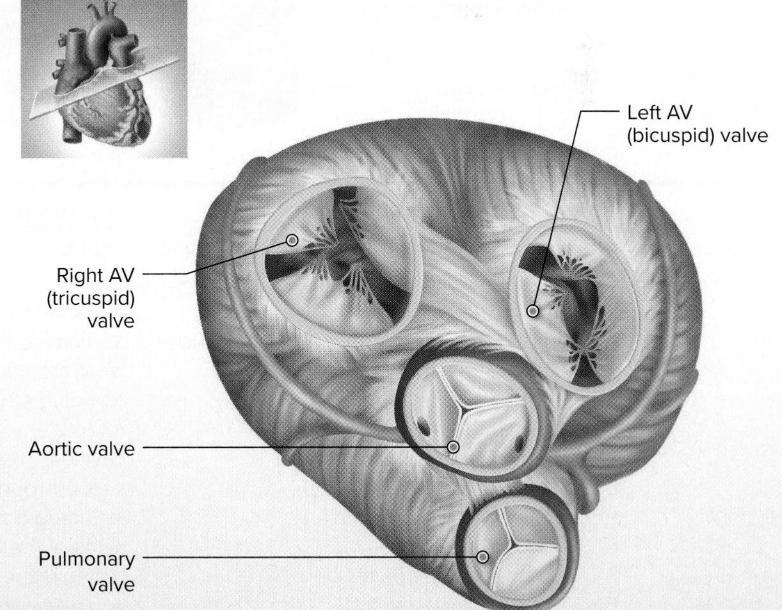

On the right side, the connector between the atrium and ventricle is the *tricuspid valve*. The *pulmonary valve* connects the right ventricle and the outgoing blood vessel, the *pulmonary artery*.

Ventricles are strong and muscular. When the heart compresses, the ventricles force the blood out into the outgoing blood vessels (*arteries*). The right ventricle sends blood to the lungs to get fresh oxygen and to discard excess carbon dioxide. The fresh blood is sent out from the heart by the left ventricle to the rest of the body to provide oxygen and collect the body's carbon dioxide waste.

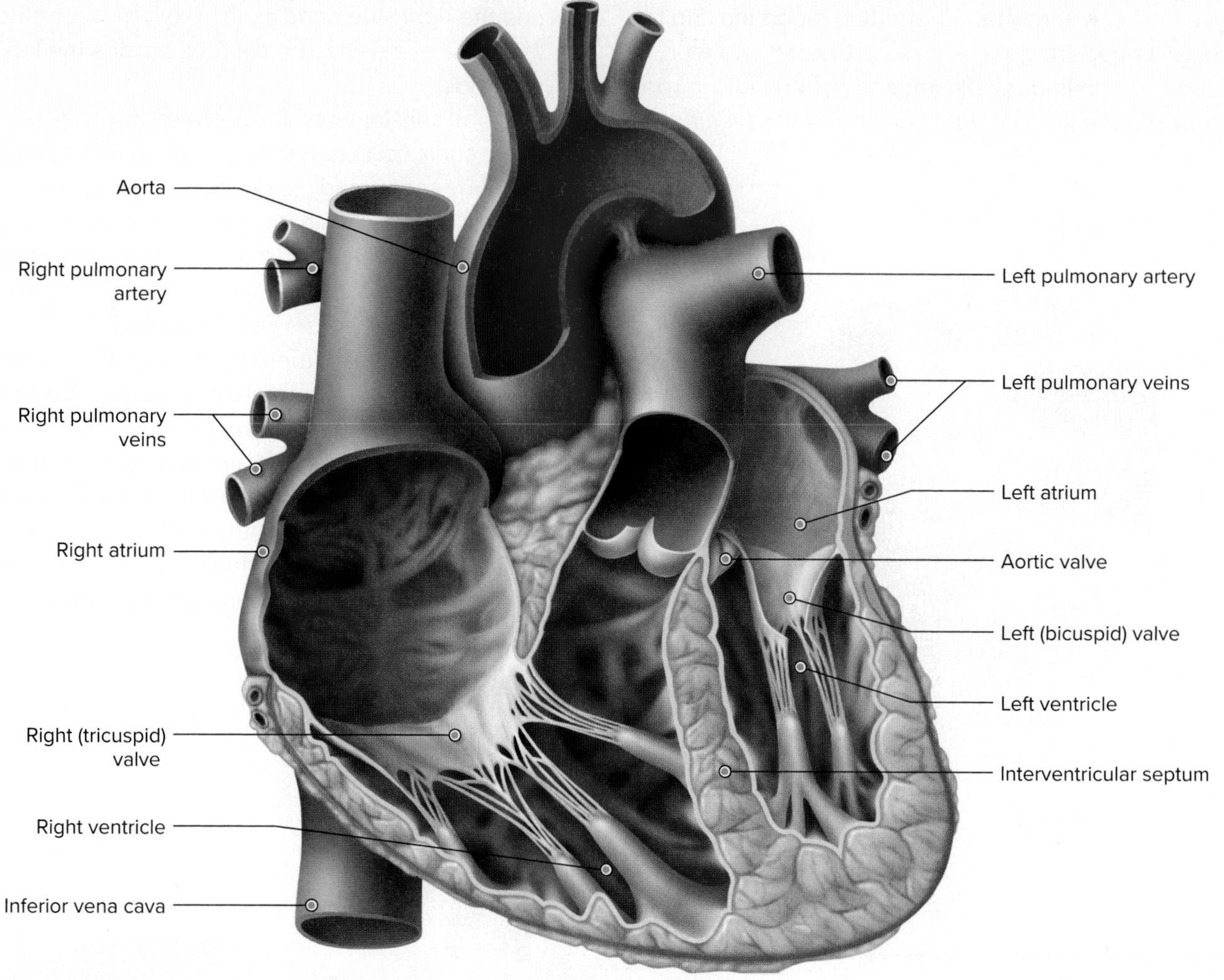

atrium (upper chamber)

ROOT: ***atri/o***

EXAMPLES: atrium, atrial fibrillation

NOTES: The *atrium* is the upper portion of each side of the heart. The term comes from Roman architecture, where it referred to the large open area that was characteristic of most Roman houses; typically, all the other rooms of the house would branch off from this center space. Even today, a large central area in a building is often called its *atrium*.

septum (plural: septa)

ROOT: ***sept/o***

EXAMPLES: atrial septal defect, septoplasty

NOTES: *Septum* comes from a Latin word meaning "partition" or "dividing structure" and can refer to any wall dividing two cavities. There are numerous septa throughout the body, including between the two sides of the heart. The easiest to find is the nasal septum. If you place an index finger in each nostril and try to make them touch, what you are feeling is the nasal septum. If you find that your nasal septum leans to one side, you have a deviated septum.

ventricle (lower chamber)

ROOT: ***ventricul/o***

EXAMPLE: ventriculotomy

NOTES: The ventricle is the lower portion of each side of the heart. The word is a combination of *venter* (stomach) plus the diminutive suffix *-icle*, and means "little stomach."

heart

ROOT: ***cardi/o***

EXAMPLES: cardiology, cardiac arrest, myocarditis

NOTES: The root *cardio* can be tricky because it ends in the double vowel *io*. You expect the *o* to go away sometimes, but when a suffix beginning with an *i* is added to this root, not just the *o*, but also an *i* disappears as well. For example: *myo* (muscle) + *cardio* (heart) + *itis* (inflammation) = myocard-*I*-itis.

heart

ROOT: ***coron/o***

EXAMPLES: coronary artery, coronary thrombosis

NOTES: The term *corona* literally means "crown" and refers to the way the blood vessels that supply the heart descend and support the heart like a crown. The term *coronary* is used in medical language to refer specifically to the heart's blood supply.

Circulation

There are miles of blood vessels in the body. From vessels the size of a garden hose down to tiny capillaries much thinner than a human hair, blood vessels make up a large transportation network that acts like a road system. This system is a closed loop.

The left ventricle forces blood into the main outgoing vessel (*aorta*). The aorta branches into smaller arteries, just as highways have exits to smaller roads. These branches break off further still. Eventually, they reach their destinations: the brain, stomach, muscles, and so on.

By this point, the blood is flowing in tiny vessels known as *capillaries*. The oxygen and other nutrients pass out into the tissues that need it, and they give back their waste.

Once the blood has made the delivery and picked up the waste, it begins its journey back to the heart through veins. Smaller veins collect into larger veins, which collect into the upper (*superior*) and lower (*inferior*) *vena cava*. These main veins return blood to the right atrium.

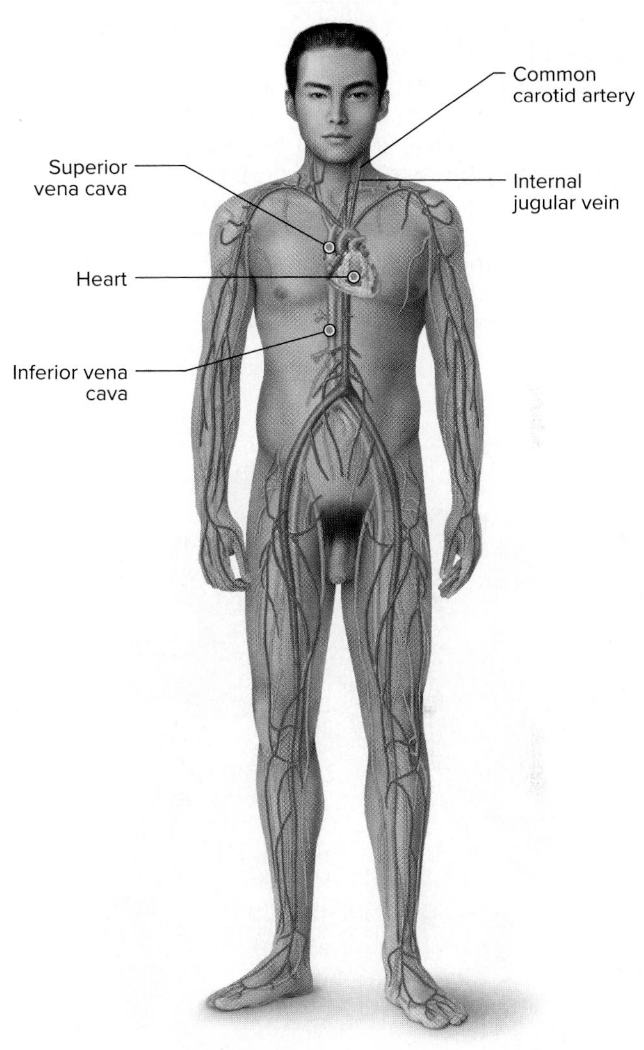

©Storman/Getty Images RF

vessel

ROOTS: ***angi/o, vas/o, vascul/o***

EXAMPLES: angioplasty, angiogram, vasodilator, vasculitis

NOTES: All these roots come from words meaning "jar" or "pitcher." *Angio* comes from Greek, and *vaso* and *vasculo* come from Latin. Although blood vessels don't look like jars, they do hold a lot of liquid—almost 6 quarts in the average man and almost 4 quarts in the average woman.

At the same time that the left ventricle pumps blood into the aorta, the right ventricle pumps blood into the *pulmonary artery*. The pulmonary artery carries blood to the lungs to attain oxygen and discard carbon dioxide. Once these gases are traded, the blood returns to the heart through a system of veins that lead to the main *pulmonary vein*. The pulmonary vein dumps the oxygen-rich blood into the left atrium. When the valve opens between the left atrium and left ventricle, the blood fills the ventricle and the cycle continues.

aorta

ROOT: ***aort/o***

EXAMPLES: aortitis, aortolith

NOTES: The *aorta* is the main artery leaving the heart and distributing oxygenated blood throughout the body. Its name means "to rise up" and refers to the fact that as the aorta leaves the heart, it rises up briefly and branches off into the arteries that supply the upper body before making what is called the *arch of the aorta* and descending into the lower body.

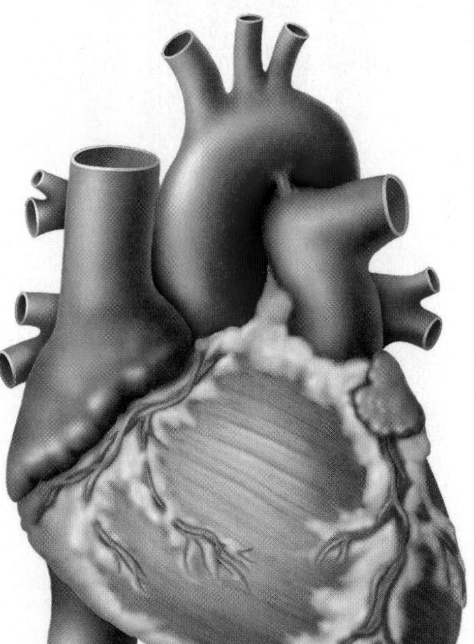

artery

ROOT: ***arteri/o***

EXAMPLES: arteriosclerosis, endarterectomy

NOTES: Arteries are the large blood vessels that carry oxygenated blood from heart to body tissue. It's funny that the word *artery* is actually a Greek word for "trachea" or "windpipe," a reference to the fact that some of the body's arteries are so large that early students of anatomy thought they carried air.

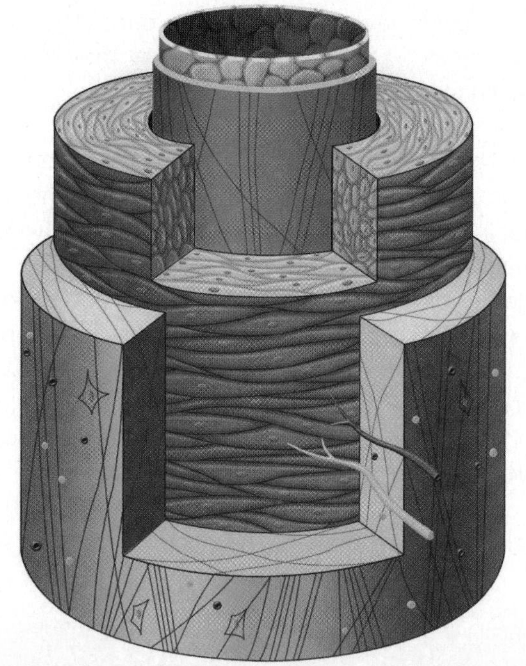

fatty plaque

ROOT: ***ather/o***

EXAMPLE: atherosclerosis

NOTES: This root comes from Greek, for "gruel" or "porridge." Be careful: This root is easily confused with *arterio*, especially in the words *arteriosclerosis* and *atherosclerosis*. There's another reason for the confusion: atherosclerosis is actually a form of arteriosclerosis. Arteriosclerosis means "hardening of an artery" and atherosclerosis means "hardening of an artery due specifically to buildup of fatty plaque."

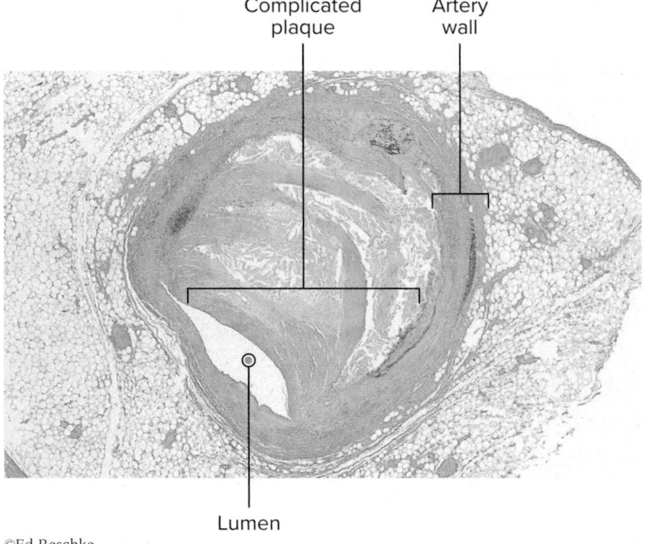

©Ed Reschke

vein

ROOTS: ***phleb/o, ven/o***

EXAMPLES: phlebotomy, venospasm

NOTES: The term *phlebotomy* comes from *phlebo* (vein) and *tomy* (incision). It's the term used for drawing blood. But always make sure you pronounce the word carefully. You don't want to go to the hospital to get some blood drawn (*phlebotomy*) and end up having a portion of your brain removed (*lobotomy*).

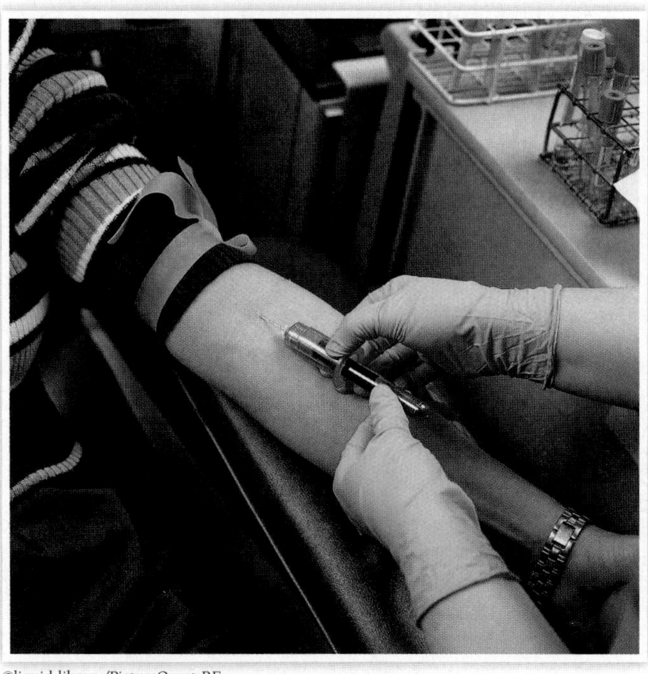

©liquid library/PictureQuest RF

Learning Outcome 9.1 Exercises

Additional exercises available in connect

TRANSLATION

EXERCISE 1 *Match the word part on the left with its definition on the right.*

_____	1. valvul/o	a. from Latin, for "partition" or "dividing structure"; can refer to any wall dividing two cavities
_____	2. atri/o	b. literally means "crown" and refers to the way the blood vessels that supply the heart descend and support the heart like a crown; the term is used in medical language to refer specifically to the heart's blood supply
_____	3. ventricul/o	c. lower chamber of the heart
_____	4. sept/o	d. upper chamber of the heart
_____	5. coron/o	e. valve

Learning Outcome 9.1 Exercises

EXERCISE 2 *Translate the following word parts.*

1. cardi/o ____________
2. atri/o ____________
3. valvul/o ____________
4. ventricul/o ____________
5. sept/o ____________
6. coron/o ____________

EXERCISE 3 *Underline and define the word parts from this chapter in the following terms.*

1. cardiac arrest ____________
2. endocarditis ____________
3. valvuloplasty ____________
4. coronary thrombosis ____________
5. ventricular septal defect (2 roots) ____________
6. atrial septal defect (2 roots) ____________

EXERCISE 4 *Break down the following words into their component parts and translate.*

EXAMPLE:	sinusitis	*sinus | itis*	*inflammation of the sinuses*

1. cardiology ____________
2. valvulotomy ____________
3. cardiomegaly ____________
4. coronary circulation ____________
5. atrial septal defect ____________
6. ventricular septal defect ____________

EXERCISE 5 *Match the word part on the left with its definition on the right. Some definitions will be used more than once.*

______	1. ven/o	a.	blood vessel
______	2. aort/o	b.	fatty plaque
______	3. phleb/o	c.	large blood vessels that carry oxygenated blood from the heart to body tissue
______	4. vas/o	d.	main artery leaving the heart and distributing oxygenated blood throughout the body
______	5. vascul/o	e.	vein
______	6. arteri/o		
______	7. angi/o		
______	8. ather/o		

Learning Outcome 9.1 Exercises

EXERCISE 6 *Translate the following word parts.*

1. arteri/o ______
2. aort/o ______
3. ven/o ______
4. vas/o ______
5. vascul/o ______
6. angi/o ______
7. phleb/o ______
8. ather/o ______

EXERCISE 7 *Underline and define the word parts from this chapter in the following terms.*

1. angiosclerosis ______
2. venosclerosis ______
3. atherosclerosis ______
4. phlebosclerosis ______
5. arteriectomy ______
6. aortolith ______
7. vasoconstrictor ______
8. vascular endoscopy ______
9. aortic stenosis ______
10. thrombophlebitis ______
11. superior vena cava ______
12. cardiovascular (2 roots) ______
13. angiocarditis (2 roots) ______
14. coronary artery bypass surgery (2 roots) ______

EXERCISE 8 *Break down the following words into their component parts and translate.*

EXAMPLE: sinusitis *sinus | itis* *inflammation of the sinuses*

1. angioplasty ______
2. aortotomy ______
3. arterioplasty ______
4. atherectomy ______
5. coronary arterectomy ______

6. phlebotomy ____
7. vasculitis ____
8. vasodilator ____
9. venectomy ____

GENERATION

EXERCISE 9 *Identify the roots for the following definitions.*

1. septum ____
2. valve ____
3. ventricle ____
4. atrium ____
5. upper chamber of the heart ____
6. lower chamber of the heart ____
7. heart (2 roots) ____

EXERCISE 10 *Build a medical term from the information provided.*

1. inflammation of the heart (use *cardi/o*) ____
2. inflammation of a heart valve ____
3. heart specialist (use *cardi/o*) ____
4. inflammation of the tissue around the heart (use *cardi/o*) ____

EXERCISE 11 *Identify the roots for the following definitions.*

1. aorta ____
2. artery ____
3. fatty plaque ____
4. vein (2 roots) ____
5. vessel (3 roots) ____

EXERCISE 12 *Build a medical term from the information provided.*

1. record of a vessel (use *angi/o*) ____
2. record of a vein (use *ven/o*) ____
3. record of the aorta ____
4. record of an artery ____
5. inflammation of a vein ____
6. involuntary contraction of a vessel (use *vas/o*) ____
7. the formation of a fatty plaque (use *-genesis*) ____

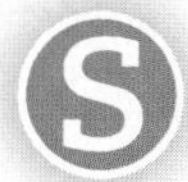

Subjective

Patient History, Problems, Complaints

Heart

Circulation

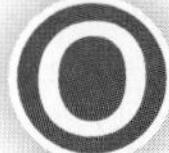

Objective

Observation and Discovery

Heart—structure

Heart

Circulation—structure

Circulation

Diagnostic procedures

Professional terms

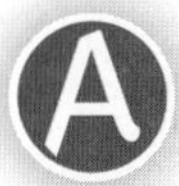

Assessment

Diagnosis and Pathology

Heart

Circulation

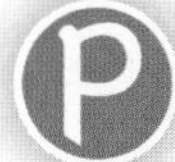

Plan

Treatments and Therapies

Drugs

Heart procedures

Circulation procedures

This section contains medical terms built from the roots presented in the previous section. The purpose of this section is to expose you to words used in cardiology that are built from the word roots presented earlier. The focus of this book is to teach you the process of learning roots and translating them in context. Each term is presented with the correct pronunciation, followed by a word analysis that breaks down the word into its component parts, a definition that provides a literal translation of the word, as well as supplemental information if the literal translation deviates from its medical use.

The terms are organized using a health care professional's SOAP note (first introduced in Chapter 2) as a model.

SUBJECTIVE

9.2 Patient History, Problems, Complaints

The most common heart problem patients report is chest pain (*pectoralgia*). The causes can range from minor issues, like muscle soreness, to the pain associated with a heart attack (*angina pectoris*). Patients can occasionally feel pain in their blood vessels. This is most common with enlarged surface veins (*phlebalgia*).

While the heart never stops beating, we are rarely aware of its rhythm. When the heart beats out of pace, a patient might feel a jumping sensation (*palpitation*). If the heart continues to beat in an odd rhythm (*arrhythmia, dysrhythmia*), a patient may notice this as well.

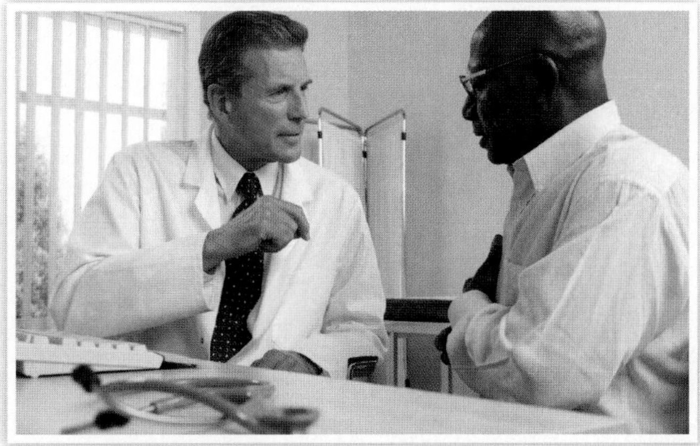

©Adam Gault/SPL/Science Photo Library/Getty Images RF

9.2 Patient History, Problems, Complaints

heart

Term	Word Analysis
angina pectoris an-JAI-nah PEK-tor-is **Definition** oppressive pain in the chest caused by irregular blood flow to the heart	**angina pectoris** to choke chest
arrhythmia ay-RITH-mee-ah **Definition** irregular heartbeat	**a / rrhythm / ia** no / rhythm / condition
dysrhythmia dis-RITH-mee-ah **Definition** irregular heartbeat (*arrhythmia* is more common)	**dys / rhythm / ia** bad / rhythm / condition
palpitation PAL-pih-TAY-shun **Definition** rapid or irregular beating of the heart	**from Latin, for** "to flutter"
pectoralgia PEK-tor-AL-jah **Definition** chest pain	**pector / algia** chest / pain

circulation

Term	Word Analysis
aortalgia AY-or-TAL-jah **Definition** pain in the aorta	**aort / algia** aorta / pain
diaphoresis DAI-ah-for-EE-sis **Definition** profuse sweating	**dia / phoresis** through / carry

9.2 Patient History, Problems, Complaints

circulation *continued*

Term	Word Analysis
hemorrhage HEM-oh-RIJ **Definition** loss of blood	**hemo / rrhage** blood / burst forth
phlebalgia fleh-BAL-jah **Definition** pain in a vein	**phleb / algia** vein / pain

Learning Outcome 9.2 Exercises

PRONUNCIATION

EXERCISE 1 *Indicate which syllable is emphasized when pronounced.*

EXAMPLE: bronchitis bron**chi**tis

1. phlebalgia ______
2. dysrhythmia ______
3. arrhythmia ______
4. angina pectoris ______
5. palpitation ______
6. pectoralgia ______
7. hemorrhage ______
8. aortalgia ______
9. diaphoresis ______

Learning Outcome 9.2 Exercises

TRANSLATION

EXERCISE 2 *Break down the following words into their component parts.*

EXAMPLE: nasopharyngoscope *naso | pharyngo | scope*

1. pectoralgia ______
2. aortalgia ______
3. phlebalgia ______
4. arrhythmia ______
5. dysrhythmia ______
6. hemorrhage ______

EXERCISE 3 *Underline and define the word parts from this chapter in the following terms.*

1. aortalgia ______
2. phlebalgia ______
3. hemorrhage ______

EXERCISE 4 *Match the term on the left with its definition on the right. Some definitions may be used more than once.*

______	1. aortalgia	a.	oppressive pain in the chest caused by irregular blood flow to the heart
______	2. phlebalgia	b.	chest pain
______	3. pectoralgia	c.	irregular heartbeat
______	4. arrhythmia	d.	loss of blood
______	5. dysrhythmia	e.	pain in a vein
______	6. palpitation	f.	pain in the aorta
______	7. hemorrhage	g.	profuse sweating
______	8. angina pectoris	h.	rapid or irregular beating of the heart
______	9. diaphoresis		

EXERCISE 5 *Translate the following terms as literally as possible.*

EXAMPLE: nasopharyngoscope *an instrument for looking at the nose and throat*

1. aortalgia ______
2. phlebalgia ______
3. pectoralgia ______
4. arrhythmia ______
5. dysrhythmia ______
6. angina pectoris ______

S Learning Outcome 9.2 Exercises

GENERATION

EXERCISE 6 *Build a medical term from the information provided.*

EXAMPLE: inflammation of the sinuses *sinusitis*

1. pain in a vein (use *phleb/o*) ____________________
2. chest pain ____________________
3. pain in the aorta ____________________
4. no rhythm condition ____________________
5. bad rhythm condition ____________________

EXERCISE 7 *Multiple-choice questions. Select the correct answer(s).*

1. Select the terms that pertain to heartbeat (select all that apply).
   a. angina pectoris
   b. aortalgia
   c. arrhythmia
   d. diaphoresis
   e. hemorrhage
   f. palpitation
   g. pectoralgia
   h. phlebalgia
2. Select the terms that pertain to pain in the heart or chest (select all that apply).
   a. angina pectoris
   b. aortalgia
   c. arrhythmia
   d. diaphoresis
   e. hemorrhage
   f. palpitation
   g. pectoralgia
   h. phlebalgia
3. Which of the following types of pain in the chest is caused by irregular blood flow to the heart?
   a. angina pectoris
   b. diaphoresis
   c. hemorrhage
   d. palpitation
   e. phlebalgia
4. Which of the following terms is from Latin, for "to flutter"?
   a. angina pectoris
   b. diaphoresis
   c. hemorrhage
   d. palpitation
   e. phlebalgia
5. Which of the following terms means "profuse sweating"?
   a. angina pectoris
   b. diaphoresis
   c. hemorrhage
   d. palpitation
   e. phlebalgia
6. Which of the following terms literally means "blood burst forth"?
   a. angina pectoris
   b. diaphoresis
   c. hemorrhage
   d. palpitation
   e. phlebalgia

OBJECTIVE

9.3 Observation and Discovery

During a patient consultation about a heart or circulation problem, the first thing the examiner might notice is a change in the color of the patient's skin. Patients with very poor circulation or low oxygen in their blood may appear a bit blue (*cyanosis*). Generally, cyanosis is seen in emergency situations; it signals the need for immediate action.

While skin color change may not be noted in most cardiac patients, hearts will almost always be examined by measuring patients' vital signs. The two vital signs most closely related to the heart are pulse and blood pressure. As a patient's heart squeezes, it is possible to feel throbbing when placing a finger over certain blood vessels. This is the *pulse*. A pulse is described as either strong or weak and can be a very helpful indicator in heart health. When a pulse is very weak, it may be an indication of dangerously low blood pressure (*hypotension*).

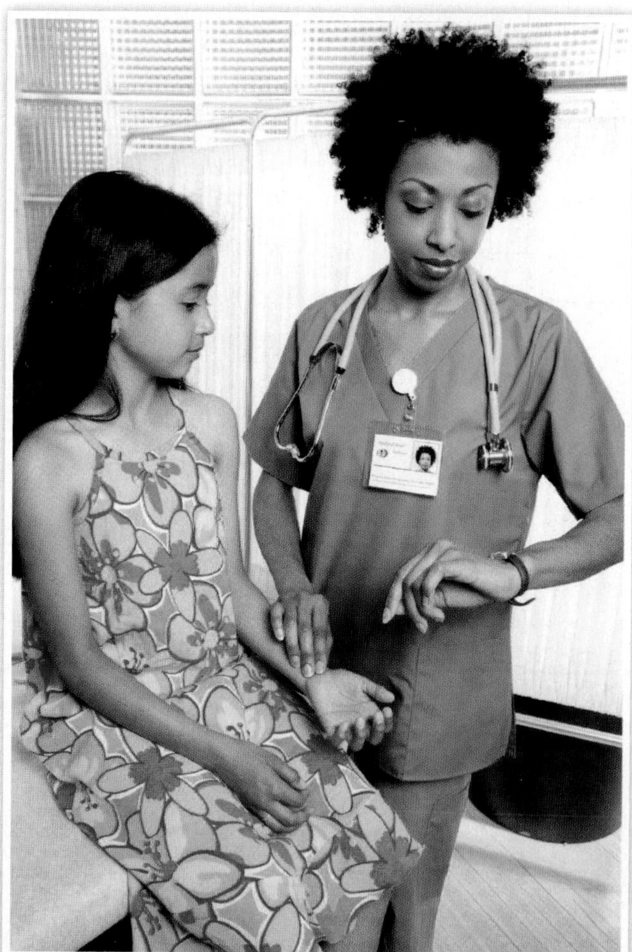

The most basic piece of observable data about the heart is the heart rate, discovered easiest through taking the patient's pulse at the wrist.

A pulse reading can also indicate how fast the patient's heart is beating (*heart rate*). If the patient's heart is beating too fast (*tachycardia*) or too slow (*bradycardia*), this may be an indication of disease. The rate at which a heart beats is controlled by electrical signals. The signals travel throughout the heart muscle fibers to get them to work together.

Have you ever noticed that in some houses the water comes out of the shower faster and harder than in others? This is due to differences in water pressure. Blood pressure works in the same way—it measures how strong the flow of blood is in the body. When a patient's heart muscle fibers are contracting and sending blood out of the ventricles, the pressure in the arteries is at its highest. This arterial pressure, the *systole*, is the first number of a blood pressure reading.

The second number of a blood pressure reading is called the *diastole*. It refers to the pressure on the vessels when the heart is relaxed and filling with blood. When a patient's blood vessels are caked with hard deposits, higher pressure is needed to force blood through them. This is the most common cause of high blood pressure (*hypertension*). The blood pressure is another vital sign and is measured by listening to changes in the sound of blood flow through an artery as a special cuff is constricted.

Chief among the means of evaluating the heart is listening directly to the heartbeat. There are two heart sounds that are caused by the closing of valves in the heart. The first heart sound (S1) is due to the closing of the valves between the atria and ventricles. This represents the beginning of heart contraction (*systole*). Systole ends with closing of the pulmonary and aortic valves, which creates the second heart sound (S2). When listening to the heart, the examiner listens for abnormal sounds (*murmurs*) or a disturbance in the rhythm.

Two very common tests are used to observe the heart: *electrocardiograms* and *echocardiograms*. An electrocardiogram measures the electrical signals in the heart. During the test, electrodes are placed on different parts of a patient's body and measure electrical signals from the heart. One important reason for this test is to check for signs of decreased blood flow to the heart

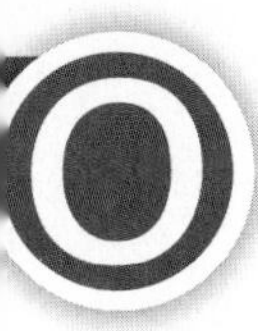

(*ischemia*). Sometimes a patient must exercise in order to exhibit these signs (*stress electrocardiogram*).

An echocardiogram uses ultrahigh sound frequencies (*ultrasound*) to watch the heart as it works. With an echocardiogram it is possible to view the layers of the heart (*pericardium, myocardium*, and *endocardium*), the *valves*, and the wall of the heart (*septum*). An examiner can also visualize the flow of blood through the heart. The flow through the valves may be tight (*stenosis*) or may flow back the wrong direction (*regurgitation*).

The most common way to examine blood vessels is to inject dye into the blood and view the results using an x-ray (*angiogram*). This type of study can show all sorts of problems, including deposits of fat (*atherosclerosis*), a floating object that blocks blood flow (*embolus*), a cutoff in blood flow (*occlusion*), or the dilation of a vessel (*ectasia*).

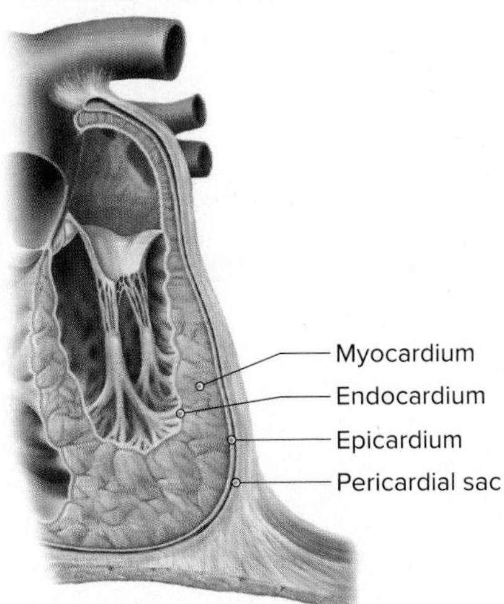

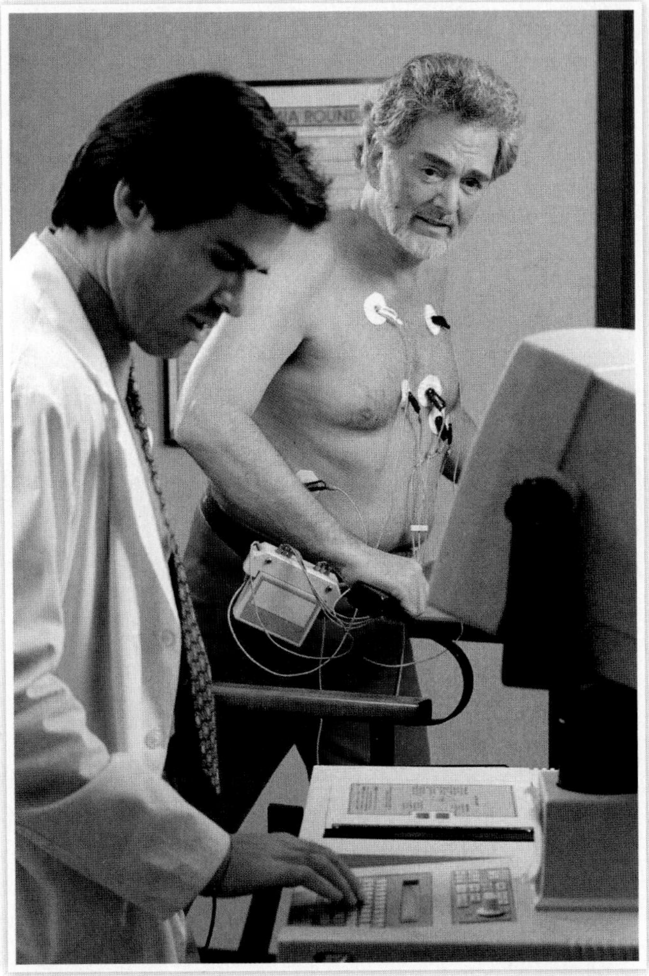

A stress electrocardiogram observes the patient's heart while the patient exercises.

heart structure

Term	Word Analysis
endocardium EN-doh-KAR-dee-um **Definition** tissue lining the inside of the heart	**endo / card / ium** inside / heart / tissue
epicardium EH-puh-KAR-dee-um **Definition** tissue lining the outside of the heart	**epi / card / ium** upon / heart / tissue
myocardium MAI-oh-KAR-dee-um **Definition** heart muscle tissue	**myo / card / ium** muscle / heart / tissue

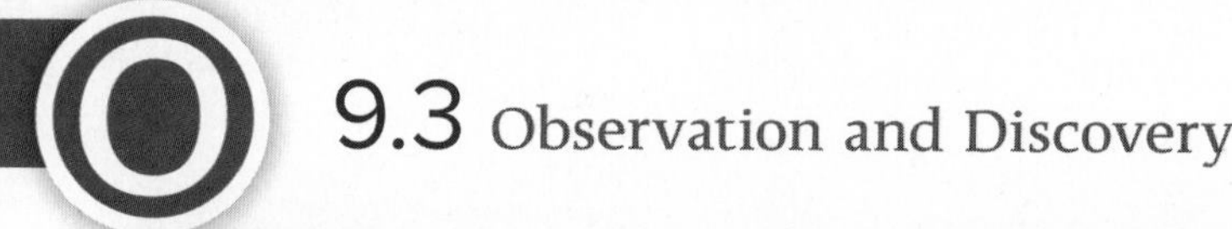

9.3 Observation and Discovery

heart structure *continued*

Term	Word Analysis
pericardium PER-uh-KAR-dee-um **Definition** tissue around the heart	**peri / card / ium** around / heart / tissue

heart

Term	Word Analysis
bradycardia BRAY-dih-KAR-dee-ah **Definition** slow heartbeat	**brady / card / ia** slow / heart / condition
cardiomegaly KAR-dee-oh-MEH-gah-lee **Definition** enlarged heart	**cardio / megaly** heart / enlargement
cardiotoxic KAR-dee-oh-TOK-sik **Definition** poisonous to the heart	**cardio / toxic** heart / poison
cyanosis SAI-ah-NOH-sis **Definition** bluish appearance to the skin—a sign that the tissue isn't receiving enough oxygen	**cyan / osis** blue / condition
murmur MIR-mir **Definition** abnormal heart sound	**from Latin, for** "to grumble" **or** "hum"
tachycardia TAK-ih-KAR-dee-ah **Definition** rapid heartbeat	**tachy / card / ia** fast / heart / condition

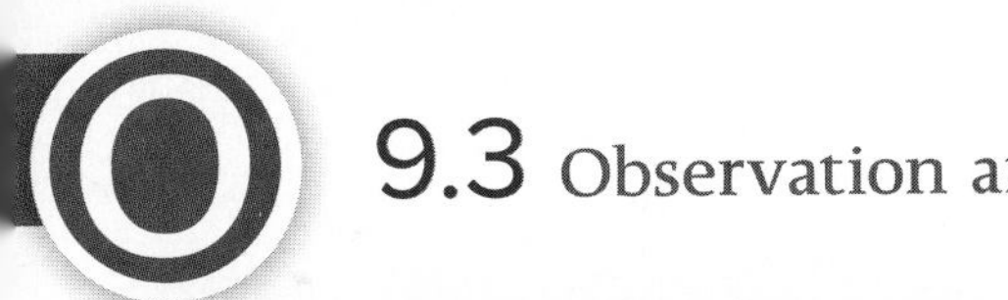

9.3 Observation and Discovery

circulation structure

Term	Word Analysis
vena cava VEE-nah CAY-vah	**vena** — vein; **cava** — hollow
Definition large-diameter vein that gathers blood from the body and returns it to the heart	
inferior vena cava in-FEER-ee-or VEE-nah CAY-vah	**inferior** — lower; **vena** — vein; **cava** — hollow
Definition portion of the vena cava that gathers blood from the lower portion of the body	
superior vena cava soo-PEER-ee-or VEE-nah CAY-vah	**superior** — upper; **vena** — vein; **cava** — hollow
Definition portion of the vena cava that gathers blood from the upper portion of the body (head and arms)	

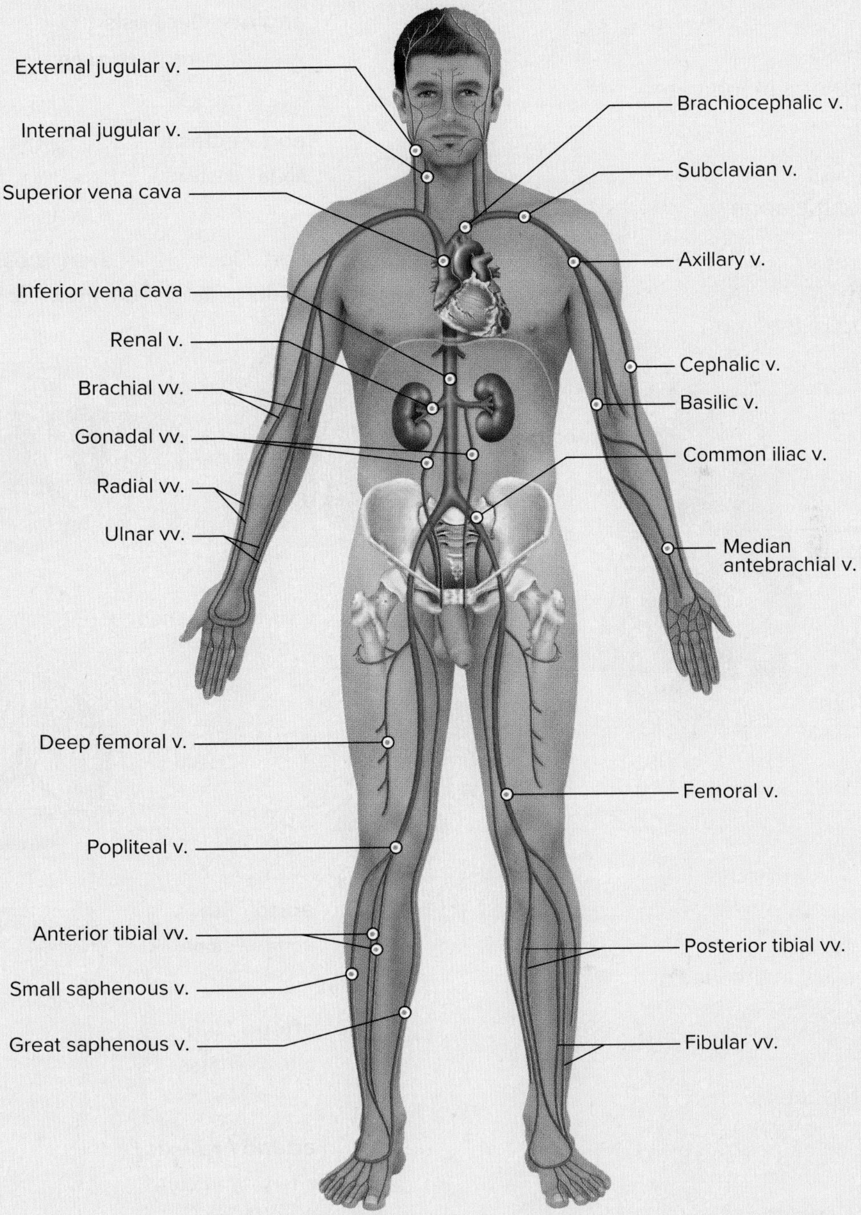

External jugular v.
Internal jugular v.
Superior vena cava
Inferior vena cava
Renal v.
Brachial vv.
Gonadal vv.
Radial vv.
Ulnar vv.
Deep femoral v.
Popliteal v.
Anterior tibial vv.
Small saphenous v.
Great saphenous v.
Brachiocephalic v.
Subclavian v.
Axillary v.
Cephalic v.
Basilic v.
Common iliac v.
Median antebrachial v.
Femoral v.
Posterior tibial vv.
Fibular vv.

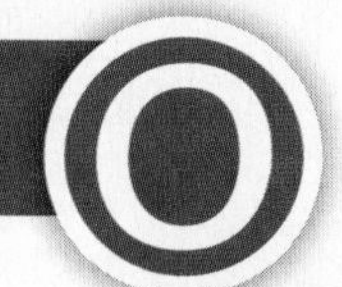

9.3 Observation and Discovery

circulation

Term	Word Analysis
angiogenesis AN-jee-oh-JIN-eh-sis **Definition** development of blood vessels	**angio / genesis** vessel / creation
angiolith AN-jee-oh-LITH **Definition** stone forming in the wall of a blood vessel	**angio / lith** vessel / stone
angiopoiesis AN-jee-oh-poh-EE-sis **Definition** formation of blood vessels	**angio / poiesis** vessel / formation
angiosclerosis AN-jee-oh-skleh-ROH-sis **Definition** hardening of a blood vessel	**angio / scler / osis** vessel / hard / condition
aortectasia ay-OR-tek-TAY-zhah **Definition** dilation of the aorta	**aort / ectasia** aorta / dilation
aortic stenosis ay-OR-tik stih-NOH-sis **Definition** narrowing of the aorta	**aort / ic sten / osis** aorta / pertaining to narrow / condition
aortolith ay-OR-toh-LITH **Definition** stone deposit in the wall of the aorta	**aorto / lith** aorta / stone
arteriolith ar-TER-ee-oh-LITH **Definition** stone in the artery	**arterio / lith** artery / stone
arteriorrhexis ar-TER-ee-oh-REK-sis **Definition** rupture of an artery	**arterio / rrhexis** artery / rupture

circulation *continued*

Term	Word Analysis
arteriosclerosis ar-TER-ee-oh-skleh-ROH-sis **Definition** hardening of an artery	**arterio / scler / osis** artery / hard / condition
atherogenesis A-ther-oh-JIN-eh-sis **Definition** formation of fatty plaque on the wall of an artery	**athero / genesis** fatty plaque / creation
atherosclerosis A-ther-oh-skleh-ROH-sis **Definition** hardening of an artery due to buildup of fatty plaque	**athero / scler / osis** fatty plaque / hard / condition
embolus EM-boh-lus **Definition** mass of matter present in the blood **NOTE:** In Greek, this word was used to mean "stopper," as in the opening of a bottle.	**em / bolus** in / throw
embolism EM-boh-LIZ-um **Definition** blockage in a blood vessel caused by an embolus	**embol / ism** embolus / condition
ischemia ih-SKEE-mee-ah **Definition** blockage of blood flow to an organ	**isch / emia** hold back / blood condition
occlusion oh-KLOO-zhun **Definition** closing or blockage of a passage	**from Latin, for** "to close off"
phlebosclerosis FLEB-oh-skleh-ROH-sis **Definition** hardening of a vein	**phlebo / scler / osis** vein / hard / condition
thrombus THROM-bus **Definition** blood clot **NOTE:** The difference between a thrombus and an embolus is twofold. A *thrombus* is a clot of blood and is stationary. An *embolus* is foreign material and is in motion. When a thrombus breaks off, it becomes a *thromboembolus*.	**from Greek, for** "lump," "clot," **or even** "curd of milk"

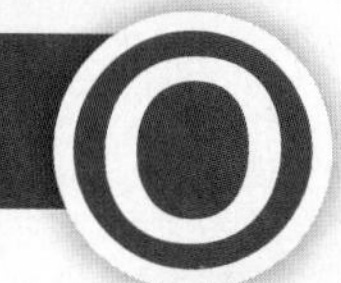

9.3 Observation and Discovery

circulation *continued*

Term	Word Analysis
varicose veins VAR-ih-kohs VAYNS **Definition** an enlarged, dilated vein toward the surface of the skin	**varicose** **veins** swollen / twisted veins
vasospasm VAS-oh-SPAZ-um **Definition** involuntary contraction of a blood vessel	**vaso / spasm** vessel / involuntary contraction
venosclerosis VEE-noh-skleh-ROH-sis **Definition** hardening of a vein	**veno / scler / osis** vein / hard / condition
venospasm VEE-noh-SPAZ-um **Definition** involuntary contraction of a vein	**veno / spasm** vein / involuntary contraction
venostasis VEE-noh-STA-sis **Definition** trapping of blood in an extremity due to compression	**veno / stasis** vein / standing

NOTE: This name refers not to the fact that the blood is trapped but, instead, to the fact that the blood is standing still and not moving.

radiology

Term	Word Analysis
angiogram AN-jee-oh-GRAM **Definition** record of the blood vessels	**angio / gram** vessel / record
angiography AN-jee-AW-grah-fee **Definition** procedure to describe the blood vessels	**angio / graphy** vessel / writing procedure

©Phanie/Alamy Stock Photo

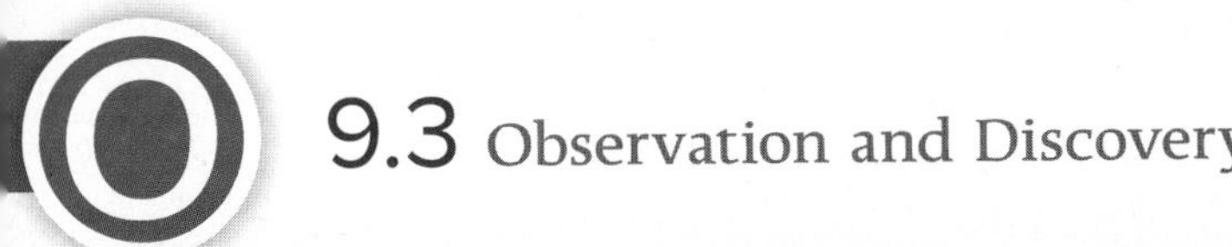

9.3 Observation and Discovery

radiology *continued*

Term	Word Analysis
aortogram ay-OR-tah-GRAM **Definition** record of the aorta	**aorto / gram** aorta / record
arteriogram ar-TER-ee-oh-GRAM **Definition** record of an artery	**arterio / gram** artery / record
venogram VEE-noh-gram **Definition** record of a vein	**veno / gram** vein / record

diagnostic procedures

Term	Word Analysis
angioscope AN-jee-oh-SKOWP **Definition** device for looking into a blood vessel	**angio / scope** vessel / device for looking
cardiac catheterization KAR-dee-ak KATH-eh-ter-ih-ZAY-shun **Definition** process of inserting a tube (catheter) into the heart **NOTE:** The word *catheter* comes from Greek words meaning "to go inside." By passing a tube through arteries, doctors are able to diagnose and treat heart problems without performing major surgery.	**cardi / ac** **catheter / ization** heart / pertaining to catheter / procedure
echocardiogram EK-oh-KAR-dee-oh-GRAM **Definition** image of the heart produced using sound waves; the same procedure as an ultrasound performed on pregnant women, but instead it is performed on a heart	**echo / cardio / gram** echo / heart / record ©Steve Allen/Brand X Pictures/Getty Images RF
echocardiography EK-oh-KAR-dee-AW-grah-fee **Definition** use of sound waves to produce an image of the heart; the same procedure as an ultrasound performed on pregnant women, but instead it is performed on a heart	**echo / cardio / graphy** echo / heart / writing procedure

diagnostic procedures *continued*

Term	Word Analysis
electrocardiogram eh-LEK-troh-KAR-dee-oh-GRAM **Definition** record of the electrical currents of the heart	**electro / cardio / gram** electricity / heart / record 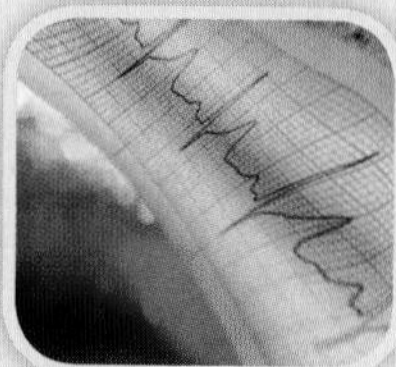 ©Brand X Pictures/Getty Images RF
electrocardiography eh-LEK-troh-KAR-dee- AW-grah-fee **Definition** procedure for recording the electrical currents of the heart	**electro / cardio / graphy** electricity / heart / writing procedure
sonography saw-NAW-grah-fee **Definition** use of sound waves to produce diagnostic images; also called ultrasound	**sono / graphy** sound / writing procedure
stress electrocardiogram STRES eh-LEK-troh-KAR-dee-oh-GRAM **Definition** records electrical signals of the heart while the patient experiences increases of exercise stress	**stress electro / cardio / gram** stress electricity / heart / record 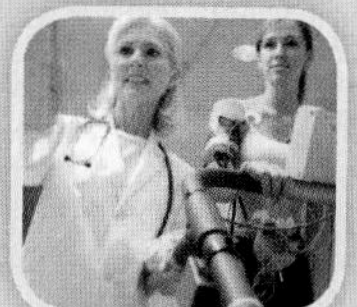 ©MBI/Alamy Stock Photo RF
transesophageal echocardiogram TRANZ-eh-SOF-ah-JEE-al EK-oh-KAR-dee-oh-GRAM **Definition** record of the heart using sound waves performed by inserting the transducer into the esophagus	**trans / esophag / eal** through / esophagus / pertaining to **echo / cardio / gram** echo / heart / record 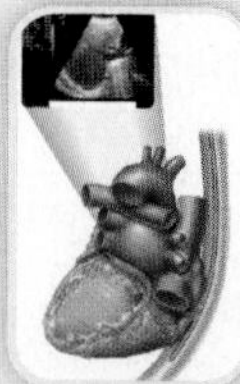 ©Steve Allen/Getty Images RF
vascular endoscopy VAS-kyoo-lar en-DAW-skoh-pee **Definition** procedure to look inside a blood vessel	**vascul / ar** **endo / scopy** vessel / pertaining to inside / looking procedure

9.3 Observation and Discovery

professional terms

Term	Word Analysis
blood pressure **BLUD** PRESH-ir **Definition** the force exerted by blood on the walls of blood vessels	**blood pressure**

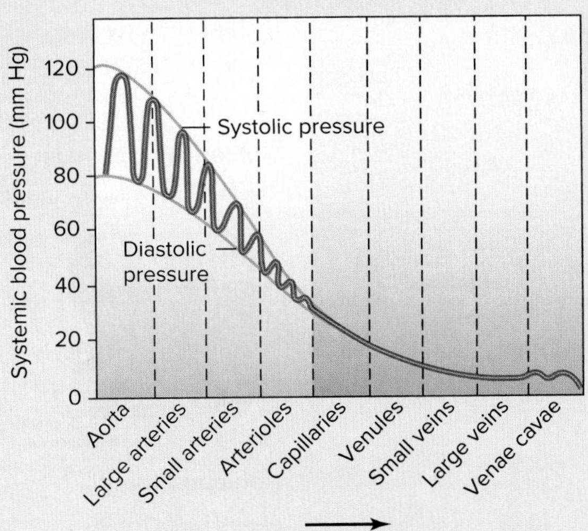

Term	Word Analysis
diastolic pressure DAI-ah-STAW-lik PRESH-ir **Definition** pressure exerted on blood vessels when heart is relaxed **NOTE:** *Stole* comes from Greek, for "to send." It can also be found in the word *epistle,* which means "letter" or "something you send someone."	**dia / stol / ic pressure** through / send / pertaining to
systolic pressure sih-STAW-lik PRESH-ir **Definition** pressure exerted on blood vessels when heart is contracting	**sys / stol / ic pressure** together / send / pertaining to
cardiologist KAR-dee-AW-loh-jist **Definition** heart specialist	**cardio / logist** heart / specialist
cardiology KAR-dee-AW-loh-jee **Definition** branch of medicine dealing with the heart	**cardio / logy** heart / study
cardiovascular KAR-dee-oh-VAS-kyoo-lar **Definition** pertaining to the heart and blood vessels	**cardio / vascul / ar** heart / vessel / pertaining to
circulation SIR-kyoo-LAY-shun **Definition** moving of blood from the heart through the vessels and back to the heart	**from Latin, for "to go in a circle"**
coronary circulation KOR-ah-NER-ee SIR-kyoo-LAY-shun **Definition** circulation of blood from the heart to the heart muscle (the heart always feeds itself first)	**coron / ary circulation** heart / pertaining to

professional terms *continued*

Term	Word Analysis
phlebologist fleb-AW-loh-jist **Definition** specialist in veins	**phlebo / logist** vein / specialist
phlebology fleb-AW-loh-jee **Definition** study of veins	**phlebo / logy** vein / study
phlebotomist fleh-BAW-toh-mist **Definition** one who draws blood	**phlebo / tom / ist** vein / incision / specialist ©Keith Brofsky/Getty Images RF
phlebotomy fleh-BAW-toh-mee **Definition** incision into a vein—the technical term for drawing blood	**phlebo / tomy** vein / incision
pulmonary circulation PUL-mon-AR-ee SIR-kyoo-LAY-shun **Definition** circulation of blood from the heart to the lungs (to oxygenate it)	**pulmon / ary circulation** lung / pertaining to
systemic circulation sih-STEM-ik SIR-kyoo-LAY-shun **Definition** circulation of blood from the heart to the rest of the body	**sys / stem / ic circulation** together / stand / pertaining to

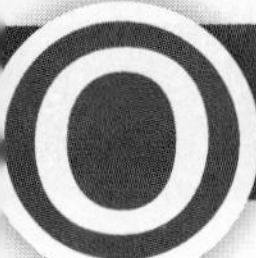

Learning Outcome 9.3 Exercises

PRONUNCIATION

EXERCISE 1 *Indicate which syllable is emphasized when pronounced.*

EXAMPLE: bronchitis bron**chi**tis

1. circulation
2. embolism
3. cardiology
4. cardiovascular
5. angiolith
6. angiogram
7. arteriogram
8. angioscope
9. aortectasia
10. atherogenesis
11. venosclerosis
12. atherosclerosis
13. phlebosclerosis
14. arteriosclerosis
15. echocardiogram
16. electrocardiogram
17. murmur
18. thrombus
19. embolus
20. venogram
21. phlebology
22. ischemia
23. occlusion
24. phlebotomist
25. phlebotomy

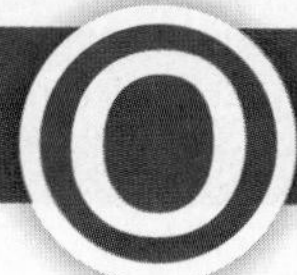

Learning Outcome 9.3 Exercises

TRANSLATION

EXERCISE 2 *Break down the following words into their component parts.*

EXAMPLE: nasopharyngoscope *naso | pharyngo | scope*

1. cardiology ______
2. phlebology ______
3. angiography ______
4. sonography ______
5. cardiotoxic ______
6. cyanosis ______
7. phlebotomist ______
8. angiogenesis ______
9. atherogenesis ______
10. aortic stenosis ______
11. echocardiography ______
12. electrocardiography ______

EXERCISE 3 *Underline and define the word parts from this chapter in the following terms.*

1. cardiologist ______
2. phlebologist ______
3. cardiomegaly ______
4. angiogram ______
5. aortogram ______
6. arteriogram ______
7. venogram ______
8. angiopoiesis ______
9. aortectasia ______
10. venostasis ______
11. phlebotomy ______
12. arteriorrhexis ______
13. atherosclerosis ______
14. vena cava ______
15. echocardiogram ______
16. electrocardiogram ______
17. stress electrocardiogram ______

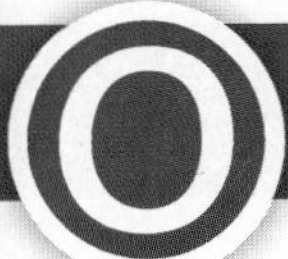

Learning Outcome 9.3 Exercises

18. transesophageal echocardiogram ______________________
19. vascular endoscopy ______________________
20. cardiovascular (2 roots) ______________________
21. coronary circulation ______________________

EXERCISE 4 *Select the correct option for each given translation.*

EXAMPLE: hypoglycemia	*hypo* over | under	*glyc* salt | sugar	*-emia* blood | urine condition

1. tachycardia = fast/slow (*tachy*) + heart condition (*cardia*)
2. bradycardia = fast/slow (*brady*) + heart condition (*cardia*)
3. venospasm = artery/blood vessel/vein (*veno*) + involuntary contraction (*spasm*)
4. vasospasm = artery/blood vessel/vein (*vaso*) + involuntary contraction (*spasm*)
5. arteriosclerosis = artery/blood vessel/vein (*arterio*) + hard condition (*sclerosis*)
6. venosclerosis = artery/blood vessel/vein (*veno*) + hard condition (*sclerosis*)
7. phlebosclerosis = artery/blood vessel/vein (*phlebo*) + hard condition (*sclerosis*)
8. angiosclerosis = artery/blood vessel/vein (*angio*) + hard condition (*sclerosis*)

EXERCISE 5 *Fill in the blanks.*

1. angioscope = device for looking into a(n) ______________________
2. aortolith = stone forming in the wall of the ______________________
3. arteriolith = stone forming in a(n) ______________________
4. angiolith = stone forming in the wall of a(n) ______________________
5. myocardium = heart ______________________ tissue
6. pericardium = tissue ______________________ the heart
7. endocardium = tissue lining the ______________________ of the heart
8. epicardium = tissue lining the ______________________ of the heart

EXERCISE 6 *Match the term on the left with its definition on the right.*

_____ 1. blood pressure

_____ 2. circulation

_____ 3. murmur

_____ 4. cyanosis

_____ 5. varicose vein

a. abnormal heart sound

b. blood clot; from Greek, for "lump," "clot," or even "curd of milk"

c. bluish appearance to the skin; a sign that the tissue isn't receiving enough oxygen

d. mass of matter present in the blood; from Greek, for "stopper," as in the opening of a bottle

e. enlarged, dilated vein toward the surface of the skin

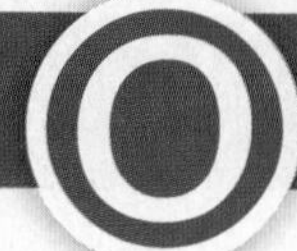

Learning Outcome 9.3 Exercises

______ 6. occlusion	f.	blockage of blood flow to an organ
______ 7. ischemia	g.	closing or blockage of a passage; from Latin, for "to close off"
______ 8. cardiac catheterization	h.	force exerted by blood on the walls of blood vessels
______ 9. embolus	i.	moving of blood from the heart through the vessels and back to the heart
______ 10. thrombus	j.	process of inserting a tube into the heart

EXERCISE 7 *Translate the following terms as literally as possible.*

EXAMPLE: nasopharyngoscope *an instrument for looking at the nose and throat*

1. cardiovascular ______
2. cardiotoxic ______
3. angiogenesis ______
4. endocardium ______
5. epicardium ______
6. myocardium ______
7. pericardium ______
8. bradycardia ______
9. tachycardia ______
10. angiography ______
11. sonography ______
12. atherosclerosis ______
13. angiopoiesis ______
14. arteriorrhexis ______
15. cyanosis ______
16. inferior vena cava ______
17. superior vena cava ______
18. vascular endoscopy ______

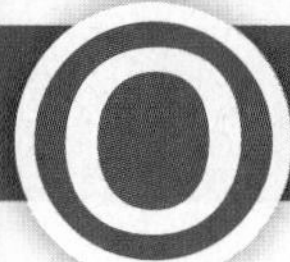

Learning Outcome 9.3 Exercises

GENERATION

EXERCISE 8 *Build a medical term from the information provided.*

EXAMPLE: inflammation of the sinuses *sinusitis*

1. study of veins (use *phleb/o*) __________
2. study of the heart __________
3. record of a vein (use *ven/o*) __________
4. record of the blood vessels (use *angi/o*) __________
5. record of the aorta __________
6. record of an artery __________
7. hardening of a blood vessel (use *angi/o*) __________
8. hardening of a vein (use *phleb/o*) __________
9. hardening of a vein (use *ven/o*) __________
10. hardening of an artery __________
11. involuntary contraction of a blood vessel (use *vas/o*) __________
12. involuntary contraction of a vein (use *ven/o*) __________
13. device for looking into a blood vessel (use *angi/o*) __________
14. vessel stone (use *angi/o*) __________
15. enlarged heart __________
16. fatty plaque creation __________
17. record of the electrical currents of the heart __________

EXERCISE 9 *Multiple-choice questions. Select the correct answer(s).*

1. A *stress electrocardiogram* is:
   a. a record of the heart using sound waves performed by inserting the sonograph into the esophagus
   b. a record of electrical signals of the heart while the patient experiences increases of exercise stress
   c. a procedure to look inside blood vessels that are currently undergoing stress
   d. none of these
2. A *transesophageal echocardiogram* is:
   a. a record of the heart using sound waves performed by inserting the transducer into the esophagus
   b. a record of electrical signals of the heart while the patient experiences increases of exercise stress
   c. a procedure to look inside blood vessels that are currently undergoing stress
   d. none of these
3. Which of the following statements about the term *echocardiogram* is true? (select all that apply)
   a. image of heart produced using sound waves
   c. procedure to look inside blood vessels
   d. ultrasound of the heart
   b. image of the heart produced using electrical currents
4. *Circulation* is: (select all that apply)
   a. from Latin, for "to go in a circle"
   b. the force exerted by blood on the walls of vessels

c. the moving of blood from the heart through the vessels and back to the heart

d. none of these

5. *Systemic circulation* is:

a. circulation of blood from the heart to the heart muscle

b. circulation of blood from the heart to the lungs

c. circulation of blood from the heart to the rest of the body

d. all of these

6. *Pulmonary circulation* is:

a. circulation of blood from the heart to the heart muscle

b. circulation of blood from the heart to the lungs

c. circulation of blood from the heart to the rest of the body

d. all of these

7. *Coronary circulation* is:

a. circulation of blood from the heart to the heart muscle

b. circulation of blood from the heart to the lungs

c. circulation of blood from the heart to the rest of the body

d. all of these

8. *Blood pressure* is: (select all that apply)

a. from Latin, for "to go in a circle"

b. the force exerted by blood on the walls of vessels

c. the moving of blood from the heart through the vessels and back to the heart

d. none of these

9. *Diastolic pressure* is:

a. the force exerted on blood vessels when the heart is contracting

b. the pressure exerted on blood vessels when the heart is relaxed

c. both the force exerted on blood vessels when the heart is contracting and the pressure exerted on blood vessels when the heart is relaxed

d. none of these

10. *Systolic pressure* is:

a. the force exerted on blood vessels when the heart is contracting

b. the pressure exerted on blood vessels when the heart is relaxed

c. both the force exerted on blood vessels when the heart is contracting and the pressure exerted on blood vessels when the heart is relaxed

d. none of these

11. The *inferior vena cava* is the: (select all that apply)

a. portion of the vena cava that gathers blood from the lower portion of the body

b. portion of the vena cava that gathers blood from the upper portion of the body (head and arms)

c. large-diameter vein that gathers blood from the body and returns it to the heart

d. none of these

12. The *superior vena cava* is the: (select all that apply)

a. portion of the vena cava that gathers blood from the lower portion of the body

b. portion of the vena cava that gathers blood from the upper portion of the body (head and arms)

c. large-diameter vein that gathers blood from the body and returns it to the heart

d. none of these

13. A blockage in a blood vessel caused by a mass of matter present in the blood is known as a(n):

a. atherosclerosis
b. embolism
c. thrombus
d. venostasis

14. The trapping of blood in an extremity due to compression is known as a(n):

a. atherosclerosis
b. embolism
c. thrombus
d. venostasis

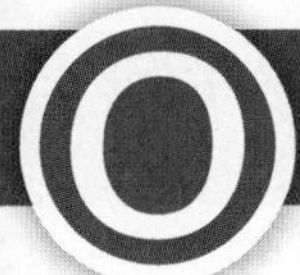

Learning Outcome 9.3 Exercises

15. An abnormal heart sound is a:
    a. cardiac anomaly
    b. cardiophony
    c. coronary anomaly
    d. murmur

16. Which of the following statements about the term *cardiac catheterization* is true? (select all that apply)
    a. It is the process of inserting a tube into the heart.
    b. Doctors are able to diagnose and treat heart problems without performing major surgery by performing this process.
    c. It comes from the root *cardio,* meaning "heart," and Greek words meaning "to go inside."
    d. None of these.

EXERCISE 10 *Briefly describe the difference between each pair of terms.*

1. cardiologist, phlebologist ____________________
2. phlebotomist, phlebotomy ____________________
3. aortolith, arteriolith ____________________
4. echocardiography, electrocardiography ____________________
5. pulmonary circulation, systemic circulation ____________________
6. diastolic pressure, systolic pressure ____________________
7. aortectasia, aortic stenosis ____________________
8. embolus, embolism ____________________
9. embolus, thrombus ____________________
10. ischemia, occlusion ____________________

9.4 Diagnosis and Pathology

Problems with the heart can begin as early as birth. Patients may be born with flaws in the structure of their heart (*congenital heart defect*). Among the most common flaws are holes in the wall of the heart (*atrial septal defect* and *ventricular septal defect*).

Another type of flaw the heart can have is in its electrical system. A problem with electrical signals can cause an abnormal rhythm in the heartbeat (*arrhythmia, dysrhythmia*). Some rhythm problems are very minor and don't even require treatment. Others, like *ventricular fibrillation*, are medical emergencies. Ventricular fibrillation occurs when the main squeezing muscle fibers of the heart do not coordinate. As a result, no blood flow occurs. Unless treated, a patient will likely die of the condition.

When the muscle fibers of the heart do not work as well as they are supposed to (*cardiomyopathy*), the heart may cease to function properly (*cardiac insufficiency*). These problems usually develop over time. Cardiomyopathies can involve muscle that is too floppy (*dilated*), too tight (*restrictive*), or too weak (*congestive*). One type involves muscle that is too thick (*hypertrophic*) and can cause sudden death while a person is playing sports. This is a major reason for physical exams prior to playing sports.

The heart is not a common site for infection, but when it does become infected, the condition is usually very serious. Infection can be inside the muscle (*myocarditis*) or along the lining of the heart and vessels (*endocarditis*).

The heart can be inflamed as a result of other illnesses as well. One site for inflammation is the thin lining on the outside of the heart (*pericarditis*), which can cause fluid to collect around the heart (*pericardial effusion*) and make it more difficult for the heart to work well.

The most common heart problem involves the blood supply to the muscle fibers of the heart. Just as the rest of the body needs blood to take in nutrients and remove harmful waste, the heart needs it too. Coronary arteries serve this purpose. Floating fat in the blood (*cholesterol*) can accumulate and harden in the arteries of the heart. This process is called *atherosclerosis*. When the coronary arteries get blocked enough that it prevents sufficient blood flow, the heart muscle fibers do not get the oxygen they need. As a result, the muscle dies—a heart attack (*myocardial infarction*).

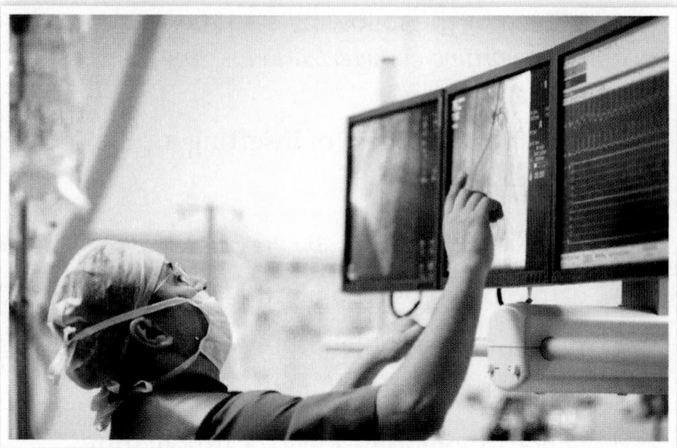

Imaging procedures are the most frequently used tools doctors use to diagnose heart issues.

Common to all heart problems is the possibility of the heart failing to adequately pump the blood to the rest of the body (*congestive heart failure*). The heart's inability to pump all the blood that reaches it creates a bottle-neck effect, which leads to fluid accumulation in the lungs or body. The symptoms of heart failure depend on which side of the heart is affected.

Other blood vessel problems include a blockage (*deep vein thrombosis*) or bulge (*aneurysm*) in the vessel. Vessels can also become inflamed. An inflamed vein (*phlebitis*) is usually a problem involving just one part of a single vein. Inflammation of several blood vessels (*vasculitis*) can present in many different ways, depending on the type of vessels affected.

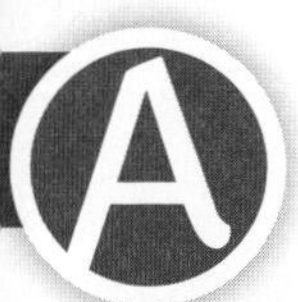

9.4 Diagnosis and Pathology

heart

Term	Word Analysis
angiocarditis AN-jee-oh-kar-DAI-tis **Definition** inflammation of the heart vessels	angio / card / itis vessel / heart / inflammation
atrial fibrillation AY-tree-al FIB-rih-LAY-shun **Definition** quivering or spontaneous contraction of muscle fibers in the heart's atrium	atri / al fibrill / ation atrium / pertaining to little fibers / process
atrial septal defect (ASD) AY-tree-al SEP-tal DEE-fekt **Definition** flaw in the septum that divides the two atria of the heart	atri / al sept / al de / fect atrium / pertaining to septum / pertaining to bad / made
cardiac arrest KAR-dee-ak ah-REST **Definition** cessation of functional circulation	cardi / ac arrest heart / pertaining to stop
cardiomyopathy KAR-dee-oh-mai-AW-pah-thee **Definition** disease of the heart muscle	cardio / myo / pathy heart / muscle / disease
congestive cardiomyopathy con-JES-tiv KAR-dee-oh-mai-AW-pah-thee **Definition** heart cavity is unable to pump all the blood out of itself (*congestive*) and becomes stretched (*dilated*), which causes weak/slow pumping of blood	con / gestive cardiomyopathy together / bring
dilated cardiomyopathy DAI-lay-ted KAR-dee-oh-mai-AW-pah-thee **Definition** another term for congestive cardiomyopathy	dilated cardio / myo / pathy expanded heart / muscle / disease

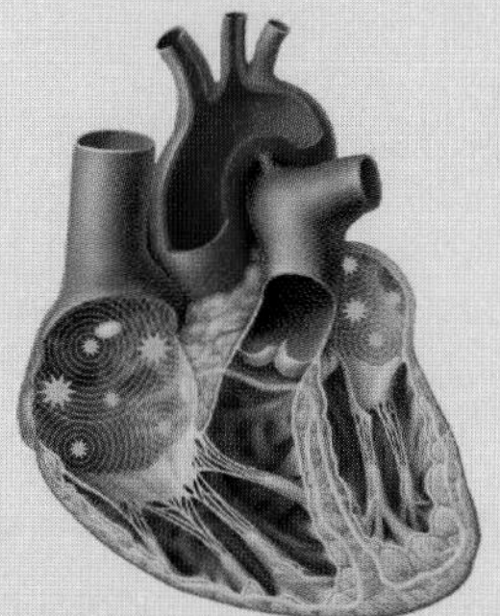

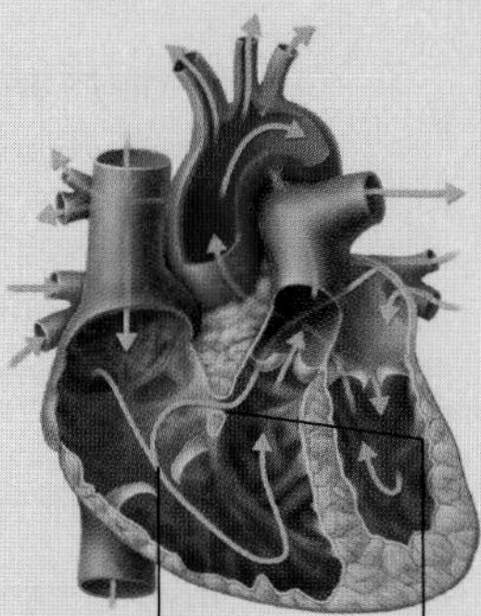

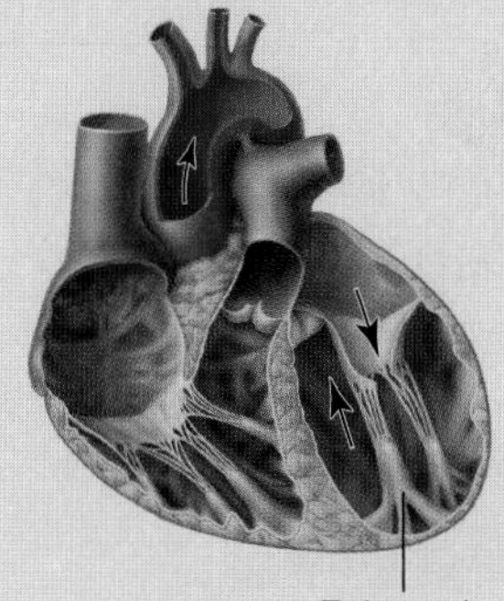

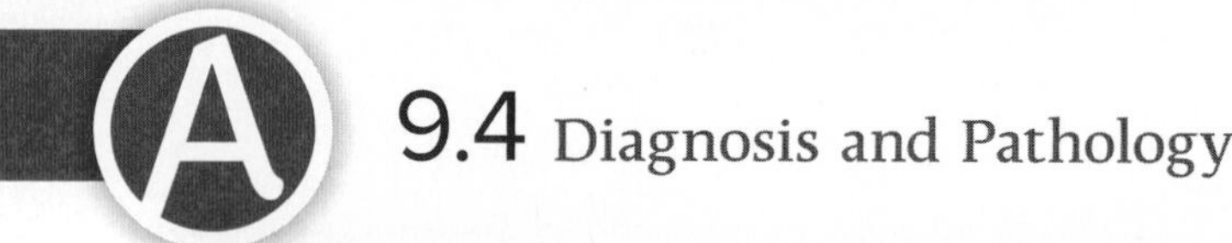

9.4 Diagnosis and Pathology

heart *continued*

Term	Word Analysis
hypertrophic cardiomyopathy HAI-per-TROH-fik KAR-dee-oh-mai-AW-pah-thee **Definition** heart muscle becomes enlarged and blocks blood flow	**hyper / troph / ic cardiomyopathy** over / developed / pertaining to
restrictive cardiomyopathy ree-STRIK-tiv KAR-dee-oh-mai-AW-pah-thee **Definition** heart muscle hardens, restricting the expansion of the heart, thus limiting the amount of blood it can pump to the rest of the body	**re / strict / ive cardiomyopathy** back / tied / pertaining to
carditis kar-DAI-tis **Definition** inflammation of the heart	**card / itis** heart / inflammation
congenital heart defect con-JEN-ih-tal HART DEE-fekt **Definition** flaw in the structure of the heart present at birth	**con / genit / al heart de / fect** together / birth / pertaining to heart bad / made
congestive heart failure (CHF) con-JES-tiv HART FAYL-yir **Definition** heart failure characterized by the heart cavity being unable to pump all the blood out of itself (*congestive*)	**con / gest / ive heart failure** together / bring / pertaining to
coronary thrombosis KOR-ah-NER-ee throm-BOH-sis **Definition** obstruction of a coronary artery by a clot	**coron / ary thromb / osis** heart / pertaining to clot / condition
endocarditis EN-doh-kar-DAI-tis **Definition** inflammation of the tissue lining the inside of the heart	**endo / card / itis** inside / heart / inflammation
myocardial infarction (MI) MAI-oh-KAR-dee-al in-FARK-shun **Definition** death of heart muscle tissue **NOTE:** The term *infarction* originally referred to a blocked blood vessel, but it came to refer to the death of tissue resulting from the blockage.	**myo / cardi / al in / farc / tion** muscle / heart / pertaining to in / stuff / condition
myocardial ischemia MAI-oh-KAR-dee-al ih-SKEE-mee-ah **Definition** blockage of blood to the heart muscle	**myo / cardi / al isch / emia** muscle / heart / pertaining to hold back / blood condition
myocarditis MAI-oh-kar-DAI-tis **Definition** inflammation of the heart muscle	**myo / card / itis** muscle / heart / inflammation

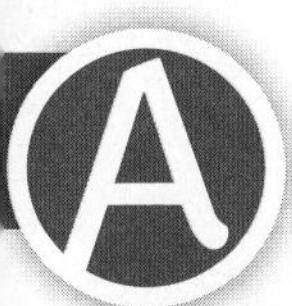

9.4 Diagnosis and Pathology

heart *continued*

Term	Word Analysis
pericardial effusion PER-ee-KAR-dee-al ee-FYOO-zhun **Definition** fluid pouring out into the tissue around the heart	**peri / cardi / al ef / fusion** around / heart / pertaining to out / pour 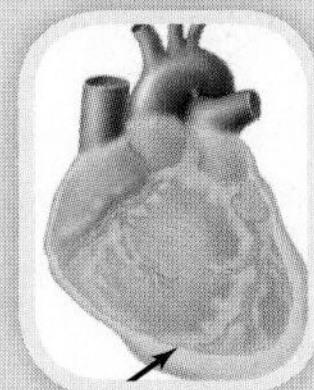
pericarditis PER-ee-kar-DAI-tis **Definition** inflammation of the tissue around the heart	**peri / card / itis** around / heart / inflammation
valvulitis VAL-vyoo-LAI-tis **Definition** inflammation of a heart valve	**valvul / itis** valve / inflammation
ventricular septal defect (VSD) ven-TRIK-yoo-lar SEP-tal DEE-fekt **Definition** flaw in the septum that divides the two ventricles of the heart	**ventricul / ar sept / al de / fect** ventricle / pertaining to septum / pertaining to bad / made

circulation

Term	Word Analysis
aneurysm AN-yir-IZ-um **Definition** bulge in a blood vessel	**an / eury / sm** up / wide / condition 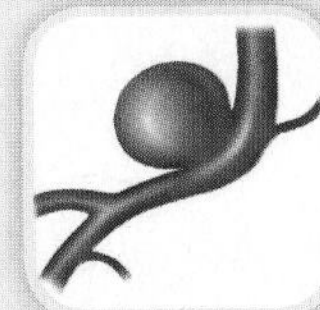

Note: The *an-* prefix here doesn't mean "not"; rather, it is short for *ana* and means "up" or "out." The "not" meaning is much more common, but there are also a few important examples of the "up/out" meaning, such as *anabolic*.

Term	Word Analysis
angioedema AN-jee-oh-eh-DEE-mah **Definition** swelling of the blood vessels	**angio / edema** vessel / swelling
angioma AN-jee-OH-mah **Definition** blood vessel tumor	**angi / oma** vessel / tumor 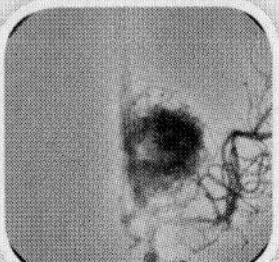 ©Simon Fraser/RNC, Newcastle upon type/Science Source
aortic aneurysm ay-OR-tik AN-yir-IZ-um **Definition** bulging or swelling of the aorta	**aort / ic an / eury / sm** aorta / pertaining to up / wide / condition

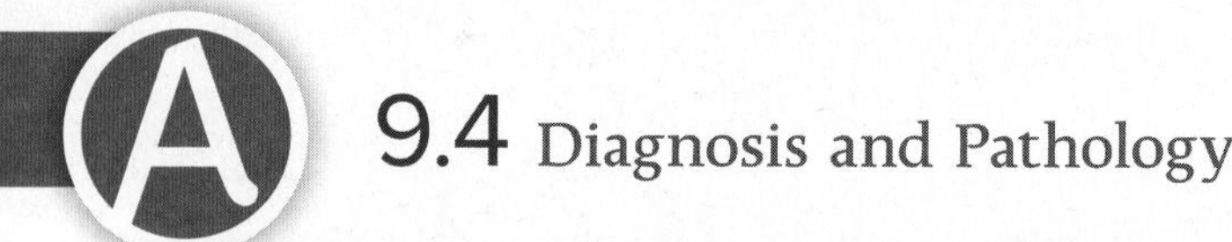

9.4 Diagnosis and Pathology

circulation *continued*

Term	Word Analysis
aortic regurgitation ay-OR-tik ree-GIR-jih-TAY-shun **Definition** flow of blood backward from the aorta into the heart; caused by a weak heart valve	**aort / ic re / gurgit / ation** aorta / pertaining to back / bubble / condition
aortitis ay-or-TAI-tis **Definition** inflammation of the aorta	**aort / itis** aorta / inflammation
arteriopathy ar-TER-ee-AW-pah-thee **Definition** disease of the arteries	**arterio / pathy** artery / disease
arteritis AR-ter-AI-tis **Definition** inflammation of the arteries	**arter / itis** artery / inflammation
deep vein thrombosis DEEP VAYN throm-BOH-sis **Definition** formation of a blood clot in a vein deep in the body, most commonly the leg	**deep vein thromb / osis** deep vein clot / condition
hypertension HAI-per-TEN-shun **Definition** high blood pressure	**hyper / tens / ion** over / stretch / condition
hypotension HAI-poh-TEN-shun **Definition** low blood pressure	**hypo / tens / ion** under / stretch / condition
normotension NOR-moh-TEN-shun **Definition** normal blood pressure	**normo / tens / ion** normal / stretch / condition
phlebitis fleh-BAI-tis **Definition** inflammation of the veins	**phleb / itis** vein / inflammation
phlebostenosis FLEB-oh-sten-OH-sis **Definition** narrowing of the veins	**phlebo / sten / osis** vein / narrow / condition
thrombophlebitis THROM-boh-fleh-BAI-tis **Definition** inflammation of vein caused by a clot	**thrombo / phleb / itis** clot / vein / inflammation
vasculitis VAS-kyoo-LAI-tis **Definition** inflammation of blood vessels	**vascul / itis** vessel / inflammation

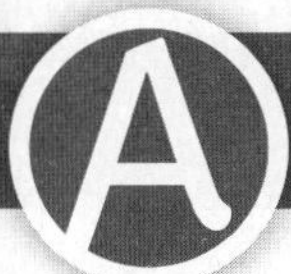

Learning Outcome 9.4 Exercises

PRONUNCIATION

EXERCISE 1 *Indicate which syllable is emphasized when pronounced.*

EXAMPLE: bronchitis bron**chi**tis

1. vasculitis
2. pericarditis
3. myocarditis
4. endocarditis
5. valvulitis
6. normotension
7. coronary thrombosis
8. pericardial effusion
9. angioedema
10. arteriopathy
11. aortic regurgitation
12. thrombophlebitis
13. aortitis
14. phlebitis
15. ventricular septal defect

TRANSLATION

EXERCISE 2 *Break down the following words into their component parts.*

EXAMPLE: nasopharyngoscope *naso | pharyngo | scope*

1. angioma
2. aortitis
3. arteritis
4. phlebitis
5. endocarditis
6. myocarditis
7. pericarditis
8. cardiomyopathy
9. dilated cardiomyopathy
10. myocardial ischemia

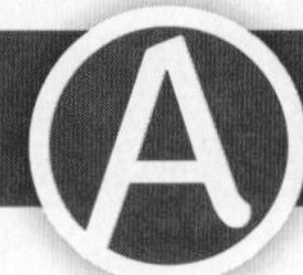

Learning Outcome 9.4 Exercises

EXERCISE 3 *Underline and define the word parts from this chapter in the following terms.*

1. carditis ______
2. valvulitis ______
3. vasculitis ______
4. cardiac arrest ______
5. angioedema ______
6. arteriopathy ______
7. aortic aneurysm ______
8. phlebostenosis ______
9. thrombophlebitis ______
10. coronary thrombosis ______
11. pericardial effusion ______
12. angiocarditis (2 roots) ______
13. myocardial infarction (2 roots) ______
14. atrial septal defect (2 roots) ______
15. ventricular septal defect (2 roots) ______

EXERCISE 4 *Match the term on the left with its definition on the right.*

______	1. normotension	a.	bulge in a blood vessel
______	2. hypertension	b.	flaw in the structure of the heart, present at birth
______	3. hypotension	c.	heart failure characterized by the heart cavity being unable to pump all the blood out of itself
______	4. deep vein thrombosis	d.	high blood pressure
______	5. atrial fibrillation	e.	low blood pressure
______	6. congestive heart failure	f.	normal blood pressure
______	7. congenital heart defect	g.	quivering or spontaneous contraction of muscle fibers in the heart's atrium
______	8. aortic regurgitation	h.	flow of blood backward from the aorta into the heart; caused by a weak heart valve
______	9. aneurysm	i.	formation of a blood clot in a vein deep in the body, most commonly the leg
______	10. restrictive cardiomyopathy	j.	heart is unable to pump all the blood out of itself and becomes stretched, which causes weak/slow blood pumping
______	11. congestive cardiomyopathy	k.	heart muscle fibers become enlarged and block blood flow
______	12. hypertropic cardiomyopathy	l.	heart muscle fibers harden, restricting the expansion of the heart and thus limiting the amount of blood it can pump to the rest of the body

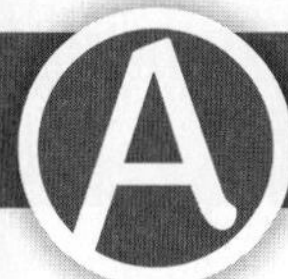

Learning Outcome 9.4 Exercises

EXERCISE 5 *Translate the following terms as literally as possible.*

EXAMPLE: nasopharyngoscope *an instrument for looking at the nose and throat*

1. arteriopathy ____________
2. angioedema ____________
3. phlebostenosis ____________
4. coronary thrombosis ____________
5. normotension ____________
6. atrial septal defect ____________
7. ventricular septal defect ____________
8. dilated cardiomyopathy ____________
9. hypertrophic cardiomyopathy ____________

GENERATION

EXERCISE 6 *Build a medical term from the information provided.*

EXAMPLE: inflammation of the sinuses *sinusitis*

1. inflammation of the veins (use *phleb/o*) ____________
2. inflammation of blood vessels (use *vascul/o*) ____________
3. blood vessel tumor (use *angi/o*) ____________
4. inflammation of the heart ____________
5. inflammation of a heart valve ____________
6. inflammation of the aorta ____________
7. inflammation of the arteries ____________
8. inflammation of the heart vessels ____________
9. inflammation of the heart muscle ____________
10. disease of the heart muscle ____________
11. inflammation of the tissue lining the inside of the heart ____________
12. inflammation of the tissue around the heart ____________
13. inflammation of a vein caused by a clot ____________

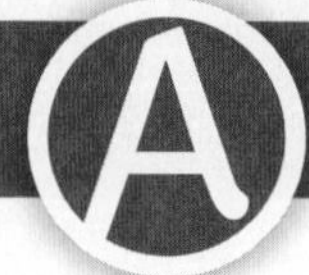

Learning Outcome 9.4 Exercises

EXERCISE 7 *Multiple-choice questions. Select the correct answer.*

1. *Cardiac arrest* is:
   a. a bulge in a blood vessel
   b. cessation of functional circulation
   c. death of heart muscle tissue
   d. fluid pouring out into the tissue around the heart
   e. the flow of blood backward from the aorta back into the heart
2. *Pericardial effusion* is:
   a. a bulge in a blood vessel
   b. cessation of functional circulation
   c. death of heart muscle tissue
   d. fluid pouring out into the tissue around the heart
   e. the flow of blood backward from the aorta back into the heart
3. An *aneurysm* is:
   a. a bulge in a blood vessel
   b. cessation of functional circulation
   c. death of heart muscle tissue
   d. fluid pouring out into the tissue around the heart
   e. the flow of blood backward from the aorta back into the heart
4. The formation of a blood clot in a vein deep in the body, most commonly the leg, is known as a(n):
   a. aneurysm
   b. angioedema
   c. angioma
   d. deep vein thrombosis
   e. thrombophlebitis
5. Quivering or spontaneous contraction of muscle fibers in the heart's upper chamber is known as:
   a. atrial fibrillation
   b. atriospasm
   c. ventricular fibrillation
   d. ventriculospasm
   e. none of these

EXERCISE 8 *Briefly describe the difference between each pair of terms.*

1. hypertension, hypotension ____________________
2. congestive cardiomyopathy, restrictive cardiomyopathy ____________________
3. congenital heart defect, congestive heart failure ____________________
4. myocardial infarction, myocardial ischemia ____________________
5. aortic aneurysm, aortic regurgitation ____________________

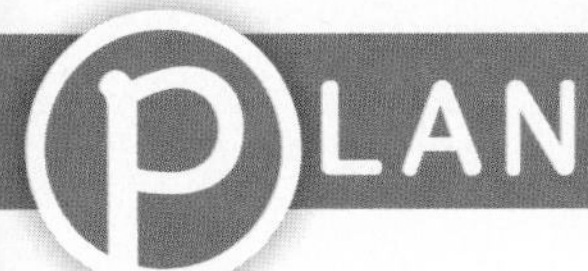

9.5 Treatments and Therapies

Medications for treating the heart deal with alleviating the pain associated with low oxygen to the heart (*antianginal*) and medicines that correct the heart's electrical signals (*antiarrhythmics*). Medicine can also work on blood vessels. They can cause the vessels to squeeze down (*vasoconstrictor, vasopressor*), which causes blood pressure to increase, or they can cause them to dilate (*vasodilator*), which lowers the blood pressure. *Thrombolytics* can work on both the heart and blood vessels. They work by breaking down dangerous accumulations that can develop in the heart or blood vessels.

In the past, the vast majority of procedures to physically correct heart problems used to include cutting open the patient's chest (*cardiothoracic surgery*) for direct access to the heart. While these more invasive means are now less common, they are still necessary for some types of surgeries like making an alternate blood vessel route (*anastomosis*) for congenital heart defects. A similar procedure is a very common treatment for blocked heart vessels. In a procedure known as coronary artery bypass graft, a blood vessel from another part of the body is used to make an alternate route for blood to get to the heart around an area of blockage. This is the most common type of heart surgery. Now, less-invasive techniques are often preferred. One such treatment for coronary artery disease involves passing instruments up a patient's blood vessels into the heart (*percutaneous coronary intervention*). Once the instrument is inside the coronary artery, there are several options for treatment. A balloon can be inflated to crush the buildup (*balloon angioplasty*), a mesh tube can be inserted (*stent*), or the buildup can be destroyed (*atherectomy*).

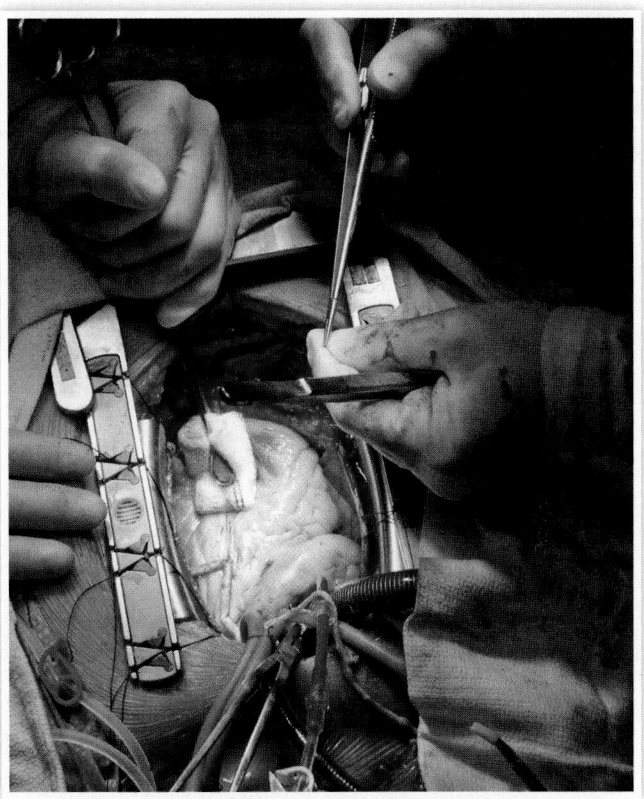

Though less-invasive techniques have been developed in recent years for a variety of heart procedures, for certain procedures—such as coronary artery bypass surgery—doctors still must employ cardiothoracic surgery.

pharmacology

Term	Word Analysis
antianginal AN-tee-AN-jih-nal	**anti / angin / al** against / *angina* (choke) / agent
Definition drug that prevents or relieves the symptoms of angina pectoris	
antiarrhythmic AN-tee-a-RITH-mik	**anti / a / rrhythm / ic** against / no / rhythm / agent
Definition drug that opposes an irregular heartbeat	

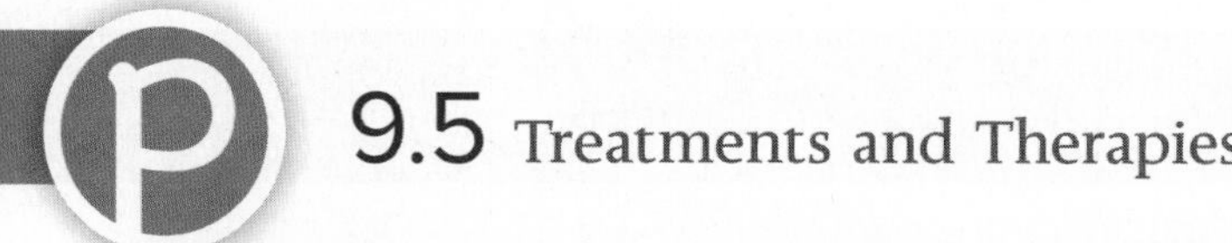

9.5 Treatments and Therapies

pharmacology *continued*

Term	Word Analysis
anticoagulant AN-tee-koh-AG-yoo-lant **Definition** drug that opposes the coagulation of the blood	**anti / coagul / ant** against / coagulation / agent
antihypertensive AN-tee-HAI-per-TEN-siv **Definition** drug that opposes high blood pressure	**anti / hyper / tens / ive** against / over / stretch / agent
cardiotonic KAR-dee-oh-TAW-nik **Definition** drug that increases the strength of the heart contractions	**cardio / ton / ic** heart / tone / agent
thrombolytic THROM-boh-LIH-tik **Definition** drug that breaks down clots	**thrombo / lyt / ic** clot / loose / agent ©Science Photo Library RF/Getty Images RF
vasoconstrictor VAS-oh-kin-STRIK-tor **Definition** drug that constricts or narrows the diameter of a blood vessel	**vaso / constrict / or** vessel / narrowing / agent
vasodilator VAS-oh-DAI-lay-tor **Definition** drug that causes the relaxation or expansion of a blood vessel	**vaso / dilat / or** vessel / expanding / agent
vasopressor VAS-oh-PRES-or **Definition** drug that constricts or narrows the diameter of a blood vessel	**vaso / press / or** vessel / press / agent

heart procedures

Term	Word Analysis
cardiomyotomy KAR-dee-oh-mai-AW-toh-mee **Definition** incision into the heart muscle	**cardio / myo / tomy** heart / muscle / incision
cardiopulmonary bypass KAR-dee-oh-PUL-mon-AR-ee BAI-pas **Definition** procedure that temporarily circulates and oxygenates a patient's blood during the portion of heart surgery where the heart is stopped	**cardio / pulmon / ary bypass** heart / lung / pertaining to

heart procedures *continued*

Term	Word Analysis
cardiopulmonary resuscitation (CPR) KAR-dee-oh-PUL-mon-AR-ee re-SUS-uh-TAY-shun **Definition** basic life support	**cardio / pulmon / ary re / suscit / ation** heart / lung / pertaining to again / stir up / procedure 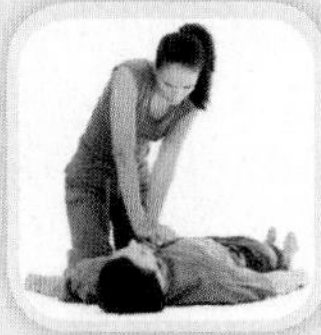 ©Stockbyte Platinum/Alamy Stock Photo RF
NOTE: Despite its name, CPR does not actually *resuscitate* an unconscious patient. Rather, through artificial breathing and chest compression, an unresponsive patient's blood circulates and is kept oxygenated until further steps can be taken.	
cardiothoracic surgery KAR-dee-oh-thoh-RA-sik SIR-jir-ee **Definition** surgery that involves cutting through the patient's chest to get to the heart	**cardio / thorac / ic surgery** heart / chest / pertaining to
NOTE: Remember, a *c* before an *a, o,* or *u* makes a *k* sound (*KAR-dee-oh*) but before an *i* or *e*, it makes an *s* sound (*thoh-RA-sik*).	
cardioversion KAR-dee-oh-VER-zhun **Definition** returning a heart to normal rhythm	**cardio / vers / ion** heart / turn / procedure
coronary arterectomy KOR-ah-NER-ee AR-ter-EK-toh-mee **Definition** surgical removal of a coronary artery	**coron / ary arter / ectomy** heart / pertaining to artery / removal
coronary artery bypass graft (CABG) KOR-ah-NER-ee AR-ter-ee BAI-pas GRAFT **Definition** borrowed piece of blood vessel used to bypass a blocked artery in the heart	**coronary artery bypass graft**
coronary artery bypass surgery KOR-ah-NER-ee AR-ter-ee BAI-pas SIR-jir-ee **Definition** surgery to bypass a blocked artery in the heart	**coronary artery bypass surgery**
percutaneous coronary intervention PER-kyoo-TAY-nee-us KOR-ah-NER-ee IN-ter-VEN-shun **Definition** alternate treatment for a coronary artery that passes instruments up a patient's blood vessels into the heart	**per / cutane / ous coron / ary** through / skin / pertaining to heart / pertaining to
pericardiocentesis PER-ee-KAR-dee-oh-sin-TEE-sis **Definition** puncture of the tissue around the heart	**peri / cardio / centesis** around / heart / puncture 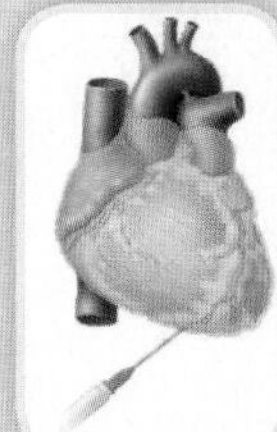
pericardiotomy PER-ee-KAR-dee-AW-toh-mee **Definition** incision into the tissue around the heart	**peri / cardio / tomy** around / heart / incision

heart procedures *continued*

Term	Word Analysis
valvectomy val-VEK-toh-mee **Definition** surgical removal of a heart valve	**valv / ectomy** valve / removal
valvotomy val-VAW-toh-mee **Definition** incision into a heart valve **NOTE:** Alternative spelling valvulotomy, using *valvulo*, is also acceptable.	**valvo / tomy** valve / incision
valvuloplasty VAL-vyoo-loh-PLAS-tee **Definition** surgical reconstruction of a heart valve	**valvulo / plasty** valve / reconstruction
ventriculotomy ven-TRIK-yoo-LAW-toh-mee **Definition** incision into a ventricle	**ventriculo / tomy** ventricle / incision

circulation procedures

Term	Word Analysis
anastomosis ah-NAS-tah-moh-sis **Definition** creation of an opening between two normally separate structures **NOTE:** The *an-* prefix here doesn't mean "not"; rather, it is short for *ana* and means "up" or "out." The "not" meaning is much more common, but there are also a few important examples of the "up/out" meaning, such as *anabolic*.	**ana / stom / osis** up / mouth / condition
aneurysmectomy AN-yir-IZ-um-EK-toh-mee **Definition** surgical removal of an aneurysm	**an / eury / sm / ectomy** up / wide / condition / removal
angioplasty AN-jee-oh-PLAS-tee **Definition** surgical reconstruction of a vessel	**angio / plasty** vessel / reconstruction
angiorrhaphy AN-jee-OR-ah-fee **Definition** suture of a vessel	**angio / rrhaphy** vessel / suture

circulation procedures *continued*

Term	Word Analysis
aortorrhaphy ay-or-TOR-ah-fee **Definition** suture of the aorta	**aorto / rrhaphy** aorta / suture
aortotomy ay-or-TAW-toh-mee **Definition** incision into the aorta	**aorto / tomy** aorta / incision
arteriectomy ar-TER-ee-EK-toh-mee **Definition** surgical removal of an artery	**arteri / ectomy** artery / removal
arterioplasty ar-TER-ee-oh-PLAS-tee **Definition** surgical reconstruction of an artery	**arterio / plasty** artery / reconstruction
arteriorrhaphy ar-TER-ee-OR-ah-fee **Definition** suture of an artery	**arterio / rrhaphy** artery / suture
atherectomy A-ther-EK-toh-mee **Definition** surgical removal of fatty plaque within an artery	**ather / ectomy** fatty plaque / removal
embolectomy EM-boh-LEK-toh-mee **Definition** surgical removal of an embolus	**embol / ectomy** embolus / removal
endarterectomy END-ar-ter-EK-toh-mee **Definition** surgical removal of the inside of an artery	**end / arter / ectomy** inside / artery / removal
phlebectomy fleb-EK-toh-mee **Definition** surgical removal of a vein	**phleb / ectomy** vein / removal
phlebophlebostomy FLEB-oh-fleb-AW-stoh-mee **Definition** procedure to create an opening between two veins	**phlebo / phlebo / stomy** vein / vein / opening

9.5 Treatments and Therapies

circulation procedures *continued*

Term	Word Analysis
varicotomy VAR-ih-KAW-toh-mee **Definition** surgical removal of a varicose vein	**varico / tomy** swollen / incision
NOTE: Normally, you would expect *-ectomy* to mean "removal," but *varicectomy* was probably too much of a mouthful.	
venectomy veh-NEK-toh-mee **Definition** surgical removal of a vein	**ven / ectomy** vein / removal

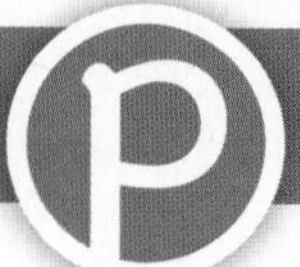

Learning Outcome 9.5 Exercises

PRONUNCIATION

EXERCISE 1 *Indicate which syllable is emphasized when pronounced.*

EXAMPLE: bronchitis bron**chi**tis

1. cardioversion ______
2. valvuloplasty ______
3. atherectomy ______
4. embolectomy ______
5. arteriectomy ______
6. arterioplasty ______
7. ventriculotomy ______
8. angiorrhaphy ______
9. arteriorrhaphy ______
10. endarterectomy ______
11. anastomosis ______
12. pericardiotomy ______
13. antiarrhythmic ______
14. pericardiocentesis ______
15. valvectomy ______
16. valvotomy ______
17. varicotomy ______
18. venectomy ______
19. phlebectomy ______
20. aortotomy ______

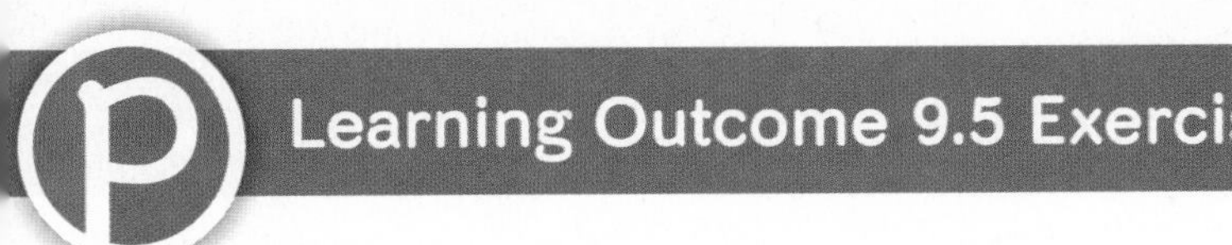

Learning Outcome 9.5 Exercises

TRANSLATION

EXERCISE 2 *Break down the following words into their component parts.*

EXAMPLE: nasopharyngoscope *naso | pharyngo | scope*

1. vasodilator ______
2. arterioplasty ______
3. angioplasty ______
4. antihypertensive ______
5. anticoagulant ______
6. thrombolytic ______
7. valvectomy ______
8. embolectomy ______
9. aortotomy ______
10. cardiomyotomy ______
11. cardioversion ______
12. pericardiotomy ______
13. phlebophlebostomy ______
14. cardiothoracic surgery ______

EXERCISE 3 *Underline and define the word parts from this chapter in the following terms.*

1. valvectomy ______
2. venectomy ______
3. atherectomy ______
4. phlebectomy ______
5. arteriectomy ______
6. endarterectomy ______
7. valvotomy ______
8. ventriculotomy ______
9. valvuloplasty ______
10. angiorrhaphy ______
11. aortorrhaphy ______
12. arteriorrhaphy ______
13. cardiotonic ______
14. vasoconstrictor ______
15. percutaneous coronary intervention ______
16. vasopressor ______
17. pericardiocentesis ______
18. cardiopulmonary bypass ______
19. coronary arterectomy (2 roots) ______

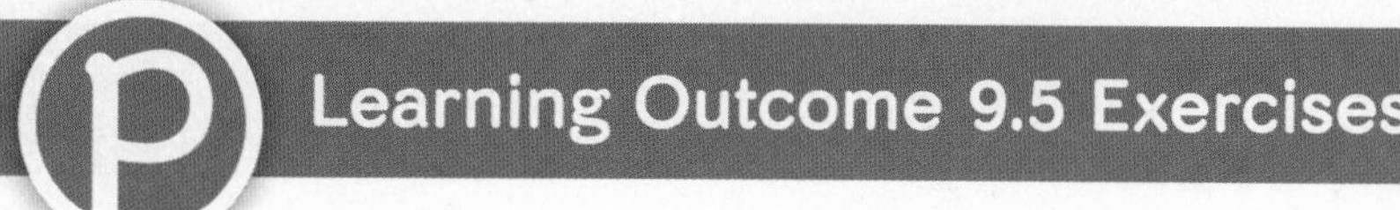

Learning Outcome 9.5 Exercises

EXERCISE 4 *Match the term on the left with its definition on the right.*

______	1. coronary artery bypass surgery	a.	borrowed piece of blood vessel used to bypass a blocked artery in the heart
______	2. coronary artery bypass graft	b.	drug that opposes an irregular heartbeat
______	3. antiarrhythmic	c.	drug that prevents or relieves the symptoms of angina pectoris
______	4. cardiopulmonary resuscitation	d.	alternate treatment for the coronary artery that passes instruments up a patient's blood vessels into the heart
______	5. percutaneous coronary intervention	e.	basic life support: artificial breathing and chest compression
______	6. antianginal	f.	surgery to bypass a blocked artery in the heart
______	7. aneurysmectomy	g.	surgical removal of a varicose vein
______	8. varicotomy	h.	surgical removal of an aneurysm
______	9. anastomosis	i.	creation of an opening between two normally separate structures

EXERCISE 5 *Translate the following terms as literally as possible.*

EXAMPLE: nasopharyngoscope *an instrument for looking at the nose and throat*

1. arterioplasty ______________________
2. valvuloplasty ______________________
3. angioplasty ______________________
4. angiorrhaphy ______________________
5. aortorrhaphy ______________________
6. arteriorrhaphy ______________________
7. vasoconstrictor ______________________
8. vasodilator ______________________
9. vasopressor ______________________
10. cardioversion ______________________
11. pericardiocentesis ______________________

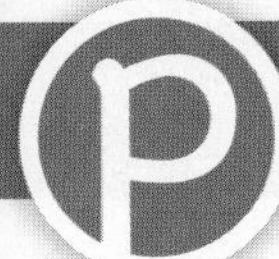

Learning Outcome 9.5 Exercises

EXERCISE 6 *Fill in the blanks.*

1. antihypertensive = drug that opposes ____________________
2. anticoagulant = drug that opposes ____________________
3. thrombolytic = drug that ____________________
4. antiarrhythmic = drug that opposes a(n) ____________________
5. antianginal = drug that prevents or relieves the symptoms of ____________________

GENERATION

EXERCISE 7 *Build a medical term from the information provided.*

EXAMPLE: inflammation of the sinuses *sinusitis*

1. surgical removal of a vein (use *phleb/o*) ____________________
2. surgical removal of a vein (use *ven/o*) ____________________
3. surgical removal of a varicose vein ____________________
4. surgical removal of a heart valve ____________________
5. incision into a heart valve ____________________
6. incision into a ventricle ____________________
7. incision into the aorta ____________________
8. incision into the heart muscle ____________________
9. incision into the tissue around the heart ____________________
10. surgical removal of an artery ____________________
11. surgical removal of a coronary artery ____________________
12. surgical removal of the inside of an artery ____________________
13. surgical removal of fatty plaque (within an artery) ____________________
14. surgical removal of an aneurysm ____________________
15. surgical removal of an embolus ____________________

Learning Outcome 9.5 Exercises

EXERCISE 8 *Multiple-choice questions. Select the correct answer.*

1. A *cardiotonic:*
   a. breaks down clots
   b. causes the relaxation of expansion of a blood vessel
   c. increases the strength of heart contractions
   d. opposes an irregular heartbeat
   e. prevents or relieves the symptoms of angina pectoris
2. A procedure that temporarily circulates and oxygenates a patient's blood during the portion of heart surgery where the heart is stopped is known as:
   a. anastomosis
   b. cardiopulmonary bypass
   c. cardiopulmonary resuscitation
   d. percutaneous coronary intervention
   e. none of these
3. Which of the following statements about the abbreviation *CPR* is *not* true?
   a. It is basic life support.
   b. It keeps a patient's blood circulating and oxygenated.
   c. It is a process of artificial breathing and chest compression.
   d. It resuscitates an unconscious patient.
   e. It stands for cardiopulmonary resuscitation.
4. The surgical removal of a varicose vein is known as:
   a. varicectomy
   b. varicotomy
   c. vasectomy
   d. venectomy
   e. none of these
5. Surgery that involves cutting through the patient's chest to get to the heart is known as:
   a. cardiopulmonary bypass surgery
   d. percutaneous coronary intervention
   b. cardiopulmonary resuscitation
   e. none of these
   c. cardiothoracic surgery

EXERCISE 9 *Briefly describe the difference between each pair of terms.*

1. vasoconstrictor, vasodilator ______
2. coronary artery bypass graft, coronary artery bypass surgery ______
3. anastomosis, phlebophlebostomy ______

9.6 Abbreviations

Abbreviations provide a shorthand way of referring to things that either recur often or are too long to write out. When dealing with the heart and circulatory system, these can refer to diseases (CAD), test data (CO, SV), test procedures (EKG, MRA), diagnoses (CHF, HTN, SCA), and treatments (CABG, PCI).

cardiovascular system abbreviations

Abbreviation	Definition
AA	abdominal aortic aneurysm
A-fib	atrial fibrillation
ASD	atrial septal defect
BP	blood pressure
CABG	coronary artery bypass graft
CAD	coronary artery disease
CHF	congestive heart failure
CO	cardiac output
CTA	computed tomographic angiography
DVT	deep vein thrombosis
ECHO	echocardiogram
EKG	electrocardiogram
HTN	hypertension
MI	myocardial infarction
MRA	magnetic resonance angiography
MVP	mitral valve prolapse
NSR	normal sinus rhythm
PCI	percutaneous coronary intervention
SCA	sudden cardiac arrest
SV	stroke volume
TEE	transesophageal echocardiogram
VSD	ventricular septal defect

Learning Outcome 9.6 Exercises

EXERCISE 1 *Define the following abbreviations.*

1. BP ____________
2. CABG ____________
3. ECHO ____________
4. EKG ____________
5. DVT ____________
6. TEE ____________
7. MRA ____________
8. NSR ____________
9. CAD ____________
10. CHF ____________
11. CO ____________
12. SCA ____________
13 A-fib ____________

EXERCISE 2 *Give the abbreviations for the following terms.*

1. atrial septal defect ____________
2. computed tomographic angiography ____________
3. hypertension ____________
4. myocardial infarction ____________
5. mitral valve prolapse ____________
6. percutaneous coronary intervention ____________
7. stroke volume ____________
8. ventricular septal defect ____________
9. coronary artery disease ____________
10. cardiac output ____________
11. normal sinus rhythm ____________
12. abdominal aortic aneurysm ____________

EXERCISE 3 *Match the abbreviation on the left with its full definition on the right.*

_____	1. BP	a. borrowed piece of blood vessel used to bypass a blocked artery in the heart
_____	2. PCI	b. alternate treatment for the coronary artery that passes instruments up a patient's blood vessels into the heart
_____	3. CABG	c. death of heart muscle tissue
_____	4. CHF	d. heart failure characterized by the heart cavity being unable to pump all the blood out of itself (*congestive*)
_____	5. MI	e. high blood pressure
_____	6. DVT	f. force exerted by blood on the walls of blood vessels
_____	7. HTN	g. formation of a blood clot deep in the body, most commonly in the leg

Learning Outcome 9.6 Exercises

EXERCISE 4 *Multiple-choice questions. Select the correct answer(s).*

1. *Stroke volume* is the volume of blood pumped from one ventricle of the heart with each beat. The abbreviation for this is:

   a. BP
   b. NSR
   c. SV
   d. Svol
   e. vol

2. *Cardiac output* is the volume of blood being pumped by the heart, in particular by a left or right ventricle, in the time interval of 1 minute. The abbreviation for this is:

   a. CAD
   b. CO
   c. CTA
   d. SCA
   e. SV

3. *MRA* is:

   a. a procedure to describe blood vessels using magnetic resonance
   b. a procedure to describe heart muscle fibers using magnetic resonance
   c. a procedure to treat blood vessels using multiple radiations
   d. a procedure to treat heart muscle fibers using multiple radiations
   e. none of these

4. *MVP* stands for:

   a. mitral valve prolapse
   b. mitral ventricle procedure
   c. mitral ventricle prolapse
   d. myocardial valve procedure
   e. myocardial valve prolapse

5. Which of the following abbreviations refer to a diagnostic procedure? (select all that apply)

   a. ASD
   b. ECHO
   c. EKG
   d. TEE
   e. VSD

6. Which of the following abbreviations refer to defects in the septa of the heart? (select all that apply)

   a. ASD
   b. ECHO
   c. EKG
   d. TEE
   e. VSD

7. *Sinus rhythm* is a term used in medicine to describe the normal beating of the heart. A person with *NSR* has:

   a. a fast heartbeat
   b. a normal heartbeat
   c. a slow heartbeat
   d. a stopped heartbeat
   e. an irregular heartbeat

9.7 Electronic Health Records

Cardiology Admission Note

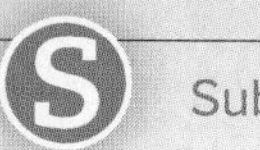 Subjective

Chief Complaint: VSD, postop.

History of Present Illness:

Sharon Jackson is a 12-month-old female with a history of **VSD** first discovered on **echocardiogram** shortly after birth. She has been followed by cardiology. She had been stable from a **cardiovascular** standpoint until the past month, when her parents noticed that she had increased difficulty eating. She would sweat after eating and become **cyanotic** with exertion. Her mother followed up with Sharon's **cardiologist**, who sent her to our office for consult.

Sharon's symptoms were consistent with **congestive heart failure**. It was decided to surgically correct her VSD. She underwent a **sternotomy** and **atriotomy** for patch placement in the ventricular septum to correct her VSD. This was performed with cardiopulmonary bypass. Sharon tolerated the procedure well and is now being admitted for postoperative observation and care.

Review of Systems: No fever, cough, congestion, vomiting, diarrhea.

Medications: IV antibiotics.

Allergies: No known drug allergies.

Past Medical History: Noncontributory.

Past Surgical History: None.

Social History: Stays at home with mother.

Two school-aged siblings.

Family History: Noncontributory.

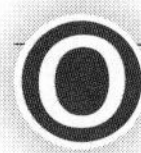 Objective

Vital Signs: Temp: 99.2; Heart rate: 94;
Respiratory rate: 26; Blood pressure: 94/64.

Physical Exam

General: Sedated and intubated.

Head: NCAT. Mucous membranes moist. PERRLA.

Cardiovascular: RRR with soft systolic murmur.

Respiratory: CTA.

Abdomen: Soft, nontender, nondistended.

Neurologic: Sedated.

Skin: No cyanosis or edema.

Labs: CBC normal.

Imaging: CXR–No **cardiomegaly**.

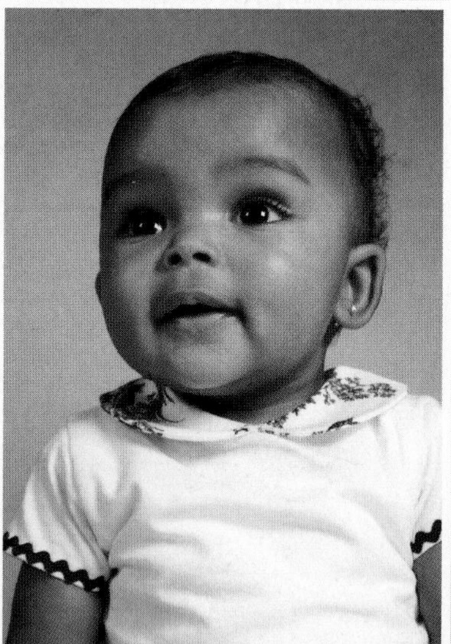

©Punchstock/Image Source RF

 Assessment

1. Postop for VSD repair–routine postop orders and care.
2. When patient switches to PO, we will d/c IV ABx, and at discharge, she will continue antibiotics as needed for **endocarditis** prophylaxis.

–Miles O'Keefe, PA

Learning Outcome 9.7 Exercises

EXERCISE 1 *Match the term on the left with its definition on the right.*

______	1. cardiology	a.	procedure that temporarily circulates and oxygenates a patient's blood during a portion of heart surgery where the heart is stopped
______	2. cardiologist	b.	image of the heart produced using sound waves; the same procedure as an ultrasound performed on pregnant women, but instead is performed on the heart
______	3. cardiomegaly	c.	branch of medicine dealing with the heart
______	4. echocardiogram	d.	enlarged heart
______	5. endocarditis	e.	flaw in the septum that divides the two ventricles of the heart
______	6. ventricular septal defect	f.	heart failure characterized by the heart cavity being unable to pump all the blood out of itself
______	7. congestive heart failure	g.	heart specialist
______	8. cardiopulmonary bypass	h.	inflammation of the tissue lining the inside of the heart

EXERCISE 2 *Fill in the blanks.*

1. Using the data recorded at the patient's physical examination, fill in the following blanks.
   a. T: ______________________________
   b. HR: ______________________________
   c. RR: ______________________________
   d. Cardiovascular (give definition: ______________________________)
      RRR (define abbreviation: ______________________________)
2. According to the history of present illness, Sharon's symptoms were consistent with *congestive heart failure* (give abbreviation: ______________________________).
3. Sharon's sternotomy (*sterno* = sternum + *tomy* = ______________________________) and atriotomy were performed with ______________________________ (a procedure that temporarily circulates and oxygenates a patient's blood during a portion of heart surgery where the heart is stopped).

EXERCISE 3 *True or false questions. Indicate true answers with a T and false answers with an F.*

1. The patient is 12 years old. ________
2. The patient has a Hx of ventricular septal defect. ________
3. The patient's VSD was first discovered on ECHO shortly after birth. ________
4. The patient has CHF. ________
5. The patient has an enlarged heart. ________
6. The patient will not need to continue her antibiotics once she is discharged. ________

Learning Outcome 9.7 Exercises

EXERCISE 4 *Multiple-choice questions. Select the correct answer(s).*

1. Sharon underwent an *atriotomy*. Which of the following is an accurate breakdown of the term?
   a. *atrio* (aorta) + *tomy* (incision) = incision into the upper chamber of the heart
   b. *atrio* (aorta) + *tomy* (removal) = incision into the lower chamber of the heart
   c. *atrio* (atrium) + *tomy* (incision) = incision into the lower chamber of the heart
   d. *atrio* (atrium) + *tomy* (incision) = incision into the upper chamber of the heart
   e. *atrio* (atrium) + *tomy* (removal) = incision into the upper chamber of the heart

2. To correct her VSD, a patch was placed on Sharon's *ventricular septum*. Select all that apply to the term *ventricular septum*.
   a. Septum comes from a Latin word meaning "partition" or "dividing structure" and can refer to any wall dividing two cavities.
   b. The term comes from Roman architecture where it referred to the large, open area in the center of every Roman house off of which all the other rooms of the house branched out.
   c. The ventricle is the lower portion of each side of the heart.
   d. The ventricle is the upper portion of each side of the heart.
   e. The word *ventricle* is a combination of *venter* (stomach) plus the diminutive suffix *-icle*, and means "little stomach"

3. Sharon will be given antibiotic as needed for *endocarditis prophylaxis*. Which of the following is an accurate breakdown of the term?
   a. *endo* (inside) + *card* (heart) + *itis* (inflammation) + *prophylaxis* (preventative treatment)
   b. *endo* (inside) + *card* (heart) + *itis* (inflammation) + *prophylaxis* (treatment of symptoms)
   c. *endo* (outside) + *card* (heart) + *itis* (inflammation) + *prophylaxis* (treatment of symptoms)
   d. *endo* (outside) + *card* (heart) + *itis* (inflammation) + *prophylaxis* (preventative treatment)
   e. none of these

4. During Sharon's physical examination, the physician noted a "soft systolic murmur," which indicates that she has:
   a. an abnormal heart rate when the heart is contracting
   b. an abnormal heart rate when the heart is relaxed
   c. an abnormal heart sound when the heart is contracting
   d. an abnormal heart sound when the heart is relaxed
   e. none of these

Cardiology Consult Note

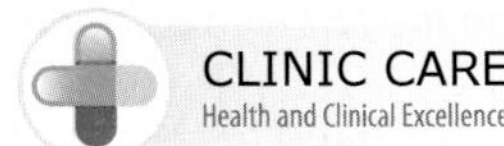

Reason for Consult: 65-year-old male with chest pain consistent with **myocardial ischemia**.

History of Present Illness: Chester Payne is a 65-year-old white male who presented to the emergency department with a 1-day history of worsening **cardiodynia**. The pain began as a dull pressure sensation 6/10 in severity. He had taken sublingual nitroglycerin at home. Despite taking two pills, Mr. Payne reported that the pain worsened to 8/10 and radiated up his neck and down his left arm. At this point, his wife insisted he seek medical attention. Upon arrival at the ED, Mr. Payne was treated according to routine cardiac protocol and the **cardiology** service was consulted.

Past Medical History:
CAD with **PTCA** in 20xx. **Hypertension.** Hypertriglyceridemia.
Medications: Beta blocker *(medicine used to decrease blood pressure)*, nitroglycerin prn, **ASA,** antilipidemic agent.
Allergies: Penicillin.
Family History: Brother deceased from an **MI** at 69 years of age.
Social: Patient does not smoke. He drinks 1–2 beers per week. Denies illicit drug use. He is married with two grown children and three grandchildren.

Review of Systems: Mr. Payne denies any new neurologic problems. Other than mild gastroesophageal reflux *(heartburn)*, which responds to OTC antacid medication, there is no GI disease. He denies asthma or any other respiratory issues.

Physical Exam:
Temp: 98.6; HR: 72; RR: 24; BP: 90/60. Pulse Ox: 99% on 3L per nasal cannula.
General: Diaphoretic, mildly uncomfortable but responsive to questions. Alert and oriented.
HEENT: Pupils equal round and reactive to light bilaterally; mucous membranes moist and pink, nares patent, no flaring.
Neck: Supple. No goiter. No **JVD** or **bruits.**
Resp: Clear to auscultation.
CV: Regular rate and rhythm. Soft **systolic** ejection **murmur**, no gallop or rub. No thrills.
Abdomen: Soft, nontender, nondistended. No abdominal bruits.
Skin: No tenting of skin. Cap refill 2 seconds.
Ext: No cyanosis, clubbing, or edema.

EKG: Ischemic changes.
Lab: Cardiac enzymes *(products of cardiac muscle breakdown)* elevated.
CXR: No **cardiomegaly.**

Impression: **Acute myocardial infarction.**

Plan: Patient has already had an emergent **coronary arteriography,** which showed three **stenotic** vessels. I have recommended **CABG** over **percutaneous catheterization** due to three-vessel involvement, and the patient agrees.

—Ramon Sinclar, MD

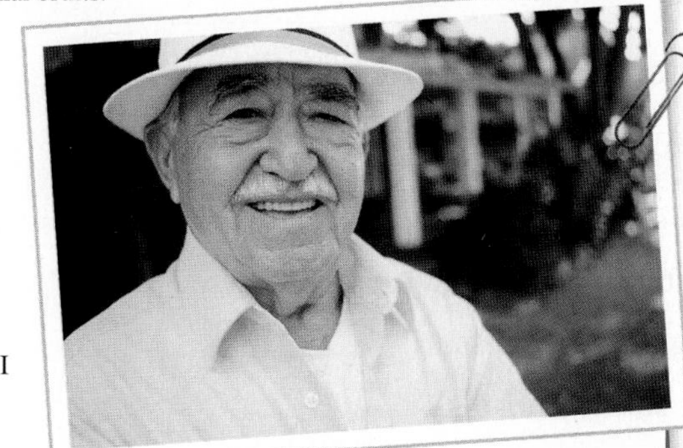

©Hillstreet Studios/Blend Images LLC RF

Learning Outcome 9.7 Exercises

EXERCISE 5 *Match the term on the left with its definition on the right.*

______	1. cardiology	a.	borrowed piece of blood vessel used to bypass a blocked artery in the heart
______	2. cardiomegaly	b.	abnormal heart sound
______	3. murmur	c.	blockage of blood flow to an organ
______	4. electrocardiogram	d.	blockage of blood to the heart muscle
______	5. coronary artery bypass graft	e.	branch of medicine dealing with the heart
______	6. ischemia	f.	death of heart muscle tissue
______	7. myocardial ischemia	g.	enlarged heart
______	8. myocardial infarction	h.	record of the electrical currents of the heart

EXERCISE 6 *Fill in the blanks.*

1. Using the data recorded at Mr. Payne's physical examination, fill in the following blanks.
   a. The patient's temperature: ______________________________
   b. The patient's heart rate: ______________________________
   c. The patient's respiratory rate: ______________________________
   d. The patient's blood pressure: ______________________________
   e. CV (give definition for abbreviation: ______________________________)
2. Past medical history: *hypertension* (give definition: ______________________________).
3. Past medical history: ______________________________ (coronary artery disease).
4. EKG (give definition for abbreviation: ______________________________): ischemic changes.
5. CXR (chest x-ray): no *cardiomegaly* (give definition: ______________________________).

EXERCISE 7 *True or false questions. Indicate true answers with a T and false answers with an F.*

1. Mr. Payne presented to the ED with cardiodynia. ________
2. Mr. Payne has high blood pressure. ________
3. Mr. Payne's heart sounds normal. ________
4. Mr. Payne has HTN. ________
5. Mr. Payne's brother died of a myocardial ischemia. ________
6. Dr. Sinclar recommends a coronary artery bypass graft. ________

Learning Outcome 9.7 Exercises

EXERCISE 8 *Multiple-choice questions. Select the correct answer.*

1. The patient's past medical history shows *coronary artery disease,* which is:
   a. a disease of the arteries
   b. a disease of the arteries of the heart
   c. a disease of the heart
   d. none of these

2. The patient has already had a *coronary arteriography*. Which of the following is an accurate breakdown of the term *coronary arteriography?*
   a. *coronary* (heart) + *arterio* (artery) + *graphy* (record)
   b. *coronary* (heart) + *arterio* (artery) + *graphy* (writing procedure)
   c. *coronary* (heart) + *arterio* (vein) + *graphy* (record)
   d. *coronary* (heart) + *arterio* (vein) + *graphy* (writing procedure)

3. The patient presented to the emergency department with *cardiodynia*. Which of the following is an accurate breakdown of the term *cardiodynia?*
   a. *cardio* (blood vessel) + *dynia* (dilation)
   b. *cardio* (blood vessel) + *dynia* (pain)
   c. *cardio* (heart) + *dynia* (dilation)
   d. *cardio* (heart) + *dynia* (pain)

4. The patient has a past medical history of *hypertriglyceridemia*. Which of the following is an accurate breakdown of the term *hypertriglyceridemia?*
   a. *hyper* (over) + *triglyceride* (fatty molecule) + *-emia* (blood condition)
   b. *hyper* (over) + *triglyceride* (fatty molecule) + *-emia* (urine condition)
   c. *hyper* (under) + *triglyceride* (fatty molecule) + *-emia* (blood condition)
   d. *hyper* (under) + *triglyceride* (fatty molecule) + *-emia* (urine condition)

5. The patient took *sublingual nitroglycerin.* Nitroglycerin is used medically as a vasodilator to treat heart conditions. A *vasodilator* is a:
   a. drug that causes the relaxation or expansion of a blood vessel
   b. drug that causes the relaxation or expansion of the heart
   c. drug that constricts or narrows the diameter of a blood vessel
   d. drug that constricts or narrows the diameter of the heart

6. The physician's impression is that the patient has *acute myocardial infarction,* which is:
   a. a blockage of blood to the heart muscle that has been going on for a while
   b. a blockage of blood to the heart muscle that just started recently
   c. a death of heart muscle tissue that has been going on for a while
   d. a death of heart muscle tissue that just started recently

7. The *percutaneous* approach is commonly used in vascular procedures. This involves a needle catheter getting access to a blood vessel, followed by the introduction of a wire through the pathway of the needle. It is over this wire that other catheters can be placed into the blood vessel. According to this medical consult:
   a. the consulting physician recommended a coronary artery bypass graft instead of a *percutaneous catheterization*
   b. the patient already had a *percutaneous catheterization*
   c. the patient refused *percutaneous catheterization*
   d. the patient will undergo a *percutaneous catheterization*

Cardiothoracic Surgery Clinic Note

Subjective

Mrs. Short presents to my office for her routine postoperative follow-up following **aortic valvuloplasty.** She has been followed by her cardiologist for known **bicuspid aortic valve** related to her Turner syndrome. She has recently had difficulty breathing with exercise and episodes of syncope. An **echocardiogram** revealed **left ventricular hypertrophy.** Since she was becoming symptomatic, she was referred to my office for surgical correction. She underwent **aortic valvuloplasty** 5 days previously and was discharged 2 days ago.

Since her surgery, she has had a few episodes of **tachycardia** and a funny feeling in her chest. She denies pain or fever.

Objective

Temp: 99.0. HR: 60. RR: 20. BP: 112/70.

General: Pleasant, responsive. No acute distress.

HEENT: Pupils equal, round, and reactive to light. Mucous membranes moist and pink.

Resp: Clear to auscultation. No wheezes, rales, rhonchi, or crackles. Good air exchange. No increased work of breathing.

Chest: **Sternotomy** incision healing well without warmth, erythema, or induration. Dressing clean and dry.

CV: Regular in rate and rhythm, no murmur. No jugulovenous distention. CR brisk. Radial pulses 2+, dorsal pedal pulses 2+.

Abd: Soft, nontender, nondistended. No hepatosplenomegaly.

Ext: No cyanosis or edema.

CXR: Unremarkable. No **cardiomegaly.**

EKG: Normal.

Labs: No elevated cardiac enzymes. Normal CBC.

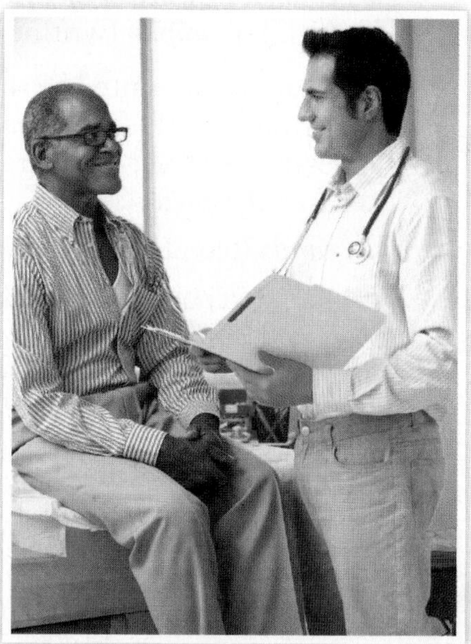

©Cathy Yeulet/123RF RF

Assessment

Given that her chest x-ray is normal, I do not believe that Mrs. Short has postoperative **pericardial effusion.** Since she is afebrile, I do not believe she has **endocarditis.** Her shortness of breath and **tachycardic** episodes are most likely postoperative **atrial flutter.**

Plan

I will admit her overnight for observation under **telemetry** and **cardioversion,** if needed.

—Anton Valentine, MD

Learning Outcome 9.7 Exercises

EXERCISE 9 *Match the term on the left with its definition on the right.*

______	1. cardiomegaly	a.	an image of the heart produced using sound waves; the same procedure as an ultrasound performed on pregnant women, but instead performed on the heart
______	2. echocardiogram	b.	enlarged heart
______	3. endocarditis	c.	fluid pouring out into the tissue around the heart
______	4. tachycardia	d.	inflammation of the tissue lining the inside of the heart
______	5. valvuloplasty	e.	rapid heartbeat
______	6. pericardial effusion	f.	returning a heart to normal rhythm
______	7. cardioversion	g.	surgical reconstruction of a heart valve

EXERCISE 10 *Fill in the blanks.*

1. Using the data recorded at Mrs. Short's physical examination, fill in the following blanks.
   a. Mrs. Short's temperature: ______________________________
   b. Mrs. Short's heart rate: ______________________________
   c. Mrs. Short's respiratory rate: ______________________________
   d. Mrs. Short's blood pressure: ______________________________
   e. CV (*cardiovascular,* give definition: ______________________________): regular rate and rhythm (give abbreviation: ______________________________)
2. An *echocardiogram* (give abbreviation: ______________________________) revealed left ventricular hypertrophy (enlargement of the ______________________________, the lower chamber of the heart).
3. Labs: no elevated cardiac enzymes. Normal ______________________________ (complete blood count).
4. Mrs. Short will be admitted overnight for observation and *cardioversion* (give definition: ______________________________) if needed.

EXERCISE 11 *True or false questions. Indicate true answers with a T and false answers with an F.*

1. Since her surgery, Mrs. Short has had a few episodes of her heart beating rapidly. ______
2. Mrs. Short has experienced cardiodynia. ______
3. Mrs. Short has a normal-sized heart. ______
4. Mrs. Short has a fever. ______
5. Mrs. Short has pericardial effusion and endocarditis. ______

Learning Outcome 9.7 Exercises

EXERCISE 12 *Multiple-choice questions. Select the correct answer(s):*

1. The patient's labs revealed no *cardiac enzymes.* The root *cardio* means:
   a. blood vessel
   b. circulation
   c. heart
   d. vein

2. Mrs. Short came into the office for a follow-up after her *aortic valvuloplasty.* The aortic valve is one of the valves of the heart. It lies between the left ventricle and the aorta. Which of the following is an accurate breakdown of the term *aortic valvuloplasty?*
   a. *aortic* (pertaining to the largest artery of the body) + *valvulo* (valve) + *plasty* (reconstruction)
   b. *aortic* (pertaining to the largest artery of the body) + *valvulo* (valve) + *plasty* (incision)
   c. *aortic* (pertaining to the largest vein of the body) + *valvulo* (valve) + *plasty* (reconstruction)
   d. *aortic* (pertaining to the largest vein of the body) + *valvulo* (valve) + *plasty* (incision)

3. Mrs. Short's echocardiogram revealed *left ventricular hypertrophy.* Which of the following is an accurate breakdown of the term *ventricular hypertrophy?*
   a. *ventricular* (pertaining to the lower chamber of the heart) + *hyper* (over) + *trophy* (nourishment)
   b. *ventricular* (pertaining to the lower chamber of the heart) + *hyper* (under) + *trophy* (nourishment)
   c. *ventricular* (pertaining to the upper chamber of the heart) + *hyper* (over) + *trophy* (nourishment)
   d. *ventricular* (pertaining to the upper chamber of the heart) + *hyper* (under) + *trophy* (nourishment)

4. Atrial flutter (AFL) is an abnormal heart rhythm that occurs in the atria of the heart. According to this clinic note: (select all that apply)
   a. AFL can possibly be treated with an antianginal medication
   b. AFL is a type of arrhythmia
   c. AFL pertains to the lower chamber of the heart
   d. AFL pertains to the upper chamber of the heart
   e. the physician believes AFL is the cause of her episodes of tachycardia
   f. the physician believes AFL is the caused by the patient's endocarditis

Additional exercises available in connect

Chapter Review exercises, along with additional practice items, are available in Connect!

Quick Reference

quick reference glossary of roots

Root	Definition	Root	Definition
angi/o	vessel	**phleb/o**	vein
aort/o	aorta	**sept/o**	septum (plural, septa)
arteri/o	artery	**valvul/o**	valve
ather/o	fatty plaque	**vas/o, vascul/o**	vessel
atri/o	atrium (upper chamber)	**ven/o**	vein
cardi/o	heart	**ventricul/o**	ventricle (lower chamber)
coron/o	heart (crown)		

quick reference glossary of terms

Term	Definition
anastomosis	creation of an opening between two normally separate structures
aneurysm	bulge in a blood vessel
aneurysmectomy	surgical removal of an aneurysm
angina pectoris	oppressive pain in the chest caused by irregular blood flow to the heart
angiocarditis	inflammation of the heart vessels
angioedema	swelling of the blood vessels
angiogenesis	development of blood vessels
angiogram	record of the blood vessels
angiography	procedure to describe the blood vessels
angiolith	stone forming in the wall of a blood vessel
angioma	blood vessel tumor
angioplasty	surgical reconstruction of a vessel
angiopoiesis	formation of blood vessels
angiorrhaphy	suture of a vessel
angiosclerosis	hardening of a blood vessel
angioscope	device for looking into a blood vessel
antianginal	drug that prevents or relieves the symptoms of angina pectoris
antiarrhythmic	drug that opposes an irregular heartbeat
anticoagulant	drug that opposes the coagulation of blood
antihypertensive	drug that opposes high blood pressure

quick reference glossary of terms *continued*

Term	Definition
aortalgia	pain in the aorta
aortectasia	dilation of the aorta
aortic aneurysm	bulging or swelling of the aorta
aortic regurgitation	flow of blood backward from the aorta into the heart; caused by a weak heart valve
aortic stenosis	narrowing of the aorta
aortitis	inflammation of the aorta
aortogram	record of the aorta
aortolith	stone deposit in the wall of the aorta
aortorrhaphy	suture of the aorta
aortotomy	incision into the aorta
arrhythmia	irregular heartbeat
arteriectomy	surgical removal of an artery
arteriogram	record of an artery
arteriolith	stone in an artery
arteriopathy	disease of the arteries
arterioplasty	surgical reconstruction of an artery
arteriorrhaphy	suture of an artery
arteriorrhexis	rupture of an artery
arteriosclerosis	hardening of an artery
arteritis	inflammation of the arteries
atherectomy	surgical removal of fatty plaque within an artery
atherogenesis	formation of fatty plaque on the wall of an artery
atherosclerosis	hardening of an artery due to buildup of fatty plaque
atrial fibrillation	quivering or spontaneous contraction of muscle fibers in the heart's atrium
atrial septal defect	flaw in the septum that divides the two atria of the heart
blood pressure	force exerted by blood on the walls of blood vessels
bradycardia	slow heartbeat
cardiac arrest	cessation of functional circulation
cardiac catheterization	the process of inserting a tube (catheter) into the heart
cardiologist	heart specialist
cardiology	branch of medicine dealing with the heart
cardiomegaly	enlarged heart

quick reference glossary of terms *continued*

Term	Definition
cardiomyopathy	disease of the heart muscle
cardiomyotomy	incision into the heart muscle
cardiopulmonary bypass	procedure that temporarily circulates and oxygenates a patient's blood during a portion of heart surgery where the heart is stopped
cardiopulmonary resuscitation	basic life support
cardiothoracic surgery	surgery that involves cutting through the patient's chest to get to the heart
cardiotonic	a drug that increases the strength of heart contractions
cardiotoxic	poisonous to the heart
cardiovascular	pertaining to the heart and blood vessels
cardioversion	returning a heart to normal rhythm
carditis	inflammation of the heart
congenital heart defect	flaw in the structure of the heart, present at birth
congestive cardiomyopathy	heart cavity is unable to pump all the blood out of it (congestive) and becomes stretched (dilated), which causes weak/slow pumping of blood
congestive heart failure	heart failure characterized by the heart cavity being unable to pump all the blood out of it (congestive)
coronary arterectomy	surgical removal of a coronary artery
coronary artery bypass graft (CABG)	borrowed piece of blood vessel used to bypass a blocked artery in the heart
coronary artery bypass surgery	surgery to bypass a blocked artery in the heart
coronary circulation	circulation of blood from the heart to the heart muscle
coronary thrombosis	obstruction of a coronary artery by a clot
cyanosis	a bluish appearance to the skin; a sign that the tissue isn't receiving enough oxygen
deep vein thrombosis	the formation of a blood clot deep in the body, most commonly in the leg
diaphoresis	profuse sweating
diastolic pressure	pressure exerted on blood vessels when the heart is relaxed
dilated cardiomyopathy	*see* congestive cardiomyopathy
dysrhythmia	irregular heartbeat
echocardiogram	image of the heart produced using sound waves; it is the same procedure as an ultrasound performed on pregnant women, but done on the heart
echocardiography	use of sound waves to produce an image of the heart

quick reference glossary of terms *continued*

Term	Definition
electrocardiogram	record of the electrical currents of the heart
electrocardiography	procedure for recording the electrical currents of the heart
embolectomy	surgical removal of an embolus
embolism	blockage in a blood vessel caused by an embolus
embolus	mass of matter present in the blood
endarterectomy	surgical removal of the inside of an artery
endocarditis	inflammation of the tissue lining the inside of the heart
endocardium	tissue lining the inside of the heart
epicardium	tissue lining the outside of the heart
hemorrhage	loss of blood
hypertension	high blood pressure
hypertropic cardiomyopathy	heart muscle becomes enlarged and blocks blood flow
hypotension	low blood pressure
ischemia	blockage of blood flow to an organ
murmur	abnormal heart sound
myocardial infarction	death of heart muscle tissue
myocardial ischemia	blockage of blood to the heart muscle
myocarditis	inflammation of the heart muscle
myocardium	heart muscle tissue
normotension	normal blood pressure
occlusion	closing or blockage of a passage
palpitation	rapid or irregular beating of the heart
pectoralgia	chest pain
percutaneous coronary intervention	alternate treatment for the coronary artery that passes instruments up a patient's blood vessels into the heart
pericardial effusion	fluid pouring out into the tissue around the heart
pericardiocentesis	puncture of the tissue around the heart
pericardiotomy	incision into the tissue around the heart
pericarditis	inflammation of the tissue around the heart
pericardium	tissue around the heart
phlebalgia	pain in a vein
phlebectomy	surgical removal of a vein

quick reference glossary of terms *continued*

Term	Definition
phlebitis	inflammation of the veins
phlebologist	specialist in veins
phlebology	study of veins
phlebophlebostomy	procedure to create an opening between two veins
phlebosclerosis	hardening of a vein
phlebostenosis	narrowing of the veins
phlebotomist	one who draws blood
phlebotomy	incision into a vein (the technical term for drawing blood)
pulmonary circulation	circulation of blood from the heart to the lungs
restrictive cardiomyopathy	heart muscle hardens, restricting the expansion of the heart and thus limiting the amount of blood it can pump to the rest of the body
sonography	use of sound waves to produce diagnostic images; also called an ultrasound
stress electrocardiogram	records electrical signals of the heart while the patient experiences increases of exercise stress
superior vena cava	portion of the vena cava that gathers blood from the upper portion of the body (head and arms)
systemic circulation	circulation of blood from the heart to the rest of the body
systolic pressure	pressure exerted on blood vessels when the heart is contracting
tachycardia	rapid heartbeat
thrombolytic	drug that breaks down clots
thrombophlebitis	inflammation of a vein caused by a clot
thrombus	blood clot (from Greek, for "lump," "clot," or "curd of milk")
transesophageal electrocardiogram	recording of the heart using sound waves performed by inserting the sonograph into the esophagus
valvectomy	surgical removal of a heart valve
valvotomy	incision into a heart valve
valvulitis	inflammation of a heart valve
valvuloplasty	surgical reconstruction of a heart valve
varicose veins	enlarged, dilated vein toward the surface of the skin
varicotomy	surgical removal of a varicose vein
vascular endoscopy	procedure to look inside a blood vessel
vasculitis	inflammation of blood vessels
vasoconstrictor	drug that constricts or narrows the diameter of a blood vessel
vasodilator	drug that causes the relaxation or expansion of a blood vessel

quick reference glossary of terms *continued*

Term	Definition
vasopressor	drug that constricts or narrows the diameter of a blood vessel
vasospasm	involuntary contraction of a blood vessel
vena cava	large-diameter vein that gathers blood from the body and returns it to the heart
vena cava inferior	portion of the vena cava that gathers blood from the lower portion of the body
venectomy	surgical removal of a vein
venogram	record of a vein
venosclerosis	hardening of a vein
venospasm	involuntary contraction of a vein
venostasis	trapping of blood in an extremity due to compression
ventricular septal defect	flaw in the septum that divides the two ventricles of the heart
ventriculotomy	incision into a ventricle

review of terms by roots

Root	Term(s)	
angi/o	angiocarditis	angioma
	angioedema	angioplasty
	angiogenesis	angiopoiesis
	angiogram	angiorrhaphy
	angiography	angiosclerosis
	angiolith	angioscope
aort/o	aortalgia	aortitis
	aortectasia	aortogram
	aortic aneurysm	aortolith
	aortic regurgitation	aortorrhaphy
	aortic stenosis	aortotomy
arteri/o	arteriectomy	arteriosclerosis
	arteriogram	arteritis
	arteriolith	coronary arterectomy
	arteriopathy	coronary artery bypass graft
	arterioplasty	coronary artery bypass surgery
	arteriorrhaphy	endarterectomy
	arteriorrhexis	
ather/o	atherectomy	atherosclerosis
	atherogenesis	

review of terms by roots *continued*

Root	Term(s)	
atri/o	atrial fibrillation atrial septal defect	
cardi/o	angiocarditis bradycardia cardiac arrest cardiac catheterization cardiologist cardiology cardiomegaly cardiomyopathy cardiomyotomy cardiopulmonary bypass	cardiopulmonary resuscitation cardiothoracic surgery cardiotonic cardiotoxic cardiovascular cardioversion carditis congestive cardiomyopathy dilated cardiomyopathy echocardiogram
cardi/o (continued)	echocardiography electrocardiogram electrocardiography endocarditis endocardium epicardium hypertropic cardiomyopathy myocardial infarction myocardial ischemia myocarditis	myocardium pericardial effusion pericardiocentesis pericardiotomy pericarditis pericardium restrictive cardiomyopathy stress electrocardiogram tachycardia transesophageal echocardiogram
coron/o	coronary arterectomy coronary artery bypass graft (CABG) coronary artery bypass surgery	coronary circulation coronary thrombosis percutaneous coronary intervention
phleb/o	phlebalgia phlebectomy phlebitis phlebologist phlebology phlebophlebostomy	phlebosclerosis phlebostenosis phlebotomist phlebotomy thrombophlebitis
sept/o	atrial septal defect ventricular septal defect	
valvul/o	valvectomy valvotomy	valvulitis valvuloplasty
varic/o	varicose veins varicotomy	

review of terms by roots *continued*

Root	Term(s)	
vas/o, vascul/o	cardiovascular	vasodilator
	vascular endoscopy	vasopressor
	vasculitis	vasospasm
	vasoconstrictor	
ven/o	superior vena cava	venogram
	vena cava	venosclerosis
	vena cava inferior	venospasm
	venectomy	venostasis
ventricul/o	ventricular septal defect	
	ventriculotomy	

other terms

anastomosis	embolism
aneurysm	embolus
aneurysmectomy	hemorrhage
angina pectoris	hypertension
antianginal	hypotension
antiarrhythmic	ischemia
anticoagulant	murmur
antihypertensive	normotension
arrhythmia	occlusion
blood pressure	palpitation
congenital heart defect	pectoralgia
congestive heart failure	pulmonary circulation
cyanosis	sonography
deep vein thrombosis	systemic circulation
diaphoresis	systolic pressure
diastolic pressure	thrombolytic
dysrhythmia	thrombus
embolectomy	

The Respiratory System—Pulmonology 10

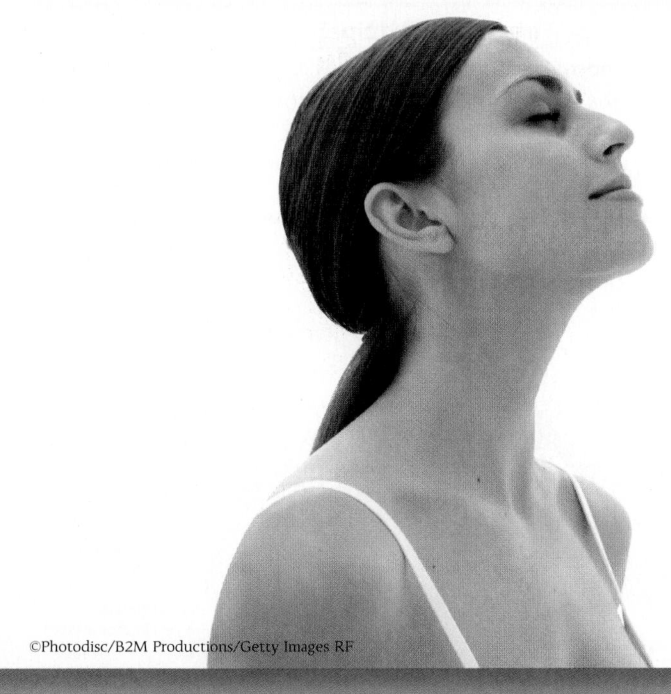

learning outcomes

Upon completion of this chapter, you will be able to:

10.1 Identify the **roots/word parts** associated with the **respiratory system**.

(S) **10.2** Translate the **Subjective** terms associated with the **respiratory system**.

(O) **10.3** Translate the **Objective** terms associated with the **respiratory system**.

(A) **10.4** Translate the **Assessment** terms associated with the **respiratory system**.

(P) **10.5** Translate the **Plan** terms associated with the **respiratory system**.

10.6 Use **abbreviations** associated with the **respiratory system**.

10.7 Distinguish terms associated with the **respiratory system** in the context of **electronic health records**.

Introduction and Overview of the Respiratory System

Spiro is the root of the word *spirit*. A person with spirit is full of enthusiasm. While we cannot actually visualize enthusiasm, we can certainly see its effect; for example, it's "team spirit" that drives sports fans to go to games shirtless in the middle of winter! In the same way, we can't see the air we breathe, but we know it gives life.

Simply put, the main job of the respiratory system is to deliver oxygen to the blood and carry carbon dioxide away from it. As we breathe in (*inhale*), we are taking in oxygen-rich air. As air passes through the respiratory tract, it is cleaned, warmed, and moistened. The air reaches its end point in the lungs, where it comes in contact with the blood. There, oxygen is exchanged for carbon dioxide. Finally, the waste air passes back out through the nose and mouth (*exhale*).

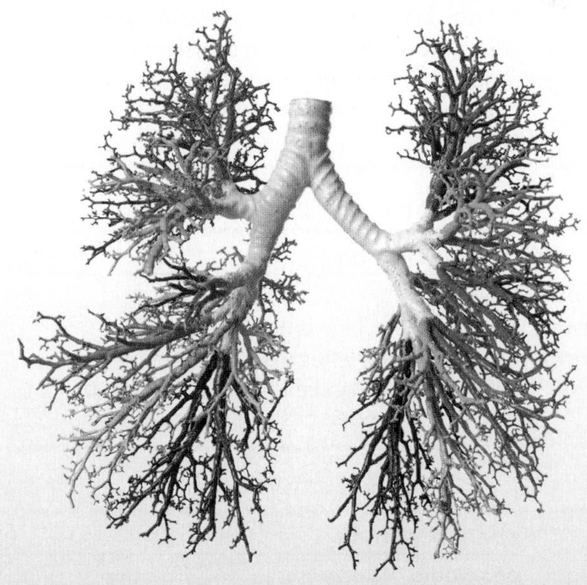

This image of the lungs shows the branching of the airways from the trachea to the bronchi, bronchioles, and down to the alveoli.

It helps to view the anatomy of the respiratory system as a tree. The mouth, nose, and throat form the tree's roots. The trachea is the tree's trunk; it leads to large branches (*bronchi*). Each branch splits into more branches (other bronchi) that further lead to twigs (*bronchioles*) and leaves (*alveoli*).

10.1 Word Parts of the Respiratory System

Upper Respiratory System

adenoid

ROOT: ***adenoid/o***

EXAMPLES: adenoidectomy, adenoiditis

NOTES: The word *adenoid* is formed by adding a suffix to the root *adeno,* which means "gland": *aden/o* + *oid* = resembling a gland.

tonsil

ROOT: ***tonsill/o***

EXAMPLES: tonsillectomy, tonsillitis

NOTES: The word *tonsil* comes from a Latin word meaning "almond." The Latin word has two *l*'s, but in English, one disappears.

nose

ROOTS: ***nas/o (Latin for* "nose"*), rhin/o (Greek for* "nose"*)***

EXAMPLES: nasogastric tube, nasendoscope, rhinorrhea, rhinoplasty

NOTES: Rhinoceros is the combination of *rhino* and *ceros* (horn), which means "horn nose." A poet named Publius Ovidius Naso (43 BC–AD 17) lived in ancient Rome. Perhaps you know him by the much shorter name Ovid. Apparently, he or one of his ancestors had quite a prominent nose—hence the root *naso*.

larynx (voice box)

ROOT: ***laryng/o***

EXAMPLES: laryngospasm, laryngitis

NOTES: Remember: the letter *g* is soft when followed by an *i* and hard when followed by an *o* (e.g., laryn**GO**spasm vs. laryn**J**Itis).

pharynx (throat)

ROOT: ***pharyng/o***

EXAMPLES: pharyngitis, pharyngostenosis

NOTES: The pharynx is the pathway used by both food and air.

trachea (windpipe)

ROOT: ***trache/o***

EXAMPLES: tracheotomy, tracheostomy

NOTES: From the Greek word for "rough," because of the bumpy ridges that line the outside of the trachea.

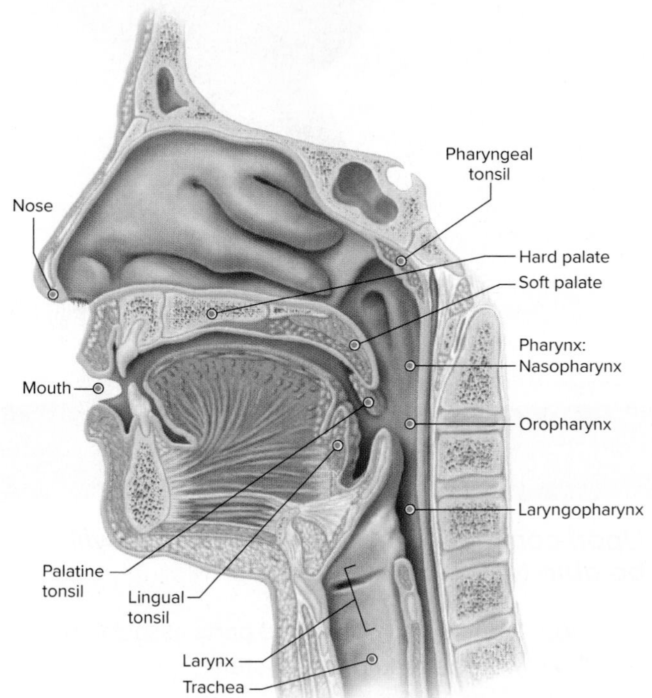

The entry point for air into the body is primarily through the nose, with some air entering through the mouth. The nose serves to warm, clean, and moisten the air. The nose consists of two nostrils (*nares*), a septum (*septum*), and tube-shaped cartilage inside the nose (*turbinates*). The nose is very vascular, which means that it contains many blood vessels, which is why the nose bleeds easily. The blood in these vessels warms the air as it enters the rest of the respiratory tract. In addition, multiple hairs line the nose and filter out dust and other particles. Finally, the nose produces mucus, which helps clean and moisten the air.

The air passes through the nose or mouth and proceeds into the throat (*pharynx*). There are three parts to the pharynx: the nasopharynx, the oropharynx, and the laryngopharynx. The laryngopharynx contains the vocal cords (*larynx*). When air passes across these cords upon exhalation, the cords vibrate at certain speeds—just like a harmonica or saxophone. These vibrations make sounds, which we use to form speech. The air continues down the windpipe (*trachea*). The trachea is surrounded by bumpy rings of cartilage that prevent it from caving in.

septum (plural: septa)

ROOT: ***sept/o***

EXAMPLES: septectomy, septoplasty

NOTES: *Septum* comes from a Latin word meaning "partition" or "dividing structure" and can refer to any wall dividing two cavities. Of the numerous septa throughout the body, the easiest to find is the nasal septum. If you place your index fingers in each nostril and press them together, you will feel the nasal septum. If your nasal septum leans to one side, you have a deviated septum.

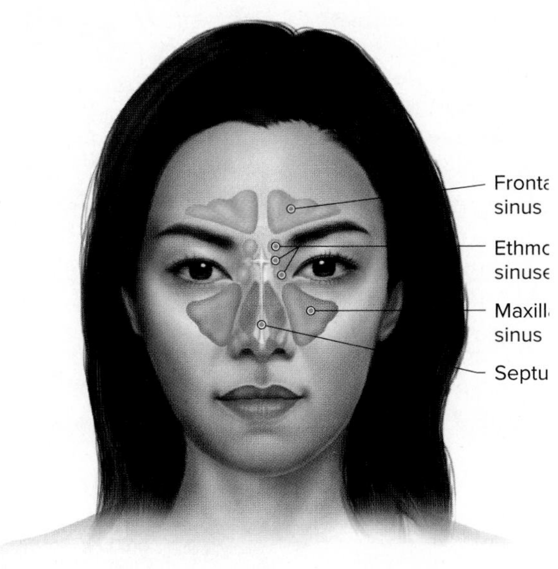

sinus

ROOTS: ***sin/o, sinus/o***

EXAMPLES: sinusitis, sinusotomy

NOTES: From a Latin word meaning "hollow" or "cavity," *sinus* refers generally to any hollow area—specifically, those in bones.

air or lungs

ROOTS: ***pneum/o, pneumat/o, pneumon/o***

EXAMPLES: pneumomelanosis, pneumatology, pneumonia

NOTES: These roots can mean either "lung" or "air." Context and familiarity will help in determining which to use. For instance, it makes more sense to translate *pneumothorax* as "air in the chest" rather than "lung in the chest."

The term *pneumatic* can also be found in the construction world. It refers to any tool that moves by forcing air into it (i.e., a pneumatic drill), as opposed to hydraulic tools, which involve the use of water instead of air (i.e., a hydraulic lift).

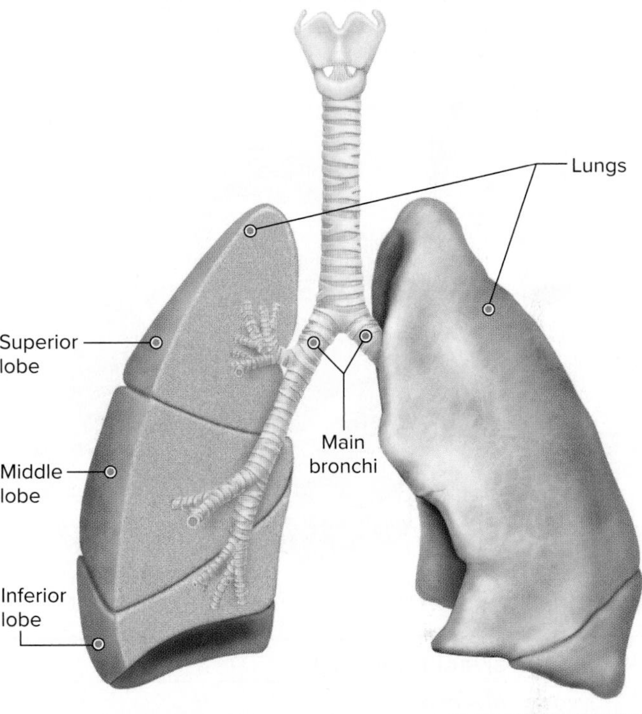

lungs

ROOT: ***pulmon/o***

EXAMPLES: pulmonologist, pulmonary

NOTES: *Pulmon/o* is listed by itself instead of with the various forms of *pneum/o* because while *pulmon/o* means only "lung," *pneum/o* can mean both "lung" (as in *pneumonia*) and "air" (as in *pneumothorax*).

lobe

ROOT: ***lob/o***

EXAMPLES: lobectomy, lobotomy

NOTES: A *lobe* is a well-defined portion of any organ. The main organs that have lobes are the lungs, brain, and liver.

What is the difference between a *lobectomy* and a *lobotomy?*

bronchus

ROOTS: ***bronch/o, bronchi/o***
EXAMPLES: bronchoscope, bronchiostenosis
NOTES: The main branches from the trachea into each lung.

bronchiole

ROOT: ***bronchiol/o***
EXAMPLES: bronchiolitis, bronchiolectasis
NOTES: The root *bronchiole* is actually formed by adding a diminutive suffix to another root: *bronch/o* + *iole* = little bronchus, which is a smaller subdivision of the bronchial tubes.

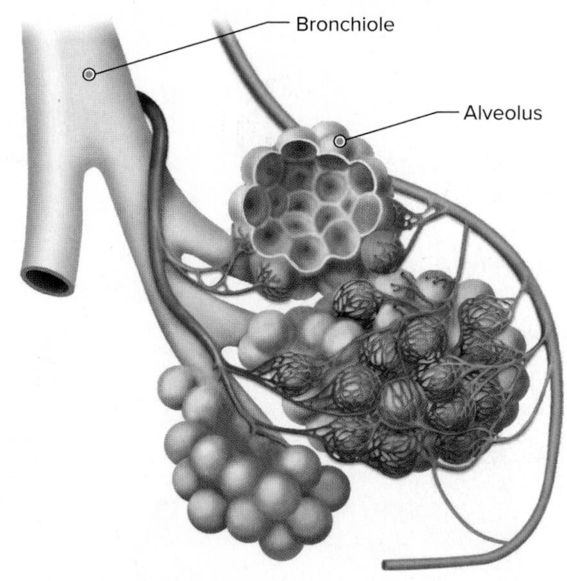

alveolus (air sac)

ROOT: ***alveol/o***
EXAMPLES: alveolitis, alveolar
NOTES: *Alveolus* comes from a Latin word meaning "hollow" or "cavity." The two main types are *pulmonary alveoli,* the air sacs in the lungs, and *dental alveoli,* the sockets in the jaw from which teeth emerge.

If you place your tongue on the roof of your mouth and move it forward, you will feel a bump called the *alveolar ridge* right before you get to your teeth.

Lower Respiratory System

After passing the *trachea,* the air finally makes its way to the lungs via two main *bronchi* (right and left). Like the trachea, rings of cartilage surround the bronchi for support. The bronchi further branch into five *lobar bronchi*—three on the right and two on the left. These branches define the five *lobes* of the lung. Each lobar bronchus breaks into smaller segments (*segmental bronchi*) that further branch into smaller airways known as *bronchioles*. The bronchioles end in clusters of *alveoli*, tiny balloon-like structures surrounded by small blood vessels. At this point, oxygen passes into the blood, and carbon dioxide passes out of the blood.

sternum

ROOT: ***stern/o***
EXAMPLES: sternocostal, sternotomy
NOTES: The *sternum* (also known as the breastbone) comes to a point at the bottom called the *xiphoid* (ZAI-foid) *process*. The term comes from the Greek word *xiphos*, meaning "sword." Therefore, *xiphoid* means "resembling a sword."

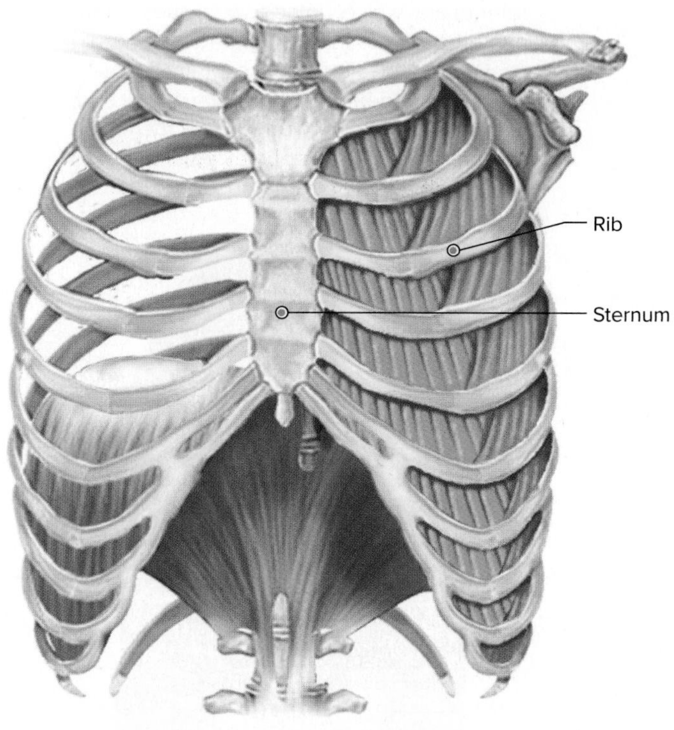

rib

ROOT: ***cost/o***
EXAMPLES: costectomy, costophrenic
NOTES: *Ribs* are sometimes grouped into three categories: true, false, and floating. The top seven ribs are called "true" ribs because they attach to both the spine and the sternum. The next three ribs are called "false" ribs because they connect to the spine and to the lowest true rib instead of the sternum. The lowest two ribs are called "floating" ribs because they attach only to the spine.

chest

ROOTS: ***thorac/o, pector/o (also pectus), steth/o***

EXAMPLES: thoracic, pectoralgia, pectus excavatum, stethoscope

NOTES: The root *pector/o* can also stand as a word by itself. When it does, however, the ending changes slightly, from *pectoro* to *pectus*. Hence, pectus excavatum.

The term *stethoscope* literally means "an instrument for looking at the chest," but of course, you do not look with a stethoscope—you listen.

pleura

ROOT: ***pleur/o***

EXAMPLES: pleuritis, pleurectomy

NOTES: The *pleura* is a membrane surrounding the lungs.

diaphragm

ROOT: ***phren/o***

EXAMPLES: phrenospasm, phrenoplegia

NOTES: In addition to the diaphragm, *phren/o* can also refer to the brain (as in the term *schizophrenia*). The rationale comes from the ancient Greek view of the mind. The Greeks believed that the chest was the seat of emotion and reason. As that view changed and the location of the mind moved from the chest to the brain, the word for mind became applied to both regions of the body.

Process of Respiration

Although air begins its journey in the nose and mouth, the work of breathing actually starts with two sets of muscles: the muscles between the ribs (*intercostal*) and a horizontal muscle (*diaphragm*) that lies between the chest and the abdomen. When these muscles shorten (*contract*), they cause the chest to enlarge, which decreases chest (*thoracic*) pressure. As a result, air is literally sucked into the lungs.

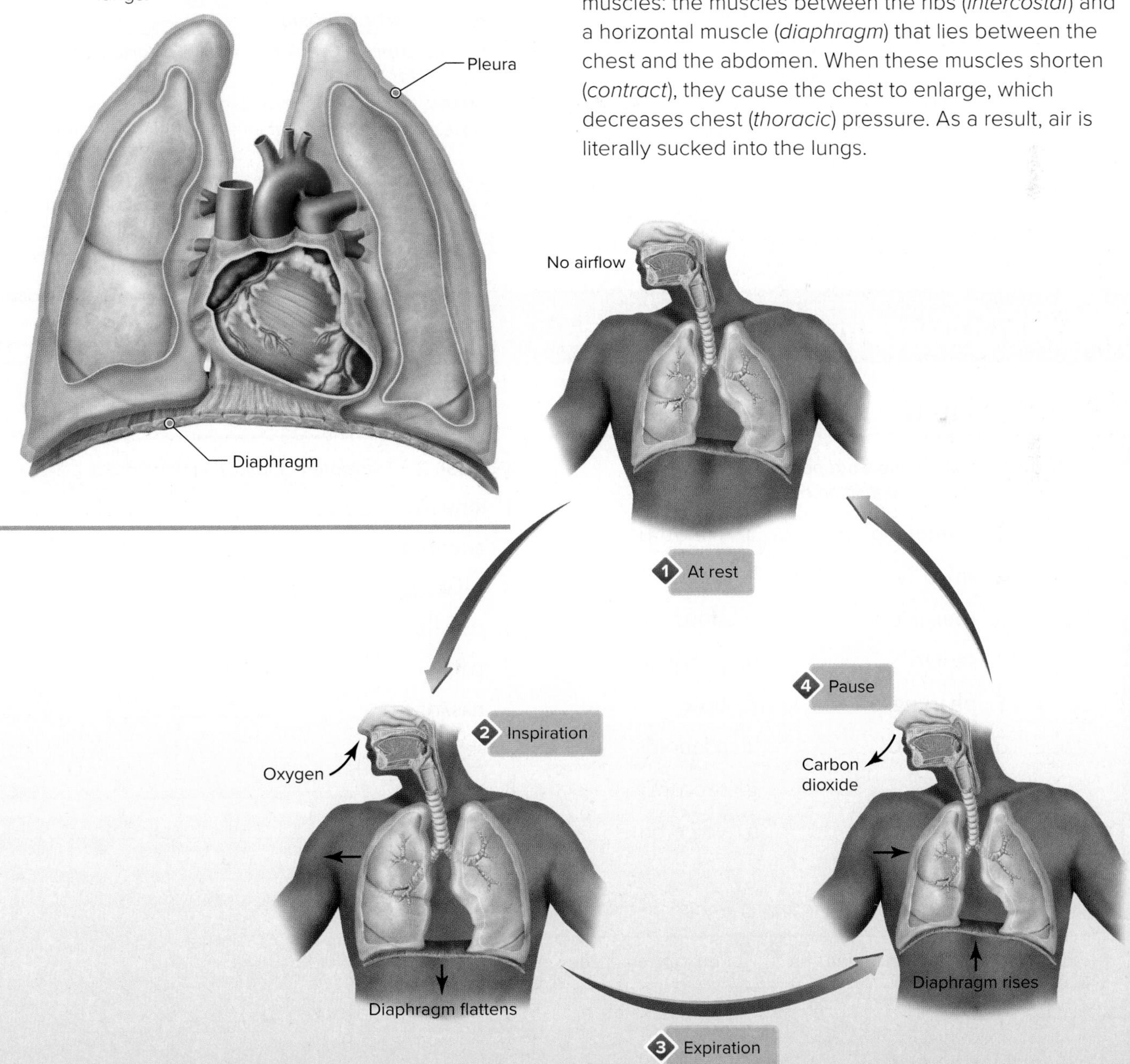

oxygen

ROOT: ***ox/o***

EXAMPLES: hypoxia, hypoxemia

NOTES: *Hypoxia* refers to a lack of oxygen in tissue cells. *Hypoxemia* refers to lack of oxygen in the blood. If a hypoxic patient is also hypoxemic, then oxygen is not getting into the blood. If the person is not hypoxemic, then the problem lies in the transfer of oxygen from blood to tissue. Diagnosing this problem is similar to tracking a package: If a customer does not receive a package, the delivery chain could have broken down in any number of places along the way. The package might never have been sent, might not have made it on the delivery truck, or might not have been delivered to the right door.

breathing

WORD PARTS: ***spir/o, -pnea***

EXAMPLES: spirometry, sleep apnea

NOTES: *Spir/o* also occurs in other words:

- *Perspire* translates as "to breathe through."
- *Conspire* translates as "to breathe together"—no doubt coming from the idea that people who are *conspiring* can be thought of as being huddled together and breathing the same air.
- *Expire* also contains the *spir/o* root and means "to breathe out." It was originally written as *exspire*, but the letter *s* was dropped because *x* is made up of two *k* sounds. To test this, say *expire* and *exspire*. They are rarely pronounced differently.

carbon dioxide

ROOTS: ***capn/o (Greek for "smoke"), carb/o (Latin for "coal")***

EXAMPLES: hypercapnia, hypocarbia

NOTES: One of the treatments for hyperventilation is to have the person breathe into a paper bag. A person who is hyperventilating has *hypocarbia* and thus needs to increase the carbon dioxide in his or her respiratory system.

Learning Outcome 10.1 Exercises

Additional exercises available in connect®

TRANSLATION

EXERCISE 1 *Match the word part on the left with its definition on the right.*

_____	1. adenoid/o	a. windpipe
_____	2. sin/o	b. tonsil
_____	3. tonsill/o	c. sinus
_____	4. sept/o	d. pharynx
_____	5. pharyng/o	e. nose
_____	6. trache/o	f. adenoids
_____	7. rhin/o	g. septum
_____	8. laryng/o	h. voice box

EXERCISE 2 *Translate the following word parts.*

1. sinus/o _____
2. adenoid/o _____
3. pharyng/o _____
4. tonsill/o _____
5. palat/o _____
6. nas/o _____
7. sept/o _____
8. trache/o _____
9. laryng/o _____

EXERCISE 3 *Break down the following words into their component parts and define.*

EXAMPLE: sinusitis *sinus | itis* *inflammation of the sinuses*

1. laryngitis _____
2. tonsillitis _____

3. septectomy ______________________________
4. nasendoscope ______________________________
5. pharyngostenosis ______________________________

EXERCISE 4 *Match the word part on the left with its definition on the right.*

______	1. bronch/o	a. air
______	2. pleur/o	b. lung
______	3. lob/o	c. lobe
______	4. alveol/o	d. sternum
______	5. stern/o	e. alveolus
______	6. pneum/o	f. chest
______	7. phren/o	g. bronchus
______	8. pulmon/o	h. pleura
______	9. thorac/o	i. rib
______	10. cost/o	j. diaphragm

EXERCISE 5 *Translate the following word parts.*

1. lob/o ______________________________
2. stern/o ______________________________
3. pleur/o ______________________________
4. bronchiol/o ______________________________
5. steth/o ______________________________
6. pneumat/o ______________________________
7. alveol/o ______________________________
8. pneumon/o ______________________________
9. pector/o ______________________________
10. pulmon/o ______________________________
11. phren/o ______________________________
12. cost/o ______________________________

EXERCISE 6 *Break down the following words into their component parts and define.*

EXAMPLE: sinusitis *sinus | itis* *inflammation of the sinuses*

1. pneumonia ______________________________
2. bronchitis ______________________________
3. pleuritis ______________________________
4. lobectomy ______________________________

5. alveolitis ______________________________
6. stethoscope ______________________________
7. phrenoplegia ______________________________
8. bronchiostenosis ______________________________

EXERCISE 7 *Match the word part on the left with its definition on the right.*

______	1. ox/o	a. oxygen
______	2. capn/o	b. breathing
______	3. spir/o	c. carbon dioxide

EXERCISE 8 *Translate the following word parts.*

1. ox/o ______________________________
2. carb/o ______________________________
3. capn/o ______________________________
4. spir/o ______________________________
5. -pnea ______________________________

GENERATION

EXERCISE 9 *Identify the roots for the following definitions.*

1. tonsil ______________________________
2. adenoid ______________________________
3. pharynx ______________________________
4. trachea ______________________________
5. nose ______________________________
6. throat ______________________________
7. voice box ______________________________

EXERCISE 10 *Build a medical term from the information provided.*

1. inflammation of the throat ______________________________
2. inflammation of the sinus ______________________________
3. incision into the trachea ______________________________
4. discharge from the nose ______________________________
5. surgical removal of the tonsils ______________________________
6. creation of an opening in the trachea ______________________________
7. surgical reconstruction of the septum ______________________________

Learning Outcome 10.1 Exercises

EXERCISE 11 *Identify the roots for the following definitions.*

1. bronchus __________
2. sternum __________
3. pleura __________
4. lobe __________
5. bronchiole __________
6. alveolus __________
7. diaphragm __________
8. lungs __________
9. chest __________
10. air or lungs __________
11. rib __________
12. air sac __________

EXERCISE 12 *Build a medical term from the information provided.*

1. chest pain __________
2. the study of the lungs __________
3. instrument to look into the bronchus __________
4. surgical removal of a rib __________
5. involuntary contraction of the diaphragm __________
6. inflammation of the smaller subdivisions of the bronchus __________
7. pertaining to the sternum and ribs __________
8. a black lung condition __________

EXERCISE 13 *Break down the following words into their component parts and define.*

EXAMPLE: sinusitis	*sinus | itis*	*inflammation of the sinuses*

1. hypercapnia __________
2. hypoxemia __________
3. apnea __________

EXERCISE 14 *Identify the roots for the following definitions.*

1. breathing __________
2. oxygen __________
3. carbon dioxide __________

EXERCISE 15 *Build a medical term from the information provided.*

1. deficient oxygen __________
2. excessive carbon dioxide __________
3. instrument for measuring breathing __________

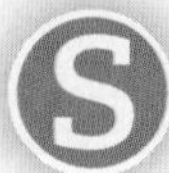

Subjective
Patient History, Problems, Complaints
Breathing processes
Upper respiratory
Lower respiratory
Discharges and secretions

Objective
Observation and Discovery
Physical findings and examination methods
Pathological findings
Laboratory data
Radiology
Diagnostic procedures

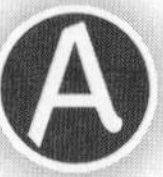

Assessment
Diagnosis and pathology
Upper respiratory
Lower respiratory

Plan
Treatments and Therapies
Upper respiratory
Lower respiratory
Drugs

The focus of this book is to teach you the process of learning roots and translating them in context. This section contains medical terms built from the roots presented in the previous section. The purpose of this section is to expose you to words used in pulmonology that are built from the word roots presented earlier in the chapter. In this section, each term is presented with the correct pronunciation. This is followed by a word analysis that breaks down the word into its component parts, a definition that provides a literal translation of the word, and supplemental information if the word's literal translation deviates from its medical use.

The terms are organized using a health care professional's SOAP note (first introduced in Chapter 2) as a model.

SUBJECTIVE

10.2 Patient History, Problems, Complaints

The most common patient respiratory complaint is coughing. Depending on whether *sputum* is present, a cough can be described as either *productive* or *nonproductive.* A productive cough is also known as *expectoration.* Coughing blood (*hemoptysis*) is generally a more worrisome symptom.

Other respiratory symptoms include changes in the breathing patterns and pain. Descriptions of the breathing pattern reflect the speed of breathing (*tachypnea, bradypnea*), the depth of breathing (*hyperventilation, hypoventilation*), or the work involved in breathing (*orthopnea, dyspnea*). While pain is a less frequent symptom in the respiratory system than in other systems, it should never be overlooked. When chest pain happens during *inspiration* or with a cough, it is known as *pleuritic chest pain.* If pain occurs at these intervals, the pain may be distinguished as respiratory in nature.

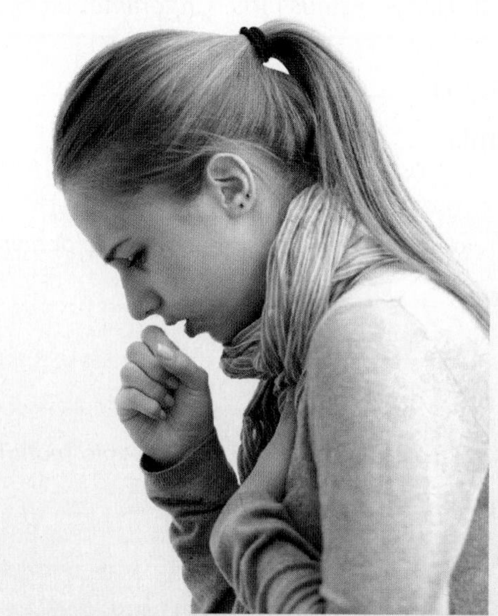

©istock/360/Alex Raths/Getty Images RF

10.2 Patient History, Problems, Complaints

breathing processes

Term	Word Analysis
apnea AP-nee-ah **Definition** cessation of breathing	a / pnea not / breathing
eupnea YOOP-nee-ah **Definition** good/normal breathing	eu / pnea good / breathing
tachypnea ta-KIP-nee-ah **Definition** rapid breathing	tachy / pnea fast / breathing
bradypnea brad-ip-NEE-ah **Definition** slow breathing	brady / pnea slow / breathing
hypopnea hai-POP-nee-ah **Definition** shallow breathing	hypo / pnea under / breathing
hyperpnea hai-perp-NEE-ah **Definition** heavy breathing	hyper / pnea over / breathing
dyspnea disp-NEE-ah **Definition** difficulty breathing	dys / pnea bad / breathing
orthopnea or-thop-NEE-ah **Definition** able to breathe only in an upright position	ortho / pnea straight / breathing
hyperventilation hai-per-ven-ti-LAY-shun **Definition** overbreathing; the condition of having too much air flowing into and out of the lungs; leads to hypocapnia	hyper / ventil / ation over / breathing / process
hypoventilation hai-po-ven-ti-LAY-shun **Definition** underbreathing; the condition of having too little air flowing into and out of the lungs; leads to hypercapnia	hypo / ventil / ation under / breathing / process

upper respiratory

Term	Word Analysis
dysphonia dis-FON-ia **Definition** bad voice condition (also known as hoarseness)	dys / phonia bad / sound / voice

10.2 Patient History, Problems, Complaints

upper respiratory *continued*

Term	Word Analysis
epistaxis ep-ee-STAKS-is **Definition** a nosebleed	**from the Greek word** *epistazo,* **meaning** "to drip out or upon"
rhinorrhagia rai-no-RAY-jah **Definition** excessive blood flow from the nose (another term for a nosebleed)	**rhino / rrhagia** nose / excessive bleeding
rhinorrhea rai-no-REE-yah **Definition** runny nose	**rhino / rrhea** nose / discharge

lower respiratory

Term	Word Analysis
bronchospasm BRON-ko-spaz-um **Definition** involuntary contraction of the bronchus	**broncho / spasm** bronchus / involuntary contraction
phrenospasm fre-no-SPAZ-um **Definition** involuntary contraction of the diaphragm (also known as the hiccups)	**phreno / spasm** diaphragm / involuntary contraction
pleuralgia plur-AL-jah **Definition** pain in the pleura	**pleur / algia** pleura / pain
pleurodynia plur-oh-DIH-nee-ah **Definition** pain in the pleura	**pleuro / dynia** pleura / pain
thoracalgia thor-a-KAL-jah **Definition** chest pain	**thorac / algia** chest / pain

discharges and secretions

Term	Word Analysis
bronchorrhea bron-koh-REE-ah **Definition** discharge from the bronchi	**broncho / rrhea** bronchus / discharge

discharges and secretions *continued*

Term	Word Analysis
expectoration eks-pec-tor-A-shun **Definition** coughing or spitting material out of the lungs	**ex / pector / ation** out / chest / process
hemoptysis heem-op-TIS-is **Definition** coughing up blood	**hemo / ptysis** blood / cough
sputum SPYOO-tum **Definition** mucus discharged from the lungs by coughing	**Latin for "spit"**

Learning Outcome 10.2 Exercises

PRONUNCIATION

EXERCISE 1 *Indicate which syllable is emphasized when pronounced.*

EXAMPLE: bronchitis bron**chi**tis

1. eupnea ____________
2. hypopnea ____________
3. dyspnea ____________
4. hypoventilation ____________
5. rhinorrhagia ____________
6. phrenospasm ____________
7. bronchospasm ____________
8. hemoptysis ____________

TRANSLATION

EXERCISE 2 *Underline and define the word parts from this chapter in the following terms.*

1. tachypnea ____________
2. hypopnea ____________
3. rhinorrhagia ____________
4. bronchospasm ____________
5. phrenospasm ____________
6. bronchorrhea ____________

Learning Outcome 10.2 Exercises

7. pleuralgia ______________________________
8. thoracalgia ______________________________
9. hyperventilation ______________________________
10. expectoration ______________________________

EXERCISE 3 *Match the term on the left with its definition on the right.*

______	1. apnea	a.	hoarseness
______	2. eupnea	b.	cessation of breathing
______	3. dyspnea	c.	pain in the pleura
______	4. orthopnea	d.	normal breathing
______	5. hyperventilation	e.	runny nose
______	6. epistaxis	f.	coughing up blood
______	7. dysphonia	g.	able to breathe only in an upright position
______	8. rhinorrhea	h.	nosebleed
______	9. pleurodynia	i.	overbreathing, or too much air flowing into and out of the lungs
______	10. hemoptysis	j.	mucus discharged from the lungs by coughing
______	11. sputum	k.	difficulty breathing

EXERCISE 4 *Break down the following words into their component parts.*

EXAMPLE: nasopharyngoscope *naso | pharyngo | scope*

1. bradypnea ______________________________
2. hyperpnea ______________________________
3. rhinorrhea ______________________________
4. phrenospasm ______________________________
5. pleurodynia ______________________________
6. thoracalgia ______________________________
7. hypoventilation ______________________________
8. hemoptysis ______________________________

EXERCISE 5 *Translate the following terms as literally as possible.*

EXAMPLE: nasopharyngoscope *an instrument for looking at the nose and throat*

1. orthopnea ______________________________
2. hyperpnea ______________________________
3. hypopnea ______________________________
4. rhinorrhagia ______________________________
5. bronchospasm ______________________________
6. pleuralgia ______________________________

7. thoracalgia ______
8. dysphonia ______
9. bronchorrhea ______
10. hyperventilation ______
11. hypoventilation ______

GENERATION

EXERCISE 6 *Build a medical term from the information provided.*

EXAMPLE: inflammation of the sinuses *sinusitis*

1. not breathing ______
2. good breathing ______
3. difficulty breathing ______
4. slow breathing ______
5. fast breathing ______
6. pain in the pleura ______
7. runny nose ______
8. involuntary contraction of the diaphragm ______
9. coughing up blood ______

EXERCISE 7 *Multiple-choice questions. Select the correct answer.*

1. *Epistaxis* comes from the Greek word meaning "to drip out or upon" and is used to indicate:
   a. a nosebleed
   b. a runny nose
   c. mucus on the lungs
   d. a wet cough

2. The Latin word for *spit*, which indicates mucus discharged by the lungs, is:
   a. spasm
   b. sputum
   c. mucus
   d. wet cough

3. Which of the following is NOT a term related to describing a breathing process?
   a. hyperventilation
   b. hypopnea
   c. bradypnea
   d. hemoptysis

4. Which of the following is NOT a term to describe pain in the lower respiratory system?
   a. pleuralgia
   b. rhinorrhagia
   c. pleurodynia
   d. thoracalgia

5. Which term describes a patient who is coughing up blood?
   a. rhinorrhagia
   b. epistaxis
   c. hemoptysis
   d. dyspnea

OBJECTIVE

10.3 Observation and Discovery

When gathering clues about the status of a patient's respiration, a health care professional may use physical findings, labs, and specialized tests or imaging. Sights and sounds are valuable tools in the physical exam of a patient with a respiratory problem. Inspection may reveal an abnormal chest shape, a patient working harder to breathe, or a change in skin color. When listening to the patient's chest (*auscultation*), an examiner may notice changes in breathing sounds.

Lab data mainly deal with the levels of carbon dioxide and oxygen in the blood. *Capnography* and *oximetry* are fast tests that provide this information, but more specialized tests examine how well the lungs work.

Spirometry measures the strength of breathing, while a *ventilation–perfusion scan* measures how effectively oxygen and blood reach different parts of the lungs. Finally, it may be necessary to get a closer look to get to the root of the problem (e.g., *bronchoscopy* and *thorascopy*).

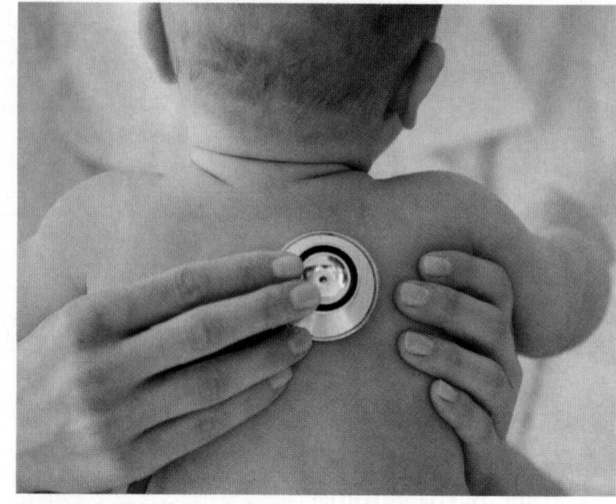

A doctor's first step in gathering data for a diagnosis is to listen to lung function using a stethoscope.

physical findings and examination methods

Term	Word Analysis
auscultation ah-skul-TAY-shun	**from the Latin word *ausculto,* meaning** "to listen"
Definition a health care professional using a stethoscope to listen to a patient's chest	
cyanosis sai-an-O-sis	**cyan / osis** blue / condition
Definition a bluish color in the skin caused by insufficient oxygen	
pectoriloquy pek-tor-IH-low-kwee	**pectori / loquy** chest / speak
Definition speaking from the chest; used as a means of finding masses in the lung. A health professional listening to a patient's chest asks the patient to whisper a word. The word will be audible in areas where fluid or a mass is present. Hence the chest "speaks" in those places. **NOTE:** A common related word is *ventriloquist,* a person who makes a puppet appear to talk. *Venter* means "stomach"; thus *ventriloquist* translates as "one who speaks from his stomach."	
pectus carinatum PEK-tus car-ee-NAH-tum	**pectus carinatum** chest keel
Definition a chest that protrudes like the keel of a ship	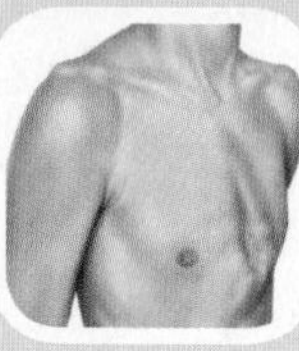

physical findings and examination methods *continued*

Term	Word Analysis
pectus excavatum PEK-tus eks-cuh-VAH-tum **Definition** a chest that is hollowed out	**pectus ex / cavatum** chest out / hollowed 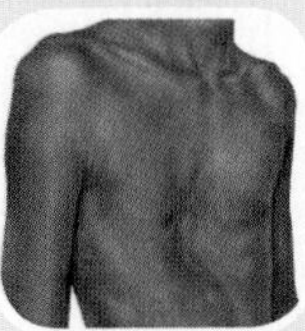
percussion per-KUH-shun **Definition** striking the body surface (in this context, to cause vibrations that can help locate fluid buildup in the chest)	**from the Latin word *percussio,* meaning "to strike"**
retraction reh-TRAK-shun **Definition** the sucking in of the skin around bones during inhalation, happens when someone is in respiratory distress	**re / trac / tion** back / drag process

pathology

Term	Word Analysis
atelectasis ah-tel-EK-ta-sis **Definition** incomplete expansion	**a / tel / ectasis** not / complete / expansion
bronchiectasis bron-key-EK-ta-sis **Definition** expansion of the bronchi	**bronchi / ectasis** bronchus / expansion
caseous necrosis KAYZ-ee-us ne-CROW-sis **Definition** the death of tissue with a cheeselike appearance	**caseous necr / osis** cheeselike death / condition
chylothorax kai-low-THOR-aks **Definition** chyle in the chest **NOTE:** Chyle is a milky bodily fluid formed in the small intestine during digestion of fatty foods and carried through the body via lymph vessels.	**chylo / thorax** chyle / chest
empyema em-pie-EE-mah **Definition** pus inside the chest	**em / py / ema** in / pus / condition
hemothorax heem-o-THOR-aks **Definition** blood in the chest	**hemo / thorax** blood / chest 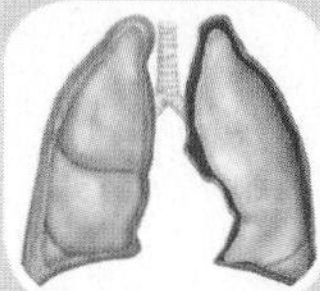

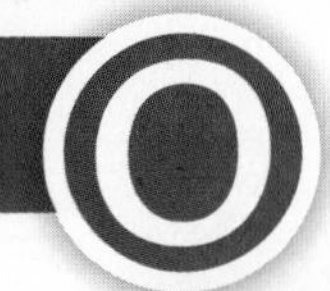

10.3 Observation and Discovery

pathology *continued*

Term	Word Analysis
phrenoplegia fre-no-PLEE-jah **Definition** paralysis of the diaphragm	**phreno / plegia** diaphragm / paralysis
phrenoptosis fre-nop-TOE-sis **Definition** drooping of the diaphragm	**phreno / ptosis** diaphragm / drooping condition
pleural effusion PLUR-al ef-YOO-zhun **Definition** fluid pouring out into the pleura **Note:** The prefix in *effusion* is actually *ex*. The *x* turns to an *f* when followed by an *f*. Why? Say *exfusion* 10 times. Most people slur *exfusion* into *effusion* because it is easier to say.	**pleur / al ex / fusion** pleura / pertaining to out / pour
pneumohemothorax new-moh-hee-moh-THOR-aks **Definition** air and blood in the chest	**pneumo / hemo / thorax** air / blood / chest
pneumothorax new-moh-THOR-aks **Definition** air in the chest	**pneumo / thorax** air / chest
pulmonary edema pul-mon-AIR-ee ah-DEE-ma **Definition** swelling in the lungs	**pulmon / ary edema** lung / pertaining to swelling
pyothorax pie-oh-THOR-aks **Definition** pus in the chest	**pyo / thorax** pus / chest
tracheostenosis tray-kee-oh-sten-OH-sis **Definition** narrowing of the trachea	**tracheo / stenosis** trachea / narrowing

10.3 Observation and Discovery

laboratory data

Term	Word Analysis
hypercapnia hai-per-CAP-nee-yah **Definition** excessive carbon dioxide	**hyper / capn / ia** over / carbon dioxide / condition
hypercarbia hai-per-CAR-bee-yah **Definition** excessive carbon dioxide	**hyper / carb / ia** over / carbon dioxide / condition
hypocapnia hai-po-CAP-nee-yah **Definition** insufficient carbon dioxide	**hypo / capn / ia** under / carbon dioxide / condition
hypocarbia hai-po-CAR-bee-yah **Definition** insufficient carbon dioxide	**hypo / carb / ia** under / carbon dioxide / condition
hypoxemia hai-poks-EEM-ee-yah **Definition** insufficient oxygen in the blood	**hypo / ox / emia** under / oxygen / blood condition
hypoxia hai-POKS-ee-yah **Definition** insufficient oxygen	**hypo / ox / ia** under / oxygen / condition

radiology

Term	Word Analysis
computed tomography com-PYOO-ted tom-O-grah-fee **Definition** an imaging procedure using a computer to cut **NOTE:** *Cut* in this context does not mean incision but rather using a computer to view "slices" of a patient's organs.	**computed tomo / graphy** cut / writing procedure
pulmonary angiography pul-mon-AIR-ee an-jee-O-grah-fee **Definition** an imaging procedure for recording pulmonary blood vessel activity	**pulmon / ary angio / graphy** lung / pertaining to vessel / writing procedure
ventilation–perfusion scan (VQ scan) ven-ti-LAY-shun–per-FYOO-shun skan **Definition** a scan that tests whether a problem in the lungs is caused by airflow (ventilation) or blood flow (perfusion) **NOTE:** Q is the abbreviation for perfusion, or blood flow, because the letter *P* is commonly used to abbreviate pulmonary. So we use the next letter in the alphabet.	**ventil / ation – per / fusion** breathing / process – through / pour

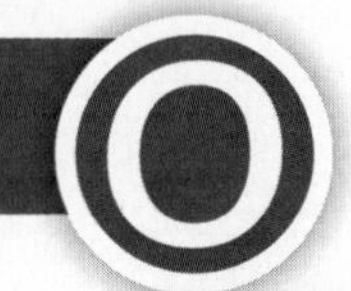

10.3 Observation and Discovery

diagnostic procedures

Term	Word Analysis
bronchoscopy bron-KOS-koh-pee **Definition** procedure to look inside the bronchi	**broncho / scopy** bronchus / looking procedure
capnography cap-NAH-gra-fee **Definition** procedure to record carbon dioxide levels	**capno / graphy** carbon dioxide / writing procedure
capnometer cap-NOM-eh-ter **Definition** instrument to measure carbon dioxide levels	**capno / meter** carbon dioxide / instrument to measure
endoscope EN-doh-SKOHP **Definition** instrument to look inside	**endo / scope** inside / instrument to look
nasopharyngoscope nay-zoh-fa-RIN-go-skope **Definition** an instrument to look at the nose and throat	**naso / pharyngo / scope** nose / throat / instrument to look
oximetry ok-SIM-ah-tree **Definition** procedure to measure oxygen levels	**oxi / metry** oxygen / measuring process
polysomnography po-lee-som-NAH-gra-fee **Definition** recording multiple aspects of sleep	**poly / somno / graphy** multiple / sleep / writing procedure

diagnostic procedures *continued*

Term	Word Analysis
pulmonary function testing (PFT) pul-mon-AIR-ee funk-shun TES-ting **Definition** a group of tests used to evaluate the condition and operation of the lungs	**pulmon / ary** **function testing** lung / pertaining to
spirometry speer-O-meh-tree **Definition** procedure to measure breathing	**spiro / metry** breathing / measuring process
thoracoscopy thor-a-KOS-koh-pee **Definition** examination of the chest **NOTE:** This word is sometimes shortened to *thorascopy* to make it easier to say.	**thoraco / scopy** chest / looking procedure

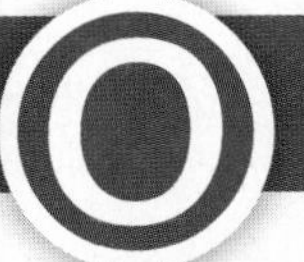

Learning Outcome 10.3 Exercises

PRONUNCIATION

EXERCISE 1 *Indicate which syllable is emphasized when pronounced.*

EXAMPLE: bronchitis bron**chi**tis

1. capnometter ________________
2. hemothorax ________________
3. hypoxia ________________
4. empyema ________________
5. phrenoptosis ________________
6. pyothorax ________________
7. pneumohemothorax ________________
8. atelectasis ________________
9. hypocarbia ________________
10. pectoriloquy ________________
11. endoscopy ________________
12. polysomnography ________________
13. thoracoscopy ________________

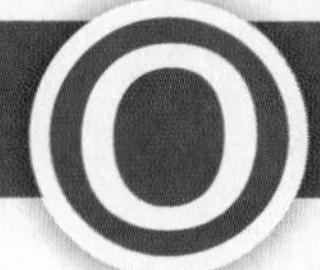

Learning Outcome 10.3 Exercises

TRANSLATION

EXERCISE 2 *Underline and define the word parts from this chapter in the following terms.*

1. pectoriloquy ______
2. pulmonary ______
3. chylothorax ______
4. hypercarbia ______
5. hypocapnia ______
6. hypoxia ______
7. capnography ______
8. bronchoscopy ______
9. spirometry ______
10. thoracoscopy ______

EXERCISE 3 *Match the term on the left with its definition on the right.*

____	1. percussion	a.	a scan that tests whether a problem in the lungs is caused by airflow or blood flow
____	2. cyanosis	b.	death of tissue with a cheeselike appearance
____	3. pectus excavatum	c.	an instrument to look at the nose and throat
____	4. pectus carinatum	d.	chest that is hollowed out
____	5. auscultation	e.	a bluish color in the skin
____	6. caseous necrosis	f.	instrument to look inside
____	7. atelectasis	g.	a recording procedure using a computer to view "cuts" of a patient's organs
____	8. pleural effusion	h.	fluid pouring out into the pleura
____	9. hypoxemia	i.	deficient oxygen in the blood
____	10. endoscope	j.	using a stethoscope to listen to the chest
____	11. nasopharyngoscope	k.	a group of tests used to evaluate the condition and operation of the lungs
____	12. ventilation-perfusion scan	l.	incomplete expansion
____	13. computed tomography	m.	striking the body surface to help locate fluid buildup in the chest
____	14. pulmonary function testing	n.	a chest that protrudes

EXERCISE 4 *Break down the following words into their component parts.*

EXAMPLE: nasopharyngoscope *naso | pharyngo | scope*

1. hemothorax ______
2. phrenoplegia ______
3. capnometer ______
4. oximetry ______
5. hypercapnia ______
6. hypocarbia ______

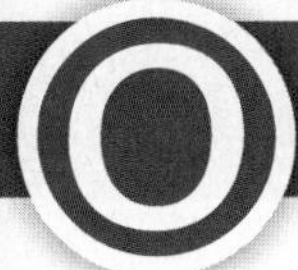

Learning Outcome 10.3 Exercises

7. pyothorax ____________________
8. pneumothorax ____________________
9. pneumohemothorax ____________________
10. empyema ____________________
11. tracheostenosis ____________________
12. bronchiectasis ____________________
13. polysomnography ____________________
14. phrenoptosis ____________________
15. pulmonary angiography ____________________

EXERCISE 5 *Translate the following terms as literally as possible.*

EXAMPLE: nasopharyngoscope *an instrument for looking at the nose and throat*

1. oximetry ____________________
2. hypercapnia ____________________
3. hypocarbia ____________________
4. hypercarbia ____________________
5. hypocapnia ____________________
6. hypoxia ____________________
7. thoracoscopy ____________________
8. capnography ____________________
9. hemothorax ____________________
10. pneumohemothorax ____________________
11. bronchiectasis ____________________
12. polysomnography ____________________
13. pulmonary angiography ____________________
14. phrenoptosis ____________________
15. pectus excavatum ____________________
16. pectoriloquy ____________________

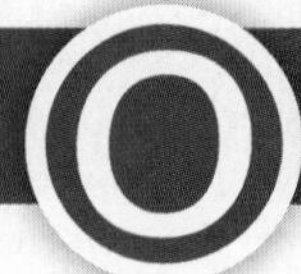

Learning Outcome 10.3 Exercises

GENERATION

EXERCISE 6 *Build a medical term from the information provided.*

EXAMPLE: inflammation of the sinuses *sinusitis*

1. swelling in the lungs ______
2. air in the chest ______
3. pus inside the chest ______
4. pus in the chest ______
5. chyle in the chest ______
6. paralysis of the diaphragm ______
7. narrowing of the trachea ______
8. instrument to measure carbon dioxide levels ______
9. procedure to look inside the bronchi ______
10. procedure to measure breathing ______

EXERCISE 7 *Multiple-choice questions. Select the correct answer.*

1. A health care professional uses a stethoscope as part of the following procedure:
   a. auscultation
   b. polysomnography
   c. endoscopy
   d. capnography
2. Which of the following terms pertains to the diaphragm?
   a. pleural effusion
   b. pulmonary edema
   c. phrenoplegia
   d. pneumothorax
3. Which procedure measures oxygen levels?
   a. spirometry
   b. capnography
   c. bronchoscopy
   d. oximetry
4. The term *hemothorax* means that there is which of the following in the chest?
   a. blood
   b. pus
   c. chyle
   d. air

ASSESSMENT

10.4 Diagnosis and Pathology

Since the upper respiratory tract is the first line of defense, infections in this area are very common. While inflammation in these areas (*rhinitis, sinusitis, pharyngitis, laryngitis,* etc.) is not *always* caused by infection, infection is certainly the most common cause. The lower respiratory tract has its share of infections as well, with the most common being *bronchitis* and *pneumonia. Asthma* and *chronic obstructive pulmonary disorder* are long-term, noninfectious causes of illness that can be serious.

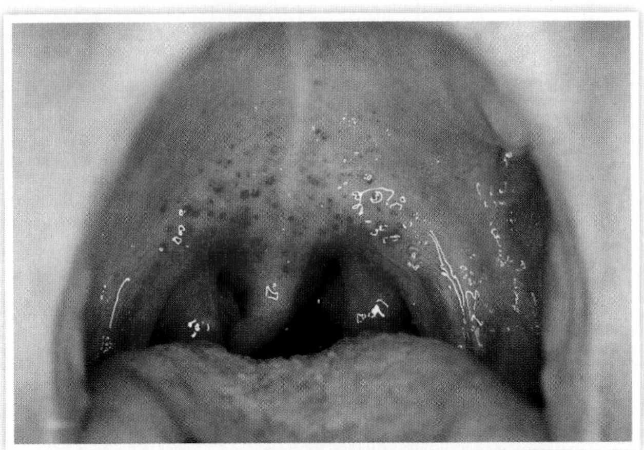

"Open up and say 'Ah' " is the way many examinations involving the respiratory system begin.

Source: Centers for Disease Control and Prevention

upper respiratory pathology

Term	Word Analysis
laryngitis la-rin-JAI-tis **Definition** inflammation of the larynx	**laryng / itis** larynx / inflammation
laryngotracheobronchitis la-rin-go-tray-key-o-bron-KAI-tis **Definition** inflammation of the larynx, trachea, and bronchi	**laryngo / tracheo / bronch / itis** larynx / trachea / bronchus / inflammation
rhinitis rai-NAI-tis **Definition** inflammation of the nasal passages	**rhin / itis** nose / inflammation
sinusitis sai-nus-AI-tis **Definition** inflammation of the sinus	**sinus / itis** sinus / inflammation
pansinusitis pan-sai-nus-AI-tis **Definition** inflammation of all sinuses	**pan / sinus / itis** all / sinus / inflammation
sleep apnea sleep AP-nee-ah **Definition** a condition where the patient ceases to breathe while asleep	**a / pnea** not / breathing

10.4 Diagnosis and Pathology

upper respiratory pathology *continued*

Term	Word Analysis
tonsillitis ton-sil-AI-tis **Definition** inflammation of the tonsils	**tonsill / itis** tonsil / inflammation Source: Centers for Disease Control and Prevention
tracheitis tray-kee-AI-tis **Definition** inflammation of the trachea	**trache / itis** trachea / inflammation
tracheomalacia tray-kee-oh-ma-LAY-shah **Definition** softening of the trachea	**tracheo / malacia** trachea / softening

lower respiratory pathology

Term	Word Analysis
asthma AZ-ma **Definition** a disease causing episodic narrowing and inflammation of the airway **NOTE:** The name describes the wheezing and shortness of breath that accompanies an attack.	**from the Greek word for "panting" or "gasping"** ©CT757fan/E+/Getty Images RF
bronchiolitis bron-kee-yo-LAI-tis **Definition** inflammation of a bronchiole	**bronchiol / itis** bronchiole / inflammation
bronchitis bron-KAI-tis **Definition** inflammation of the bronchi	**bronch / itis** bronchus / inflammation
chronic obstructive pulmonary disease (COPD) KRON-ik ob-STRUKT-iv pul-mon-AIR-ee diz-EEZ **Definition** a group of lung diseases characterized by the continual blockage of lung passages	**chron / ic ob / struct / ive** time / pertaining to in the way / build / pertaining to **pulmon / ary** lung / pertaining to

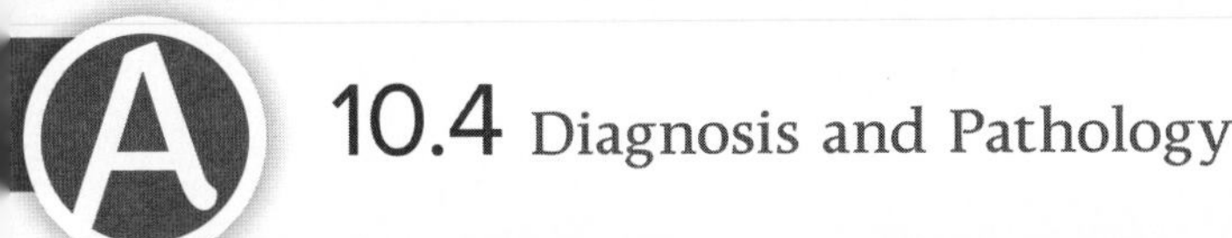

10.4 Diagnosis and Pathology

lower respiratory pathology *continued*

Term	Word Analysis
cystic fibrosis SIS-tik fai-BROH-sis **Definition** a disease causing thick mucous buildup in the lungs and pancreas, named after the changes it causes to the lungs	**cyst / ic** — cyst / pertaining to **fibr / osis** — fiber / condition
diaphragmatocele dai-a-frag-MAT-o-seel **Definition** hernia of the diaphragm	**diaphragmato / cele** diaphragm / pouch / tumor / hernia
emphysema im-fi-ZEE-ma **Definition** a disease that causes the alveoli to lose elasticity; emphysema patients can inhale but have difficulty exhaling	**from the Greek word *emphysan*, meaning "to inflate"**
obstructive lung disorder ob-STRUKT-iv **Definition** a lung disorder caused by a blockage	**ob / struct / ive** — in the way / build / pertaining to **lung disorder**
pleuritis plur-AI-tis **Definition** inflammation of the pleura	**pleur / itis** pleura / inflammation
pleurisy PLUR-ih-see **Definition** another word for pleuritis	**pleur / isy** pleura / inflammation
pneumatocele new-MAT-o-seel **Definition** hernia of the lung	**pneumato / cele** lung / pouch / tumor / hernia
pneumoconiosis new-moh-con-i-O-sis **Definition** a lung condition caused by dust	**pneumo / coni / osis** lung / dust / condition
pneumonia new-MOH-nee-yah **Definition** a lung condition	**pneumon / ia** lung / condition
pneumonitis new-moh-NAI-tis **Definition** inflammation of the lung	**pneumon / itis** lung / inflammation
pulmonary embolism pul-mon-AIR-ee em-bol-IZ-um **Definition** blockage in the pulmonary blood supply	**pulmon / ary** — lung / pertaining to **embol / ism** — embolus / condition

10.4 Diagnosis and Pathology

lower respiratory pathology *continued*

Term	Word Analysis
pulmonary neoplasm pul-mon-AIR-ee nee-oh-PLAZ-sum **Definition** new growth (tumor) in the lung	**pulmon / ary** — lung / pertaining to; **neo / plasm** — new / formation 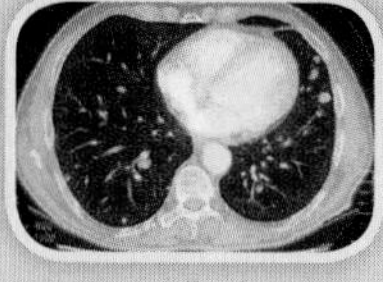 ©McGraw-Hill Education
restrictive lung disorder re-STRIKT-iv **Definition** a lung disorder caused by the limiting of air into the lungs	**re / strict / ive** — back / bind / tie / pertaining to; **lung disorder**

oncology

Term	Word Analysis
bronchiogenic carcinoma bron-kee-oh-JEN-ic car-si-NO-ma **Definition** a cancerous tumor originating in the bronchi	**bronchio / genic** — bronchus / beginning in; **carcin / oma** — cancer / tumor 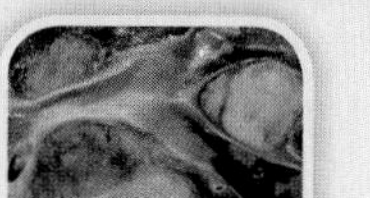 ©BSP/Science Source
mesothelioma mee-zoh-thee-lee-OH-mah **Definition** a cancerous tumor of the mesothelial cells lining the lungs **NOTE:** Mesothelium refers to a type of cell that lines the inside of several hollow cavities in the body. The term is derived from its relationship to epithelium, which is the outer layer of cells on most inner and outer surfaces in the body.	**meso / theli / oma** — middle / nipple / tumor

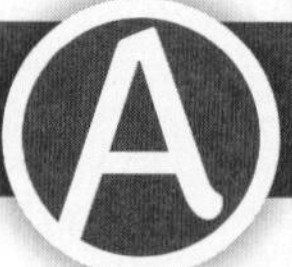

Learning Outcome 10.4 Exercises

PRONUNCIATION

EXERCISE 1 *Indicate which syllable is emphasized when pronounced.*

EXAMPLE: bronchitis bron**chi**tis

1. rhinitis ______
2. pleuritis ______
3. pleurisy ______
4. asthma ______
5. pneumonia ______
6. sinusitis ______
7. emphysema ______

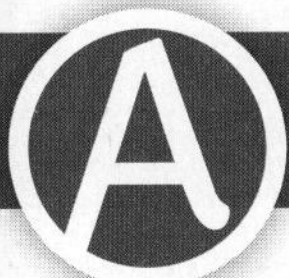

Learning Outcome 10.4 Exercises

TRANSLATION

EXERCISE 2 *Break down the following words into their component parts.*

EXAMPLE: nasopharyngoscope *naso | pharyngo | scope*

1. bronchiolitis ____________
2. pansinusitis ____________
3. tracheomalacia ____________
4. pneumoconiosis ____________
5. pulmonary embolism ____________
6. laryngotracheobronchitis ____________
7. bronchiogenic carcinoma ____________

EXERCISE 3 *Underline and define the word parts from this chapter in the following terms.*

1. laryngitis ____________
2. rhinitis ____________
3. sinusitis ____________
4. tonsillitis ____________
5. bronchitis ____________
6. pulmonary ____________
7. tracheitis ____________
8. pleuritis ____________

EXERCISE 4 *Match the term on the left with its definition on the right.*

______	1. sleep apnea	a.	a disease that causes the alveoli to lose their elasticity
______	2. obstructive lung disorder	b.	blockage in the pulmonary blood supply
______	3. restrictive lung disorder	c.	a lung disease caused by the continual blocking of lung passages
______	4. asthma	d.	a condition where the patient ceases to breathe while asleep
______	5. emphysema	e.	inflammation of the pleura
______	6. chronic obstructive pulmonary disease (COPD)	f.	a lung disorder caused by a blockage
______	7. pleurisy	g.	a disease causing episodic narrowing and inflammation of the airway
______	8. pulmonary embolism	h.	a lung disorder caused by the limiting of air into the lungs

EXERCISE 5 *Translate the following terms as literally as possible.*

EXAMPLE: nasopharyngoscope *an instrument for looking at the nose and throat*

1. pneumonia ____________
2. pleuritis ____________
3. rhinitis ____________
4. pansinusitis ____________
5. tracheomalacia ____________

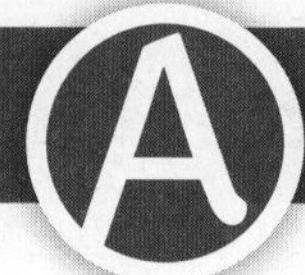

6. pneumatocele ____________
7. diaphragmatocele ____________
8. pulmonary neoplasm ____________
9. laryngotracheobronchitis ____________
10. bronchiogenic carcinoma ____________

GENERATION

EXERCISE 6 *Build a medical term from the information provided.*

EXAMPLE: inflammation of the sinuses *sinusitis*

1. inflammation of the larynx ____________
2. inflammation of all sinuses ____________
3. inflammation of the tonsils ____________
4. inflammation of the lung ____________
5. inflammation of the trachea ____________
6. inflammation of the bronchi ____________
7. a lung condition caused by dust ____________

EXERCISE 7 *Multiple-choice questions. Select the correct answer(s).*

1. The Greek word for "panting" or "gasping" is:
   a. emphysema
   b. asthma
   c. pleurisy
   d. embolism
2. *Emphysema* comes from the Greek word meaning ____________ and describes a disease that causes the alveoli to lose their elasticity.
   a. to deflate
   b. to stretch
   c. to inflate
   d. to loosen
3. Select the terms that pertain to the upper respiratory system.
   a. bronchitis
   b. laryngitis
   c. laryngotracheobronchitis
   d. pansinusitis
   e. pleuritis
   f. pneumonitis
   g. rhinitis
   h. sinusitis
   i. tonsillitis
   j. tracheitis
4. Select the terms that pertain to the lower respiratory system.
   a. bronchitis
   b. laryngitis
   c. laryngotracheobronchitis
   d. pansinusitis
   e. pleuritis
   f. pneumonitis
   g. rhinitis
   h. sinusitis
   i. tonsillitis
   j. tracheitis

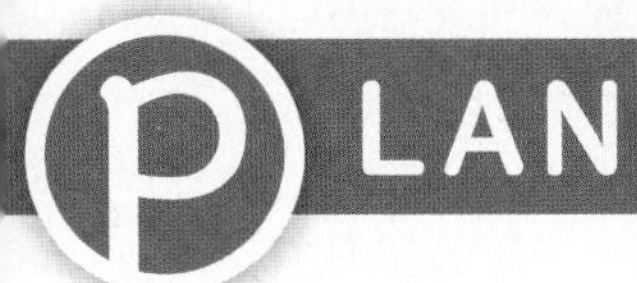

10.5 Treatments and Therapies

Most respiratory illnesses respond to medicines. Bronchi-opening medicines (*bronchodilators*) given through an *inhaler device* or a machine (*nebulizer*) help people with asthma or chronic obstructive pulmonary disorder. Cough-stopping (*antitussive*) medicines are popular, but not necessarily very helpful.

With some illnesses, more aggressive intervention is needed. Surgeries of the upper airway are among the most common procedures. Lower airway surgeries, such as cutting out part of the lung (*lobectomy*), are less common. Very ill patients or patients who are undergoing surgery may need to have a tube placed in the mouth and into the windpipe (*endotracheal tube*). The tube is then attached to a breathing machine.

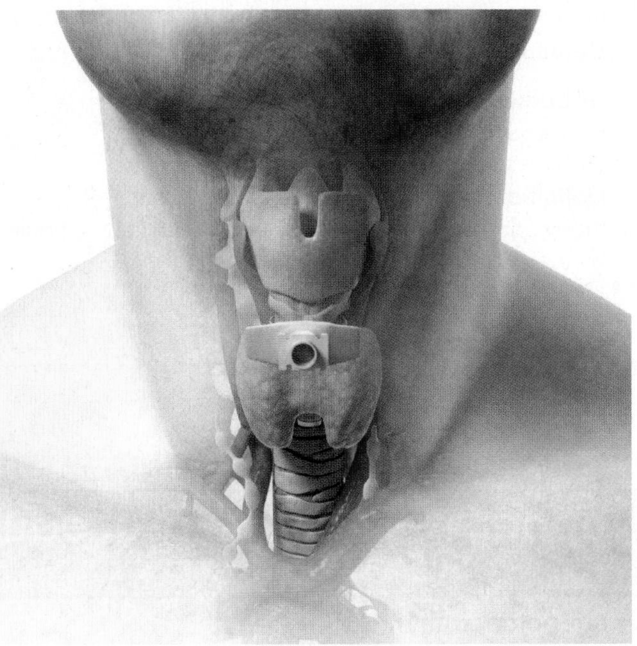

One way of bypassing a patient's obstructed airway is through a tracheostomy, creating an artificial opening in the trachea to allow air to enter the lungs easier.

©MedicalRF.com RF

pharmacology

Term	Word Analysis
antitussive an-tee-TUSS-iv **Definition** a drug that prevents coughing	**anti / tuss / ive** against / cough / agent ©PhotoDisc/Getty Images RF
bronchodilator bron-koh-DAI-lay-tor **Definition** a drug that expands the walls of the bronchi	**broncho / dilator** bronchus / expander
expectorant eks-PEK-tor-ant **Definition** a drug that encourages the expulsion of material from the lungs	**ex / pector / ant** out / chest / agent

pharmacology *continued*

Term	Word Analysis
mucolytic myoo-koh-LIT-ik **Definition** a drug that aids in the breakdown of mucus	**muco / lytic** mucus / breakdown agent
nebulizer neh-byoo-LAI-zir **Definition** a machine that administers respiratory medication by creating a "cloud" or mist that is inhaled by the patient	**from the Latin word *nebula*, meaning "cloud"** ©Stockbyte/Punchstock RF

upper respiratory procedures

Term	Word Analysis
adenoidectomy a-din-oid-EK-toe-mee **Definition** removal of the adenoids	**adenoid / ectomy** adenoid / removal
intubate IN-tub-ate **Definition** to insert a breathing tube from the mouth down into the trachea, to provide breathing support	**in / tub / ate** in / tube / process
laryngectomy la-rin-JEK-toe-mee **Definition** removal of the larynx	**laryng / ectomy** larynx / removal
laryngoplasty la-rin-GO-plas-tee **Definition** reconstruction of the larynx	**laryngo / plasty** larynx / reconstruction
palatoplasty pal-e-toe-PLAS-tee **Definition** reconstruction of a palate	**palato / plasty** palate / reconstruction
septoplasty sep-toe-PLAS-tee **Definition** reconstruction of a septum	**septo / plasty** septum / reconstruction
tonsillectomy ton-sil-EK-toe-mee **Definition** removal of the tonsils	**tonsill / ectomy** tonsil / removal
tracheostomy tray-kee-AH-stoh-mee **Definition** creation of an opening in the trachea	**tracheo / stomy** trachea / opening

upper respiratory procedures *continued*

Term	Word Analysis
tracheotomy tray-kee-AH-toe-mee **Definition** incision into the trachea	**tracheo / tomy** trachea / incision 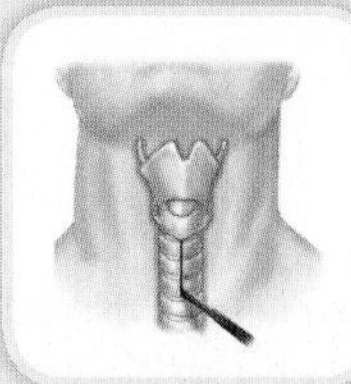
endotracheal intubation en-doh-TRAY-kee-al in-too-BAY-shun **Definition** insertion of a tube inside the trachea	**endo / trache / al** **in / tub / ation** inside / trachea / pertaining to in / tube / process

lower respiratory procedures

Term	Word Analysis
bronchoplasty bron-koh-PLAS-tee **Definition** reconstruction of a bronchus	**broncho / plasty** bronchus / reconstruction
cardiopulmonary resuscitation (CPR) kar-dee-oh-pul-mon-AIR-ee ree-sus-i-TAY-shun **Definition** method of artificially maintaining blood flow and airflow when breathing and pulse have stopped **NOTE:** *Suscit* is formed by adding the prefix *sub-* to the Latin word *cito,* which means "to move." *Suscit* = *sub* + *cito* = to move from beneath, and thus "to raise" or "awaken." The *cito* root is found in other words like *excite, incite,* and *recite.*	**cardio / pulmon / ary** lung / heart / pertaining to **re / suscit / ation** again / awaken / process 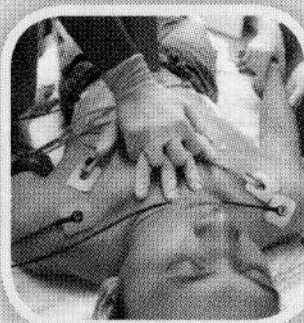 ©ERproductions Ltd/Blend Images LLC RF
lobectomy loh-BEK-toe-mee **Definition** removal of a lobe	**lob / ectomy** lobe / removal 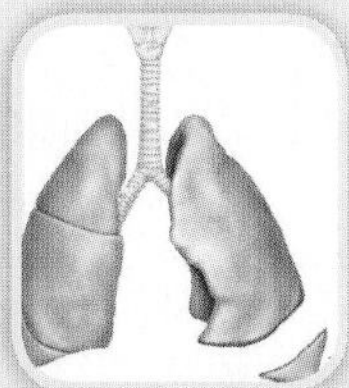 ©Stockbyte/Punchstock RF
pleuropexy ploo-rah-PEK-see **Definition** reattachment of the pleura	**pleuro / pexy** pleura / fixation

10.5 Treatments and Therapies

lower respiratory procedures *continued*

Term	Word Analysis
pneumonectomy new-mon-EK-toe-mee **Definition** removal of a lung	**pneumon / ectomy** lung / removal
thoracentesis thor-a-sin-TEE-sis **Definition** puncture of the chest **NOTE:** This word drops a syllable from *thoracocentesis* to make it easier to say.	**thora [co] / centesis** chest / puncture
thoracocentesis thor-a-koh-sin-TEE-sis **Definition** puncture of the chest	**thoraco / centesis** chest / puncture 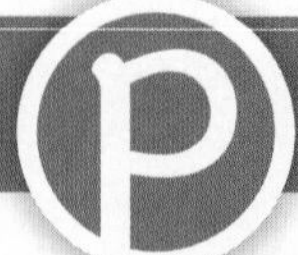
thoracoplasty thor-a-koh-PLAS-tee **Definition** reconstruction of the chest	**thoraco / plasty** chest / reconstruction
thoracostomy thor-a-KOS-toe-mee **Definition** creation of an opening in the chest	**thoraco / stomy** chest / opening
thoracotomy thor-a-KAH-toe-mee **Definition** incision into the chest	**thoraco / tomy** chest / incision

Learning Outcome 10.5 Exercises

PRONUNCIATION

EXERCISE 1 *Indicate which syllable is emphasized when pronounced.*

EXAMPLE: bronchitis bron**chi**tis

1. lobectomy ______
2. antitussive ______
3. adenoidectomy ______
4. palatoplasty ______
5. tracheostomy ______
6. thoracentesis ______
7. thoracostomy ______

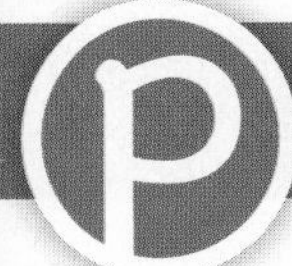

Learning Outcome 10.5 Exercises

TRANSLATION

EXERCISE 2 *Break down the following words into their component parts.*

EXAMPLE: nasopharyngoscope *naso | pharyngo | scope*

1. septoplasty ______
2. laryngoplasty ______
3. tracheotomy ______
4. adenoidectomy ______
5. pneumonectomy ______
6. thoracostomy ______
7. tracheostomy ______
8. pleuropexy ______
9. thoracocentesis ______
10. antitussive ______
11. expectorant ______
12. mucolytic ______

EXERCISE 3 *Underline and define the word parts from this chapter in the following terms.*

1. laryngectomy ______
2. bronchoplasty ______
3. thoracocentesis ______
4. expectorant ______
5. endotracheal ______

EXERCISE 4 *Match the term on the left with its definition on the right.*

______ 1. thoracotomy
______ 2. nebulizer
______ 3. thoracentesis
______ 4. endotracheal intubation
______ 5. cardiopulmonary resuscitation

a. insertion of a tube inside the trachea
b. a machine that administers respiratory medication by creating a "cloud" or mist that is inhaled by the patient
c. a puncture of the chest
d. a method of artificially maintaining blood flow and airflow when breathing and pulse have stopped
e. incision into the chest

EXERCISE 5 *Translate the following terms as literally as possible.*

EXAMPLE: nasopharyngoscope *an instrument for looking at the nose and throat*

1. antitussive ______
2. expectorant ______
3. laryngoplasty ______
4. septoplasty ______
5. adenoidectomy ______
6. pneumonectomy ______
7. tracheotomy ______
8. tracheostomy ______
9. thoracostomy ______
10. pleuropexy ______
11. thoracocentesis ______
12. mucolytic ______

Learning Outcome 10.5 Exercises

GENERATION

EXERCISE 6 *Build a medical term from the information provided.*

EXAMPLE: inflammation of the sinuses *sinusitis*

1. removal of the larynx ____________
2. removal of the tonsils ____________
3. removal of a lobe ____________
4. reconstruction of a palate ____________
5. reconstruction of a bronchus ____________
6. reconstruction of the chest ____________
7. a drug that expands the walls of the bronchi ____________

EXERCISE 7 *Multiple-choice questions. Select the correct answer(s).*

1. A *nebulizer* administers medication by creating a mist to be inhaled by a patient. It comes from the Latin word *nebula,* meaning:
   a. mist
   b. smoke
   c. cloud
   d. medication
2. Select the terms that pertain to the upper respiratory system.
   a. adenoidectomy
   b. bronchoplasty
   c. laryngectomy
   d. laryngoplasty
   e. lobectomy
   f. palatoplasty
   g. pneumonectomy
   h. septoplasty
   i. thoracoplasty
   j. tonsillectomy
3. Select the terms that pertain to the lower respiratory system.
   a. adenoidectomy
   b. bronchoplasty
   c. laryngectomy
   d. laryngoplasty
   e. lobectomy
   f. palatoplasty
   g. pneumonectomy
   h. septoplasty
   i. thoracoplasty
   j. tonsillectomy
4. Select the terms that involve removal of a part of the respiratory system.
   a. adenoidectomy
   b. bronchoplasty
   c. laryngectomy
   d. laryngoplasty
   e. lobectomy
   f. palatoplasty
   g. pneumonectomy
   h. septoplasty
   i. thoracoplasty
   j. tonsillectomy
5. Select the terms that involve reconstruction of a part of the respiratory system.
   a. adenoidectomy
   b. bronchoplasty
   c. laryngectomy
   d. laryngoplasty
   e. lobectomy
   f. palatoplasty
   g. pneumonectomy
   h. septoplasty
   i. thoracoplasty
   j. tonsillectomy
6. Which drug is used to break down mucus?
   a. antitussive
   b. bronchodilator
   c. expectorant
   d. mucolytic

10.6 Abbreviations

Abbreviations provide a shorthand way of referring to things that either recur often or are too long to write out. When dealing with the respiratory system, those terms include clinical observations (CTA), diagnostic tests (CXR, V/Q), diagnoses (LTB, COPD, URI), and treatments (T&A, CPAP).

respiratory system abbreviations

Abbreviation	Definition
ABG	arterial blood gas analysis of the gases in the blood; used to determine the effectiveness of the lungs in exchanging gases occasionally they use capillary blood from a finger stick, at which point it's known as a capillary blood gas (CBG)
ARDS	acute respiratory distress syndrome
Bx	biopsy
CF	cystic fibrosis
COPD	chronic obstructive pulmonary disease
CPAP	continuous positive airway pressure a treatment for apnea involving keeping a patient's airways open using air pressure delivered via a face mask
CPR	cardiopulmonary resuscitation
CT	computed tomography
CTA	clear to auscultation when an examination reveals nothing abnormal about a patient's lung
CXR	chest x-ray ©Getty Images/Brand X RF
DOE	dyspnea on exertion
ETT	endotracheal tube
LRTI	lower respiratory tract infection
LTB	laryngotracheobronchitis
MRI	magnetic resonance imaging

respiratory system abbreviations *continued*

Abbreviation	Definition
OSA	obstructive sleep apnea
PE	pulmonary embolism
PET	positron emission tomography
PFT	pulmonary function test
PSG	polysomnography
SOB	shortness of breath
T&A	tonsillectomy and adenoidectomy
TB	tuberculosis
URI/URTI	upper respiratory infection, upper respiratory tract infection
V/Q	ventilation–perfusion scan

Learning Outcome 10.6 Exercises

TRANSLATION

EXERCISE 1 *Define the following abbreviations.*

1. CPR ______
2. MRI ______
3. PET ______
4. CT ______
5. CTA ______
6. URI ______
7. T&A ______
8. ABG ______
9. CXR ______
10. CPAP ______
11. SOB ______
12. ARDS ______
13. CF ______
14. DOE ______
15. ETT ______

EXERCISE 2 *Give the abbreviations for the following terms.*

1. biopsy ______
2. pulmonary embolism ______
3. clear to auscultation ______

Learning Outcome 10.6 Exercises

4. ventilation–perfusion scan ______
5. chronic obstructive pulmonary disease ______
6. laryngotracheobronchitis ______
7. polysomnography ______
8. obstructive sleep apnea ______
9. cystic fibrosis ______
10. pulmonary function test ______
11. endotracheal ______
12. tuberculosis ______
13. lower respiratory tract infection ______

EXERCISE 3 *Multiple-choice questions. Select the correct answer.*

1. CPAP is a treatment for:
   a. bronchitis
   b. thoracalgia
   c. apnea
   d. hyperventilation
2. A patient with an infection in the upper respiratory system has a(n):
   a. CTA
   b. URI
   c. PSG
   d. ABG
3. A patient with a blockage in the blood supply to the lungs has a(n):
   a. URI
   b. PE
   c. LTB
   d. T&A
4. A T&A involves the removal of:
   a. tonsils and adenoids
   b. trachea and adenoids
   c. tonsils and alveolus
   d. trachea and alveolus
5. LTB is an inflammation of the:
   a. larynx, trachea, and bronchi
   b. lobe, trachea, and bronchi
   c. lung, trachea, and breathing
   d. larynx, tonsil, and bronchi
6. A patient with OSA:
   a. has difficulty sleeping due to obstructive sputum
   b. has overactive sinuses when awake
   c. has obstructive adenoids when asleep
   d. stops breathing when asleep
7. An analysis of gases in the blood to determine the effectiveness of the lungs in exchanging gases is:
   a. ABG
   b. AGB
   c. LGE
   d. GBLE
8. Which of the following is NOT a diagnostic procedure?
   a. V/S
   b. CT
   c. PFT
   d. LTB

10.7 Electronic Health Records

Primary Care Visit

S Subjective

The patient is 4 months old with a 4-day history of **nasal** congestion, **rhinorrhea,** and a dry cough. He also has been **wheezing** for the past 2 days. His congestion is getting worse. He has had a fever up to 103.4°F. His parents say he has not had any **apnea, cyanosis,** or trouble breathing. No one in his family has **asthma.** His mother was recently diagnosed with **bronchitis.**

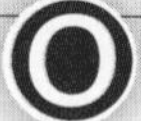

Objective

Objective:	Temp: 101.1°F; HR: 110; **RR:** 32; BP: 84/60; **Pulse ox:** 93%
Gen:	He is alert and in no apparent distress.
HEENT:	His ear canals are clear. There is no evidence of an ear infection. There is congestion in his **nares.** His lips and mouth are moist. He does not have any **pharyngeal exudate.**
Resp:	He is wheezing **bilaterally** on **auscultation.**
CV:	His heart is beating with a regular rate and rhythm and without a murmur.
Skin:	His skin is warm, dry, and pink.
CXR:	There is **peribronchial** (*around the bronchi*) fluid with mild **hyperinflation** of his lungs. An opacity (*an opaque area on x-ray*) is seen on one x-ray view but not the other. This is likely from **atelectasis.**

Assessment

Since he is wheezing, his cough is probably **bronchospastic.** He did not improve after using a bronchodilator in the office. Therefore, I believe the patient has a URI and **bronchiolitis.**

Plan

Use a humidifier in his room at night and clean his nose with a suction bulb.

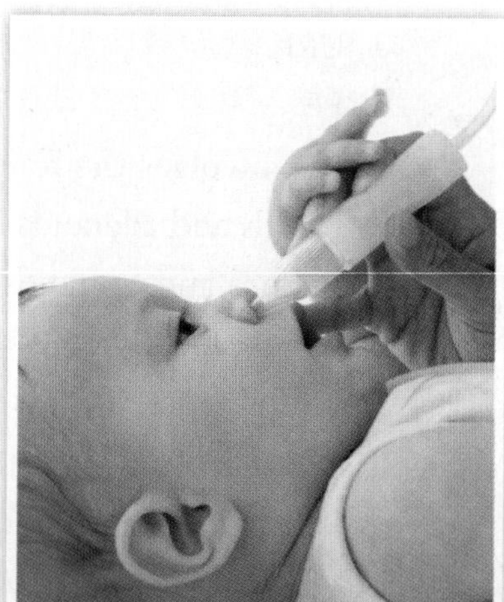

Learning Outcome 10.7 Exercises

EXERCISE 1 *Fill in the blanks.*

1. The patient has a history of *rhinorrhea* (define rhinorrhea: ______________________________).
2. The parents deny ____________________ (that the patient is not breathing) or *cyanosis* (define cyanosis: ______________________________).
3. Respiratory observation revealed bilateral wheezing on auscultation (define auscultation: ______________________________).
4. The cough is most likely caused by ____________________ (involuntary contraction of the bronchus).
5. The patient did not respond to ____________________ (drug that expands the walls of the bronchi).
6. The patient has URI (____________________) and ____________________ (inflammation of the bronchioles).

EXERCISE 2 *True or false questions. Indicate true answers with a T and false answers with an F.*

1. The doctor noticed the patient had cyanosis. ____________________
2. The parents claim the patient had stopped breathing. ____________________
3. The doctor attempted to open the patient's bronchial tubes using medication. ____________________

EXERCISE 3 *Multiple-choice questions. Select the correct answer.*

1. What test indicated incomplete expansion of the bronchial tubes?
   a. chest x-ray
   b. CT scan
   c. ABG
   d. auscultation

2. The patient's cough is probably caused by:
   a. overexpansion of the bronchial tubes
   b. incomplete expansion of the bronchial tubes
   c. involuntary contraction of the bronchial tubes
   d. blockage of the bronchial tubes

Emergency Department Visit

Chief Complaint: **Hemoptysis**

History of Present Illness: The patient has been brought to the emergency department by her mother. She is a 22-year-old female with **cystic fibrosis.** She has had a 1-day history of **hemoptysis.** She has been feeling tired for 5 days. Her mother says that the patient has had mild **dyspnea** and cough. The patient's last **PFTs** were much worse than normal for her. She has not had any **epistaxis,** bleeding from her gums, bloody stool, or easy bruising.

Past Medical History: Cystic fibrosis; bronchiectasis.

Medications: **Inhaled** antibiotic (tobramycin inhaled); **mucolytic** agent (pulmozyme); vitamins ADEK; **bronchodilator** (albuterol).

Allergies: NKDA.

Social: She is a nonsmoker. She is a sophomore in college and lives with her parents.

Surgical History: None.

Physical Exam: RR: 30; HR: 92; Temp: 102.1°F; BP: 90/57; **Pulse ox:** 89%

Gen: Mildly **cyanotic.** In mild **respiratory distress.**

Her nose and mouth are a little dry.

HEENT: Her eardrums and ear canals are normal.

CV: Mildly **tachycardic.** No murmur. Her pulses are a little weak.

Resp: **Tachypneic,** shallow breaths, breath sounds are weaker than normal **bilaterally.**

GI: Normal. Her liver and spleen are not large.

Emergency Department Course: When she came to the **ED,** the patient was in **acute respiratory distress.** She was **intubated** with an **endotracheal tube** and placed on a ventilator. A **CXR** verified correct placement in her trachea. She had poor circulation, so she was given **IVF** and transfused with 2 units of blood **(prbcs)**. An **ABG** showed **hypoxemia** and **hypercapnia,** both of which improved on follow-up **ABG** after she was intubated. The **pulmonology** team was contacted; the team decided **bronchoscopy** would be best. The team found that she was bleeding in her **bronchi** and treated her with **endobronchial electrocautery.** Afterward, she was transferred to the **ICU** for further care.

Learning Outcome 10.7 Exercises

EXERCISE 4 *Fill in the blanks.*

1. The patient has cystic fibrosis and a 1-day history of ____________________ (coughing up blood).
2. The patient has had *dyspnea* (give definition: ____________________).
3. Her recent PFTs (give definition: ____________________) were significantly worse than previously.
4. Her medical history includes cystic fibrosis as well as ____________________ (expansion of the bronchi).
5. Among her medications is albuterol, a *bronchodilator* (give definition: ____________________).
6. Her physical exam revealed that she has mild cyanosis (give definition: ____________________) and her breathing was rapid or ____________________.
7. The patient was then intubated with a tube in her ____________________. They used a bedside CXR (give definition: ____________________) to confirm correct placement.
8. ABG (give definition: ____________________) revealed *hypoxemia* (give definition: ____________________) and ____________________ (excessive carbon dioxide).
9. The pulmonologist performed a bronchoscopy (give definition: ____________________).
10. A(n) ____________________ (inside the bronchi) electrocautery was used for hemostasis.

EXERCISE 5 *Multiple-choice questions. Select the correct answer.*

1. Which is a symptom mentioned by the patient?
   a. coughing up blood
   b. runny nose
   c. sleeplessness
   d. sore throat
2. How was the patient breathing when examined in the ED?
   a. rapidly
   b. slowly
   c. not at all
   d. heavily
3. The chart says the patient was taking shallow breaths. What is another term for that?
   a. hyperpnea
   b. hypopnea
   c. orthopnea
   d. apnea
4. Where was a tube placed in the patient?
   a. nowhere
   b. into the nose
   c. into the trachea
   d. into the nose and throat
5. What did the analysis of the patient's arterial blood gases reveal?
   a. deficient oxygen levels
   b. excessive carbon dioxide
   c. both
   d. neither

EXERCISE 6 *True or false questions. Indicate true answers with a T and false answers with an F.*

1. The patient has had a recent nosebleed. ______
2. The patient takes medication for constricted bronchial tubes. ______
3. The patient takes medication for insufficient mucus secretion. ______
4. The doctor noted the patient's skin had a slight blue color. ______
5. An examination of the patient's bronchial tubes was performed. ______

Pulmonology Consult

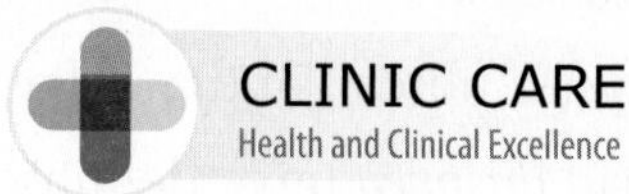

Reason for Consult: Cough and dyspnea.

The patient is a 64-year-old male who has had a cough for 2 months. His cough has had a lot of sputum in it. Now he also has **dyspnea**. He has been sweating at night and has lost 5 pounds in the past 2 months. He does not have any **hemoptysis, dysphonia,** or fever. He is a 2-pack-per-day smoker.

On physical exam, the patient is alert. He takes occasional pauses when he says long sentences, but otherwise, he is not in any distress. He has an occasional cough during his exam. His skin is pink and dry, and his lips are moist. His heartbeat is regular in rate and rhythm, without a murmur. On lung examination, he has **pectoriloquy** on the right side while whispering with decreased breath sounds. He does not have any **retractions**. His liver and spleen are not large.

A **CT** of his lungs revealed opacities (*opaque areas on x-ray*) in his right upper lobe, with a small area of **pleural effusion** on the right. There are also two large **thoracic** lymph nodes.

An **ABG** shows mild **hypoxemia**. I believe this is from the large amount of **bronchorrhea.**

Thoracoscopy with **biopsy** was then done under sedation in the surgical suite. The biopsy sample was sent to the pathology lab. The results showed **bronchioloalveolar carcinoma** (carcinoma of the bronchi and alveoli).

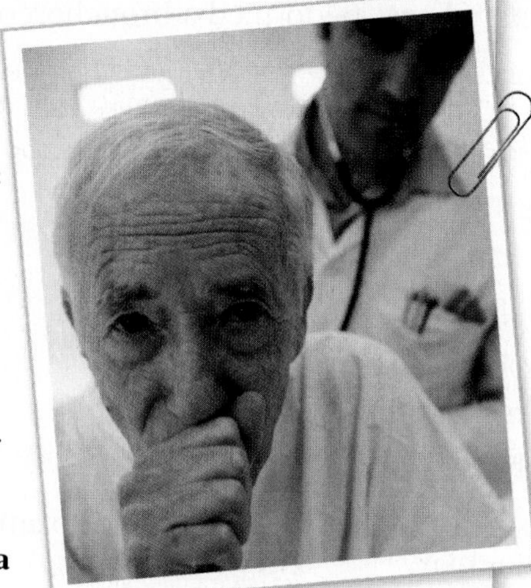
©Fuse/Getty Images RF

I have discussed the results with the patient, including his treatment options. I explained he would need a partial **lobectomy.** He is scheduled for a surgical consultation later this week. After surgical resection of the tumor and lobectomy, he will need to begin chemotherapy.

Learning Outcome 10.7 Exercises

EXERCISE 7 *Fill in the blanks.*

1. The patient's cough has clear ________________ and progressed to *dyspnea* (give definition: ________________).
2. He denies ________________ (coughing up blood), dysphonia, and fever.
3. The CT, or ________________, of his lungs revealed a small area of fluid pouring into the pleura, or a(n) ________________.
4. Arterial blood gases, or ________________, revealed *hypoxemia* (give definition: ________________).
5. Treatment will include partial removal of a lobe of the lung, or ________________.

EXERCISE 8 *True or false questions. Indicate true answers with a T and false answers with an F.*

1. *Thorascopy* is a shortening of the word *thoracoscopy*. ________
2. The patient was diagnosed with cancer. ________
3. The patient had a lung removed. ________
4. The patient has sufficient oxygen in his blood. ________
5. The patient's lung was CTA. ________
6. The patient has been coughing up blood. ________
7. The patient complains of hoarseness. ________
8. The lining of the patient's lungs has excess fluid in it. ________

Quick Reference

quick reference glossary of roots

Root	Definition	Root	Definition
adenoid/o	adenoid	**pleur/o**	pleura
bronch/o, bronchi/o	bronchus	**-pnea**	breathing
bronchiol/o	bronchiole	**pneum/o, pneumat/o, pneumon/o**	air or lungs
capn/o	carbon dioxide	**pulmon/o**	lungs
carb/o	carbon dioxide	**rhin/o**	nose
laryng/o	larynx (voice box)	**sept/o**	septum
lob/o	lobe	**sin/o, sinus/o**	sinus
nas/o	nose	**spir/o**	breathing
ox/o	oxygen	**thorac/o**	chest
pector/o	chest	**tonsill/o**	tonsil
pharyng/o	pharynx (throat)	**trache/o**	trachea (windpipe)
phren/o	diaphragm		

quick reference glossary of terms

Term	Definition
adenoidectomy	removal of the adenoids
antitussive	a drug that prevents coughing
apnea	cessation of breathing
asthma	a disease caused by episodic narrowing and inflammation of the airway
atelectasis	incomplete expansion
auscultation	from the Latin word *ausculto,* meaning "to listen"; a doctor using a stethoscope is performing an auscultation
bradypnea	slow breathing
bronchiectasis	expansion of the bronchi
bronchiogenic carcinoma	a cancerous tumor originating in the bronchi
bronchiolitis	inflammation of the bronchiole
bronchioplasty	reconstruction of a bronchus
bronchitis	inflammation of the bronchi
bronchodilator	a drug that expands the walls of the bronchi

quick reference glossary of terms *continued*

Term	Definition
bronchorrhea	discharge from the bronchi
bronchoscopy	a procedure to look inside the bronchi
bronchospasm	involuntary contraction of the bronchi
capnography	a procedure to record carbon dioxide levels
capnometer	instrument to measure carbon dioxide levels
cardiopulmonary resuscitation (CPR)	a method of artificially maintaining blood flow and airflow when breathing and pulse have stopped
caseous necrosis	the death of tissue with a cheeselike appearance
chronic obstructive pulmonary disease (COPD)	a lung disease caused by the continual blockage of lung passages
chylothorax	chyle in the chest
computed tomography	a recording procedure using a computer to "cut" or view "slices" of a patient's organs
cyanosis	a bluish color in the skin caused by insufficient oxygen
cystic fibrosis	a genetic disease primarily affecting the lungs
diaphragmatocele	hernia of the diaphragm
dysphonia	"bad voice condition"; hoarseness
dyspnea	difficulty breathing
emphysema	a disease that causes the alveoli to lose their elasticity; patients can inhale but have difficulty exhaling
empyema	pus inside (the chest)
endoscope	instrument to look inside
endotracheal intubation	insertion of a tube inside the trachea
epistaxis	nosebleed
eupnea	good/normal breathing
expectorant	a drug that encourages that expulsion of material from the lungs
expectoration	coughing or spitting material out of the lungs
hemoptysis	coughing up blood
hemothorax	blood in the chest
hypercapnia	condition of having excessive carbon dioxide in the blood
hypercarbia	excessive carbon dioxide
hyperpnea	heavy breathing
hyperventilation	overbreathing; condition of having too much air flowing into and out of the lungs; leads to hypocapnia

quick reference glossary of terms *continued*

Term	Definition
hypocapnia	insufficient carbon dioxide
hypocarbia	insufficient carbon dioxide
hypopnea	shallow breathing
hypoventilation	underbreathing; condition of having too little air flowing into and out of the lungs; leads to hypercapnia
hypoxemia	insufficient oxygen in the blood
hypoxia	insufficient oxygen
laryngectomy	removal of the larynx
laryngitis	inflammation of the larynx
laryngoplasty	reconstruction of the larynx
laryngotracheobronchitis	inflammation of the larynx, trachea, and bronchi
lobectomy	removal of a lobe
mesothelioma	a cancerous tumor of the mesothelium cells lining the lungs
mucolytic	a drug that aids in the breakdown of mucus
nasopharyngoscope	an instrument to look at the nose and throat
nebulizer	a machine that administers respiratory medication by creating a "cloud" or mist that is inhaled by the patient
obstructive lung disorder	a lung disorder caused by a blockage
orthopnea	able to breathe only in an upright position
oximetry	a procedure to measure oxygen levels
palatoplasty	reconstruction of the palate
pansinusitis	inflammation of all sinuses
pectoriloquy	"speaking from the chest"; used as a means of finding masses in the lung
pectus carinatum	a chest that protrudes like the keel of a ship
pectus excavatum	a chest that is hollowed out
percussion	the body surface; in this context, to cause vibrations that can help locate fluid buildup in the chest
phrenoplegia	paralysis of the diaphragm
phrenoptosis	drooping of the diaphragm
phrenospasm	involuntary contraction of the diaphragm
pleuradynia	pain in the pleura
pleural effusion	fluid pouring out into the pleura
pleuralgia	pain in the pleura
pleurisy	inflammation of the pleura; another word for pleuritis

quick reference glossary of terms *continued*

Term	Definition
pleuritis	inflammation of the pleura
pleuropexy	reattachment of the pleura
pneumatocele	hernia of the lung
pneumoconiosis	a lung condition caused by dust
pneumohemothorax	air and blood in the chest
pneumonectomy	removal of a lung
pneumonia	a lung condition
pneumonitis	inflammation of the lung
pneumothorax	air in the chest
polysomnography	recording multiple aspects of sleep
pulmonary angiography	a procedure for recording pulmonary blood vessel activity
pulmonary edema	swelling in the lungs
pulmonary embolism	blockage in the pulmonary blood supply
pulmonary function testing	a group of tests used to evaluate the condition of the lungs
pulmonary neoplasm	new growth (tumor) in the lung
pyothorax	pus in the chest
restrictive lung disorder	a lung disorder caused by the limiting of air into the lungs
retraction	the sucking in of the skin around bones during inhalation, happens when someone is in respiratory distress
rhinitis	inflammation of the nasal passages
rhinorrhagia	excessive blood flow from the nose (another term for nosebleed)
rhinorrhea	runny nose
septoplasty	reconstruction of a septum
sinusitis	inflammation of the sinus
sleep apnea	a condition where the patient ceases to breathe while asleep
spirometry	a procedure to measure breathing
sputum	mucus discharged from the lungs by coughing
tachypnea	rapid breathing
thoracalgia	chest pain
thoracentesis	puncture of the chest
thoracocentesis	puncture of the chest
thoracoplasty	reconstruction of the chest
thoracoscopy	examination of the chest

quick reference glossary of terms *continued*

Term	Definition
thoracostomy	creation of an opening in the chest
thoracotomy	incision into the chest
tonsillectomy	removal of the tonsils
tonsillitis	inflammation of the tonsils
tracheitis	inflammation of the trachea
tracheomalacia	softening of the trachea
tracheostenosis	narrowing of the trachea
tracheostomy	creation of an opening in the trachea
tracheotomy	incision into the trachea
ventilation–perfusion scan	a scan that tests whether a problem in the lungs is caused by airflow (ventilation) or blood flow (perfusion)

review of terms by roots

Root	Term(s)	
adenoid/o	adenoidectomy	
bronch/o, bronchi/o	bronchiectasis bronchiogenic carcinoma bronchioplasty bronchitis bronchodilator	bronchorrhea bronchoscopy bronchospasm laryngotracheobronchitis
bronchiol/o	bronchiolitis	
capn/o	capnography capnometer	hypercapnia hypocapnia
carb/o	hypercarbia hypocarbia	
laryng/o	laryngectomy laryngitis	laryngoplasty laryngotracheobronchitis
lob/o	lobectomy	
nas/o	nasopharyngoscope	
ox/o	hypoxemia hypoxia	oximetry
palat/o	palatoplasty	
pector/o	expectorant expectoration pectoriloquy	pectus carinatum pectus excavatum

review of terms by roots *continued*

Root	Term(s)	
pharyng/o	nasopharyngoscope	
phren/o	phrenoplegia phrenoptosis	phrenospasm
pleur/o	pleural effusion pleuralgia pleuritis	pleurodynia pleuropexy
-pnea	apnea bradypnea dyspnea eupnea hyperpnea	hypopnea orthopnea sleep apnea tachypnea
pneum/o, pneumat/o, pneumon/o	pneumatocele pneumoconiosis pneumohemothorax pneumonectomy	pneumonia pneumonitis pneumothorax
pulmon/o	cardiopulmonary resuscitation chronic obstructive pulmonary disease pulmonary angiography pulmonary edema	pulmonary embolism pulmonary function testing pulmonary neoplasm
rhin/o	rhinitis rhinorrhagia	rhinorrhea
sept/o	septoplasty	
sin/o, sinus/o	pansinusitis sinusitis	
spir/o	spirometry	
thorac/o	chylothorax hemothorax laryngotracheobronchitis pneumohemothorax pneumothorax pyrothorax thoracalgia	thoracentesis thoracocentesis thoracoplasty thoracoscopy thoracostomy thoracotomy
tonsill/o	tonsillectomy tonsillitis	
trache/o	endotracheal intubation tracheitis tracheomalacia	tracheostenosis tracheostomy tracheotomy

The Gastrointestinal System—Gastroenterology

11

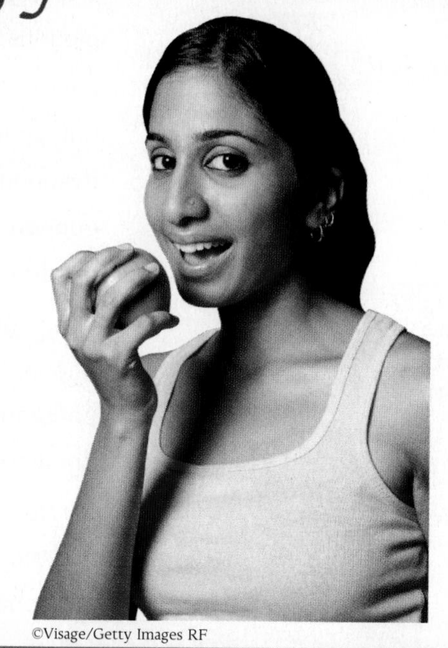
©Visage/Getty Images RF

Introduction and Overview of the Gastrointestinal System

Energy is necessary to make machines work, whether it comes from gasoline, batteries, or electricity. The body is the same way–it constantly needs energy. The gastrointestinal (GI) system is responsible for turning food into energy. As a first step, it digests the food. *Digest* comes from *di* (short for dia), meaning "through," and *gest*, meaning "to carry." *Digestion* is the process of carrying food through the body and breaking it apart into usable and unusable parts. There are three main types of usable food fuel: *protein, fat,* and *carbohydrates.* As food passes through the digestive system, the body breaks down and absorbs the usable parts and discards any unusable parts.

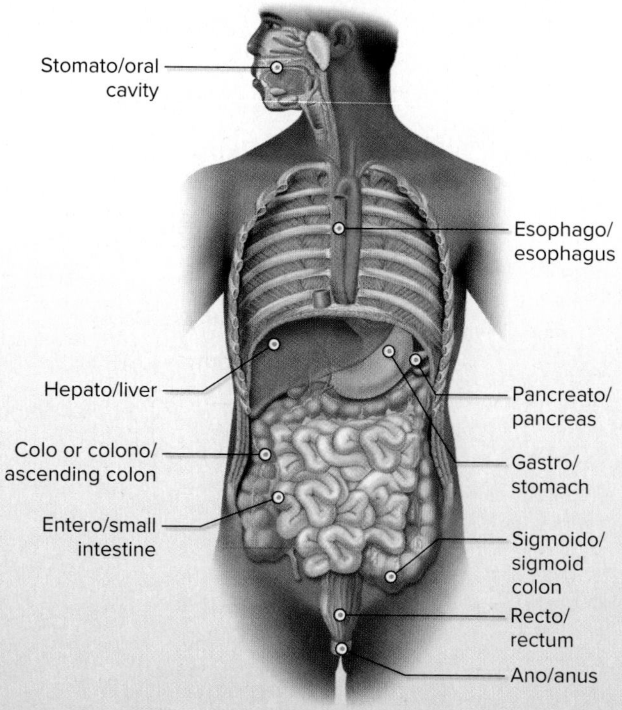

learning outcomes

Upon completion of this chapter, you will be able to:

11.1 Identify the **roots/word parts** associated with the **gastrointestinal system.**

(S) **11.2** Translate the **Subjective** terms associated with the **gastrointestinal system.**

(O) **11.3** Translate the **Objective** terms associated with the **gastrointestinal system.**

(A) **11.4** Translate the **Assessment** terms associated with the **gastrointestinal system.**

(P) **11.5** Translate the **Plan** terms associated with the **gastrointestinal system.**

11.6 Use **abbreviations** associated with the **gastrointestinal system.**

11.7 Distinguish terms associated with the **gastrointestinal system** in the context of **electronic health records.**

The gastrointestinal system is mainly one long tube. Health care providers often talk about the system's two parts: the *upper* and *lower gastrointestinal (GI) tracts*. The upper GI tract includes the mouth, esophagus, and stomach. The lower GI tract is made up of the small and large intestines. In addition to the stomach and intestines, there are other organs that help in dealing with our nutrition. These organs are the liver, pancreas, and gallbladder.

11.1 Word Parts of the Gastrointestinal System

Upper Gastrointestinal Tract

The process of digestion begins in the mouth. When people eat, they start with chewing their food. When chewing, teeth (*dento*) tear food into smaller parts. At the same time, the salivary glands make saliva (*sialo*). The saliva helps to moisten the food to help it pass down the throat. Saliva also has chemicals that help to break the food apart.

mouth

ROOTS: ***or/o, stomat/o***

EXAMPLES: oral, stomatosis

NOTES: Most people tend to chew on the side of the mouth that corresponds to the hand with which they write. Right-handed folks use the right side of their mouth, and left-handed folks—well, you get the idea.

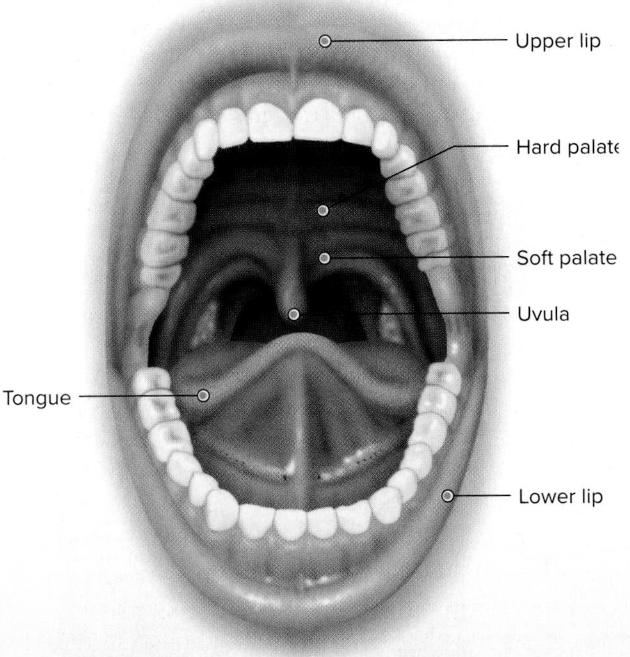

gums

ROOT: ***gingiv/o***

EXAMPLES: gingivitis, gingivostomatitis

NOTES: This root comes from the Latin word for *gums*. Healthy gums are a pinkish-red color, but the color can vary depending on the lightness or darkness of the patient's skin.

tooth

ROOTS: ***dent/o, odont/o***

EXAMPLES: dentist, odontalgia

NOTES: The enamel on the outside of the *tooth* is the hardest thing in the human body. Adult humans have 32 teeth (or they're supposed to, anyway). An opossum has 50 teeth, a mosquito has 47 teeth, and sharks have as many as 40 sets of teeth in their lifetime.

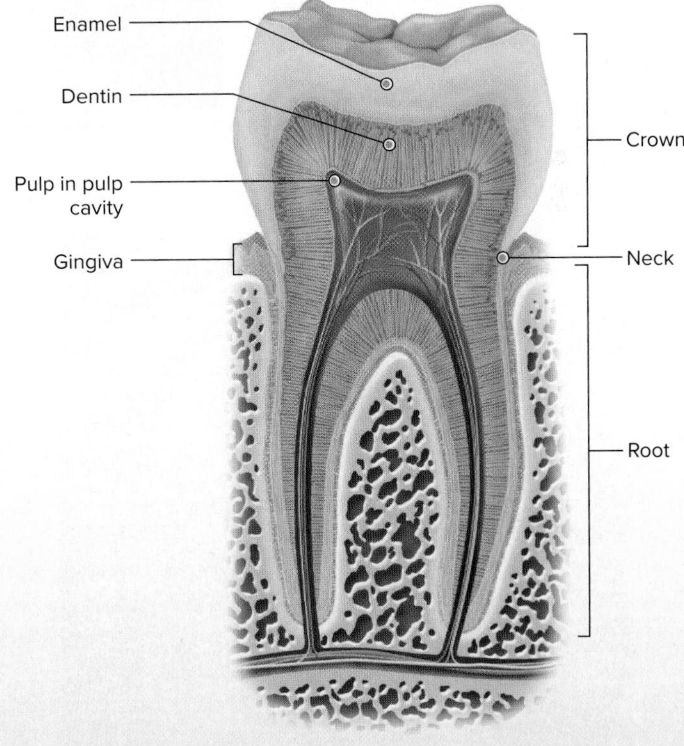

The food is passed from the mouth down a tube (*esophagus*) that leads to the stomach (*gastro*). The esophagus has two gates that keep the food moving the right way. The first gate keeps out air from the stomach and the second gate keeps food from leaving the stomach in the wrong direction.

As we eat, food collects in the stomach. The stomach makes acid, which breaks down protein. The stomach acts almost like a blender. Through muscle contractions, the stomach mixes the food with stomach juices, including acid. This mixing process physically and chemically softens the food into a paste-like substance known as *chyme*. Food then passes through a muscle at the end of the stomach, the *pylorus*, and into the small intestine.

stomach

ROOT: ***gastr/o***

EXAMPLES: gastritis, gastropexy

NOTES: Here are two things you probably don't know about the *stomach:* It must produce a new layer of mucus every 2 weeks or it will digest itself, and when you blush, your stomach changes colors, too.

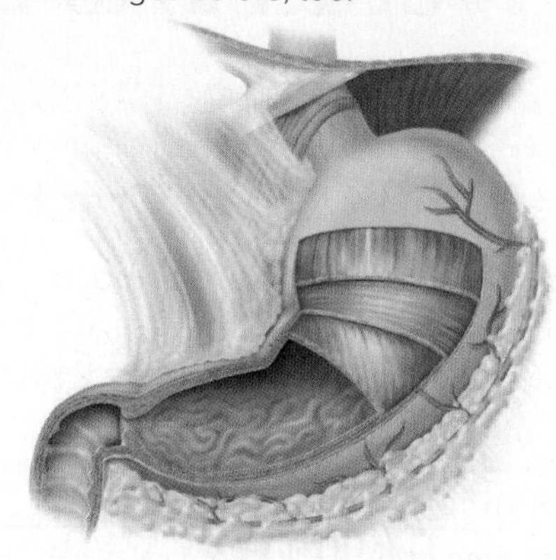

tongue

ROOTS: ***gloss/o, lingu/o***

EXAMPLES: glossopathy, hypoglossal, sublingual

NOTES: The strongest muscle in the human body, relative to its size, is the *tongue*. It is also the only muscle in the human body that is attached at only one end. Here's an interesting fact: Whether or not you can roll your tongue into a tube or other shapes is predetermined by your genetics.

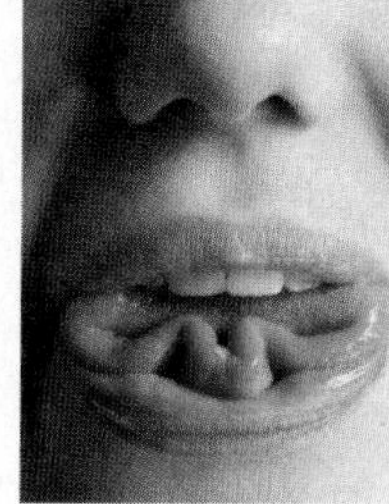

©Christopher Robbins/Getty Images RF

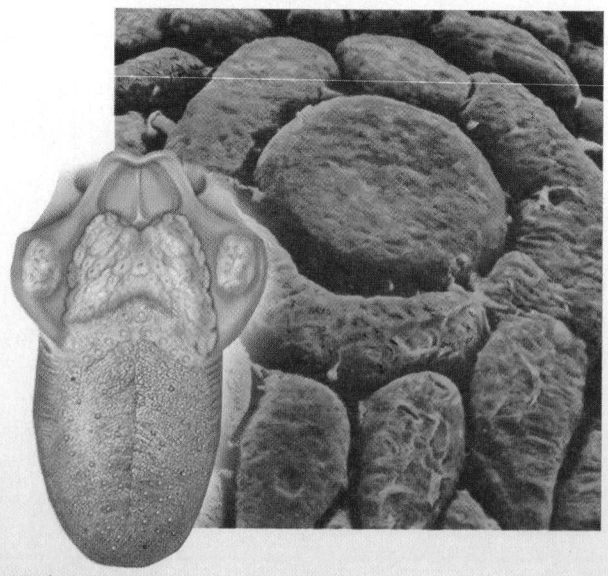

©Omikron/Science Source

esophagus

ROOT: ***esophag/o***

EXAMPLES: esophageal, esophagitis

NOTES: The *esophagus* is a tube that is about the diameter of a quarter; it connects your mouth to your stomach. The name breaks down into *eso* (carry) and *phagus* (eat) and literally means "the thing that carries what you eat," presumably to the stomach.

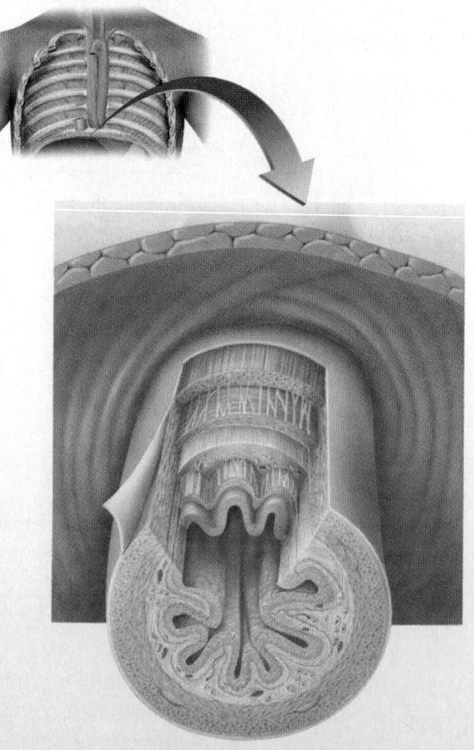

Cross section of the esophagus

Lower Gastrointestinal Tract

The lower GI tract is made up of the small and large intestines. The small intestine is the longest part of the gastrointestinal system. It is made up of three parts: the *duodenum, jejunum*, and *ileum*. Most of the chemical breakdown in the small intestine happens in its first part, the duodenum. In the duodenum, chemicals from the liver (*bile*) and the pancreas mix with the food. The food continues digestion throughout the rest of the long path of the jejunum and ileum.

From here, the food then passes into the large intestine. By this point, most of the nutrients have been absorbed. The main role of the large intestine is to absorb the water from the remaining food. The stool passes through the *ascending, transverse, descending*, and *sigmoid colon* into the *rectum*, where it waits to be excreted.

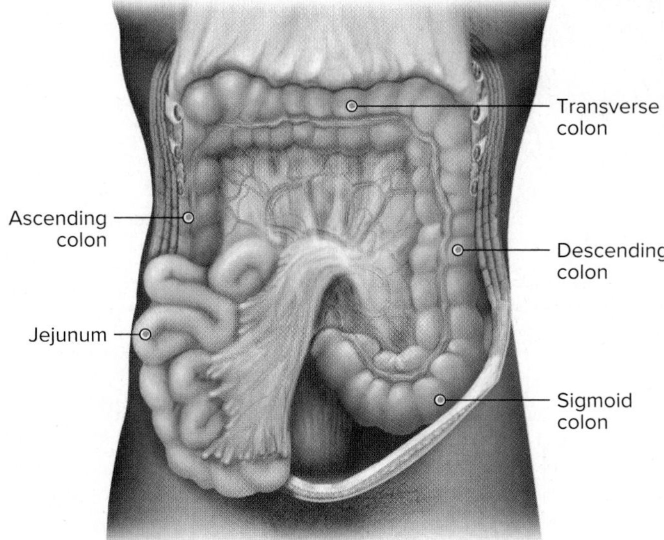

intestines

ROOT: ***enter/o***

EXAMPLES: gastroenterology, dysentery

NOTES: This combining form refers to the intestines in general. It comes from a Greek word meaning "inside." It's appropriate, because your intestines take up a great deal of space inside you. The average adult has over 20 feet of intestines.

duodenum

ROOT: ***duoden/o***

EXAMPLES: gastroduodenoscope, duodenectomy

NOTES: The small intestine is divided into three sections: the *duodenum, jejunum*, and *ileum*. The duodenum is the first of the three sections. Its name means "twelve" and refers to the fact that its length is about the same as the width of 12 fingers.

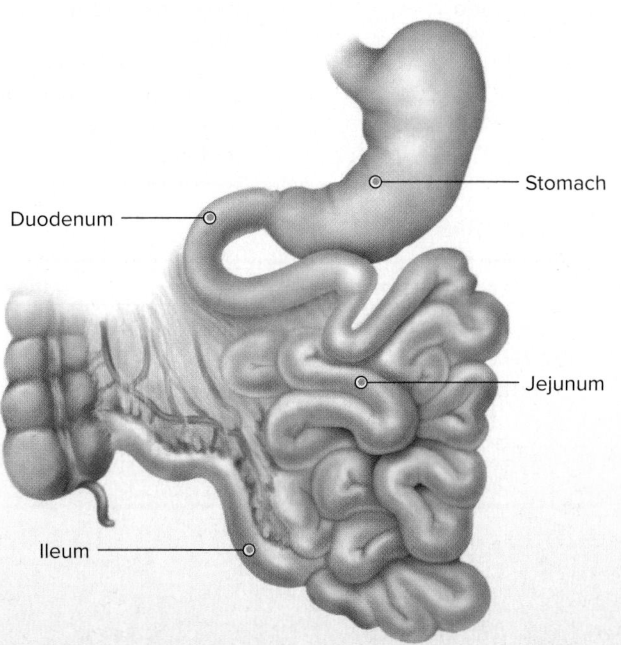

jejunum

ROOT: ***jejun/o***

EXAMPLES: jejunotomy, jejunitis

NOTES: The jejunum is the second of the small intestine's three sections. Its name means "empty" and refers to the fact that it is found empty during dissections.

ileum

ROOT: ***ile/o***

EXAMPLES: ileotomy, ileitis

NOTES: The ileum is the third of the small intestine's three sections. Its name means "groin" and refers to the fact that it is located in the lower abdomen.

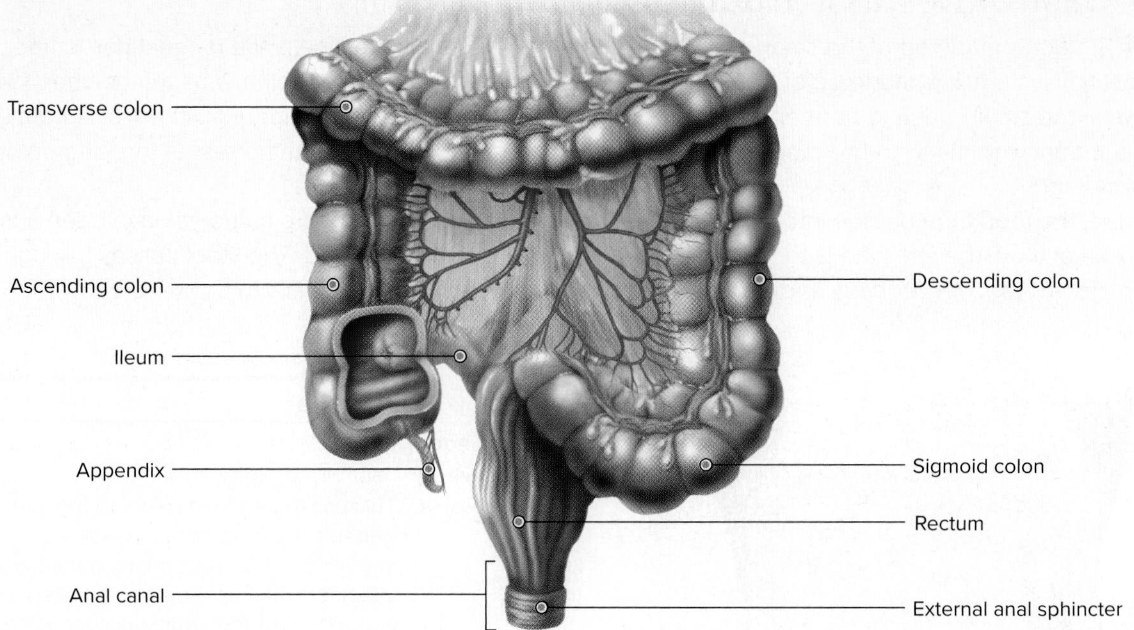

colon (large intestine)

ROOTS: ***col/o, colon/o***

EXAMPLES: colorectal carcinoma, colitis, colonoscopy, colonectomy

NOTES: The colon starts at the bottom of the abdomen (remember, that's where the ileum ends) and is divided into three main sections: the ascending (*going up*) colon, the transverse (*going across*) colon, and the descending (*going down*) colon.

sigmoid colon

ROOT: ***sigmoid/o***

EXAMPLE: sigmoidoscope

NOTES: The sigmoid colon is at the end of the colon, before the rectum begins. Its name is derived from the Greek letter *sigma* (Σ, related to the letter *s*) + *oid* (resembling). It refers to the fact it has an *s*-shaped curve.

rectum

ROOT: ***rect/o***

EXAMPLES: rectoplasty, rectitis

NOTES: *Rectum* is Latin for "straight" and refers to the final portion of the colon before it arrives at the anus. Although it is straight in comparison to the rest of the intestines, the human rectum really isn't straight. It got its name from an ancient doctor named Galen, who dissected animals that really did have straight rectums.

anus

ROOT: ***an/o***

EXAMPLES: anoplasty, anal fistula

NOTES: The *anus* is the sphincter or muscle at the end of the intestines that allows for the passage of feces. Its name comes from the Latin word for "ring."

anus and rectum

ROOT: ***proct/o***

EXAMPLES: proctology, proctitis

NOTES: The root *ano* refers specifically to the anus and the root *recto* refers specifically to the rectum, but *procto* refers to both the anus and rectum.

Supporting Structures/Digestive Organs

The gastrointestinal system also includes other organs that help to break down food, including the liver and pancreas. The *liver* is the largest gland in the body. It has many roles in nutrition. It helps get rid of dangerous toxins, plays a role in energy storage, and makes a substance used to break down fat in the GI tract, called *bile*.

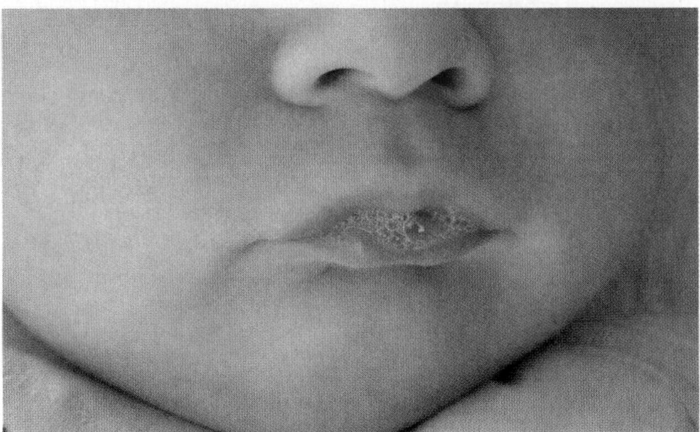

Bile is sent to two places: the small intestine and a storage gland called the *gallbladder*. Bile enters the small intestine by the common bile duct. Bile breaks big pieces of fat into smaller pieces of fat.

The *pancreas* is an important organ in the endocrine system. It also is part of the gastrointestinal system. The pancreas makes chemicals known as enzymes that break apart proteins, fats, and carbohydrates.

saliva

ROOT: ***sial/o***
EXAMPLE: sialoadenitis
NOTES: The average human produces between 1 and 3 pints of saliva a day. In addition to beginning the process of digestion, saliva is necessary to taste food. You cannot taste food until it is mixed with saliva.

bile (gall)

ROOTS: ***bil/i, chol/e***
EXAMPLES: biligenesis, cholelith
NOTES: *Bile*, which is sometimes called *gall*, is a substance produced in the liver that is required for the body to digest food.

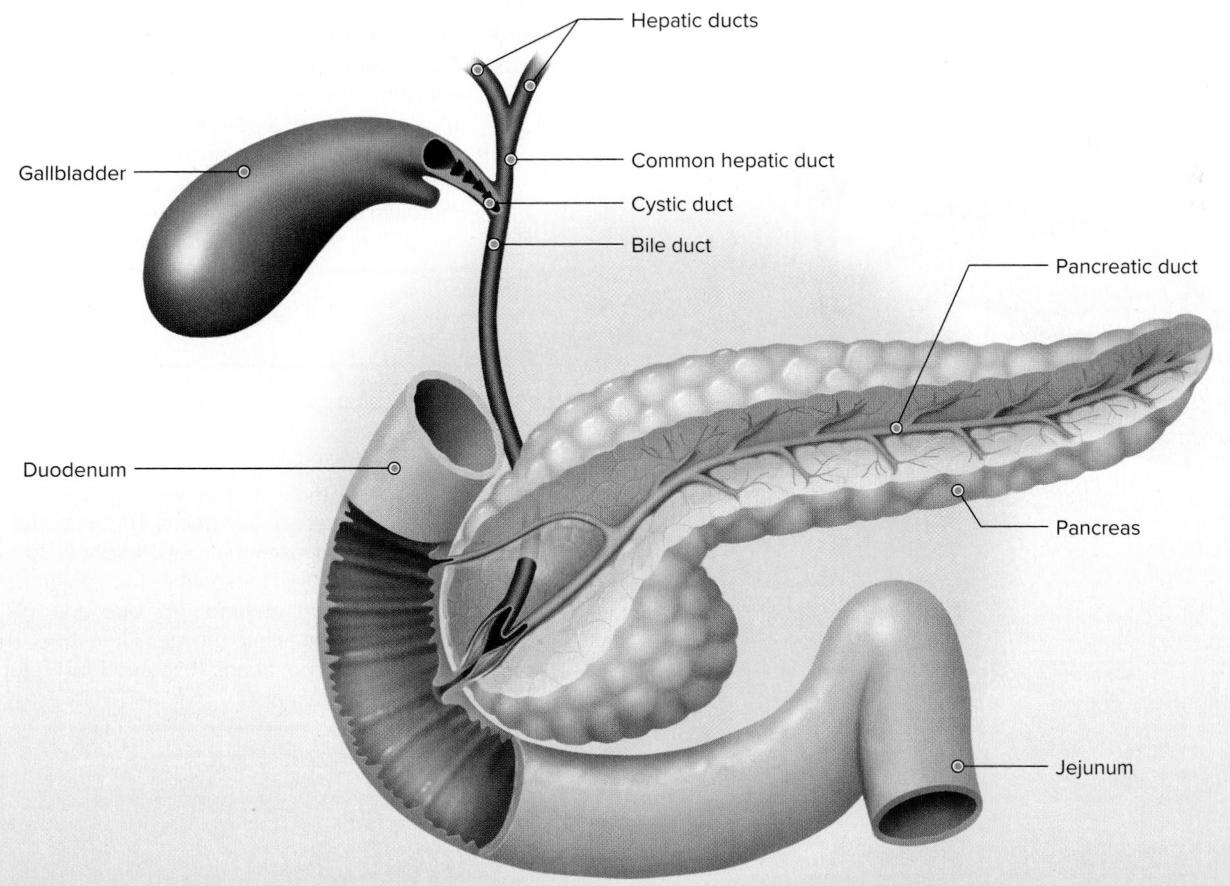

The gastrointestinal organs are located in the part of the body known as the *abdomen* and are surrounded by a membrane that keeps everything in place. This membrane is called the *peritoneum*. It has more specific nerve fibers than the organs it surrounds. If infection or inflammation spreads to the peritoneum, the pain is usually more specific in its nature. This is very helpful when examining a patient with gastrointestinal pain.

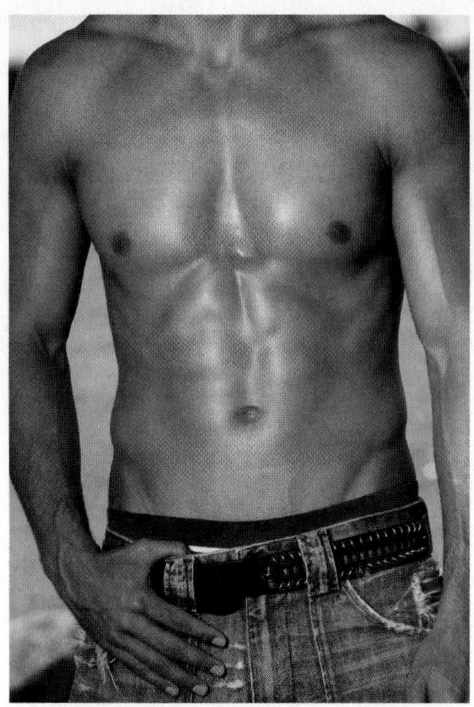

©Hola Images/Getty Images RF

abdomen

ROOTS: ***abdomin/o, celi/o, lapar/o***

EXAMPLES: abdominocentesis, celiopathy, laparoscope

NOTES: Laparoscopic surgery is a way to perform surgery on the *abdomen* without making lengthy incisions. In fact, it is so minimally invasive that it is sometimes referred to as *Band-Aid* or *keyhole* surgery because the incisions are so small. One unique aspect of this procedure, though, is that in order to have enough room to work, surgeons must fill the abdomen with air, or blow it up like a balloon.

bladder

ROOT: ***cyst/o***

EXAMPLES: cholecystogram, cholecystectomy

NOTES: Once bile is produced in the liver, some of it is stored in the *gallbladder*, a small organ about the size of a pear that's located under the liver. While it is being stored, the bile becomes more concentrated in order to increase its potency. It is stored until the body needs it to help digest fatty foods.

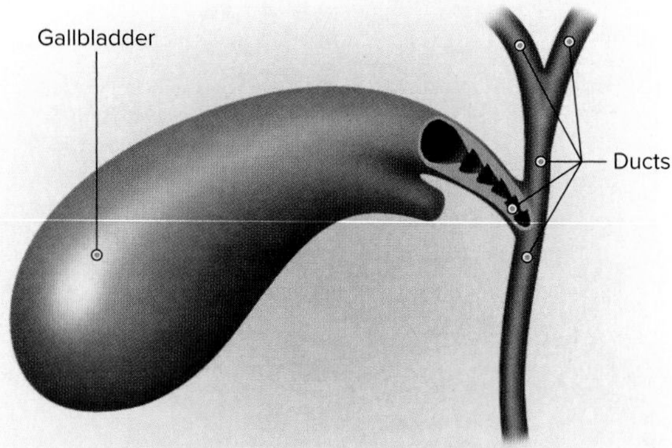

duct

ROOT: ***doch/o***

EXAMPLE: choledocholithiasis

NOTES: Okay, this is tricky. Bile leaves the liver through numerous bile *ducts*. The name for these, though, uses the root *cholangio*, for *bile vessels*. All of these little ducts eventually unite to form the *common bile duct*, a single tube that empties into the small intestine. The root *choledocho* means "bile duct" but refers to only this main duct.

liver

ROOTS: ***hepat/o, hepatic/o***

EXAMPLES: hepatitis, hepaticotomy

NOTES: The *liver*, which is located on the right side of your abdomen just below your rib cage, is the largest organ in the human body (except the skin); it can filter more than a liter of blood every minute.

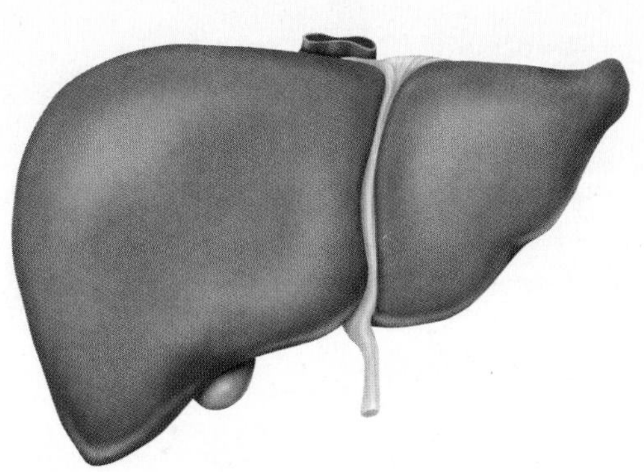

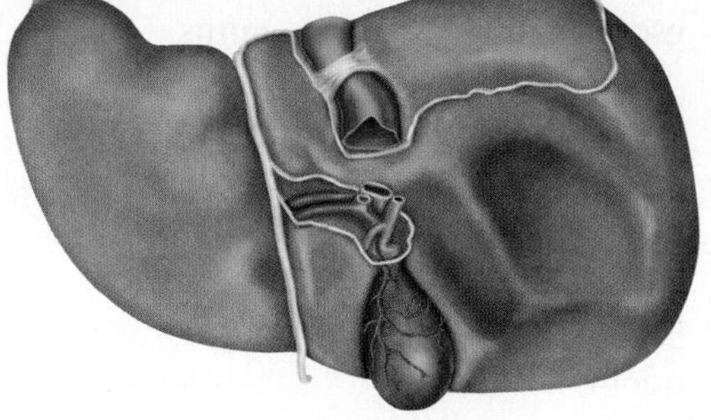

pancreas

ROOT: ***pancreat/o***

EXAMPLES: pancreatitis, pancreatolith

NOTES: The term *pancreas* comes from two Greek words: *pan* (all) and *kreas* (flesh). People debate the reason why, but some think it is because of the organ's fleshy consistency. If you are in a restaurant and are tempted to order *sweetbreads*, be careful. It's a term used by chefs to mean *cooked pancreas*.

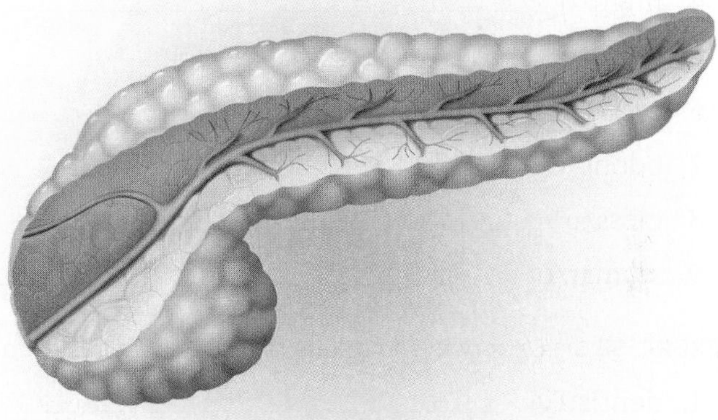

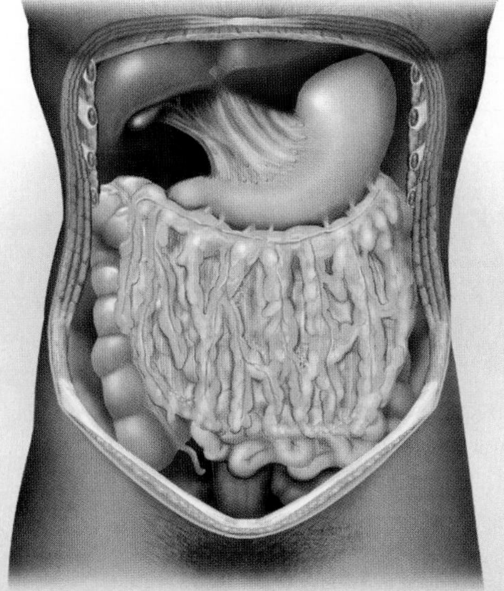

peritoneum

ROOT: ***peritone/o***

EXAMPLE: peritoneotomy

NOTES: The peritoneum is a membrane that lines the abdominal cavity and covers most of the abdominal organs. The name comes from *peri* (around) and *teneo* (stretch) and refers to the fact that it appears to be *stretched around* the abdominal organs.

Learning Outcome 11.1 Exercises

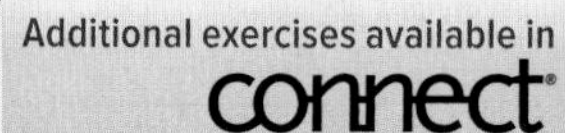

TRANSLATION

EXERCISE 1 *Match the root on the left with its definition on the right. Some definitions will be used more than once.*

______	1. dent/o	a. esophagus
______	2. esophag/o	b. gums
______	3. gingiv/o	c. mouth
______	4. lingu/o	d. stomach
______	5. or/o	e. tongue
______	6. gastr/o	f. tooth
______	7. odont/o	
______	8. gloss/o	
______	9. stomat/o	

EXERCISE 2 *Translate the following roots.*

1. dent/o ______________________________
2. esophag/o ______________________________
3. gingiv/o ______________________________
4. lingu/o ______________________________
5. or/o ______________________________
6. gastr/o ______________________________
7. odont/o ______________________________
8. gloss/o ______________________________
9. stomat/o ______________________________

EXERCISE 3 *Underline and define the roots from this chapter in the following terms.*

1. dentistry ______________________________
2. orthodontics ______________________________
3. esophageal carcinoma ______________________________
4. gingival hyperplasia ______________________________
5. nasogastric tube ______________________________
6. glossorrhaphy ______________________________
7. stomatomycosis ______________________________
8. stomatogastric (2 roots) ______________________________
9. esophagogastroplasty (2 roots) ______________________________

Learning Outcome 11.1 Exercises

EXERCISE 4 *Break down the following words into their component parts and translate.*

EXAMPLE: sinusitis *sinus | itis* *inflammation of the sinuses*

1. dentalgia ____
2. odontalgia ____
3. stomatoplasty ____
4. esophagalgia ____
5. gastralgia ____
6. gastroplasty ____
7. gingivoplasty ____
8. glossoplasty ____

EXERCISE 5 *Match the root on the left with its definition on the right.*

____	1. proct/o	a. sphincter or muscle at the end of the intestines that allows for the passage of feces; its name comes from the Latin word for "ring"
____	2. enter/o	b. anus and rectum
____	3. an/o	c. end of the colon before it enters the rectum; its name is derived from the Greek letter *sigma* (Σ, related to the letter *s*) + *oid* (resembling), and it refers to the fact it has an *s*-shaped curve
____	4. rect/o	d. first of three sections of the small intestine; the name means "twelve" and refers to the fact that its length is about the same as the width of 12 fingers
____	5. ile/o	e. intestines
____	6. jejun/o	f. Latin for "straight" and refers to the final portion of the colon, before it arrives at the anus
____	7. duoden/o	g. starts at the bottom of the abdomen and is divided into three main sections: the ascending, the transverse, and the descending
____	8. col/o	h. the second of three sections of the small intestine, its name means "empty," a reference to the fact that it is found empty during dissections
____	9. sigmoid/o	i. the third of three sections of the small intestine, its name means "groin," a reference to the fact that it is located in the lower abdomen

EXERCISE 6 *Translate the following roots.*

1. proct/o ____
2. an/o ____
3. rect/o ____
4. colon/o ____
5. enter/o ____
6. col/o ____
7. jejun/o ____
8. duoden/o ____
9. ile/o ____
10. sigmoid/o ____

Learning Outcome 11.1 Exercises

EXERCISE 7 *Underline and define the roots from this chapter in the following terms.*

1. anal fistula ______
2. colovaginal fistula ______
3. colostomy ______
4. jejunostomy ______
5. sigmoidoscopy ______
6. rectopexy ______
7. enterorrhaphy ______
8. proctoptosis ______
9. colorectal carcinoma (2 roots) ______
10. anosigmoidoscopy (2 roots) ______
11. gastroduodenostomy (2 roots) ______
12. gastroenterostomy (2 roots) ______

EXERCISE 8 *Break down the following words into their component parts and translate.*

EXAMPLE: sinusitis *sinus | itis* *inflammation of the sinuses*

1. rectalgia ______
2. anoplasty ______
3. proctology ______
4. colectomy ______
5. duodenectomy ______
6. enterectomy ______
7. ileotomy ______
8. jejunotomy ______
9. sigmoidoscope ______

Learning Outcome 11.1 Exercises

EXERCISE 9 *Match the root on the left with its definition on the right. Some definitions will be used more than once.*

_____ 1. pancreat/o
_____ 2. abdomin/o
_____ 3. lapar/o
_____ 4. sial/o
_____ 5. bil/i
_____ 6. chol/e
_____ 7. hepat/o
_____ 8. cyst/o
_____ 9. choledoch/o
_____ 10. cholangi/o
_____ 11. peritone/o
_____ 12. celi/o

a. membrane that lines the abdominal cavity and covers most of the abdominal organs; the name comes from *peri* (around) and *teneo* (stretch) and refers to the fact that it appears to be *stretched around* the abdominal organs
b. a substance produced in the liver and required for the body to digest food
c. abdomen
d. begins the process of digestion; required to taste food
e. bladder
f. located on the right side of your abdomen just below your rib cage, this, the largest organ in the human body (except the skin), can filter over a liter of blood every minute
g. main bile duct
h. pancreas
i. bile vessels through which bile leaves the liver

EXERCISE 10 *Translate the following roots.*

1. abdomin/o _____
2. pancreat/o _____
3. bil/i _____
4. peritone/o _____
5. celi/o _____
6. chol/e _____
7. hepatic/o _____
8. hepat/o _____
9. lapar/o _____
10. doch/o _____
11. cyst/o _____
12. sial/o _____

EXERCISE 11 *Underline and define the roots from this chapter in the following terms.*

1. abdominocentesis _____
2. biligenesis _____
3. celiomyositis _____
4. cholelithotripsy _____
5. peritoneoscopy _____
6. laparoscopic surgery _____
7. sialolithiasis _____
8. hepatomalacia _____
9. pancreatolithiasis _____
10. cholecystectomy (2 roots) _____

Learning Outcome 11.1 Exercises

11. choledocholithiasis (2 roots) ____________
12. hepaticogastrostomy (2 roots) ____________
13. laparoenterostomy (2 roots) ____________
14. cholangiopancreatography (2 roots) ____________

EXERCISE 12 *Break down the following words into their component parts and translate.*

> EXAMPLE: sinusitis *sinus | itis* *inflammation of the sinuses*

1. cholelith ____________
2. celiotomy ____________
3. cholelithotomy ____________
4. cholecystalgia ____________
5. choledochotomy ____________
6. sialolith ____________
7. abdominoplasty ____________
8. hepaticotomy ____________
9. laparotomy ____________
10. pancreatolith ____________
11. peritonitis ____________
12. sialolithotomy ____________

GENERATION

EXERCISE 13 *Identify the roots for the following definitions.*

1. esophagus ____________
2. gums ____________
3. stomach ____________
4. tooth (2 roots) ____________
5. tongue (2 roots) ____________
6. mouth (2 roots) ____________

EXERCISE 14 *Build a medical term from the information provided.*

> EXAMPLE: inflammation of the sinuses *sinusitis*

1. inflammation of the mouth (use *stomat/o*) ____________
2. inflammation of the esophagus ____________
3. inflammation of the stomach ____________
4. inflammation of the gums ____________

5. tooth specialist (use *dent/o*) ______
6. straight teeth specialist (use *odont/o*) ______
7. inflammation of the gums and tongue (use *gloss/o*) ______
8. around tooth inflammation (use *odont/o*) ______

EXERCISE 15 *Identify the roots for the following definitions.*

1. anus ______
2. rectum ______
3. anus and rectum ______
4. ileum ______
5. jejunum ______
6. duodenum ______
7. intestines ______
8. colon (2 roots) ______
9. sigmoid colon ______

EXERCISE 16 *Build a medical term from the information provided.*

EXAMPLE: inflammation of the sinuses *sinusitis*

1. inflammation of the colon (use *col/o*) ______
2. inflammation of the duodenum ______
3. inflammation of the ileum ______
4. inflammation of the jejunum ______
5. inflammation of the rectum ______
6. surgical reconstruction of the anus ______
7. instrument to look into the sigmoid colon ______
8. inflammation of the anus and rectum (use *proct/o*) ______
9. inflammation of the ileum and colon (use *col/o*) ______
10. inflammation of the jejunum and ileum ______
11. inflammation of the stomach, intestines, and colon (use *col/o*) ______

EXERCISE 17 *Identify the roots for the following definitions.*

1. peritoneum ______
2. pancreas ______
3. bladder ______
4. duct ______
5. saliva ______
6. liver (2 roots) ______
7. bile (2 roots) ______
8. abdomen (3 roots) ______

Learning Outcome 11.1 Exercises

EXERCISE 18 *Build a medical term from the information provided.*

EXAMPLE: inflammation of the sinuses *sinusitis*

1. inflammation of the liver (use *hepat/o*) ______
2. inflammation of the pancreas ______
3. inflammation of the peritoneum ______
4. inflammation of the bile bladder (use *chol/e*) ______
5. incision into the bile duct (use *chol/e*) ______
6. incision into the abdomen (use *lapar/o*) ______
7. surgical reconstruction of the abdomen (use *abdomin/o*) ______
8. disease of the abdomen (use *celi/o*) ______

EXERCISE 19 *Multiple-choice questions. Select the correct answer(s).*

1. Select all of the roots below that pertain to the supporting structures/digestive organs.
   a. abdomin/o
   b. chol/e
   c. colon/o
   d. enter/o
   e. esophag/o
   f. gastr/o
   g. gingiv/o
   h. hepatic/o
   i. pancreat/o
   j. proct/o
   k. sial/o
   l. stomat/o

2. Select all of the roots below that pertain to the lower GI tract.
   a. abdomin/o
   b. chol/e
   c. colon/o
   d. enter/o
   e. esophag/o
   f. gastr/o
   g. gingiv/o
   h. hepatic/o
   i. pancreat/o
   j. proct/o
   k. sial/o
   l. stomat/o

3. Select all of the roots below that pertain to the upper GI tract.
   a. abdomin/o
   b. chol/e
   c. colon/o
   d. enter/o
   e. esophag/o
   f. gastr/o
   g. gingiv/o
   h. hepatic/o
   i. pancreat/o
   j. proct/o
   k. sial/o
   l. stomat/o

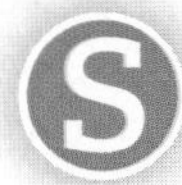

Subjective

Patient History, Problems, Complaints

Upper gastro tract

Lower gastro tract

Supporting organs

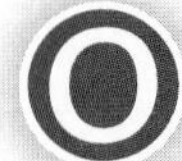

Objective

Observation and Discovery

Upper gastro tract

Lower gastro tract

Supporting organs

Diagnostic procedures

Professional terms

Anatomical regions

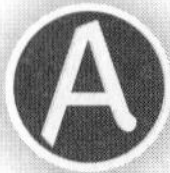

Assessment

Diagnosis and Pathology

Upper gastro tract

Lower gastro tract

Supporting organs

Plan

Treatments and Therapies

Drugs

Upper gastro tract

Lower gastro tract

Supporting organs

This section contains medical terms built from the roots presented in the previous section. The purpose of this section is to expose you to words used in gastroenterology that are built from the word roots presented earlier. The focus of this book is to teach you the process of learning roots and translating them in context. Each term is presented with the correct pronunciation, followed by a word analysis that breaks down the word into its component parts, a definition that provides a literal translation of the word, as well as supplemental information if the literal translation deviates from its medical use.

The terms are organized using a health care professional's SOAP note (first introduced in Chapter 2) as a model.

SUBJECTIVE

11.2 Patient History, Problems, Complaints

Gastrointestinal complaints are a very common reason for patient visits to a health care provider. Problems of the upper gastrointestinal tract differ a bit from problems of the lower gastrointestinal tract. Pain in the upper GI tract is much more common than in the lower GI tract.

A patient may have pain in his or her mouth (*stomatodynia*). This is common with inflammation of the mouth (*stomatitis*), which may include ulcers. Esophageal pain (*esophalgia*) is very common in patients who have acid reflux disease, where stomach acid comes up the wrong way from the stomach. Stomach pain (*gastralgia*) can be from a hole in the lining of the stomach or from inflammation.

The other common type of upper GI complaint is change in function. A patient may have discomfort with eating (*dyspepsia*); this may either be pain or general

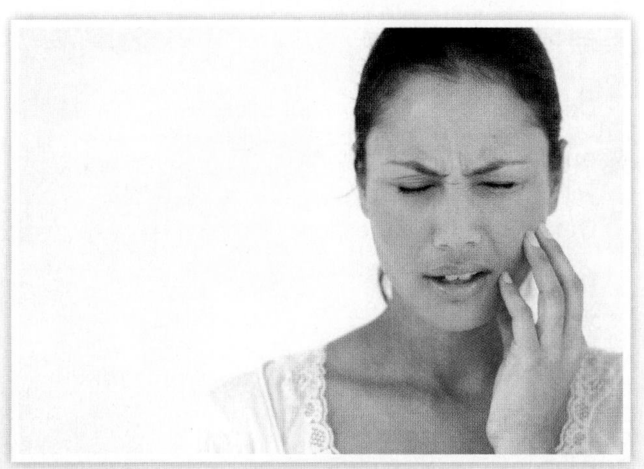

It might not seem like it, but dentalgia, or tooth pain, can be a sign of a gastroenterology problem as well as a dentistry problem.

©Stockbyte/Punchstock RF

11.2 Patient History, Problems, Complaints

nausea. If nausea becomes severe, the body may vomit (*emesis*) the stomach's contents.

Symptoms of the lower GI tract generally relate to problems with how food moves through the tract. If food moves too fast, less of the water in it is absorbed into the body, and stools may become very watery (*diarrhea*). If food moves too slowly, the stool may become hard, causing constipation. If food doesn't move at all, there may be a blockage (*obstruction*). If the obstruction blocks even gas from passing, it's known as *obstipation*.

The supporting organs of the digestive system can cause pain as well. Gallbladder pain (*cholecystalgia*) is among the more common GI complaints in adult patients. It can be caused by blockage, infection, or both. Pancreatic pain is usually very severe and often requires strong pain medicine for relief. While diseases of the liver can also cause pain, they more often first present as yellow discoloration of the eyes and skin (*jaundice*). This is due to an accumulation of *bilirubin*.

upper gastro tract

Term	Word Analysis
aerodontalgia ER-oh-dawn-TAL-jah **Definition** tooth pain caused by exposure to air	**aer / odont / algia** air / tooth / pain
aphagia a-FAY-jah **Definition** inability to eat	**a / phagia** no / eat
dentalgia den-TAL-jah **Definition** tooth pain	**dent / algia** tooth / pain ©Karin Dreyer/Blend Images LLC RF
dyspepsia dis-PEP-see-ah **Definition** bad digestion	**dys / peps / ia** bad / digestion / condition
esophagalgia eh-SAWF-ah-GAL-jah **Definition** pain in the esophagus	**esophag / algia** esophagus / pain
eupepsia yoo-PEP-see-ah **Definition** good digestion	**eu / peps / ia** good / digestion / condition
gastralgia gas-TRAL-jah **Definition** stomach pain	**gastr / algia** stomach / pain
gastrodynia GAS-troh-DIH-nee-ah **Definition** stomach pain	**gastro / dynia** stomach / pain

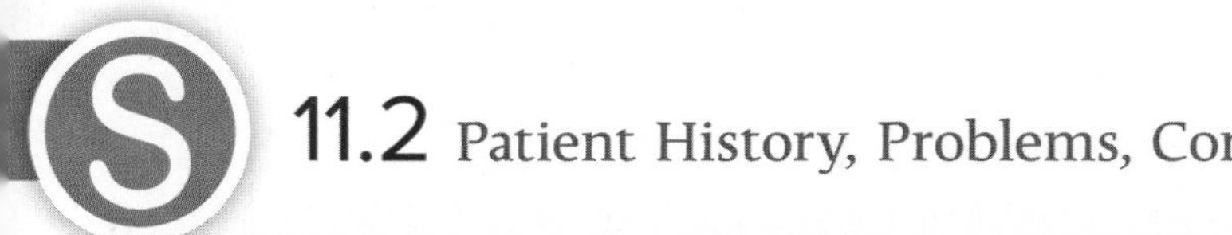

11.2 Patient History, Problems, Complaints

upper gastro tract *continued*

Term	Word Analysis
gingivalgia JIN-jih-VAL-jah **Definition** gum pain	**gingiv / algia** gum / pain
gingivostomatitis JIN-jih-voh-STOH-mah-TAI-tis **Definition** inflammation of the mouth and gums	**gingivo / stomat / itis** gum / mouth / inflammation
hematemesis HEM-at-EM-eh-sis **Definition** vomiting blood	**hemat / emesis** blood / vomiting
hyperemesis HAI-per-EM-eh-sis **Definition** excessive vomiting	**hyper / emesis** over / vomiting
odontalgia OH-dawn-TAL-jah **Definition** tooth pain	**odont / algia** tooth / pain
odontodynia oh-DAWN-toh-DAI-nee-ah **Definition** tooth pain	**odonto / dynia** tooth / pain
stomatitis STOH-mah-TAI-tis **Definition** inflammation of the mouth	**stomat / itis** mouth / inflammation
stomatodynia stoh-MAT-oh-DAI-nee-ah **Definition** mouth pain	**stomato / dynia** mouth / pain

lower gastro tract

Term	Word Analysis
constipation KAWN-stih-PAY-shun **Definition** difficulty passing feces	**from Latin, for "to crowd together"**

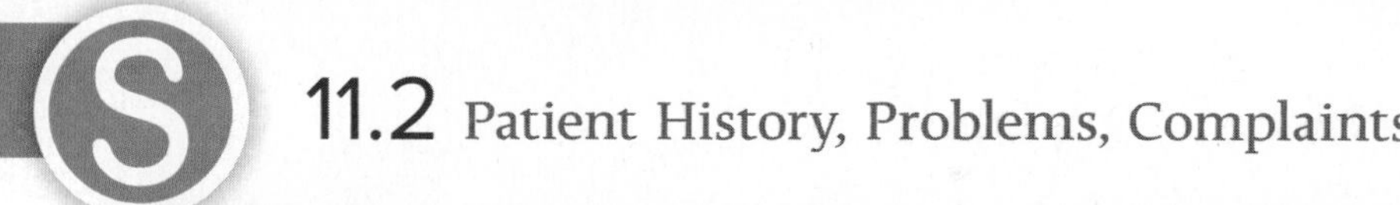

lower gastro tract *continued*

Term	Word Analysis
diarrhea DAI-ah-REE-ah **Definition** passing of fluid or unformed feces	dia / rrhea through / discharge
dysentery DIS-en-TER-ee **Definition** another name for diarrhea	dys / enter / y bad / intestine / condition
enterodynia EN-ter-oh-DIH-nee-ah **Definition** pain in the intestines	entero / dynia intestine / pain
hemorrhoid HEM-oh-ROID **Definition** inflammation of the veins surrounding the anus	from a Greek word referring to veins likely to discharge blood
rectalgia rek-TAL-jah **Definition** rectal pain	rect / algia rectum / pain

supporting organs

Term	Word Analysis
cholecystalgia KOH-lay-sis-TAL-jah **Definition** pain in the gallbladder	chole / cyst / algia bile / bladder / pain
jaundice JAWN-dis **Definition** yellowing of skin, tissue, and fluids caused by increased levels of bilirubin in the blood	from French, meaning "yellow"
icterus IK-ter-us **Definition** another name for jaundice **NOTE:** This word has its origins in the name of a bird with a yellow breast; it was once believed that seeing the bird would cure jaundice.	from Greek, for "jaundice" Source: Centers for Disease Control and Prevention

11.2 Patient History, Problems, Complaints

supporting organs *continued*

Term	Word Analysis
sialorrhea SAI-ah-loh-REE-ah **Definition** excessive salivation	**sialo / rrhea** saliva / excessive discharge

Learning Outcome 11.2 Exercises

PRONUNCIATION

EXERCISE 1 *Indicate which syllable is emphasized when pronounced.*

EXAMPLE: bronchitis bron**chi**tis

1. jaundice ____________
2. hemorrhoid ____________
3. stomatitis ____________
4. diarrhea ____________
5. gastralgia ____________
6. enterodynia ____________
7. sialorrhea ____________
8. gingivalgia ____________
9. hematemesis ____________
10. odontodynia ____________
11. aphagia ____________
12. dentalgia ____________
13. rectalgia ____________
14. dyspepsia ____________

Learning Outcome 11.2 Exercises

TRANSLATION

EXERCISE 2 *Break down the following words into their component parts.*

EXAMPLE: nasopharyngoscope *naso | pharyngo | scope*

1. stomatitis ______
2. gastrodynia ______
3. odontodynia ______
4. enterodynia ______
5. hematemesis ______
6. hyperemesis ______
7. gingivalgia ______
8. dyspepsia ______
9. eupepsia ______
10. aerodontalgia ______
11. cholecystalgia ______
12. gingivostomatitis ______

EXERCISE 3 *Underline and define the roots from this chapter in the following terms.*

1. dentalgia ______
2. odontalgia ______
3. gastralgia ______
4. esophagalgia ______
5. rectalgia ______
6. stomatodynia ______
7. enterodynia ______
8. sialorrhea ______
9. aerodontalgia ______
10. dysentery ______
11. gingivostomatitis (2 roots) ______
12. cholecystalgia (2 roots) ______

Learning Outcome 11.2 Exercises

EXERCISE 4 *Match the term on the left with its definition on the right.*

______	1. constipation	a.	inability to eat
______	2. diarrhea	b.	bad digestion
______	3. hemorrhoid	c.	good digestion
______	4. dyspepsia	d.	difficulty passing feces
______	5. eupepsia	e.	passing of fluid or unformed feces
______	6. jaundice	f.	inflammation of the veins surrounding the anus
______	7. aphagia	g.	yellowing of the skin, tissue, and fluids caused by increased levels of bilirubin in the blood

EXERCISE 5 *Fill in the blanks.*

1. rectalgia = pain in the ______________________________
2. esophagalgia = pain in the ______________________________
3. gastralgia = pain in the ______________________________
4. gingivalgia = pain in the ______________________________
5. dentalgia = pain in the ______________________________
6. odontalgia = pain in the ______________________________

EXERCISE 6 *Translate the following terms as literally as possible.*

EXAMPLE: nasopharyngoscope *an instrument for looking at the nose and throat*

1. odontodynia ______________________________
2. stomatodynia ______________________________
3. enterodynia ______________________________
4. aerodontalgia ______________________________
5. dyspepsia ______________________________
6. eupepsia ______________________________
7. hematemesis ______________________________
8. hyperemesis ______________________________
9. aphagia ______________________________

Learning Outcome 11.2 Exercises

GENERATION

EXERCISE 7 *Build a medical term from the information provided.*

EXAMPLE: inflammation of the sinuses *sinusitis*

1. inflammation of the mouth (use *stomat/o*) ____________
2. inflammation of the mouth and gums (use *stomat/o*) ____________
3. stomach pain (use *-dynia*) ____________
4. bad intestine condition ____________
5. excessive salivation ____________

EXERCISE 8 *Multiple-choice questions. Select the correct answer(s).*

1. Select all of the terms below that pertain to the lower GI tract.
   a. constipation
   b. dentalgia
   c. diarrhea
   d. hematemesis
   e. hemorrhoid
   f. rectalgia
   g. stomatitis
2. Select all of the terms below that pertain to the upper GI tract.
   a. constipation
   b. dentalgia
   c. diarrhea
   d. hematemesis
   e. hemorrhoid
   f. rectalgia
   g. stomatitis
3. Which of the terms below literally means "through excessive discharge" and is the passing of fluid or unformed feces?
   a. constipation
   b. diarrhea
   c. dysentery
   d. hemorrhoid
   e. icterus
4. Which of the terms below is generally considered the OPPOSITE of *diarrhea*?
   a. constipation
   b. diarrhea
   c. dysentery
   d. hemorrhoid
   e. icterus
5. Which of the definitions below is the correct definition of the term *hemorrhoid*?
   a. inflammation of the skin surrounding the anus
   b. inflammation of the skin surrounding the rectum
   c. inflammation of the veins surrounding the anus
   d. inflammation of the veins surrounding the rectum
   e. none of these
6. Which of the terms below means "pain in the gallbladder"?
   a. bilemesis
   b. bilidynia
   c. cholecystalgia
   d. choledynia
   e. hematemesis

OBJECTIVE

11.3 Observation and Discovery

The first component to examining a patient with gastrointestinal complaints is visual inspection. Color changes, like jaundice, can indicate problems with the GI system. Another visual finding could be a very large, fluid-filled abdomen (*ascites*). This is usually associated with serious liver problems.

After visually inspecting the patient, the next step is to touch, or *palpate*, the abdomen. During abdominal palpation, an examiner may notice masses, pain, or tensing of the abdominal muscles in response to pain, which is known as *guarding*.

It is important to know where a patient has tenderness during the exam. The abdomen is divided into different regions to help distinguish the types of problems a patient may have. One specific goal of palpation is locating the liver's edge. An enlarged liver (*hepatomegaly*) can be a sign of disease.

Many laboratory tests for the digestive system involve examining the waste product of the digestion—that is, the stool. Some tests look for nutrients that have not been broken down or absorbed correctly. For example, fat in the stool (*steatorrhea*) indicates disease. Other tests look for blood (*fecal occult blood test*) or pus in the stool, and still others look for bacteria (*stool culture*) in the stool.

A few blood tests specifically relate to the GI system. These tests involve the chemicals that organs make to break down food (*enzymes*) and include liver enzymes and pancreatic enzymes.

As with all parts of the body, images can be very helpful in diagnosing disease. X-rays, CT scans, and ultrasounds are all very common ways of assessing the abdomen and GI structures. Because the GI system is one long tube, visual inspection with a camera is also possible (*endoscopy*). Common examples include camera inspection of the entire colon (*colonoscopy*) or just the end part (*sigmoidoscopy*), as well as inspection of the esophagus, stomach, and duodenum (*esophagogastroduodenoscopy*). There are also more specialized tests that examine vessels and ducts. One common example studies the release of bile from the gallbladder (*cholangiogram*).

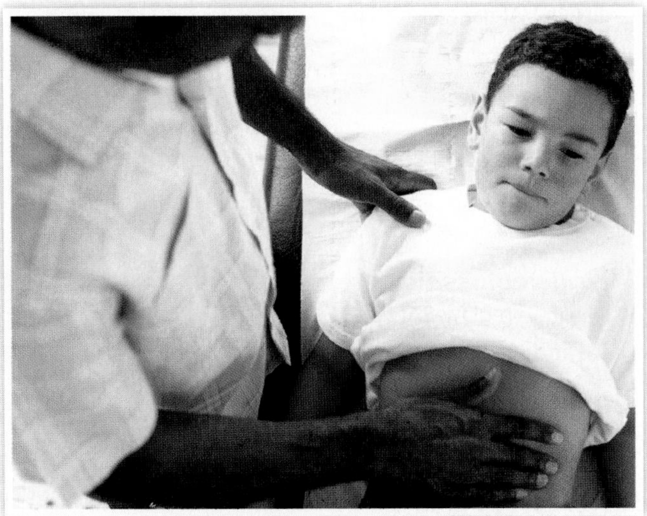

A doctor pressing on a patient's abdomen during a physical exam is checking for hepatomegaly.

upper gastro tract

Term	Word Analysis
gastromalacia GAS-troh-mah-LAY-shah **Definition** softening of the stomach	**gastro / malacia** stomach / softening
gastroparesis GAS-troh-par-EE-sis **Definition** partial paralysis of the stomach	**gastro / paresis** stomach / partial paralysis

11.3 Observation and Discovery

upper gastro tract *continued*

Term	Word Analysis
gingivitis JIN-jih-VAI-tis **Definition** inflammation of the gums	**gingiv / itis** gum / inflammation Source: CDC/Minnesota Department of Health, R.N. Barr Library; Librarians Melissa Rethlefsen and Marie Jones
gingivoglossitis JIN-jih-voh-glaw-SAI-tis **Definition** inflammation of the gums and tongue	**gingivo / gloss / itis** gum / tongue / inflammation
glossoplegia GLAW-soh-PLEE-jah **Definition** paralysis of the tongue	**glosso / plegia** tongue / paralysis
odontoclasis OH-dawn-TAWK-lah-sis **Definition** breaking of a tooth	**odonto / clasis** tooth / break
stomatogastric stoh-MAH-toh-GAS-trik **Definition** pertaining to the mouth and stomach	**stomato / gastr / ic** mouth / stomach / pertaining to
stomatosis STOH-mah-TOH-sis **Definition** mouth condition	**stomat / osis** mouth / condition

lower gastro tract

Term	Word Analysis
anophony an-AW-foh-nee **Definition** sound from the anus	**ano / phony** anus / sound
flatus FLAH-tus **Definition** medical term for passing gas	**from Latin, for "to blow"**

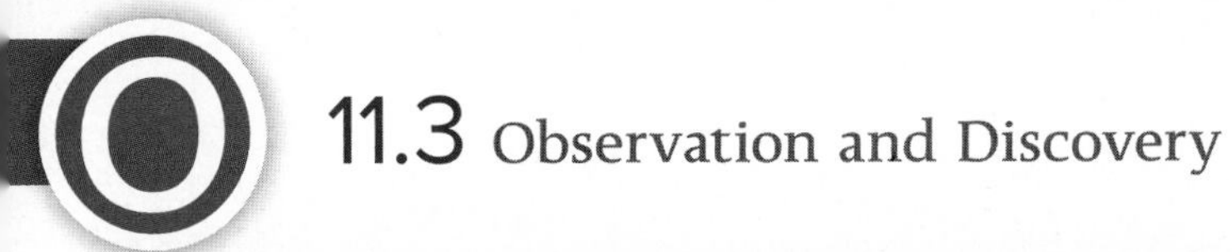

11.3 Observation and Discovery

lower gastro tract *continued*

Term	Word Analysis
hernia HER-nee-ah **Definition** rupture or protrusion of an organ through the wall that normally contains it	**from Latin, for "rupture"**
steatorrhea STAY-at-oh-REE-ah **Definition** excessive fat discharged in the feces	**steato / rrhea** fat / discharge

supporting organs

Term	Word Analysis
ascites ah-SAI-teez **Definition** retention of fluid in the peritoneum **NOTE:** The name comes from the patient's resemblance to an *askos*.	**from the Greek word *askos*, referring to a bag made from the skin of a goat that was used to hold wine**
biligenesis bih-lih-JIN-eh-sis **Definition** formation of bile	**bili / genesis** bile / creation
cholelith KOH-lay-lith **Definition** gallstone; literally "a stone in the bile"	**chole / lith** bile / stone
hepatomalacia heh-PAT-oh-mah-LAY-shah **Definition** softening of the liver	**hepato / malacia** liver / softening
hepatomegaly heh-PAT-oh-MEG-ah-lee **Definition** enlargement of the liver	**hepato / megaly** liver / enlargement
hepatoptosis heh-PAT-op-TOH-sis **Definition** downward displacement of the liver	**hepato / ptosis** liver / drooping condition
pancreatolith pan-kree-AT-oh-lith **Definition** stone in the pancreas	**pancreato / lith** pancreas / stone

supporting organs *continued*

Term	Word Analysis
sialoangiectasis SAI-ah-loh-AN-jee-EK-tah-sis **Definition** overexpansion of the salivary vessels	sialo / angi / ectasis saliva / vessel / expansion
sialolith sai-AL-oh-lith **Definition** stone in the saliva	sialo / lith saliva / stone
sialostenosis SAI-ah-loh-steh-NOH-sis **Definition** narrowing of the salivary glands	sialo / sten / osis saliva / narrowing / condition

radiology

Term	Word Analysis
cholangiogram koh-LAN-jee-oh-gram **Definition** record of the bile vessels (ducts)	chol / angio / gram bile / vessel / record
cholangiography koh-LAN-jee-AW-grah-fee **Definition** procedure for mapping the bile vessels (ducts)	chol / angio / graphy bile / vessel / writing procedure
cholangiopancreatography koh-LAN-jee-oh-PAN-kree-ah-TAW-grah-fee **Definition** procedure for mapping the bile vessels (ducts) and pancreas **Note:** This can be performed either by endoscope (ERCP) or by MRI (MRCP).	chol / angio / pancreato / graphy bile / vessel / pancreas / writing procedure
cholecystogram KOH-lay-SIS-toh-gram **Definition** record of the bile (gall) bladder	chole / cysto / gram bile / bladder / record
pancreatography PAN-kree-ah-TAW-graw-FEE **Definition** procedure for mapping the pancreas	pancreato / graphy pancreas / writing procedure

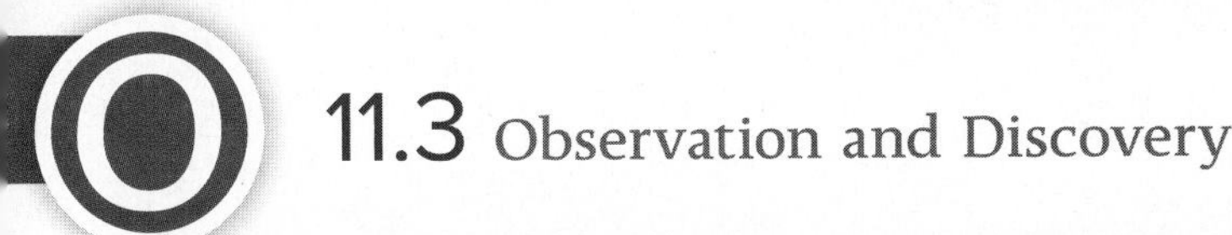

11.3 Observation and Discovery

diagnostic procedures

Term	Word Analysis
anosigmoidoscopy AN-oh-SIG-moid-AW-skoh-pee **Definition** procedure for looking at the anus and sigmoid colon	**ano / sigmoido / scopy** anus / sigmoid / looking procedure
colonoscopy COH-lon-AW-skoh-pee **Definition** procedure for looking at the colon	**colono / scopy** colon / looking procedure
endoscope EN-doh-SKOHP **Definition** instrument used to look inside	**endo / scope** inside / instrument to look
endoscopy en-DAW-skoh-pee **Definition** procedure of looking inside	**endo / scopy** inside / looking procedure
esophagogastroduodenoscopy eh-SAW-fah-goh-GAS-stroh-DOO-aw-den-AW-skoh-pee **Definition** procedure for looking inside the esophagus, stomach, and duodenum	**esophago / gastro / duodeno / scopy** esophagus / stomach / duodenum / looking procedure
esophagoscopy eh-SAW-fah-GAW-skoh-pee **Definition** procedure for looking inside the esophagus	**esophago / scopy** esophagus / looking procedure
fecal occult blood test (FOBT) FEE-kal ah-KULT BLUD TEST **Definition** test of feces to discover blood not visibly apparent	**fec / al occult blood test** feces / pertaining to hidden
gastroscope GAS-troh-SKOHP **Definition** instrument for looking at the stomach	**gastro / scope** stomach / instrument to look
gastroscopy gas-TRAW-skoh-pee **Definition** procedure for looking at the stomach	**gastro / scopy** stomach / looking procedure

diagnostic procedures *continued*

Term	Word Analysis
laparoscope LAP-ar-roh-skohp **Definition** instrument for looking inside the abdomen	**laparo / scope** abdomen / instrument to look 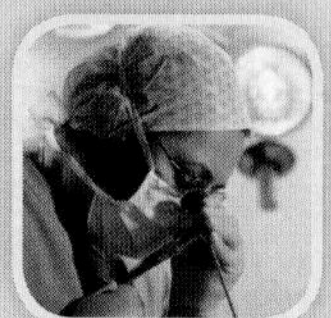 ©Corbis/VCG/Getty Images RF
laparoscopy LAP-ah-RAWS-koh-pee **Definition** procedure for looking inside the abdomen	**laparo / scopy** abdomen / looking procedure
nasogastric tube NAY-soh-GAS-trik TOOB **Definition** tube inserted through the nose into the stomach	**naso / gastr / ic tube** nose / stomach / pertaining to 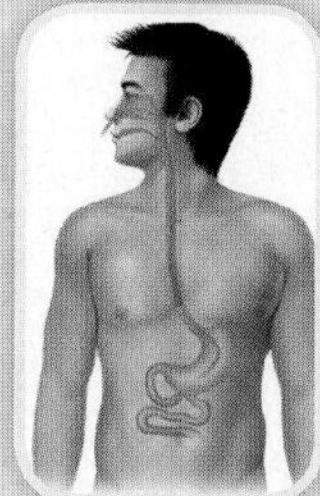
peritoneoscopy PER-ih-TOH-nee-AW-skoh-pee **Definition** procedure for looking at the peritoneum	**peritoneo / scopy** peritoneum / looking procedure
proctoscope PRAWK-toh-skohp **Definition** instrument for looking at the anus and rectum	**procto / scope** anus/rectum / instrument to look
proctoscopy prawk-TAW-skoh-pee **Definition** procedure for looking at the anus and rectum	**procto / scopy** anus/rectum / looking procedure
sigmoidoscope sig-MOY-doh-skohp **Definition** instrument for looking at the sigmoid colon	**sigmoido / scope** sigmoid / looking procedure
sigmoidoscopy sig-moy-DAW-skoh-pee **Definition** procedure for looking at the sigmoid colon	**sigmoido / scopy** sigmoid / looking procedure

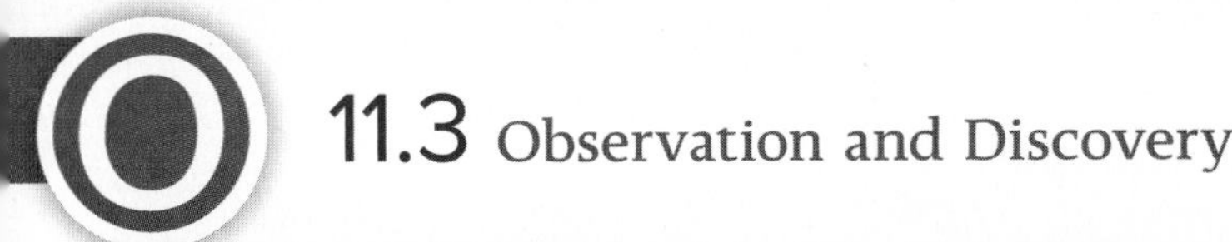

11.3 Observation and Discovery

professional terms

Term	Word Analysis
bariatrics BAR-ee-at-riks **Definition** branch of medicine dealing with weight issues **Note:** In weather forecasts, the atmospheric pressure is called *barometric pressure*.	**bar / iatr / ics** heavy / doctor / pertaining to
dentifrice DEN-ti-fris **Definition** toothpaste **Note:** The suffix *-frice* also gives us the word *friction*.	**denti / frice** tooth / rub ©dumrongsak/123RF RF
dentist DEN-tist **Definition** specialist in teeth	**dent / ist** tooth / specialist
dentistry DEN-tis-tree **Definition** branch of medicine dealing with teeth	**dent / istry** tooth / specialty ©Karin Dreyer/Blend Images LLC RF
gastroenterologist GAS-troh-EN-ter-AW-loh-jist **Definition** specialist in the stomach and intestines	**gastro / entero / logist** stomach / intestines / specialist
gastroenterology GAS-troh-EN-ter-AW-loh-jee **Definition** study of the stomach and intestines	**gastro / entero / logy** stomach / intestines / study
orthodontics or-thoh-DAWN-tiks **Definition** branch of medicine dealing with the straightening of teeth	**ortho / dont / ics** straight / teeth / pertaining to ©Keith Brofsky/Photodisc/Getty Images RF
orthodontist or-thoh-DAWN-tist **Definition** specialist in straightening teeth	**ortho / dont / ist** straight / teeth / specialist
proctologist prok-TAW-loh-jist **Definition** specialist in the anus, rectum, and colon	**procto / logist** anus/rectum / specialist
proctology prok-TAW-loh-jee **Definition** branch of medicine dealing with the anus, rectum, and colon	**procto / logy** anus/rectum / study

11.3 Observation and Discovery

anatomical regions

Term	Word Analysis
epigastric eh-pee-GAS-trik **Definition** upper center portion of the abdomen	epi / gastr / ic upon / stomach / pertaining to
hypochondriac hai-poh-KON-dree-ak **Definition** upper side portions of the abdomen	hypo / chondr / iac beneath / cartilage / pertaining to
hypogastric hai-poh-GAS-trik **Definition** lower center portion of the abdomen	hypo / gastr / ic beneath / stomach / pertaining to
inguinal IN-gwin-al **Definition** lower side portions of the abdomen	inguin / al groin / pertaining to
lumbar LUM-bar **Definition** middle side portions of the abdomen	lumb / ar loin / pertaining to
umbilical um-BIL-ih-kal **Definition** middle center portion of the abdomen	umbilic / al belly button / pertaining to

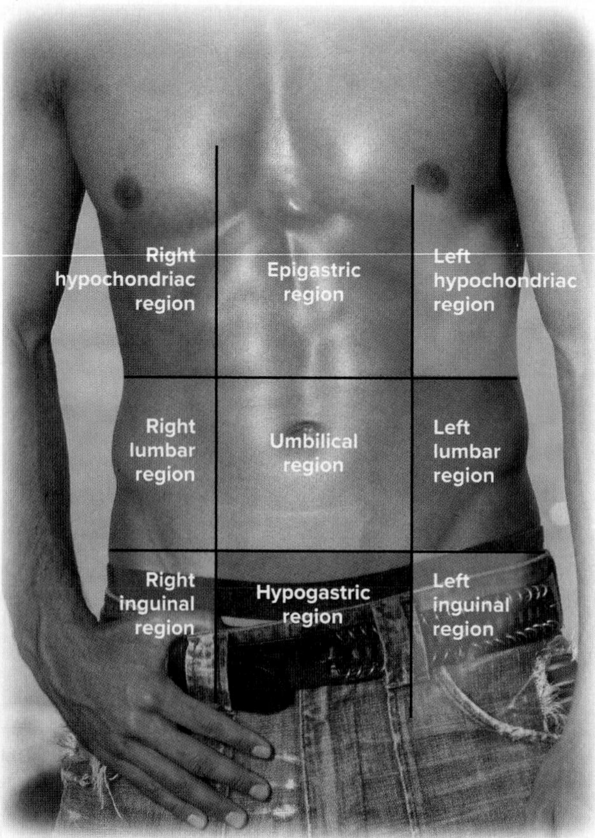

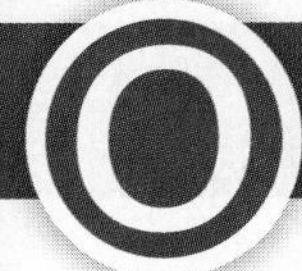

Learning Outcome 11.3 Exercises

PRONUNCIATION

EXERCISE 1 *Indicate which syllable is emphasized when pronounced.*

EXAMPLE: bronchitis bron**chi**tis

1. hepatomegaly ______
2. endoscope ______
3. gastroscope ______
4. stomatosis ______
5. hepatomalacia ______
6. gastroparesis ______
7. glossoplegia ______
8. laparoscopy ______
9. cholangiogram ______
10. sigmoidoscope ______
11. pancreatography ______
12. ascites ______
13. hepatoptosis ______
14. sialostenosis ______
15. cholangiography ______
16. orthodontist ______
17. proctologist ______
18. umbilical ______
19. anophony ______
20. gastroscopy ______
21. proctoscopy ______
22. pancreatolith ______
23. laparoscope ______
24. proctoscope ______
25. bariatrics ______

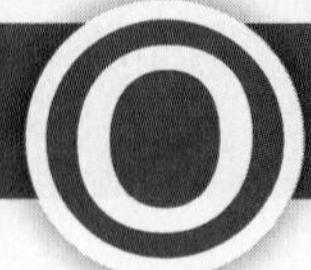

Learning Outcome 11.3 Exercises

TRANSLATION

EXERCISE 2 *Break down the following words into their component parts.*

EXAMPLE: nasopharyngoscope *naso | pharyngo | scope*

1. gastroscope __________
2. laparoscope __________
3. proctoscope __________
4. sigmoidoscope __________
5. endoscope __________
6. endoscopy __________
7. proctology __________
8. dentist __________
9. dentifrice __________
10. gastromalacia __________
11. pancreatolith __________
12. sialostenosis __________
13. hepatomegaly __________
14. anophony __________
15. steatorrhea __________
16. nasogastric tube __________
17. gastroenterology __________
18. orthodontics __________
19. hypochondriac __________
20. cholangiogram __________
21. cholangiography __________
22. hepatoptosis __________
23. sialoangiectasis __________
24. cholangiopancreatography __________

EXERCISE 3 *Underline and define the roots from this chapter in the following terms.*

1. dentistry __________
2. orthodontist __________
3. proctologist __________

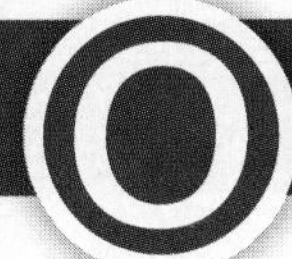

Learning Outcome 11.3 Exercises

4. gingivitis ____________________
5. epigastric ____________________
6. hypogastric ____________________
7. gastroparesis ____________________
8. biligenesis ____________________
9. glossoplegia ____________________
10. odontoclasis ____________________
11. stomatosis ____________________
12. anophony ____________________
13. cholelith ____________________
14. hepatomalacia ____________________
15. sialolith ____________________
16. cholecystogram ____________________
17. pancreatography ____________________
18. colonoscopy ____________________
19. esophagoscopy ____________________
20. gastroscopy ____________________
21. laparoscopy ____________________
22. peritoneoscopy ____________________
23. proctoscopy ____________________
24. sigmoidoscopy ____________________
25. stomatogastric (2 roots) ____________________
26. gastroenterologist (2 roots) ____________________
27. gingivoglossitis (2 roots) ____________________
28. anosigmoidoscopy (2 roots) ____________________
29. esophagogastroduodenoscopy (3 roots) ____________________

EXERCISE 4 *Match the term on the left with its definition on the right.*

______	1. hernia	a.	branch of medicine dealing with weight issues
______	2. fecal occult blood test	b.	lower side portions of the abdomen
______	3. bariatrics	c.	medical term for passing gas; from the Latin word meaning "to blow"
______	4. flatus	d.	middle center portion of the abdomen
______	5. lumbar	e.	middle side portions of the abdomen
______	6. umbilical	f.	retention of fluid in the peritoneum
______	7. inguinal	g.	rupture or protrusion of an organ through the wall that normally contains it
______	8. ascites	h.	test of feces to discover blood not visibly apparent

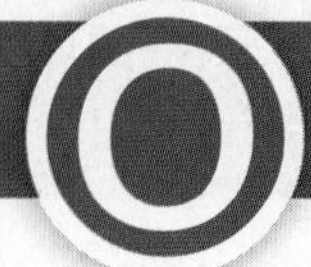

Learning Outcome 11.3 Exercises

EXERCISE 5 *Fill in the blanks.*

1. dentist = specialist in ____________________
2. proctologist = specialist in ____________________
3. orthodontist = specialist in ____________________
4. gastroenterologist = specialist in ____________________
5. colonoscopy = procedure for looking at the ____________________
6. gastroscopy = procedure for looking at the ____________________
7. esophagoscopy = procedure for looking at the ____________________
8. peritoneoscopy = procedure for looking at the ____________________
9. proctoscopy = procedure for looking at the ____________________
10. laparoscopy = procedure for looking at the ____________________
11. sigmoidoscopy = procedure for looking at the ____________________
12. anosigmoidoscopy = procedure for looking at the ____________________
13. esophagogastroduodenoscopy = procedure for looking at the ____________________

EXERCISE 6 *Translate the following terms as literally as possible.*

EXAMPLE: nasopharyngoscope *an instrument for looking at the nose and throat*

1. biligenesis ____________________
2. pancreatography ____________________
3. stomatosis ____________________
4. gastroparesis ____________________
5. glossoplegia ____________________
6. odontoclasis ____________________
7. stomatogastric ____________________
8. anophony ____________________
9. sialostenosis ____________________
10. hepatoptosis ____________________
11. nasogastric tube ____________________
12. dentistry ____________________
13. orthodontics ____________________
14. steatorrhea ____________________
15. sialoangiectasis ____________________
16. cholangiopancreatography ____________________

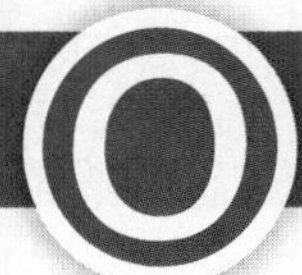

Learning Outcome 11.3 Exercises

GENERATION

EXERCISE 7 *Build a medical term from the information provided.*

EXAMPLE: inflammation of the sinuses *sinusitis*

1. enlargement of the liver ____
2. softening of the liver ____
3. softening of the stomach ____
4. inflammation of the gums ____
5. stone in the pancreas ____
6. stone in the saliva ____
7. gall (bile) stone ____
8. record of the bile (gall) bladder ____
9. instrument for looking at the sigmoid colon ____
10. instrument for looking at the stomach ____
11. instrument for looking inside the abdomen ____
12. instrument for looking at the anus and rectum ____
13. inflammation of the gums and tongue ____
14. study of the stomach and intestines ____
15. study of the anus, rectum, and colon ____

EXERCISE 8 *Multiple-choice questions. Select the correct answer(s).*

1. Which of the terms below is the technical term for *toothpaste*?
   a. bariatric
   b. dentifrice
   c. inguinal
   d. odontoclasis
   e. none of these
2. A person with *ascites* has fluid retention in which part of the GI system?
   a. esophagus
   b. ileum
   c. mouth
   d. peritoneum
   e. sigmoid colon
3. An FOBT tests the feces for what?
   a. allergies
   b. bile
   c. blood
   d. sugar
   e. undigested materials
4. *Bariatrics* is a:
   a. branch of medicine dealing with the anus, rectum, and colon
   b. branch of medicine dealing with digestive disorders
   c. branch of medicine dealing with intestinal issues
   d. branch of medicine dealing with weight issues
   e. none of these
5. Which of the terms below comes from the Latin word meaning "to blow"?
   a. anophony
   b. ascites
   c. dentifrice
   d. flatus
   e. hernia
6. Which of the terms below comes from the Latin word meaning "to rupture"?
   a. anophony
   b. ascites
   c. dentifrice
   d. flatus
   e. hernia

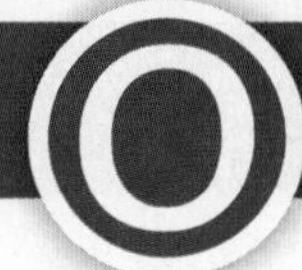

Learning Outcome 11.3 Exercises

EXERCISE 9 *Briefly describe the difference between each pair of terms.*

1. cholangiogram, cholangiography ______
2. endoscope, endoscopy ______
3. gingivitis, gingivoglossitis ______
4. sialoangiectasis, sialostenosis ______
5. gastroparesis, glossoplegia ______
6. epigastric, hypochondriac ______
7. epigastric, hypogastric ______
8. hypochondriac, inguinal ______
9. lumbar, umbilical ______

ASSESSMENT

11.4 Diagnosis and Pathology

GI problems include infection or inflammation, change in function, and problems in the GI tract's structure. Infection of the GI tract is perhaps the most common GI problem seen in the office setting. *Acute gastroenteritis* is infection of the entire tract; it presents with vomiting and/or diarrhea. Most cases are caused by a virus and require no treatment. However, food poisoning can possibly lead to life-threatening illness.

Less-common infections include infection of the liver (*hepatitis*) or pancreas (*pancreatitis*). Infectious hepatitis is generally caused by a virus and presents with pain, jaundice, and/or vomiting. The chief symptom of pancreatitis is intense pain. Inflammation of GI organs can also be caused by inherited disorders like *ulcerative colitis* or acquired due to stress or reaction to a medication, such as stomach inflammation (*gastritis*).

When the GI tract isn't working the way it should, food might travel in the wrong direction. For instance, when food passes from the stomach back up the esophagus (*gastroesophageal reflux*), the result can be a painful burning sensation. While medicine often helps, this problem can become severe enough to require surgery.

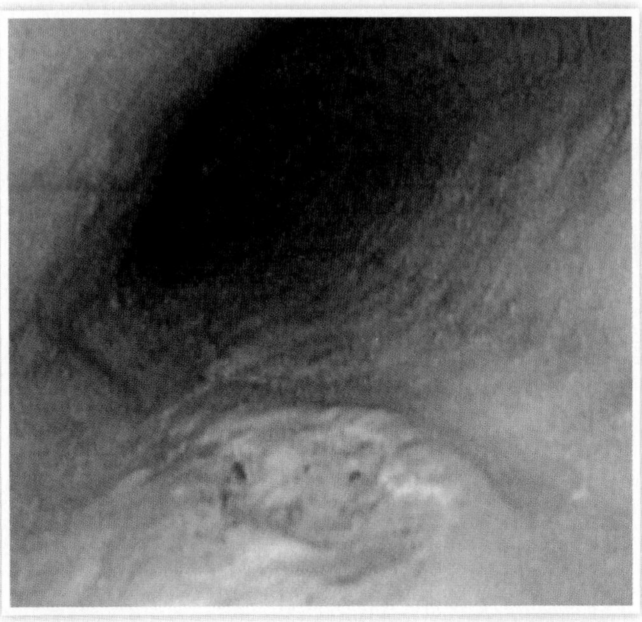

Endoscopes are invaluable tools in diagnosing problems in the digestive tract.

upper gastro tract

Term	Word Analysis
esophagitis eh-SAWF-ah-JAI-tis **Definition** inflammation of the esophagus	**esophag / itis** esophagus / inflammation
gastritis gas-TRAI-tis **Definition** inflammation of the stomach	**gastr / itis** stomach / inflammation
gastroenteritis GAS-troh-EN-ter-AI-tis **Definition** inflammation of the stomach and intestines	**gastro / enter / itis** stomach / intestine / inflammation
gastroenterocolitis GAS-troh-EN-ter-oh-coh-LAI-tis **Definition** inflammation of the stomach, intestine, and colon	**gastro / entero / col / itis** stomach / intestine / colon / inflammation

A 11.4 Diagnosis and Pathology

upper gastro tract *continued*

Term	Word Analysis
gastroesophageal reflux disease (GERD) GAS-troh-eh-SOF-ah-JEE-al REE-fluks dih-ZEEZ **Definition** disease in which acid comes up from the stomach and damages the esophagus	**gastro / esophag / eal re / flux** stomach / esophagus / pertaining to back / flow 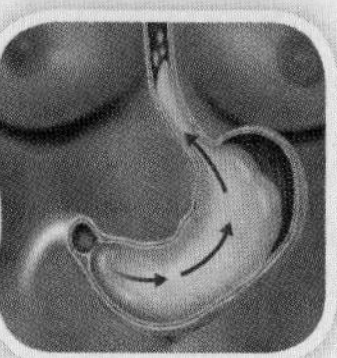
gingival hyperplasia JIN-jih-val HAI-per-PLAY-zhah **Definition** overformation of gum tissue	**gingiv / al hyper / plasia** gum / pertaining to over / formation
glossopathy glaws-AW-pah-thee **Definition** disease of the tongue	**glosso / pathy** tongue / disease
glossotrichia GLAWS-oh-TRIK-ee-ah **Definition** overdevelopment of bumps on the tongue, making the tongue appear to be hairy	**glosso / trich / ia** tongue / hair / condition
periodontitis PER-ee-OH-don-TAI-tis **Definition** inflammation of region around the teeth	**peri / odont / itis** around / tooth / inflammation
pyloric stenosis PAI-lor-ik steh-NOH-sis **Definition** narrowing of the sphincter at the base of the stomach	**pylor / ic sten / osis** gatekeeper / pertaining to narrowing / condition 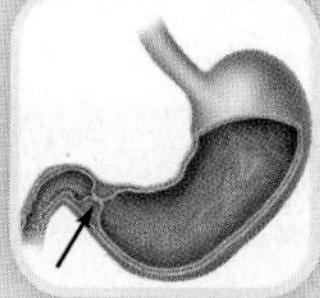
Note: The body has three muscles called *sphincters* that open and close to allow the passage of fluid and solids—the esophageal (between the esophagus and the stomach), the pyloric (between the stomach and the intestines), and the anus. *Pyloric* comes from Greek, for "gatekeeper."	
stomatomycosis stoh-MAT-oh-mai-KOH-sis **Definition** fungus condition of the mouth	**stomato / myc / osis** mouth / fungus / condition
stomatosis STOH-mah-TOH-sis **Definition** mouth condition	**stomat / osis** mouth / condition

A

11.4 Diagnosis and Pathology

lower gastro tract

Term	Word Analysis
colitis coh-LAI-tis **Definition** inflammation of the colon	**col / itis** colon / inflammation
duodenitis doo-AH-den-AI-tis **Definition** inflammation of the duodenum	**duoden / itis** duodenum / inflammation
enterocele EN-ter-oh-seel **Definition** hernia of the intestines	**entero / cele** intestine / tumor 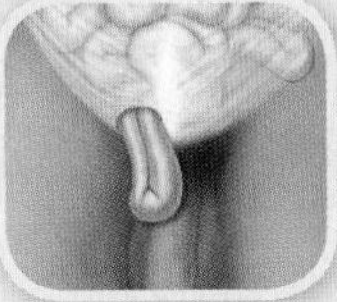
enteropathy EN-ter-AW-pah-thee **Definition** disease of the intestines	**entero / pathy** intestine / disease
fistula FIS-tyoo-la **Definition** any abnormal passageway in the body that shouldn't be there	**from Latin, for "pipe"** 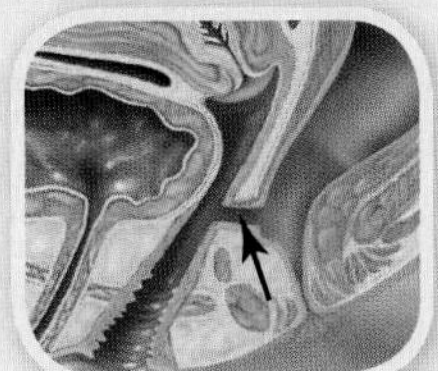
anal fistula AY-nal FIS-tyoo-la **Definition** abnormal opening between the rectum and the exterior perianal skin	**an / al fistula** anus / pertaining to pipe
colovaginal fistula COH-loh-VAJ-in-al FIS-tyoo-la **Definition** abnormal opening between the colon and vagina	**colo / vagin / al fistula** colon / vagina / pertaining to pipe
diverticulitis dai-ver-tik-yoo-LAI-tis **Definition** the inflammation of diverticula in the colon	**diverticul / itis** diverticulum / inflammation 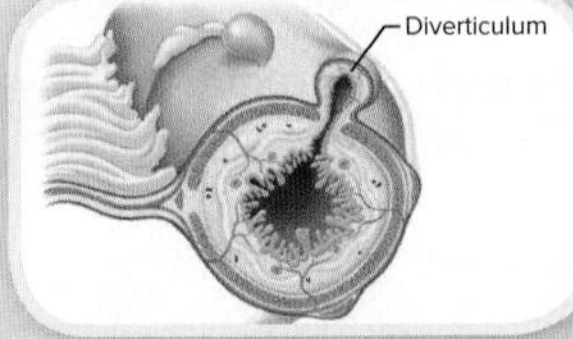
NOTE: *Diverticulum* (plural: *diverticula*) comes from a Latin word that means "little side road" *di* (away) *vert* (turn) *icle* (little). It literally means "a little place to turn aside." It refers to a bulge, hernia, or pouch that forms off of the colon.	
diverticulosis dai-ver-tik-yoo-LOH-sis **Definition** the condition of having diverticula in the colon	**diverticul / osis** diverticulum / inflammation
NOTE: The presence and development of diverticula in the colon is called *diverticulosis*. When those divertulca cause problems, it becomes diverticulitis.	

lower gastro tract *continued*

Term	Word Analysis
celiac disease SEE-lee-ak dih-ZEEZ **Definition** disease of the intestines due to an adverse reaction to gluten **NOTE:** The name refers to the chief symptom experienced by people who suffer from it—intense abdominal pain. In recent years, another term, *gluten-sensitive enteropathy,* has emerged.	celi / ac disease abdomen / pertaining to disease
ileitis IH-lee-AI-tis **Definition** inflammation of the ileum	ile / itis ileum / inflammation
ileocolitis IH-lee-oh-koh-LAI-tis **Definition** inflammation of the ileum and colon	ileocol / itis ileum / inflammation
jejunitis JE-joo-NAI-tis **Definition** inflammation of the jejunum	jejun / itis jejunum / inflammation
jejunoileitis je-JOO-noh-IH-lee-AI-tis **Definition** inflammation of the jejunum and ileum	jejuno / ile / itis jejunum / ileum / inflammation
malabsorption **Definition** incomplete or lack of absorbing nutrients from the intestines	mal / absorption bad / absorption
proctitis prok-TAI-tis **Definition** inflammation of the anus and rectum	proct / itis anus/rectum / inflammation
proctoptosis prok-TOP-toh-sis **Definition** downward displacement of the rectum and anus	procto / ptosis anus/rectum / drooping condition
rectitis rek-TAI-tis **Definition** inflammation of the rectum	rect / itis rectum / inflammation
ulcerative colitis UL-sir-ah-tiv koh-LAI-tis **Definition** inflammation of the colon, characterized by ulcers	ulcer / ative col / itis ulcer / characterized colon / inflammation

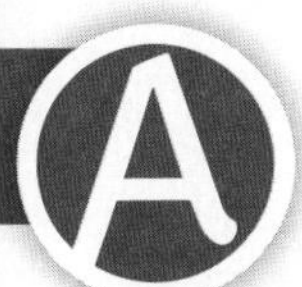

11.4 Diagnosis and Pathology

supporting organs

Term	Word Analysis
celiomyositis SEE-lee-oh-MAI-oh-SAI-tis **Definition** inflammation of the abdominal muscle	**celio / myos / itis** abdomen / muscle / inflammation
celiopathy see-lee-AW-pah-thee **Definition** disease of the abdomen	**celio / pathy** abdomen / disease
cholangitis KOH-lan-JAI-tis **Definition** inflammation of the bile vessels (ducts)	**cholang / itis** bile vessels / inflammation
cholecystitis KOH-lay-sis-TAI-tis **Definition** inflammation of the bile (gall) bladder	**chole / cyst / itis** bile / bladder / inflammation
choledochocele koh-lay-DOH-koh-seel **Definition** hernia of the (common) bile duct	**chole / docho / cele** bile / duct / tumor
choledocholithiasis koh-lay-DOH-koh-lith-AI-ah-sis **Definition** presence of a stone in the (common) bile duct	**chole / docho / lith / iasis** bile / duct / stone / presence
cholelithiasis KOH-lay-lih-THAI-ah-sis **Definition** presence of a gallstone	**chole / lith / iasis** bile / stone / presence
cirrhosis sir-OH-sis **Definition** liver disease named for the change of color in the liver **NOTE:** The standard Greek root for "yellow" is *xantho*. This word uses a much rarer root for yellow.	**from the Greek word *cirrho*, for "yellow"**
hepatitis HEH-pah-TAI-tis **Definition** inflammation of the liver **NOTE:** There are five types of viral hepatitis, named Hepatitis A through E. The most serious are Hep B and Hep C because they can lead to chronic hepatitis and cancer.	**hepat / itis** liver / inflammation 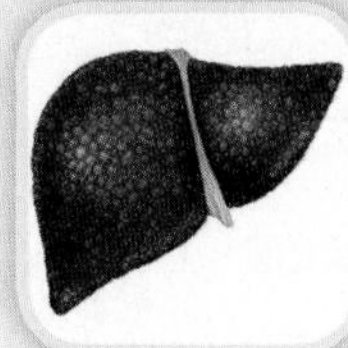

11.4 Diagnosis and Pathology

supporting organs *continued*

Term	Word Analysis
hepatosclerosis heh-PAT-oh-skleh-ROH-sis **Definition** hardening of the liver	**hepato / scler / osis** liver / hardening / condition
laparocele LAP-ar-oh-seel **Definition** abdominal hernia	**laparo / cele** abdomen / tumor ©Biophoto Associates/Science Source/Getty Images RF
pancreatitis PAN-kree-ah-TAI-tis **Definition** inflammation of the pancreas	**pancreat / itis** pancreas / inflammation
pancreatolithiasis PAN-kree-AH-toh-lih-THAI-ah-sis **Definition** presence of a stone in the pancreas	**pancreato / lith / iasis** pancreas / stone / presence
peritonitis PER-ih-toh-NAI-tis **Definition** inflammation of the peritoneum	**periton / itis** peritoneum / inflammation
sclerosing cholangitis skleh-ROH-sing KOH-lan-JAI-tis **Definition** inflammation and hardening of the bile vessels (ducts)	**scleros / ing chol / ang / itis** harden / ing bile / vessel / inflammation
sialoadenitis sai-AL-oh-AD-en-AI-tis **Definition** inflammation of the salivary glands	**sialo / aden / itis** saliva / gland / inflammation
sialoadenosis sai-AL-oh-AD-en-OH-sis **Definition** a condition of the salivary glands	**sialo / aden / osis** saliva / gland / condition
sialolithiasis sai-AL-oh-lih-THAI-ah-sis **Definition** presence of salivary stones	**sialo / lith / iasis** saliva / stone / presence

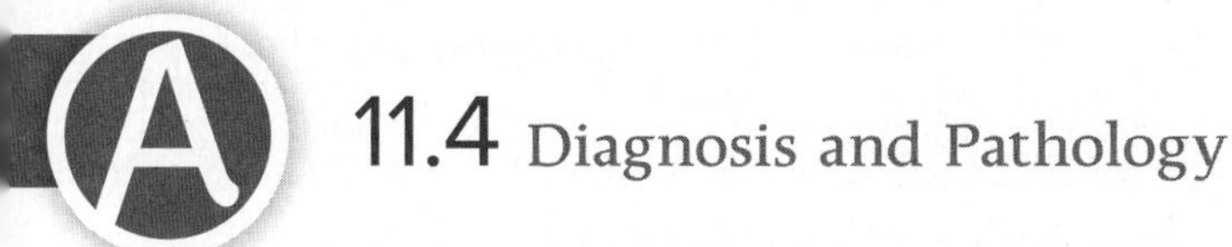

11.4 Diagnosis and Pathology

oncology

Term	Word Analysis
cholangioma koh-lan-jee-OH-mah **Definition** tumor of the bile vessels (ducts)	**chol / angi / oma** bile / vessel / tumor
colorectal carcinoma COH-loh-REK-tal KAR-sih-NOH-mah **Definition** cancerous tumor of the colon or rectum	**colo / rect / al** colon / rectum / pertaining to **carcin / oma** cancer / tumor
esophageal carcinoma eh-SAWF-ah-JEE-al KAR-sih-NOH-mah **Definition** cancerous tumor of the esophagus	**esophag / eal** **carcin / oma** esophagus / pertaining to cancer / tumor
hepatocarcinoma heh-PAT-oh-KAR-sih-NOH-mah **Definition** cancerous tumor of the liver	**hepato / carcin / oma** liver / cancer / tumor
hepatoma HEH-pah-TOH-mah **Definition** tumor of the liver	**hepat / oma** liver / tumor

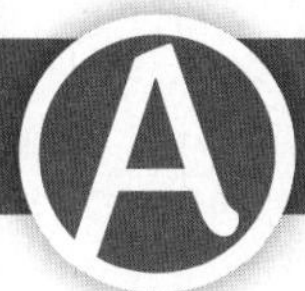

Learning Outcome 11.4 Exercises

PRONUNCIATION

EXERCISE 1 *Indicate which syllable is emphasized when pronounced.*

EXAMPLE: bronchitis bron**chi**tis

1. hepatitis ______
2. enteropathy ______
3. pancreatitis ______
4. gastroenteritis ______
5. ileocolitis ______
6. jejunoileitis ______
7. sialoadenitis ______
8. gastroenterocolitis ______
9. proctoptosis ______
10. cholelithiasis ______

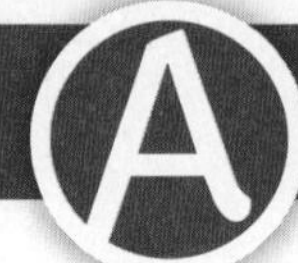

Learning Outcome 11.4 Exercises

11. pancreatolithiasis ______
12. celiopathy ______
13. gastritis ______
14. rectitis ______
15. proctitis ______
16. fistula ______
17. cirrhosis ______
18. diverticulosis ______
19. laparocele ______
20. enterocele ______
21. cholangioma ______
22. diverticulitis ______
23. celiac disease ______
24. ulcertative colitis ______

TRANSLATION

EXERCISE 2 *Break down the following words into their component parts.*

EXAMPLE: nasopharyngoscope *naso | pharyngo | scope*

1. gastritis ______
2. colitis ______
3. esophagitis ______
4. cholangitis ______
5. hepatoma ______
6. enteropathy ______
7. stomatosis ______
8. glossotrichia ______
9. ileocolitis ______
10. jejunoileitis ______
11. celiomyositis ______
12. hepatosclerosis ______
13. proctoptosis ______
14. sialoadenitis ______
15. sialolithiasis ______
16. cholelithiasis ______
17. pancreatolithiasis ______
18. choledocholithiasis ______

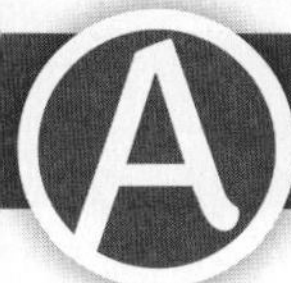

Learning Outcome 11.4 Exercises

EXERCISE 3 *Underline and define the roots from this chapter in the following terms.*

1. pancreatitis ______
2. rectitis ______
3. peritonitis ______
4. ileitis ______
5. jejunitis ______
6. duodenitis ______
7. hepatitis ______
8. proctitis ______
9. cholangitis ______
10. periodontitis ______
11. gingival hyperplasia ______
12. esophageal carcinoma ______
13. hepatocarcinoma ______
14. enterocele ______
15. laparocele ______
16. celiopathy ______
17. glossopathy ______
18. stomatomycosis ______
19. sclerosing cholangitis ______
20. sialoadenosis ______
21. gastroesophageal reflux disease (2 roots) ______
22. gastroenteritis (2 roots) ______
23. colorectal carcinoma (2 roots) ______
24. cholecystitis (2 roots) ______
25. choledochocele (2 roots) ______
26. gastroenterocolitis (3 roots) ______

EXERCISE 4 *Match the term on the left with its definition on the right.*

______	1. cirrhosis	a.	abnormal opening between the colon and vagina
______	2. colovaginal fistula	b.	abnormal opening between the rectum and the exterior perianal skin
______	3. anal fistula	c.	any abnormal passageway in the body that shouldn't be there
______	4. fistula	d.	liver disease named for the change in color in the liver
______	5. pyloric stenosis	e.	narrowing of the sphincter at the base of the stomach

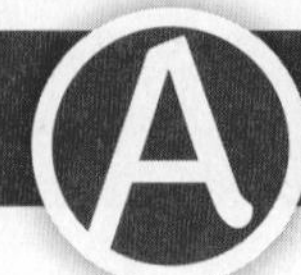

Learning Outcome 11.4 Exercises

EXERCISE 5 *Translate the following terms as literally as possible.*

EXAMPLE: nasopharyngoscope *an instrument for looking at the nose and throat*

1. laparocele __________
2. glossopathy __________
3. stomatosis __________
4. cholangitis __________
5. celiopathy __________
6. hepatosclerosis __________
7. esophageal carcinoma __________
8. colorectal carcinoma __________
9. gingival hyperplasia __________
10. stomatomycosis __________
11. celiomyositis __________
12. proctoptosis __________
13. choledocholithiasis __________
14. sclerosing cholangitis __________

GENERATION

EXERCISE 6 *Build a medical term from the information provided.*

EXAMPLE: inflammation of the sinuses *sinusitis*

1. inflammation of the esophagus __________
2. inflammation of the pancreas __________
3. inflammation of the rectum __________
4. inflammation of the colon __________
5. inflammation of the duodenum __________
6. inflammation of the jejunum __________
7. inflammation of the ileum __________
8. inflammation of the peritoneum __________
9. inflammation of the stomach __________
10. inflammation of the liver __________
11. inflammation of the anus and rectum __________
12. inflammation of the stomach and intestines __________
13. inflammation of the ileum and colon __________

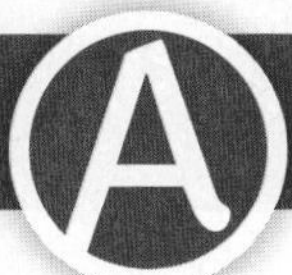

Learning Outcome 11.4 Exercises

14. inflammation of the jejunum and ileum ______
15. inflammation of the region around the teeth ______
16. inflammation of the bile (gall) bladder ______
17. inflammation of the salivary glands ______
18. inflammation of the stomach, intestine, and colon ______

EXERCISE 7 *Multiple-choice questions. Select the correct answer(s).*

1. A person suffering from *cirrhosis* has: (select all that apply)
   a. a liver disease
   b. a purple liver
   c. a yellow liver
   d. liver cancer
   e. liver inflammation
2. The pyloric sphincter is located between the stomach and the intestines. A patient with *pyloric stenosis* has:
   a. hardening of the sphincter at the base of the stomach
   b. narrowing of the sphincter at the base of the stomach
   c. softening of the sphincter at the base of the stomach
   d. widening of the sphincter at the base of the stomach
   e. none of these
3. GERD is:
   a. a disease in which acid comes up from the intestines and damages the esophagus
   b. a disease in which acid comes up from the intestines and damages the stomach
   c. a disease in which acid comes up from the stomach and damages the esophagus
   d. a disease in which acid comes up from the stomach and damages the intestines
   e. none of these
4. A person with *glossotrichia* has:
   a. abnormal hair growth in the mouth
   b. hair growing on the tongue
   c. overdevelopment of bumps on the tongue, making the tongue appear to be hairy
   d. hair from the nose long enough to touch the tongue
   e. none of these
5. An abnormal passageway (one that shouldn't be there) in the body is called a:
   a. carcinoma
   b. cirrhosis
   c. fistula
   d. laparocele
   e. stenosis

EXERCISE 8 *Briefly describe the difference between each pair of terms.*

1. cholelithiasis, pancreatolithiasis ______
2. enterocele, enteropathy ______
3. anal fistula, colovaginal fistula ______
4. cholangioma, choledochocele ______
5. sialoadenosis, sialolithiasis ______
6. hepatocarcinoma, hepatoma ______

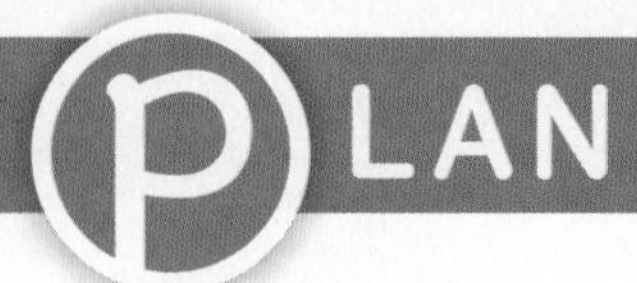

11.5 Treatments and Therapies

Medicines that are utilized to help patients with GI problems generally treat issues with stomach acid and the movement of food through their GI tracts. Patients with gastroesophageal reflux and ulcers may need medicine to decrease levels of stomach acid (*antacids*). Medicines also help with food movement, including medicine to stop vomiting (*antiemetics*) or medicine to help accelerate the movement of food or aid with constipation (*cathartics*).

Nonmedication methods are also commonly used to treat GI problems. Among the most common treatments is keeping the patient from eating or drinking anything (*NPO*), which helps the GI tract rest. Another form of assistance includes inserting a tube into part of the GI tract. The most common tube is the nasogastric tube (*NGT*). This tube can either send food into the stomach, bypassing the throat, or it can be used to suck out (*aspirate*) the contents of the stomach. A tube can also be passed through the anus into the colon to administer fluid (*enema*) to help flush out stool that is stuck there.

There are two types of surgical approaches when operating on the gastrointestinal system: cutting a patient open (*laparotomy*) and inserting a camera and instruments through small holes (*laparoscopic*). The most common type of surgery involves removing part of the GI tract. When a section of the GI tract is removed, the remaining ends need to be reconnected (*anastomosis*). Occasionally, one end is attached to an opening to the outside of the body (*ostomy*), and the part past this is left disconnected. Usually, this is a temporary procedure to give time for the GI tract to heal. The most common of all gastrointestinal surgeries is removal of the appendix (*appendectomy*). The appendix is a small extension off the large intestine with little to no function. If blocked, it can become infected and possibly rupture.

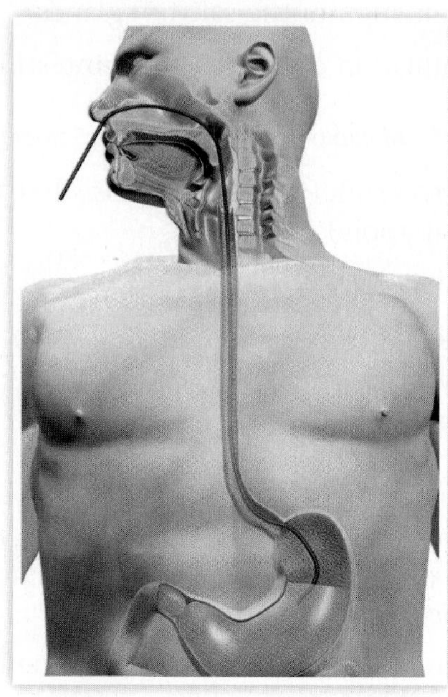

A nasograstric tube can either send food into the stomach, bypassing the throat, or can suck out (aspirate) the contents of the stomach.

pharmacology

Term	Word Analysis
antacid ant-AS-id **Definition** agent that neutralizes acid	**ant / acid** against / acid

pharmacology *continued*

Term	Word Analysis
antiemetic AN-tih-EE-met-ik **Definition** agent that prevents or relieves nausea or vomiting	**anti / emet / ic** against / vomiting / pertaining to ©McGraw-Hill Education/Pat Watson, photographer
cathartic kah-THAR-tik **Definition** agent that produces bowel movements	**cathart / ic** cleansing / pertaining to
sialagogic sai-AL-ah-GAW-jik **Definition** agent that causes salivation	**sial / agog / ic** saliva / leading / pertaining to

upper gastro tract procedures

Term	Word Analysis
esophagectomy eh-SAW-fah-JEK-toh-mee **Definition** surgical removal of the esophagus	**esophag / ectomy** esophagus / removal
esophagogastroplasty eh-SAW-fah-goh-GAS-troh-PLAS-tee **Definition** surgical reconstruction of the esophagus and stomach	**esophago / gastro / plasty** esophagus / stomach / reconstruction
gastrectomy gas-TREK-toh-mee **Definition** surgical removal of the stomach	**gastr / ectomy** stomach / removal
gastroduodenostomy GAS-troh-doo-AH-den-AW-stoh-mee **Definition** creation of an opening between the stomach and the duodenum	**gastro / duodeno / stomy** stomach / duodenum / opening
gastroenterostomy GAS-troh-EN-ter-AW-stoh-mee **Definition** creation of an opening between the stomach and the intestines	**gastro / entero / stomy** stomach / intestine / opening
gastrojejunostomy GAS-troh-JEH-joo-NAW-stoh-mee **Definition** creation of an opening between the stomach and the jejunum	**gastro / jejuno / stomy** stomach / jejunum / opening

upper gastro tract procedures *continued*

Term	Word Analysis
gastropexy GAS-troh-PEK-see **Definition** surgical fixation of the stomach	**gastro / pexy** stomach / fixation
gastroplasty GAS-troh-PLAS-tee **Definition** surgical reconstruction of the stomach	**gastro / plasty** stomach / reconstruction
gingivectomy JIN-jih-VEK-toh-mee **Definition** surgical removal of gum tissue	**gingiv / ectomy** gum / removal
gingivoplasty JIN-jih-voh-PLAS-tee **Definition** surgical reconstruction of gum tissue	**gingivo / plasty** gum / reconstruction
glossoplasty GLAWS-oh-PLAS-tee **Definition** surgical reconstruction of the tongue	**glosso / plasty** tongue / reconstruction
glossorrhaphy glaws-OR-ah-fee **Definition** suture of the tongue	**glosso / rrhaphy** tongue / suture
glossotomy glaws-AW-toh-mee **Definition** incision into the tongue	**glosso / tomy** tongue / incision
odontectomy oh-dawn-TEK-toh-mee **Definition** surgical removal of a tooth	**odont / ectomy** tooth / removal

lower gastro tract procedures

Term	Word Analysis
anastomosis ah-NAS-toh-MOH-sis **Definition** creation of an opening; a surgical procedure connecting two previously unconnected hollow tubes	**ana / stom / osis** up / out / mouth / condition 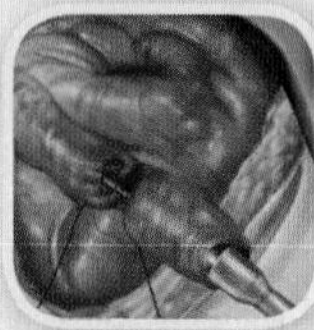

NOTE: The prefix *ana-* here means "out" or "up" instead of "no" or "not." This is the same type of usage as in the word *aneurysm.*

11.5 Treatments and Therapies

lower gastro tract procedures *continued*

Term	Word Analysis
anoplasty AN-noh-PLAS-tee **Definition** surgical reconstruction of the anus	**ano / plasty** anus / recontruction
colectomy koh-LEK-toh-mee **Definition** surgical removal of the colon	**col / ectomy** colon / removal
colostomy koh-LAW-stoh-mee **Definition** creation of an opening in the colon	**colo / stomy** colon / opening
duodenectomy doo-AW-den-EK-toh-mee **Definition** surgical removal of the duodenum	**dudoden / ectomy** duodenum / removal
enterectomy en-ter-EK-toh-mee **Definition** surgical removal of the intestines	**enter / ectomy** intestine / removal
enterorrhaphy en-ter-OR-ah-fee **Definition** suture of the intestines	**entero / rrhaphy** intestine / suture
enterotomy en-ter-AW-toh-mee **Definition** incision into the intestines	**entero / tomy** intestine / incision
hemicolectomy HEH-mee-koh-LEK-toh-mee **Definition** surgical removal of half (a portion) of the colon	**hemi / col / ectomy** half / colon / removal
hemorrhoidectomy HEM-oh-roi-DEK-toh-mee **Definition** surgical removal of hemorrhoids	**hemorrhoid / ectomy** hemorrhoid / removal
herniorrhaphy her-nee-OR-ah-fee **Definition** suture of a hernia	**hernio / rrhaphy** hernia / suture
ileocolostomy IHL-ee-oh-koh-LAW-stoh-mee **Definition** creation of an opening between the ileum and colon	**ileo / colo / stomy** ileum / colon / opening

lower gastro tract procedures *continued*

Term	Word Analysis
ileorrhaphy IHL-ee-OR-ah-fee **Definition** suture of the ileum	**ileo / rrhaphy** ileum / suture
ileostomy IHL-ee-AWS-toh-mee **Definition** creation of an opening in the ileum	**ileo / stomy** ileum / opening
ileotomy IHL-ee-AW-toh-mee **Definition** incision into the ileum	**ileo / tomy** ileum / incision
jejunorrhaphy JE-joo-NOR-ah-fee **Definition** suture of the jejunum	**jejuno / rrhaphy** jejunum / suture
jejunostomy JE-joo-NAW-stoh-mee **Definition** creation of an opening in the jejunum	**jejuno / stomy** jejunum / opening
jejunotomy JE-joo-NAW-toh-mee **Definition** incision into the jejunum	**jejuno / tomy** jejunum / incision
proctoplasty PROK-toh-PLAS-tee **Definition** surgical reconstruction of the anus and rectum	**procto / plasty** anus/rectum / reconstruction
rectopexy REK-toh-PEK-see **Definition** surgical fixation of the rectum	**recto / pexy** rectum / fixation

supporting organs procedures

Term	Word Analysis
abdominocentesis ab-DAW-min-oh-sin-TEE-sis **Definition** puncture of the abdomen (usually for the purpose of withdrawing fluid)	**abdomino / centesis** abdomen / puncture ©Stockbyte/PunchStock RF
abdominoplasty ab-DAW-min-oh-PLAS-tee **Definition** surgical reconstruction of the abdomen	**abdomino / plasty** abdomen / reconstruction

supporting organs procedures *continued*

Term	Word Analysis
celiotomy SEE-lee-AW-toh-mee **Definition** incision into the abdomen	**celio / tomy** abdomen / incision
cholangiogastrostomy kohl-AN-jee-oh-gas-TRAW-stoh-mee **Definition** creation of an opening between the bile vessel (ducts) and the stomach	**cholangio / gastro / stomy** bile vessel / stomach / opening
cholecystectomy KOH-lay-sis-TEK-toh-me **Definition** surgical removal of the bile (gall) bladder	**chole / cyst / ectomy** bile / bladder / removal
choledochoenterostomy KOH-leh-DOH-koh-EN-ter-AW-stoh-mee **Definition** creation of an opening between (common) bile duct and the intestines	**chole / docho / entero / stomy** bile / duct / intestine / opening
choledocholithectomy KOH-leh-DOH-koh-lih-THEK-toh-mee **Definition** surgical removal of a stone from the (common) bile duct	**chole / docho / lith / ectomy** bile / duct / stone / removal
choledochotomy KOH-leh-doh-KAW-toh-mee **Definition** incision into the (common) bile duct	**chole / docho / tomy** bile / duct / incision
cholelithotomy KOH-lay-lih-THAW-toh-mee **Definition** incision to remove bile (gall) stones	**chole / litho / tomy** bile / stone / incision
cholelithotripsy KOH-lay-lih-THOH-trip-see **Definition** crushing of bile (gall) stones	**chole / litho / trips / y** bile / stone / rub / procedure
hepatectomy HEP-ah-TEK-toh-me **Definition** surgical removal of the liver	**hepat / ectomy** liver / removal
hepaticogastrostomy heh-PAT-ih-koh-gas-TRAW-stoh-mee **Definition** creation of an opening between the liver and the stomach	**hepatico / gastro / stomy** liver / stomach / opening
hepaticotomy heh-PAT-ih-KAW-toh-me **Definition** incision into the liver	**hepatico / tomy** liver / incision
hepatopexy heh-PAT-oh-PEK-see **Definition** surgical fixation of the liver	**hepato / pexy** liver / fixation

supporting organs procedures *continued*

Term	Word Analysis
laparoenterostomy LAP-ah-roh-EN-ter-AWS-toh-me **Definition** creation of an opening between the abdomen and the intestines	**laparo / entero / stomy** abdomen / intestine / opening
laparoscopic surgery LAP-ah-roh-SKAW-pik SIR-jir-ee **Definition** the use of a laparoscope to perform minimally invasive surgery	**laparo / scop / ic surgery** abdomen / device to look / pertaining to
laparotomy LAP-ah-RAW-toh-mee **Definition** incision into the abdomen	**laparo / tomy** abdomen / incision
pancreatectomy PAN-kree-ah-TEK-toh-mee **Definition** surgical removal of the pancreas	**pancreat / ectomy** pancreas / removal
pancreatoduodenectomy PAN-kree-at-oh-DOO-aw-den-EK-toh-mee **Definition** surgical removal of the pancreas and duodenum	**pancreato / duoden / ectomy** pancreas / duodenum / removal
pancreatolithectomy PAN-kree-at-oh-lih-THECK-toh-mee **Definition** surgical removal of stones in the pancreas	**pancreato / lith / ectomy** pancreas / stone / removal
sialoadenectomy sai-AL-oh-AD-en-EK-toh-mee **Definition** surgical removal of a salivary gland	**sialo / aden / ectomy** saliva / gland / removal
sialolithotomy sai-AL-oh-lih-THAW-toh-mee **Definition** incision to remove salivary stones	**sialo / litho / tomy** saliva / stone / incision
stomatoplasty stoh-MAH-toh-PLAS-tee **Definition** surgical reconstruction of the mouth	**stomato / plasty** mouth / reconstruction

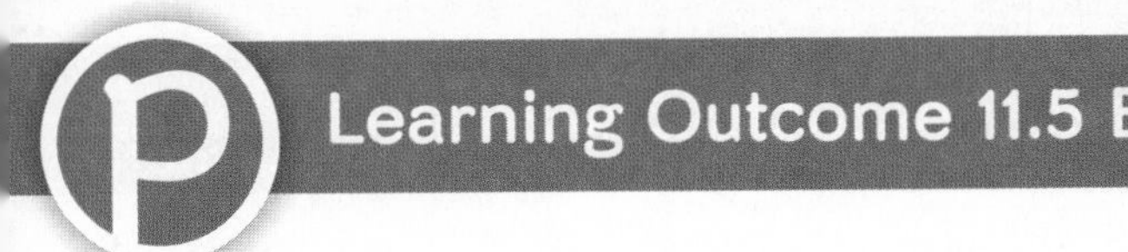

Learning Outcome 11.5 Exercises

PRONUNCIATION

EXERCISE 1 *Indicate which syllable is emphasized when pronounced.*

EXAMPLE: bronchitis bron**chi**tis

1. gastroplasty _______________
2. gastropexy _______________
3. antiemetic _______________
4. ileostomy _______________
5. hepatopexy _______________
6. laparotomy _______________
7. jejunostomy _______________
8. gingivoplasty _______________
9. ileorrhaphy _______________
10. anastomosis _______________
11. duodenectomy _______________
12. abdominoplasty _______________
13. cholelithotomy _______________
14. cholelithotripsy _______________
15. pancreatolithectomy _______________
16. laparoenterostomy _______________
17. antacid _______________
18. cathartic _______________
19. glossotomy _______________
20. colectomy _______________
21. colostomy _______________
22. gastrectomy _______________
23. odontectomy _______________
24. herniorrhaphy _______________

TRANSLATION

EXERCISE 2 *Break down the following words into their component parts.*

EXAMPLE: nasopharyngoscope *naso | pharyngo | scope*

1. hepatopexy _______________
2. laparotomy _______________
3. ileostomy _______________
4. colostomy _______________
5. gastropexy _______________
6. jejunostomy _______________
7. gingivoplasty _______________
8. abdominoplasty _______________
9. glossorrhaphy _______________
10. herniorrhaphy _______________
11. enterorrhaphy _______________
12. hemorrhoidectomy _______________
13. ileocolostomy _______________
14. sialolithotomy _______________
15. pancreatolithectomy _______________
16. laparoenterostomy _______________
17. gastroduodenostomy _______________

Learning Outcome 11.5 Exercises

18. gastroenterostomy ______
19. gastrojejunostomy ______
20. hepaticogastrostomy ______
21. choledochotomy ______
22. cholelithotripsy ______
23. anastomosis ______
24. cholangiogastrostomy ______
25. choledochoenterostomy ______

EXERCISE 3 *Underline and define the roots from this chapter in the following terms.*

1. glossoplasty ______
2. proctoplasty ______
3. stomatoplasty ______
4. gastroplasty ______
5. anoplasty ______
6. glossotomy ______
7. enterotomy ______
8. ileotomy ______
9. jejunotomy ______
10. celiotomy ______
11. hepaticotomy ______
12. cholelithotomy ______
13. ileorrhaphy ______
14. jejunorrhaphy ______
15. rectopexy ______
16. esophagectomy ______
17. gastrectomy ______
18. gingivectomy ______
19. odontectomy ______
20. colectomy ______
21. duodenectomy ______
22. enterectomy ______
23. hemicolectomy ______
24. hepatectomy ______
25. pancreatectomy ______
26. sialoadenectomy ______

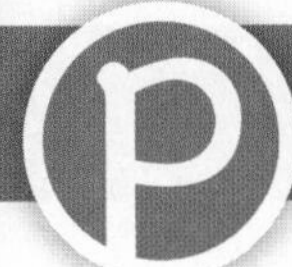

Learning Outcome 11.5 Exercises

27. abdominocentesis ____________________
28. laparoscopic surgery ____________________
29. esophagogastroplasty (2 roots) ____________________
30. cholecystectomy (2 roots) ____________________
31. choledocholithectomy (2 roots) ____________________
32. pancreatoduodenectomy (2 roots) ____________________

EXERCISE 4 *Match the term on the left with its definition on the right.*

______	1. antacid	a.	agent that causes salivation
______	2. sialagogic	b.	agent that neutralizes acid
______	3. antiemetic	c.	agent that prevents/relieves nausea or vomiting
______	4. cathartic	d.	agent that produces bowel movements

EXERCISE 5 *Translate the following terms as literally as possible.*

> EXAMPLE: nasopharyngoscope *an instrument for looking at the nose and throat*

1. enterotomy ____________________
2. jejunotomy ____________________
3. laparotomy ____________________
4. celiotomy ____________________
5. esophagectomy ____________________
6. herniorrhaphy ____________________
7. glossorrhaphy ____________________
8. enterorrhaphy ____________________
9. ileorrhaphy ____________________
10. jejunorrhaphy ____________________
11. gastropexy ____________________
12. duodenectomy ____________________
13. hemorrhoidectomy ____________________
14. abdominocentesis ____________________
15. laparoscopic surgery ____________________

EXERCISE 6 *Fill in the blanks.*

1. colostomy = creation of an opening in the ____________________
2. ileostomy = creation of an opening in the ____________________
3. jejunostomy = creation of an opening in the ____________________
4. ileocolostomy = creation of an opening between ____________ and ____________

5. gastroduodenostomy = creation of an opening between ______________ and ______________
6. gastroenterostomy = creation of an opening between ______________ and ______________
7. gastrojejunostomy = creation of an opening between ______________ and ______________
8. hepaticogastrostomy = creation of an opening between ______________ and ______________
9. laparoenterostomy = creation of an opening between ______________ and ______________
10. cholangiogastrostomy = creation of an opening between ______________ and ______________
11. choledochoenterostomy = creation of an opening between ______________ and ______________

GENERATION

EXERCISE 7 *Build a medical term from the information provided.*

EXAMPLE: inflammation of the sinuses *sinusitis*

1. surgical reconstruction of the stomach ______________
2. surgical reconstruction of gum tissue ______________
3. surgical reconstruction of the tongue ______________
4. surgical reconstruction of the anus ______________
5. surgical reconstruction of the abdomen ______________
6. surgical reconstruction of the mouth ______________
7. surgical reconstruction of the anus and rectum ______________
8. surgical reconstruction of the esophagus and stomach ______________
9. incision into the ileum ______________
10. incision into the tongue ______________
11. incision into the (common) bile duct ______________
12. surgical removal of the stomach ______________
13. surgical removal of the duodenum ______________
14. surgical fixation of the rectum ______________
15. surgical fixation of the liver ______________

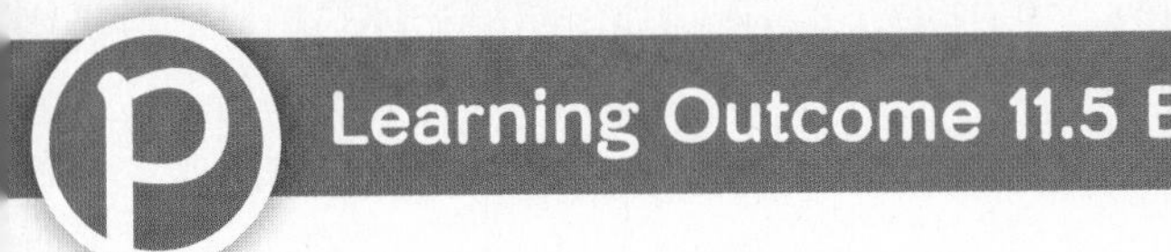

Learning Outcome 11.5 Exercises

EXERCISE 8 *Multiple-choice questions. Select the correct answer(s).*

1. Select all of the terms below that pertain to the upper GI tract.
   a. cholecystectomy
   b. choledocholithectomy
   c. colectomy
   d. duodenectomy
   e. enterectomy
   f. esophagectomy
   g. gastrectomy
   h. gingivectomy
   i. hepatectomy
   j. odontectomy
2. Select all of the terms below that pertain to the lower GI tract.
   a. cholecystectomy
   b. choledocholithectomy
   c. colectomy
   d. duodenectomy
   e. enterectomy
   f. esophagectomy
   g. gastrectomy
   h. gingivectomy
   i. hepatectomy
   j. odontectomy
3. Select all of the terms below that pertain to the supporting organs for the GI system.
   a. cholecystectomy
   b. choledocholithectomy
   c. colectomy
   d. duodenectomy
   e. enterectomy
   f. esophagectomy
   g. gastrectomy
   h. gingivectomy
   i. hepatectomy
   j. odontectomy

EXERCISE 9 *Briefly describe the difference between each pair of terms.*

1. gingivectomy, odontectomy ______________________
2. colectomy, hemicolectomy ______________________
3. hepatectomy, hepaticotomy ______________________
4. pancreatectomy, pancreatolithectomy ______________________
5. cholelithotomy, cholelithotripsy ______________________
6. cholecystectomy, choledocholithectomy ______________________
7. sialoadenectomy, sialolithotomy ______________________
8. antacid, antiemetic ______________________
9. cathartic, sialagogic ______________________

11.6 Abbreviations

Abbreviations provide a shorthand way of referring to things that either recur often or are too long to write out. When dealing with the digestive system, these abbreviations can refer to regions of the abdomen (RLQ, LUQ), organs (GB), systems (N&V), diseases (PUD), and procedures (PEG, FOBT).

gastrointestinal system abbreviations

Abbreviation	Definition
BE	barium enema
BM	bowel movement
CCE	cholecystectomy
EGD	esophagogastroduodenoscopy
ERCP	endoscopic retrograde cholangiopancreatography
EUS	endoscopic ultrasound
FOBT	fecal occult blood test
GERD	gastroesophageal reflux disease
GI	gastrointestinal
HAV, HBV, HCV	Hepatitis A virus, Hepatitis B virus, Hepatitis C virus
IBD	inflammatory bowel disease
IBS	irritable bowel syndrome
LFT	liver function test
NGT	nasogastric tube
NPO	nothing by mouth (nihil per os)
N&V	nausea and vomiting
PEG	percutaneous endoscopic gastrostomy
PEJ	percutaneous endoscopic jejunostomy
PUD	peptic ulcer disease
RLQ	right lower quadrant
RUQ	right upper quadrant
LLQ	left lower quadrant
LUQ	left upper quadrant
UGI	upper gastrointestinal

Learning Outcome 11.6 Exercises

EXERCISE 1 *Define the following abbreviations.*

1. GERD ______
2. BM ______
3. N&V ______
4. BE ______
5. FOBT ______
6. NPO ______
7. CCE ______
8. PUD ______
9. EUS ______
10. RUQ ______
11. LFT ______

EXERCISE 2 *Give the abbreviations for the following definitions.*

1. right lower quadrant ______
2. left upper quadrant ______
3. left lower quadrant ______
4. nasogastric tube ______
5. gastrointestinal ______
6. esophagogastroduodenoscopy ______
7. percutaneous endoscopic gastrostomy ______
8. endoscopic retrograde cholangiopancreatography ______
9. percutaneous endoscopic jejunostomy ______
10. upper gastrointestinal ______

EXERCISE 3 *Multiple-choice questions. Select the correct answer.*

1. The abbreviation EUS stands for "endoscopic ultrasound." Which of the descriptions below is an accurate breakdown of the term *endoscopic*?
   a. *endo* (inside) + *scopic* (pertaining to looking)
   b. *endo* (outside) + *scopic* (pertaining to looking)
   c. *endo* (around) + *scopic* (pertaining to looking)
   d. *endo* (beneath) + *scopic* (pertaining to looking)
   e. *endo* (above) + *scopic* (pertaining to looking)
2. Which of the terms below pertains to the CCE?
   a. cholangitis
   b. cholecystalgia
   c. choledochocele
   d. cholelithiasis
   e. cholecystectomy

Learning Outcome 11.6 Exercises

3. *PEJ* stands for *percutaneous endoscopic jejunostomy*. Which of the definitions below is correct for *jejunostomy?*
   a. creation of an opening in the jejunum
   b. incision into the jejunum
   c. narrowing of the jejunum
   d. removal of the jejunum
   e. suture of the jejunum

EXERCISE 4 *Match the abbreviation on the left with its full definition on the right.*

_____	1. RLQ	a. tube inserted through the nose into the stomach
_____	2. LUQ	b. disease in which acid comes up from the stomach and damages the esophagus
_____	3. LLQ	c. nothing by mouth
_____	4. RUQ	d. procedure for looking inside the esophagus, stomach, and duodenum
_____	5. GERD	e. test of feces to discover blood not visibly apparent
_____	6. FOBT	f. left upper quadrant
_____	7. NGT	g. left lower quadrant
_____	8. EGD	h. right upper quadrant
_____	9. NPO	i. right lower quadrant

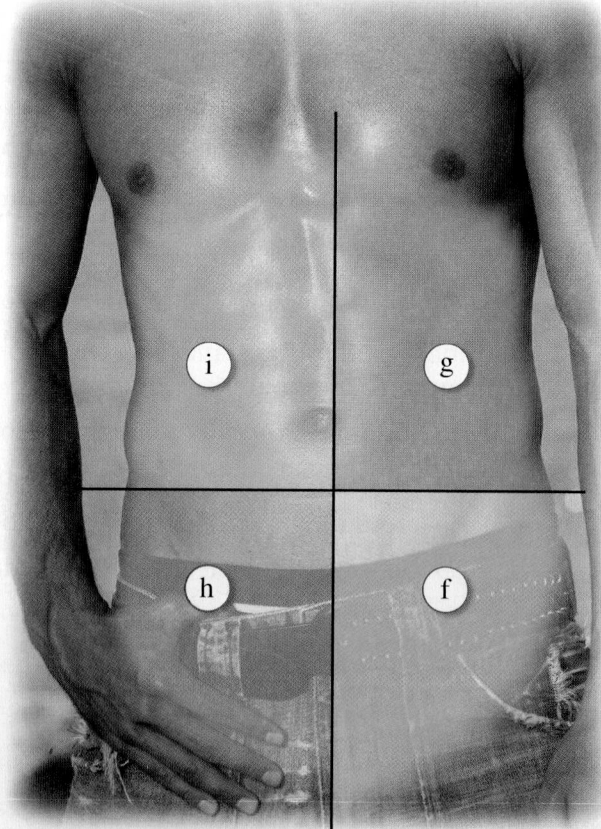

11.7 Electronic Health Records

Clinic Note

S Subjective

Mr. Robert Luno presents to our clinic with a 2-month history of intermittent postprandial **gastralgia** and **dyspepsia**. It has become more and more frequent. He also reports occasional **emesis** as well, but denies **hematemesis** and cholemesis. He denies **diarrhea** and **constipation**.

O Objective

Temp: 98.6; HR: 64; RR: 16; BP: 120/80.
General: Overweight, middle-aged man in no apparent distress.
HEENT: PERRLA. No conjunctival injection.
No scleral icterus. Mucous membranes moist and pink. TMs normal.
CV: RRR without murmur.
Resp: CTA. Good air entry.
Abd: Soft, nontender, nondistended.
No HSM. Normative bowel sounds.

A Assessment

I suspect Mr. Luno is suffering from **gastroesophageal reflux**. Other possibilities include **gastritis**, **cholelithiasis**, and **PUD**.

P Plan

I will begin a trial of **antacid** therapy along with recommended dietary adjustments.
If he does not respond to treatment in 1 month, I will schedule him for an **EGD**.

–Constance Stiles, NP

Learning Outcome 11.7 Exercises

EXERCISE 1 *Match the term on the left with its definition on the right.*

______	1. constipation	a.	agent that neutralizes acid
______	2. antacid	b.	bad digestion
______	3. diarrhea	c.	difficulty passing feces
______	4. gastritis	d.	disease in which acid comes up from the stomach and damages the esophagus
______	5. dyspepsia	e.	inflammation of the stomach
______	6. hematemesis	f.	passing of fluid or unformed feces
______	7. cholemesis	g.	procedure for looking inside the esophagus, stomach, and duodenum
______	8. emesis	h.	presence of a gallstone
______	9. cholelithiasis	i.	vomiting
______	10. gastroesophageal reflux	j.	vomiting bile
______	11. esophagogastroduodenoscopy	k.	vomiting blood

Learning Outcome 11.7 Exercises

EXERCISE 2 *Fill in the blanks.*

1. Using the data recorded in the patient's clinic note, fill in the following blanks.
   a. The patient's temperature: ______________________
   b. The patient's heart rate: ______________________
   c. The patient's respiratory rate: ______________________
   d. The patient's blood pressure: ______________________
   e. Abd: No ______________________ (hepatosplenomegaly)
2. Mr. Luno presents to the clinic with a 2-month history of intermittent *gastralgia* (give definition: ______________________) and *dyspepsia* (give definition: ______________________).
3. He occasionally vomits, but has not vomited ______________________ (*hematemesis*) or vomited ______________________ (*cholemesis*).

EXERCISE 3 *True or false questions. Indicate true answers with a T and false answers with an F.*

1. The medical professional suspects the patient has GERD. ________
2. The patient has stomach pain and poor digestion. ________
3. The patient has vomited both blood and bile. ________
4. The patient has difficulty passing feces. ________
5. The patient may have a gallstone. ________
6. The patient may have peptic ulcer disease. ________

EXERCISE 4 *Multiple-choice questions. Select the correct answer.*

1. Which of the following symptoms did Mr. Luno report to the medical professional?
   a. cholemesis
   b. constipation
   c. diarrhea
   d. gastralgia
   e. hematemesis
2. Which of the following is NOT a possible diagnosis?
   a. cholelithiasis
   b. gastritis
   c. gastroesophageal reflux disease
   d. hepatosplenomegaly
   e. peptic ulcer disease
3. Which is the correct definition for the abbreviation *EGD*?
   a. epigastricduodenectomy
   b. epigastrodynia
   c. esophagogastroduodenoscopy
   d. esophagogastrodynia
   e. none of these

GI Consult

Subjective

Reason for Consult: Jaundice, RUQ pain.

History of Present Illness: Ms. Renata Mendel is a 22-year-old woman well-known to the **gastroenterology** service. She was initially diagnosed with **ulcerative colitis** 2 years previously. She had presented to her primary care provider at the time with a history of recurring bloody stools and **constipation**. The symptoms progressed to include fatigue and purulent **rectal** discharge, and she was referred to our clinic. **Colonoscopy** confirmed the diagnosis of ulcerative colitis. One year ago, she developed **toxic megacolon**, which eventually led to surgical intervention. She had been doing well until 3 months ago, when she started reporting fatigue, general pruritis, and pain in her **RUQ**. Her primary provider referred her again for evaluation. She reports some history of **steatorrhea**, but denies bright red blood.

Objective

Past Medical History: **Ulcerative colitis. Toxic megacolon.**
Past Surgical History: **Total colectomy with ilieorectal anastomosis.**
Family History: Mother with **ulcerative colitis.**
Medications: Daily vitamin.

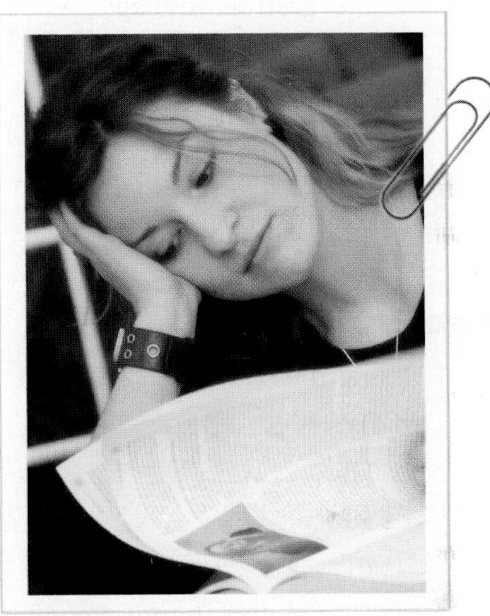

©Design Pics/Kristy-Anne Glubish RF

Physical Exam:
Temp: 98.6; Heart Rate: 76; Respiratory Rate: 22;
Blood Pressure: 108/72; Pulse Ox: 98%.

General: **Jaundiced, cachectic**-appearing young woman in no apparent distress. Alert and oriented x3.
HEENT: PERRLA. Scleral **icterus**. Moist mucous membranes. Normal dentition.
Neck: Supple. No LAD.
CV: RRR without murmur, gallop, or rub.
Resp: CTA.
Abd: Soft, nontender, nondistended. **Hepatomegaly** two-finger breadths below ribs. No **splenomegaly.**
Ext: No cyanosis, clubbing, or edema. Capillary refill brisk.

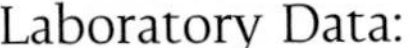

Laboratory Data:
Significant for increased **LFTs, hypoalbuminemia,** and **hyperbilirubinemia.**

Assessment

Ms. Mendel's symptoms are concerning for primary **sclerosing cholangitis**. Other possibilities include **hepatitis**, **cholelithiasis**, and biliary obstruction.

Plan

Recommendation:
We need to perform an **endoscopic retrograde cholangiopancreatogram** (**ERCP**) or **magnetic resonance cholangiopancreatogram** (**MRCP**). Given the less-invasive nature, I recommended Ms. Mendel have an MR cholangiogram, which is scheduled for later this week. If the results confirm primary sclerosing cholangitis, we will begin medical treatment and then schedule a **percutaneous hepatic biopsy.**

Thank you for your help with our mutual patient. I will keep your office up to date with further findings.

–Susan Marsden, MD

Learning Outcome 11.7 Exercises

EXERCISE 5 *Match the term on the left with its definition on the right.*

______	1. constipation	a.	creation of an opening; a surgical procedure connecting two previously unconnected hollow tubes
______	2. hepatitis	b.	difficulty passing feces
______	3. jaundice	c.	excessive fat discharged in the feces
______	4. colonoscopy	d.	inflammation and hardening of the bile vessels (ducts)
______	5. colitis	e.	inflammation of the colon
______	6. colectomy	f.	inflammation of the liver
______	7. cholangiogram	g.	procedure for looking at the colon
______	8. gastroenterology	h.	record of the bile vessels (ducts)
______	9. sclerosing cholangitis	i.	surgical removal of the colon
______	10. anastomosis	j.	presence of a gallstone
______	11. cholelithiasis	k.	study of the stomach and intestines
______	12. steatorrhea	l.	yellowing of skin, tissue, and fluids caused by increased levels of bilirubin in the blood

EXERCISE 6 *Fill in the blanks.*

1. Using the data recorded in the patient's GI consult note, fill in the following blanks.
   a. T: ______________________________
   b. HR: ______________________________
   c. RR: ______________________________
   d. BP: ______________________________
   e. CV: (give definition for abbreviation: ______________________________):
   RRR (give definition for abbreviation: ______________________________
   and ______________________________)
   f. Abd: *hepatomegaly* (give definition: ______________________________),
   no ______________________________ (enlarged spleen)
2. The patient reports some history of ______________________________ (excessive fat discharged in the feces).
3. Past surgical history: Total *colectomy* (give definition: ______________________________) with *ileorectal anastomosis* (creation of an opening between the ______________________________ and ______________________________).
4. Ms. Mendel's symptoms are concerning for primary *sclerosing cholangitis* (give definition: ______________________________).
5. Other possible diagnoses include *hepatitis* (inflammation of the ______________________________), *cholelithiasis* (presence of ______________________________), and biliary obstruction.
6. Given the less-invasive nature, Dr. Marsden recommends an MR *cholangiogram* (give definition: ______________________________).

Learning Outcome 11.7 Exercises

EXERCISE 7 *True or false questions. Indicate true answers with a T and false answers with an F.*

1. Ms. Mendel has an enlarged spleen and liver. ________
2. Ms. Mendel experienced pain in the lower left quadrant of her abdomen. ________
3. Ms. Mendel has too much bilirubin in her blood. ________
4. Ms. Mendel presented to her PCP with an Hx of hematemesis. ________
5. Ms. Mendel will undergo medical treatment and then will be scheduled for a biopsy of her liver. ________

EXERCISE 8 *Multiple-choice questions. Select the correct answer.*

1. Which of the following is NOT a possible diagnosis?
   a. enlarged liver and spleen
   b. inflammation and hardening of the bile vessels (ducts)
   c. inflammation of the liver
   d. the presence of a gallstone
   e. yellowing of skin, tissue, and fluids caused by increased levels of bilirubin in the blood
2. The conjunctivas of the eye are among the first tissues to change color as bilirubin levels rise. This is sometimes referred to as *scleral icterus*. The yellowing of skin, tissue, and fluids caused by increased levels of bilirubin in the blood is commonly known as:
   a. cholangitis
   b. hepatitis
   c. icterus
   d. jaundice
   e. jejunitis
3. The patient developed *toxic megacolon*. Which of the following descriptions is a correct breakdown of the term?
   a. damaging (*toxic*) + enlarged (*mega-*) + colon (*colon*)
   b. damaging (*toxic*) + small (*mega-*) + colon (*colon*)
   c. harmless (*toxic*) + enlarged (*mega-*) + colon (*colon*)
   d. harmless (*toxic*) + small (*mega-*) + colon (*colon*)
4. The patient's laboratory data revealed *hypoalbuminemia*. Which of the following descriptions is a correct breakdown of the term?
   a. high (*hypo*) + albumin (*albumin*) + blood condition (*-emia*)
   b. high (*hypo*) + albumin (*albumin*) + urine condition (*-emia*)
   c. low (*hypo*) + albumin (*albumin*) + blood condition (*-emia*)
   d. low (*hypo*) + albumin (*albumin*) + urine condition (*-emia*)
5. The medical professional writing this GI consult recommends an ERCP or an MRCP. MRCP stands for "magnetic resonance cholangiopancreatogram." Which of the following descriptions is a correct definition for *cholangiopancreatogram?*
   a. procedure for mapping the bile vessels (ducts) and pancreas
   b. record of the bile vessels (ducts) and pancreas
   c. procedure for mapping the gallbladder and pancreas
   d. record of the gallbladder and pancreas

Discharge Summary

Date of Admission: 4/13/2015
Date of Discharge: 4/16/2015

Admission Diagnosis

1. Acute abdominal pain
2. **Pancreatitis**

Discharge Diagnosis

1. **Choledocholithiasis**
2. S/p **choledocholithectomy** and **cholecystectomy**
3. Pancreatitis, resolved

Discharge Condition
Stable

Consultations
General surgery

Procedures

1. **Laparoscopic choledocholithectomy** and **cholecystectomy**

Labs
Admission labs: Elevated **LFTs**, **hyperbilirubinemia**, leukocytosis, elevated pancreatic enzymes.
Discharge labs: Everything had returned to normal levels.
Imaging
Ultrasound of the upper abdomen revealed **cholelithiasis** and **choledocholithiasis** with bile duct dilation.

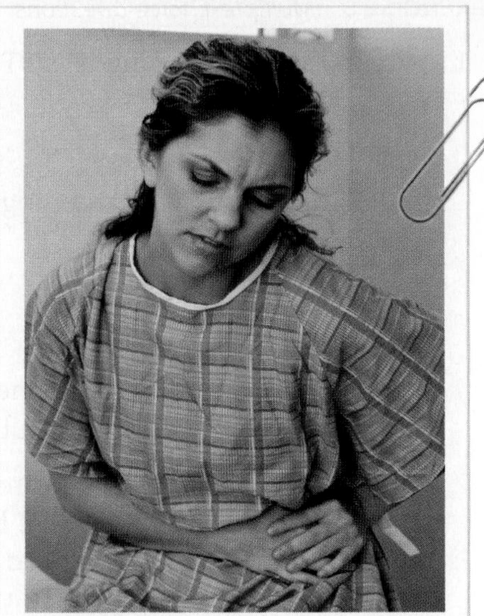

©PhotoAlto/Michele Constantini/Getty Images RF

HPI
Mrs. Roxana Collach presented to the ED with a 2-day history of increasing **epigastric** pain. She described the pain as constant and dull with radiation to her back. She also had progressive anorexia. She denied nausea, emesis, or diarrhea. She was febrile in the ED and had marked epigastric tenderness on exam with guarding. Her abdomen was slightly distended and she was mildly jaundiced. Her elevated pancreatic enzyme levels confirmed the suspicion of acute **pancreatitis**. She was admitted for pain control and IVF.

Hospital Course
Mrs. Collach was admitted to the medical service. She was placed on NPO status and given IVF and analgesics. An ultrasound revealed gallstones in the common bile duct as the etiology for Mrs. Collach's pancreatitis. Surgery was consulted. On hospital day 2, Mrs. Collach was taken to the OR for laparoscopic choledocholithectomy and cholecystectomy. She tolerated the procedure well. She began a postoperative refeeding plan with a low-protein, low-fat diet. She tolerated advancing the diet, and 2 days after her surgery, her pain had improved enough that she was discharged home.

Discharge Physical Examination
Temp: 98.6; RR: 24; HR: 86; BP: 100/64.
Gen: WDWN. Alert.
CV: RRR.
Resp: CTA.
GI: Abdomen soft, nondistended, mild tenderness to palpation over the surgical incisions.
Three small horizontal surgical wounds in her abdomen. Wounds clean, dry, and intact.

Discharge Summary *(continued)*

Activity
No restrictions.

Diet
Low protein, low fat.

Meds
Analgesics prn.

Follow-Up Appointments
Primary care provider: Dr. Primo, 1 week.
Surgery: Dr. Sleiss, 1 month.

Learning Outcome 11.7 Exercises

EXERCISE 9 *Match the term on the left with its definition on the right.*

______	1. diarrhea	a.	inflammation of the pancreas
______	2. pancreatitis	b.	passing of fluid or unformed feces
______	3. jaundice	c.	surgical removal of a stone from the (common) bile duct
______	4. emesis	d.	surgical removal of the bile (gall) bladder
______	5. laparascopic	e.	presence of a gallstone
______	6. epigastric	f.	presence of a stone in the (common) bile duct
______	7. cholecystectomy	g.	use of a laparoscope to perform minimally invasive surgery
______	8. choledocholithectomy	h.	upper center portion of the abdomen
______	9. choledocholithiasis	i.	vomiting
______	10. cholelithiasis	j.	yellowing of skin, tissue, and fluids caused by increased levels of bilirubin in the blood

EXERCISE 10 *Fill in the blanks.*

1. Using the data recorded in Mrs. Collach's discharge summary, fill in the following blanks.
   a. ______________________ (the presence of a stone in the [common] bile duct).
   b. S/p *choledocholithectomy* (surgical removal of a(n) ______________________ from the ______________________) and *cholecystectomy* (surgical removal of the ______________________).
   c. ______________________ (inflammation of the pancreas), resolved.
2. Using the data recorded for the history of the present illness, fill in the following blanks.
   a. Mrs. Collach presented to the ED (give definition for abbreviation: ______________________) with a 2-day history of increasing *epigastric* (give definition: ______________________) pain.
   b. Mrs. Collach was admitted for pain control and IVF (give definition for abbreviation: ______________________).

Learning Outcome 11.7 Exercises

3. Using the data recorded at Mrs. Collach's discharge physical examination, fill in the following blanks.
   a. Mrs. Collach's temperature: ______________________________
   b. Mrs. Collach's heart rate: ______________________________
   c. Mrs. Collach's respiratory rate: ______________________________
   d. Mrs. Collach's blood pressure: ______________________________

EXERCISE 11 *True or false questions. Indicate true answers with a T and false answers with an F.*

1. Mrs. Collach presented to the emergency department with nausea, vomiting, and diarrhea. ________
2. Mrs. Collach had a fever upon admission. ________
3. Mrs. Collach still has pancreatitis. ________
4. Mrs. Collach was admitted with enterodynia. ________
5. Mrs. Collach had a gallstone removed using a celiotomy. ________
6. As part of the hospital course, Mrs. Collach was given a regular diet of food and drink. ________

EXERCISE 12 *Multiple-choice questions. Select the correct answer.*

1. Mrs. Collach's laboratory data revealed *hyperbilirubinemia.* Which is a correct breakdown of the term?
   a. high (*hyper*) + bilirubin (*bilirubin*) + blood condition (*-emia*)
   b. high (*hyper*) + bilirubin (*bilirubin*) + urine condition (*-emia*)
   c. low (*hyper*) + bilirubin (*bilirubin*) + blood condition (*-emia*)
   d. low (*hyper*) + bilirubin (*bilirubin*) + urine condition (*-emia*)
2. Which of the following is the correct definition for the term *laparoscopic choledocholithectomy?*
   a. surgical removal of a stone from the (common) bile duct with the use of a laparoscope to perform minimally invasive surgery
   b. surgical removal of the bile (gall) bladder with the use of a laparoscope to perform minimally invasive surgery
   c. surgical removal of a stone from the (common) bile duct with the use of a laparoscope to create a large incision in the abdomen
   d. surgical removal of the bile (gall) bladder with the use of a laparoscope to create a large incision in the abdomen
3. The abbreviation NPO means:
   a. nihil per os
   b. nothing by mouth
   c. the patient shouldn't eat
   d. all of these

Quick Reference

quick reference glossary of roots

Root	Definition	Root	Definition
abdomin/o	abdomen	**hepatic/o**	liver
an/o	anus	**hepat/o**	liver
bil/i	bile (gall)	**ile/o**	ileum
celi/o	abdomen	**jejun/o**	jejunum
chol/e	bile (gall)	**lapar/o**	abdomen
col/o	colon (large intestine)	**lingu/o**	tongue
colon/o	colon (large intestine)	**odont/o**	tooth
cyst/o	bladder	**or/o**	mouth
dent/o	tooth	**pancreat/o**	pancreas
doch/o	duct	**peritone/o**	peritoneum
duoden/o	duodenum	**proct/o**	anus and rectum
enter/o	intestines	**rect/o**	rectum
esophag/o	esophagus	**sial/o**	saliva
gastr/o	stomach	**sigmoid/o**	sigmoid colon
gingiv/o	gums	**stomat/o**	mouth
gloss/o	tongue		

quick reference glossary of terms

Term	Definition
abdominocentesis	puncture of the abdomen (usually for the purpose of withdrawing fluid)
abdominoplasty	surgical reconstruction of the abdomen
aerodontalgia	tooth pain caused by exposure to air
anal fistula	abnormal opening between the rectum and the exterior perianal skin
anastomosis	creation of an opening; a surgical procedure connecting two previously unconnected hollow tubes
anophony	sound from the anus
anoplasty	surgical reconstruction of the anus
anosigmoidoscopy	procedure for looking at the anus and sigmoid colon
antacid	agent that neutralizes acid
antiemetic	agent that prevents/relieves nausea or vomiting
aphagia	inability to eat

quick reference glossary of terms *continued*

Term	Definition
ascites	retention of fluid in the peritoneum
bariatrics	branch of medicine dealing with weight issues
biligenesis	formation of bile
cathartic	agent that produces bowel movements
celiac disease	disease of the intestines due to an adverse reaction to gluten
celiomyositis	inflammation of the abdominal muscle
celiopathy	disease of the abdomen
celiotomy	incision into the abdomen
cholangiogram	record of the bile vessels (ducts)
cholangiography	procedure for mapping the bile vessels (ducts)
cholangioma	tumor of the bile vessels (ducts)
cholangiopancreatography	procedure for mapping the bile vessels (ducts) and pancreas
cholangitis	inflammation of the bile vessels (ducts)
choleangiogastrostomy	creation of an opening between the bile vessel (ducts) and the stomach
cholecystalgia	pain in the gallbladder
cholecystectomy	surgical removal of the bile (gall) bladder
cholecystitis	inflammation of the bile (gall) bladder
cholecystogram	record of the bile (gall) bladder
choledochocele	hernia of the (common) bile duct
choledochoenterostomy	creation of an opening between (common) bile duct and the intestines
choledocholithectomy	surgical removal of a stone from the (common) bile duct
choledocholithiasis	presence of a stone in the (common) bile duct
choledochotomy	incision into the (common) bile duct
cholelith	gallstone; literally, a stone in the bile
cholelithiasis	presence of a gallstone
cholelithotomy	incision to remove bile (gall) stones
cholelithotripsy	crushing of bile (gall) stones
cholemesis	vomiting bile
cirrhosis	liver disease named for the change of color in the liver
colectomy	surgical removal of the colon
colitis	inflammation of the colon
colonoscopy	procedure for looking at the colon
colorectal carcinoma	cancerous tumor of the colon or rectum

quick reference glossary of terms *continued*

Term	Definition
colostomy	creation of an opening in the colon
colovaginal fistula	abnormal opening between the colon and vagina
constipation	difficulty passing feces
dentalgia	tooth pain
dentifrice	toothpaste
dentist	specialist in teeth
dentistry	branch of medicine dealing with teeth
diarrhea	passing of fluid or unformed feces
diverticulitis	the inflammation of diverticula in the colon
diverticulosis	the condition of having diverticula in the colon
duodenectomy	surgical removal of the duodenum
duodenitis	inflammation of the duodenum
dysentery	another name for diarrhea
dyspepsia	bad digestion
endoscope	instrument used to look inside
endoscopy	procedure of looking inside
enterectomy	surgical removal of the intestines
enterocele	hernia of the intestines
enterodynia	pain in the intestines
enteropathy	disease of the intestines
enterorrhaphy	suture of the intestines
enterotomy	incision into the intestines
epigastric	upper center portion of the abdomen
esophagalgia	pain in the esophagus
esophageal carcinoma	cancerous tumor of the esophagus
esophagectomy	surgical removal of the esophagus
esophagitis	inflammation of the esophagus
esophagogastroduodenoscopy	procedure for looking inside the esophagus, stomach, and duodenum
esophagogastroplasty	surgical reconstruction of the esophagus and stomach
esophagoscopy	procedure for looking inside the esophagus
eupepsia	good digestion
fecal occult blood test (FOBT)	test of feces to discover blood not visibly apparent
fistula	any abnormal passageway in the body that shouldn't be there

quick reference glossary of terms *continued*

Term	Definition
flatus	medical term for passing gas
gastralgia	stomach pain
gastrectomy	surgical removal of the stomach
gastritis	inflammation of the stomach
gastroduodenostomy	creation of an opening between the stomach and the duodenum
gastrodynia	stomach pain
gastroenteritis	inflammation of the stomach and intestines
gastroenterocolitis	inflammation of the stomach, intestine, and colon
gastroenterologist	specialist in the stomach and intestines
gastroenterology	study of the stomach and intestines
gastroenterostomy	creation of an opening between the stomach and the intestines
gastroesophageal reflux disease (GERD)	disease in which acid comes up from the stomach and damages the esophagus
gastrojejunostomy	creation of an opening between the stomach and the jejunum
gastromalacia	softening of the stomach
gastroparesis	partial paralysis of the stomach
gastropexy	surgical fixation of the stomach
gastroplasty	surgical reconstruction of the stomach
gastroscope	instrument for looking at the stomach
gastroscopy	procedure for looking at the stomach
gingival hyperplasia	overformation of gum tissue
gingivalgia	gum pain
gingivectomy	surgical removal of gum tissue
gingivitis	inflammation of the gums
gingivoglossitis	inflammation of the gums and tongue
gingivoplasty	surgical reconstruction of gum tissue
gingivostomatitis	inflammation of the mouth and gums
glossopathy	disease of the tongue
glossoplasty	surgical reconstruction of the tongue
glossoplegia	paralysis of the tongue
glossorrhaphy	suture of the tongue
glossotomy	incision into the tongue
glossotrichia	overdevelopment of bumps on the tongue, making the tongue appear to be hairy

quick reference glossary of terms *continued*

Term	Definition
hematemesis	vomiting blood
hemicolectomy	surgical removal of half (a portion) of the colon
hemorrhoid	inflammation of the veins surrounding the anus
hemorrhoidectomy	surgical removal of hemorrhoids
hepatectomy	surgical removal of the liver
hepaticogastrostomy	creation of an opening between the liver and the stomach
hepaticotomy	incision into the liver
hepatitis	inflammation of the liver
hepatocarcinoma	cancerous tumor of the liver
hepatoma	tumor of the liver
hepatomalacia	softening of the liver
hepatomegaly	enlargement of the liver
hepatopexy	surgical fixation of the liver
hepatoptosis	downward displacement of the liver
hepatosclerosis	hardening of the liver
hernia	rupture or protrusion of an organ through the wall that normally contains it
herniorrhaphy	suture of a hernia
hyperemesis	excessive vomiting
hypochondriac	upper side portions of the abdomen
hypogastric	lower center portion of the abdomen
icterus	another name for jaundice
ileitis	inflammation of the ileum
ileocolitis	inflammation of the ileum and colon
ileocolostomy	creation of an opening between the ileum and colon
ileorrhaphy	suture of the ileum
ileostomy	creation of an opening in the ileum
ileotomy	incision into the ileum
inguinal	lower side portions of the abdomen
jaundice (icterus)	yellowing of skin, tissue, and fluids caused by increased levels of bilirubin in the blood
jejunitis	inflammation of the jejunum
jejunoileitis	inflammation of the jejunum and ileum

quick reference glossary of terms *continued*

Term	Definition
jejunorrhaphy	suture of the jejunum
jejunostomy	creation of an opening in the jejunum
jejunotomy	incision into the jejunum
laparocele	abdominal hernia
laparoenterostomy	creation of an opening between the abdomen and the intestines
laparoscope	instrument for looking inside the abdomen
laparoscopic surgery	use of a laparoscope to perform minimally invasive surgery
laparoscopy	procedure for looking inside the abdomen
laparotomy	incision into the abdomen
lumbar	middle side portions of the abdomen
nasogastric tube	tube inserted through the nose into the stomach
odontalgia	tooth pain
odontectomy	surgical removal of a tooth
odontoclasis	breaking of a tooth
odontodynia	tooth pain
orthodontics	branch of medicine dealing with the straightening of teeth
orthodontist	specialist in straightening teeth
pancreatectomy	surgical removal of the pancreas
pancreatitis	inflammation of the pancreas
pancreatoduodenectomy	surgical removal of the pancreas and duodenum
pancreatography	procedure for mapping the pancreas
pancreatolith	stone in the pancreas
pancreatolithectomy	surgical removal of stones in the pancreas
pancreatolithiasis	presence of a stone in the pancreas
periodontitis	inflammation of region around the teeth
peritoneoscopy	procedure for looking at the peritoneum
peritonitis	inflammation of the peritoneum
proctitis	inflammation of the anus and rectum
proctologist	specialist in the anus, rectum, and colon
proctology	branch of medicine dealing with the anus, rectum, and colon
proctoplasty	surgical reconstruction of the anus and rectum
proctoptosis	downward displacement of the rectum and anus
proctoscope	instrument for looking at the anus and rectum

quick reference glossary of terms *continued*

Term	Definition
proctoscopy	procedure for looking at the anus and rectum
pyloric stenosis	narrowing of the sphincter at the base of the stomach
rectalgia	rectum pain
rectitis	inflammation of the rectum
rectopexy	surgical fixation of the rectum
sclerosing cholangitis	inflammation and hardening of the bile vessels (ducts)
sialagogic	agent that causes salivation
sialoadenectomy	surgical removal of a salivary gland
sialoadenitis	inflammation of the salivary glands
sialoadenosis	condition of the salivary glands
sialoangiectasis	overexpansion of the salivary vessels
sialolith	stone in the saliva
sialolithiasis	presence of salivary stones
sialolithotomy	incision to remove salivary stones
sialorrhea	excessive salivation
sialostenosis	narrowing of the salivary glands
sigmoidoscope	instrument for looking at the sigmoid colon
sigmoidoscopy	procedure for looking at the sigmoid colon
steatorrhea	excessive fat discharged in the feces
stomatitis	inflammation of the mouth
stomatodynia	mouth pain
stomatogastric	pertaining to the mouth and stomach
stomatomycosis	fungus condition of the mouth
stomatoplasty	surgical reconstruction of the mouth
stomatosis	mouth condition
ulcerative colitis	inflammation of the colon, characterized by ulcers
umbilical	middle center portion of the abdomen

review of terms by roots

Root	Term(s)	
abdomin/o	abdominocentesis	
	abdominoplasty	
an/o	anal fistula	anoplasty
	anophony	anosigmoidoscopy
bil/i	biligenesis	
celi/o	celiac disease	celiopathy
	celiomyositis	celiotomy
chol/e	cholangiogram	choledochoenterostomy
	cholangiography	choledocholithectomy
	cholangioma	choledocholithiasis
	cholangiopancreatography	choledochotomy
	cholangitis	cholelith
	choleangiogastrostomy	cholelithiasis
	cholecystalgia	cholelithotomy
	cholecystectomy	cholelithotripsy
	cholecystitis	cholemesis
	cholecystogram	sclerosing cholangitis
	choledochocele	
col/o, colon/o	colectomy	gastroenterocolitis
	colitis	hemicolectomy
	colonoscopy	ileocolitis
	colorectal carcinoma	ileocolostomy
	colostomy	ulcerative colitis
	colovaginal fistula	
cyst/o	cholecystalgia	cholecystitis
	cholecystectomy	cholecystogram
dent/o	dentalgia	dentist
	dentifrice	dentistry
doch/o	choledochocele	choledocholithiasis
	choledochoenterostomy	choledochotomy
	choledocholithectomy	
duoden/o	duodenectomy	gastroduodenostomy
	duodenitis	pancreatoduodenectomy
	esophagogastroduodenoscopy	

review of terms by roots *continued*

Root	Term(s)	
enter/o	choledochoenterostomy	enterotomy
	dysentery	gastroenteritis
	enterectomy	gastroenterocolitis
	enterocele	gastroenterologist
	enterodynia	gastroenterology
	enteropathy	gastroenterostomy
	enterorrhaphy	laparoenterostomy
esophag/o	esophagalgia	esophagogastroplasty
	esophageal carcinoma	esophagogastroduodenoscopy
	esophagectomy	esophagoscopy
	esophagitis	gastroesophageal reflux disease (GERD)
gastr/o	cholangiogastrostomy	gastroenterostomy
	epigastric	gastroesophageal reflux disease (GERD)
	esophagogastroduodenoscopy	gastrojejunostomy
	esophagogastroplasty	gastromalacia
	gastralgia	gastroparesis
	gastrectomy	gastropexy
	gastritis	gastroplasty
	gastroduodenostomy	gastroscope
	gastrodynia	gastroscopy
	gastroenteritis	hepaticogastrostomy
	gastroenterocolitis	hypogastric
	gastroenterologist	nasogastric tube
	gastroenterology	stomatogastric
gingiv/o	gingival hyperplasia	gingivoglossitis
	gingivalgia	gingivoplasty
	gingivectomy	gingivostomatitis
	gingivitis	
gloss/o	gingivoglossitis	glossorrhaphy
	glossopathy	glossotomy
	glossoplasty	glossotrichia
	glossoplegia	

review of terms by roots *continued*

Root	Term(s)	
hepat/o	hepatectomy	hepatomalacia
	hepaticogastrostomy	hepatomegaly
	hepaticotomy	hepatopexy
	hepatitis	hepatoptosis
	hepatocarcinoma	hepatosclerosis
	hepatoma	
ile/o	ileitis	ileostomy
	ileocolitis	ileotomy
	ileocolostomy	jejunoileitis
	ileorrhaphy	
jejun/o	gastrojejunostomy	jejunorrhaphy
	jejunitis	jejunostomy
	jejunoileitis	jejunotomy
lapar/o	laparocele	laparoscopic surgery
	laparoenterostomy	laparoscopy
	laparoscope	laparotomy
odont/o	aerodontalgia	odontodynia
	odontalgia	orthodontics
	odontectomy	orthodontist
	odontoclasis	periodontitis
pancreat/o	cholangiopancreatography	pancreatography
	pancreatectomy	pancreatolith
	pancreatitis	pancreatolithectomy
	pancreatoduodenectomy	pancreatolithiasis
peritone/o	peritoneoscopy	
	peritonitis	
proct/o	proctitis	proctoptosis
	proctologist	proctoscope
	proctology	proctoscopy
	proctoplasty	
rect/o	colorectal carcinoma	rectitis
	rectalgia	rectopexy
sial/o	sialagogic	sialolith
	sialoadenectomy	sialolithiasis

review of terms by roots *continued*

Root	Term(s)	
	sialoadenitis	sialolithotomy
	sialoadenosis	sialorrhea
	sialoangiectasis	sialostenosis
sigmoid/o	anosigmoidoscopy	sigmoidoscopy
	sigmoidoscope	
stomat/o	anastomosis	jejunostomy
	choledochoenterostomy	laparoenterostomy
	colostomy	stomatitis
	gastroduodenostomy	stomatodynia
	gastroenterostomy	stomatogastric
	gastrojejunostomy	stomatomycosis
	gingivostomatitis	stomatoplasty
	hepaticogastrostomy	stomatosis
	ileocolostomy	
	ileostomy	

other terms

antacid	fistula
antiemetic	flatus
aphagia	hematemesis
ascites	hemorrhoid
bariatrics	hemorrhoidectomy
cathartic	hernia
cirrhosis	herniorrhaphy
constipation	hyperemesis
diarrhea	hypochondriac
diverticulitis	icterus
diverticulosis	inguinal
dyspepsia	jaundice (icterus)
endoscope	lumbar
endoscopy	pyloric stenosis
eupepsia	steatorrhea
fecal occult blood test (FOBT)	umbilical

The Urinary and Male Reproductive Systems—Urology

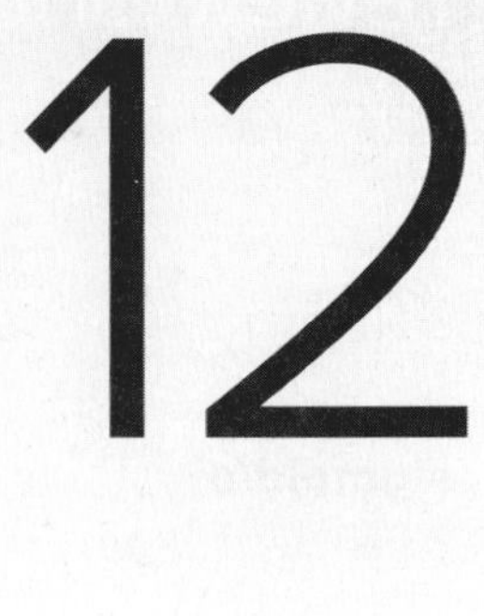

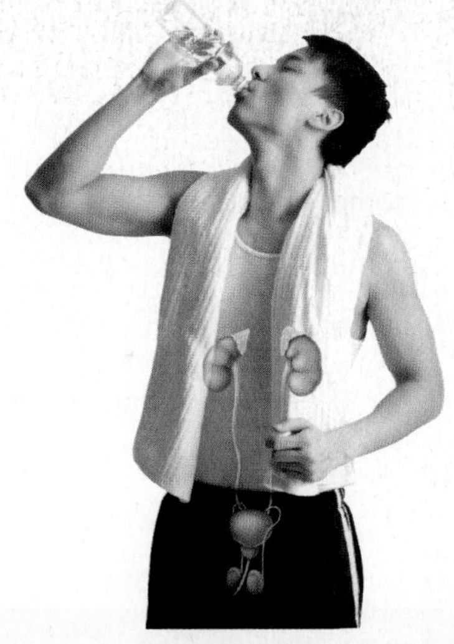

©Asia selects/Getty Images RF

learning outcomes

Upon completion of this chapter, you will be able to:

12.1 Identify the **roots/word parts** associated with the **urinary system.**

12.2 Identify the **roots/word parts** associated with the **male reproductive system.**

(S) **12.3** Translate the **Subjective** terms associated with the **urinary and male reproductive systems.**

(O) **12.4** Translate the **Objective** terms associated with the **urinary and male reproductive systems.**

(A) **12.5** Translate the **Assessment** terms associated with the **urinary and male reproductive systems.**

(P) **12.6** Translate the **Plan** terms associated with the **urinary and male reproductive systems.**

12.7 Use **abbreviations** associated with the **urinary and male reproductive systems.**

12.8 Distinguish terms associated with the **urinary and male reproductive systems** in the context of **electronic health records.**

Introduction and Overview of the Urinary and Male Reproductive Systems

So far, we have addressed body systems that are identical in men and women. What separates the sexes, of course, is their reproductive systems. Both men and women produce half the blueprints for new life, which are found in *sperm* and *eggs.* The reproductive systems are responsible for making these code carriers and also for helping to bring the two together.

In medicine, the male and female reproductive systems are cared for by different specialties. The next two chapters deal with those specialties. This chapter deals with the specialty of *urology.* Since the male reproductive system shares structures with the urinary system, urology deals with both the urinary tract and the male reproductive system. The next chapter deals with the specialty of *obstetrics* and *gynecology,* which focuses specifically on the female reproductive system.

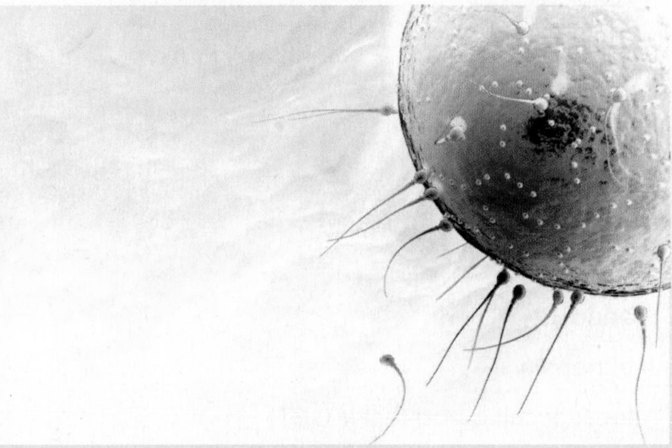

Sperm attempting to fertilize an egg.

©MedicalRF.com/Getty Images, RF

12.1 Word Parts of the Urinary System

Many homes and businesses have aquariums. People enjoy watching fish swim peacefully around in the water. In fact, some studies have shown that watching fish in an aquarium can lower a person's blood pressure.

While the fish are the main attraction, a great deal of hard work goes into keeping the water in their tank just right. The water must be cleaned and maintained with a balance of chemicals to keep a safe and clean environment for the fish to live in. Otherwise, the water becomes unsuitable for life.

The kidneys, the unsung heroes of the body, perform a similar function for the blood. The cells of the body are in constant contact with the blood, just like fish are always in contact with the water in an aquarium. Cells require just the right balance of pH, minerals, water, and sugar, and the kidneys monitor and regulate these levels. If they did not perform their job, blood would soon become toxic.

The basic working unit of the kidney is called the *nephron.* There are more than two million nephrons in a single kidney. Blood passes through the kidneys into a cluster of small blood vessels known as the *glomerulus.* Here, the blood is filtered, with water and nutrients being forced into the surrounding capsule around the glomerulus. This filtered liquid (filtrate) then flows through a series of small tubes.

These tubes flow next to blood vessels. As the filtrate passes through this series of tubes, much of the water and nutrients in it are reabsorbed back into the bloodstream. At the same time, the remaining unfiltered waste is forced into the last part of the tubes.

These tubes containing waste dump into a basin known as the *renal pelvis.* Long vessels from each kidney, called *ureters,* drain these collecting areas into the *bladder,* a large holding bag for urine. When the bladder becomes full, a signal is sent to the muscle that is holding the urine in the bladder. When this muscle relaxes, the urine empties out of the body through the *urethra.*

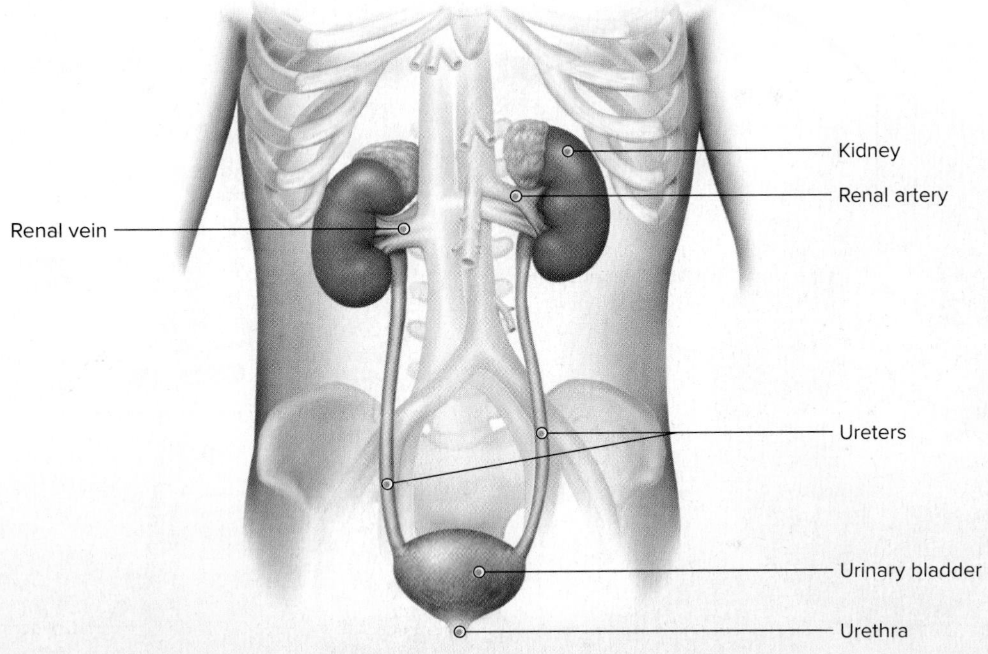

glomerulus (plural: glomeruli)

ROOT: ***glomerul/o***

EXAMPLES: glomerulopathy, glomerulonephritis

NOTES: *Glomerulus* comes from a Latin word meaning "little ball" and refers to the little balls of blood vessels inside the kidney. These serve as the primary place for filtering the blood to form urine.

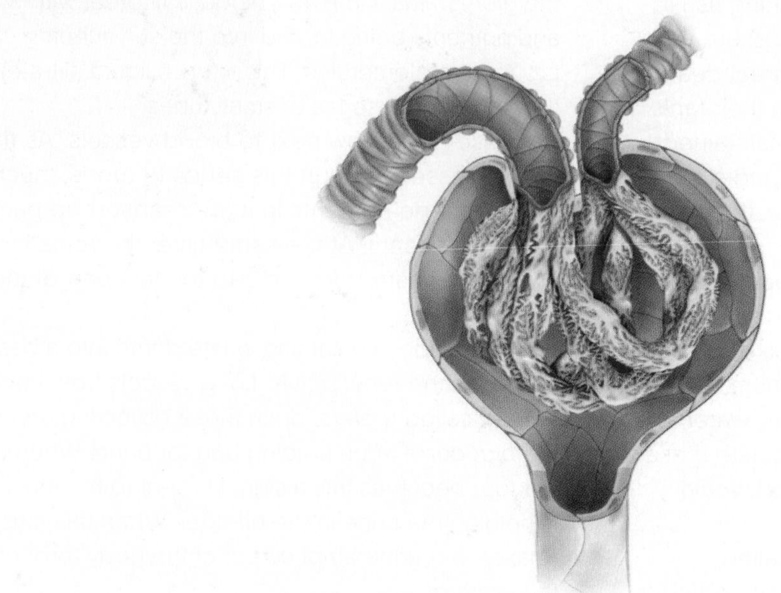

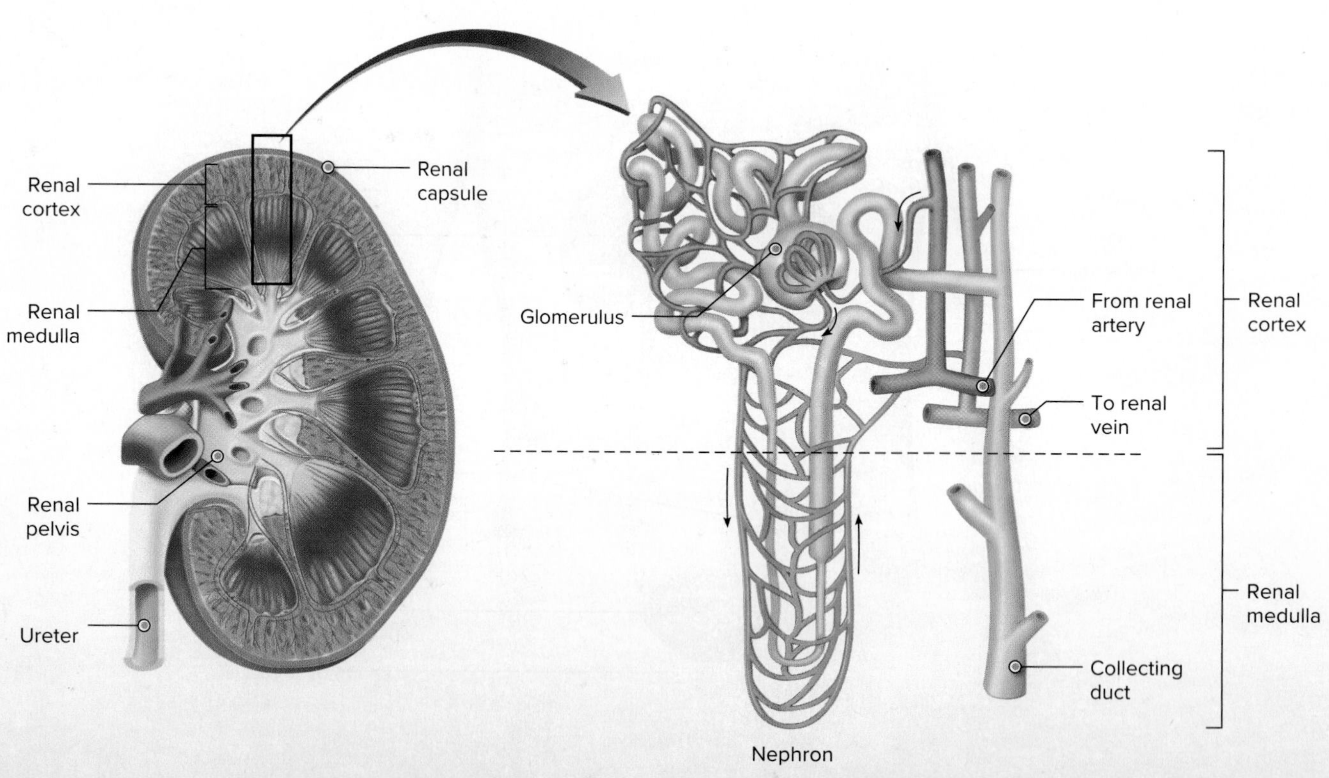

kidney

ROOTS: ***nephr/o, ren/o***

EXAMPLES: nephrology, nephritis, renal failure

NOTES: Kidneys perform the necessary task of filtering the blood—at a rate of 200 quarts per day. If you lose or donate a kidney, your remaining kidney can adjust and perform the work of two by increasing the amount it filters and by increasing in size. If you are born with only one kidney, your kidney may grow to be the size of two normal kidneys.

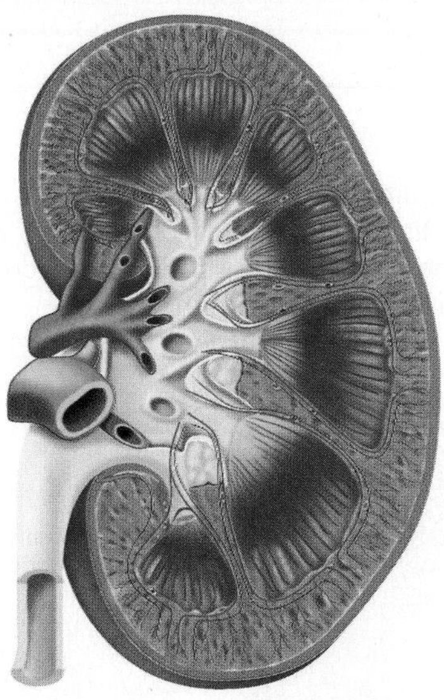

renal pelvis

ROOT: ***pyel/o***

EXAMPLES: pyelonephritis, pyelitis

NOTES: *Pyelo* is a root meaning "pelvis." There are two things that the word *pelvis* can apply to: the *skeletal pelvis,* which is where your legs and your spine attach to one another; and the *renal pelvis,* which is a series of tubes that funnel urine out of the kidneys and into the ureters and on to the bladder. *Pyelo* is used most commonly for the renal pelvis.

urine

ROOTS: ***ur/o, urin/o***

EXAMPLES: urology, hematuria

NOTES: Healthy urine is completely sterile and contains ammonia molecules. This latter fact led the ancient Romans to use urine in two odd ways: to wash clothes (in fact, Romans set up large urinals outside laundries to gather urine free of charge) and to whiten teeth. It served both functions really well . . . but *gross.*

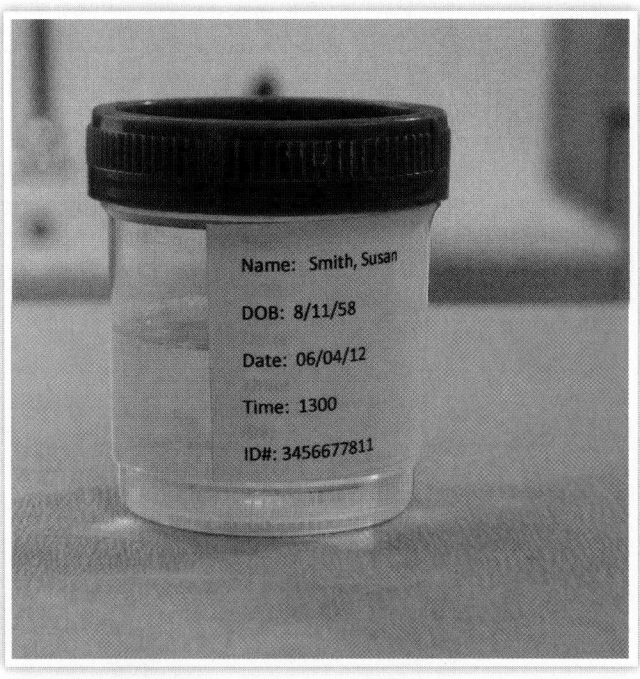

©McGraw-Hill Education

stone

ROOT: ***lith/o***

EXAMPLES: lithiasis, lithotripsy

NOTES: Kidney stones aren't "stones"; instead, they are accumulations of mineral salts and calcium. To make sure people don't mistakenly think they are little rocks, health care professionals sometimes translate *litho* as *calculus,* a Latin word meaning—you guessed it—"little rocks."

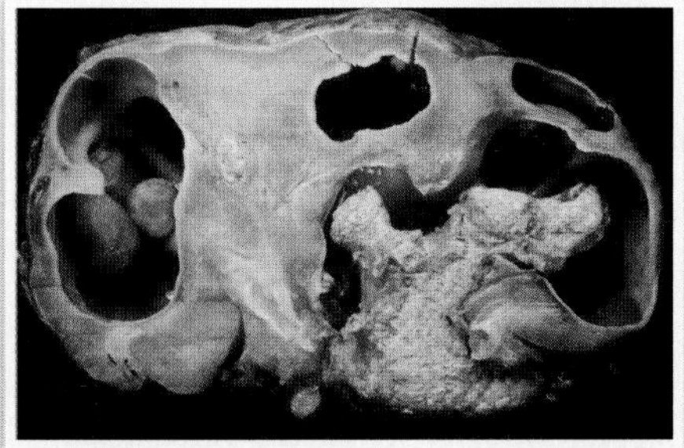

©Biophoto Associates/Science Source

bladder

ROOTS: ***cyst/o, vesic/o***

EXAMPLES: cystotomy, cystitis, vesiculotomy, vesiculitis

NOTES: When completely full, the urinary bladder is roughly the size of a softball and can hold about 18 ounces of liquid. But it rarely reaches capacity. When the bladder is only about a quarter full, most people can't "hold it" anymore and feel an urgent need to urinate.

urethra

ROOT: ***urethr/o***

EXAMPLES: urethrostenosis, urethritis

NOTES: The length of the urethra differs depending on sex. The average male urethra is about 8 inches long, and the average female urethra is 1.5 to 2 inches long. This difference is sometimes mentioned as the reason why kidney stones are more painful for men than women; in fact, some say that the pain of kidney stones is the closest men can come to the pain of giving birth. Others argue that men are just big babies. You be the judge.

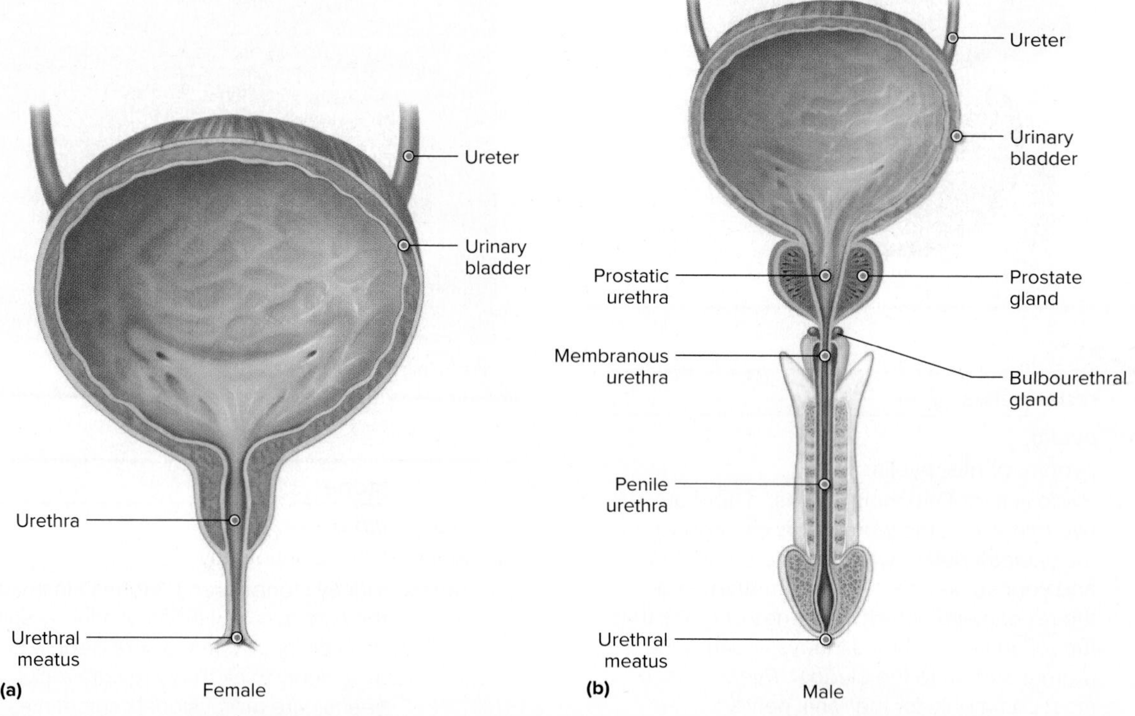

ureter

ROOT: ***ureter/o***

EXAMPLES: ureterocele, ureterectomy

NOTES: *Ureters* are the thick-walled tubes about 10 inches in length that carry urine from the kidneys to the bladder. Don't confuse ureters with the *urethra,* a tube that runs from the bladder to the outside world. You have two ureters, but only one urethra.

opening

ROOT: ***meat/o***

EXAMPLES: meatoscope, meatal stenosis

NOTES: *Meatus* comes from a word meaning "to go through"; it means "opening." The English word *permeate* comes from the same term. There are meatuses in several places in the body: nasal meatuses, aural meatuses, and a urethral meatus.

Learning Outcome 12.1 Exercises

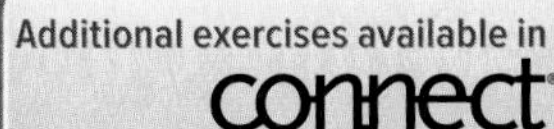

TRANSLATION

EXERCISE 1 *Translate the following roots.*

1. ureter/o ______
2. urethr/o ______
3. urin/o ______
4. lith/o ______
5. glomerul/o ______
6. nephr/o ______
7. ur/o ______
8. cyst/o ______
9. vesic/o ______
10. ren/o ______
11. pyel/o ______
12. meat/o ______

EXERCISE 2 *Match the root on the left with its definition on the right. Some definitions will be used more than once.*

______	1. cyst/o	a.	bladder
______	2. vesic/o	b.	comes from a word meaning "to go through"
______	3. ur/o	c.	from Latin, for "little ball"; refers to little balls of blood vessels inside the kidney that serve as the primary place for filtering the blood to form urine
______	4. pyel/o	d.	organ that filters the blood
______	5. glomerul/o	e.	series of tubes that funnel urine out of the kidneys and into the ureter and on to the bladder
______	6. ren/o	f.	thick-walled tubes about 10 inches in length that carry urine from the kidneys to the bladder
______	7. ureter/o	g.	urine
______	8. meat/o		

EXERCISE 3 *Underline and define the roots from this chapter in the following terms.*

1. glucosuria ______
2. cystodynia ______
3. ureterocele ______
4. urethroscopy ______
5. renal angiogram ______
6. pyelogram ______
7. vesicocele ______
8. meatal stenosis ______
9. uroxanthin ______
10. glomerulosclerosis ______
11. laparonephrectomy ______
12. cystolithectomy (2 roots) ______
13. nephroureterectomy (2 roots) ______

Learning Outcome 12.1 Exercises

EXERCISE 4 *Fill in the blanks.*

1. ureteralgia: pain in the ______
2. urethroplasty: surgical reconstruction of the ______
3. nephralgia: pain in the ______
4. lithectomy: removal of a(n) ______
5. glomerulopathy: disease of the ______
6. cystalgia: pain in the ______
7. uropathy: disease of the ______
8. meatoscope: device for examining the ______ of the urethra
9. pyeloplasty: surgical reconstruction of the ______
10. renal ischemia: deficiency of blood in the ______

EXERCISE 5 *Break down the following words into their component parts and translate.*

EXAMPLE: sinusitis *sinus | itis* *inflammation of the sinuses*

1. urologist ______
2. ureteroplasty ______
3. urethrectomy ______
4. cystostomy ______
5. nephrologist ______
6. renal failure ______
7. pyeloplasty ______
8. vesicotomy ______
9. meatotomy ______
10. nephrolithotomy ______

GENERATION

EXERCISE 6 *Identify the roots for the following definitions.*

1. ureter ______
2. urethra ______
3. glomerulus ______
4. stone ______
5. opening ______
6. urine (2 roots) ______
7. bladder (2 roots) ______
8. kidney (2 roots) ______

Learning Outcome 12.1 Exercises

EXERCISE 7 *Build a medical term from the information provided.*

EXAMPLE: inflammation of the sinuses *sinusitis*

1. inflammation of the bladder (use *cyst/o*) ____________________
2. inflammation of the kidney (use *nephr/o*) ____________________
3. inflammation of the urethra ____________________
4. inflammation of the ureter ____________________
5. inflammation of the renal pelvis ____________________
6. inflammation of a stone in the kidney (use *nephr/o*) ____________________
7. inflammation of the glomerulus and kidney (use *nephr/o*) ____________________
8. inflammation of the renal pelvis and bladder (use *cyst/o*) ____________________
9. inflammation of the urethra and bladder (use *cyst/o*) ____________________
10. inflammation of the bladder and ureter (use *cyst/o*) ____________________
11. inflammation of the ureter and renal pelvis ____________________
12. stone in the bladder (use *cyst/o*) ____________________
13. surgical reconstruction of the opening (of the urethra) ____________________

12.2 Word Parts of the Male Reproductive System

The male reproductive system shares structures with the urinary system. For this reason, *urologists* deal with both urinary tract problems and male genital problems. The male reproductive system is made up of the *testicles,* the *epididymis,* the *seminiferous tubules,* the *prostate gland,* and the *penis.*

The structures of the male genital system can be divided by their function into three categories: those that make and store *sperm,* those that make special carrier fluid for sperm, and the outer parts. The first category makes and stores sperm. Each sperm carries half of the blueprint for a human life (23 chromosomes). The organ that makes these blueprint carriers is called a *gonad.* The male gonads are testicles and the female gonads are the *ovaries.*

In addition to making sperm, the testicles also produce *testosterone,* the male hormone that causes male character traits like muscle growth and facial hair. While sperm cells are made in the testicles, they are stored in the *epididymis.* During sexual intercourse, the sperm cells travel out of the epididymis via ducts called the *vas*

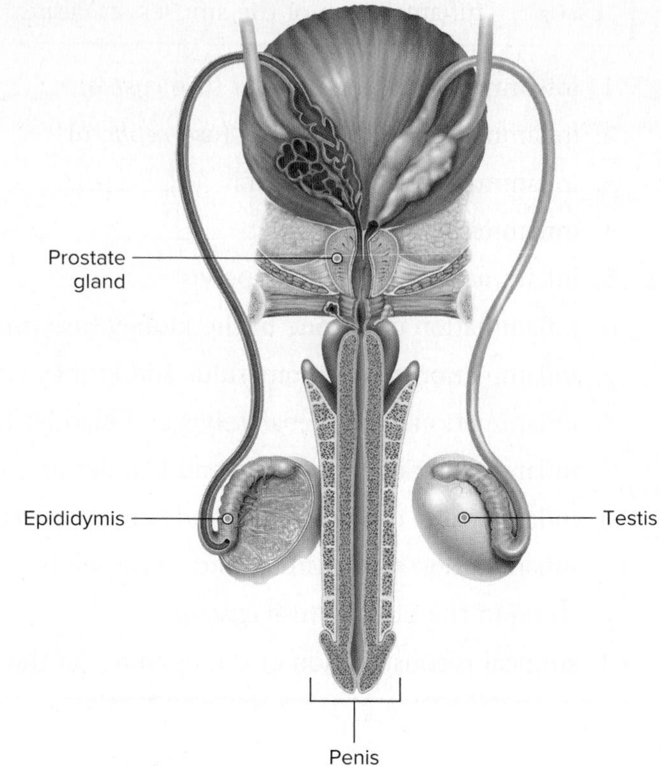

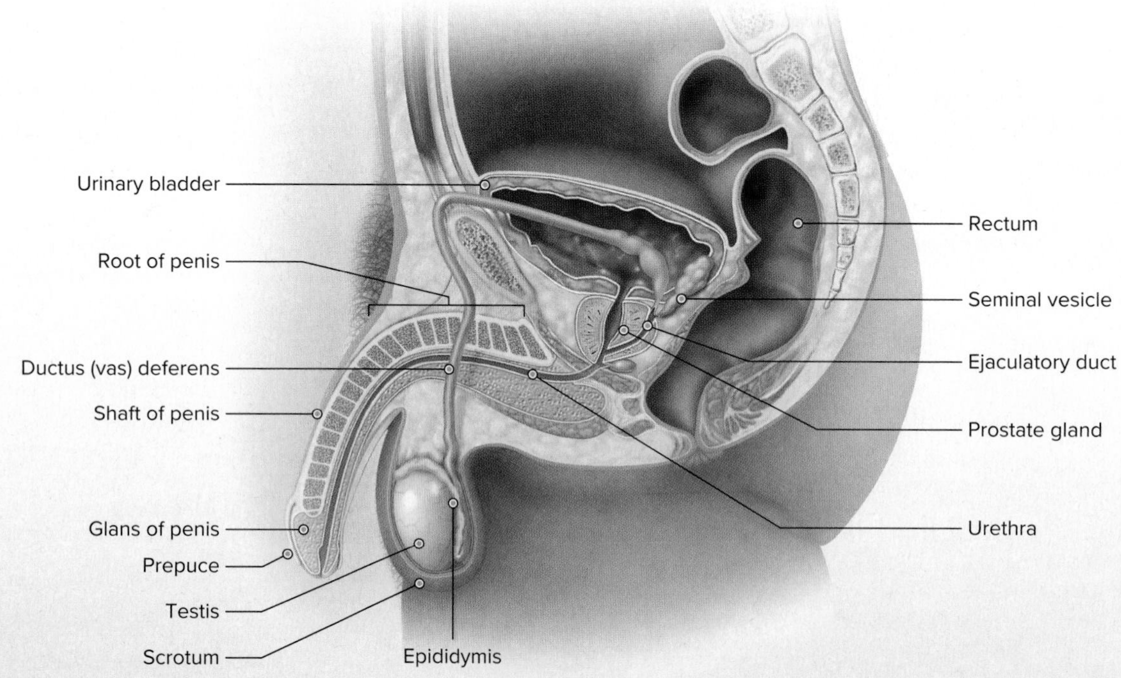

deferens. Sperm cells mix with a carrier fluid known as *semen.*

The majority of this fluid is made in the *seminal vesicles* and the prostate gland. At climax, the semen is ejected out of the body (*ejaculation*) through the penis.

The third category of structures is the visible parts of the male reproductive system: the penis and the *scrotum.* These are also known as the male *genitals.* The penis is the organ for directing urine and sperm outside the body, and the scrotum is the external sac that holds the testicles in place outside the body.

penis

ROOT: ***balan/o***

EXAMPLES: balanorrhea, balanitis

NOTES: The root *balano* comes from a Greek word meaning "acorn"; this is an allusion to the shape of the tip of the penis. It was also the word the Greeks used to refer to a deadbolt lock on a door.

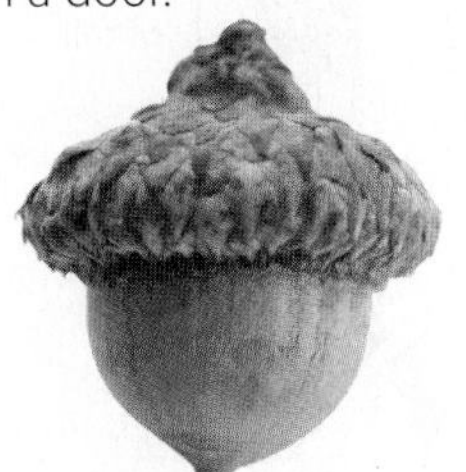

©Enigma/Alamy Stock Photo RF

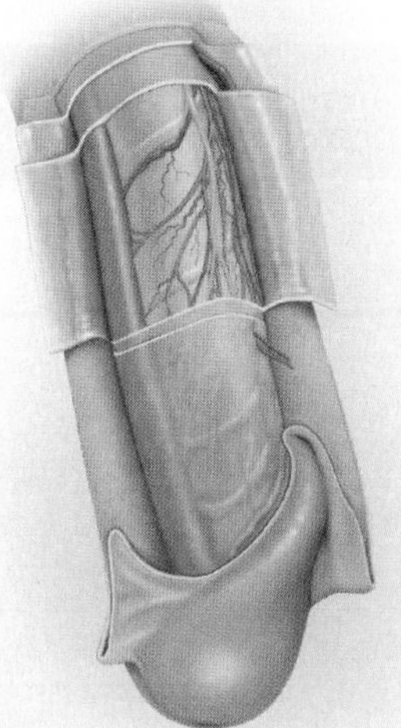

epididymis

ROOT: ***epididym/o***

EXAMPLES: epididymotomy, epididymectomy

NOTES: The *epididymis,* an oblong organ that sits on top of each testicle, is the place where sperm cells complete their final level of development and are stored. Interestingly, the root *didymis* means "twins," so the name of this organ is literally "upon the twins."

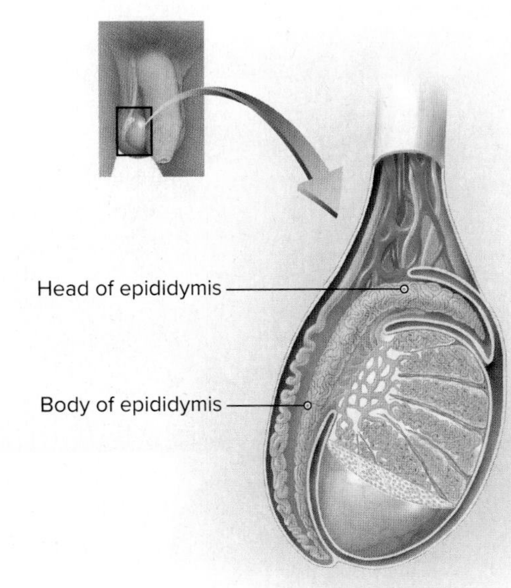

testicle

ROOTS: ***orch/o, orchi/o, orchid/o, test/o, testicul/o***

EXAMPLES: orchitis, orchiopexy, anorchidism, testitis

NOTES: You likely noticed right away that one of the main roots for *testicle* is similar to the word *orchid.* Believe or not, the flower is named for the organ, and not the other way around. The plant was called an *orchid* because some believed that its roots looked like a pair of testicles.

prostate

ROOT: ***prostat/o***

EXAMPLES: prostatitis, prostatomegaly

NOTES: The *prostate* is an organ in the male reproductive tract that surrounds the urethra. The name *prostate* breaks down into *pro* (before) and *state* (stand) and literally translates to mean "the one that stands before or in front of." It was so named because of its position in front of the urinary bladder.

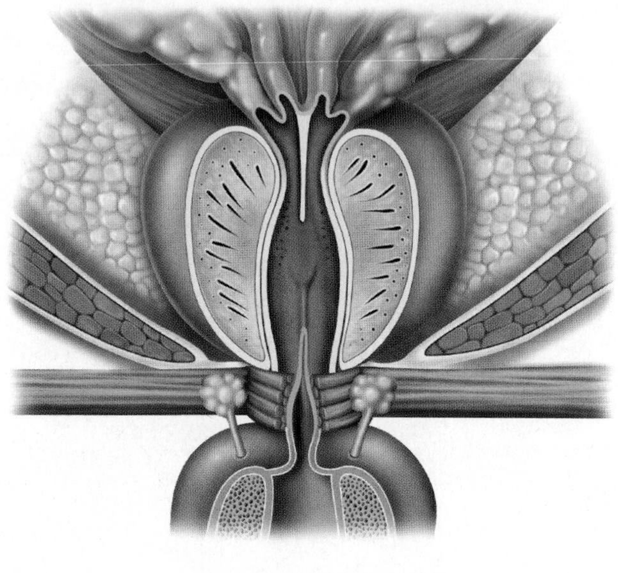

sperm

ROOTS: ***sperm/o, spermat/o, sperm/i***

EXAMPLES: aspermia, spermicide, spermatocele

NOTES: *Sperm* (from Greek, for "seed") is produced in the testicles. It takes roughly 10 weeks to produce a single sperm. Sperm can sit in the epididymis for as long as 2 weeks before being ejaculated. These sperm can survive in the female reproductive tract for as long as 5 days. Because the male's sperm determines the sex of a baby, sperm can be either male or female. Male sperm are faster swimmers, but weaker. Female sperm are slower, but stronger.

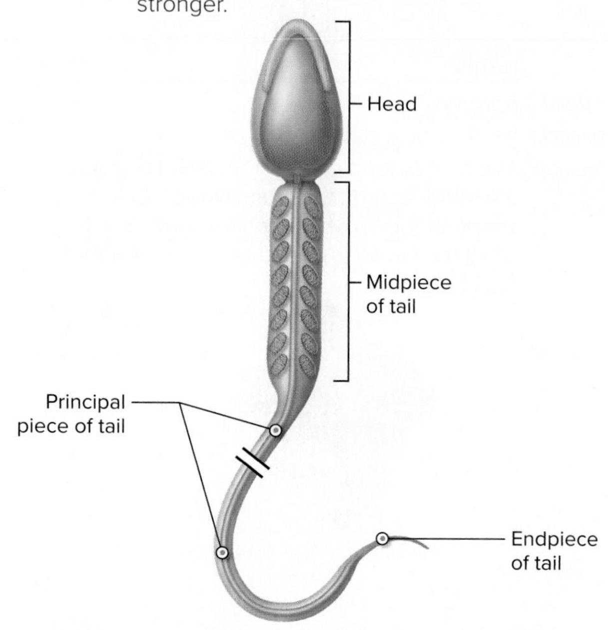

Learning Outcome 12.2 Exercises

TRANSLATION

EXERCISE 1 *Translate the following roots.*

1. prostat/o ______
2. test/o ______
3. spermat/o ______
4. epididym/o ______
5. orchid/o ______
6. orch/o ______
7. balan/o ______

Learning Outcome 12.2 Exercises

EXERCISE 2 *Match the root on the left with its definition on the right. Some definitions will be used more than once.*

_____ 1. test/o

_____ 2. prostat/o

_____ 3. sperm/o

_____ 4. balan/o

_____ 5. orchi/o

_____ 6. epididym/o

a. organ in the male reproductive tract surrounding the urethra; the name literally translates into "the one that stands before or in front of"

b. from Greek, for "acorn," an allusion to the shape of its tip

c. from Greek, for "seed"; produced in the testicles

d. organ that sits on top of each testicle; the place where sperm cells complete their final level of development and are stored

e. testicle

EXERCISE 3 *Underline and define the roots from this chapter in the following terms.*

1. spermicide ________________
2. testicular carcinoma ________________
3. epididymectomy ________________
4. balanorrhea ________________
5. anorchidism ________________
6. prostatovesiculectomy (2 roots) ________________

EXERCISE 4 *Break down the words into their component parts and translate.*

EXAMPLE: sinusitis *sinus | itis* *inflammation of the sinuses*

1. epididymotomy ________________
2. orchidectomy ________________
3. orchiodynia ________________
4. prostatectomy ________________
5. aspermia ________________

GENERATION

EXERCISE 5 *Identify the roots for the following definitions.*

1. prostate ________________
2. epididymis ________________
3. penis ________________
4. sperm (2 roots) ________________
5. testicle (5 roots) ________________

Learning Outcome 12.2 Exercises

EXERCISE 6 *Fill in the blanks.*

1. testitis: inflammation of the ______________________
2. prostatorrhea: discharge from the ______________________
3. spermatogenesis: creation of ______________________
4. orchitis: inflammation of the ______________________
5. balanoplasty: surgical reconstruction of the ______________________
6. epididymo-orchitis: inflammation of the ______________________ and ______________________

EXERCISE 7 *Build a medical term from the information provided.*

1. inflammation of the testicle (use *orchid/o*) ______________________
2. inflammation of a testicle (use *test/o*) ______________________
3. inflammation of the prostate ______________________
4. inflammation of the epididymis ______________________
5. inflammation of the penis ______________________
6. inflammation of the prostate and bladder (use *cyst/o*) ______________________
7. inflammation of the testicle (use *orch/o*) and epididymis ______________________

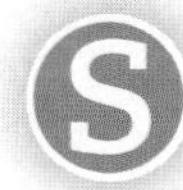
Subjective
Patient History, Problems, Complaints
Urinary tract
Male genitalia

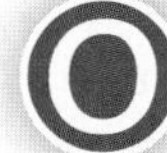
Objective
Observation and Discovery
Urinary tract
Diagnostic procedures
Professional terms
Male genitalia
Diagnostic procedures
Professional terms

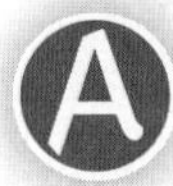
Assessment
Diagnosis and Pathology
Urinary tract
Male genitalia

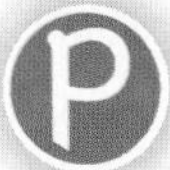
Plan
Treatments and Therapies
Urinary tract
Male genitalia

This section contains medical terms built from the roots presented in the previous section. The purpose of this section is to expose you to words used in urology that are built from the word roots presented earlier. The focus of this book is to teach you the process of learning roots and translating them in context. Each term is presented with the correct pronunciation, followed by a word analysis that breaks down the word into its component parts, a definition that provides a literal translation of the word, as well as supplemental information if the literal translation deviates from its medical use.

The terms are organized using a health care professional's SOAP note (first introduced in Chapter 2) as a model.

SUBJECTIVE

12.3 Patient History, Problems, Complaints

Patients with urinary system problems frequently seek medical care with one of two types of problems: pain or problems with urinating. Pain is a very common symptom of infections of the urinary system.

Pain with urination (*dysuria*) is the most common symptom of an infection in the urinary tract. A simple urinary tract infection also may cause pain in the bladder (*cystalgia*). If the infection spreads to the kidney(s), the patient may have kidney pain (*nephralgia*). Severe kidney pain that comes in waves (*renal colic*) is a very good indicator of a kidney stone. The urethra is also a common source of pain (*urethralgia*) when infected or irritated by chemicals. Difficulty with urination may present with inability to hold urine in (*incontinence, enuresis*). Patients may also urinate too frequently (*polyuria*) or not enough (*oliguria*). Complete lack of urination (*anuria*) is a serious symptom that represents either a blockage or kidney failure. A patient's urine itself may be a concern, as he or she may notice blood (*hematuria*) or pus (*pyuria*) in the urine.

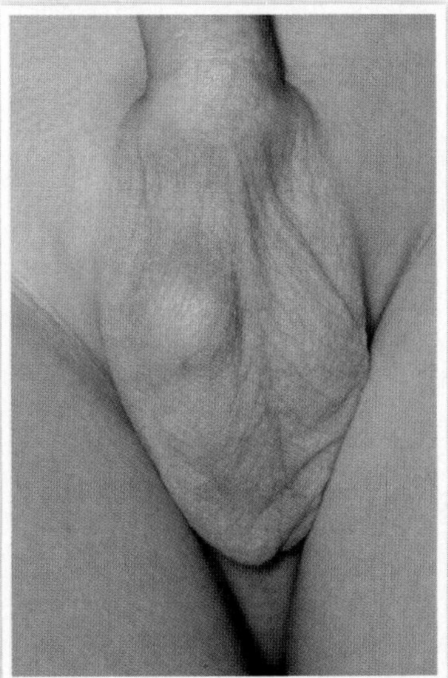

Though a patient might notice only one testicle, usually a medical exam is required to determine whether the missing testicle is not there *(anorchidism)* or is hidden *(cryptorchidism)*.

12.3 Patient History, Problems, Complaints

Male patients may have special genitourinary issues that are unique to them. When genital pain is a concern, the testicle (*orchialgia, orchiodynia*) is the most common site. Male patients may also have problems with erections. They can be painful and prolonged (*priapism*) or may not last long enough for sexual intercourse (*impotence*). Finally, a male patient may have concerns with penile discharge (*balanorrhea, urethrorrhea*). This is often an indicator of a sexually transmitted infection.

urinary tract

Term	Word Analysis
anuria an-YUR-ee-ah **Definition** lack of urination	**an / ur / ia** no / urine / condition
cystalgia sis-TAL-jah **Definition** pain in the bladder	**cyst / algia** bladder / pain
cystodynia SIS-toh-DAI-nee-ah **Definition** pain in the bladder	**cysto / dynia** bladder / pain
cystoplegia SIS-toh-PLEE-jah **Definition** bladder paralysis	**cysto / plegia** bladder / paralysis
dysuria dis-YUR-ee-ah **Definition** painful urination	**dys / ur / ia** bad / urine / condition
enuresis EN-yur-EE-sis **Definition** involutary urination	**from Greek, for** "to urinate"
hematuria HEE-mah-TUR-ee-ah **Definition** bloody urination	**hemat / ur / ia** blood / urine / condition
incontinence in-CON-tih-nentz **Definition** inability to control urination	**in / con / tinence** not / together / hold
nephralgia neh-FRAL-jah **Definition** pain in the kidney	**nephr / algia** kidney / pain
nocturia nok-TUR-ee-ah **Definition** nighttime urination	**noct / ur / ia** night / urine / condition
nocturnal enuresis nok-TIR-nal EN-yur-EE-sis **Definition** nighttime involuntary urination	**nocturnal enuresis** nighttime involuntary urination

12.3 Patient History, Problems, Complaints

urinary tract *continued*

Term	Word Analysis
oliguria aw-lih-GYIR-ee-ah **Definition** low urine output	**olig / ur / ia** few / urine / condition
polydipsia PAW-lee-DIP-see-ah **Definition** excessive thirst	**poly / dips / ia** many / thirst / condition
polyuria PAW-lee-YUR-ee-ah **Definition** excessive urination	**poly / ur / ia** many / urine / condition
pyuria pai-YUR-ee-ah **Definition** pus in the urine	**py / ur / ia** pus / urine / condition
ureteralgia yur-EE-ter-AL-jah **Definition** pain in the ureter	**ureter / algia** ureter / pain
urethrodynia yoo-REE-throh-DAI-nee-ah **Definition** pain in the urethra	**urethro / dynia** urethra / pain
urethrorrhea yoo-REE-throh-REE-ah **Definition** discharge from the urethra	**urethro / rrhea** urethra / discharge
urocyanosis YUR-oh-SAI-ah-NOH-sis **Definition** blue urine	**uro / cyan / osis** urine / blue / condition
urodynia YUR-oh-DAI-nee-ah **Definition** painful urination	**uro / dynia** urine / pain

male genitalia

Term	Word Analysis
balanorrhea BAL-ah-noh-REE-ah **Definition** discharge from the penis	**balano / rrhea** penis / discharge
orchialgia OR-kee-AL-jah **Definition** testicle pain	**orchi / algia** testicle / pain
orchidoptosis OR-kih-dop-TOH-sis **Definition** downward displacement of a testicle	**orchido / ptosis** testicle / drooping condition

12.3 Patient History, Problems, Complaints

male genitalia *continued*

Term	Word Analysis
orchiodynia OR-kee-oh-DIH-nee-ah **Definition** testicle pain	**orchio / dynia** testicle / pain
priapism PREE-ap-izm **Definition** persistent and painful erection	from ancient Greek, minor fertility god named Priapus, who is always shown with a large and permanently erect penis

Learning Outcome 12.3 Exercises

PRONUNCIATION

EXERCISE 1 *Indicate which syllable is emphasized when pronounced.*

EXAMPLE: bronchitis bron**chi**tis

1. polyuria ______
2. urodynia ______
3. pyuria ______
4. enuresis ______
5. orchialgia ______
6. ureteralgia ______
7. oliguria ______
8. orchiodynia ______
9. incontinence ______
10. cystalgia ______
11. nephralgia ______
12. nocturia ______
13. dysuria ______
14. priapism ______

TRANSLATION

EXERCISE 2 *Break down the following words into their component parts.*

EXAMPLE: nasopharyngoscope *naso | pharyngo | scope*

1. anuria ______
2. dysuria ______
3. nocturia ______
4. cystodynia ______
5. orchiodynia ______
6. urocyanosis ______
7. incontinence ______

Learning Outcome 12.3 Exercises

EXERCISE 3 *Underline and define the root from this chapter in the following terms.*

1. cystoplegia ______
2. urethrorrhea ______
3. balanorrhea ______
4. ureteralgia ______
5. nephralgia ______
6. orchidoptosis ______
7. enuresis ______

EXERCISE 4 *Match the term on the left with its definition on the right.*

______	1. incontinence	a.	bloody urination
______	2. hematuria	b.	inability to control urination
______	3. pyuria	c.	low urine output
______	4. nocturnal enuresis	d.	nighttime involuntary urination
______	5. oliguria	e.	pain in the bladder
______	6. cystodynia	f.	persistent and painful erection
______	7. priapism	g.	pus in the urine

EXERCISE 5 *Fill in the blanks.*

1. cystalgia: pain in the ______
2. orchialgia: pain in the ______
3. urethrodynia: pain in the ______
4. urodynia: pain in ______
5. polydipsia: excessive ______
6. polyuria: excessive ______

EXERCISE 6 *Translate the following terms as literally as possible.*

EXAMPLE: nasopharyngoscope *an instrument for looking at the nose and throat*

1. cystalgia ______
2. hematuria ______
3. oliguria ______
4. pyuria ______
5. urocyanosis ______
6. orchialgia ______

Learning Outcome 12.3 Exercises

GENERATION

EXERCISE 7 *Build a medical term from the information provided.*

EXAMPLE: inflammation of the sinuses *sinusitis*

1. pain in the ureter ______________________
2. discharge from the urethra ______________________
3. discharge from the penis ______________________
4. downward displacement of a testicle ______________________
5. bladder paralysis ______________________
6. pain in the kidney ______________________
7. nighttime urination ______________________

EXERCISE 8 *Briefly describe the difference between each pair of terms.*

1. urethrodynia, urodynia ______________________
2. anuria, dysuria ______________________
3. polydipsia, polyuria ______________________
4. enuresis, nocturnal enuresis ______________________
5. orchiodynia, priapism ______________________

OBJECTIVE

12.4 Observation and Discovery

When evaluating a patient with urinary concerns, the examiner will first need to determine whether the patient is alert and oriented. Kidney failure can cause confusion and delirium and may also cause swelling (*edema*) in the feet.

The abdominal exam may uncover pain in the lower abdomen (*suprapubic tenderness*), which may be an indication of inflammation of the bladder. Pain when pushing on the lower back (*costovertebral angle*) can warn of kidney infection.

When examining male patients, the examiner will inspect the head of the penis. Does the foreskin pull back normally, or is it stuck (*phimosis*)? The exam also includes visualizing the hole through which the urine comes out (*urethral meatus*). The hole may be too small (*meatal stenosis*) or in the wrong position (*hypospadias*).

A testicular exam includes ensuring that both testes are present in the scrotum. If one is absent, it could mean that the patient is missing a testicle (*anorchid*) or that the testicle is hidden (*cryptorchid*). Palpation of the testicles may reveal a mass, which could be fluid (*hydrocele*), misplaced intestines (*hernia*), or a tumor.

The last part of a urologist's physical exam is the insertion of a finger in the patient's anus to feel his prostate (*digital rectal exam*). While unpleasant, this exam is very important in detecting an enlarged prostate.

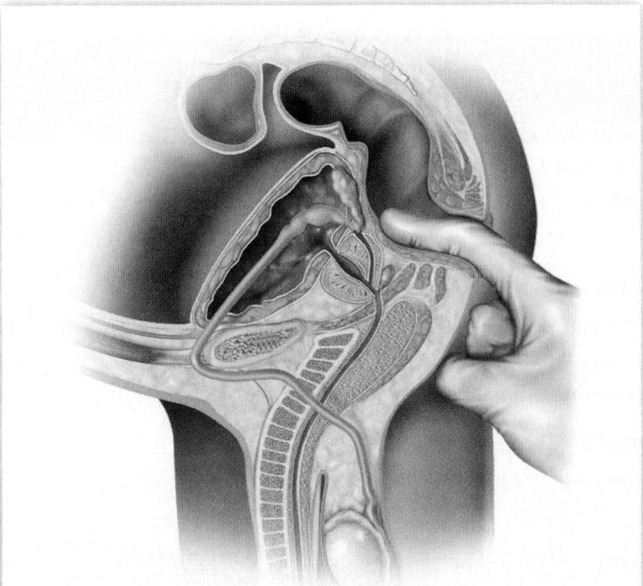

The principal way to examine the prostate is with a digital rectal exam (DRE).

Not surprisingly, laboratory testing for urinary problems focuses mostly on testing the urine directly (*urinalysis*). A routine urinalysis reveals a lot about a patient. For example, how concentrated the urine is reveals how well hydrated the patient is.

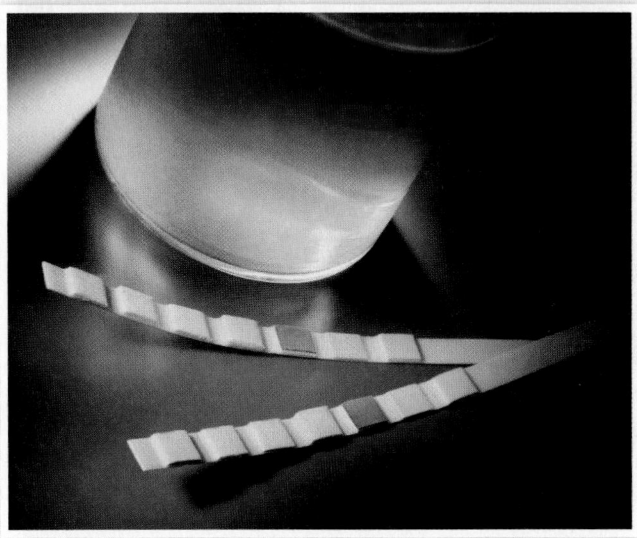

Test strips help in analyzing urine samples.

Urinalysis can also show things that are in the urine that don't belong there. Protein in the urine (*proteinuria*) is always abnormal. One specific protein that may show up in the urine is albumin (*albuminuria*). Protein spilling into the urine is a sign that the kidneys are not functioning properly. The presence of sugar (*glucosuria/glycosuria*) is also always abnormal; usually, sugar in the urine indicates that the patient has diabetes. If the patient's diabetes is severe or if he or she is dehydrated, the urine may include a by-product of fat breakdown called *ketones* (*ketonuria*). This can also happen in fasting states. Blood in the urine (*hematuria*) may not have been noticed by the patient but can be seen with lab testing. This type of hematuria is called *microscopic hematuria* (as opposed to *gross hematuria,* which can be seen by the naked eye).

When a patient's kidneys do not work properly, there may be some abnormalities in his or her blood work, too. The patient's blood may have high potassium (*hyperkalemia*) or low sodium (*hyponatremia*) levels. Also, the blood may have an overaccumulation of a waste product known as *blood urea nitrogen (BUN).* When the BUN is too high, the condition is called *azotemia.*

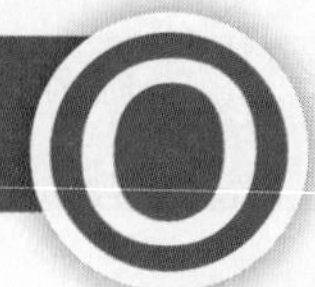

12.4 Observation and Discovery

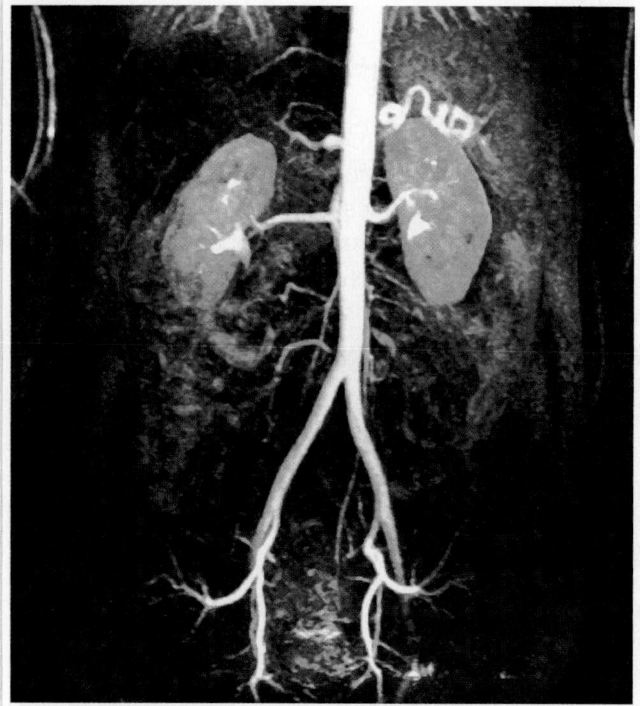

An image of the abdomen with the kidneys and bladder prominent.

There are also a few laboratory tests related to genital function. The main male-specific lab test in the field of urology is *sperm count,* a test of how many sperm cells are present in a patient's *semen.* This test can help detect low sperm counts (*oligospermia*) in an infertile male or confirm that there is no sperm (*aspermia, azoospermia*) in the semen of a patient who has undergone surgery to become sterile.

Sometimes, it may be necessary to examine parts of the urinary tract either with images or a camera to get a clearer understanding of the problem. *Ultrasound* offers the least invasive way of looking at many parts of the urinary system. A renal ultrasound, or *nephrosonography*, is a very common test that can help determine if the kidneys are filled with fluid (*hydronephrosis*). This is often a good indicator of an anatomical problem of the urinary tract. A bladder ultrasound can be helpful to show if a patient is retaining urine.

Among the most common types of images of the urinary tract is an *intravenous pyelogram.* In this test, the patient receives an intravenous injection of a special dye and then undergoes a CT scan of the urinary tract. This test can be very useful in showing kidney stones (*nephrolithiasis*) or problems with the anatomy of the urinary tract. For example, the CT may show that the patient's ureter is narrowing (*ureterostenosis*) or that the ureter has developed a pouch (*ureterocele*). Some patients are allergic to the special dye used in the intravenous pyelogram. In such a case, it may be necessary to insert a special camera into the bladder (*cystoscope*) or ureter (*ureteroscope*).

At times, a physician may want to watch the flow of urine (*urodynamic testing*). The most common of these types of tests involves putting dye in the patient's bladder and watching the direction of the urine as the patient urinates (*voiding cystourethrogram*).

urinary tract

Term	Word Analysis
albuminuria al-byoo-mih-NUR-ee-ah **Definition** protein in the urine	**albumin / ur / ia** protein / urine / condition
azotemia AZ-oh-TEE-mee-ah **Definition** excess nitrogen in the blood	**azot / emia** nitrogen / blood condition
Note: The *azot* root comes from the two roots *a* (not) and *zo* (living). It was applied to nitrogen because things cannot live in it.	
azotorrhea AZ-oh-toh-REE-ah **Definition** excessive discharge of nitrogen	**azoto / rrhea** nitrogen / discharge
azoturia AZ-oh-TUR-ee-ah **Definition** excess nitrogen in the urine	**azot / ur / ia** nitrogen / urine / condition

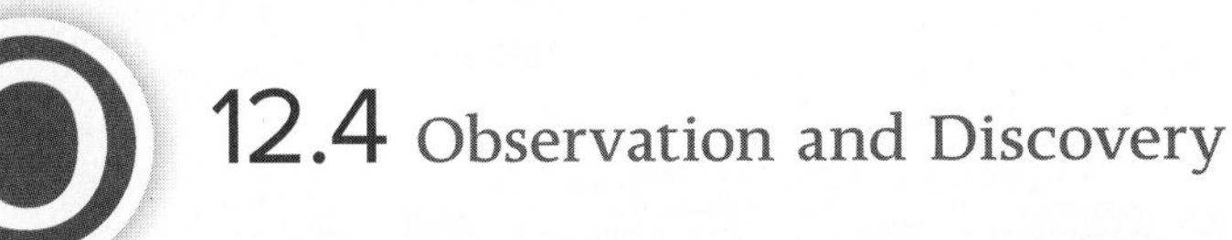

12.4 Observation and Discovery

urinary tract *continued*

Term	Word Analysis
cystorrhexis SIS-toh-REK-sis **Definition** rupture of the bladder	**cysto / rrhexis** bladder / rupture
dipsogenic DIP-soh-JIN-ik **Definition** creating thirst	**dipso / genic** thirst / creating
glucosuria GLOO-koh-shur-EE-ah **Definition** sugar in the urine	**glucos / ur / ia** sugar / urine / condition
glycosuria GLAI-koh-shur-EE-ah **Definition** sugar in the urine	**glycos / ur / ia** sugar / urine / condition
hyperkalemia HAI-per-kah-LEE-mee-ah **Definition** excessive potassium in the blood	**hyper / kal / emia** over / potassium / blood condition
hyponatremia HAI-poh-nah-TREE-mee-ah **Definition** low sodium in the blood	**hypo / natr / emia** under / sodium / blood condition
ketolysis kee-TAW-lih-sis **Definition** breakdown of ketones	**keto / lysis** ketones / loose
ketonuria kee-toh-NUR-ee-ah **Definition** presence of ketones in the urine	**keton / ur / ia** ketones / urine / condition
meatal stenosis mee-AY-tal steh-NOH-sis **Definition** narrowing of the opening of the urethra	**meat / al** **sten / osis** opening / pertaining to narrow / condition
nephroptosis nef-rop-TOH-sis **Definition** downward displacement of a kidney	**nephro / ptosis** kidney / drooping condition
nephrosis neh-FROH-sis **Definition** kidney condition	**nephr / osis** kidney / condition

urinary tract *continued*

Term	Word Analysis
uremia ur-EE-mee-ah **Definition** urine in the blood	**ur / emia** urine / blood condition
ureterocele yoo-REE-ter-oh-SEEL **Definition** hernia of a ureter	**uretero / cele** ureter / hernia
ureterolithiasis yoo-REE-ter-oh-lih-THAI-ah-sis **Definition** presence of stones in a ureter	**uretero / lith / iasis** ureter / stone / presence
ureterostenosis yoo-REE-ter-oh-steh-NOH-sis **Definition** narrowing of a ureter	**uretero / sten / osis** ureter / narrow / condition
urethrospasm yoo-REE-throh-SPAZ-um **Definition** involuntary contraction of the urethra	**urethro / spasm** urethra / involuntary contraction
urethrostenosis yoo-REE-throh-steh-NOH-sis **Definition** narrowing of the urethra	**urethro / sten / osis** urethra / narrowing / condition

urinary diagnostic procedures

Term	Word Analysis
cystoscopy sis-TAW-skoh-pee **Definition** process for examining the bladder	**cysto / scopy** bladder / looking procedure
meatoscope mee-AT-oh-SKOHP **Definition** instrument for examining the opening of the urethra	**meato / scope** opening / instrument to look
meatoscopy MEE-ah-TAW-skoh-pee **Definition** process for examining the opening of the urethra	**meato / scopy** opening / looking procedure
nephroscopy ne-FRAW-skoh-pee **Definition** procedure for examining a kidney	**nephro / scopy** kidney / looking procedure

urinary diagnostic procedures *continued*

Term	Word Analysis
resectoscope rih-SEK-toh-SKOHP **Definition** instrument for examining and cutting (usually the prostate)	**re / secto / scope** back / cut / instrument to look
ureteroscopy yoo-REE-ter-AW-skoh-pee **Definition** process of examining a ureter	**uretero / scopy** ureter / looking procedure
urethroscope yoo-REE-throh-SKOHP **Definition** instrument for examining the urethra	**urethro / scope** urethra / instrument to look
urethroscopy yoo-ree-THRAW-skoh-pee **Definition** process of examining the urethra	**urethro / scopy** urethra / looking procedure
urinalysis (UA) YUR-ih-NAL-ih-sis **Definition** analysis of the urine to determine presence of abnormal elements **NOTE:** The *-in* sound at the end of *urine* combines with an *an-* sound at the beginning of *analysis* to make a single sound.	*urinalysis* is actually a shortened form of *urine analysis* 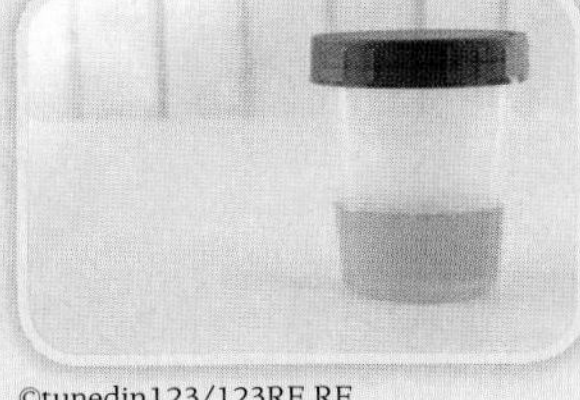 ©tunedin123/123RF RF

professional terms

Term	Word Analysis
blood urea nitrogen (BUN) BLUD yoo-REE-ah NAI-troh-jun **Definition** nitrogen in the blood in the form of urea; it is the product of the breakdown of amino acids for energy **NOTE:** The level of urea in the blood can be an indicator of kidney function.	**blood urea nitrogen**
diuresis DAI-yur-EE-sis **Definition** excessive urination **NOTE:** The prefix for this word is actually *dia*, but when the next word part starts with a vowel (as does *uresis*), the *dia* shortens to *di*.	**di / uresis** through / urination
nephrologist neh-FRAW-loh-jist **Definition** specialist in the kidneys	**nephro / logist** kidney / specialist
nephrology neh-FRAW-loh-jee **Definition** study of the kidneys	**nephro / logy** kidney / study

professional terms *continued*

Term	Word Analysis
urologist yur-AW-loh-jist **Definition** specialist in the urinary tract	**uro / logist** urine / specialist ©McGraw-Hill Education/Rick Brady, photographer
urology yur-AW-loh-jee **Definition** study of the urinary tract	**uro / logy** urine / study
uropoiesis YUR-oh-poh-EE-sis **Definition** formation of urine	**uro / poiesis** urine / formation
uroxanthin YUR-oh-ZAN-thin **Definition** substance in urine that makes it yellow	**uro / xanthin** urine / yellow
voiding VOI-ding **Definition** another term for urination	**from a term meaning** "empty"

male genitalia

Term	Word Analysis
anorchidism an-OR-kih-DIZ-um **Definition** lack of a testicle	**an / orchid / ism** no / testicle / condition
aspermia ay-SPER-mee-ah **Definition** condition characterized by lack of sperm	**a / sperm / ia** no / sperm / condition
azoospermia ay-ZOH-aw-SPER-mee-ah **Definition** condition characterized by lack of living sperm	**a / zoo / sperm / ia** no / living / sperm / condition
cryptorchidism krip-TOR-kih-DIZ-um **Definition** hidden testicle	**crypt / orchid / ism** hidden / testicle / condition

male genitalia *continued*

Term	Word Analysis
hydrocele HAI-droh-SEEL **Definition** fluid-filled mass in a testicle	**hydro / cele** water / hernia
hypospadias HAI-poh-SPAY-dee-as **Definition** birth defect in which the opening of the urethra is on the underside, instead of the end, of the penis	**from Greek, for** "to tear underneath"
oligospermia AW-lih-goh-SPER-mee-ah **Definition** condition characterized by low sperm production	**oligo / sperm / ia** low / sperm / condition
phimosis fih-MOH-sis **Definition** contraction of the foreskin of the penis, preventing it from being retracted	**from Greek, for** "muzzle"
prostatolith pros-TAT-oh-lith **Definition** stone in the prostate	**prostato / lith** prostate / stone
prostatomegaly PROS-ta-toh-MEH-gah-lee **Definition** abnormal enlargement of the prostate	**prostato / megaly** prostate / enlargement
prostatorrhea PROS-ta-toh-REE-ah **Definition** discharge from the prostate	**prostato / rrhea** prostate / discharge
seminoma SEM-ih-NOH-mah **Definition** type of testicular cancer arising from sperm-forming tissue	**semin / oma** sperm / tumor
spermatocele sper-MAH-toh-SEEL **Definition** hernia or distention of the epididymis caused by sperm cells	**spermato / cele** sperm / hernia
spermatolysis SPER-mah-TAW-lih-sis **Definition** destruction of sperm cells	**spermato / lysis** sperm / loose

12.4 Observation and Discovery

male genitalia diagnostic procedure

Term	Word Analysis
digital rectal exam (DRE) DIJ-ih-tal REK-tal ek-ZAM **Definition** examination of the prostate using a finger inserted into the rectum	**digit / al** — finger / pertaining to **rect / al exam** — rectum / pertaining to exam 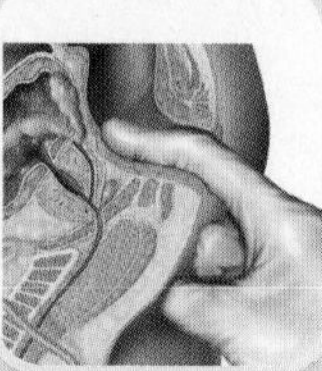

professional terms

Term	Word Analysis
ejaculation ee-JAK-yoo-LAY-shun **Definition** emission of semen from the urethra	**e / jacul / ation** out / throw / process
gonads GOH-nadz **Definition** pair of organs used for sexual reproduction; in males, they are the testicles, and in females, they are the ovaries	**gon / ads** creation / pair
spermatogenesis sper-MAT-oh-JIN-eh-sis **Definition** creation of sperm	**spermato / genesis** sperm / creation
vas deferens VAS DEH-frenz **Definition** vessel carrying sperm from the testicles **NOTE:** The word *vessel* can cause confusion. Most people hear "vessel" and think "blood vessel." "Vessel" simply means "tube or duct." So the vas deferens is a vessel; it just carries sperm instead of blood.	**vas de / ferens** vessel away / carrying

radiology

Term	Word Analysis
urinary tract	
cystogram SIS-toh-gram **Definition** image of the bladder	**cysto / gram** bladder / record
cystography sis-TAW-grah-fee **Definition** process for recording/imaging the bladder	**cysto / graphy** bladder / writing procedure

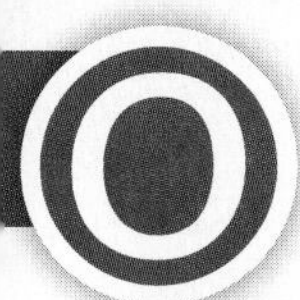

12.4 Observation and Discovery

radiology *continued*

Term	Word Analysis
nephrogram NEF-roh-gram **Definition** image of a kidney	**nephro / gram** kidney / record ©James Cavallini/Science Source
nephrography neh-FRAW-grah-fee **Definition** procedure for imaging a kidney	**nephro / graphy** kidney / writing procedure
nephrosonography NEF-roh-soh-NAW-grah-fee **Definition** procedure for imaging a kidney using sound waves	**nephro /sono /graphy** kidney / sound / writing procedure
pyelogram PAI-el-oh-GRAM **Definition** image of the renal pelvis	**pyelo / gram** pelvis / record
renal angiogram REE-nal AN-jee-oh-GRAM **Definition** image of a kidney blood vessel	**ren / al angio / gram** kidney / pertaining to vessel / record
renal angiography REE-nal AN-jee-AW-grah-fee **Definition** process of imaging a kidney blood vessel	**ren / al angio / graphy** kidney / pertaining to vessel / writing procedure
renal arteriogram REE-nal ar-TER-ee-oh-GRAM **Definition** image of a kidney artery	**ren / al arterio / gram** kidney / pertaining to artery / record
retrograde pyelogram REH-troh-grayd PAI-el-oh-GRAM **Definition** image of the renal pelvis produced by injecting a contrast dye from the bladder to the kidney **NOTE:** The term *retrograde* is used because the contrast goes in the opposite direction of normal urine flow.	**retro / grade pyelo / gram** backward / walk pelvis / record
ultrasonography UL-trah- soh-NAW-grah-fee **Definition** imaging procedure using high-frequency sound waves	**ultra / sono / graphy** high / sound / writing procedure
voiding cystourethrogram (VCUG) VOI-ding SIS-toh-yoo-REE-throh-GRAM **Definition** imaging procedure of the bladder and urethra produced during urination	**voiding cysto / urethro / gram** urinating bladder / urethra / record

radiology *continued*

Term	Word Analysis
male genitalia	
transrectal ultrasonography TRANZ-REK-tal UL-trah-soh-NAW-grah-fee	**trans / rect / al** — through / rectum / pertaining to; **ultra / sono / graphy** — high / sound / writing procedure
Definition procedure using a probe inserted into the rectum using high-frequency sound waves to scan through the rectum to nearby tissue (most commonly, the prostate)	
urethrogram yoo-REE-throh-GRAM	**urethro / gram** — urethra / record
Definition image of the urethra	

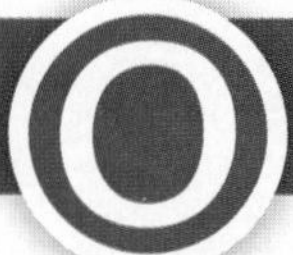

Learning Outcome 12.4 Exercises

PRONUNCIATION

EXERCISE 1 *Indicate which syllable is emphasized when pronounced.*

EXAMPLE: bronchitis bron**chi**tis

1. gonads ______
2. aspermia ______
3. nephrosis ______
4. ketolysis ______
5. ketonuria ______
6. prostatolith ______
7. nephroptosis ______
8. cryptorchidism ______
9. urology ______
10. urologist ______
11. nephrology ______
12. nephrologist ______
13. cystography ______
14. cystoscopy ______
15. nephroscopy ______
16. nephrogram ______
17. nephrography ______
18. hydrocele ______
19. seminoma ______
20. dipsogenic ______
21. glucosuria ______
22. azotemia ______
23. azoturia ______
24. resectoscope ______
25. urinalysis ______
26. urethrogram ______
27. spermatocele ______
28. cystorrhexis ______
29. prostatorrhea ______
30. prostatomegaly ______

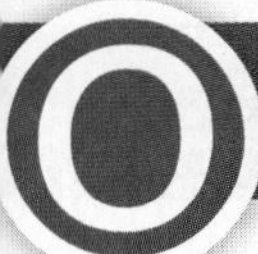

Learning Outcome 12.4 Exercises

TRANSLATION

EXERCISE 2 *Break down the following words into their component parts.*

EXAMPLE: nasopharyngoscope *naso | pharyngo | scope*

1. urology ______
2. nephrology ______
3. nephrogram ______
4. cystogram ______
5. spermatocele ______
6. ureterocele ______
7. hydrocele ______
8. meatoscope ______
9. urethroscope ______
10. pyelogram ______
11. nephrosis ______
12. prostatomegaly ______
13. urethrospasm ______
14. albuminuria ______
15. dipsogenic ______
16. aspermia ______
17. nephrosonography ______
18. ultrasonography ______
19. resectoscope ______
20. anorchidism ______

EXERCISE 3 *Underline and define the roots from this chapter in the following terms.*

1. urinalysis ______
2. nephrologist ______
3. urologist ______
4. urethrogram ______
5. spermatolysis ______
6. nephroptosis ______
7. cystorrhexis ______
8. meatal stenosis ______
9. ureterostenosis ______
10. urethrostenosis ______
11. oligospermia ______
12. azoospermia ______
13. uroxanthin ______
14. azoturia ______
15. glucosuria ______
16. retrograde pyelogram ______
17. diuresis ______
18. cryptorchidism ______
19. prostatolith (2 roots) ______
20. ureterolithiasis (2 roots) ______

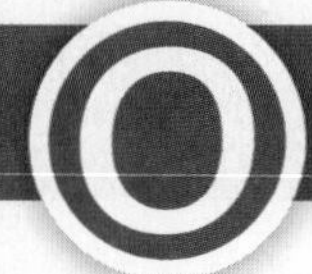

Learning Outcome 12.4 Exercises

EXERCISE 4 *Match the term on the left with its definition on the right.*

_____ 1. ejaculation
_____ 2. gonads
_____ 3. blood urea nitrogen
_____ 4. digital rectal exam
_____ 5. voiding
_____ 6. transrectal ultrasonography
_____ 7. vas deferens
_____ 8. seminoma
_____ 9. hypospadias
_____ 10. phimosis

a. birth defect in which the opening of the urethra is on the underside, instead of the end, of the penis
b. contraction of the foreskin of the penis, preventing it from being retracted
c. procedure using a probe inserted into the rectum using high-frequency sound waves to scan through the rectum to nearby tissue (most commonly, the prostate)
d. type of testicular cancer arising from sperm-forming tissue
e. another term for urination
f. exam of the prostate using a finger inserted into the rectum
g. nitrogen in the blood in the form of urea; can be an indicator of kidney function
h. emission of semem from the urethra
i. pair of organs used for sexual reproduction (testicles in males; ovaries in females)
j. vessel carrying sperm from the testicles

EXERCISE 5 *Underline the correct option for each given translation.*

EXAMPLE: hypoglycemia *hypo* over/**under** *pharyngo* salt/**sugar** -emia **blood**/urine condition

1. albuminuria = *albumin* protein/nitrogen + *uria* urine/blood condition
2. azotemia = *azot* protein/nitrogen + *emia* urine/blood condition
3. glucosuria = *glucos* sugar/sodium + *uria* urine/blood condition
4. glycosuria = *glycos* sugar/potassium + *uria* urine/blood condition
5. hyperkalemia = *hyper* over/under + *kal* sugar/potassium + *emia* urine/blood condition
6. hyponatremia = *hypo* over/under + *natr* sugar/sodium + *emia* urine/blood condition

EXERCISE 6 *Fill in the blanks.*

1. ureteroscopy: process for examining the ______________________________
2. urethroscopy: process for examining the ______________________________
3. cystoscopy: process for examining the ______________________________
4. nephroscopy: process for examining the ______________________________
5. meatoscopy: process for examining the ______________________________
6. cystography: process for recording/imaging the ______________________________
7. nephrography: process for recording/imaging the ______________________________

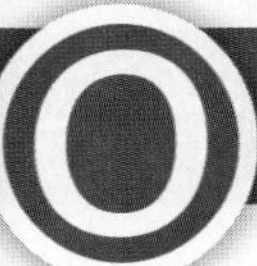

Learning Outcome 12.4 Exercises

8. renal angiogram: image of a(n) ______
9. renal arteriogram: image of a(n) ______
10. renal angiography: process of imaging a(n) ______

EXERCISE 7 *Translate the following terms as literally as possible.*

EXAMPLE: nasopharyngoscope *an instrument for looking at the nose and throat*

1. nephrology ______
2. cystoscopy ______
3. meatoscope ______
4. urethroscope ______
5. pyelogram ______
6. spermatogenesis ______
7. urinalysis ______
8. prostatorrhea ______
9. cryptorchidism ______
10. glucosuria ______
11. ketonuria ______
12. uropoiesis ______
13. uroxanthin ______
14. cystorrhexis ______
15. uremia ______
16. anorchidism ______
17. azoospermia ______
18. resectoscope ______
19. ketolysis ______
20. dipsogenic ______
21. azotorrhea ______

GENERATION

EXERCISE 8 *Build a medical term from the information provided.*

EXAMPLE: inflammation of the sinuses *sinusitis*

1. kidney condition (use *nephr/o*) ______
2. image of the urethra ______
3. procedure for imaging a kidney (use *nephr/o*) ______

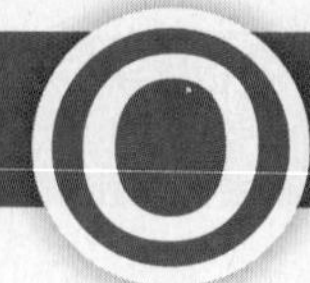

Learning Outcome 12.4 Exercises

4. process for recording/imaging the bladder (use *cyst/o*) ________________
5. process of imaging a kidney blood vessel (use *ren/o*) ________________
6. process for examining the opening of the urethra ________________
7. procedure for examining a kidney ________________
8. specialist in the kidneys ________________
9. abnormal enlargement of the prostate ________________
10. involuntary contraction of the urethra ________________
11. downward displacement of a kidney ________________
12. low-sperm condition ________________
13. urine formation ________________
14. hernia of a ureter ________________
15. stone in the prostate ________________
16. presence of stones in the ureter ________________
17. low sodium in the blood ________________
18. excessive potassium in the blood ________________
19. imaging procedure using high-frequency sound waves ________________
20. procedure for imaging a kidney using sound waves ________________

EXERCISE 9 *Multiple-choice questions. Select the correct answer(s).*

1. The emission of semen from the urethra is known as:
   a. aspermia
   b. ejaculation
   c. phimosis
   d. seminoma
   e. spermatolysis
2. The breakdown of ketones is known as:
   a. azotemia
   b. azotorrhea
   c. hyperkalemia
   d. ketolysis
   e. ketonuria
3. The narrowing of the opening of the urethra is called:
   a. meatal stenosis
   b. meatorrhaphy
   c. ureterostenosis
   d. urethrospasm
   e. urethrostenosis
4. Which of the choices below are true of the term *blood urea nitrogen*?
   a. abbreviated BUN
   b. nitrogen in the blood in the form of urea
   c. product of the breakdown of amino acids for energy
   d. level of urea in the blood can be an indicator of kidney function
   e. all of these
5. The medical term for *excessive urination* is:
   a. diuresis
   b. uremia
   c. uropoiesis
   d. uroxanthin
   e. voiding
6. A hernia or distention of the epididymis caused by sperm cells is called a(n):
   a. epididymitis
   b. epididymocele
   c. hydrocele
   d. seminoma
   e. spermatocele
7. A *hydrocele* is a fluid-filled mass in the:
   a. bladder
   b. kidney
   c. prostate
   d. testicle
   e. none of these

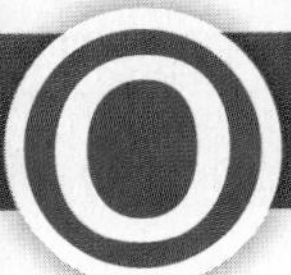

Learning Outcome 12.4 Exercises

8. The *digital rectal exam* and the *transrectal ultrasonography* are both procedures for examining the:
   a. bladder
   b. kidney
   c. prostate
   d. testicle
   e. none of these

9. Which of the statements below are true of the term *retrograde pyelogram?* (select all that apply)
   a. image of the kidney
   b. image of the renal pelvis
   c. image produced by injecting a contrast dye from the bladder to the kidney
   d. image produced by injecting a contrast dye from the bladder to the urethra
   e. literally means "backward walk pelvis record"

10. Which of the statements below are true of the term *seminoma?* (select all that apply)
    a. a type of prostate cancer
    b. a type of testicular cancer
    c. arises from sperm-forming tissue
    d. literally means "sperm condition"
    e. literally means "sperm tumor"

11. Which of the statements below are true of the term *hypospadias?* (select all that apply)
    a. birth defect
    b. from Greek, for "to tear underneath"
    c. literally means "over sperm"
    d. opening of the urethra is on the end of the penis
    e. opening of the urethra is on the underside of the penis

12. Select all of the terms below that pertain to male genitalia.
    a. aspermia
    b. phimosis
    c. uremia
    d. ureterolithiasis
    e. voiding

13. Select all of the terms below that pertain to the urinary tract.
    a. aspermia
    b. phimosis
    c. uremia
    d. ureterolithiasis
    e. voiding

EXERCISE 10 *Briefly describe the difference between each pair of terms.*

1. urologist, urology ______
2. cystogram, nephrogram ______
3. ureteroscopy, urethroscopy ______
4. ureterostenosis, urethrostenosis ______
5. spermatolysis, spermatogenesis ______
6. azotorrhea, prostatorrhea ______
7. azotemia, azoturia ______
8. renal angiogram, renal arteriogram ______
9. gonads, vas deferens ______

ASSESSMENT

12.5 Diagnosis and Pathology

Just like all the other body systems, the urinary system can have problems with its anatomy, infection, tumors, and blood supply. On a large scale, the vessels in patients' urinary tracts can have abnormal pouches (for example, *cystoceles*). These pouches can be harmless or cause a blockage of urine. In the case of the ureter (*ureterocele*), this pouching intrudes into the bladder. Patients may also have large cysts in the kidneys (*polycystic kidney disease*). These don't cause blockage, but they can prevent the kidneys from working correctly.

On a microscopic level, the kidneys can have all manner of problems. These general kidney problems (*nephropathy*) fall into two general types with (*nephritis*) or without (*nephrosis*) inflammation. Often, the difference is seen in a urinalysis. Nephritis will most often cause white blood cells and red blood cells to show up in the urine. Both types of diseases can be severe enough to lead to kidney failure. Kidney failure is marked by the kidney's inability to filter waste out of the blood. If this problem is not fixed, the patient will die.

The urinary tract is vulnerable to infection. Urinary tract infections (UTIs) are often divided into lower urinary tract and upper urinary tract infections, depending on whether the kidneys are involved. Lower urinary tract infections generally refer to infections of the bladder (*cystitis*). They are much more common in females than in males, and they are also frequently seen in patients whose urine flows back toward the kidneys from the bladder (*vesicoureteral reflux*).

When infection spreads to the kidneys (*pyelonephritis*), it generally becomes more severe. A patient with pyelonephritis may have back pain and high fever, and may appear very ill. Another common infection of the urinary tract involves just the urethra (*urethritis*). The usual cause is *gonorrhea,* a sexually transmitted infection.

Tumors of the urinary tract are most common in the larger structures of the tract: the kidney (*nephroma*) or bladder (*cystoma*). The most usual presenting symptom is blood in the urine. By far, the most common cancer of the kidney is *renal cell carcinoma.* Often, there are few early warning symptoms for this cancer.

Kidneys need a constant supply of blood. Poor blood supply to the kidneys (*renal ischemia*) is usually caused by cholesterol deposits in the arteries. Another cause is narrowing of the arteries that lead to the kidney (*renal artery stenosis*). When the blood supply to the kidneys is low, the kidneys release signals to the rest of the body to increase the blood's pressure (*renovascular hypertension*). Any time a patient's high blood pressure doesn't respond to typical medical management, a renal cause should be considered.

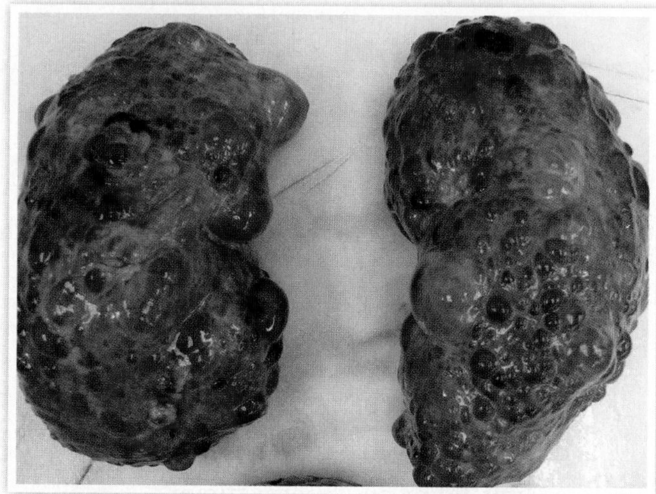

A pair of kidneys with polycystic kidney disease.

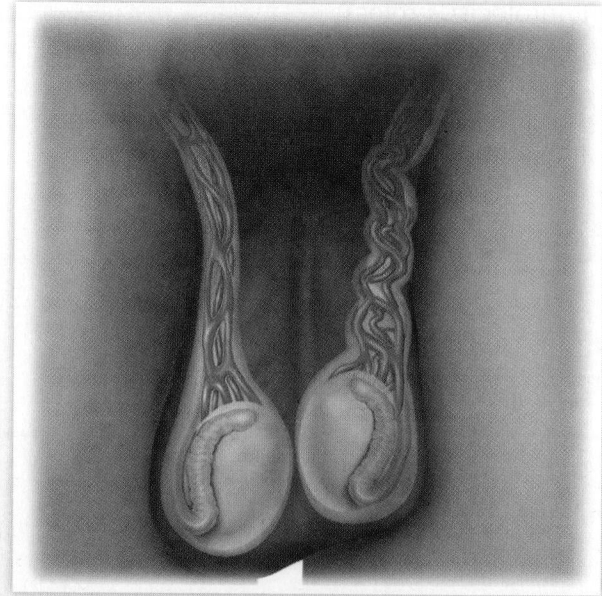

Testicular torsion—when a testicle becomes twisted—is considered a medical emergency.

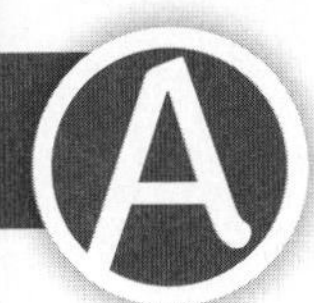

12.5 Diagnosis and Pathology

Male patients can have specific problems with their genitourinary systems. The prostate gland is a common cause of problems in older men. The prostate gland may become enlarged (*benign prostate hypertrophy*), infected (*prostatitis*), or cancerous. Prostate symptoms include pain and blocked flow of urine, leading to a weak urine stream or difficulty starting a urine stream at all.

The testicles can cause problems in any age group. *Testicular carcinoma* is the most common form of cancer in young adult men. It usually presents as a painful lump on the testicle. The testicle can also become infected (*orchitis*), a problem usually associated with the mumps.

Since testicles hang from the body, it is possible for one of them to become twisted (*testicular torsion*). This can cut off the blood supply to the testicle and is considered a medical emergency. Concerns in other parts of the reproductive system include infection of the epididymis (*epididymitis*) and swelling of the veins in the scrotum (*varicocele*).

urinary tract

Term	Word Analysis
cystitis sis-TAI-tis **Definition** inflammation of the bladder	**cyst / itis** bladder / inflammation
cystocele SIS-toh-seel **Definition** hernia of the bladder	**cysto / cele** bladder / tumor
cystolith SIS-toh-lith **Definition** stone in the bladder	**cysto / lith** bladder / stone
cystoptosis sis-TOP-toh-sis **Definition** downward displacement of the bladder	**cysto / ptosis** bladder / drooping condition
cystospasm SIS-toh-SPAZ-um **Definition** involuntary contraction of the bladder	**cysto / spasm** bladder / involuntary contraction
cystoureteritis SIS-toh-yoo-REE-ter-AI-tis **Definition** inflammation of the bladder and ureter	**cysto / ureter / itis** bladder / ureter / inflammation
cystourethrocele SIS-toh-yoo-REE-throh-seel **Definition** hernia of the bladder and urethra	**cysto / urethro / cele** bladder / urethra / hernia
glomerulonephritis gloh-MER-yoo-loh-neh-FRAI-tis **Definition** inflammation of the kidneys involving primarily the glomeruli	**glomerulo / nephr / itis** glomerulus / kidney / inflammation
glomerulopathy gloh-MER-yoo-LAW-pah-thee **Definition** disease of the kidney involving primarily the glomeruli	**glomerulo / pathy** glomerulus / disease

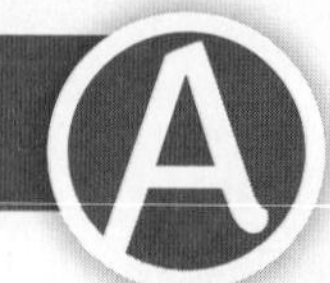

12.5 Diagnosis and Pathology

urinary tract *continued*

Term	Word Analysis
glomerulosclerosis gloh-MER-yoo-loh-skleh-ROH-sis **Definition** hardening of the glomeruli	**glomerulo / sclerosis** glomerulus / hardening
hydronephrosis HAI-droh-neh-FROH-sis **Definition** kidney condition caused by the obstruction of urine flow	**hydro / nephr / osis** water / kidney / condition
lithonephritis LIH-thoh-neh-FRAI-tis **Definition** inflammation of the kidneys caused by stones	**litho / nephr / itis** stone / kidney / inflammation
nephritis neh-FRAI-tis **Definition** inflammation of the kidney	**nephr / itis** kidney / inflammation
nephrocele NEH-froh-seel **Definition** hernia of a kidney	**nephro / cele** kidney / hernia
nephrohypertrophy NEH-froh-hai-PER-troh-fee **Definition** overdevelopment of the kidney	**nephro / hyper / trophy** kidney / over / nourishment
nephrolithiasis NEH-froh-lih-THAI-ah-sis **Definition** presence of stones in the kidney	**nephro / lith / iasis** kidney / stone / presence ©McGraw-Hill Education
nephromalacia NEH-froh-mah-LAY-shah **Definition** abnormal softening of a kidney	**nephro / malacia** kidney / softening
nephromegaly NEH-froh-MEG-ah-lee **Definition** abnormal enlargement of a kidney	**nephro / megaly** kidney / enlargement

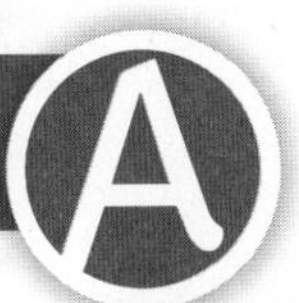

12.5 Diagnosis and Pathology

urinary tract *continued*

Term	Word Analysis
nephropathy neh-FRAW-pah-thee **Definition** any kidney disease	**nephro / pathy** kidney / disease
nephroptosis NEH-frop-TOH-sis **Definition** downward displacement of a kidney	**nephro / ptosis** kidney / drooping condition
nephrosclerosis NEH-froh-skleh-ROH-sis **Definition** abnormal hardening of a kidney	**nephro / scler / osis** kidney / hardening / condition
polycystic kidney disease (PKD) PAW-lee-SIS-tik KID-nee dih-ZEEZ **Definition** disease characterized by the formation of many fluid-filled cysts in the kidneys	**poly / cyst / ic kidney disease** many / cysts / pertaining to ©McGraw-Hill Education
pyelitis PAI-el-AI-tis **Definition** inflammation of the renal pelvis	**pyel / itis** pelvis / inflammation
pyelocystitis PAI-el-oh-sis-TAI-tis **Definition** inflammation of the renal pelvis and bladder	**pyelo / cyst / itis** pelvis / bladder / inflammation
pyelocystostomosis PAI-el-oh-SIS-toh-staw-MOH-sis **Definition** creation of an opening between the renal pelvis and bladder	**pyelo / cysto / stom / osis** pelvis / bladder / mouth / condition
pyelonephritis PAI-el-oh-neh-FRAI-tis **Definition** inflammation of the kidney and renal pelvis	**pyelo / nephr / itis** pelvis / kidney / inflammation
pyelopathy PAI-el-AW-pah-thee **Definition** disease of the renal pelvis	**pyelo / pathy** pelvis / disease

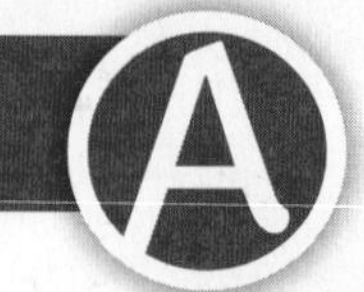

12.5 Diagnosis and Pathology

urinary tract *continued*

Term	Word Analysis
pyeloureterectasia PAI-el-oh-yoo-REE-ter-ek-TAY-zhah **Definition** dilation of the renal pelvis and ureter	**pyelo / ureter / ectasia** pelvis / ureter / dilation Normal Diseased
pyonephritis PAI-oh-neh-FRAI-tis **Definition** inflammation of the kidney caused by pus	**pyo / nephr / itis** pus / kidney / inflammation
pyonephrolithiasis PAI-oh-NEH-froh-lih-THAI-ah-sis **Definition** presence of pus and stones in the kidney	**pyo / nephro / lith / iasis** pus / kidney / stone / presence
pyopyeloectasis PAI-oh-PAI-el-oh-EK-tah-sis **Definition** pus in a dilated renal pelvis	**pyo / pyelo / ectasis** pus / pelvis / expansion
renal failure REE-nal FAY-el-yur **Definition** kidney failure	**ren / al failure** kidney / pertaining to failure
renal ischemia REE-nal ih-SKEE-mee-ah **Definition** deficiency of blood in a kidney	**ren / al isch / emia** kidney / pertaining to hold back / blood condition
stress urinary incontinence (SUI) STRESS YUR-ih-NAR-ee in-CON-tih-nentz **Definition** loss of bladder control caused by the application of external pressure **Note:** This is the medical term for loss of bladder control due to excessive laughing, a hard cough, or similar motion.	**stress urin / ary in / con / tinence** stress urine / pertaining to not / together / holding
ureteritis yoo-REE-ter-AI-tis **Definition** inflammation of a ureter	**ureter / itis** ureter / inflammation
ureteropyelitis yoo-REE-ter-oh-PAI-el-AI-tis **Definition** inflammation of a ureter and renal pelvis	**uretero / pyel / itis** ureter / pelvis / inflammation

urinary tract *continued*

Term	Word Analysis
ureteropyelonephritis yoo-REE-ter-oh-PAI-el-oh-neh-FRAI-tis **Definition** inflammation of a kidney, renal pelvis, and ureter	**uretero / pyelo / nephr / itis** ureter / pelvis / kidney / inflammation
urethritis yoo-ree-THRAI-tis **Definition** inflammation of the urethra	**urethr / itis** urethra / inflammation
urethrocystitis yoo-REE-throh-sis-TAI-tis **Definition** inflammation of the urethra and bladder	**urethro / cyst / itis** urethra / bladder / inflammation
urinary tract infection (UTI) YUR-ih-NAR-ee TRAKT in-FEK-shun **Definition** infection of the urinary tract	**urinary tract infection**
uropathy yur-AW-pah-thee **Definition** disease of the urinary tract	**uro / pathy** urine / disease
vesicocele VES-ih-koh-SEEL **Definition** hernia of the bladder	**vesico / cele** bladder / hernia
vesicoureteral reflux (VUR) VES-ih-koh-yoo-REE-ter-al REE-fluks **Definition** abnormal flow of urine from the bladder back into the ureters	**vesico / ureter / al re / flux** bladder / ureter / pertaining to back / flow

male genitalia

Term	Word Analysis
balanitis bal-ah-NAI-tis **Definition** inflammation of the penis	**balan / itis** penis / inflammation
benign prostate hyperplasia (BPH) beh-NAIN PROS-tayt HAI-per-PLAY-zhah **Definition** noncancerous overdevelopment of the prostate, also known as *enlarged prostate*	**benign prostate hyper / plas / ia** friendly prostate over / formation / condition ©McGraw-Hill Education
benign prostate hypertrophy beh-NAIN PROS-tayt hai-PER-troh-fee **Definition** another term for benign prostate hyperplasia	**benign prostate hyper / trophy** friendly prostate over / nourishment
epididymitis EP-ih-DID-ih-MAI-tis **Definition** inflammation of the epididymis	**epididym / itis** epididymis / inflammation

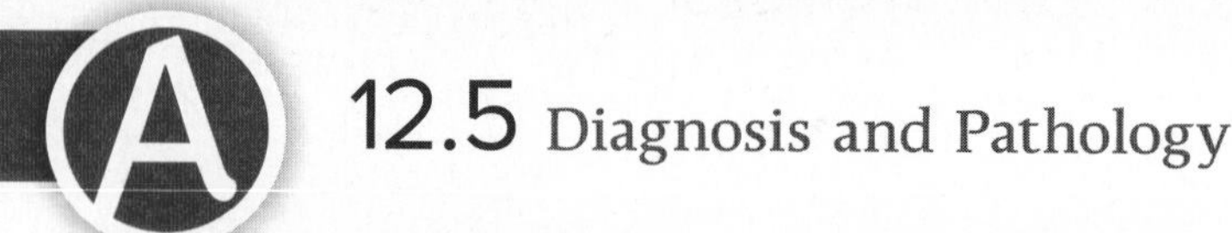

12.5 Diagnosis and Pathology

male genitalia *continued*

Term	Word Analysis
epididymo-orchitis EP-ih-DID-ih-moh-or-KAI-tis **Definition** inflammation of the testicles and epididymis	**epididymo / orch / itis** epididymis / testicle / inflammation
orchiditis OR-kih-DAI-tis **Definition** inflammation of the testicles	**orchid / itis** testicle / inflammation
orchiepididymitis OR-kee-EP-ih-DID-ih-MAI-tis **Definition** inflammation of the testicles and epididymis	**orchi / epididym / itis** testicle / epididymis / inflammation
orchiopathy OR-kee-AW-pah-thee **Definition** disease of the testicles	**orchio / pathy** testicle / disease
orchitis or-KAI-tis **Definition** inflammation of the testicles	**orch / itis** testicle / inflammation
prostatitis PRAWS-tah-TAI-tis **Definition** inflammation of the prostate	**prostat / itis** prostate / inflammation
prostatocystitis PROS-ta-toh-sis-TAI-tis **Definition** inflammation of the prostate and bladder	**prostato / cyst / itis** prostate / bladder / inflammation
prostatovesiculitis PROS-ta-toh-veh-SIK-yoo-LAI-tis **Definition** inflammation of the prostate and seminal vesicles	**prostato / vesicul / itis** prostate / bladder / inflammation
testitis tes-TAI-tis **Definition** inflammation of a testicle	**test / itis** testicle / inflammation
varicocele VAR-ih-koh-SEEL **Definition** overexpansion of the blood vessels of the testicles, leading to a soft tumor	**varico / cele** twisted / hernia

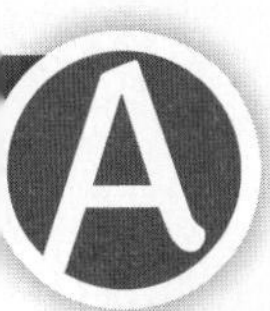

12.5 Diagnosis and Pathology

oncology

Term	Word Analysis
cystoma sis-TOH-mah **Definition** tumor of the bladder	**cyst / oma** bladder / tumor ©McGraw-Hill Education
hypernephroma HAI-per-neh-FROH-mah **Definition** another name for renal cell carcinoma	**hyper / nephr / oma** over / kidney / tumor
nephroma neh-FROH-mah **Definition** kidney tumor	**nephr / oma** kidney / tumor
renal cell carcinoma REE-nal SELL KAR-sih-NOH-mah **Definition** cancer of the kidneys	**ren / al** — kidney / pertaining to; **cell carcin / oma** — cell cancer / tumor ©McGraw-Hill Education
seminoma SEM-ih-NOH-mah **Definition** type of testicular cancer arising from sperm-forming tissue	**semin / oma** sperm / tumor
testicular carcinoma tes-TIK-yoo-lar KAR-sih-NOH-mah **Definition** testicular cancer	**testicul / ar** — testicle / pertaining to; **carcin / oma** — cancer / tumor

sexually transmitted diseases

Term	Word Analysis
chlamydia klah-MIH-dee-ah **Definition** sexually transmitted disease characterized by genital discharge and painful urination, caused by the bacterium *Chlamydia trachomatis*	**from Greek, for "cloak"**

sexually transmitted diseases *continued*

Term	Word Analysis
gonorrhea GAW-noh-REE-ah **Definition** a sexually transmitted disease characterized by discharge from the gonads, caused by the bacterium *Neisseria gonorrhoeae*	**gono / rrhea** gonad / discharge 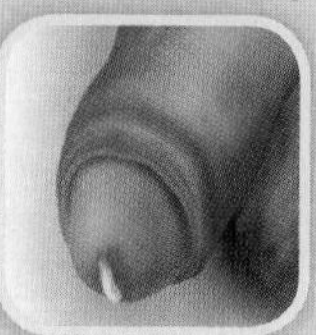
herpes simplex virus (HSV) HER-peez SIM-pleks VAI-rus **Definition** a family of highly contagious viruses that effect mucous membranes and produce watery blisters that eventually scab over **NOTE:** Herpes Simplex 1 (HSV-1) affects the mouth and nose and is commonly called "cold sore." Herpes Simplex 2 (HSV-2) affects the genital areas and is commonly called "herpes" or "genital herpes."	**herpes comes from Greek, for "to creep"**
human immunodeficiency virus (HIV) HYOO-man ih-myoo-noh-deh-FIH-shun-see VAI-rus **Definition** a disease that compromises a patient's immune system leaving them open to other opportunistic infections. The late stage of this disease is referred to as AIDS (acquired immune deficiency syndrome).	**human immuno / deficiency virus** immune / deficiency
human papilloma virus (HPV) HYOO-man pap-ih-LOH-ma VAI-rus **Definition** a virus that can cause warts and precancerous lesions in genital areas **NOTE:** The name refers to the "nipple-like" appearance of the precancerous lesions. Nearly all cervical cancers are HPV.	**human papill / oma virus** nipple / tumor
syphilis SIH-fih-lis **Definition** a sexually transmitted disease characterized at first by skin irritations then later developing into neurological and heart symptoms, caused by the bacterium *Treponema pallidum*	Syphilis is derived from a poem published in the 1500s called "Syphilis, or the French Disease," which tells the story of a shepherd named Syphilis who was supposedly the first to suffer with the disease.
trichomoniasis tri-koh-moh-NAI-ah-sis **Definition** a sexually transmitted disease characterized by genital itching, painful urination, and genital discharge, caused by the parasite *Trichomonas vaginalis* **NOTE:** As you might notice in the name, the parasite *Trichomonas* is named after the fact that it has a hairlike flagellum that is used for movement.	**trichomon / iasis** trichomonas presence of 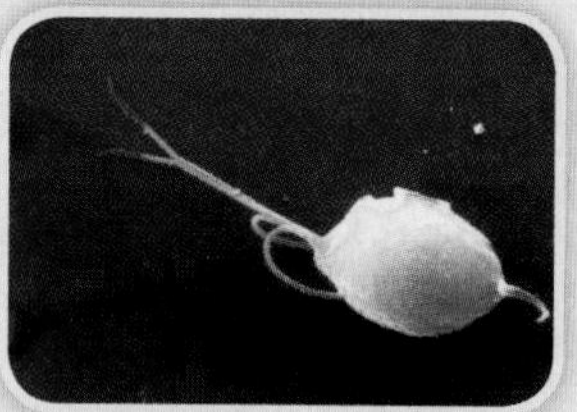 *Trichomonas* parasite ©BSIP/Universal Images Group/Getty Images

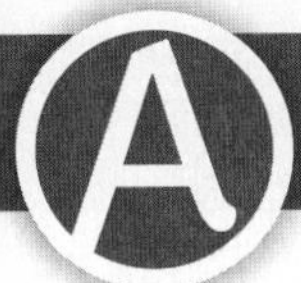

Learning Outcome 12.5 Exercises

PRONUNCIATION

EXERCISE 1 *Indicate which syllable is emphasized when pronounced.*

EXAMPLE: bronchitis bron**chi**tis

1. cystitis ____________
2. orchitis ____________
3. testitis ____________
4. nephritis ____________
5. balanitis ____________
6. urethritis ____________
7. cystoma ____________
8. nephroma ____________
9. uropathy ____________
10. nephropathy ____________
11. cystocele ____________
12. nephrocele ____________
13. cystolith ____________
14. cystospasm ____________
15. cystoptosis ____________
16. nephroptosis ____________
17. pyelitis ____________
18. ureteritis ____________
19. orchiditis ____________
20. prostatitis ____________
21. pyonephritis ____________
22. pyelopathy ____________
23. nephromegaly ____________
24. nephrolithiasis ____________
25. glomerulonephritis ____________

TRANSLATION

EXERCISE 2 *Break down the following words into their component parts.*

EXAMPLE: nasopharyngoscope *naso | pharyngo | scope*

1. cystitis ____________
2. testitis ____________
3. nephritis ____________
4. vesicocele ____________
5. gonorrhea ____________
6. orchiopathy ____________
7. epididymitis ____________
8. nephromalacia ____________
9. hydronephritis ____________
10. ureteropyelitis ____________
11. urethrocystitis ____________
12. pyelonephritis ____________
13. pyonephritis ____________
14. prostatocystitis ____________
15. orchiepididymitis ____________
16. glomerulosclerosis ____________
17. nephrolithiasis ____________
18. pyopyeloectasis ____________
19. ureteropyelonephritis ____________
20. pyelocystostomosis ____________

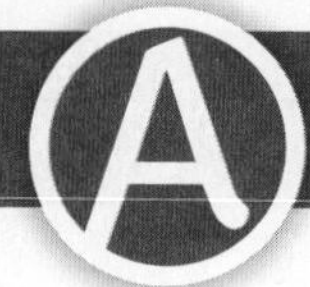

Learning Outcome 12.5 Exercises

EXERCISE 3 *Underline and define the roots from this chapter in the following terms.*

1. prostatitis ______
2. ureteritis ______
3. urethritis ______
4. orchitis ______
5. orchiditis ______
6. balanitis ______
7. cystocele ______
8. nephrocele ______
9. uropathy ______
10. pyelopathy ______
11. glomerulopathy ______
12. renal failure ______
13. cystoptosis ______
14. nephromegaly ______
15. hypernephroma ______
16. renal cell carcinoma ______
17. testicular carcinoma ______
18. cystourethrocele (2 roots) ______
19. lithonephritis (2 roots) ______
20. pyeloureterectasia (2 roots) ______
21. pyonephrolithiasis (2 roots) ______
22. vesicoureteral reflux (2 roots) ______
23. epididymo-orchitis (2 roots) ______
24. prostatovesiculitis (2 roots) ______

EXERCISE 4 *Match the term on the left with its definition on the right.*

______	1. urinary tract infection	a.	deficiency of blood in a kidney
______	2. stress urinary incontinence disease	b.	disease characterized by the formation of many fluid-filled cysts in the kidneys
______	3. polycystic kidney disease	c.	infection of the urinary tract
______	4. benign prostate hypertrophy	d.	kidney condition caused by obstruction of urine flow
______	5. hydronephrosis	e.	literally, "friendly prostate overformation condition"; noncancerous overdevelopment of the prostate or *enlarged prostate*
______	6. benign prostate hyperplasia	f.	literally, "friendly prostate overnourishment condition"; noncancerous overdevelopment of the prostate or enlarged prostate

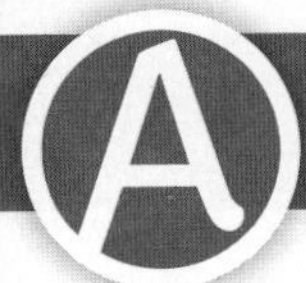

Learning Outcome 12.5 Exercises

_____ 7. nephrohypertrophy

_____ 8. varicocele

_____ 9. renal ischemia

g. loss of bladder control caused by the application of external pressure

h. overdevelopment of the kidney

i. overexpansion of the blood vessels of the testicles, leading to a soft tumor

EXERCISE 5 *Match the term on the left with its definition on the right.*

_____ 1. chlamydia

_____ 2. gonorrhea

_____ 3. herpes simplex virus

_____ 4. human immunodeficiency virus

_____ 5. human papilloma virus

_____ 6. syphilis

_____ 7. trichomoniasis

a. a sexually transmitted disease characterized by genital itching, painful urination, and genital discharge, caused by the parasite *Trichomonas vaginalis*

b. sexually transmitted disease characterized by genital discharge and painful urination, caused by the bacterium *Chlamydia trachomatis*

c. a sexually transmitted disease characterized at first by skin irritations then later developing into neurological and heart symptoms

d. a virus that can cause warts and precancerous lesions in genital areas

e. a disease that compromises a patient's immune system leaving them open to other opportunistic infections

f. a sexually transmitted disease characterized by discharge from the gonads

g. a family of highly contagious viruses that affect mucous membranes and produce watery blisters that eventually scab over

EXERCISE 6 *Fill in the blanks.*

1. testitis: inflammation of the ____________________
2. prostatitis: inflammation of the ____________________
3. urethritis: inflammation of the ____________________
4. nephritis: inflammation of the ____________________
5. ureteritis: inflammation of the ____________________
6. orchiditis: inflammation of the ____________________
7. cystitis: inflammation of the ____________________
8. pyelitis: inflammation of the ____________________
9. balanitis: inflammation of the ____________________
10. orchitis: inflammation of the ____________________
11. epididymitis: inflammation of the ____________________
12. cystoureteritis: inflammation of the ____________ and ____________

13. urethrocystitis: inflammation of the __________ and __________
14. ureteropyelitis: inflammation of the __________ and __________
15. prostatocystitis: inflammation of the __________ and __________
16. pyelocystitis: inflammation of the __________ and __________
17. pyelonephritis: inflammation of the __________ and __________
18. epididymo-orchitis: inflammation of the __________ and __________
19. ureteropyelonephritis: inflammation of the __________, __________ and __________

EXERCISE 7 *Translate the following terms as literally as possible.*

EXAMPLE: nasopharyngoscope *an instrument for looking at the nose and throat*

1. cystolith __________
2. pyelopathy __________
3. gonorrhea __________
4. glomerulopathy __________
5. nephromegaly __________
6. pyonephritis __________
7. prostatovesiculitis __________
8. orchiepididymitis __________
9. nephrolithiasis __________
10. nephrohypertrophy __________
11. testicular carcinoma __________
12. pyelocystostomosis __________
13. pyeloureterectasia __________
14. pyopyeloectasis __________
15. renal ischemia __________
16. benign prostate hyperplasia __________

GENERATION

EXERCISE 8 *Build a medical term from the information provided.*

EXAMPLE: inflammation of the sinuses *sinusitis*

1. hernia of the bladder (use *cyst/o*) __________
2. hernia of the bladder (use *vesic/o*) __________
3. hernia of a kidney __________
4. kidney failure (use *ren/o*) __________
5. kidney tumor (use *nephr/o*) __________
6. kidney disease (use *nephr/o*) __________
7. involuntary contraction of the bladder (use *cyst/o*) __________
8. disease of the testicles (use *orchi/o*) __________
9. disease of the urinary tract __________
10. abnormal hardening of a kidney __________
11. hardening of the glomeruli __________
12. downward displacement of a kidney __________

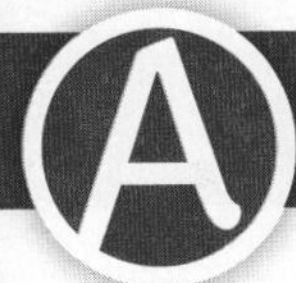

Learning Outcome 12.5 Exercises

13. inflammation of the kidneys involving primarily the glomeruli (use *nephr/o*)
14. inflammation of the kidney and renal pelvis
15. inflammation of the kidneys caused by stones
16. inflammation of the bladder and urethra
17. presence of pus and stones in the kidney (use *nephr/o*)

EXERCISE 9 *Multiple-choice questions. Select the correct answer(s).*

1. Select all of the terms below that pertain to the urinary tract.
   a. cystoma
   b. cystospasm
   c. epididymitis
   d. glomerulopathy
   e. hypernephroma
   f. nephroma
   g. orchitis
   h. testicular carcinoma
2. Select all of the terms below that pertain to the male genitalia.
   a. cystoma
   b. cystospasm
   c. epididymitis
   d. glomerulopathy
   e. hypernephroma
   f. nephroma
   g. orchitis
   h. testicular carcinoma
3. The term *nephropathy* refers to:
   a. any cancer of the kidney
   b. any cancer of the urinary tract
   c. any disease of the bladder
   d. any disease of the kidney
   e. any disease of the urinary tract
4. Which of the following statements is true of the term *stress urinary incontinence*?
   a. abbreviated SUI
   b. loss of bladder control caused by the application of external pressure
   c. medical term for loss of bladder control due to excessive laughing, a hard cough, or something like that
   d. would apply to the common phrase "I peed in my pants"
   e. all of these
5. An infection of the urinary tract is known as a:
   a. urinary tract infection
   b. uropathy
   c. UTI
   d. urinary tract infection and UTI
   e. uropathy and UTI
6. A disease characterized by the formation of many fluid-filled cysts in the kidneys is known as:
   a. hypernephroma
   b. nephrohypertrophy
   c. nephrolithiasis
   d. polycystic kidney disease
   e. renal cell carcinoma

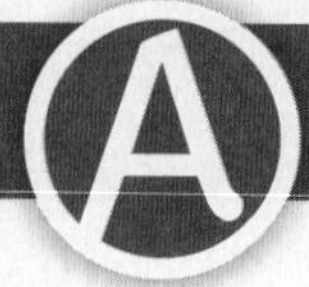

Learning Outcome 12.5 Exercises

7. The abnormal flow of urine from the bladder back into the ureter is known as:
   a. urethrocystitis
   b. urinary tract infection
   c. uropathy
   d. vesicocele
   e. vesicoureteral reflux
8. The overexpansion of the blood vessels of the testicles, leading to a soft tumor, is called:
   a. epididymo-orchitis
   b. pyeloureterectasia
   c. renal ischemia
   d. varicocele
   e. vesicocele
9. Select all of the choices below that pertain to the term *renal cell carcinoma.*
   a. also known as hypernephroma
   b. also known as nephrohypertrophy
   c. also known as polycystic kidney disease
   d. benign growth in the kidneys
   e. cancer of the kidneys
10. Select all of the choices below that pertain to the term *benign prostate hypertrophy.*
    a. also known as benign prostate hyperplasia
    b. also known as enlarged prostate
    c. literally, "friendly prostate overformation condition"
    d. literally, "friendly prostate overnourishment condition"
    e. noncancerous overdevelopment of the prostate

EXERCISE 10 *Briefly describe the difference between each pair of terms.*

1. cystolith, cystoma ______
2. cystoptosis, nephroptosis ______
3. nephromalacia, nephrosclerosis ______
4. pyelitis, pyelocystitis ______
5. prostatocystitis, prostatovesiculitis ______

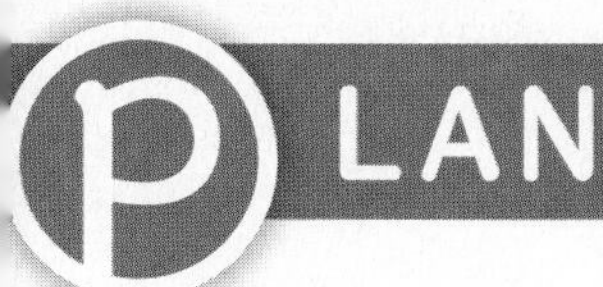

12.6 Treatments and Therapies

The main medicines used to treat the kidneys and urinary tract are focused on helping the patient urinate more (*diuretic*) or less (*antidiuretic*) often. If urinary control is a problem due to twitching of the muscle that holds back urine flow, an *antispasmodic* may be helpful.

Medicines that are specifically for men are very limited. They include medicine to help correct erectile dysfunction and testosterone, the male hormone, which is used in patients with low levels of the hormone. Patients may also choose to use liquids designed to kill sperm (*spermicides*) as a method of birth control; spermicides are available over the counter.

The most common nonsurgical procedure involving the urinary tract is bladder *catheterization.* A *catheter* is a small tube inserted into the bladder to help with urination or to get a urine sample.

The main nonsurgical treatment for the urinary tract is *dialysis.* Dialysis does the work of the kidneys when they have failed. Dialysis must be done regularly or the patient will die. The two types of dialysis involve either the inner lining of the abdomen (*peritoneal dialysis*) or a machine outside the body (*hemodialysis*). Another nonsurgical treatment in the urinary system is the use of sound waves to break up a stone in the urinary tract (*extracorporeal shock wave lithotripsy*).

Often, surgeries of the urinary tract help correct anatomical problems and restore normal urine flow. This can involve direct work on a part of the tract like the ureter (*ureteroplasty*) or urethra (*urethroplasty*). It could also involve making a new connection between two points in the tract, like a connection between the kidney and bladder (*nephrocystanastomosis*).

Another surgery of the kidneys is their complete removal (*nephrectomy*), which is often the main treatment for renal cell carcinoma. In men, the prostate is another organ that can be completely removed (*prostatectomy*) if cancerous. Part of the prostate may be removed through the urethra (*transurethral resection of the prostate*) when the prostate is enlarged and blocking urine flow. Newer, less-invasive procedures for this include using a heated needle (*transurethral needle ablation*) to remove part of the prostate.

When a testicle rides high in the scrotum it may need to be fixed (*orchiopexy*) or removed altogether (*orchiectomy*). When removed, a fake testicle (*testicular prosthesis*) is sometimes placed in the scrotum.

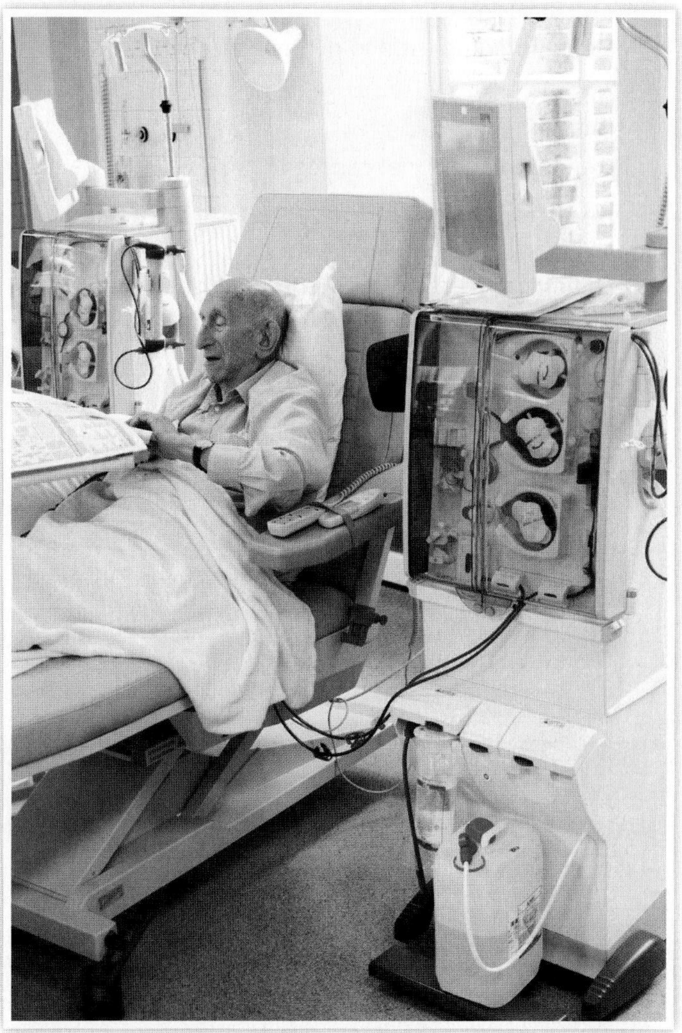

Hemodialysis uses a machine to do the work of kidneys that do not function as they should.

The most common procedure in males is the removal of the foreskin at birth (*circumcision*). While there are small medical benefits, the surgery is generally chosen for cultural or religious reasons. Circumcision is not recommended in patients with hypospadias or epispadias because the foreskin is used to surgically correct those conditions (*balanoplasty*). *Vasectomy* is another very common procedure. In the procedure, a surgeon cuts the vas deferens as a means of birth control. Occasionally, situations change, so a patient may want to reverse the procedure. Doing so is simple—reconnecting the two ends of the vas deferens (*vasovasotomy*).

12.6 Treatments and Therapies

pharmacology

Term	Word Analysis
antispasmodic AN-tee-spaz-MAWD-ik **Definition** drug used to prevent spasms	**anti / spasmod / ic** against / involuntary contraction / pertaining to
diuretic DAI-yur-IT-ik **Definition** agent that causes urination	**di / uret / ic** through / urine / pertaining to
nephrotoxin NEH-froh-TOK-sin **Definition** agent poisonous to the kidney	**nephro / toxin** kidney / poison
spermicide SPER-mih-sahyd **Definition** agent that kills sperm	**spermi / cide** sperm / kill
spermolytic SPER-moh-LIH-tik **Definition** agent that kills sperm	**spermo / lytic** sperm / breakdown agent

urinary tract procedures

Term	Word Analysis
cystectomy sis-TEK-toh-mee **Definition** surgical removal of the bladder	**cyst / ectomy** bladder / removal
cystolithectomy sis-toh-lih-THEK-toh-mee **Definition** surgical removal of a stone in the bladder	**cysto / lith / ectomy** bladder / stone / removal
cystostomy sis-TAW-stoh-mee **Definition** creation of an opening in the bladder	**cysto / stomy** bladder / opening
extracorporeal shock wave lithotripsy (ESWL) EKS-trah-cor-POR-ee-al SHOK WAYV LIH-thoh-TRIP-see **Definition** breakdown of kidney stones using sound waves generated outside the body	**extra / corpor / eal** outside / body / pertaining to **shock wave litho / tripsy** shock wave stone / wear down procedure

12.6 Treatments and Therapies

urinary tract procedures *continued*

Term	Word Analysis
fulguration FUL-gur-AY-shun **Definition** use of electric current to destroy tissue	**from Latin, for "lightning"**
heminephrectomy HEH-mee-neh-FREK-toh-mee **Definition** surgical removal of half a kidney	**hemi / nephr / ectomy** half / kidney / removal
heminephroureterectomy HEH-mee-NEH-froh-yoo-REE-ter-EK-toh-mee **Definition** surgical removal of half a kidney and a ureter	**hemi / nephro / ureter / ectomy** half / kidney / ureter / removal
hemodialysis HEE-moh-dai-AL-ah-sis **Definition** procedure for removing waste from the bloodstream	**hemo / dia / lysis** blood / through / loose
intracorporeal lithotripsy IN-trah-cor-POR-ee-al LIH-thoh-TRIP-see **Definition** breakdown of kidney stones using a device placed inside the body	**intra / corpore / al** **litho / tripsy** inside / body / pertaining to stone / wear down procedure
kidney dialysis KID-nee dai-AL-ah-sis **Definition** procedure for removing waste from the blood (a shorter name for hemodialysis) **Note:** The name comes from the fact that the procedure separates or loses (*lysis*) blood from waste by passing it through (*dia*) an external filter.	**dia / lysis** through / loose 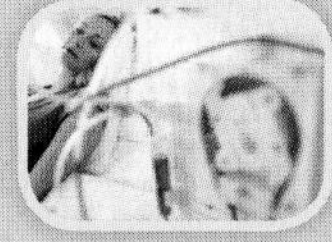 ©Science Photo Library/Getty Images RF
laparonephrectomy LAP-ah-roh-neh-FREK-toh-mee **Definition** surgical removal of a kidney through the abdomen	**laparo / nephr / ectomy** abdomen / kidney / removal
lithectomy lih-THEK-toh-mee **Definition** surgical removal of a stone	**lith / ectomy** stone / removal
lithocystotomy LIH-thoh-SIS-TAW-toh-mee **Definition** incision into the bladder to remove a stone	**litho / cysto / tomy** stone / bladder / incision
lithonephrotomy LIH-thoh-neh-FRAW-toh-mee **Definition** incision into a kidney to remove a stone	**litho / nephro / tomy** stone / kidney / incision

urinary tract procedures *continued*

Term	Word Analysis
lithotripsy LIH-thoh-TRIP-see **Definition** breakdown of a stone	**litho / tripsy** stone / wear down procedure 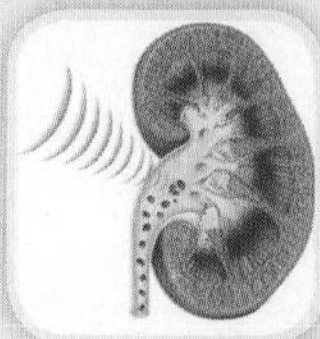
meatoplasty mee-AT-toh-PLAS-tee **Definition** surgical reconstruction of the opening of the urethra	**meato / plasty** opening / reconstruction
meatorrhaphy MEE-ah-TOR-ah-fee **Definition** suture of the opening of the urethra	**meato / rrhaphy** opening / suture
meatotomy MEE-ah-TAW-toh-mee **Definition** incision into the opening of the urethra	**meato / tomy** opening / incision
nephrectomy neh-FREK-toh-mee **Definition** surgical removal of a kidney through the abdomen	**nephr / ectomy** kidney / removal 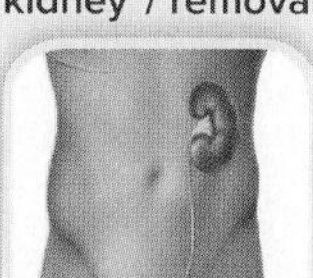
nephrocystanastomosis NEH-froh-SIST-ah-NAS-tah-MOH-sis **Definition** opening of a passageway between a kidney and the bladder	**nephro / cyst / ana / stom / osis** kidney / bladder / up / mouth / condition
nephrolithotomy NEH-froh-lih-THAW-toh-mee **Definition** incision into a kidney to remove a stone	**nephro / litho / tomy** kidney / stone / incision 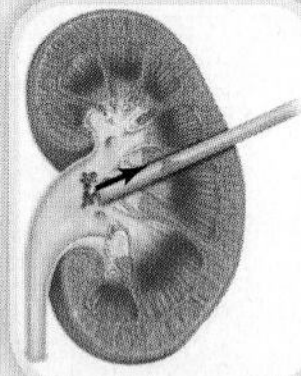
nephropexy NEH-froh-PEK-see **Definition** surgical fixation of a kidney	**nephro / pexy** kidney / fixation
nephrorrhaphy neh-FROR-ah-fee **Definition** suture of a kidney	**nephro / rrhaphy** kidney / suture

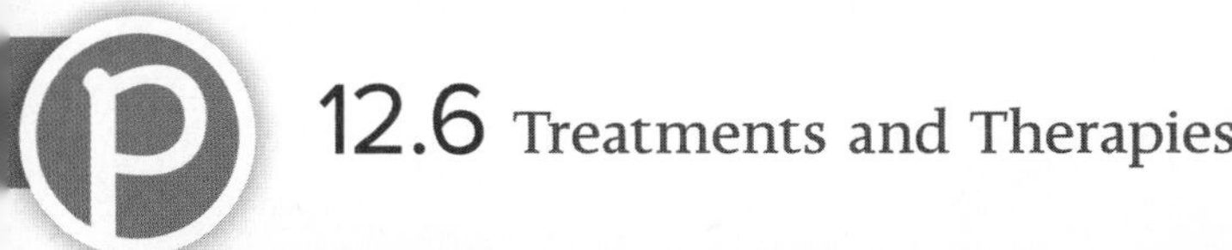

12.6 Treatments and Therapies

urinary tract procedures *continued*

Term	Word Analysis
nephrostomy neh-FRAW-stoh-mee **Definition** creation of an opening in a kidney	**nephro / stomy** kidney / opening 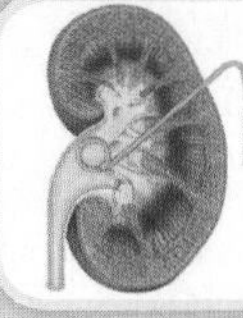
nephrotomy neh-FRAW-toh-mee **Definition** incision into a kidney	**nephro / tomy** kidney / incision
nephroureterectomy NEH-froh-yoo-REE-ter-EK-toh-mee **Definition** surgical removal of a kidney and ureter	**nephro / ureter / ectomy** kidney / ureter / removal
pyelolithotomy PAI-el-oh-lih-THAW-toh-mee **Definition** incision into a renal pelvis to remove a stone	**pyelo / litho / tomy** pelvis / stone / incision 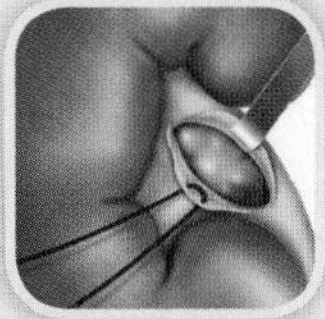
pyeloplasty PAI-el-oh-PLAS-tee **Definition** surgical reconstruction of a renal pelvis	**pyelo / plasty** pelvis / reconstruction
pyelostomy PAI-el-AW-stoh-mee **Definition** creation of an opening in a renal pelvis	**pyelo / stomy** pelvis / opening
pyelotomy PAI-el-AW-toh-mee **Definition** incision into a renal pelvis	**pyelo / tomy** pelvis / incision
renal angioplasty REE-nal AN-jee-oh-PLAS-tee **Definition** surgical reconstruction of a kidney blood vessel	**ren / al** **angio / plasty** kidney / pertaining to vessel / reconstruction
ureteroileostomy yoo-REE-ter-oh-IL-ee-AWS-toh-mee **Definition** creation of an opening between a ureter and the ileum (a portion of the small intestine)	**uretero / ileo / stomy** ureter / ileum / opening
ureteronephrectomy yoo-REE-ter-oh-neh-FREK-toh-mee **Definition** surgical removal of a kidney and ureter	**uretero / nephr / ectomy** ureter / kidney / removal 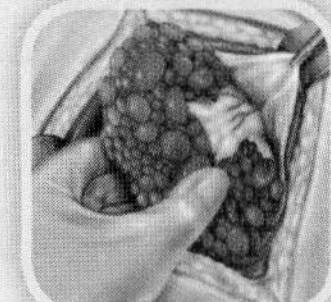

urinary tract procedures *continued*

Term	Word Analysis
ureteroplasty yoo-REE-ter-oh-PLAS-tee **Definition** surgical reconstruction of a ureter	**uretero / plasty** ureter / reconstruction
ureterorrhaphy yoo-REE-ter-OR-ah-fee **Definition** suture of a ureter	**uretero / rrhaphy** ureter / suture
urethrectomy yoo-ree-THREK-toh-mee **Definition** surgical removal of the urethra	**urethr / ectomy** urethra / removal
urethropexy yoo-REE-throh-PEK-see **Definition** surgical fixation of the urethra	**urethro / pexy** urethra / fixation
urethroplasty yoo-REE-throh-PLAS-tee **Definition** surgical reconstruction of the urethra	**urethro / plasty** urethra / reconstruction
urethrotomy yoo-ree-THRAW-toh-mee **Definition** incision into the urethra	**urethro / tomy** urethra / incision
urinary catheterization YUR-ih-NAR-ee KATH-eh-ter-ih-ZAY-shun **Definition** insertion of a catheter into the bladder to drain urine **Note:** The word *catheter* comes from Greek, for "to go inside."	**urin / ary** **catheter / ization** urine / pertaining to catheter / procedure
urostomy yur-AW-stoh-mee **Definition** creation of an opening in the urinary tract, normally to divert urine flow away from a diseased bladder	**uro / stomy** urine / opening
vesicostomy VEH-sih-KAWS-toh-mee **Definition** creation of an opening in the bladder	**vesico / stomy** bladder / opening
vesicotomy VEH-sih-KAW-toh-mee **Definition** incision into the bladder	**vesico / tomy** bladder / incision

male genitalia procedures

Term	Word Analysis
balanoplasty BAL-ah-noh-PLAS-tee **Definition** surgical reconstruction of the penis	**balano / plasty** penis / reconstruction
circumcision SIR-kum-SIH-zhun **Definition** surgical removal of the foreskin of the penis	**circum / cision** around / cut
epididymectomy EP-ih-DID-ih-MEK-toh-mee **Definition** surgical removal of the epididymis	**epididym / ectomy** epididymis / removal
epididymotomy EP-ih-DID-ih-MAW-toh-mee **Definition** incision into the epididymis	**epididymo / tomy** epididymis / incision
hydrocelectomy HAI-droh-seel-EK-toh-mee **Definition** surgical removal of a hydrocele	**hydro / cel / ectomy** water / hernia / removal
orchidectomy OR-kid-EK-toh-mee **Definition** surgical removal of a testicle	**orchid / ectomy** testicle / removal
orchidopexy OR-kid-oh-PEK-see **Definition** surgical fixation of a testicle	**orchido / pexy** testicle / fixation
orchidotomy OR-kid-AW-toh-mee **Definition** incision into a testicle	**orchido / tomy** testicle / incision
orchiectomy OR-kee-EK-mee **Definition** surgical removal of a testicle	**orchi / ectomy** testicle / removal
orchiopexy OR-kee-oh-PEK-see **Definition** surgical fixation of a testicle	**orchio / pexy** testicle / fixation
orchioplasty OR-kee-oh-PLAS-tee **Definition** surgical reconstruction of a testicle	**orchio / plasty** testicle / reconstruction

male genitalia procedures *continued*

Term	Word Analysis
prostatectomy PROS-tah-TEK-toh-mee **Definition** surgical removal of the prostate	**prostat / ectomy** prostate / removal
prostatolithotomy pros-TAT-oh-lih-THAW-toh-mee **Definition** incision into the prostate to remove a stone	**prostato / litho / tomy** prostate / stone / incision
prostatovesiculectomy pros-TAT-oh-veh-SIK-yoo-LEK-toh-mee **Definition** surgical removal of the prostate and seminal vesicles **NOTE:** Here, the root *vesicul* refers *not* to the urinary bladder but instead to the small seminal vesicles, or bladders, that hold seminal fluid.	**prostato / vesicul / ectomy** prostate / bladder / removal
transurethral resection of the prostate (TURP) **Definition** procedure of removing all or part of the prostate by the insertion of a resectoscope into the urethra	**trans / urethr / al** — through / urethra / pertaining to **re / sect / ion** — back / cut / procedure
vasectomy vah-SEK-toh-mee **Definition** surgical removal of the vas deferens	**vas / ectomy** vessel / removal
vasovasostomy VAS-oh-vah-SAWS-toh-mee **Definition** creation of an opening between two vessels; this is the technical term for a vasectomy reversal	**vaso / vaso / stomy** vessel / vessel / opening
vesiculectomy veh-SIK-yoo-LEK-toh-mee **Definition** surgical removal of the seminal vesicles **NOTE:** See the note for prostatovesiculectomy above to see how *vesiculo* refers not to the bladder but to seminal vesicles.	**vesicul / ectomy** bladder / removal

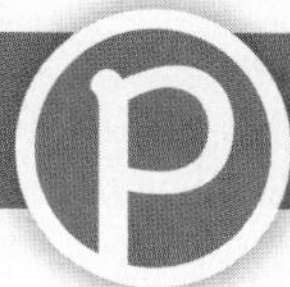

Learning Outcome 12.6 Exercises

PRONUNCIATION

EXERCISE 1 *Indicate which syllable is emphasized when pronounced.*

EXAMPLE: bronchitis bron**chi**tis

1. spermicide ______
2. vasectomy ______
3. lithectomy ______
4. cystectomy ______
5. nephrectomy ______
6. urostomy ______
7. cystostomy ______
8. nephrostomy ______
9. nephrotomy ______
10. cystolithectomy ______
11. nephrorrhaphy ______
12. orchiopexy ______
13. urethropexy ______
14. nephropexy ______
15. orchidopexy ______
16. lithotripsy ______
17. nephrotoxin ______
18. urethrotomy ______
19. vesicostomy ______
20. ureteroplasty ______
21. balanoplasty ______
22. urethrectomy ______
23. vesiculectomy ______
24. prostatectomy ______
25. heminephrectomy ______
26. nephrolithotomy ______
27. vasovasostomy ______
28. ureteroileostomy ______
29. ureterorrhaphy ______
30. epididymotomy ______

TRANSLATION

EXERCISE 2 *Break down the following words into their component parts.*

EXAMPLE: nasopharyngoscope *naso | pharyngo | scope*

1. nephrotoxin ______
2. urostomy ______
3. orchiopexy ______
4. urethroplasty ______
5. antispasmodic ______
6. meatorrhaphy ______
7. nephrorrhaphy ______
8. ureterorrhaphy ______
9. spermolytic ______
10. vesiculectomy ______
11. hydrocelectomy ______
12. vasovasostomy ______
13. pyelolithotomy ______
14. lithonephrotomy ______
15. nephrolithotomy ______
16. prostatolithotomy ______
17. ureteroileostomy ______
18. heminephrectomy ______
19. laparonephrectomy ______
20. cystolithectomy ______
21. hemodialysis ______
22. circumcision ______

Learning Outcome 12.6 Exercises

EXERCISE 3 *Underline and define the roots from this chapter in the following terms.*

1. spermicide ______
2. lithotripsy ______
3. ureteroplasty ______
4. orchioplasty ______
5. balanoplasty ______
6. meatoplasty ______
7. urethropexy ______
8. nephropexy ______
9. orchidopexy ______
10. cystostomy ______
11. nephrostomy ______
12. pyelostomy ______
13. vesicostomy ______
14. epididymotomy ______
15. diuretic ______
16. renal angioplasty ______
17. intracorporeal lithotripsy ______
18. transurethral resection ______
19. urinary catheterization ______
20. extracorporeal shock wave lithotripsy ______
21. heminephroureterectomy (2 roots) ______
22. prostatovesiculectomy (2 roots) ______
23. nephrocystanastomosis (2 roots) ______

EXERCISE 4 *Match the term on the left with its definition on the right.*

______	1. circumcision	a.	agent that causes urination
______	2. kidney dialysis	b.	insertion of a catheter into the bladder to drain urine
______	3. urinary catheterization	c.	procedure for removing waste from the bloodstream
______	4. diuretic	d.	procedure for removing waste from the blood (a shorter name for hemodialysis)
______	5. hemodialysis	e.	procedure of removing all or part of the prostate by the insertion of a resectoscope into the urethra
______	6. vasovasostomy	f.	surgical removal of the foreskin of the penis
______	7. transurethral resection of the prostate	g.	breakdown of kidney stones using a device placed inside the body

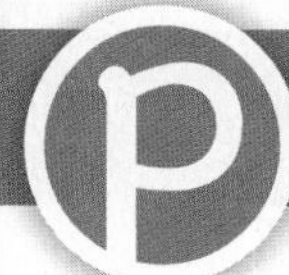

_____	8. intracorporeal lithotripsy	h.	breakdown of kidney stones using sound waves generated outside the body
_____	9. extracorporeal shock wave lithotripsy	i.	creation of an opening between two vessels; the technical term for a vasectomy reversal
_____	10. fulguration	j.	use of electric current to destroy tissue

EXERCISE 5 *Fill in the blanks.*

1. meatotomy: incision into _____
2. nephrotomy: incision into _____
3. pyelotomy: incision into _____
4. urethrotomy: incision into _____
5. vesicotomy: incision into _____
6. epididymotomy: incision into _____
7. orchidotomy: incision into _____
8. cystectomy: surgical removal of the _____
9. lithectomy: surgical removal of the _____
10. nephrectomy: surgical removal of the _____
11. urethrectomy: surgical removal of the _____
12. epididymectomy: surgical removal of the _____
13. orchidectomy: surgical removal of the _____
14. orchiectomy: surgical removal of the _____
15. prostatectomy: surgical removal of the _____
16. vasectomy: surgical removal of the _____
17. nephroureterectomy: surgical removal of a(n) _____ and _____
18. ureteronephrectomy: surgical removal of a(n) _____ and _____
19. prostatovesiculectomy: surgical removal of a(n) _____ and _____

EXERCISE 6 *Translate the following terms as literally as possible.*

EXAMPLE: nasopharyngoscope *an instrument for looking at the nose and throat*

1. urethrotomy _____
2. vasectomy _____
3. orchidopexy _____
4. meatorrhaphy _____
5. ureterorrhaphy _____
6. pyelostomy _____
7. lithotripsy _____
8. vesiculectomy _____
9. epididymotomy _____
10. spermicide _____
11. antispasmodic _____
12. cystolithectomy _____

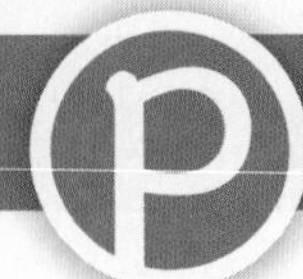

Learning Outcome 12.6 Exercises

13. prostatolithotomy ____________
14. prostatovesiculectomy ____________
15. renal angioplasty ____________
16. hydrocelectomy ____________
17. ureteroileostomy ____________
18. heminephroureterectomy ____________
19. nephrocystanastomosis ____________

GENERATION

EXERCISE 7 *Build a medical term from the information provided.*

EXAMPLE: inflammation of the sinuses *sinusitis*

1. incision into the bladder (use *vesic/o*) ____________
2. incision into a testicle (use *orchid/o*) ____________
3. incision into the opening (of the urethra) ____________
4. creation of an opening in the bladder (use *cyst/o*) ____________
5. creation of an opening in the bladder (use *vesic/o*) ____________
6. surgical removal of the epididymis ____________
7. surgical removal of the urethra ____________
8. surgical removal of the prostate ____________
9. surgical removal of a kidney and ureter ____________
10. surgical reconstruction of a ureter ____________
11. surgical reconstruction of the opening (of the urethra) ____________
12. surgical reconstruction of a renal pelvis ____________
13. surgical reconstruction of the penis ____________
14. surgical fixation of the urethra ____________

EXERCISE 8 *Multiple-choice questions. Select the correct answer(s).*

1. The surgical removal of a kidney through the abdomen is known as:
   a. abdominonephrectomy
   b. fulguration
   c. heminephrectomy
   d. laparonephrectomy
   e. meatonephrectomy
2. An incision into the renal pelvis is called a:
   a. renal incision
   b. pyelectomy
   c. pyelotomy
   d. nephrotomy
   e. nephrectomy
3. A *spermolytic* is:
   a. an agent that assists in conception by making sperm meet with an egg for fertilization
   b. an agent that assists the testicles in the formation of sperm
   c. an agent that creates sperm
   d. an agent that kills sperm
   e. none of these

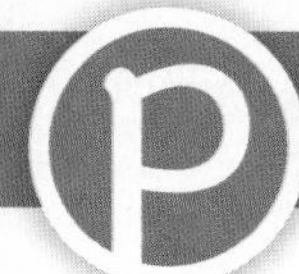

Learning Outcome 12.6 Exercises

4. Which of the following statements is true of the term *kidney dialysis*?
   a. procedure for removing waste from the blood
   b. shorter name for hemodialysis
   c. its name comes from the fact that the procedure separates or loses (*lysis*) blood from waste by passing it through (*dia*) an external filter
   d. all of these
   e. none of these
5. Select all of the following choices that pertain to the term *urostomy*.
   a. creation of an opening in the bladder
   b. creation of an opening in the urinary tract
   c. literally, "bladder opening"
   d. literally, "urine opening"
   e. procedure normally used to divert urine flow away from a diseased bladder
6. Select all of the following choices that pertain to the term *fulguration*.
   a. from Latin, for "coffee"
   b. from Latin, for "lightning"
   c. the use of electric current to destroy tissue
   d. the use of electric current to repair tissue
   e. none of these
7. Select all of the following terms that pertain to the urinary tract.
   a. cystectomy
   b. epididymectomy
   c. lithectomy
   d. nephrectomy
   e. orchidectomy
   f. prostatectomy
   g. urethrectomy
   h. vesicotomy
8. Select all of the following terms that pertain to the male genitalia.
   a. cystectomy
   b. epididymectomy
   c. lithectomy
   d. nephrectomy
   e. orchidectomy
   f. prostatectomy
   g. urethrectomy
   h. vesicotomy

EXERCISE 9 *Briefly describe the difference between each pair of terms.*

1. ureteroplasty, urethroplasty ____________________
2. balanoplasty, orchioplasty ____________________
3. nephrostomy, nephrotomy ____________________
4. orchiectomy, orchiopexy ____________________
5. heminephrectomy, nephrectomy ____________________
6. lithocystotomy, lithonephrotomy ____________________
7. nephrolithotomy, pyelolithotomy ____________________

12.7 Abbreviations

Abbreviations provide a shorthand way of referring to things that either recur often or are too long to write out. When dealing with the urinary tract and male genitalia, these terms can include lab work (UA), diagnostic procedures (DRE), common complaints (SUI), diagnoses (UTI, BPH), or treatments (ESWL, TURP).

urinary tract

Abbreviation	Definition
BUN	blood urea nitrogen
Bx	biopsy
cath	catheter
ESWL	extracorporeal shock wave lithotripsy
HD	hemodialysis
I&O	intake and output
IVP	intravenous pyelogram
IVU	intravenous urogram
KUB	kidneys, ureters, bladder
OAB	overactive bladder
PKD	polycystic kidney disease
RP	retrograde pyelogram
SUI	stress urinary incontinence
UA	urinalysis ©McGraw-Hill Education
UTI	urinary tract infection
VCUG	voiding cystourethrogram
VUR	vesicoureteral reflux

male genitalia

Abbreviation	Definition
AIDS	acquired immunodeficiency syndrome
BPH	benign prostate hyperplasia

male genitalia *continued*

Abbreviation	Definition
DRE	digital rectal exam
ED	erectile dysfunction
HIV	human immunodeficiency virus
HPV	human papilloma virus
HSV	herpes simplex virus
PSA	prostate-specific antigen
STD/STI	sexually transmitted disease, sexually transmitted infection
TURP	transurethral resection of the prostate

Learning Outcome 12.7 Exercises

EXERCISE 1 *Define the following abbreviations.*

1. STD ______
2. STI ______
3. cath ______
4. ED ______
5. UTI ______
6. IVP ______
7. IVU ______
8. UA ______
9. HD ______
10. KUB ______
11. RP ______
12. VCUG ______
13. PSA ______
14. OAB ______

EXERCISE 2 *Give the abbreviations for the following definitions.*

1. biopsy ______
2. catheter ______
3. digital rectal exam ______
4. blood urea nitrogen ______
5. intravenous urogram ______
6. kidneys, ureters, bladder ______

Learning Outcome 12.7 Exercises

7. polycystic kidney disease ____________________
8. stress urinary incontinence ____________________
9. benign prostate hyperplasia ____________________
10. transurethral resection of the prostate ____________________
11. voiding cystourethrogram ____________________
12. extracorporeal shock wave lithotripsy ____________________
13. intake and output ____________________

EXERCISE 3 *Match the abbreviation on the left with its full definition on its right.*

______	1. UTI	a. abnormal flow of urine from the bladder back into the ureters
______	2. UA	b. analysis of the urine
______	3. DRE	c. disease characterized by the formation of many fluid-filled cysts in the kidneys
______	4. HD	d. examination of the prostate using a finger inserted into the rectum
______	5. BPH	e. image of the renal pelvis produced by injecting a contrast dye from the bladder to the kidney
______	6. PKD	f. infection of the urinary tract
______	7. BUN	g. loss of bladder control caused by the application of external pressure
______	8. RP	h. nitrogen in the blood in the form of urea; it is the product of the breakdown of amino acids for energy
______	9. SUI	i. noncancerous overdevelopment of the prostate, also known as an enlarged prostate
______	10. VUR	j. procedure for removing waste from the bloodstream

EXERCISE 4 *Multiple-choice questions. Select the correct answer(s).*

1. IVP stands for *intravenous pyelogram.* Which is the correct breakdown of the term?
   a. *intra* (inside) + *venous* (vein) + *pyelo* (renal pelvis) + *gram* (record)
   b. *intra* (outside) + *venous* (vein) + *pyelo* (renal pelvis) + *gram* (record)
   c. *intra* (outside) + *venous* (vein) + *pyelo* (bladder) + *gram* (record)
   d. *intra* (inside) + *venous* (vein) + *pyelo* (bladder) + *gram* (record)
   e. *intra* (inside) + *venous* (vein) + *pyelo* (kidney) + *gram* (record)
2. VUR stands for *vesicoureteral flux.* Which is the correct breakdown of the term?
   a. *vesico* (bladder) + *ureteral* (testicle) + *reflux* (flow back)
   b. *vesico* (bladder) + *ureteral* (ureter) + *reflux* (flow back)
   c. *vesico* (kidney) + *ureteral* (ureter) + *reflux* (flow back)
   d. *vesico* (seminal vesicle) + *ureteral* (testicle) + *reflux* (flow back)
   e. *vesico* (seminal vesicle) + *ureteral* (ureter) + *reflux* (flow back)
3. TURP stands for:
   a. topographical ureteral retrograde procedure
   b. topographical urethral retrograde procedure
   c. transureteral resection of the prostate
   d. transurethral resection of the prostate
   e. transurethral retrograde pyelogram

12.8 Electronic Health Records

Consult Note

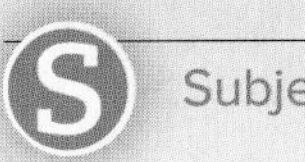

Subjective

Reason for Consult: **urinary retention**

HPI: Mr. Johnson is a 57-year-old male with a 2-month history of difficulty **voiding.** He reports **urgency** and **frequency.** He has had increasing problems with a weak urinary stream. The symptoms have progressed to include mild abdominal discomfort and **erectile dysfunction.** He denies any **incontinence, hematuria, balanorrhea, orchiodynia,** or trauma. He has not tried any medicines at this point. PMHx: Hypercholesterolemia–currently controlled with diet. Positive history of gonococcal **urethritis** 3 years previously. No history of **urolithiasis.**

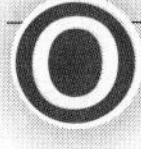

Objective

Physical Exam

Vitals: T 98.6; HR: 84; RR: 24; BP: 124/90.

Gen: Alert, well-appearing man in no apparent distress.

HEENT: Normocephalic. Pupils equal, round, and reactive to light and accommodation. Tympanic membranes normal. Mucous membranes moist and pink.

Neck: Supple. No lymphadenopathy. No jugulovenous distention.

Cardiovascular: Regular in rate and rhythm without murmur, gallops, or rubs.

Resp: Clear to auscultation bilaterally.

Abd: Mild distention. Fullness and discomfort of **suprapubic** area.

Neuro: Normal reflexes and strength of the lower extremities, normal sphincter tone.

Gross appearance of penis: No **meatal stenosis,** easily retractable foreskin, no penile ulcers.

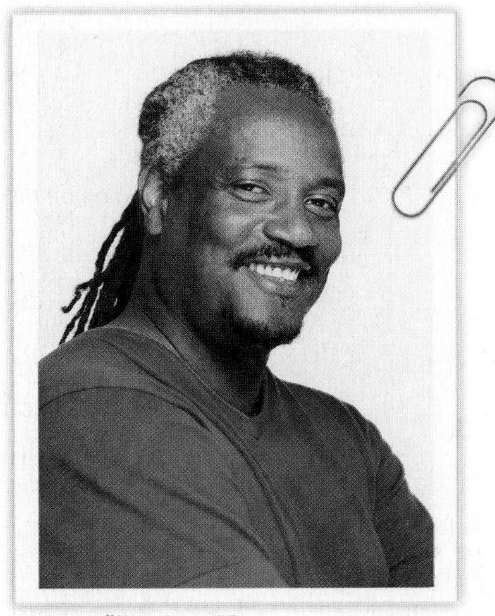

©Tom Le Goff/Getty Images RF

DRE: Enlarged prostate of 3 finger breadths. No **prostatorrhea.** Labs: Elevated **PSA**. **UA** normal. UCx negative. BMP normal.

Imaging:

Transabdominal ultrasound revealed significant **postvoid** residual. Consistent with **bladder outlet obstruction.**

Cystoscopy to r/o **urethral stricture** was normal.

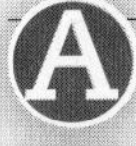

Assessment

Mr. Johnson has **benign prostatic hyperplasia.**

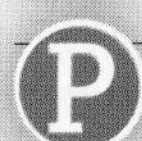

Plan

Plan:

We will be starting initial treatment of fluid intake restriction and medicine. I explained to Mr. Johnson that if he fails this therapy, the next step would be surgical. There are several options available. I discussed these options, including **TURP** versus open **prostatectomy** versus **transurethral incision** of **prostate** (TUIP). Mr. Johnson will return to my clinic for follow-up in 6 weeks.

–Jonas Wallin, MD

Learning Outcome 12.8 Exercises

EXERCISE 1 *Match the term on the left with its definition on the right.*

_____ 1. urethritis
_____ 2. prostatomegaly
_____ 3. voiding
_____ 4. incontinence
_____ 5. prostatectomy
_____ 6. orchiodynia
_____ 7. benign prostate hyperplasia
_____ 8. hematuria
_____ 9. balanorrhea
_____ 10. meatal stenosis

a. abnormal enlargement of the prostate
b. another term for urination
c. bloody urination
d. discharge from the penis
e. inability to control urination
f. inflammation of the urethra
g. narrowing of the opening of the urethra
h. noncancerous overdevelopment of the prostate, also known as an enlarged prostate
i. surgical removal of the prostate
j. testicle pain

EXERCISE 2 *Match the abbreviation on the left with its definition on the right.*

_____ 1. ED
_____ 2. UA
_____ 3. BPH
_____ 4. DRE
_____ 5. TURP

a. benign prostate hyperplasia
b. digital rectal exam
c. erectile dysfunction
d. transurethral resection of the prostate
e. urinalysis

EXERCISE 3 *Fill in the blanks.*

1. _____ _____ _____: History of present illness
   a. The patient's name: _____
   b. The patient's age: _____
   c. The patient's gender: _____
   d. The patient's CC: difficulty _____ (urinating), the symptoms of which have progressed to include abdominal discomfort and *erectile dysfunction* (give abbreviation: _____)
   e. The patient denies *incontinence* (give definition: _____), *hematuria* (give definition: _____), *balanorrhea* (give definition: _____), or *orchiodynia* (give definition: _____)
2. PMHx: Past Medical
   a. Positive history of gonococcal *urethritis* (inflammation of the _____)
   b. No history of *urolithiasis* (presence of _____ in the urinary system)
3. PE: _____ Exam
   a. DRE: (define abbreviation: _____ _____ _____)
   b. No _____ (discharge from the prostate)

Learning Outcome 12.8 Exercises

EXERCISE 4 *True or false questions. Indicate true answers with a T and false answers with an F.*

1. Mr. Johnson is experiencing ED. ______________
2. Mr. Johnson complains of blood in the urine as well as an inability to control his urination. ________________
3. Mr. Johnson's prostate is a normal size. ________
4. The patient's urinalysis was abnormal. ________
5. The patient has BPH. _______
6. The patient has cancer and will need to have his prostate removed. ________

EXERCISE 5 *Multiple-choice questions. Select the correct answer(s).*

1. A *cystoscopy* is a:
   a. procedure for examining the bladder
   b. procedure for examining the urinary tract
   c. recording or image of the bladder
   d. recording or image of the urinary tract
2. Mr. Johnson's imaging revealed "significant *postvoid* residual." The term *postvoid* refers to:
   a. after urination
   b. before urination
   c. the urinary tract
   d. the urine itself
3. The patient does not have a past medical history of *urolithiasis*. Which of the following is a correct breakdown of this term?
   a. *uro* (urinary tract) + *lith* (stones) + *iasis* (inflammation)
   b. *uro* (urinary tract) + *lith* (stones) + *iasis* (presence)
   c. *uro* (urinary tract) + *lith* (tumor) + *iasis* (inflammation)
   d. *uro* (urinary tract) + *lith* (tumor) + *iasis* (presence)
4. One of the patient's surgical options includes a *transurethral incision of prostate* (TUIP). Which of the following is a correct breakdown of the term *transurethral*?
   a. *trans* (through) + *urethral* (urethra)
   b. *trans* (around) + *urethral* (urethra)
   c. *trans* (out) + *urethral* (urethra)
   d. *trans* (inside) + *urethral* (urethra)
5. The patient has a history of *hypercholesterolemia*. Which of the following is a correct breakdown of this term?
   a. *hyper* (over) + *cholesterol* (cholesterol) + *emia* (blood condition)
   b. *hyper* (over) + *cholesterol* (cholesterol) + *emia* (urine condition)
   c. *hyper* (under) + *cholesterol* (cholesterol) + *emia* (blood condition)
   d. *hyper* (under) + *cholesterol* (cholesterol) + *emia* (urine condition)

Urology Clinic Note

Subjective:
Mr. Hector Joules presents to the office today for swelling in his right testicle. The swelling has been present for the past month. He reports **orchialgia,** described as a dull ache in the testicle. He also has had a feeling of heaviness in his abdomen. He hasn't had any recent injury to the area. He denies risky sexual behavior, **urethrorrhea, dysuria, nocturia, polyuria.**

PMHx: **Cryptorchidism** as a child.
PSHx: **Orchipexy** at 4 years.

Objective:
Vital signs: Temp: 100.0; HR: 62; RR: 22; BP: 102/72.
General: Well developed, well nourished, in no acute distress. Alert and oriented.
HEENT: Normocephalic atraumatic. Pupils equal, round, and reactive to light and accommodation. Mucous membranes moist and pink. Nares patent. Normal ear canals and tympanic membranes.
CV: Regular in rate and rhythm without murmurs.
Resp: Clear to auscultation bilaterally. No wheezes, rales, or rhonchi.
Abd: Soft, nontender, nondistended. Hepatomegaly 2 cm below costal margin. No splenomegaly.
GU: Right-sided 2.5 cm solid, firm testicular mass. Immobile and fixed to testicle. Nontender to palpation.
Lymph nodes: Enlarged supraclavicular and inguinal nodes.
Radiology: Testicular U/S: hypoechoic (*areas that show darker on ultrasound*), solid **intratesticular** mass

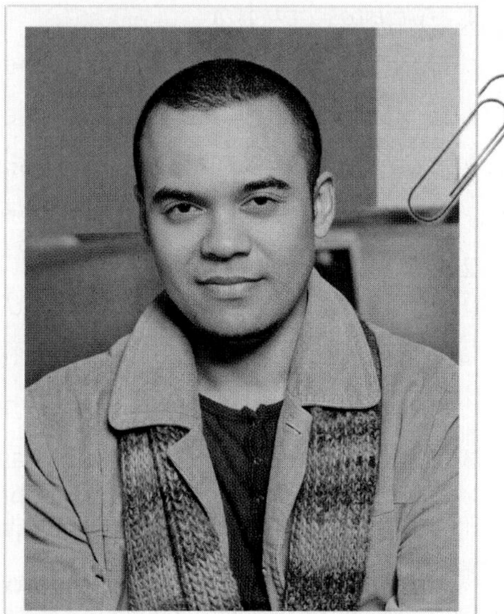

Assessment:
This is a 24-year-old male with a right-sided testicular mass. Given the u/s results, this is most likely testicular carcinoma. The differential diagnosis also includes **epididymitis, testicular torsion, hydrocele, spermatocele,** and **varicocele.**

Plan:
Since there is significant risk for cancer, we will schedule Mr. Joules for a radical **orchidectomy.** We will send samples to Pathology to confirm the diagnosis and staging. I outlined the general treatment and follow-up plan with Mr. Joules. Today, we will check a sperm count to establish a baseline, as **azoospermia/oligospermia** are risks of surgery.

–**Priscilla Pascal, MD**

Learning Outcome 12.8 Exercises

EXERCISE 6 *Match the term on the left with its definition on the right.*

	Term		Definition
______ 1.	testicular carcinoma	a.	fluid-filled mass in a testicle
______ 2.	orchialgia	b.	hernia or distention of the epididymis caused by sperm cells
______ 3.	orchidectomy	c.	condition characterized by lack of living sperm
______ 4.	urethrorrhea	d.	condition characterized by low sperm production
______ 5.	epididymitis	e.	discharge from the urethra
______ 6.	dysuria	f.	excessive urination
______ 7.	nocturia	g.	hidden testicle
______ 8.	polyuria	h.	inflammation of the epididymis
______ 9.	cryptorchidism	i.	nighttime urination
______ 10.	orchiopexy	j.	overexpansion of the blood vessels of the testicles, leading to a soft tumor
______ 11.	hydrocele	k.	painful urination
______ 12.	varicocele	l.	surgical fixation of a testicle
______ 13.	spermatocele	m.	surgical removal of a testicle
______ 14.	azoospermia	n.	testicle pain
______ 15.	oligospermia	o.	testicular cancer

EXERCISE 7 *Fill in the blanks.*

1. The patient's name:______________________
2. The patient's age:______________________
3. The patient's gender:______________________
4. The patient's temperature:______________________
5. Subjective
   a. The patient reports *orchialgia* (give definition: ______________________)
   b. The patient denies *urethrorrhea* (give definition: ______________________),
   dysuria (give definition: ______________________),
   nocturia (give definition: ______________________),
   or *polyuria* (give definition: ______________________)
6. PMHx: Past Medical______________________
   a. ______________________ (hidden testicle) as a child
7. PSHX: Past ______________________ History
   a. *orchiopexy* (give definition: ______________________) at 4 years

EXERCISE 8 *True or false questions. Indicate true answers with a T and false answers with an F.*

1. The patient does not have painful or excessive urination. __________
2. Mr. Joules most likely has testicular cancer. __________

3. The patient will be able to keep both of his testicles. ________
4. Lack of living sperm is one risk of the recommended surgery. ________

EXERCISE 9 *Multiple-choice questions. Select the correct answer(s).*

1. Which of the following symptoms is the patient reporting?
   a. discharge from the urethra
   b. excessive urination
   c. nighttime urination
   d. pain in the testicle
   e. painful urination
2. Which of the following choices is NOT part of the differential diagnosis?
   a. fluid-filled mass in the testicle
   b. hernia or distention of the epididymis caused by sperm cells
   c. inflammation of the epididymis
   d. noncancerous overdevelopment of the prostate
   e. overexpansion of the blood vessels of the testicles, leading to a soft tumor
3. Which of the following choices is NOT part of the patient's plan?
   a. a test to determine the patient's live sperm count
   b. a test to determine the patient's sperm production
   c. biopsy of a testicle
   d. surgical removal of a testicle
   e. none of these

Discharge Summary

Patient: Susan Nesbit
Date of Admission: 7/7/2015
Date of Discharge: 7/17/2015

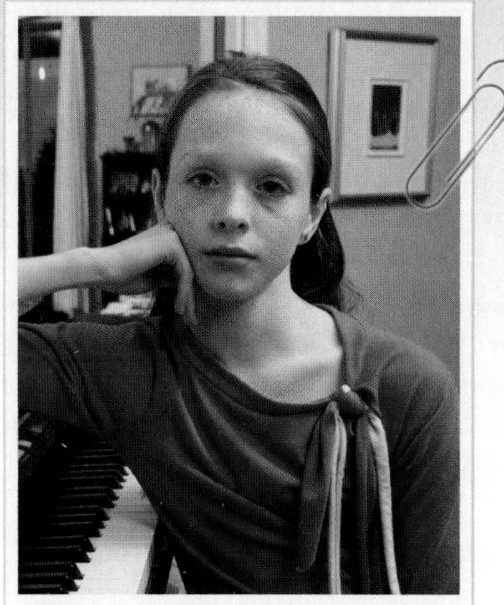
©Pixtal/AGE Fotostock RF

Admission Diagnosis
1. **Dysuria**
2. Fever

Discharge Diagnosis
1. **Pyelonephritis**
2. **Perinephric Abscess**

Discharge Condition:
Stable

Consultations:
Nephrology
Urology

Procedures
1. U/S guided percutaneous **renal** needle aspiration with drain placement.

Labs
Admission labs: UA: **Pyuria:** >20 wbcs; **Hematuria:** 3+ blood; **Albuminuria:** 1+ protein.
Urine culture: *E. coli.*
Blood culture: *E. coli.*
Discharge labs: UA normal. Urine culture normal.

Imaging
VCUG: No **vesicoureteral reflux** noted.
RUS: No **hydronephrosis** noted. Normal.
Spiral CT of kidneys on day 3 of admission revealed perinephric abscess formation of the left kidney.

HPI
Miss Susan Nesbit is a 12-year-old female who first visited her primary care provider for **dysuria.** A **UA** was ordered, but the patient could not urinate in the office. She took the UA cup home, but did not return with the sample. The next day, Susan's dysuria worsened, and she developed a fever of 102.3°F, as well as vomiting and **hematuria,** so she returned to the clinic. A urinalysis performed in the office revealed significant **pyuria, hematuria,** and **albuminuria.** Since Susan was not able to keep any fluids down, her primary care provider sent her to the emergency department for evaluation for admission.

Hospital Course
On arrival at the ED, Susan was alert and oriented, but she looked a little pale and tired. She was treated with IVF for dehydration and given antipyretics for her fever. Within an hour, she had improved some, but given her inability to tolerate PO, the pediatric on-call physician recommended that she be admitted. She was admitted for a **UTI** and treated with IV antibiotics, and a urine culture was sent. On hospital day 2,

Discharge Summary *(continued)*

her fever had improved, and she was looking better overall. Unfortunately, on hospital day 3, Susan's fever returned, and she looked acutely ill.

A spiral CT (*a more detailed type of CT*) of Susan's abdomen and pelvis showed a developing perinephric abscess. Both nephrology and urology were consulted at that time, and they both agreed that the best treatment option would be needle aspiration with drain placement. She was taken to the OR, and the drain was placed. Fluid collection from the abscess was sent for culture.

Susan tolerated the procedure well and was admitted to the PICU. She continued IV antibiotics through her PICU course. After 5 days with the drain, the discharge had decreased significantly, so we repeated a spiral CT to confirm clearing of the abscess. The CT was normal, so the drain was removed and Susan was transferred to the regular pediatric wing. A renal ultrasound was also normal, as was a **voiding cystourethrogram**. Susan switched to oral antibiotics and was discharged home.

Discharge Physical Examination
VS
Temp: 98.6; RR: 24; HR: 86; BP: 100/64.
General: WDWN. Alert.
HEENT: PERRLA, TMs normal. Mucous membranes moist and pink.
CV: RRR.
RESP: CTA.
Abdomen: Soft, nondistended, no CVA tenderness. No suprapubic tenderness.
Skin: Warm, pink.

Activity
No restrictions. Diet: No restrictions.

Meds
Antibiotics.

Follow-Up Appointments
Primary care provider: 1 week
Urology: 2 weeks
Nephrology: 1 month

–Dictated by Jennifer Wong, DO

Learning Outcome 12.8 Exercises

EXERCISE 10 *Match the term on the left with its definition on the right.*

	Term		Definition
_____	1. urology	a.	abnormal flow of urine from the bladder back into the ureters
_____	2. nephrology	b.	bloody urination
_____	3. dysuria	c.	inflammation of the kidney and renal pelvis
_____	4. hematuria	d.	kidney condition caused by the obstruction of urine flow
_____	5. pyuria	e.	painful urination
_____	6. albuminuria	f.	protein in the urine
_____	7. pyelonephritis	g.	pus in the urine
_____	8. hydronephrosis	h.	study of the kidneys
_____	9. vesicoureteral reflux	i.	study of the urinary tract

EXERCISE 11 *Fill in the blanks.*

1. Admission diagnosis
   a. *Dysuria* (give definition: ________________________)
2. Discharge diagnosis
   a. *Pyelonephritis* (give definition: ________________________)
3. Consultations
   a. *Nephrology* (study of the ________________________)
   b. *Urology* (study of the ________________________)
4. Labs: UA (give definition for abbreviation: ________________________)
   a. *pyuria* (________________________ in urine)
   b. *hematuria* (________________________ in urine)
   c. *albuminuria* (________________________ in urine)

EXERCISE 12 *True or false questions. Indicate true answers with a T and false answers with an F.*

1. Susan's imaging revealed that she has vesicoureteral reflux. ________
2. On arrival at the ED, Susan was treated with intravenous fluids. ________
3. Susan could tolerate oral food and drink upon her arrival at the ED. ________
4. Susan was admitted to the hospital for a urinary tract infection. ________
5. Susan's imaging revealed a kidney condition caused by the obstruction of urine flow. ________

Learning Outcome 12.8 Exercises

EXERCISE 13 *Multiple-choice questions. Select the correct answer(s).*

1. According to the in-clinic urinalysis, which of the following was NOT present in Susan's urine?
   a. blood
   b. protein
   c. pus
   d. sugar
   e. all of these were present in Susan's urine
2. According to the discharge diagnosis, Susan had a *perinephric abscess.* Which of the following choices is a correct breakdown of the term *perinephric?*
   a. *peri* (around) + *nephric* (bladder)
   b. *peri* (around) + *nephric* (kidney)
   c. *peri* (inside) + *nephric* (bladder)
   d. *peri* (inside) + *nephric* (kidney)
   e. *peri* (outside) + *nephric* (kidney)
3. The hospital course reports that Susan's *renal ultrasound* was normal. A *renal ultrasound* is an:
   a. image of the bladder using high-frequency sound waves
   b. image of the kidney using high-frequency sound waves
   c. image of the renal pelvis using high-frequency sound waves
   d. image of the urinary tract using high-frequency sound waves
   e. none of these

Urology Consult

Chief Complaint: **Hematuria.**

History of Present Illness: Doug Harper is a 5-year-old boy with a 2-day history of gross **hematuria.** Doug's parents noted that Doug had had **oliguria** the past 2 days and had very dark, tea-colored urine. They took Doug to his primary care provider, Nelda Lopez, NP. Ms. Lopez tested a **urinalysis,** and the results showed **hematuria** and **albuminuria.** She also noted Doug had periorbital edema and that he was **hypertensive** in the office. The parents report that Doug had a recent throat infection (last week) that resolved on its own.

Review of Systems: Positive for nausea, but no emesis. Otherwise negative.

Medications: None.

Allergies: No known drug allergies.

Past Medical History: Noncontributory.

Past Surgical History: **Balanoplasty** for **hypospadias** at age 1.

Social History: Doug lives with his parents and older sister. He is going into kindergarten in the fall.

Family History: Paternal grandfather with **polycystic kidney disease.**

Vital Signs

Temp: 98.6; Heart Rate: 100; Respiratory Rate: 24; Blood Pressure: 118/86.

Physical Exam

General: WDWN. Nontoxic. NAD.

Head: PERRLA. EOMI bilaterally. Periorbital edema. No erythema. No proptosis. Mucous membranes moist and pink. TMs normal.

Cardiovascular: Regular in rate and rhythm without murmurs, gallop, or rubs. No JVD.

Respiratory: Clear to auscultation.

Abdomen: Soft, nontender, nondistended, no hepatosplenomegaly. No **CVA tenderness.** Neurologic: Alert, oriented.

Skin: Pink, warm.

Extremities: Edema of feet. Dorsal pedal pulses present.

Labs: Elevated **BUN** and creatinine. **Hypocomplementemia.** Antistreptolysin O and antiDNAase B.

Imaging: None.

Assessment/Plan

1. Hematuria/albuminuria: Doug clearly has a **nephropathy.** The differential diagnosis includes **post streptococcal glomerulonephritis,** basement membrane disease, lupus **nephritis, membranoproliferative glomerulonephritis.** Since he had a recent throat infection, post streptococcal glomerulonephritis is the most likely cause. We will wait for the labs to confirm a recent strep infection.
2. Hypertension, edema: We will begin Doug on **diuretics** and **fluid restriction,** as well as a low-sodium diet.

–William Hunter, MD

Learning Outcome 12.8 Exercises

EXERCISE 14 *Match the term on the left with its definition on the right.*

_____ 1. nephritis
_____ 2. nephropathy
_____ 3. urinalysis
_____ 4. diuretic
_____ 5. polycystic kidney disease
_____ 6. hematuria
_____ 7. albuminuria
_____ 8. oliguria
_____ 9. glomerulonephritis
_____ 10. balanoplasty
_____ 11. hypospadias

a. birth defect in which the opening of the urethra is on the underside, instead of the end, of the penis
b. agent that causes urination
c. analysis of the urine
d. any kidney disease
e. bloody urination
f. disease characterized by the formation of many fluid-filled cysts in the kidneys
g. inflammation of the kidney
h. inflammation of the kidneys, involving primarily the glomeruli
i. low urine output
j. protein in the urine
k. surgical reconstruction of the penis

EXERCISE 15 *Fill in the blanks.*

1. HPI (define abbreviation: ____________________ of ____________________)
   a. Patient's name: ____________________
   b. Patient's age: ____________________
   c. Patient's gender: ____________________
   d. 2-day history of *hematuria* (give definition: ____________________)
   e. Patient had ____________________ (low urine output)
   f. *Urinalysis* (give abbreviation: ____________________) showed ____________________ (blood in the urine) and *albuminuria* (give definition: ____________________)
2. PMHx (define abbreviation: ______________ ______________ ______________): noncontributory
3. ____________________ ____________________ ____________________ (Past Surgical History)
   a. *Balanoplasty* (give definition: ____________________) for ____________________ (a birth defect in which the opening of the urethra is on the underside, instead of the end, of the penis
4. Assessment/Plan
   a. The patient clearly has a(n) ____________________ (disease of the kidney)
   b. The patient will begin fluid restriction and the use of ____________________ (agent that causes urination)

EXERCISE 16 *True or false questions. Indicate true answers with a T and false answers with an F.*

1. According to Dr. Hunter, Doug has a disease of the kidney. _______
2. Doug's CC is PKD. _______
3. Doug is nauseous and vomiting. _______

Learning Outcome 12.8 Exercises

EXERCISE 17 *Multiple-choice questions. Select the correct answer(s).*

1. Doug's grandfather has which of the following medical conditions?
   a. disease characterized by the formation of many fluid-filled cysts in the kidneys
   b. PKD
   c. polycystic kidney disease
   d. all of these
   e. none of these
2. Doug's physical exam revealed *hepatosplenomegaly*. Which of the following is a correct breakdown of the term *hepatosplenomegaly*?
   a. *hepato* (bladder) + *spleno* (spleen) + *megaly* (enlarged)
   b. *hepato* (kidney) + *spleno* (spleen) + *megaly* (reduced)
   c. *hepato* (liver) + *spleno* (spleen) + *megaly* (enlarged)
   d. *hepato* (prostate) + *spleno* (spleen) + *megaly* (enlarged)
   e. *hepato* (testicle) + *spleno* (spleen) + *megaly* (reduced)
3. According to Dr. Hunter's differential diagnosis, Doug may have a form of *glomerulonephritis.* Which of the following is a correct breakdown of the term?
   a. *glomerulo* (glomerulus) + *nephr* (bladder) + *itis* (disease)
   b. *glomerulo* (glomerulus) + *nephr* (bladder) + *itis* (inflammation)
   c. *glomerulo* (glomerulus) + *nephr* (kidney) + *itis* (disease)
   d. *glomerulo* (glomerulus) + *nephr* (kidney) + *itis* (inflammation)
   e. *glomerulo* (glomerulus) + *nephr* (kidney) + *itis* (tumor)

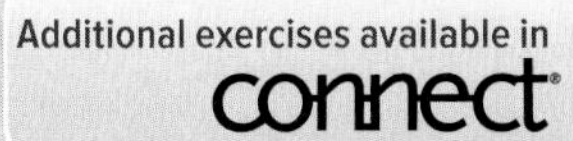

Chapter Review exercises, along with additional practice items, are available in Connect!

Quick Reference

quick reference glossary of roots

Root	Definition	Root	Definition
balan/o	penis	**pyel/o**	renal pelvis
cyst/o	bladder	**ren/o**	kidney
epididym/o	epididymis	**sperm/o, spermat/o**	sperm
glomerul/o	glomerulus	**test/o**	testicle
lith/o	stone	**ur/o, urin/o**	urine
meat/o	opening	**ureter/o**	ureter
nephr/o	kidney	**urethr/o**	urethra
orch/o, orchi/o, orchid/o	testicle	**vesic/o**	bladder
prostat/o	prostate		

quick reference glossary of terms

Term	Definition
albuminuria	protein in the urine
anorchidism	absence of a testicle
antispasmodic	drug used to prevent spasms
anuria	lack of urination
aspermia	condition characterized by a lack of sperm
azoospermia	condition characterized by lack of living sperm
azotemia	excess nitrogen in the blood
azotorrhea	excessive discharge of nitrogen
azoturia	excess nitrogen in the urine
balanitis	inflammation of the penis
balanoplasty	surgical reconstruction of the penis
balanorrhea	discharge from the penis
benign prostate hyperplasia	noncancerous overdevelopment of the prostate; also known as *enlarged prostate*
benign prostate hypertrophy	another term for benign prostate hyperplasia
blood urea nitrogen	nitrogen in the blood in the form of urea; it is the product of the breakdown of amino acids for energy
circumcision	surgical removal of the foreskin of the penis
cryptorchidism	hidden testicle

quick reference glossary of terms *continued*

Term	Definition
cystalgia	pain in the bladder
cystectomy	surgical removal of the bladder
cystitis	inflammation of the bladder
cystocele	hernia of the bladder
cystodynia	pain in the bladder
cystogram	image of the bladder
cystography	process for recording/imaging the bladder
cystolith	stone in the bladder
cystolithectomy	surgical removal of a stone in the bladder
cystoma	tumor of the bladder
cystoplegia	bladder paralysis
cystoptosis	downward displacement of the bladder
cystorrhexis	rupture of the bladder
cystoscopy	process for examining the bladder
cystospasm	involuntary contraction of the bladder
cystostomy	creation of an opening in the bladder
cystoureteritis	inflammation of the bladder and ureter
cystourethrocele	hernia of the bladder and urethra
digital rectal exam	examination of the prostate using a finger inserted into the rectum
dipsogenic	creating thirst
diuresis	excessive urination
diuretic	agent that causes urination
dysuria	painful urination
ejaculation	emission of semen from the urethra
enuresis	involutary urination
epididymectomy	surgical removal of the epididymis
epididymitis	inflammation of the epididymis
epididymo-orchitis	inflammation of the testicles and epididymis
epididymotomy	incision into the epididymis
extracorporeal shock wave lithotripsy (ESWL)	breakdown of kidney stones using sound waves generated outside the body
fulguration	use of electric current to destroy tissue
glomerulonephritis	inflammation of the kidneys involving primarily the glomeruli

quick reference glossary of terms *continued*

Term	Definition
glomerulopathy	disease of the kidney involving primarily the glomeruli
glomerulosclerosis	hardening of the glomeruli
glucosuria	sugar in the urine
glycosuria	sugar in the urine
gonads	the pair of organs used for sexual reproduction; testicles in males and ovaries in females
gonorrhea	discharge from the gonads
hematuria	bloody urination
heminephrectomy	surgical removal of half a kidney
heminephroureterectomy	surgical removal of half a kidney and a ureter
hemodialysis	procedure for removing waste from the bloodstream
hydrocele	fluid-filled mass in a testicle
hydrocelectomy	surgical removal of a hydrocele
hydronephrosis	kidney condition caused by the obstruction of urine flow
hyperkalemia	excessive potassium in the blood
hypernephroma	cancer of the kidneys
hyponatremia	low sodium in the blood
hypospadias	birth defect in which the opening of the urethra is on the underside, instead of the end, of the penis
incontinence	inability to control urination
intracorporeal lithotripsy	breakdown of kidney stones using a device placed inside the body
ketolysis	breakdown of ketones
ketonuria	presence of ketones in the urine
kidney dialysis	procedure for removing waste from the blood (a shorter name for hemodialysis)
laparonephrectomy	surgical removal of a kidney through the abdomen
lithectomy	surgical removal of a stone in the bladder
lithocystotomy	incision into the bladder to remove a stone
lithonephritis	inflammation of the kidneys caused by stones
lithonephrotomy	incision into a kidney to remove a stone
lithotripsy	breakdown of a stone
meatal stenosis	narrowing of the opening of the urethra
meatoplasty	surgical reconstruction of the opening of the urethra
meatorrhaphy	suture of the opening of the urethra

quick reference glossary of terms *continued*

Term	Definition
meatoscope	instrument for examining the opening of the urethra
meatoscopy	process for examining the opening of the urethra
meatotomy	incision into the opening of the urethra
nephralgia	pain in the kidney
nephrectomy	surgical removal of a kidney
nephritis	inflammation of the kidney
nephrocele	hernia of a kidney
nephrocystanastomosis	opening of a passageway between kidney and bladder
nephrogram	image of a kidney
nephrography	procedure for imaging a kidney
nephrohypertrophy	overdevelopment of the kidney
nephrolithiasis	the presence of stones in the kidney
nephrolithotomy	incision into a kidney to remove a stone
nephrologist	specialist in the kidneys
nephrology	study of the kidneys
nephroma	kidney tumor
nephromalacia	abnormal softening of a kidney
nephromegaly	abnormal enlargement of a kidney
nephropathy	any kidney disease
nephropexy	surgical fixation of a kidney
nephroptosis	downward displacement of a kidney
nephrorrhaphy	suture of a kidney
nephrosclerosis	abnormal hardening of a kidney
nephroscopy	procedure for examining a kidney
nephrosis	kidney condition
nephrosonography	procedure for imaging a kidney using sound waves
nephrostomy	creation of an opening in a kidney
nephrotomy	incision into a kidney to remove a stone
nephrotoxin	an agent poisonous to the kidney
nephroureterectomy	surgical removal of a kidney and ureter
nocturia	nighttime urination
nocturnal enuresis	nighttime involuntary urination
oligospermia	condition characterized by low sperm production

quick reference glossary of terms *continued*

Term	Definition
oliguria	low urine output
orchialgia	testicle pain
orchidectomy	surgical removal of a testicle
orchiditis	inflammation of the testicles
orchidopexy	surgical fixation of a testicle
orchidoptosis	downward displacement of a testicle
orchidotomy	incision into a testicle
orchiectomy	surgical removal of a testicle
orchiepididymitis	inflammation of the testicles and epididymis
orchiodynia	testicle pain
orchiopathy	disease of the testicles
orchiopexy	surgical fixation of a testicle
orchioplasty	surgical reconstruction of a testicle
orchitis	inflammation of the testicles
phimosis	contraction of the foreskin of the penis, preventing it from being retracted
polycystic kidney disease	disease characterized by the formation of many fluid-filled cysts in the kidneys
polydipsia	excessive thirst
polyuria	excessive urination
priapism	persistent and painful erection
prostatectomy	surgical removal of the prostate
prostatitis	inflammation of the prostate
prostatocystitis	inflammation of the prostate and bladder
prostatolith	a stone in the prostate
prostatolithotomy	incision into a prostate to remove a stone
prostatomegaly	abnormal enlargement of the prostate
prostatorrhea	discharge from the prostate
prostatovesiculectomy	surgical removal of the prostate and seminal vesicles
prostatovesiculitis	inflammation of the prostate and seminal vesicles
pyelitis	inflammation of the renal pelvis
pyelocystitis	inflammation of the renal pelvis and bladder
pyelocystostomosis	creation of an opening between the renal pelvis and bladder
pyelogram	image of the renal pelvis

quick reference glossary of terms *continued*

Term	Definition
pyelolithotomy	incision into a renal pelvis to remove a stone
pyelonephritis	inflammation of the kidney and renal pelvis
pyelopathy	disease of the renal pelvis
pyeloplasty	surgical reconstruction of a renal pelvis
pyelostomy	creation of an opening in a renal pelvis
pyelotomy	incision into a renal pelvis
pyeloureterectasia	dilation of the renal pelvis and ureter
pyonephritis	inflammation of the kidney caused by pus
pyonephrolithiasis	the presence of pus and stones in the kidney
pyopyeloectasis	pus in a dilated renal pelvis
pyuria	pus in the urine
renal angiogram	image of a kidney blood vessel
renal angiography	process of imaging a kidney blood vessel
renal angioplasty	surgical reconstruction of a kidney blood vessel
renal arteriogram	image of a kidney artery
renal cell carcinoma (hypernephroma)	cancer of the kidneys
renal failure	kidney failure
renal ischemia	deficiency of blood in a kidney
resectoscope	instrument for examining and cutting (usually the prostate)
retrograde pyelogram	image of the renal pelvis produced by injecting a contrast dye from the bladder to the kidney
seminoma	type of testicular cancer arising from sperm-forming tissue
spermatocele	hernia or distention of the epididymis caused by sperm cells
spermatogenesis	creation of sperm
spermatolysis	destruction of sperm cells
spermicide	agent that kills sperm
spermolytic	agent that kills sperm
stress urinary incontinence (SUI)	loss of bladder control caused by the application of external pressure
testicular carcinoma	testicular cancer
testitis	inflammation of the testicles and epididymis
transrectal ultrasonography	procedure involving a probe inserted into the rectum using high-frequency sound waves to scan through the rectum to nearby tissue (most commonly, the prostate)

quick reference glossary of terms *continued*

Term	Definition
transurethral resection of the prostate (TURP)	procedure of removing all or part of the prostate by the insertion of a resectoscope into the urethra
ultrasonography	imaging procedure using high-frequency sound waves
uremia	urine in the blood
ureteralgia	pain in the ureter
ureteritis	inflammation of a ureter
ureterocele	hernia of the ureter
ureteroileostomy	creation of an opening between a ureter and the ileum, a portion of the small intestine
ureterolithiasis	presence of stones in a ureter
ureteronephrectomy	surgical removal of a kidney and ureter
ureteroplasty	surgical reconstruction of a ureter
ureteropyelitis	inflammation of a ureter and renal pelvis
ureteropyelonephritis	inflammation of a kidney, renal pelvis, and ureter
ureterorrhaphy	suture of the ureter
ureteroscopy	process of examining a ureter
ureterostenosis	narrowing of a ureter
urethrectomy	surgical removal of the urethra
urethritis	inflammation of the urethra
urethrocystitis	inflammation of the urethra and bladder
urethrodynia	pain in the urethra
urethrogram	image of the urethra
urethropexy	surgical fixation of the urethra
urethroplasty	surgical reconstruction of the urethra
urethrorrhea	discharge from the urethra
urethroscope	instrument for examining the urethra
urethroscopy	process of examining the urethra
urethrospasm	involuntary contraction of the urethra
urethrostenosis	narrowing of the urethra
urethrotomy	incision into the urethra
urinalysis	analysis of the urine to determine presence of abnormal elements
urinary catheterization	insertion of a catheter into the bladder to drain urine
urinary tract infection (UTI)	infection of the urinary tract
urocyanosis	blue urine

quick reference glossary of terms *continued*

Term	Definition
urodynia	painful
urologist	specialist in the urinary tract
urology	study of the urinary tract
uropathy	disease of the urinary tract
uropoiesis	formation of urine
urostomy	creation of an opening in the urinary tract, normally to divert urine flow away from a diseased bladder
uroxanthin	substance in urine that makes it yellow
varicocele	overexpansion of the blood vessels of the testicles, leading to a soft tumor
vas deferens	vessel carrying sperm from the testicles
vasectomy	surgical removal of the vas deferens
vasovasostomy	creation of an opening between two vessels; technical term for a vasectomy reversal
vesicocele	hernia of the bladder
vesicostomy	creation of an opening in the bladder
vesicotomy	incision into the bladder
vesicoureteral reflux	abnormal flow of urine from the bladder back into the ureters
vesiculectomy	surgical removal of the seminal vesicles
voiding	another term for urination

review of terms by roots

Root	Term(s)	
balan/o	balanitis balanoplasty	balanorrhea
cyst/o	cystalgia cystectomy cystitis cystocele cystodynia cystogram cystography cystolith cystolithectomy cystoma cystoplegia cystoptosis cystorrhexis	cystoscopy cystospasm cystostomy cystoureteritis cystourethrocele lithocystotomy nephrocystanastomosis polycystic kidney disease prostatocystitis pyelocystitis pyelocystostomosis urethrocystitis voiding cystourethrogram

review of terms by roots *continued*

Root	Term(s)	
epididym/o	epididymectomy	epididymotomy
	epididymitis	orchiepididymitis
	epididymo-orchitis	
glomerul/o	glomerulonephritis	glomerulosclerosis
	glomerulopathy	
lith/o	cystolith	lithotripsy
	cystolithectomy	nephrolithiasis
	extracorporeal shock wave lithotripsy (ESWL)	nephrolithotomy
	intracorporeal lithotripsy	prostatolithotomy
	lithectomy	pyelolithotomy
	lithocystotomy	pyonephrolithiasis
	lithonephritis	ureterolithiasis
	lithonephrotomy	
meat/o	meatal stenosis	meatoscope
	meatoplasty	meatoscopy
	meatorrhaphy	meatotomy
nephr/o	glomerulonephritis	nephroma
	heminephrectomy	nephromalacia
	heminephroureterectomy	nephromegaly
	hydronephrosis	nephropathy
	hypernephroma	nephropexy
	laparonephrectomy	nephroptosis
	lithonephritis	nephrorrhaphy
	lithonephrotomy	nephrosclerosis
	nephralgia	nephroscopy
	nephrectomy	nephrosis
	nephritis	nephrosonography
	nephrocele	nephrostomy
	nephrocystanastomosis	nephrotomy
	nephrogram	nephrotoxin
	nephrography	nephroureterectomy
	nephrohypertrophy	pyelonephritis
	nephrolithiasis	pyonephritis
	nephrolithotomy	pyonephrolithiasis
	nephrologist	ureteronephrectomy
	nephrology	ureteropyelonephritis

review of terms by roots *continued*

Root	Term(s)	
orch/o, orchi/o, orchid/o	anorchidism	orchidotomy
	cryptorchidism	orchiectomy
	epididymo-orchitis	orchiepididymitis
	orchialgia	orchiodynia
	orchidectomy	orchiopathy
	orchiditis	orchiopexy
	orchidopexy	orchioplasty
	orchidoptosis	orchitis
prostat/o	benign prostate hyperplasia	prostatolithotomy
	benign prostate hypertrophy	prostatomegaly
	prostatectomy	prostatorrhea
	prostatitis	prostatovesiculectomy
	prostatocystitis	prostatovesiculitis
	prostatolith	transurethral resection of the prostate (TURP)
pyel/o	pyelitis	pyelostomy
	pyelocystitis	pyelotomy
	pyelocystostomosis	pyeloureterectasia
	pyelogram	pyopyeloectasis
	pyelolithotomy	retrograde pyelogram
	pyelonephritis	ureteropyelitis
	pyelopathy	ureteropyelonephritis
	pyeloplasty	
ren/o	renal angiogram	renal cell carcinoma (hypernephroma)
	renal angiography	renal failure
	renal angioplasty	renal ischemia
	renal arteriogram	
sperm/o, spermat/o	aspermia	spermatogenesis
	azoospermia	spermatolysis
	oligospermia	spermicide
	spermatocele	spermolytic
test/o	testicular carcinoma	
	testitis	

review of terms by roots *continued*

Root	Term(s)	
ureter/o	cystoureteritis	ureteronephrectomy
	heminephroureterectomy	ureteroplasty
	nephroureterectomy	ureteropyelitis
	pyeloureterectasia	ureteropyelonephritis
	ureteralgia	ureterorrhaphy
	ureteritis	ureteroscopy
	ureterocele	ureterostenosis
	ureteroileostomy	vesicoureteral reflux
	ureterolithiasis	
urethr/o	cystourethrocele	urethroplasty
	transurethral resection of the prostate (TURP)	urethrorrhea
	urethrectomy	urethroscope
	urethritis	urethroscopy
	urethrocystitis	urethrospasm
	urethrodynia	urethrostenosis
	urethrogram	urethrotomy
	urethropexy	
ur/o	albuminuria	pyuria
	anuria	stress urinary incontinence
	azoturia	uremia
	diuresis	urinalysis
	diuretic	urinary catheterization
	dysuria	urinary tract infection
	enuresis	urocyanosis
	glucosuria	urodynia
	glycosuria	urologist
	hematuria	urology
	ketonuria	uropathy
	nocturia	uropoiesis
	nocturnal enuresis	urostomy
	oliguria	uroxanthin
	polyuria	
vesic/o	prostatovesiculectomy	vesicotomy
	prostatovesiculitis	vesicoureteral reflux
	vesicocele	vesiculectomy
	vesicostomy	

other terms

antispasmodic
azotemia
azotorrhea
blood urea nitrogen
circumcision
digital rectal exam
dipsogenic
ejaculation
fulguration
gonads
gonorrhea
hemodialysis
hydrocele
hydrocelectomy
hyperkalemia
hyponatremia
hypospadiast
incontinence
ketolysis
kidney dialysis
phimosis
polydipsia
priapism
resectoscope
seminoma
transrectal ultrasonography
ultrasonography
varicocele
vas deferens
vasectomy
vasovasostomy
voiding

The Female Reproductive System—Gynecology, Obstetrics, and Neonatology 13

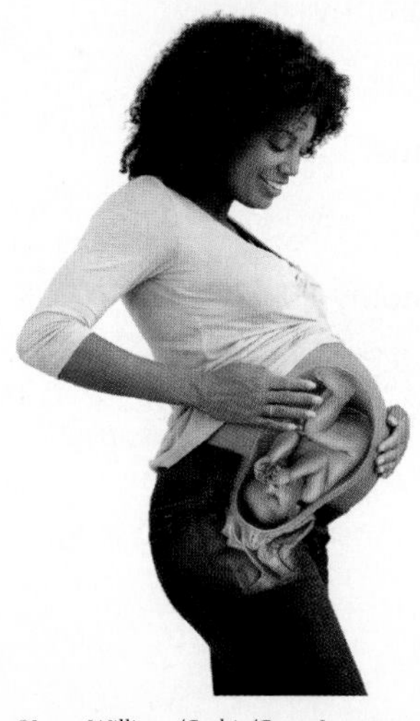

©Larry Williams/Corbis/Getty Images

learning outcomes

Upon completion of this chapter, you will be able to:

13.1 Identify the **roots/word parts** associated with the **female reproductive system.**

S **13.2** Translate the **Subjective** terms associated with the **female reproductive system.**

O **13.3** Translate the **Objective** terms associated with the **female reproductive system.**

A **13.4** Translate the **Assessment** terms associated with the **female reproductive system.**

P **13.5** Translate the **Plan** terms associated with the **female reproductive system.**

13.6 Use **abbreviations** associated with the **female reproductive system.**

13.7 Distinguish terms associated with the **female reproductive system** in the context of **electronic health records.**

Introduction and Overview of the Female Reproductive System

With few exceptions, everyone is born with the basic equipment to help bring new life into the world. Both sexes contain reproductive organs that produce half the code for a human life. The female reproductive system is much more active and complex. While the main function of the male reproductive system is the production and the delivery of sperm cells, the female reproductive system is responsible for much more. Females not only provide half the code for a human life, but also provide the environment and nutrition to sustain and grow that life until birth.

13.1 Word Parts of the Female Reproductive System

Gynecology, External

The outer structures of the female reproductive system are collectively known as the *vulva.* The vulva includes the clitoris, the labia majora and labia minora, the urethral meatus, and the vaginal opening.

The *clitoris* is the most sensitive part of a woman's anatomy. In this way, it is similar to the head of a man's penis. The *labia* are the folds of tissue around the opening of the vagina. The outer folds, which are larger, are the *labia majora,* and the inner folds, which are thinner, are the *labia minora.* The urethral opening is located within the labia minora superior to the vaginal opening.

While not directly connected to the rest of the reproductive parts, the *breasts* are a very important outside structure. While they are very sensitive and provide stimulation that plays a part in sexual intercourse, their main purpose is to provide a food supply for a newborn baby.

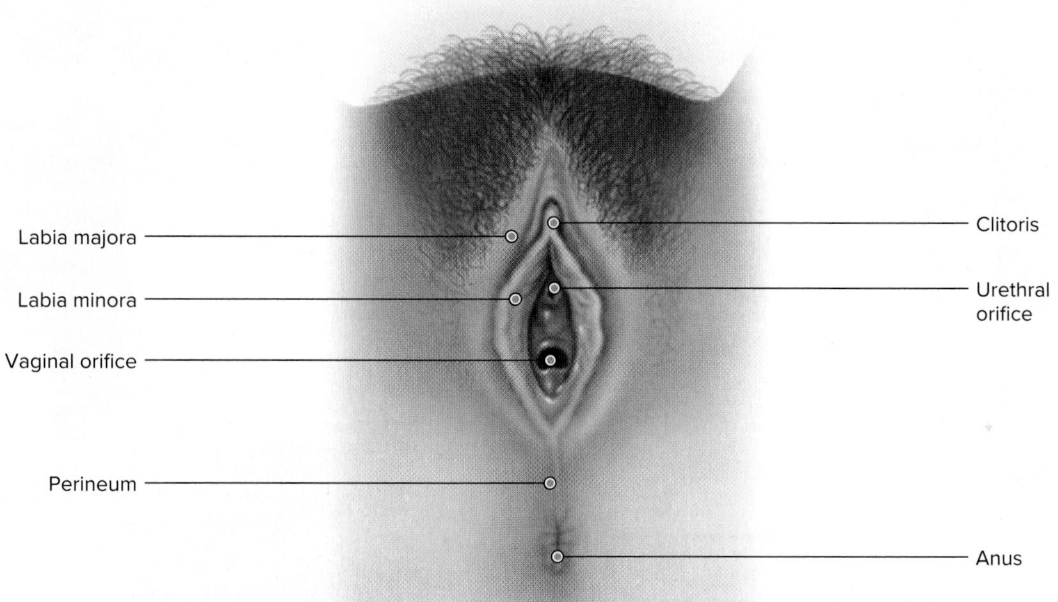

vagina

ROOTS: ***colp/o, vagin/o***
EXAMPLES: colposcope, vaginitis
NOTES: The word *vagina* comes from Latin and means the "sheath" or "scabbard of a sword."

vulva

ROOTS: ***episi/o, vulv/o***
EXAMPLES: episiotomy, vulvodynia
NOTES: *Vulva* is the term for the external genital organs of a female.

perineum

ROOT: ***perine/o***
EXAMPLES: perineoplasty, perineorrhaphy
NOTES: *Perineum* is the term for the region between the genital organs and the anus. No one is really sure where the term came from, but one easy way to remember what it means is to think *peri* (around) + *anus* = "region around the anus." It's not 100 percent accurate, but it's enough to help you remember.

woman

ROOTS: ***gynec/o, gyn/o***

EXAMPLES: gynecology, gynecologist

NOTES: This root comes from Greek, for *woman.* If you are afraid of women, you have *gynophobia.* Believe it or not, this root is where the English words *queen* and *goon* come from.

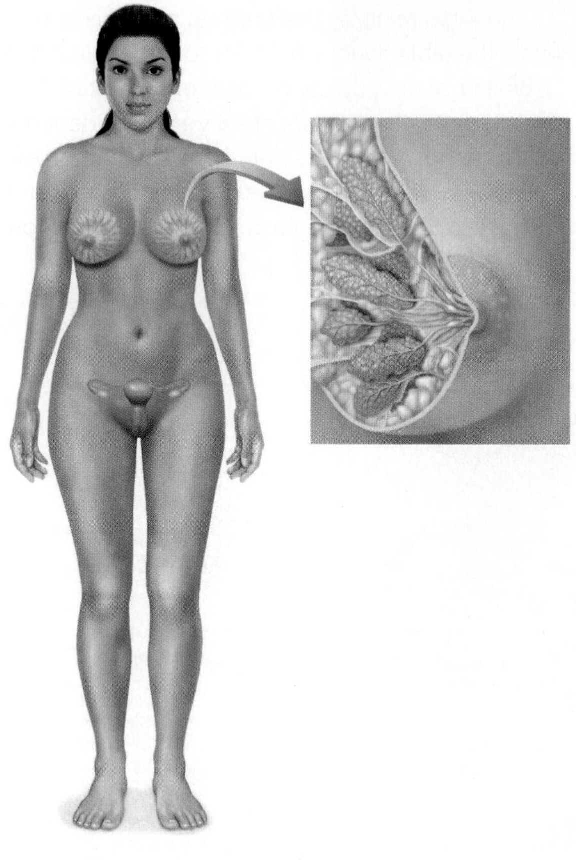

breast

ROOTS: ***mast/o, mamm/o***

EXAMPLES: mastopexy, mastectomy, mammogram

NOTES: Believe it or not, the name of the *mastodon,* a long-extinct type of elephant similar to a mammoth, actually breaks down as *mast* (breast) and *odon* (tooth). The mastodon got its name from a scientist who thought that the animal's molar teeth had nipple-like tops, which gave them the appearance of breasts.

milk

ROOT: ***lact/o***

EXAMPLES: lactation, lactorrhea

NOTES: The root for milk, *lacto,* is also the root for the English word *galaxy.* Have you ever looked at the stars from a really dark spot out in the country? If so, you've seen stars that you'd never be able to see near a city. One thing you can see is the Milky Way, the thick band of stars that makes up our galaxy. It's called the Milky Way because the ancient Greeks thought the dense cloud of stars looked like milk sprayed in the night sky. A Greek myth tells how the hero Hercules, who was breast-fed by the goddess Hera, once bit down so hard that milk sprayed everywhere—creating the Milky Way.

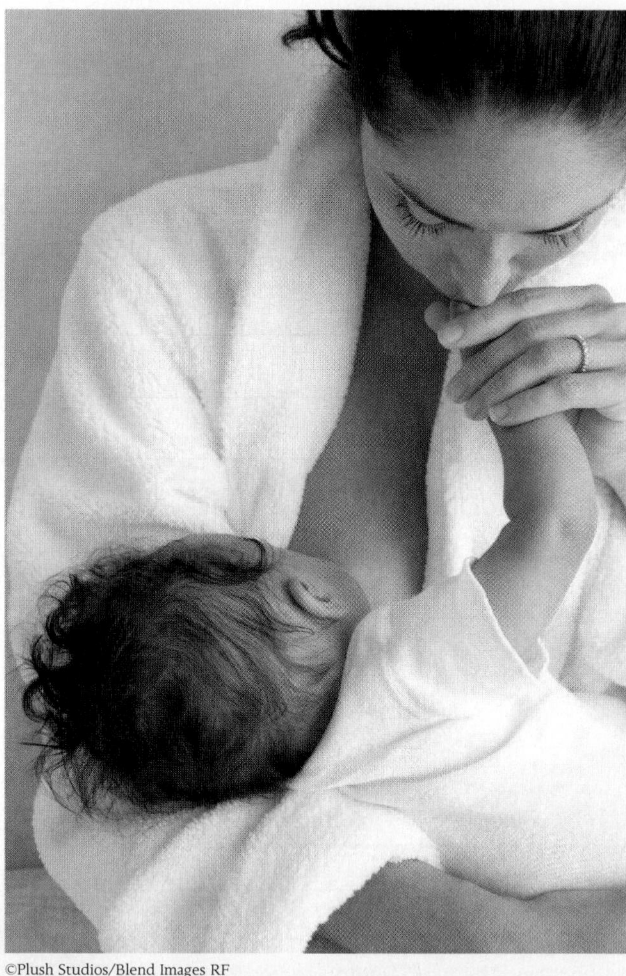

Gynecology, Internal

A woman's inner reproductive system is shaped like a capital "T." On either end of the horizontal part of the "T" rest the ovaries. The *ovaries* hold all of the woman's eggs (*ova*). Roughly every 28 to 30 days during a woman's adult years, an ovary will allow an egg to mature and then releases it (*ovulation*). The ova travel along tubes (*fallopian tubes*) to the uterus.

The *uterus* is a pear-shaped organ in the vertical part of the "T," along with the vagina. The uterus is the incubator for growing and developing new life. Every month, the walls of the uterus grow and become rich in blood supply. If the woman's egg is fertilized by a sperm, it travels to the uterus and implants itself in the walls. If a new life is not implanted in the walls of the uterus, the tissues are shed and the process starts all over again. This cycle of building and shedding nutritive tissues in the uterus is known as the *menstrual cycle*. It is driven by the female hormones *estrogen* and *progesterone*. Both of these hormones are made in the ovaries.

At the end of the uterus is a connection to the vagina known as the *cervix*. It is smaller and thicker than the rest of the uterus. Further down the vertical part of the "T" is the vagina, the reproductive system's main point of contact with the outside world. It is the part of a woman's body that is involved in sexual intercourse. Additionally, the opening of the urethra, which drains the bladder, is found in front of the anterior wall of the vagina.

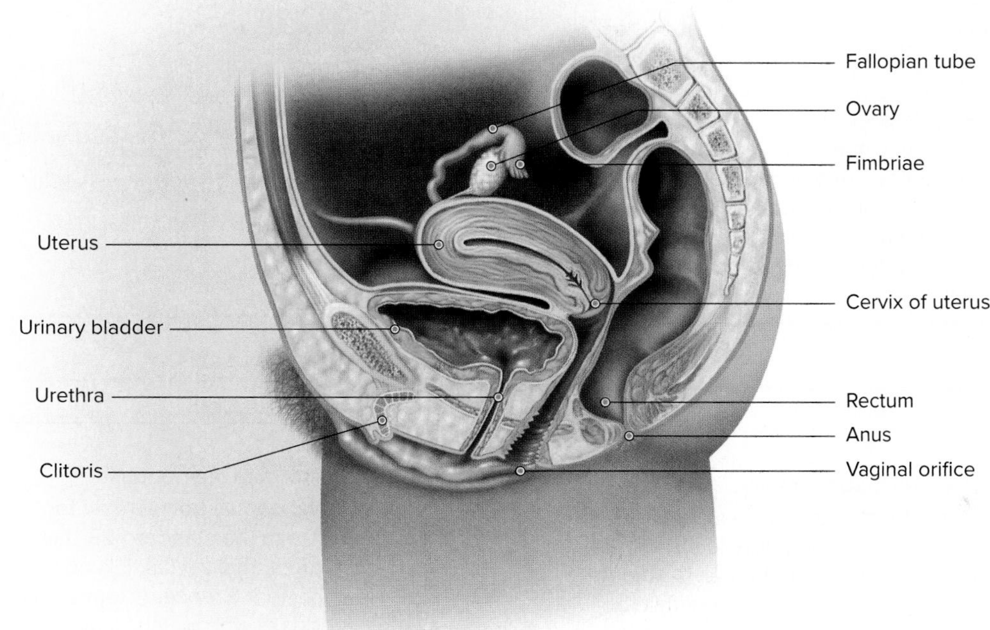

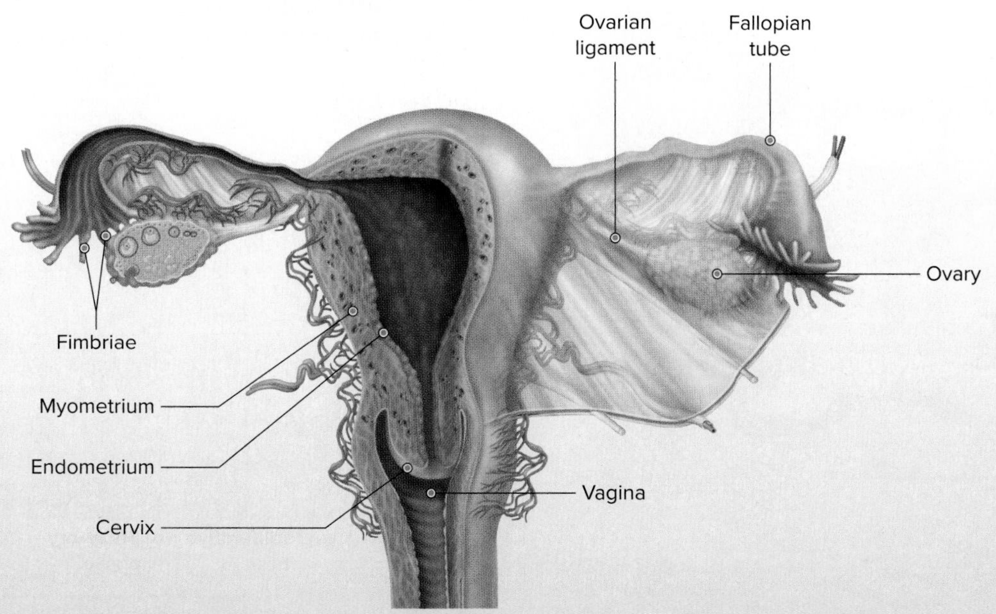

cervix

ROOT: ***cervic/o***

EXAMPLES: cervicodynia, cervicitis

NOTES: *Cervix* means "neck" and refers not to the neck connecting your head to your body but to the opening between the uterus and the vagina.

REMEMBER: The letter *c* changes sounds depending on what vowel follows it. Before *e* or *i,* the letter *c* makes an *s* sound (**ce**rvi**ci**tis—**SE**R-vih-**SAI**-tis). Before *a, o,* or *u,* the letter *c* makes a *k* sound (**ce**rvi**co**dynia—**SE**R-vih-**ko**h-DAI-nee-ah).

uterus

ROOTS: ***hyster/o, metr/o, uter/o***

EXAMPLES: hysterectomy, endometrium, uterus

NOTES: Break down the word *hysteria* as a medical term. It means "a uterus condition," right (*hyster* + *ia*)? Believe it or not, that is exactly where the term came from. It was used to refer to a medical condition (usually neurological) occurring in women and caused by a malfunctioning uterus. Think about that the next time you refer to a friend or a movie as "hysterical."

pelvis

ROOT: ***pelv/i***

EXAMPLES: pelvimetry, pelvic sonography

NOTES: *Pelvis* comes from a Latin word meaning "basin" or "washtub" and refers to the shape of the bones that make up the pelvis. Another root, *pyelo,* also means "pelvis," but this root is used exclusively for the portion of the kidney called the *renal pelvis.*

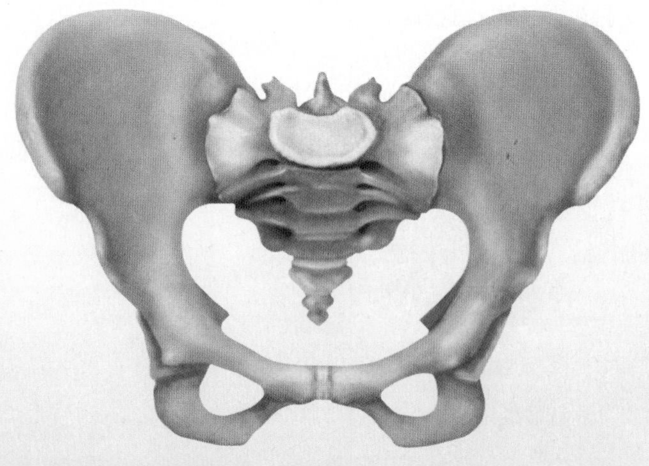

ovary

ROOTS: ***oophor/o, ovari/o***

EXAMPLES: oophorectomy, ovariocentesis

NOTES: *Oophoro* can be broken down into two words: *oo,* meaning "egg," and *phor,* meaning "to carry." Thus, *oophor* literally means "the thing that carries the eggs."

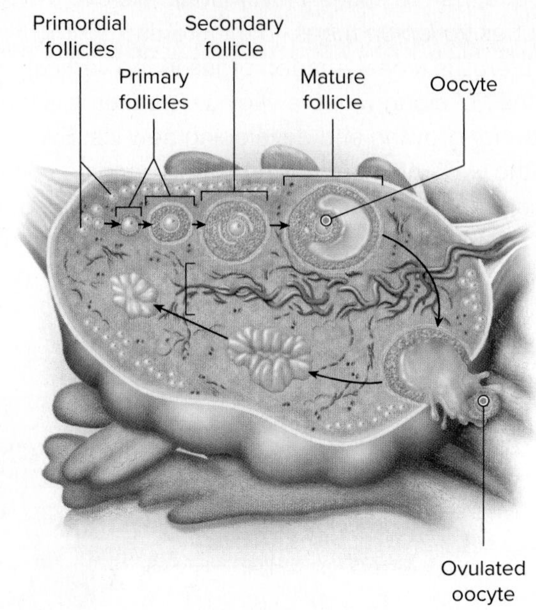

menstruation

ROOT: ***men/o***

EXAMPLES: menorrhea, menopause

NOTES: *Meno* comes from Greek, for "month," and refers to the standard 28-day recurrence of menstrual cycles. It is no wonder that in ancient Greece, Artemis was both the goddess who watched over young girls entering womanhood and the goddess associated with the moon, which goes through its phases roughly every 28 days.

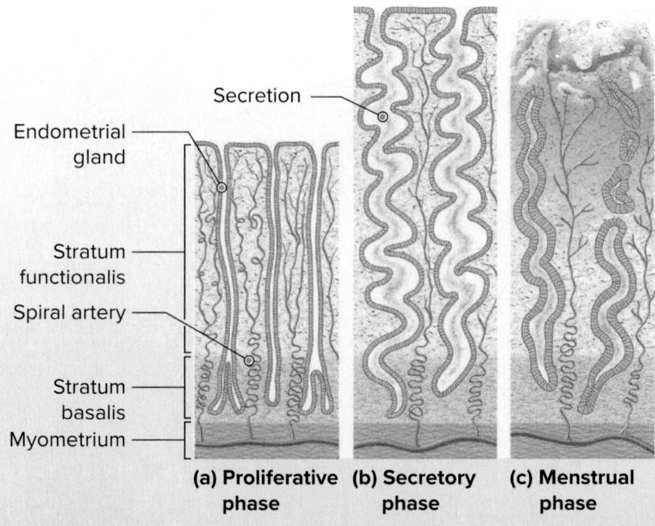

fallopian tube

ROOT: ***salping/o***

EXAMPLES: salpingectomy, salpingoscope

NOTES: *Salpingo* comes from the Latin word for "trumpet." Four sites in the body use this term due to their resemblance to a long, straight Roman trumpet: the ear canals and the fallopian tubes, which connect the ovaries to the uterus. The fallopian tubes are named for Gabriello Fallopio, an Italian specialist in anatomy who first described them in the 1500s.

REMEMBER: The letter *g* changes sounds depending on what vowel follows it. Before *e* or *i,* the letter *g* makes a *j* sound (salpin**gi**tis—SAL-pin-**JAI**-tis). Before *a, o,* or *u,* the letter *g* makes a *g* sound (salpin**go**scope—sal-PING-**goh**-SKOHP).

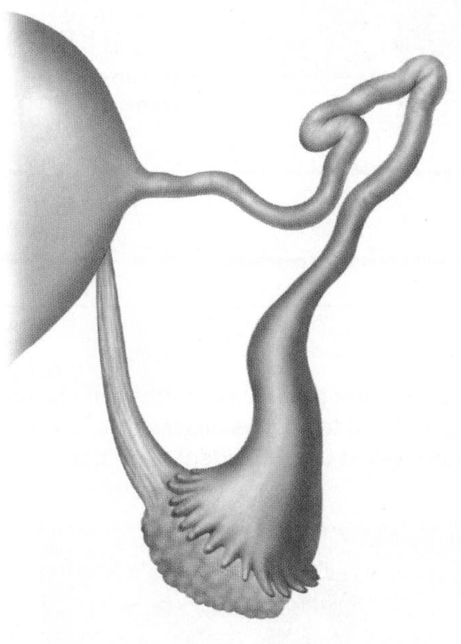

Obstetrics

Pregnancy is the amazing process of a human life growing inside a woman. During pregnancy, a baby is called a *fetus.* The fetus grows and develops in the mother's *uterus.* The fetus is connected to the uterus via the *placenta.* The placenta is an important source for feeding the fetus. There, nutrients provided by the mother's blood vessels cross into the blood vessels of the fetus.

The fetus is attached to the placenta through the *umbilical cord,* which is cut at birth. This is where the belly button comes from. The fetus is surrounded by a fluid-filled sac (*amnion* or *amniotic sac*) that helps act as a shock absorber to protect it. Outside the amnion is another membrane, the *chorion,* which helps anchor the baby to the walls of the uterus and provides nutrition.

When the fetus is ready for birth, the woman's body goes through the painful process known as *labor.* During labor, the woman's *cervix* widens and the muscles of the uterus squeeze to push the baby out.

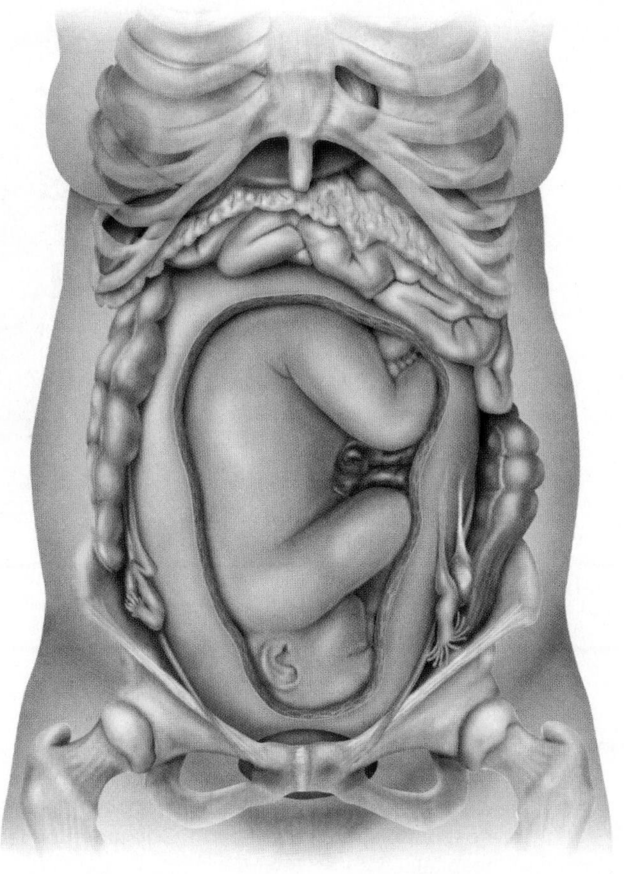

amnion

ROOT: ***amni/o***

EXAMPLE: amniocentesis

NOTES: The *amnion* is the innermost membrane covering the fetus.

pregnancy

SUFFIX: ***-cyesis***

EXAMPLE: pseudocyesis

NOTES: Although women experience pregnancy firsthand, there is a documented medical condition called Couvade syndrome, or sympathetic pregnancy, in which a man experiences some of the symptoms of pregnancy, including weight gain, morning sickness, and, in some cases, labor "pains."

chorion

ROOTS: ***chori/o, chorion/o***

EXAMPLE: choriocarcinoma, chorionitis

NOTES: The *chorion* is the outer membrane covering the fetus. It connects the fetus to the wall of the uterus.

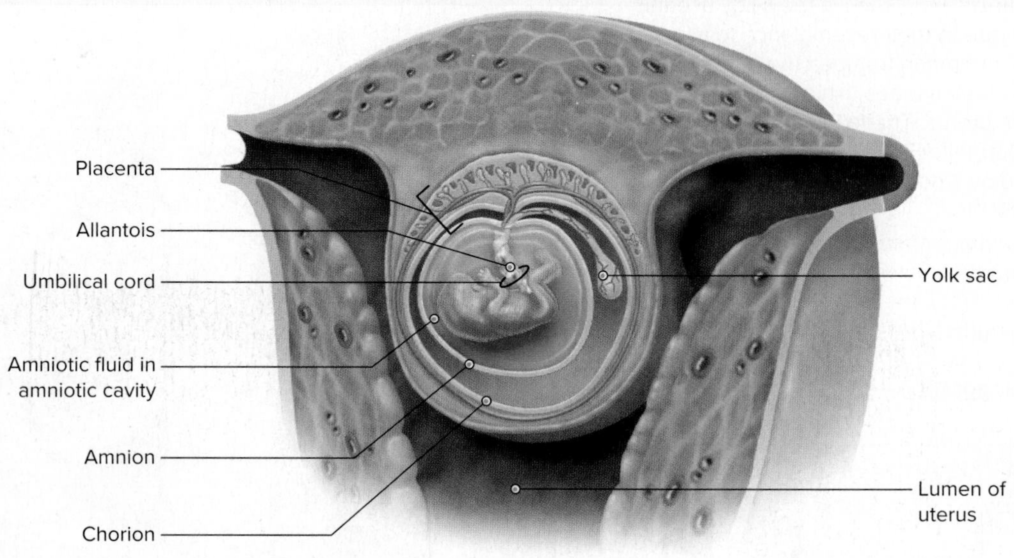

labor

ROOT: ***toc/o***

EXAMPLES: dystocia, tocograph

NOTES: In the United States, there are more boy babies born than girl babies. For the past 60 years, the ratio has been about the same: 105 male births for every 100 female births. Also, according to some statistics, Tuesday is the most popular day to give birth. One more fun fact: Jimmy Carter was the first U.S. president to be born in a hospital.

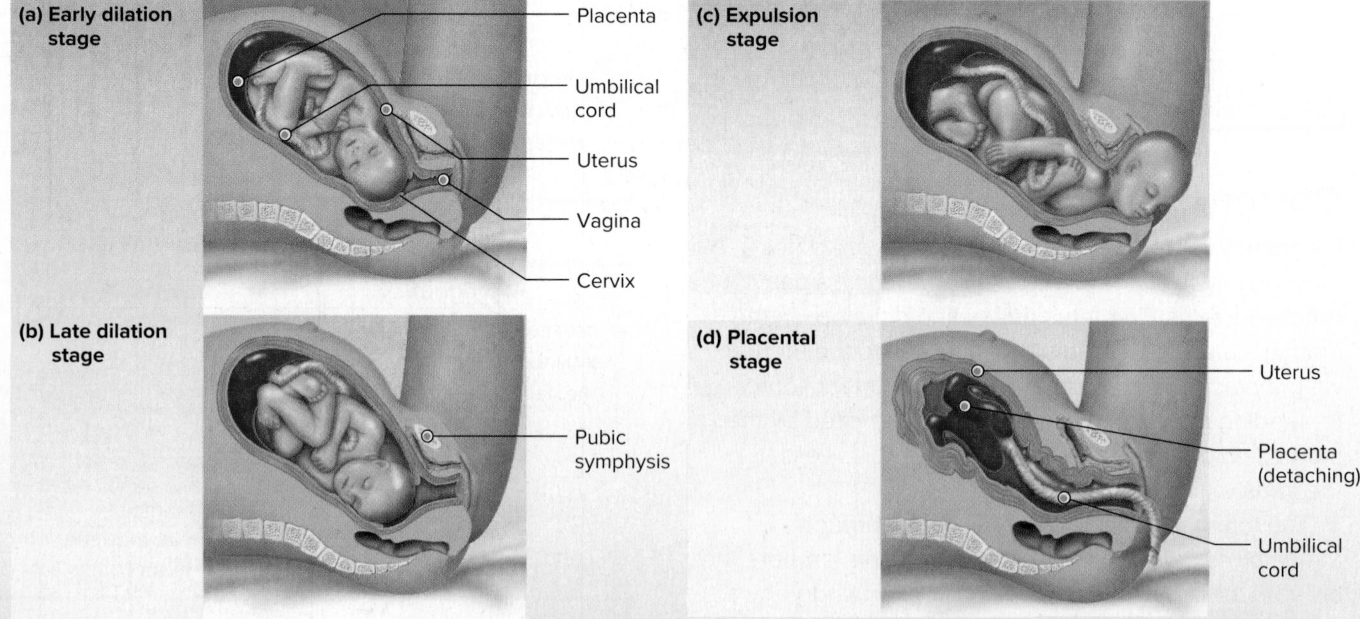

fetus

ROOT: ***fet/o***

EXAMPLE: fetometry

NOTES: *Fetus* is a Latin word that means "offspring." The Greek word is *embryo.* In current medical usage, a fetus is an unborn child after the eighth week of pregnancy. Before that time, it is referred to as an embryo. Before the fertilization of an egg, the sperm and egg are called *gametes* (Greek for "husband" and "wife"). Once they join, a separate, distinct, and genetically unique creature is created that is called a *zygote* (Greek for "joined together"). Once the unborn child becomes implanted in the wall of the uterus, it is called an embryo.

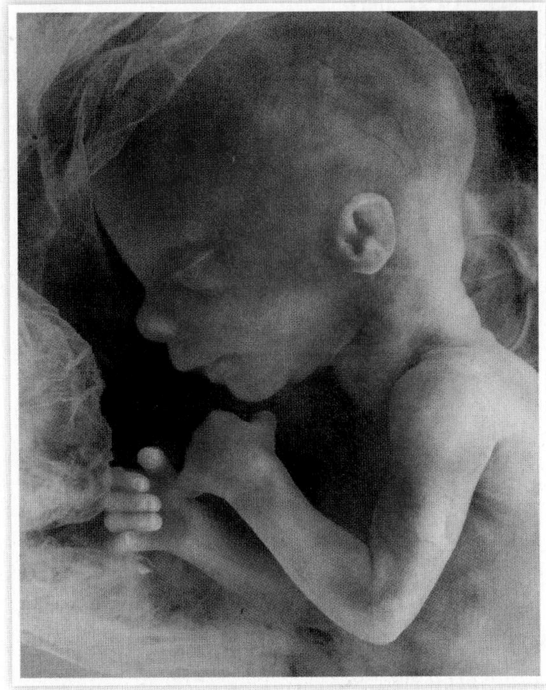

birth

ROOTS: ***part/o, nat/o***

EXAMPLES: postpartum, neonatal

NOTES: Both roots mean "birth," but their focus is different. *Parto* means more accurately "to give birth" and therefore focuses on the mother. *Nato* means more literally "to be born" and therefore focuses on the baby. Hence, a mother gets *postpartum depression* and a baby is cared for by a *neonatologist.*

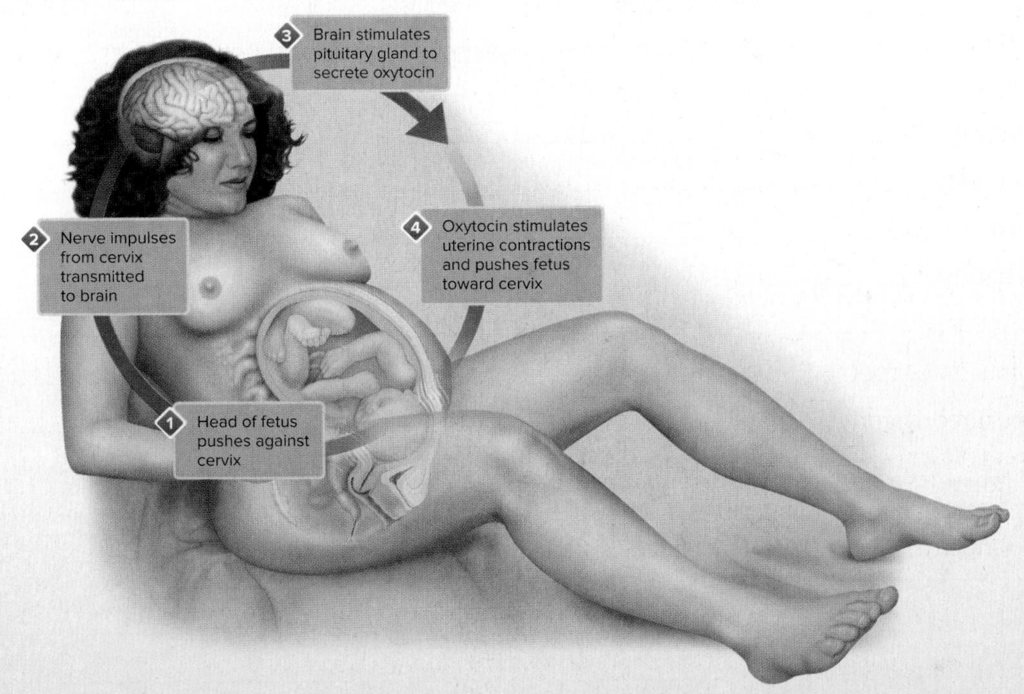

Learning Outcome 13.1 Exercises

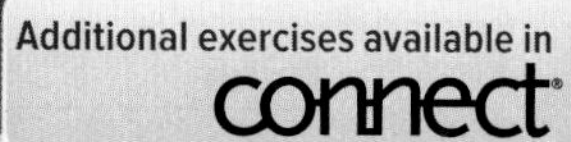

TRANSLATION

EXERCISE 1 *Match the root on the left with its definition on the right. Some definitions will be used more than once.*

_____	1. vagin/o	a. breast
_____	2. vulv/o	b. external genital organs of a female
_____	3. mamm/o	c. milk
_____	4. lact/o	d. region between the genital organs and the anus
_____	5. gynec/o	e. vagina
_____	6. perine/o	f. woman
_____	7. gyn/o	
_____	8. colp/o	
_____	9. episi/o	
_____	10. mast/o	

EXERCISE 2 *Translate the following roots.*

1. vagin/o _____
2. vulv/o _____
3. gynec/o _____
4. lact/o _____
5. perine/o _____
6. mamm/o _____
7. gyn/o _____
8. episi/o _____
9. mast/o _____
10. colp/o _____

EXERCISE 3 *Underline and define the roots from this chapter in the following terms.*

1. vulvitis _____
2. lactation _____
3. perineocele _____
4. colpocystitis _____
5. mammoplasty _____
6. mastoptosis _____
7. episiorrhaphy _____
8. vaginomycosis _____
9. gynecomastia (2 roots) _____
10. vaginoperineorrhaphy (2 roots) _____

EXERCISE 4 *Break down the following words into their component parts and translate.*

EXAMPLE: sinusitis *sinus | itis* *inflammation of the sinuses*

1. vaginitis _____
2. vulvitis _____
3. mastitis _____

4. colpitis ____________________
5. gynecologist ____________________
6. mammogram ____________________
7. lactogenic ____________________
8. perineorrhaphy ____________________
9. episiostenosis ____________________
10. vulvovaginitis ____________________

EXERCISE 5 *Match the root on the left with its definition on the right. Some definitions will be used more than once.*

_____	1. uter/o	a. fallopian tube
_____	2. ovari/o	b. menstruation
_____	3. cervic/o	c. opening between the uterus and the vagina
_____	4. pelv/i	d. ovary
_____	5. men/o	e. pelvis
_____	6. hyster/o	f. uterus
_____	7. metr/o	
_____	8. oophor/o	
_____	9. salping/o	

EXERCISE 6 *Translate the following roots.*

1. ovari/o ____________________
2. cervic/o ____________________
3. pelv/i ____________________
4. uter/o ____________________
5. men/o ____________________
6. hyster/o ____________________
7. salping/o ____________________
8. oophor/o ____________________
9. metr/o ____________________

EXERCISE 7 *Underline and define the roots from this chapter in the following terms.*

1. ovariocentesis ____________________
2. uterine prolapse ____________________
3. cervical dysplasia ____________________
4. menorrhagia ____________________
5. salpingectomy ____________________
6. endometritis ____________________
7. hysteroptosis ____________________
8. oophorocystectomy ____________________
9. cephalopelvic disproportion ____________________
10. metromenorrhagia (2 roots) ____________________

Learning Outcome 13.1 Exercises

11. metrocolpocele (2 roots) ______
12. salpingo-oophorectomy (2 roots) ______
13. hysterosalpingectomy (2 roots) ______

EXERCISE 8 *Break down the following words into their component parts and translate.*

EXAMPLE: sinusitis *sinus | itis* *inflammation of the sinuses*

1. ovaritis ______
2. cervicography ______
3. hysterography ______
4. oophoroma ______
5. perimetritis ______
6. dysmenorrhea ______
7. hysterosalpingogram ______
8. sonohysterography ______

EXERCISE 9 *Match the word part on the left with its definition on the right. Some definitions will be used more than once.*

______	1. fet/o	a. "to be born"; focus on the baby
______	2. nat/o	b. "to give birth"; focus on the mother
______	3. amni/o	c. innermost membrane covering the fetus
______	4. part/o	d. labor
______	5. chorion/o	e. outer membrane covering the fetus; connects the fetus to the wall of the uterus
______	6. chori/o	f. pregnancy
______	7. -cyesis	g. unborn child after the eighth week of pregnancy
______	8. toc/o	

EXERCISE 10 *Translate the following word parts.*

1. amni/o ______
2. chori/o, chorion/o ______
3. fet/o ______
4. nat/o ______
5. part/o ______
6. toc/o ______
7. -cyesis ______

EXERCISE 11 *Underline and define the word parts from this chapter in the following terms.*

1. fetometry ______
2. amniorrhexis ______
3. choriocarcinoma ______
4. pseudocyesis ______
5. perinatologist ______
6. intrapartum ______
7. eutocia ______

Learning Outcome 13.1 Exercises

EXERCISE 12 *Break down the following words into their component parts and translate.*

EXAMPLE:	sinusitis	*sinus | itis*	*inflammation of the sinuses*

1. amnioscopy ______________________
2. chorioamnionitis ______________________
3. ovariocyesis ______________________
4. fetometry ______________________
5. neonatal ______________________
6. antepartum ______________________
7. tocography ______________________

GENERATION

EXERCISE 13 *Identify the roots for the following definitions.*

1. perineum ______________________
2. milk ______________________
3. woman (2 roots) ______________________
4. breast (2 roots) ______________________
5. vagina (2 roots) ______________________
6. vulva (2 roots) ______________________

EXERCISE 14 *Build a medical term from the information provided.*

EXAMPLE:	inflammation of the sinuses	*sinusitis*

1. pain in the vulva (use *vulv/o*) ______________________
2. surgical removal of a breast (use *mast/o*) ______________________
3. incision into the vulva (use *episi/o*) ______________________
4. the discharge of milk (use *-rrhea*) ______________________
5. surgical reconstruction of a breast (use *mamm/o*) ______________________
6. surgical reconstruction of the vagina (use *vagin/o*) ______________________
7. surgical reconstruction of the vagina (use *colp/o*) ______________________
8. surgical reconstruction of the perineum ______________________
9. the study of medical issues specific to women ______________________
10. surgical reconstruction of the vagina and perineum (use *vagin/o*) ______________________

Learning Outcome 13.1 Exercises

EXERCISE 15 *Identify the roots for the following definitions.*

1. cervix ______
2. pelvis ______
3. menstruation ______
4. fallopian tube ______
5. ovary (2 roots) ______
6. uterus (3 roots) ______

EXERCISE 16 *Build a medical term from the information provided.*

1. instrument for examining the uterus (use *hyster/o*) ______
2. inflammation of an ovary (use *oophor/o*) ______
3. pain in the ovary (use *ovari/o*) ______
4. inflammation of the cervix ______
5. procedure for measuring the pelvis ______
6. inflammation of the fallopian tube ______
7. inflammation of the fallopian tube and ovary (use *oophor/o*) ______

EXERCISE 17 *Identify the roots for the following definitions.*

1. fetus ______
2. amnion ______
3. pregnancy ______
4. labor ______
5. chorion (2 roots) ______
6. birth (2 roots) ______

EXERCISE 18 *Build a medical term from the information provided.*

1. pertaining to after the birth (use *nat/o*) ______
2. pertaining to after the birth (use *part/o*) ______
3. inflammation of the chorion ______
4. instrument for examining the amnion ______
5. instrument for recording the strength of labor (contractions) ______
6. pregnancy in a fallopian tube ______

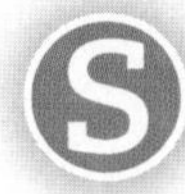

Subjective

Patient History, Problems, Complaints

Gynecology

Obstetrics

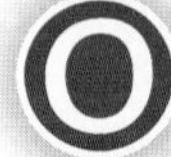

Objective

Observation and Discovery

Gynecology

Gynecology—diagnostic procedures

Gynecology—professional terms

Obstetrics

Obstetrics—diagnostic procedures

Obstetrics—professional terms

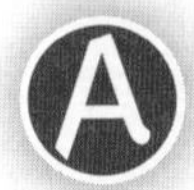

Assessment

Diagnosis and Pathology

Gynecology

Obstetrics

Plan

Treatments and Therapies

Gynecology

Obstetrics

This section contains medical terms built from the roots presented in the previous section. The purpose of this section is to expose you to words used in gynecology, obstetrics, and neonatology that are built from the word roots presented earlier. The focus of this book is to teach you the process of learning roots and translating them in context. Each term is presented with the correct pronunciation, followed by a word analysis that breaks down the word into its component parts, a definition that provides a literal translation of the word, as well as supplemental information if the literal translation deviates from its medical use.

The terms are organized using a health care professional's SOAP note (first introduced in Chapter 2) as a model.

SUBJECTIVE

13.2 Patient History, Problems, Complaints

Pain is always a common symptom in medicine, and the female reproductive system is no exception. The nerve fibers of the interior reproductive system share nerves with the lower gastrointestinal tract, so pain originating from this area can be hard to distinguish from gastrointestinal pain.

Pain in the vulva (*vulvodynia*) is often a condition without a known cause. Pain in the vagina (*vaginodynia*) is a common complication of infections, including fungal infections. More commonly, women will present to a medical office with pain that recurs at specific times, such as during menses (*dysmenorrhea*) or sexual intercourse (*dyspareunia*). Many times, women have both symptoms. These can be complications of *endometriosis* or *pelvic inflammatory disorder*.

Both females and males can present with pain in the breast (*mastalgia*). Women often suffer from this condition during breastfeeding. In males, this usually happens during puberty, when they may develop a small amount of breast tissue (*gynecomastia*).

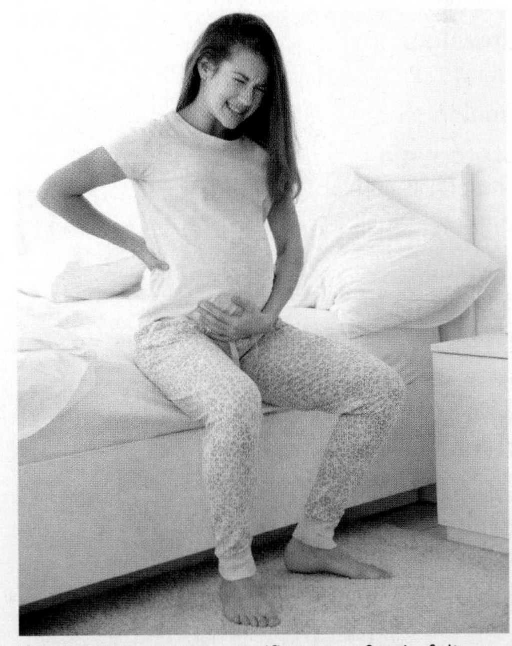

Contractions are a specific type of pain felt during pregnancy.

13.2 Patient History, Problems, Complaints

Women often come to health care providers with problems with menses. Their menses can be too frequent (*metrorrhagia*), too heavy (*menorrhagia*), or both (*metromenorrhagia*). Patients also may experience skipped periods (*oligomenorrhea*) or none at all (*amenorrhea*).

Women may also present with complaints of *abnormal discharge*. The discharge's odor and color can be good indicators of its cause. Sexually transmitted infections, such as *gonorrhea*, are a common cause of abnormal discharge.

During pregnancy, a woman's "water" breaking is also a discharge (*amniorrhea*). It is a good indicator that delivery is near.

gynecology

Term	Word Analysis
amenorrhea AY-men-oh-REE-ah **Definition** no menstruation	**a / meno / rrhea** no / menstruation / discharge
colpostenosis KOL-poh-steh-NOH-sis **Definition** narrowing in the vaginal opening	**colpo / sten / osis** vagina / narrow / condition
dysmenorrhea DIS-men-oh-REE-ah **Definition** painful menstruation	**dys / meno / rrhea** bad / menstruation / discharge
dyspareunia dis-pah-ROO-nee-ah **Definition** painful sexual intercourse	**dys / par / eun / ia** bad / alongside / couch / condition
gynecomastia GAI-neh-koh-MAS-tee-a **Definition** development of breast tissue in males NOTE: This term applies to men and not women, but it is included in this chapter because of the root it uses.	**gyneco / mast / ia** woman / breast / condition ©Dr. P. Marazzi/Science Source
hysteralgia HIS-ter-AL-jah **Definition** pain in the uterus	**hyster / algia** uterus / pain
hysterodynia HIS-ter-oh-DIH-nee-ah **Definition** pain in the uterus	**hystero / dynia** uterus / pain
leukorrhea LOO-koh-REE-ah **Definition** white vaginal discharge	**leuko / rrhea** white / discharge
mastalgia mas-TAL-jah **Definition** breast pain	**mast / algia** breast / pain
mastoptosis MAS-top-TOH-sis **Definition** downward displacement (drooping) of the breast	**masto / ptosis** breast / drooping condition

13.2 Patient History, Problems, Complaints

gynecology *continued*

Term	Word Analysis
menorrhagia MEN-oh-RAY-jah **Definition** excessive menstrual flow	**meno / rrhagia** menstruation / excessive discharge
menorrhalgia MEN-oh-RAL-jah **Definition** painful menstruation	**meno / rrh / algia** uterus / discharge / pain
NOTE: The difference between the last two words is only one letter—but that one letter makes a big difference.	
metromenorrhagia MEH-troh-MEN-oh-RAY-jah **Definition** excessive menstrual bleeding at irregular intervals	**metro / meno / rrhagia** uterus / menstruation / excessive discharge
metrorrhagia MEH-troh-RAY-jah **Definition** menstrual bleeding at irregular times	**metro / rrhagia** uterus / excessive discharge
oligomenorrhea AW-lih-goh-MEN-oh-REE-ah **Definition** infrequent or light menstrual periods	**oligo / meno / rrhea** few / menstruation / discharge
ovaralgia OH-var-AL-jah **Definition** pain of the ovaries	**ovar / algia** ovary / pain
ovarialgia oh-VAR-ee-AL-jah **Definition** pain of the ovaries	**ovari / algia** ovary / pain
NOTE: Both ovaralgia and ovarialgia are acceptable spellings and mean the same thing.	
perineocele PER-ih-NEE-oh-seel **Definition** hernia in the perineal region	**perineo / cele** perineum / pouch / tumor / hernia
polymenorrhea PAW-lee-MEN-oh-REE-ah **Definition** menstrual periods occurring with greater-than-normal frequency	**poly / meno / rrhea** many / menstruation / discharge
vaginodynia VAJ-ih-noh-DIH-nee-ah **Definition** vaginal pain	**vagino / dynia** vagina / pain
vulvodynia VUL-voh-DIH-nee-ah **Definition** pain in the vulva	**vulvo / dynia** vulva / pain

13.2 Patient History, Problems, Complaints

obstetrics

Term	Word Analysis
amniorrhea AM-nee-oh-REE-ah **Definition** discharge of amniotic fluid	**amnio / rrhea** amnion / discharge
amniorrhexis AM-nee-oh-REK-sis **Definition** rupture of the amniotic sac	**amnio / rrhexis** amnion / rupture
Braxton Hicks contraction BRAKS-ton HIKS con-TRAK-shun **Definition** sporadic contractions of the uterine muscles of women not in labor; also known as false labor	*named after John Braxton Hicks, the doctor who first noted them, in 1872*
contraction con-TRAK-shun **Definition** shortening or tightening of a muscle; during labor, the uterine muscles contract	**from Latin, for** "to draw together" **or** "shorten"

Learning Outcome 13.2 Exercises

PRONUNCIATION

EXERCISE 1 *Indicate which syllable is emphasized when pronounced.*

EXAMPLE: bronchitis bron**chi**tis

1. mastoptosis ______
2. hysterodynia ______
3. colpostenosis ______
4. metrorrhagia ______
5. menorrhalgia ______
6. perineocele ______
7. metromenorrhagia ______
8. dyspareunia ______
9. mastalgia ______
10. contraction ______
11. menorrhagia ______
12. ovarialgia ______
13. ovaralgia ______
14. amenorrhea ______
15. amniorrhexis ______

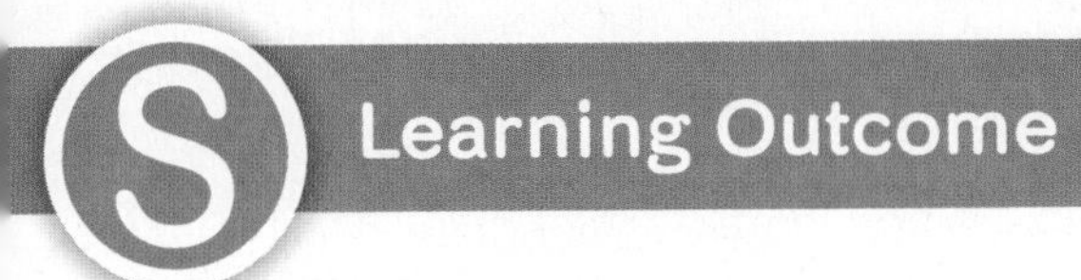

Learning Outcome 13.2 Exercises

TRANSLATION

EXERCISE 2 *Break down the following words into their component parts.*

EXAMPLE: nasopharyngoscope *naso | pharyngo | scope*

1. ovaralgia ______
2. leukorrhea ______
3. hysterodynia ______
4. menorrhagia ______
5. menorrhalgia ______
6. perineocele ______
7. amniorrhexis ______
8. gynecomastia ______
9. mastoptosis ______
10. amenorrhea ______

EXERCISE 3 *Underline and define the word parts from this chapter in the following terms.*

1. ovarialgia ______
2. vaginodynia ______
3. vulvodynia ______
4. amniorrhea ______
5. hysteralgia ______
6. mastalgia ______
7. metrorrhagia ______
8. colpostenosis ______
9. dysmenorrhea ______
10. oligomenorrhea ______
11. metromenorrhagia (2 roots) ______

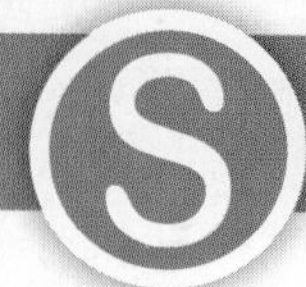

Learning Outcome 13.2 Exercises

EXERCISE 4 *Match the term on the left with its definition on the right.*

_____	1. contraction	a.	discharge of amniotic fluid
_____	2. Braxton Hicks contraction	b.	excessive menstrual bleeding at irregular intervals
_____	3. amenorrhea	c.	infrequent or light menstrual periods
_____	4. leukorrhea	d.	menstrual periods occurring with greater-than-normal frequency
_____	5. amniorrhea	e.	no menstruation
_____	6. polymenorrhea	f.	painful menstruation
_____	7. dysmenorrhea	g.	painful sexual intercourse
_____	8. oligomenorrhea	h.	sporadic contraction of the uterine muscles of women in labor; also known as false labor
_____	9. dyspareunia	i.	shortening or tightening of a muscle
_____	10. metromenorrhagia	j.	white vaginal discharge

EXERCISE 5 *Translate the following terms as literally as possible.*

EXAMPLE: nasopharyngoscope *an instrument for looking at the nose and throat*

1. vaginodynia ____________________
2. vulvodynia ____________________
3. hysterodynia ____________________
4. ovaralgia ____________________
5. hysteralgia ____________________
6. mastalgia ____________________
7. colpostenosis ____________________
8. perineocele ____________________
9. amniorrhexis ____________________
10. metrorrhagia ____________________
11. oligomenorrhea ____________________

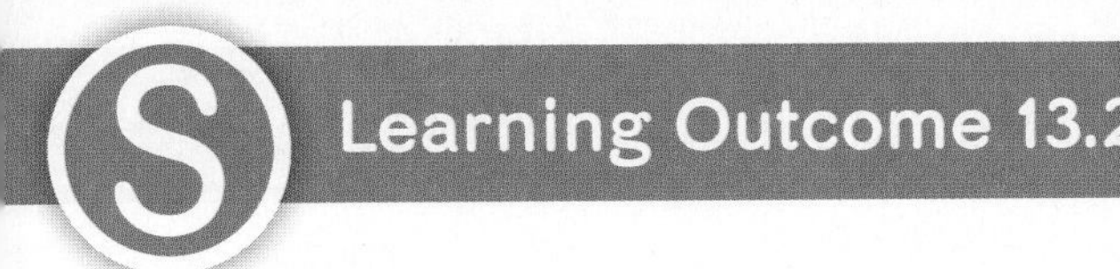

Learning Outcome 13.2 Exercises

GENERATION

EXERCISE 6 *Build a medical term from the information provided.*

EXAMPLE: inflammation of the sinuses *sinusitis*

1. discharge of amniotic fluid ____________
2. no menstruation ____________
3. excessive menstrual flow ____________
4. painful menstruation ____________
5. white discharge ____________
6. downward displacement (drooping) of the breast ____________
7. development of breast tissue in males ____________
8. menstrual periods occurring with greater-than-normal frequency ____________

EXERCISE 7 *Multiple-choice questions. Select the correct answer.*

1. Sporadic contractions of the uterine muscles of women not in labor are known as:
   a. Braxton Hicks contractions
   b. dyspareunia
   c. pseudocyesis
   d. pseudotocoria
2. Which of the following statements about the term *contraction* is FALSE?
   a. from Greek, for "to ball up"
   b. from Latin, for "to draw together" or "shorten"; means the shortening or tightening of a muscle
   c. occurs during labor
3. The term *dyspareunia* means:
   a. painful menstruation
   b. painful sexual intercourse
   c. unusual menstruation
   d. unusual sexual intercourse
4. Which of the following words is the correct medical term for "pain in the ovaries"?
   a. oopharalgia
   b. oophorodynia
   c. ovarialgia
   d. ovariodynia

OBJECTIVE

13.3 Observation and Discovery

A physical exam of the female reproductive system includes a breast exam, an external genital exam, and a pelvic exam. When examining a patient's breast, the examiner must pay close attention to color changes, skin texture, any lumps in the breast, and the nipple. In an external genital exam, examiners must take into consideration the patient's developmental stage (if she is a child) and the general appearance of the vulvar area.

The most important part of a female reproductive (*gynecologic*) exam is the pelvic exam. This involves placing an instrument called a *speculum* in the opening of the vagina. This instrument spreads open the walls of the vagina to make it easier to visualize the cervix.

An exam of the cervix (*colposcopy*) is a routine exam for all adult females. A critical part of this exam is the Pap smear, which involves removing a sample of tissue from the cervix and examining it with a microscope to screen for cancer.

Feeling the uterus and ovaries requires a *bimanual* exam, which involves placing fingers from one hand inside the vagina and one hand on the abdomen and feeling the structures between both hands. This type of exam aids in detecting any lumps or painful areas.

Finally, the examiner may need to perform a *rectovaginal* exam to best feel the walls of the vagina. The exam involves placing one or two fingers in the patient's rectum and the other in her vagina to search for any abnormalities.

Two common types of imaging studies are used to analyze a woman's reproductive system. One is the *mammogram,* a special x-ray that looks for cancer in the breast. The other common image type is an *ultrasound.* An ultrasound placed inside the vagina (*transvaginal ultrasound*) is a common way of looking at the ovaries, uterus, and cervix. During pregnancy, ultrasound is commonly used to screen the health of the uterus and baby (*prenatal ultrasound*). Many times, a more direct visual inspection of a patient's reproductive tract can help a physician determine the nature of a patient's problem. For a more in-depth view of the vulva, vagina, and cervix, the physician may need to use a special magnifying instrument (*colposcope*). This procedure is known as *colposcopy.* Similarly, he or she may use a special device to visualize the inside of the uterus (*hysteroscopy*).

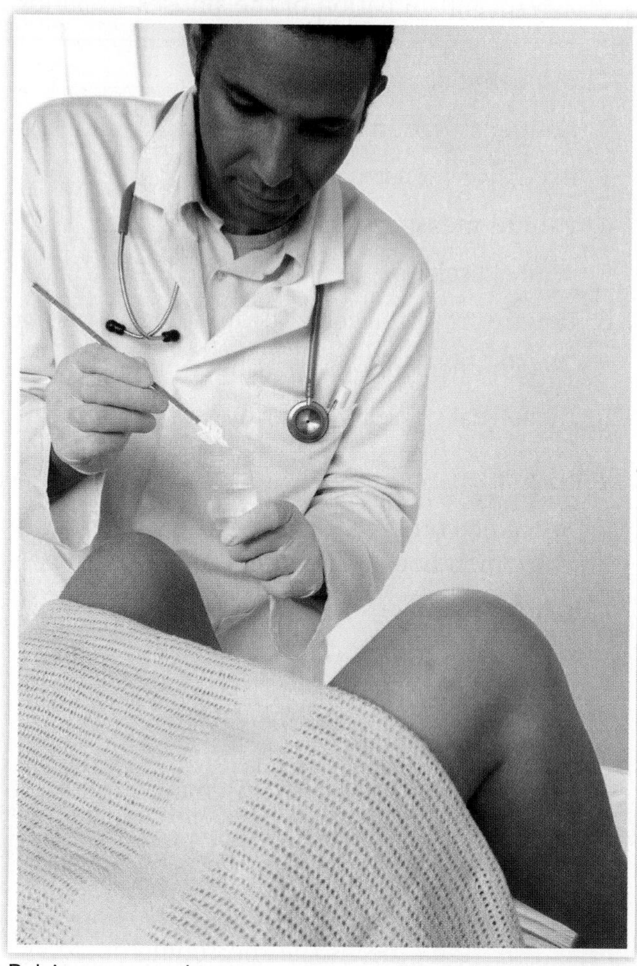

Pelvic exams and mammograms provide vital information for diagnosing gynecological issues.

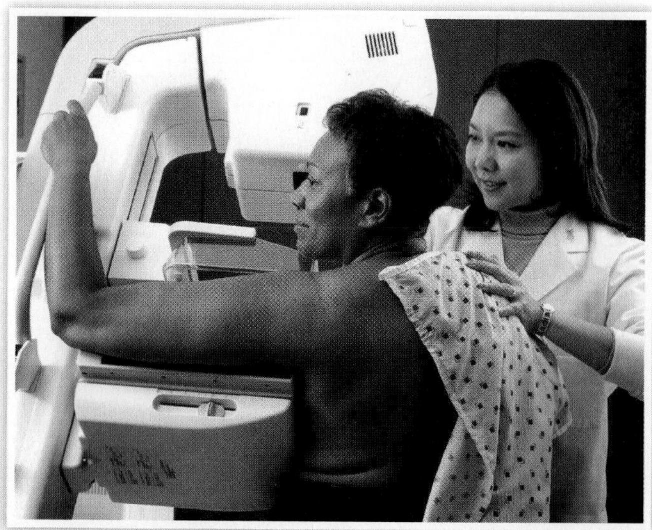

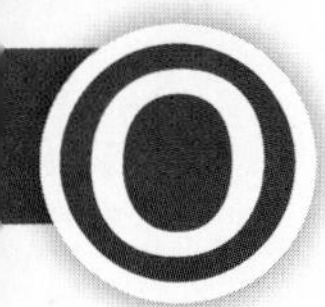

13.3 Observation and Discovery

Women frequently see health care providers for *prenatal care* throughout a pregnancy. Just prior to delivery (*antepartum*), it is important to determine how the baby is positioned inside the mother (*presentation*). By the time the baby is ready for delivery, its head should be facing downward (*cephalic*), but at times a baby's bottom or legs will be near the birth canal (*breech*). Because it is harder to deliver a baby in breech presentation, most obstetricians will choose to deliver the baby surgically (*cesarean section*).

During the antepartum visits, a health care worker will also need to determine the baby's size (*fetometry*), whether or not any birth defects (*congenital anomalies*) are present, and the womb's fluid (*amniotic fluid*) level. A large (*macrocephaly*) or small (*microcephaly*) head could indicate a problem with the brain. Too little amniotic fluid (*oligohydramnios*) generally indicates kidney problems in the baby. Too much fluid (*polyhydramnios*) can have numerous causes, including diabetes in the mother or gastrointestinal or urinary problems in the baby.

During delivery, the goal is a normal, uncomplicated delivery (*eutocia*). However, the delivery can be unusually painful (*dystocia*), perhaps if the baby's head is larger than the delivery canal (*cephalopelvic disproportion*). This condition is another common reason for a cesarean section delivery.

After delivery (*postpartum*), the mother will have follow-up exams to ensure that she is recovering well and to determine whether she has begun producing breast milk (*lactorrrhea*). This usually happens by 3 to 4 days after delivery.

The laboratory data collected when diagnosing female reproductive problems include results from a test called the *Pap smear,* which screens for cancer. It is among the most common labs specific to females. Another common lab is the wet mount. A *wet mount* involves collecting some vaginal discharge and putting it on a slide to examine with a microscope and look for signs of infection.

Pregnant patients often need lab tests to evaluate the fluid that surrounds the baby (*amniocentesis*). The test's results can reveal information on the baby's lung maturity, the presence of certain birth defects involving the spinal cord, and certain genetic conditions.

gynecology

Term	Word Analysis
amastia ay-MAS-tee-ah **Definition** absence of breast	**a / mast / ia** no / breast / condition
cervical dysplasia SER-vih-kal dis-PLAY-zhah **Definition** bad formation of cervical cells	**cervic / al dys / plasia** cervix / pertaining to bad / formation
colpoptosis KOL-pawp-TOH-sis **Definition** downward displacement of the vagina	**colpo / ptosis** vagina / drooping condition
episiostenosis eh-PEE-zee-oh-stih-NOH-sis **Definition** narrowing of the vulvar opening	**episio / sten / osis** vulva / narrow / condition

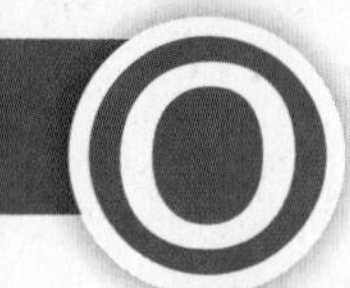

13.3 Observation and Discovery

gynecology *continued*

Term	Word Analysis
hematosalpinx heh-MAT-oh-SAL-pinks **Definition** blockage in a fallopian tube caused by blood	**hemato / salpinx** blood / fallopian tube
hydrosalpinx HAI-droh-SAL-pinks **Definition** blockage in a fallopian tube caused by water (or any clear fluid)	**hydro / salpinx** water / fallopian tube
hypermastia HAI-per-MAS-tee-ah **Definition** excessively large breasts **NOTE:** This term can also refer to an abnormal number of breasts.	**hyper / mast / ia** over / breast / condition
hypomastia HAI-poh-MAS-tee-ah **Definition** abnormally small breasts	**hypo / mast / ia** under / breast / condition
hysteroptosis HIS-ter-awp-TOH-sis **Definition** downward displacement of the uterus into the vagina	**hystero / ptosis** uterus / drooping condition
macromastia MAK-roh-MAS-tee-ah **Definition** abnormally large breasts	**macro / mast / ia** big / breast / condition
micromastia MAI-kroh-MAS-tee-ah **Definition** abnormally small breasts	**micro / mast / ia** small / breast / condition
oophorocystosis OH-aw-FOR-oh-SIS-toh-sis **Definition** ovarian cysts	**oophoro / cyst / osis** ovary / cyst / condition
pyosalpinx PAI-oh-SAL-pinks **Definition** blockage in a fallopian tube caused by pus	**pyo / salpinx** pus / fallopian tube
uterine prolapse YOO-ter-in PROH-laps **Definition** downward displacement of the uterus into the vagina	**uter / ine pro / lapse** uterus / pertaining to forward / fall

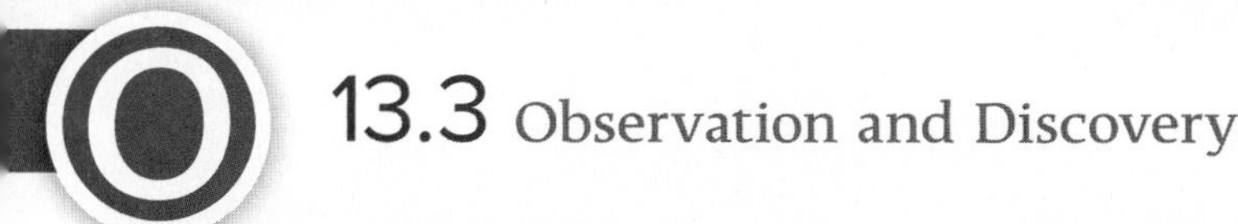

13.3 Observation and Discovery

gynecology—diagnostic procedures

Term	Word Analysis
colposcope KOL-poh-SKOHP **Definition** instrument used to examine the vagina	**colpo / scope** vagina / instrument to look
colposcopy kol-PAW-skoh-pee **Definition** procedure for examining the vagina	**colpo / scopy** vagina / looking procedure 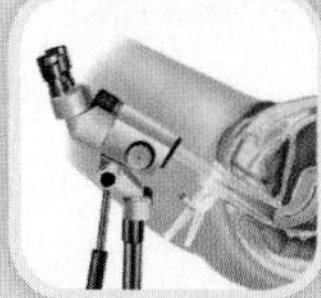
hysteroscope HIS-ter-oh-SKOHP **Definition** instrument for examining the uterus	**hystero / scope** uterus / instrument to look
hysteroscopy HIS-ter-AW-skoh-pee **Definition** procedure for examining the uterus	**hystero / scopy** uterus / looking procedure
Pap smear PAP SMEER **Definition** test used to detect cancer cells, most commonly in the cervix	*named after the inventor of the procedure, Dr. Georgios Papanicolaou* 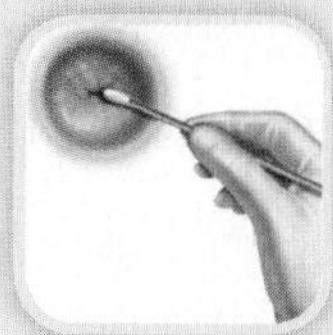
vaginoscope VAJ-ih-noh-SKOHP **Definition** instrument used to examine the vagina	**vagino / scope** vagina / instrument to look

gynecology—professional terms

Term	Word Analysis
endometrium EN-doh-MEE-tree-um **Definition** inner layer of uterine tissue	**endo / metr / ium** inside / uterus / tissue 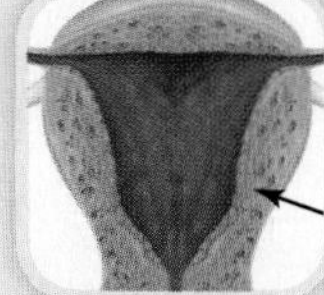
gynecologist GAI-neh-KAW-loh-jist **Definition** specialist in medical issues specific to women	**gyneco / logist** woman / specialist 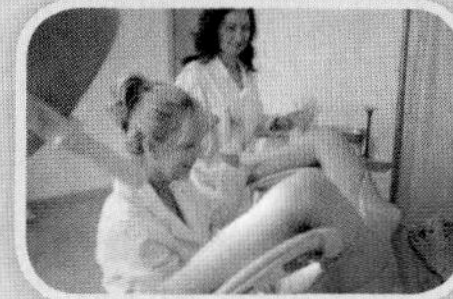 ©Maya/Getty Images RF

gynecology—professional terms *continued*

Term	Word Analysis
gynecology GAI-neh-KAW-loh-jee **Definition** study of medical issues specific to women	**gyneco / logy** woman / study
menarche MEN-ar-kee **Definition** beginning or first menstruation	**men / arche** menstruation / beginning
myometrium MAI-oh-MEE-tree-um **Definition** middle layer of uterine muscle tissue	**myo / metr / ium** muscle / uterus / tissue ©McGraw-Hill Education/Al Telser, photographer
perimetrium PER-ee-MEE-tree-um **Definition** tissue on the outside of the uterus, the outer layer of the uterus	**peri / metr / ium** around / uterus / tissue
speculum SPEH-kyoo-lum **Definition** device for examining a body cavity, most commonly the vagina	**from Latin, for** "mirror"

obstetrics

Term	Word Analysis
bradytocia BRAY-dih-TOH-shee-ah **Definition** slow labor	**brady / toc / ia** slow / birth / condition
cephalopelvic disproportion (CPD) SEE-fah-loh-PEL-vik DIS-proh-POR-shun **Definition** condition characterized by the inability of the mother's pelvis to allow the baby to pass through the birth canal **Note:** This can be caused by either a small pelvis or a large baby, or both.	**cephalo / pelv / ic disproportion** head / pelvic / pertaining to
congenital anomaly con-JIN-ih-tal ah-NAW-moh-lee **Definition** irregular condition that is present at the time of birth	**con / genit / al anomaly** with / birth / pertaining to irregularity
dystocia dis-TOH-shee-ah **Definition** difficult labor	**dys / toc / ia** bad / birth / condition

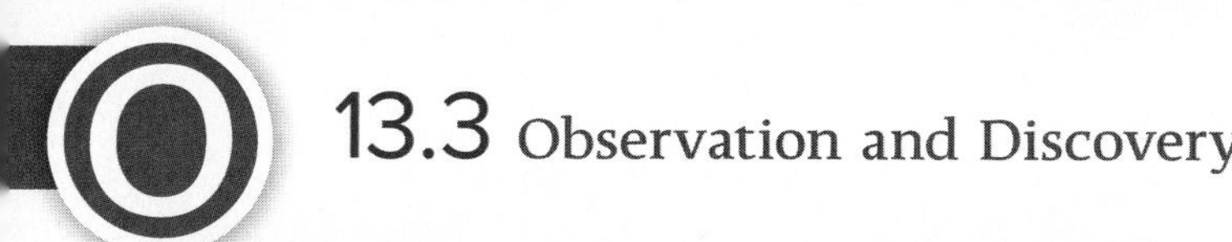

13.3 Observation and Discovery

obstetrics *continued*

Term	Word Analysis
eutocia yoo-TOH-shee-ah **Definition** normal labor	**eu / toc / ia** good / birth / condition
gravida GRAH-vid-ah **Definition** another term for pregnant **NOTE:** This word, which is also where the word gravity comes from, means "heavy" and is similar to an old expression about pregnancy that a woman is "great with child."	**gravida** heavy
hysterocele HIS-ter-oh-SEEL **Definition** hernia of the uterus	**hystero / cele** uterus / pouch / tumor / hernia
hysterorrhexis HIS-ter-oh-REK-sis **Definition** rupture of the uterus	**hystero / rrhexis** uterus / rupture
lactogenic LAK-toh-JIN-ik **Definition** causing the formation of milk	**lacto / gen / ic** milk / creation / pertaining to
lactorrhea LAK-toh-REE-ah **Definition** discharge of milk	**lacto / rrhea** milk / discharge
macrosomia MAK-roh-SOH-mee-ah **Definition** baby with a large body	**macro / som / ia** large / body / condition
microcephalus MAI-kroh-SEF-ah-lus **Definition** baby with a small head	**micro / cephalus** small / head
oligohydramnios AW-lih-goh-hai-DRAM-nee-ohs **Definition** not enough amniotic fluid	**oligo / hydr / amnios** few / water / amnion
polyhydramnios PAW-lee-hai-DRAM-nee-ohs **Definition** excessive amniotic fluid	**poly / hydr / amnios** a lot / water / amnion
teratogenic TER-ah-toh-JIN-ik **Definition** causing the formation of birth defects	**terato / gen / ic** monster / creation / pertaining to

13.3 Observation and Discovery

obstetrics—diagnostic procedures

Term	Word Analysis
amniocentesis AM-nee-oh-sin-TEE-sis **Definition** surgical puncture of the amnion	**amnio / centesis** amnion / puncture 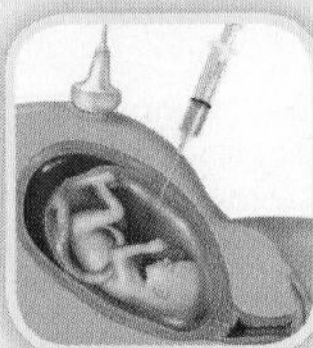
amnioscope AM-nee-oh-SKOHP **Definition** instrument for examining the amnion	**amnio / scope** amnion / instrument to look
amnioscopy AM-nee-AWS-koh-pee **Definition** procedure for examining the amnion	**amnio / scopy** amnion / looking procedure
cardiotocograph KAR-dee-oh-TOH-koh-GRAF **Definition** instrument for recording the baby's heart rate during contractions; also known as a fetal heart monitor	**cardio / toco / graph** heart / birth / instrument to record 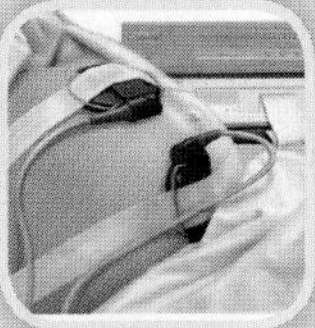
fetometry fee-TAW-meh-tree **Definition** procedure for measuring the fetus	**feto / metry** fetus / measuring process
pelvicephalometry PEL-vih-SEF-eh-LAW-meh-tree **Definition** procedure for measuring the head size of the baby and the pelvis size of the mother	**pelvi / cephalo / metry** pelvis / head / measuring process
pelvimetry pel-VIM-eh-tree **Definition** procedure for measuring the pelvis	**pelvi / metry** pelvis / measuring process
tocodynagraph TOH-koh-DAI-nah-GRAF **Definition** instrument for recording the strength of labor contractions	**toco / dyna / graph** birth / power / instrument to record
tocography toh-KAW-grah-fee **Definition** procedure for recording the strength of labor contractions	**toco / graphy** birth / writing procedure

13.3 Observation and Discovery

obstetrics—process of conception

Term	Word Analysis
conception kon-SEP-shun **Definition** the process of conceiving a child **NOTE:** The root *cept* means "to take or gather." It also appears in words like *accept* and *capture.*	**concept / tion** conceive / process
contraception con-trah-SEP-shun **Definition** a process that prevents or hinders the conception of a child **NOTE:** This word is formed as a negation of conception. The prefix *contra* is added while *con* is dropped and *cept* carries the meaning of "conception."	**contra / cept / tion** against / conception / process
fertilization fir-tih-lih-ZAY-shun **Definition** the process of an egg and sperm joining to form	**fertiliz / ation** fertile / process 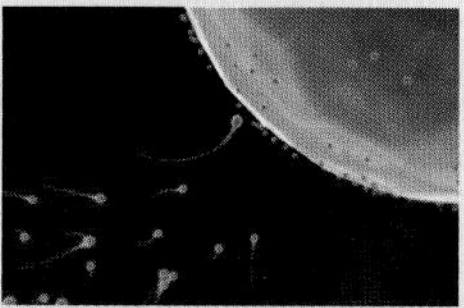 ©MedicalRF.com RF
gestation jes-TAY-shun **Definition** the process of carrying a child from conception until birth	**gest / ation** carry / process
implantation im-plan-TAY-shun **Definition** the process of a fertilized egg attaching or adhering to the uterus; this enables it to begin to receive oxygen and nutrients from the mother to continue to grow **NOTE:** Notice how *in* turns to *im* when put next to *plant.* It's because you make a *p* sound by putting your lips together. Thus, it is easier to say if you change the *n* to an *m*, which is also made by putting your lips together.	**im / plant / ation** in / plant / process
ovulation aw-vyoo-LAY-shun **Definition** the process of an egg being released from an ovary **NOTE:** Recall the diminutive suffixes from Chapter 1 (*ule*, *icle*, etc.). They make things little. *Ovum* means "egg." *Ovulum* means "small egg."	**ov / ul / ation** egg / small / process

obstetrics—professional terms

Term	Word Analysis
antepartum AN-tee-PAR-tum **Definition** time before birth	**ante / partum** before / birth
intrapartum IN-trah-PAR-tum **Definition** time during birth	**intra / partum** during / birth

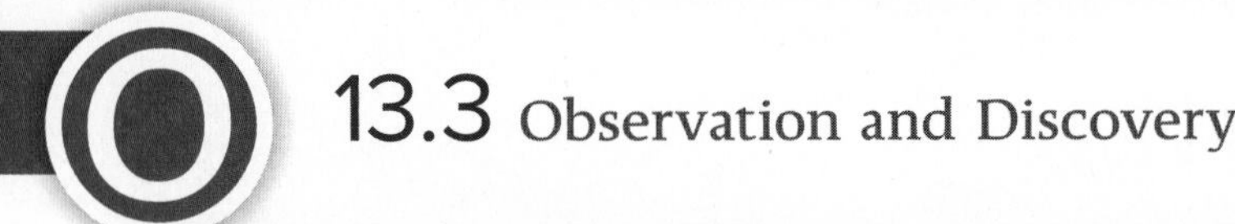

13.3 Observation and Discovery

obstetrics—professional terms *continued*

Term	Word Analysis
lactation lak-TAY-shun **Definition** production of milk	**lact / ation** milk / formation 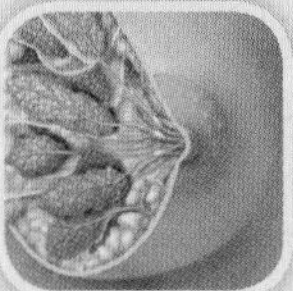
natal NAY-tal **Definition** pertaining to birth	**nat / al** birth / pertaining to
neonatal NEE-oh-NAY-tal **Definition** pertaining to new birth; normally the first 28 days after birth	**neo / nat / al** new / birth / pertaining to
neonatologist NEE-oh-nay-TAW-loh-jist **Definition** specialist in the neonatal period	**neo / nato / logist** new / birth / specialist
neonatology NEE-oh-nay-TAW-loh-jee **Definition** study of the neonatal period	**neo / nato / logy** new / birth / study 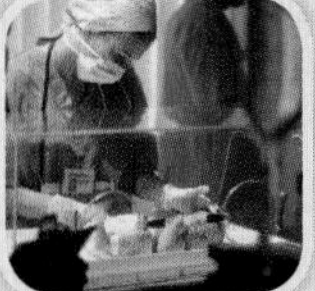 ©Flying Colours Ltd/Getty Images RF
obstetrician OB-steh-TRIH-shun **Definition** specialist in pregnancy, labor, and delivery of newborns	**from Latin, for** "midwife" **or literally** "one who stands beside"
obstetrics ob-STEH-triks **Definition** branch of medicine dealing with pregnancy, labor, and delivery of newborns	**from Latin, for** "midwife" **or literally** "one who stands beside"
perinatal PEH-ree-NAY-tal **Definition** time around the birth, normally ranging from 28 weeks of pregnancy to 28 days after pregnancy	**peri / nat / al** around / birth / pertaining to
perinatologist PEH-ree-nay-TAW-loh-jist **Definition** specialist in the perinatal period	**peri / nato / logist** around / birth / specialist
perinatology PER-ee-nay-TAW-loh-jee **Definition** branch of medicine dealing with the perinatal period	**peri / nato / logy** around / birth / study
postnatal post-NAY-tal **Definition** pertaining to after birth	**post / nat / al** after / birth / pertaining to

obstetrics—professional terms *continued*

Term	Word Analysis
postpartum POST-PAR-tum **Definition** pertaining to after birth **NOTE:** The difference between this word and *postnatal* is the focus. Normally, *nato* words focus on the baby and *partum* words focus on the mother.	**post / partum** after / birth
prenatal pree-NAY-tal **Definition** pertaining to before birth	**pre / natal** before / birth
teratology TER-ah-TAW-loh-jee **Definition** branch of medicine dealing with the study of birth defects and their causes	**terato / logy** monster / study

radiology

Term	Word Analysis
Gynecology	
cervicography SER-vih-KAW-grah-fee **Definition** procedure for imaging the cervix	**cervico / graphy** cervix / writing procedure
hysterosalpingogram HIS-ter-oh-sal-PING-goh-gram **Definition** record of the uterus and fallopian tubes	**hystero / salpingo / gram** uterus / fallopian tube / record
mammogram MAM-oh-GRAM **Definition** record of a breast exam	**mammo / gram** breast / record Source: Rhoda Baer/National Cancer Institute (NCI)
sonohysterography SOH-noh-HIS-ter-AW-grah-fee **Definition** procedure using sound waves to examine the uterus	**sono / hystero / graphy** sound / uterus / writing procedure ©Banana Stock/Punchstock RF

13.3 Observation and Discovery

radiology *continued*

Term	Word Analysis
transvaginal sonography TRANZ-VAJ-ih-nal soh-NAW-grah-fee	trans / vagin / al sono / graphy through / vagina / pertaining to sound / writing procedure
Definition imaging procedure using sound waves emitted from a device inserted in the vagina	
Obstetrics	
hysterography HIS-ter-AW-grah-fee	hystero / graphy uterus / writing procedure
Definition procedure for imaging the uterus	
pelvic sonograph PEL-vik SAW-noh-GRAF	pelv / ic sono / graph pelvis / pertaining to sound / instrument to record
Definition instrument for imaging the pelvis using sound waves	

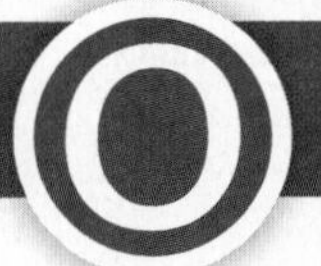

Learning Outcome 13.3 Exercises

PRONUNCIATION

EXERCISE 1 *Indicate which syllables are emphasized when pronounced.*

EXAMPLE: bronchitis bron**chi**tis

1. amastia ____________
2. perinatal ____________
3. macromastia ____________
4. macrosomia ____________
5. antepartum ____________
6. endometrium ____________
7. teratogenic ____________
8. amnioscope ____________
9. amnioscopy ____________
10. hysterography ____________
11. cardiotocograph ____________
12. neonatology ____________
13. obstetrician ____________
14. hysterorrhexis ____________
15. oligohydramnios ____________
16. polyhydramnios ____________
17. natal ____________
18. postnatal ____________
19. prenatal ____________
20. speculum ____________
21. dystocia ____________
22. fetometry ____________
23. pelvimetry ____________
24. tocography ____________
25. lactation ____________
26. obstetrics ____________

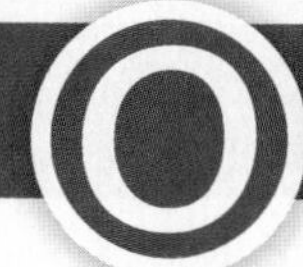

Learning Outcome 13.3 Exercises

TRANSLATION

EXERCISE 2 *Break down the following words into their component parts.*

EXAMPLE: nasopharyngoscope *naso | pharyngo | scope*

1. vaginoscope ______
2. fetometry ______
3. lactorrhea ______
4. hysterocele ______
5. gynecology ______
6. neonatal ______
7. postnatal ______
8. intrapartum ______
9. dystocia ______
10. eutocia ______
11. amniocentesis ______
12. cervical dysplasia ______
13. pelvic sonograph ______
14. neonatology ______
15. perinatologist ______
16. hematosalpinx ______
17. pyosalpinx ______
18. colpoptosis ______
19. hysteroptosis ______
20. sonohysterography ______
21. tocodynagraph ______
22. polyhydramnios ______
23. teratology ______
24. microcephalus ______

EXERCISE 3 *Underline and define the word parts from this chapter in the following terms.*

1. natal ______
2. amnioscope ______
3. cervicography ______
4. gynecologist ______
5. lactogenic ______
6. mammogram ______
7. pelvimetry ______
8. prenatal ______
9. postpartum ______
10. cardiotocograph ______
11. perinatal ______
12. colposcope ______
13. hysteroscope ______
14. episiostenosis ______
15. neonatologist ______
16. antepartum ______
17. amastia ______
18. perinatology ______
19. bradytocia ______

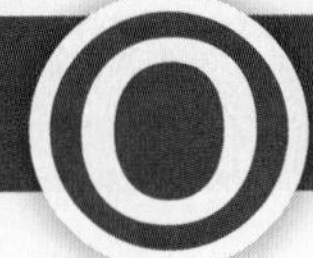

Learning Outcome 13.3 Exercises

20. menarche ______
21. oligohydramnios ______
22. hysterorrhexis ______
23. hydrosalpinx ______
24. myometrium ______
25. oophorocystosis ______
26. transvaginal sonography ______
27. pelvicephalometry ______
28. hysterosalpingogram (2 roots) ______

EXERCISE 4 *Match the term on the left with its definition on the right.*

______	1. Pap smear	a.	baby with a large body
______	2. obstetrics	b.	condition characterized by the inability of the mother's pelvis to allow the baby to pass through the birth canal
______	3. obstetrician	c.	device for examining a body cavity, most commonly the vagina
______	4. speculum	d.	specialist in pregnancy, labor, and delivery of newborns
______	5. congenital anomaly	e.	test used to detect cancer cells, most commonly in the cervix
______	6. cephalopelvic disproportion	f.	irregular condition that is present at the time of birth
______	7. uterine prolapse	g.	branch of medicine dealing with pregnancy, labor, and delivery of newborns
______	8. macrosomia	h.	causing the formation of birth defects
______	9. teratogenic	i.	downward displacement of the uterus into the vagina
______	10. gravida	j.	pregnant

EXERCISE 5 *Fill in the blanks.*

1. amnioscopy: procedure for examining the ______
2. cervicography: procedure for imaging the ______
3. hysterography: procedure for imaging the ______
4. colposcopy: procedure for examining the ______
5. hysteroscopy: procedure for examining the ______
6. tocography: procedure for recording the strength of ______
7. mammography: procedure for imaging the ______
8. vaginoscopy: procedure for examining the ______

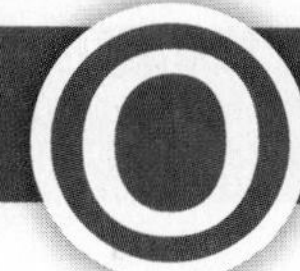

Learning Outcome 13.3 Exercises

EXERCISE 6 *Translate the following terms as literally as possible.*

EXAMPLE: nasopharyngoscope *an instrument for looking at the nose and throat*

1. natal ______
2. lactation ______
3. gynecology ______
4. tocograph ______
5. colposcope ______
6. hysteroscope ______
7. hysterocele ______
8. lactorrhea ______
9. pyosalpinx ______
10. hypomastia ______
11. micromastia ______
12. amniocentesis ______
13. perinatology ______
14. hysterorrhexis ______
15. perimetrium ______
16. colpoptosis ______
17. oophorocystosis ______
18. cervical dysplasia ______
19. tocodynagraph ______
20. cardiotocograph ______
21. transvaginal sonography ______
22. pelvicephalometry ______
23. macrosomia ______
24. teratology ______

EXERCISE 7 *Match the term on the left with its definition on the right.*

______	1. ovulation	a.	the process of conceiving a child
______	2. fertilization	b.	a process that prevents or hinders the conception of a child.
______	3. conception	c.	the process of an egg and sperm joining to conceive a child
______	4. implantation	d.	the process of carrying a child from conception until birth
______	5. gestation	e.	the process of an egg being released from an ovary
______	6. contraception	f.	the process of a fertilized egg attaching or adhering to the uterus. This enables it to begin to receive oxygen and nutrients from the mother to continue to grow.

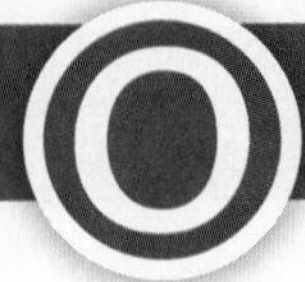

Learning Outcome 13.3 Exercises

GENERATION

EXERCISE 8 *Build a medical term from the information provided.*

EXAMPLE: inflammation of the sinuses *sinusitis*

1. instrument used to examine the vagina (use *vagin/o*) ______
2. procedure for examining the vagina (use *colp/o*) ______
3. procedure for imaging the uterus (use *hyster/o*) ______
4. procedure for examining the uterus (use *hyster/o*) ______
5. procedure using sound waves to examine the uterus (use *hyster/o*) ______
6. record of a breast exam (use *mamm/o*) ______
7. procedure for examining the amnion ______
8. procedure for measuring the fetus ______
9. instrument for imaging the pelvis using sound waves ______
10. study of the neonatal period ______
11. specialist in medical issues specific to women ______
12. slow labor ______
13. narrowing of the vulvar opening (use *episi/o*) ______
14. causing the formation of milk ______
15. absence of breasts (use *mast/o*) ______
16. beginning or first menstruation ______
17. excessively large breasts (use *hyper-*) ______
18. downward displacement of the uterus ______
19. inner layer of uterine tissue ______
20. time during birth (use *part/o*) ______
21. record of the uterus and fallopian tubes ______
22. procedure for recording the strength of labor contractions ______
23. baby with a small head ______

EXERCISE 9 *Multiple-choice questions. Select the correct answer(s).*

1. The production of milk is called:
   a. intrapartum
   b. lactation
   c. lactogenic
   d. lactorrhea
   e. none of these
2. The downward displacement of the uterus into the vagina is known as:
   a. uterine prolapse
   b. hysteroptosis
   c. vesicovaginal fistula
   d. uterine prolapse and hysteroptosis
   e. hysteroptosis and vesicovaginal fistula
3. The middle layer of uterine muscle tissue is the:
   a. endometrium
   b. intrametrium
   c. myometrium
   d. perimetrium
   e. none of these

Learning Outcome 13.3 Exercises

4. A condition characterized by the inability of the mother's pelvis to allow the baby to pass through the birth canal is known as:
   a. cephalopelvic disproportion
   b. microcephalus
   c. pelvicephalometry
   d. teratogenic
   e. none of these

5. Another term for *pregnant* is:
   a. amastia
   b. gravida
   c. menarche
   d. prenatal
   e. teratogenic

6. Select all of the following statements that apply to the term *Pap smear*.
   a. a diagnostic procedure used in gynecology
   b. a diagnostic procedure used in obstetrics
   c. a test used to detect cancer cells, most commonly in the cervix
   d. a test used to detect cancer cells, most commonly in the vulva
   e. named after the inventor of the procedure, Dr. Georgios Papanicolaou

7. A device for examining a body cavity, most commonly the vagina, is called a(n):
   a. episiostenosis
   b. gravida
   c. hysterocele
   d. mammogram
   e. speculum

8. Select all of the following terms that pertain to obstetrics.
   a. amnioscope
   b. colposcope
   c. hysteroscope
   d. pelvimetry
   e. tocodynagraph
   f. vaginoscope

9. Select all of the following terms that pertain to gynecology.
   a. amnioscope
   b. colposcope
   c. hysteroscope
   d. pelvimetry
   e. tocodynagraph
   f. vaginoscope

EXERCISE 10 *Briefly describe the difference between each pair of terms.*

1. postnatal, prenatal ______
2. obstetrics, obstetrician ______
3. macromastia, micromastia ______
4. hypermastia, hypomastia ______
5. antepartum, postpartum ______
6. endometrium, perimetrium ______
7. neonatal, perinatal ______
8. neonatologist, perinatologist ______
9. dystocia, eutocia ______
10. hematosalpinx, hydrosalpinx ______
11. congenital anomaly, teratogenic ______

13.4 Diagnosis and Pathology

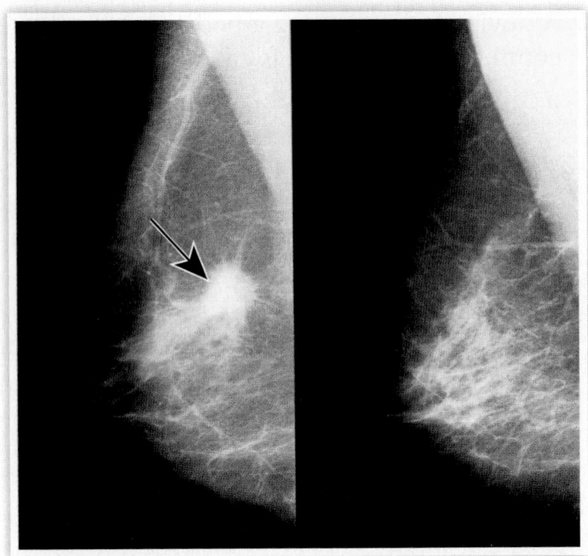
Mammogram of a breast with a tumor at the arrow (left), compared with the appearance of normal fibrous connective tissue of the breast (right).

Problems with periods are very routine causes for females to seek medical help. The normal range for a female's first period (*menarche*) is 10 to 16 years of age. An early or delayed start for periods may indicate an underlying problem. Missing one or more periods (*amenorrhea*) is a common reason for a medical visit. This can be caused by pregnancy, hormone problems, or problems with anatomy.

Unfortunately, cancers of the female reproductive system are common problems. Breast cancer (*adenocarcinoma of the breast*) is the most common cancer in women. For this reason, routine exams and mammograms are very important in female health care.

The uterus, cervix, and ovaries are also common areas for cancer. The Pap smear helps detect early evidence of cancer or precancerous changes in the cervix (*cervical intraepithelial neoplasia*).

Infection or inflammation of the female reproductive system happens more frequently in the outer parts of the reproductive system. Irritation of the vagina (*vaginitis*) or the vagina and its surrounding area (*vulvovaginitis*) can present with pain and/or itching. Both bacteria (*bacterial vaginosis*) and fungi (*vaginomycosis*) are frequent causes.

Many bacterial and viral infections of the female reproductive tract are spread through sexual intercourse. If infection spreads higher into the reproductive tract, such as to the fallopian tubes (salpingitis) and cervix (cervicitis), the patient may become quite ill; these infections can even lead to scarring and infertility. Another common infection in females is infection of the breast (mastitis), particularly in nursing mothers. Mastitis can make the breastfeeding process very painful.

Pregnancy can cause its own set of medical issues. A fertilized egg that implants anywhere other than the uterus is known as an *ectopic pregnancy*. Examples of ectopic locations include the fallopian tubes (*salpingocyesis*) and ovaries (*ovariacyesis*). Ectopic pregnancies are not viable, and they can cause pain and bleeding, infertility, and even death in some extreme circumstances.

During pregnancy, many women experience nausea and vomiting, a condition commonly known as *morning sickness*. In some cases, the vomiting can become quite severe (*hyperemesis gravidarum*) and need medical treatment.

Another problem encountered by some women during pregnancy is *preeclampsia*. This condition is marked by high blood pressure and protein in the urine. It can progress to include seizures (*eclampsia*).

The connection point between the mother and the baby (*placenta*) can also be a source of medical problems. A placenta in the wrong position can block the opening in the uterus (*placenta previa*), making delivery problematic. If the blood supply to the placenta is interrupted (*abruptio placentae*), the baby may be at risk of not getting enough blood, and the mother could suffer severe blood loss.

The membranes of the womb can develop tumors or infection. Tumors of the womb actually arise from fetal tissue. Rarely, this can become cancerous (*choriocarcinoma*). Infections in the womb (*chorioamnionitis*) routinely occur just prior to delivery and are treated with antibiotics.

Not every pregnancy produces a baby capable of survival. In fact, upward of 25 percent of all known pregnancies result in the mother's body ending the pregnancy. This is mainly the mother's body's response to a fetus with severe problems that would prevent survival. Commonly known as a *miscarriage*, the medical term is *spontaneous abortion*. This is opposed to common lay use of the term *abortion*, which usually refers to an *induced abortion*. An induced abortion is when a pregnancy is deliberately ended by artificial means. Induced abortions can be performed by taking a medication or via surgery.

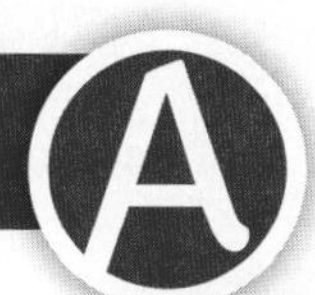

13.4 Diagnosis and Pathology

gynecology

Term	Word Analysis
cervicitis SER-vih-SAI-tis **Definition** inflammation of the cervix	**cervic / itis** cervix / inflammation
cervicocolpitis SER-vih-koh-kol-PAI-tis **Definition** inflammation of the cervix and vagina	**cervico / colp / itis** cervix / vagina / inflammation
cervicovaginitis SER-vih-koh-VAJ-ih-NAI-tis **Definition** inflammation of the cervix and vagina	**cervico / vagin / itis** cervix / vagina / inflammation
colpitis kol-PAI-tis **Definition** inflammation of the vagina	**colp / itis** vagina / inflammation
colpocystitis KOL-poh-sis-TAI-tis **Definition** inflammation of the vagina and urinary bladder	**colpo / cyst / itis** vagina / bladder / inflammation
cystocele SIS-toh-seel **Definition** hernia of the urinary bladder into the vagina	**cysto / cele** bladder / pouch / tumor / hernia
endocervicitis EN-doh-SER-vih-SAI-tis **Definition** inflammation of the inside of the cervix	**endo / cervic / itis** inside / cervix / inflammation
endometriosis EN-doh-MEE-tree-OH-sis **Definition** condition in which endometrium cells appear and grow outside the uterus	**endo / metri / osis** inside / uterus / condition
endometritis EN-doh-meh-TRAI-tis **Definition** inflammation of the endometrium	**endo / metr / itis** inside / uterus / inflammation
mastitis mas-TAI-tis **Definition** inflammation of the breast	**mast / itis** breast / inflammation

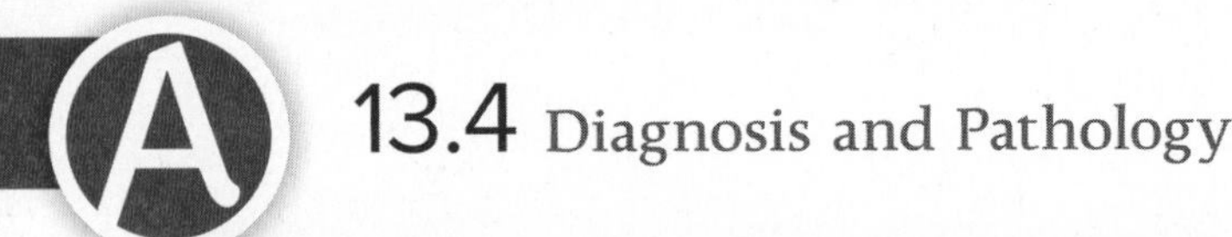

13.4 Diagnosis and Pathology

gynecology *continued*

Term	Word Analysis
menopause MEN-oh-pawz **Definition** cessation of menstruation	**meno / pause** menstruation / stop
metrocolpocele MEH-troh-KOL-poh-seel **Definition** hernia of the uterus and prolapse into the vagina	**metro / colpo / cele** uterus / vagina / pouch / tumor / hernia
metrophlebitis MEH-troh-fleh-BAI-tis **Definition** inflammation of the blood vessels of the uterus	**metro / phleb / itis** uterus / vein / inflammation
myometritis MAI-oh-meh-TRAI-tis **Definition** inflammation of the myometrium	**myo / metr / itis** muscle / uterus / inflammation
oophoritis OH-aw-for-AI-tis **Definition** inflammation of an ovary	**oophor / itis** ovary / inflammation
oophoroma OH-aw-for-OH-mah **Definition** ovarian tumor	**oophor / oma** ovary / tumor
ovariorrhexis oh-VAR-ee-oh-REK-sis **Definition** rupture of an ovary	**ovario / rrhexis** ovary / rupture
ovaritis OH-vah-RAI-tis **Definition** inflammation of an ovary	**ovar / itis** ovary / inflammation
perimetritis PER-ee-meh-TRAI-tis **Definition** inflammation of the perimetrium	**peri / metr / itis** around / uterus / inflammation
rectocele REK-toh-seel **Definition** hernia or protrusion of the rectum into the vagina	**recto / cele** rectum / pouch / tumor / hernia
salpingitis SAL-pin-JAI-tis **Definition** inflammation of a fallopian tube	**salping / itis** tube / inflammation

13.4 Diagnosis and Pathology

gynecology *continued*

Term	Word Analysis
salpingocele sal-PING-goh-seel **Definition** hernia of a fallopian tube	**salpingo / cele** fallopian tube / pouch / tumor / hernia
salpingo-oophoritis sal-PIN-goh-OH-aw-for-AI-tis **Definition** inflammation of a fallopian tube and ovary	**salpingo / oophor / itis** fallopian tube / ovary / inflammation
urethrocele yur-EE-throh-seel **Definition** hernia or prolapse of the urethra into the vagina	**urethro / cele** urethra / pouch / tumor / hernia
vaginitis VAJ-ih-NAI-tis **Definition** inflammation of the vagina	**vagin / itis** vagina / inflammation
vaginomycosis VAJ-ih-noh-MAI-koh-sis **Definition** fungal condition of the vagina	**vagino / myc / osis** vagina / fungus / condition
vaginosis VAJ-ih-NOH-sis **Definition** condition of the vagina	**vagin / osis** vagina / condition
vesicovaginal fistula VES-ih-koh-VAJ-ih-nal FIS-tyoo-lah **Definition** abnormal opening between the urinary bladder and the vagina	**vesico / vagin / al fistula** bladder / vagina / pertaining to pipe
vulvitis vul-VAI-tis **Definition** inflammation of the vulva	**vulv / itis** vulva / inflammation
vulvovaginitis VUL-voh-VAJ-ih-NAI-tis **Definition** inflammation of the vulva and vagina	**vulvo / vagin / itis** vulva / vagina / inflammation

obstetrics

Term	Word Analysis
abortion ah-BOR-shun **Definition** termination of pregnancy	**from Latin, for** "an untimely birth or miscarriage"

NOTE: There are two general categories of abortion: spontaneous (when the body does it of its own accord) and *induced* (when there is an external cause). Outside the medical world, many people commonly use the term miscarriage to refer to a spontaneous abortion and abortion to refer exclusively to an induced abortion.

13.4 Diagnosis and Pathology

obstetrics *continued*

Term	Word Analysis
abruptio placentae ah-BRUP-shee-oh plah-SIN-tee **Definition** separation of the placenta from the wall of the uterus	**abruptio placentae** tear away placenta 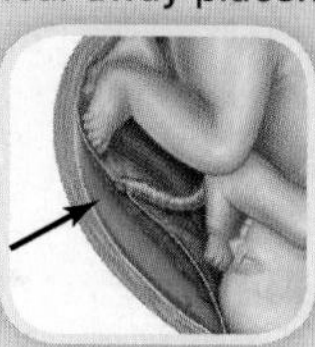
chorioamnionitis KOR-ee-oh-AM-nee-oh-NAI-tis **Definition** inflammation of the chorion and amnion	**chorio / amnion / itis** chorion / amnion / inflammation
chorionitis KOR-ee-aw-NAI-tis **Definition** inflammation of the chorion	**chorion / itis** chorion / inflammation
eclampsia eh-KLAMP-see-ah **Definition** severe, life-threatening complication of pregnancy characterized by seizures **NOTE:** The term probably comes from the fact that seizures strike suddenly, like lightning.	**from Greek, for "to shine" or "lightning"**
ectopic pregnancy ek-TOP-ik PREG-nan-see **Definition** implantation of a fertilized egg in a place other than the uterus	**ec / top / ic pregnancy** outside / place / pertaining to pregnancy
hyperemesis gravidarum HAI-per-eh-MEE-sis GRAV-ih-DAR-um **Definition** pregnancy-related vomiting; an extreme form of the more common *morning sickness*	**hyper / emesis gravidarum** over / vomit pregnancy
hysterorrhexis HIS-ter-oh-REK-sis **Definition** rupture of the uterus	**hystero / rrhexis** uterus / rupture
ovariocyesis oh-VAR-ee-oh-sai-EE-sis **Definition** ectopic pregnancy in an ovary	**ovario / cyesis** ovary / pregnancy
placenta previa plah-SIN-tah PREE-vee-ah **Definition** condition in which the placenta is attached to the uterus near the cervix	**placenta previa** placenta first 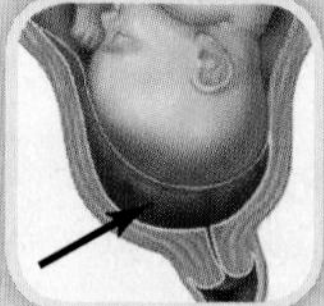
preeclampsia PREE-eh-KLAMP-see-ah **Definition** condition characterized by high blood pressure and high protein in the urine **NOTE:** See *eclampsia* for the origin of the term. The term comes from the fact that without proper treatment, a patient will develop eclampsia.	**pre / eclampsia** before / eclampsia
pseudocyesis SOO-doh-sai-EE-sis **Definition** false pregnancy	**pseudo / cyesis** false / pregnancy

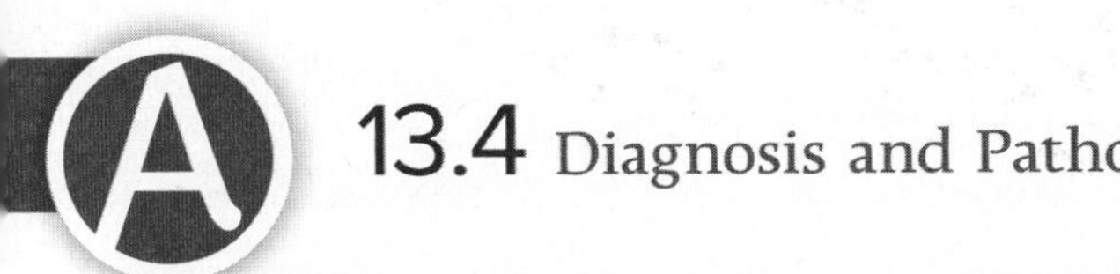

13.4 Diagnosis and Pathology

obstetrics *continued*

Term	Word Analysis
salpingocyesis sal-PING-goh-sai-EE-sis **Definition** ectopic pregnancy in a fallopian tube	**salpingo / cyesis** fallopian tube / pregnancy
spontaneous abortion spawn-TAY-nee-is ah-BOR-shun **Definition** naturally occurring termination of pregnancy; also known as a *miscarriage* **NOTE:** See *abortion* for the origin of the term.	

oncology

Term	Word Analysis
adenocarcinoma of the breast AD-en-oh-KAR-sih-NOH-mah **Definition** glandular tumor in the breast	**adeno / carcin / oma of the breast** gland / cancer / tumor 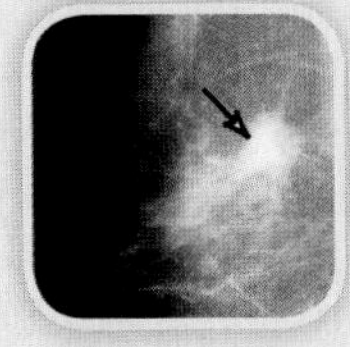 ©UHB Trust/The Image Bank/Getty Images
cervical intraepithelial neoplasia SER-vih-kal IN-trah-EP-ih-THEE-lee-al NEE-oh-PLAY-zhah **Definition** abnormal growth of cervical cells **NOTE:** Epithelial cells are a type of tissue that lines the surface of the skin and other membranes.	**cervic / al intra / epithelial neo / plasia** cervix / pertaining to inside / epithelial new / formation
chorioangioma KOR-ee-oh-AN-jee-OH-mah **Definition** blood vessel tumor of the chorion	**chorio / angi / oma** chorion / vessel / tumor
choriocarcinoma KOR-ee-oh-KAR-sih-NOH-mah **Definition** cancerous tumor of the chorion	**chorio / carcin / oma** chorion / cancer / tumor
dermoid cyst DER-moyd SIST **Definition** ovarian cyst containing skin and sometimes hair, teeth, bone, or cartilage	**derm / oid cyst** skin / resembling cyst 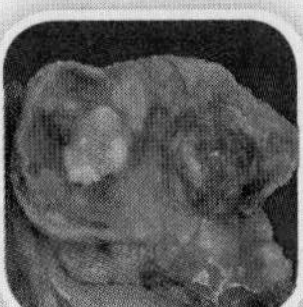 ©McGraw-Hill Education
teratoma TER-ah-TOH-mah **Definition** another term for a dermoid cyst; the name derives from the contents of the cyst	**terat / oma** monster / tumor

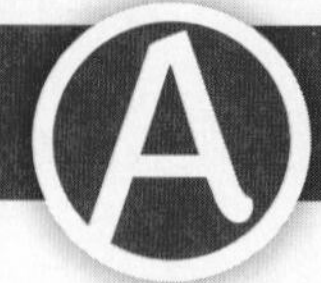

Learning Outcome 13.4 Exercises

PRONUNCIATION

EXERCISE 1 *Indicate which syllable is emphasized when pronounced.*

EXAMPLE: bronchitis bron**chi**tis

1. teratoma ____________
2. vaginitis ____________
3. vaginosis ____________
4. chorionitis ____________
5. myometritis ____________
6. perimetritis ____________
7. endometriosis ____________
8. metrocolpocele ____________
9. hysterorrhexis ____________
10. preeclampsia ____________
11. pseudocyesis ____________
12. salpingocyesis ____________
13. vulvovaginitis ____________
14. colpitis ____________
15. mastitis ____________
16. vulvitis ____________
17. salpingitis ____________
18. cystocele ____________
19. rectocele ____________
20. menopause ____________

TRANSLATION

EXERCISE 2 *Break down the following words into their component parts.*

EXAMPLE: nasopharyngoscope *naso | pharyngo | scope*

1. vaginosis ____________
2. cystocele ____________
3. rectocele ____________
4. teratoma ____________
5. urethrocele ____________
6. pseudocyesis ____________
7. ovariorrhexis ____________
8. hysterorrhexis ____________
9. colpocystitis ____________
10. endocervicitis ____________
11. metrocolpocele ____________
12. myometritis ____________
13. choriocarcinoma ____________
14. vaginomycosis ____________

EXERCISE 3 *Underline and define the word parts from this chapter in the following terms.*

1. chorioangioma ____________
2. menopause ____________
3. metrophlebitis ____________
4. cervical intraepithelial neoplasia ____________
5. oophoroma ____________
6. salpingocele ____________
7. endometriosis ____________
8. vesicovaginal fistula ____________
9. vulvovaginitis (2 word parts) ____________
10. ovariocyesis (2 word parts) ____________
11. salpingocyesis (2 word parts) ____________

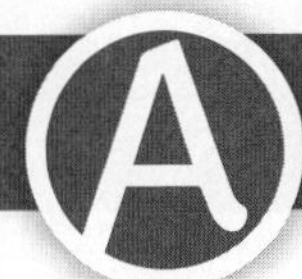

Learning Outcome 13.4 Exercises

EXERCISE 4 *Match the term on the left with its definition on the right.*

_____ 1. abortion

_____ 2. spontaneous abortion

_____ 3. ectopic pregnancy

_____ 4. adenocarcinoma of the breast

_____ 5. dermoid cyst

_____ 6. abruptio placentae

_____ 7. placenta previa

_____ 8. eclampsia

_____ 9. hyperemesis gravidarum

_____ 10. preeclampsia

a. condition characterized by high blood pressure and high level of protein in the urine

b. condition in which the placenta is attached to the uterus near the cervix

c. glandular tumor in the breast

d. ovarian cyst containing skin and sometimes hair, teeth, bone, or cartilage

e. characterized by seizures

f. pregnancy-related vomiting; an extreme form of the more common *morning sickness*

g. implantation of a fertilized egg in a place other than the uterus

h. termination of pregnancy

i. naturally occurring termination of pregnancy; also known as a miscarriage

j. separation of the placenta from the wall of the uterus

EXERCISE 5 *Fill in the blanks.*

1. vaginitis: inflammation of the _______________
2. vulvitis: inflammation of the _______________
3. cervicitis: inflammation of the _______________
4. ovaritis: inflammation of the _______________
5. chorionitis: inflammation of the _______________
6. mastitis: inflammation of the _______________
7. colpitis: inflammation of the _______________
8. endometritis: inflammation of the _______________
9. perimetritis: inflammation of the _______________
10. oophoritis: inflammation of the _______________
11. salpingitis: inflammation of the _______________
12. cervicocolpitis: inflammation of the _______________ and _______________
13. cervicovaginitis: inflammation of the _______________ and _______________
14. chorioamnionitis: inflammation of the _______________ and _______________
15. salpingo-oophoritis: inflammation of the _______________ and _______________
16. vulvovaginitis: inflammation of the _______________ and _______________

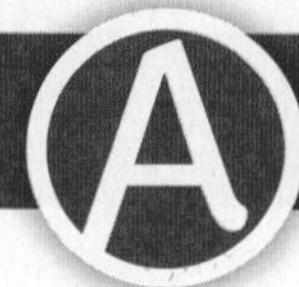

Learning Outcome 13.4 Exercises

EXERCISE 6 *Translate the following terms as literally as possible.*

EXAMPLE: nasopharyngoscope *an instrument for looking at the nose and throat*

1. chorionitis ____________
2. oophoritis ____________
3. salpingitis ____________
4. ovariorrhexis ____________
5. menopause ____________
6. myometritis ____________
7. colpocystitis ____________
8. endocervicitis ____________
9. cervicocolpitis ____________
10. cervicovaginitis ____________
11. salpingo-oophoritis ____________
12. adenocarcinoma of the breast ____________

GENERATION

EXERCISE 7 *Build a medical term from the information provided.*

EXAMPLE: inflammation of the sinuses *sinusitis*

1. inflammation of the vagina (use *vagin/o*) ____________
2. inflammation of the vulva (use *vulv/o*) ____________
3. inflammation of the ovary (use *ovari/o*) ____________
4. inflammation of the vagina (use *colp/o*) ____________
5. inflammation of the cervix ____________
6. false pregnancy ____________
7. rupture of the uterus ____________
8. hernia of a fallopian tube ____________
9. tumor of the ovary ____________
10. inflammation of the breast ____________
11. inflammation of the chorion and amnion ____________
12. inflammation of the blood vessels of the uterus (use *metr/o*) ____________
13. a blood vessel tumor of the chorion ____________
14. cancerous tumor of the chorion ____________

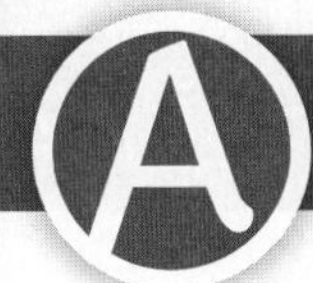

Learning Outcome 13.4 Exercises

EXERCISE 8 *Multiple-choice questions. Select the correct answer(s).*

1. The implantation of a fertilized egg in a place other than the uterus is called a(n):
   a. ectopic pregnancy
   b. ovariocyesis
   c. pseudocyesis
   d. salpingocyesis
   e. none of these
2. Which of the following options is the correct breakdown of the term *hyperemesis gravidarum*?
   a. over (*hyper*) + throw up (*emesis*) + pregnancy (*gravidarum*)
   b. under (*hyper*) + throw up (*emesis*) + pregnancy (*gravidarum*)
   c. over (*hyper*) + grow (*emesis*) + pregnancy (*gravidarum*)
   d. under (*hyper*) + grow (*emesis*) + pregnancy (*gravidarum*)
   e. none of these
3. Which of the following statements is the correct definition of the term *rectocele*?
   a. hernia or protrusion of the rectum into the vagina
   b. hernia or protrusion of the uterus into the rectum
   c. abnormal opening between the vagina and the rectum
   d. abnormal opening between the uterus and rectum
   e. none of these
4. Which of the following statements is the correct definition of the term *cervical intraepithelial neoplasia*?
   a. abnormal growth of cervical cells
   b. abnormal growth of ovarian cells
   c. abnormal growth of uterine cells
   d. new growth in the ovaries that extends into the uterus
   e. new growth in the uterus that extends into the cervix
5. Which of the following statements is the correct definition of *endometriosis*?
   a. a condition in which endometrium cells appear and grow outside the uterus
   b. condition of the inside of the cervix
   c. inflammation of the endometrium
   d. inflammation of the inside of the cervix
   e. none of these
6. Which of the following statements is the correct definition of the term *metrocolpocele*?
   a. an abnormal opening between the urinary bladder and the vagina
   b. hernia of the uterus and prolapse into the vagina
   c. an abnormal opening between the uterus and the vagina
   d. hernia of the urinary bladder into the vagina
   e. none of these
7. Which of the following statements is the correct definition of the term *vesicovaginal fistula*?
   a. an abnormal opening between the urinary bladder and the vagina
   b. hernia of the uterus and prolapse into the vagina
   c. an abnormal opening between the uterus and the vagina
   d. hernia of the urinary bladder into the vagina
   e. none of these
8. Select all of the following that apply to the term *dermoid cyst*.
   a. a uterine cyst
   b. also called a *teratoma*
   c. an ovarian cyst
   d. contains skin and sometimes hair, teeth, bone, or cartilage
   e. literally means "monster tumor"
   f. literally means "skin resembling cyst"

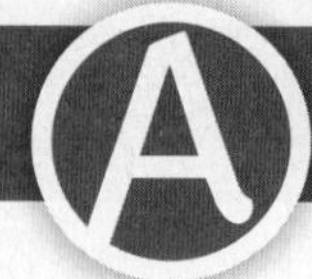

Learning Outcome 13.4 Exercises

9. Select all of the following that apply to the term *teratoma*.
   a. a uterine cyst
   b. also called a *dermoid cyst*
   c. an ovarian cyst
   d. contains skin and sometimes hair, teeth, bone, or cartilage
   e. literally means "monster tumor"
   f. literally means "skin resembling cyst"

EXERCISE 9 *Briefly describe the difference between each pair of terms.*

1. induced abortion, spontaneous abortion ______________________
2. endometritis, perimetritis ______________________
3. vaginomycosis, vaginosis ______________________
4. ovariocyesis, salpingocyesis ______________________
5. cystocele, urethrocele ______________________
6. eclampsia, preeclampsia ______________________
7. abruptio placentae, placenta previa ______________________

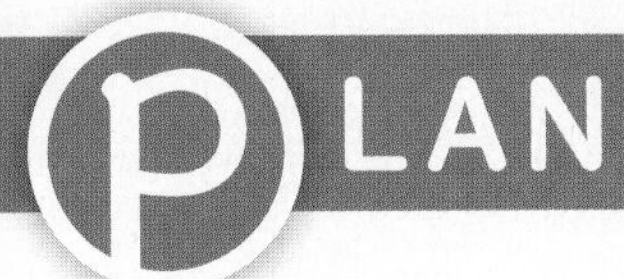

13.5 Treatments and Therapies

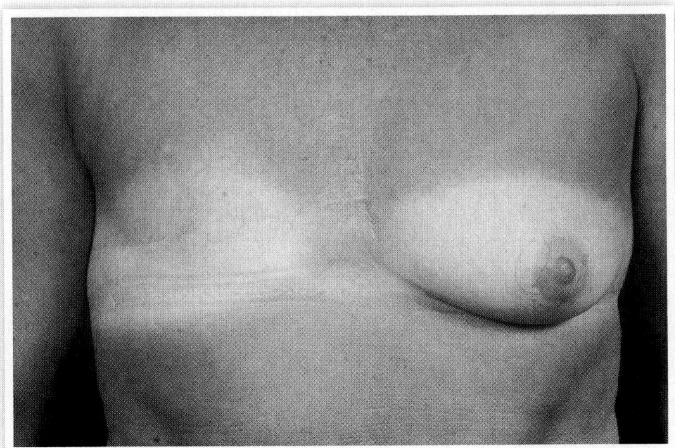

Breast cancer is a common reason a doctor might recommend a mastectomy.

One unique attribute of physicians trained in obstetrics and gynecology is that they are primary care providers for many women's health issues, but they are also surgeons. *Gynecologic surgeries* involve the interior structures of the female reproductive tract, such as the ovaries, fallopian tubes, and uterus. Ovarian surgeries can include the removal of an ovary (*oophorectomy*) to treat ovarian cancer or just the removal of a cyst on the ovary (*ovarian cystectomy*). At times, a fallopian tube is removed along with an ovary (*salpingo-oophorectomy*).

The fallopian tubes are common sites for ectopic pregnancies, and their standard treatment involves surgically opening the fallopian tube (*salpingotomy*) and removing the developing embryo. This procedure can maintain fertility and proper function of the reproductive system, but sometimes, as with a ruptured ectopic pregnancy, the tube must be removed altogether (*salpingectomy*). Another procedure involving the fallopian tubes involves blocking them (*tubal ligation*) as a means of preventing future pregnancies (*sterilization*).

Among the most frequently performed surgeries in gynecology is removal of the uterus (*hysterectomy*). Numerous medical problems are treated with hysterectomy, including cancer, fibroid tumors, and endometriosis. Prolapse of the uterus can be treated by surgically securing the uterus to another structure (*hysteropexy* or *colpopexy*).

Another very common procedure involving the uterus is *dilation and curettage* (commonly referred to as *D&C*). In this procedure, the opening of the cervix is gradually dilated with special instruments. Then, tissues lining the uterus are removed. D&C is commonly used to evaluate and treat problems of the uterus, such as abnormal bleeding. This may be due to benign problems, such as polyps, or fibroid tumors, which can be removed by cutting them out of the muscular wall of the uterus (*myomectomy*). D&C is also utilized following a miscarriage when the uterus fails to fully shed the nonviable tissue.

Defects of the vagina, whether they originate from birth or from abuse, can be corrected by a plastic surgeon (*vaginoplasty*).

Surgeries involving the breast are much more common procedures, with breast cancer being the leading reason. In some instances, the breast can be spared and just the cancer is removed (*mastotomy* with *lumpectomy*). Many times, the entire breast is removed (*mastectomy*). In these cases, breast reconstruction surgery can help restore the normal appearance of the breast. Other breast surgeries include breast reduction (*mammoplasty*) and breast lift (*mastopexy*).

The science of obstetrics is focused on keeping both mother and baby healthy during pregnancy. One important aspect is making sure that the mother avoids substances that can harm the growth of the baby (*teratogen*).

In a healthy pregnancy, delivery involves the muscles of the uterus squeezing to push the baby through the

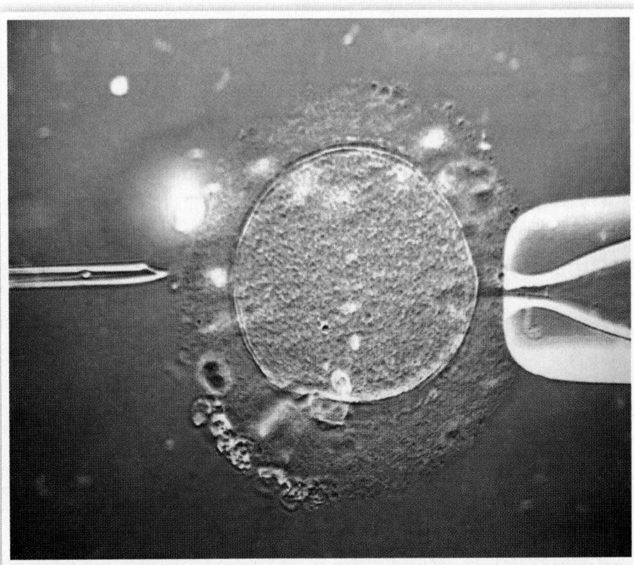

For couples struggling with fertility issues, in vitro fertilization provides possibility.

canal. If her contractions come too early, before her baby is ready to be born, a patient can take medicines that can help stop them (*tocolytic*). There are also medicines, such as oxytocin, that can be used to bring on contractions and induce labor.

Once it is time for delivery, there are two possibilities. The most common is a vaginal delivery, which involves delivering the baby naturally through the birth canal. It may be necessary to make a small cut in the mother's perineum (*episiotomy*) to help prevent tearing of skin during delivery. In cases where a baby is positioned in the wrong direction or is not moving quickly through the birth canal, the baby might need to be delivered surgically (*cesarean section*). This surgery, the most common one in medicine, involves first cutting the abdomen of the mother (*laparotomy*) and then cutting open her uterus (*hysterotomy*) to gain access to the baby.

Another procedure unique to women's health is in vitro fertilization, the fertilization of a female's egg by a male's sperm outside the body (*in vitro*). After the fertilization is complete, the *zygote* is then transferred into the woman's uterus.

gynecology procedures

Term	Word Analysis
cervicectomy SER-vih-SEK-toh-mee **Definition** surgical removal of the cervix	**cervic / ectomy** cervix / removal
colpopexy KOL-poh-PEK-see **Definition** surgical fixation of the vagina	**colpo / pexy** vagina / fixation
colpoplasty KOL-poh-PLAS-tee **Definition** surgical reconstruction of the vagina	**colpo / plasty** vagina / reconstruction
episiorrhaphy eh-PEE-zee-OR-ah-fee **Definition** suture of the vulva	**episio / rrhaphy** vulva / suture
hysterectomy HIS-ter-EK-toh-mee **Definition** surgical removal of the uterus	**hyster / ectomy** uterus / removal
hysteropexy HIS-ter-oh-PEK-see **Definition** surgical fixation of the uterus	**hystero / pexy** uterus / fixation
hysterosalpingectomy HIS-ter-oh-SAL-pin-JEK-toh-mee **Definition** surgical removal of the uterus and fallopian tube(s)	**hystero / salping / ectomy** uterus / tube / removal
mammoplasty MAM-oh-PLAS-tee **Definition** surgical reconstruction of a breast	**mammo / plasty** breast / reconstruction ©Biophoto Associates/Science Source

13.5 Treatments and Therapies

gynecology procedures *continued*

Term	Word Analysis
mastectomy mas-TEK-toh-mee **Definition** surgical removal of a breast	**mast / ectomy** breast / removal
mastopexy MAS-toh-PEK-see **Definition** surgical fixation of a breast	**masto / pexy** breast / fixation
myomectomy MAI-oh-MEK-toh-mee **Definition** surgical removal of a tumor in the muscle (usually refers to the muscle of the uterine wall)	**my / om / ectomy** muscle / tumor / removal
oophorectomy OH-aw-for-EK-toh-mee **Definition** surgical removal of an ovary	**oophor / ectomy** ovary / removal
oophorocystectomy oh-AW-for-oh-sis-TEK-toh-mee **Definition** surgical removal of an ovarian cyst	**oophoro / cyst / ectomy** ovary / cyst / removal
oophorotomy oh-AW-for-AW-toh-mee **Definition** incision into an ovary	**oophoro / tomy** ovary / incision
ovarian cystectomy oh-VEH-ree-an sis-TEK-toh-mee **Definition** surgical removal of an ovarian cyst	**ovari / an cyst / ectomy** ovary / pertaining to cyst / removal
ovariocentesis oh-VAW-ree-oh-sin-TEE-sis **Definition** surgical puncture of an ovary	**ovario / centesis** ovary / puncture
ovariostomy oh-VAW-ree-AW-stoh-me **Definition** creation of an opening into an ovary	**ovario / stomy** ovary / opening
perineoplasty PER-ih-NEE-oh-PLAS-tee **Definition** surgical reconstruction of the perineum	**perineo / plasty** perineum / reconstruction
perineorrhaphy PER-ih-nee-OR-ah-fee **Definition** suture of the perineum	**perineo / rrhaphy** perineum / suture
perineotomy PER-ih-nee-AW-toh-mee **Definition** incision into the perineum	**perineo / tomy** perineum / incision
salpingectomy SAL-pin-JEK-toh-mee **Definition** surgical removal of a fallopian tube	**salping / ectomy** fallopian tube / removal

gynecology procedures *continued*

Term	Word Analysis
salpingo-oophorectomy sal-PING-goh-OH-aw-for-EK-toh-mee **Definition** surgical removal of a fallopian tube and ovary	**salpingo / oophor / ectomy** fallopian tube / ovary / removal
salpingopexy sal-PING-goh-PEK-see **Definition** surgical fixation of a fallopian tube	**salpingo / pexy** fallopian tube / fixation
vaginoperineorrhaphy VAJ-ih-noh-PER-ih-nee-OR-ah-fee **Definition** suture of the vagina and perineum	**vagino / perineo / rrhaphy** vagina / perineum / suture
vaginoperineoplasty VAJ-ih-noh-PER-ih-NEE-oh-PLAS-tee **Definition** surgical reconstruction of the vagina and perineum	**vagino / perineo / plasty** vagina / perineum / reconstruction
vaginoperineotomy VAJ-ih-noh-PER-ih-nee-AW-toh-mee **Definition** incision into the vagina and perineum	**vagino / perineo / tomy** vagina / perineum / incision
vaginoplasty vah-JI-noh-PLAS-tee **Definition** surgical reconstruction of the vagina	**vagino / plasty** vagina / reconstruction

obstetrics procedures

Term	Word Analysis
abortifacient ah-BOR-tih-FAY-shunt **Definition** drug or device that causes the termination of pregnancy	**aborti / facient** abortion / do
amniotomy AM-nee-AW-toh-mee **Definition** incision into the amnion	**amnio / tomy** amnion / incision
cesarean section sih-SER-ee-an SEK-shun **Definition** delivery of a baby through an incision made in the uterus **NOTE:** This term does *not* refer to Julius Caesar's method of delivery. Rather, it refers to an ancient Roman law that required a child to be cut from a mother's womb if the mother died in childbirth.	**cesarean section**

obstetrics procedures *continued*

Term	Word Analysis
episiotomy eh-PEE-zee-AW-toh-mee **Definition** incision into the vulva	**episio / tomy** vulva / incision
hysterotomy HIS-ter-AW-toh-mee **Definition** incision into the uterus	**hystero / tomy** uterus / incision
induced abortion in-DOOST ah-BOR-shun **Definition** intentional termination of pregnancy	***see note on abortion***
in vitro fertilization in VEE-troh FER-tih-lih-ZAY-shun **Definition** fertilization of an egg done in a test tube	**in vitro fertilization** in glass fertilization ©Science Photo Library RF/Getty Images RF
oxytocin OK-see-TOH-sin **Definition** agent that stimulates uterine contractions and accelerates labor	**oxy / toc / in** swift / birth / agent
tocolytic TOH-koh-LIH-tik **Definition** agent that stops or delays premature labor and contractions	**toco / lytic** labor / breakdown agent

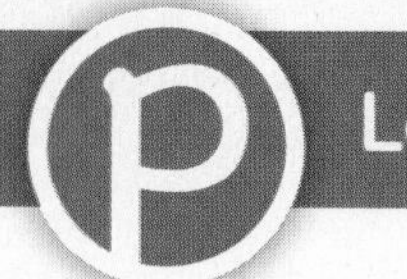

Learning Outcome 13.5 Exercises

PRONUNCIATION

EXERCISE 1 *Indicate which syllables are emphasized when pronounced.*

EXAMPLE: bronchitis bron**chi**tis

1. colpopexy ______
2. mastopexy ______
3. colpoplasty ______
4. episiotomy ______
5. amniotomy ______
6. mastectomy ______
7. hysterotomy ______
8. vaginoplasty ______
9. hysterectomy ______
10. salpingectomy ______
11. mammoplasty ______
12. perineoplasty ______
13. cervicectomy ______
14. oophorotomy ______
15. ovariostomy ______
16. salpingectomy ______
17. perineotomy ______
18. oxytocin ______

TRANSLATION

EXERCISE 2 *Break down the following words into their component parts.*

EXAMPLE: nasopharyngoscope *naso | pharyngo | scope*

1. mammoplasty ______
2. ovariocentesis ______
3. perineotomy ______
4. hysterotomy ______
5. colpoplasty ______
6. episiorrhaphy ______
7. vaginoperineorrhaphy ______
8. oophorocystectomy ______

EXERCISE 3 *Underline and define the word parts from this chapter in the following terms.*

1. amniotomy ______
2. vaginoplasty ______
3. cervicectomy ______
4. ovariostomy ______
5. perineoplasty ______
6. colpopexy ______
7. episiotomy ______
8. hysteropexy ______
9. mastopexy ______
10. salpingopexy ______
11. oophorotomy ______
12. vaginoperineoplasty (2 roots) ______

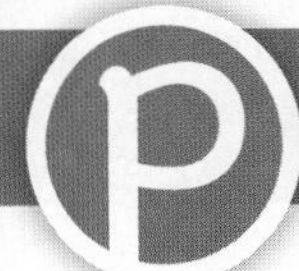

Learning Outcome 13.5 Exercises

EXERCISE 4 *Match the term on the left with its definition on the right.*

______	1. cesarean section	a.	drug or device that causes the termination of a pregnancy
______	2. in vitro fertilization	b.	agent that stimulates uterine contractions and accelerates labor
______	3. induced abortion	c.	delivery of a baby through an incision made in the uterus
______	4. perineorrhaphy	d.	fertilization of an egg done in a test tube
______	5. vaginoperineotomy	e.	incision into the vagina and perineum
______	6. abortifacient	f.	suture of the perineum
______	7. oxytocin	g.	intentional termination of pregnancy

EXERCISE 5 *Fill in the blanks.*

1. cervicectomy: surgical removal of the ______________________
2. hysterectomy: surgical removal of the ______________________
3. mastectomy: surgical removal of a(n) ______________________
4. oophorectomy: surgical removal of a(n) ______________________
5. salpingectomy: surgical removal of a(n) ______________________
6. oophorcystectomy: surgical removal of a(n) ______________________
7. ovarian cystectomy: surgical removal of a(n) ______________________
8. salpingo-oophorectomy: surgical removal of a(n) ______________ and ______________
9. hysterosalpingectomy: surgical removal of the ______________ and ______________
10. myomectomy: surgical removal of a(n) ______________________

EXERCISE 6 *Translate the following terms as literally as possible.*

> EXAMPLE: nasopharyngoscope *an instrument for looking at the nose and throat*

1. vaginoplasty ______________________
2. perineoplasty ______________________
3. colpoplasty ______________________
4. episiotomy ______________________
5. mastectomy ______________________
6. ovariocentesis ______________________
7. hysteropexy ______________________
8. salpingopexy ______________________
9. oophorocystectomy ______________________
10. ovarian cystectomy ______________________
11. vaginoperineorrhaphy ______________________
12. myomectomy ______________________
13. in vitro fertilization ______________________

Learning Outcome 13.5 Exercises

GENERATION

EXERCISE 7 *Build a medical term from the information provided.*

EXAMPLE: inflammation of the sinuses *sinusitis*

1. surgical removal of the uterus (use *hyster/o*) ______
2. surgical removal of an ovary (use *oophor/o*) ______
3. surgical removal of the cervix ______
4. surgical removal of the fallopian tube ______
5. surgical reconstruction of a breast (use *mamm/o*) ______
6. surgical fixation of the vagina (use *colp/o*) ______
7. surgical fixation of a breast (use *mast/o*) ______
8. incision into the amnion ______
9. suture of the vulva (use *episi/o*) ______
10. suture of the perineum ______
11. creation of an opening into an ovary (use *ovari/o*) ______
12. suture of the vagina and perineum ______
13. surgical removal of a fallopian tube and ovary ______
14. surgical removal of the uterus and fallopian tube ______

EXERCISE 8 *Multiple-choice questions. Select the correct answer(s).*

1. A drug or device that causes the termination of a pregnancy is called a(n):
   a. abortifacient
   b. oxytocin
   c. amniotomy
   d. cesarean section
   e. episiorrhaphy
2. An *induced abortion* is:
   a. the intentional termination of pregnancy
   b. the naturally occurring termination of pregnancy
   c. a drug or device that causes the termination of a pregnancy
   d. the separation of the placenta from the wall of the uterus
   e. none of these
3. Select all of the following statements that apply to the term *cesarean section.*
   a. a term common in obstetrics
   b. delivery of a baby through an incision in the perineum
   c. delivery of a baby through an incision made in the uterus
   d. refers to an ancient Roman law that required a child to be cut from its mother's womb if the mother died in childbirth
   e. the way in which Julius Caesar was delivered

Learning Outcome 13.5 Exercises

4. Select all of the following terms that pertain to internal gynecology.
   a. amniotomy
   b. episiotomy
   c. hysterotomy
   d. oophorotomy
   e. oxytocin
   f. perineotomy
   g. vaginoperineotomy

5. Select all of the following terms that pertain to external gynecology.
   a. amniotomy
   b. episiotomy
   c. hysterotomy
   d. oophorotomy
   e. oxytocin
   f. perineotomy
   g. vaginoperineotomy

6. Select all of the following terms that pertain to obstetrics.
   a. amniotomy
   b. episiotomy
   c. hysterotomy
   d. oophorotomy
   e. oxytocin
   f. perineotomy
   g. vaginoperineotomy

13.6 Abbreviations

Abbreviations provide a shorthand way of referring to things that either recur often or are too long to write out. When dealing with gynecology and obstetrics, these abbreviations can refer to things ranging from body parts (Cx) to diagnostic procedures (SHG, TVS), diagnoses (CIPP, PMS, TSS), and treatments (LEEP, HRT, TAH).

gynecology

Abbreviation	Definition
CIPP	chronic idiopathic pelvic pain
Cx	cervix
GYN	gynecology
HPV	human papillomavirus
HRT	hormone replacement therapy
HSG	hysterosalpingogram
LEEP	loop electrosurgical excision procedure
PID	pelvic inflammatory disease
PMS	premenstrual syndrome
SHG	sonohysterography
STD/STI	sexually transmitted disease/infection
TAH/BSO	total abdominal hysterectomy/bilateral salpingo-oophorectomy
TSS	toxic shock syndrome
TVS	transvaginal sonography
VH	vaginal hysterectomy

obstetrics

Abbreviation	Definition
CPD	cephalopelvic disproportion
CS, C-section	cesarean section ©Antonia Reeve/Science Source
DOB	date of birth
EDD	expected date of delivery
FAS	fetal alcohol syndrome

obstetrics *continued*

Abbreviation	Definition
FOB	father of the baby (or fecal occult blood)
G	gravida
IVF	in vitro fertilization
LGA	large for gestational age
LMP	last menstrual period
P	births (comes from the word *para,* which means "birth") ©ERproductions Ltd/Getty Images RF
RDS	respiratory distress syndrome
SGA	small for gestational age

Learning Outcome 13.6 Exercises

EXERCISE 1 *Define the following abbreviations.*

1. HRT ______
2. PID ______
3. PMS ______
4. TSS ______
5. HPV ______
6. STD ______
7. DOB ______
8. EDD ______
9. FAS ______
10. LMP ______
11. CPD ______
12. CS ______
13. G ______
14. FOB ______
15. HSG ______

EXERCISE 2 *Give the abbreviations for the following definitions.*

1. chronic idiopathic pelvic pain ______
2. loop electrosurgical excision procedure ______
3. respiratory distress syndrome ______

Learning Outcome 13.6 Exercises

4. small for gestational age ________________
5. large for gestational age ________________
6. para ________________
7. father of the baby ________________
8. sexually transmitted infection ________________
9. cesarean section ________________
10. total abdominal hysterectomy ________________
11. bilateral salpingo-oophorectomy ________________
12. transvaginal sonography ________________
13. sonohysterography ________________
14. vaginal hysterectomy ________________
15. in vitro fertilization ________________

EXERCISE 3 *Match the abbreviation on the left with its full definition on the right.*

______	1. GYN	a. condition characterized by the inability of the mother's pelvis to allow the baby to pass through the birth canal
______	2. CS	b. delivery of a baby through an incision made in the uterus
______	3. Cx	c. imaging procedure using sound waves emitted from a device inserted in the vagina
______	4. CPD	d. pregnant
______	5. TVS	e. opening between the uterus and the vagina
______	6. G	f. procedure using sound waves to examine the uterus
______	7. TAH	g. surgical removal of both of the ovaries and adjacent fallopian tubes; often performed as part of a total abdominal hysterectomy
______	8. VH	h. surgical removal of the uterus through an incision in the abdomen; usually includes the removal of both ovaries and fallopian tubes
______	9. BSO	i. surgical removal of the uterus through an incision in the vagina
______	10. SHG	j. study of medical issues specific to women

EXERCISE 4 *Multiple-choice questions. Select the correct answer(s).*

1. HPV is a type of:
   a. STD
   b. STI
   c. sexually transmitted disease
   d. sexually transmitted infection
   e. all of these

2. Pelvic pain that persists for a period of more than 3 months and has arisen spontaneously or from an obscure or unknown cause is known as:
   a. CIPP
   b. CPD
   c. EDD
   d. RDS
   e. SGA

Learning Outcome 13.6 Exercises

3. Which of the following abbreviations does NOT pertain to obstetrics?

   a. DOB
   b. EDD
   c. G
   d. GYN
   e. LGA

4. A baby whose birth weight lies above the 90th percentile for its *gestational age*, or the length of time the baby has been in the womb, would be considered:

   a. CPD
   b. EDD
   c. LGA
   d. LMP
   e. SGA

5. The term *para* comes from the Latin term *parere*, meaning "to bring forth" or "to bear." In medical terminology, this refers to a woman who has given birth to a viable infant (weighing at least 1 pound or of more than 20 weeks' gestation), regardless of whether that infant was alive at birth. The abbreviation for *para* is:

   a. P
   b. PAR
   c. PR
   d. PRA
   e. none of these

6. EDD stands for:

   a. electrodilator development
   b. expected date of delivery
   c. expected developmental delay
   d. expected due date
   e. none of these

13.7 Electronic Health Records

Postoperative Note

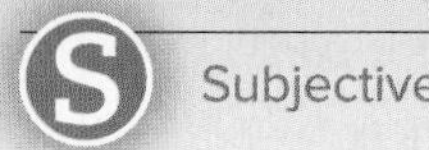

Subjective

Preoperative Diagnosis:

1. **Abruptio placentae**
2. **Chorioamnionitis**
3. **Fetal distress**

Postoperative Diagnosis:

1. Abruptio placentae
2. Chorioamnionitis
3. Fetal distress

Procedure: Emergency cesarean section
Anesthesia: General
Estimated blood loss: 750 mL
Complications: None
Findings: Male infant with cephalic presentation. Normal uterus, fallopian tubes, and ovaries.

Indications: The patient, Mrs. Jenna Friedman, is a 23-year-old **gravida** 2 **para** 1 female who presents at 37 4/7 weeks' **gestation** with **bleeding** and painful **uterine contractions** for 4 hours. An emergent ultrasound was performed to rule out **placenta previa**. The ultrasound showed a **retroplacental** hematoma. She was admitted for evaluation and treatment for **abruptio placentae**. Her physical exam on admission was significant for fever to 101.2°F, as well as abdominal and uterine tenderness.

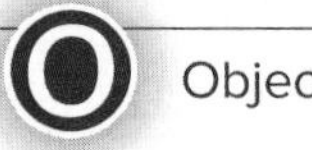

Objective

She was 3 cm dilated and effaced. Initial lab work included a CBC that showed an elevated white blood cell count but no anemia. Fibrinogen and PT/PTT were all normal, which reassured us that she did not have DIC or a coagulopathy. The patient was placed on IV fluids and antibiotics for presumed **chorioamnionitis** and was placed under continuous monitoring. Two hours after admission, fetal heart rate monitors alerted us to **fetal bradycardia** and late decelerations. The decision was made to proceed with **emergency cesarean section**.

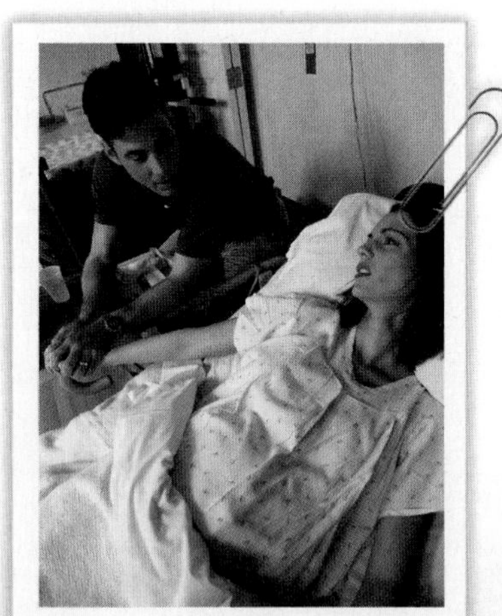

©Florian Franke/Purestock/SuperStock RF

Input: 2 L normal saline via peripheral IV.
Output: 750 mL blood, 500 mL urine.

Postoperative Note (*continued*)

HR: 76; RR: 22; BP: 102/72.
General: Sedated. Nasal cannula O_2 at 0.5 lpm.
HEENT: PERRLA. Mucous membranes moist and pink. Nares patent. No nasal flaring.
CV: RRR with murmur.
Resp: CTA.
Abd: Midline surgical wound. Dressing is clean, dry, and intact.
GU: Grossly normal, no bleeding.

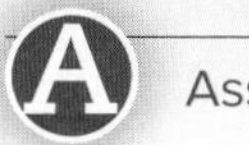

Assessment

1. Postop cesarean section–stable.
2. Chorioamnionitis.
3. Abruptio placentae–resolved. Hemodynamically stable.

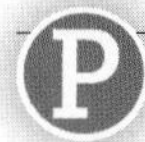

Plan

1. Continue IV fluids and progress to PO as patient becomes more alert.
2. Continue IV antibiotics.
3. Monitor blood pressure. Follow-up CBC.

–Patricia Collingsworth, PA

Learning Outcome 13.7 Exercises

EXERCISE 1 *Match the term on the left with its definition on the right.*

______	1. cesarean section	a. condition in which the placenta is attached to the uterus near the cervix
______	2. contraction	b. another term for pregnant
______	3. choriamnionitis	c. delivery of a baby through an incision made in the uterus
______	4. abruptio placentae	d. inflammation of the chorion and amnion
______	5. placenta previa	e. separation of the placenta from the wall of the uterus
______	6. gravida	f. shortening or tightening of a muscle

EXERCISE 2 *Fill in the blanks.*

1. Using the data recorded at the patient's physical examination, fill in the following blanks.
   a. Mrs. Friedman's heart rate: ______________________
   b. Mrs. Friedman's respiratory rate: ______________________
   c. Mrs. Friedman's blood pressure: ______________________
2. Preoperative diagnosis:
   a. *Abruptio placentae*–give definition: ______________________
   b. ______________________: inflammation of the chorion and amnion
   c. *Fetal distress:* presence of signs in a pregnant woman either *prepartum* (give definition: ______________________) or *intrapartum* (give definition: ______________________) that suggest the fetus may not be well.
3. Plan:
   a. Continue IV fluids (give definition for abbreviation: ______________________) and progress to (*per os*–give definition: ______________________) as patient becomes more alert.
   b. Continue ______________________ (intravenous) antibiotics.
   c. Monitor BP (give definition for abbreviation: ______________________). Follow-up ______________________ (complete blood count).

EXERCISE 3 *True or false questions. Indicate true answers with a T and false answers with an F.*

1. Mrs. Friedman is a 23-year-old pregnant woman. ______________________
2. Mrs. Friedman is afebrile. ______________________
3. Mrs. Friedman has placenta previa. ______________________
4. Mrs. Friedman was placed on intravenous antibiotics. ______________________
5. Mrs. Friedman had a vaginal birth. ______________________
6. Mrs. Friedman was given 2 L of saline through an IV. ______________________

Learning Outcome 13.7 Exercises

EXERCISE 4 *Multiple-choice questions. Select the correct answer.*

1. The ultrasound performed on Mrs. Friedman showed *retroplacental hematoma.* Which of the following options is the correct breakdown of this term?
   a. *retro* (behind) + *placental* (placenta) + *hemat* (blood) + *oma* (tumor)
   b. *retro* (behind) + *placental* (position) + *hemat* (blood) + *oma* (tumor)
   c. *retro* (behind) + *placental* (position) + *hemat* (urine) + *oma* (tumor)
   d. *retro* (behind) + *placental* (uterus) + *hemat* (blood) + *oma* (hole)
   e. *retro* (behind) + *placental* (uterus) + *hemat* (urine) + *oma* (hole)
2. Two hours after admission, heart rate monitors alerted the medical staff to *fetal bradycardia.* Which of the following options is the correct breakdown of this term?
   a. *fetal* (pertaining to the fetus) + *brady* (fast) + *cardia* (blood flow)
   b. *fetal* (pertaining to the fetus) + *brady* (fast) + *cardia* (heartbeat)
   c. *fetal* (pertaining to the fetus) + *brady* (slow) + *cardia* (heartbeat)
   d. *fetal* (pertaining to the uterus) + *brady* (fast) + *cardia* (blood flow)
   e. *fetal* (pertaining to the uterus) +*brady* (slow) + *cardia* (heartbeat)
3. Which of the following options is the correct abbreviation for *cesarean section?*
   a. CS
   b. C-sec
   c. C-section
   d. CS and C-sec
   e. CS and C-section

Emergency Department Note

Chief Complaint: Abdominal pain, fever.

History of Present Illness

Ms. Sara Miller, a 25-year-old woman, has had a 3-day history of worsening lower abdominal pain. The pain is a constant dull ache. The pain began a few days after her last **menstrual** cycle ended. The pain worsens with movement. Ms. Miller also reports **dyspareunia** and purulent **vaginal discharge.** She has tried over-the-counter ibuprofen, which yielded mild relief of the pain. The pain has worsened and now she also has nausea. She denies vomiting, diarrhea, or dysuria.

Past Medical History: Recent treatment for chlamydia **vulvovaginitis. Menarche** at 13 years of age. **LMP** 1 week ago.

Past Surgical History: None.

Social History: High-risk sexual behavior. Sexually active with multiple partners, inconsistent use of protection via condoms with her partners. 1-pack-per-day smoker.

Family History: Noncontributory.

Medications: None.

Allergies: No known drug allergies.

Physical Exam

Vital Signs: Temperature: 102.3; Heart Rate: 90; Respiratory Rate: 20; BP: 112/84.
General: Well developed and nourished, in mild discomfort. Alert and oriented x 3.
Head: Normocephalic atraumatic, slightly dry mucous membranes. Pupils equal, round, and reactive to light. TMs normal.
Neck: Supple.
Cardiovascular: Mild tachycardia. No murmur, gallop, or rub.
Respiratory: Normal effort. Clear to auscultation. No retractions.
Abdomen: Generalized tenderness to palpation. Rebound and guarding present, especially over suprapubic region. Spleen and liver edge not palpable.
Skin: Dry. Cap refill 2 seconds.
Extremities: No cyanosis, clubbing, or edema.
Pelvic exam: Adnexal tenderness and cervical motion tenderness.

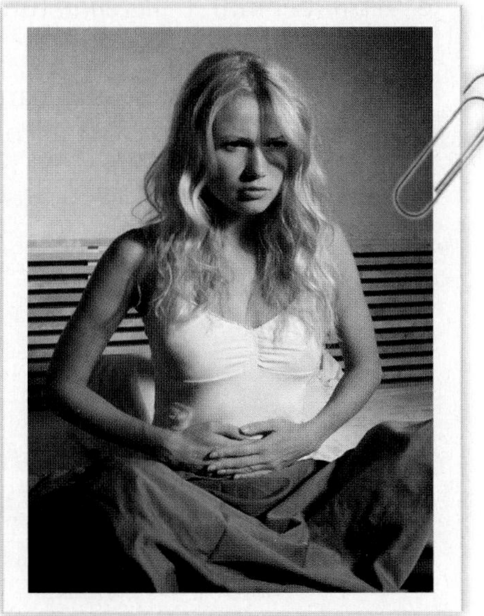

Emergency Department Course

Ms. Miller arrived at the emergency department in mild discomfort. An IV was started, and she was treated with IV fluids for mild dehydration. Ms. Miller was also given an antiemetic and ibuprofen. A rapid **hCG** test to rule out **ectopic pregnancy** was negative. A swab of Ms. Miller's purulent vaginal discharge revealed **leukorrhea.** We performed a **transvaginal sonography.** Suspicion for **pelvic inflammatory disorder** was confirmed by findings of enlarged ovaries consistent with **oophoritis, endometritis,** and **hydrosalpinx.** Results for chlamydia reinfection and gonorrhea are still pending.

Ms. Miller tolerated PO fluids and looked a little better. We educated Ms. Miller on the risks of **STIs** and the need for barrier protection. We also explained the complications of **PID,** including **tubo-ovarian abscess** and tubal **infertility.** She was sent home for outpatient management.

Disposition

Discharge to home with prescription for oral antibiotics.

–Sal Kaye, MD

Learning Outcome 13.7 Exercises

EXERCISE 5 *Match the term on the left with its definition on the right.*

Term	Definition
_____ 1. menarche	a. blockage in a fallopian tube caused by water or any clear fluid
_____ 2. ectopic pregnancy	b. imaging procedure using sound waves emitted from a device inserted in the vagina
_____ 3. transvaginal sonography	c. inflammation of an ovary
_____ 4. vulvovaginitis	d. inflammation of the endometrium
_____ 5. leukorrhea	e. inflammation of the vulva and vagina
_____ 6. endometritis	f. painful sexual intercourse
_____ 7. oophoritis	g. beginning or first menstruation
_____ 8. dyspareunia	h. implantation of a fertilized egg in a place other than the uterus
_____ 9. hydrosalpinx	i. white vaginal discharge

EXERCISE 6 *Fill in the blanks.*

1. Using the data recorded at Ms. Miller's physical examination, fill in the following blanks.
   a. T: _______________
   b. HR: _______________
   c. RR: _______________
   d. BP: _______________
   e. General: well developed, well nourished (give abbreviation: _______________)
2. Past Medical History:
   a. Recent treatment for chlamydia *vulvovaginitis* (inflammation of the _______________ and _______________)
   b. *Menarche* (give definition: _______________) at 13 years of age
   c. *LMP* (define abbreviation: _______________)
3. Emergency Department Course:
   a. A rapid hCG test to rule out _______________ (the implantation of a fertilized egg in a place other than the uterus) was negative.
   b. Suspicion for *pelvic inflammatory disorder* (give abbreviation: _______________) was confirmed by findings of enlarged ovaries consistent with *oophoritis* (inflammation of _______________), *endometritis* (inflammation of the tissue on the _______________ of the _______________), and _______________ (blockage in a fallopian tube caused by water [or any clear fluid]).

Learning Outcome 13.7 Exercises

EXERCISE 7 *True or false questions. Indicate true answers with a T and false answers with an F.*

1. Ms. Miller is experiencing painful sexual intercourse. ________
2. Ms. Miller has trouble urinating. ________
3. Ms. Miller has a slightly faster heart rate than normal. ________
4. Ms. Miller arrived at the ED in mild discomfort. ________
5. Ms. Miller was given a medication to help prevent nausea. ________
6. The TVS confirmed PID. ________
7. Ms. Miller could not hold down any fluids. ________

EXERCISE 8 *Multiple-choice questions. Select the correct answer.*

1. A swab of Ms. Miller's vaginal discharge revealed:
   a. leukorrhea
   b. lactorrhea
   c. amenorrhea
   d. none of these
2. The root word in *menstrual cycle* is the Greek word *meno,* which refers to:
   a. fallopian tubes
   b. menstruation
   c. ovaries
   d. the uterus
3. *Pelvic inflammatory disorder* is a generic term for inflammation of the uterus, fallopian tubes, and/or ovaries. Which of the following medical terms is NOT included in this definition?
   a. colpitis
   b. endometritis
   c. oophoritis
   d. salpingitis

Gynecology Clinic Note

Subjective

Mrs. Lana Pecos is a 47-year-old **premenopausal** woman with a chief complaint of heavy **menses.** For more than a year, she has experienced menstrual flow for 9 to 10 days every 2 to 3 weeks. She denies vaginal discharge and bleeding from her gums or in her stool. No easy bruising.

PMHx: Last **mammogram** 6 years ago, normal. Pap smear 10 years ago: **cervical intraepithelial neoplasia** II treated with **LEEP.** Last **Pap smear** 5 years ago: Normal.

ROS: She denies visual changes.

Objective

Physical Exam

Weight: 270 lbs; Temp: 98.6; HR: 62; BP: 102/74; RR: 22.

General: Obese, pale. Alert and in NAD.

HEENT: Pale conjunctiva. PERRLA. TMs normal. Normal dentition. Mucous membranes moist.

Neck: Supple. No goiter.

CV: RRR without murmur.

Resp: CTA.

Skin: Acanthosis nigricans. Abdominal striae.

Abdomen: Soft, nontender, nondistended.

Pelvic: Uniformly large **uterus.**

Labs: Hgb 10.4. Microcytosis. Hypochromia. Otherwise normal CBC, PT/PTT.

Endometrial Bx: Hyperplasia with atypia.

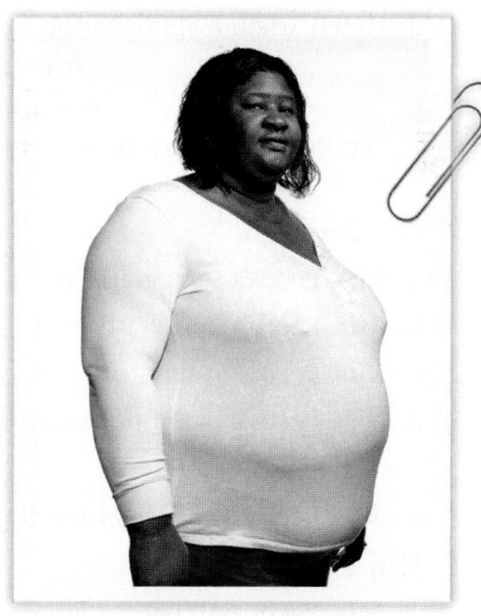

©Troy Aossey/The Image Bank/Getty Images

Assessment

Given her preliminary **endometrial biopsy** results, Mrs. Pecos's **metromenorrhagia** is due to **endometrial hyperplasia.** We will send the tissue sample to pathology to confirm the finding of atypia, but it is likely that she also has **myoinvasive endometrioid adenocarcinoma.**

Plan

Mrs. Pecos will need a **hysterectomy** and a referral to oncology. I will also begin her on iron supplementation.

–Mary Clary, DO

Learning Outcome 13.7 Exercises

EXERCISE 9 *Match the term on the left with its definition on the right.*

	Term		Definition
______	1. Pap smear	a.	record of a breast exam
______	2. menopause	b.	test used to detect cancer cells, most commonly in the cervix
______	3. mammogram	c.	abnormal growth of cervical cells
______	4. hysterectomy	d.	cessation of menstruation
______	5. endometrium	e.	excessive menstrual bleeding at irregular intervals
______	6. cervical intraepithelial neoplasia	f.	surgical removal of the uterus
______	7. metromenorrhagia	g.	inner layer of uterine tissue

EXERCISE 10 *Fill in the blanks.*

1. Subjective
   a. PMHx (define abbreviation: ____________________): last *mammogram* (give definition: ____________________) 6 years ago: normal
   b. ____________________(a test used to detect cancer cells, most commonly in the cervix): 10 years ago: *cervical intraepithelial neoplasia* II (give definition: ____________________) treated with LEEP (define abbreviation: ____________________)
2. Objective
   a. Mrs. Pecos's temperature: ____________________
   b. Mrs. Pecos's heart rate: ____________________
   c. Mrs. Pecos's respiratory rate: ____________________
   d. Mrs. Pecos's blood pressure: ____________________
3. Assessment
   a. Mrs. Pecos has *metromenorrhagia* (give definition: ____________________)
4. Plan
   a. Mrs. Pecos will need a *hysterectomy* (give definition: ____________________) and a likely referral to ____________________ (the branch of medicine dealing with tumors).

EXERCISE 11 *True or false questions. Indicate true answers with a T and false answers with an F.*

1. Mrs. Pecos is also experiencing leukorrhea. ____________________
2. According to her pelvic exam, Mrs. Pecos has macromastia. ____________________
3. Mrs. Pecos was given a biopsy. ____________________
4. Mrs. Pecos will likely have her uterus removed. ____________________

EXERCISE 12 *Multiple-choice questions. Select the correct answer.*

1. *Menses* is the term for a woman's monthly flow during her menstrual cycle. In this health record, the patient's chief complaint is:
   a. heavy menses
   b. irregular menses
   c. lack of menses
   d. light menses
   e. none of these
2. The *endometrium* is:
   a. another term for "uterus"
   b. the middle layer of uterine tissue
   c. the muscular layer of the uterus
   d. the inner layer of uterine tissue
   e. the tissue on the outside of the uterus

Learning Outcome 13.7 Exercises

3. Mrs. Pecos is a 47-year-old *premenopausal* woman, which means that:
   a. her menstrual flow has not ceased
   b. her menstrual flow is heavy
   c. her menstrual flow is irregular
   d. her menstrual flow is just beginning
   e. none of these

4. The medical professional believes the patient has *endometrial hyperplasia*. Which of the following options is a correct breakdown of this term?
   a. *endo* (inside) + *metrial* (fallopian tube) + *hyper* (under) + *plasia* (new formation)
   b. *endo* (inside) + *metrial* (pelvis) + *hyper* (over) + *plasia* (new formation)
   c. *endo* (inside) + *metrial* (uterus) + *hyper* (over) + *plasia* (new formation)
   d. *endo* (outside) + *metrial* (cervix) + *hyper* (under) + *plasia* (new formation)
   e. *endo* (outside) + *metrial* (perineum) + *hyper* (over) + *plasia* (new formation)

Quick Reference

quick reference glossary of roots

Root	Definition	Root	Definition
amni/o	amnion	**men/o**	menstruation
cervic/o	cervix	**metr/o**	uterus
chori/o	chorion	**nat/o**	birth
chorion/o	chorion	**oophor/o**	ovary
colp/o	vagina	**ovari/o**	ovary
-cyesis	pregnancy	**part/o**	birth
episi/o	vulva	**pelv/i**	pelvis
fet/o	fetus	**perine/o**	perineum
gyn/o	woman	**toc/o**	labor
gynec/o	woman	**salping/o**	fallopian tube
hyster/o	uterus	**uter/o**	uterus
lact/o	milk	**vagin/o**	vagina
mamm/o	breast	**vulv/o**	vulva
mast/o	breast		

quick reference glossary of terms

Term	Definition
abortifacient	drug or device that causes the termination of a pregnancy
abortion	termination of pregnancy
abruptio placentae	separation of the placenta from the wall of the uterus
adenocarcinoma of the breast	glandular tumor in the breast
amastia	absence of breasts
amenorrhea	no menstruation
amniocentesis	surgical puncture of the amnion
amniorrhea	discharge of amniotic fluid
amniorrhexis	rupture of the amniotic sac
amnioscope	instrument for examining the amnion
amnioscopy	procedure for examining the amnion
amniotomy	incision into the amnion
antepartum	time before birth

quick reference glossary of terms *continued*

Term	Definition
bradytocia	slow labor
Braxton Hicks contraction	sporadic contractions of the uterine muscles of women in labor; also known as false labor
cardiotocograph	instrument for recording the fetal heart rate during labor
cephalopelvic disproportion (CPD)	condition characterized by the inability of the mother's pelvis to allow the baby to pass through the birth canal
cervical dysplasia	bad formation of cervical cells
cervical intraepithelial neoplasia	abnormal growth of cervical cells
cervicectomy	surgical removal of the cervix
cervicitis	inflammation of the cervix
cervicocolpitis	inflammation of the cervix and vagina
cervicography	procedure for imaging the cervix
cervicovaginitis	inflammation of the cervix and vagina
cesarean section	delivery of a baby through an incision made in the uterus
chorioamnionitis	inflammation of the chorion and amnion
chorioangioma	blood vessel tumor of the chorion
choriocarcinoma	cancerous tumor of the chorion
chorionitis	inflammation of the chorion
colpitis	inflammation of the vagina
colpocystitis	inflammation of the vagina and urinary bladder
colpopexy	surgical fixation of the vagina
colpoplasty	surgical reconstruction of the vagina
colpoptosis	downward placement of the vagina
colposcope	instrument used to examine the vagina
colposcopy	procedure for examining the vagina
colpostenosis	narrowing in the vaginal opening
conception	the process of conceiving a child
congenital anomaly	irregular condition that is present at the time of birth
contraception	a process that prevents or hinders the conception of a child
contraction	shortening or tightening of a muscle (during labor, uterine muscles contract)
cystocele	hernia of the urinary bladder into the vagina
dermoid cyst	ovarian cyst containing skin and sometimes hair, teeth, bone, or cartilage

quick reference glossary of terms *continued*

Term	Definition
dysmenorrhea	painful menstruation
dyspareunia	painful sexual intercourse
dystocia	difficult labor
eclampsia	severe, life-threatening complication of pregnancy characterized by seizures
ectopic pregnancy	implantation of a fertilized egg in a place other than the uterus
endocervicitis	inflammation of the inside of the cervix
endometriosis	condition in which endometrium cells appear and grow outside the uterus
endometritis	inflammation of the endometrium
endometrium	inner layer of uterine tissue
episiorrhaphy	suture of the vulva
episiostenosis	narrowing of the vulvar opening
episiotomy	incision into the vulva
eutocia	normal labor
fertilization	the process of an egg and sperm joining to conceive a child
fetometry	procedure for measuring the fetus
gestation	the process of carrying a child from conception until birth
gravida	another term for *pregnant*
gynecologist	specialist in medical issues specific to women
gynecology	study of medical issues specific to women
gynecomastia	development of breast tissue in males
hematosalpinx	blockage in a fallopian tube caused by blood
hydrosalpinx	blockage in a fallopian tube caused by water (or any clear fluid)
hyperemesis gravidarum	pregnancy-related vomiting; an extreme form of the more common *morning sickness*
hypermastia	excessively large breasts (can also refer to an abnormal number of breasts)
hypomastia	abnormally small breasts
hysteralgia	pain in the uterus
hysterectomy	surgical removal of the uterus
hysterocele	hernia of the uterus
hysterodynia	pain in the uterus
hysterography	procedure for imaging the uterus

quick reference glossary of terms *continued*

Term	Definition
hysteropexy	surgical fixation of the uterus
hysteroptosis	downward displacement of the uterus into the vagina
hysterorrhexis	rupture of the uterus
hysterosalpingectomy	surgical removal of the uterus and fallopian tube
hysterosalpingogram	record of the uterus and fallopian tubes
hysteroscope	instrument for examining the uterus
hysteroscopy	procedure for examining the uterus
hysterotomy	incision into the uterus
implantation	the process of a fertilized egg attaching or adhering to the uterus. This enables it to begin to receive oxygen and nutrients from the mother to continue to grow.
in vitro fertilization	fertilization of an egg done in a test tube
induced abortion	intentional termination of pregnancy
intrapartum	time during birth
lactation	production of milk
lactogenic	causing the formation of milk
lactorrhea	discharge of milk
leukorrhea	white vaginal discharge
macromastia	abnormally large breasts
macrosomia	baby with a large body
mammogram	record of a breast exam
mammoplasty	surgical reconstruction of a breast
mastalgia	breast pain
mastectomy	surgical removal of a breast
mastitis	inflammation of the breast
mastopexy	surgical fixation of a breast
mastoptosis	downward displacement (drooping) of the breast
menarche	beginning or first menstruation
menopause	cessation of menstruation
menorrhagia	excessive menstrual flow
menorrhalgia	painful menstruation
metrocolpocele	hernia of the uterus and prolapse into the vagina
metromenorrhagia	excessive menstrual bleeding at irregular intervals

quick reference glossary of terms *continued*

Term	Definition
metrophlebitis	inflammation of the blood vessels of the uterus
metrorrhagia	menstrual bleeding at irregular times
microcephalus	baby with a small head
micromastia	abnormally small breasts
myomectomy	surgical removal of a tumor in the muscle (usually refers to the muscle of the uterine wall)
myometritis	inflammation of the myometrium
myometrium	middle layer of uterine muscle tissue
natal	pertaining to birth
neonatal	pertaining to new birth (normally the first 28 days after birth)
neonatologist	specialist in the neonatal period
neonatology	study of the neonatal period
obstetrician	specialist in pregnancy, labor, and delivery of newborns
obstetrics	branch of medicine dealing with pregnancy, labor, and delivery of newborns
oligohydramnios	not enough amniotic fluid
oligomenorrhea	infrequent or light menstrual periods
oophorectomy	surgical removal of an ovary
oophoritis	inflammation of an ovary
oophorocystectomy	surgical removal of an ovarian cyst
oophorocystosis	ovarian cysts
oophoroma	ovarian tumor
oophorotomy	incision into an ovary
ovaralgia	pain in the ovaries
ovarialgia	pain in the ovaries
ovarian cystectomy	surgical removal of an ovarian cyst
ovariocentesis	surgical puncture of an ovary
ovariocyesis	ectopic pregnancy in an ovary
ovariorrhexis	rupture of an ovary
ovariostomy	creation of an opening into an ovary
ovaritis	inflammation of an ovary
ovulation	the process of an egg being released from an ovary
oxytocin	agent that stimulates uterine contractions and accelerates labor

quick reference glossary of terms *continued*

Term	Definition
Pap (Papanicolaou) smear	test used to detect cancer cells, most commonly in the cervix
pelvic sonograph	instrument for imaging the pelvis using sound waves
pelvicephalometry	procedure for measuring the head size of the baby and the pelvis size of the mother
pelvimetry	procedure for measuring the pelvis
perimetritis	inflammation of the perimetrium
perimetrium	tissue on the outside of the uterus, the outer layer of the uterus
perinatal	time around birth (normally ranging from 28 weeks of pregnancy to 28 days after pregnancy)
perinatologist	specialist in the perinatal period
perinatology	branch of medicine dealing with the perinatal period
perineocele	hernia in the perineum region
perineoplasty	surgical reconstruction of the perineum
perineorrhaphy	suture of the perineum
perineotomy	incision into the perineum
placenta previa	condition in which the placenta is attached to the uterus near the cervix
polyhydramnios	excessive amniotic fluid
polymenorrhea	menstrual periods occurring with greater-than-normal frequency
postnatal	pertaining to after birth
postpartum	pertaining to after birth
preeclampsia	condition characterized by high blood pressure and high protein levels in the urine
prenatal	pertaining to before birth
pseudocyesis	false pregnancy
pyosalpinx	blockage in a fallopian tube caused by pus
rectocele	hernia or protrusion of the rectum into the vagina
salpingectomy	surgical removal of a fallopian tube
salpingitis	inflammation of a fallopian tube
salpingocele	hernia of a fallopian tube
salpingocyesis	ectopic pregnancy in a fallopian tube
salpingo-oophorectomy	surgical removal of a fallopian tube and ovary
salpingo-oophoritis	inflammation of a fallopian tube and ovary
salpingopexy	surgical fixation of a fallopian tube

quick reference glossary of terms *continued*

Term	Definition
sonohysterography	procedure using sound waves to examine the uterus
speculum	device for examining a body cavity, most commonly the vagina
spontaneous abortion	the naturally occurring termination of pregnancy; also known as a *miscarriage*
teratogenic	causing the formation of birth defects
teratology	branch of medicine dealing with the study of birth defects and their causes
teratoma	*see* dermoid cyst
tocodynagraph	instrument for recording the strength of labor contractions
tocography	procedure for recording the strength of labor contractions
transvaginal sonography	imaging procedure using sound waves emitted from device inserted in the vagina
urethrocele	hernia or prolapse of the urethra into the vagina
uterine prolapse	downward displacement of the uterus into the vagina
vaginitis	inflammation of the vagina
vaginodynia	vaginal pain
vaginomycosis	fungal condition of the vagina
vaginoperineoplasty	surgical reconstruction of the vagina and perineum
vaginoperineorrhaphy	suture of the vagina and perineum
vaginoperineotomy	incision into the vagina and perineum
vaginoplasty	surgical reconstruction of the vagina
vaginoscope	instrument used to examine the vagina
vaginosis	condition of the vagina
vesicovaginal fistula	abnormal opening between the urinary bladder and the vagina
vulvitis	inflammation of the vulva
vulvodynia	pain in the vulva
vulvovaginitis	inflammation of the vulva and vagina

review of terms by roots

Root	Term(s)	
amni/o	amniocentesis	amniotomy
	amniorrhea	chorioamnionitis
	amniorrhexis	oligohydramnios
	amnioscope	polyhydramnios
	amnioscopy	
cervic/o	cervical dysplasia	cervicocolpitis
	cervical intraepithelial neoplasia	cervicography
	cervicectomy	cervicovaginitis
	cervicitis	endocervicitis
chori/o	chorioamnionitis	choriocarcinoma
	chorioangioma	chorionitis
colp/o	cervicocolpitis	colpoptosis
	colpitis	colposcope
	colpocystitis	colposcopy
	colpopexy	colpostenosis
	colpoplasty	metrocolpocele
-cyesis	ovariocyesis	salpingocyesis
	pseudocyesis	
episi/o	episiorrhaphy	episiotomy
	episiostenosis	
fet/o	fetometry	
gynec/o	gynecologist	
	gynecology	
hyster/o	hysteralgia	hysterorrhexis
	hysterectomy	hysterosalpingectomy
	hysterocele	hysterosalpingogram
	hysterodynia	hysteroscope
	hysterography	hysteroscopy
	hysteropexy	hysterotomy
	hysteroptosis	sonohysterography
lact/o	lactation	lactorrhea
	lactogenic	

review of terms by roots *continued*

Root	Term(s)	
mamm/o	mammogram	mammoplasty
mast/o	amastia	mastectomy
	gynecomastia	mastitis
	hypermastia	mastopexy
	hypomastia	mastoptosis
	macromastia	micromastia
	mastalgia	
men/o	amenorrhea	menorrhagia
	dysmenorrhea	menorrhalgia
	menarche	metromenorrhagia
	menopause	oligomenorrhea
metr/o	endometriosis	metrorrhagia
	endometritis	myometritis
	endometrium	myometrium
	metrocolpocele	perimetritis
	metromenorrhagia	perimetrium
	metrophlebitis	
nat/o	natal	perinatologist
	neonatal	perinatology
	neonatologist	postnatal
	neonatology	prenatal
	perinatal	
oophor/o	oophorectomy	oophoroma
	oophoritis	oophorotomy
	oophorocystectomy	salpingo-oophorectomy
	oophorocystosis	salpingo-oophoritis
ovari/o	ovaralgia	ovariocyesis
	ovarialgia	ovariorrhexis
	ovarian cystectomy	ovariostomy
	ovariocentesis	ovaritis
part/o	antepartum	postpartum
	intrapartum	

review of terms by roots *continued*

Root	Term(s)	
pelv/i	cephalopelvic disproportion	pelvicephalometry
	pelvic sonograph	pelvimetry
perine/o	perineocele	vaginoperineoplasty
	perineoplasty	vaginoperineorrhaphy
	perineorrhaphy	vaginoperineotomy
	perineotomy	
salping/o	hematosalpinx	salpingitis
	hydrosalpinx	salpingocele
	hysterosalpingectomy	salpingocyesis
	hysterosalpingogram	salpingo-oophorectomy
	pyosalpinx	salpingo-oophoritis
	salpingectomy	salpingopexy
toc/o	bradytocia	oxytocin
	cardiotocograph	tocodynagraph
	dystocia	tocography
	eutocia	
uter/o	uterine prolapse	
vagin/o	cervicovaginitis	vaginoperineotomy
	transvaginal sonography	vaginoplasty
	vaginitis	vaginoscope
	vaginodynia	vaginosis
	vaginomycosis	vesicovaginal fistula
	vaginoperineoplasty	vulvovaginitis
	vaginoperineorrhaphy	
vulv/o	vulvitis	vulvovaginitis
	vulvodynia	

other terms

abortifacient	implantation
abortion	in vitro fertilization
abruptio placentae	induced abortion
adenocarcinoma of the breast	leukorrhea

other terms *continued*

Braxton Hicks contraction	macrosomia
cesarean section	microcephalus
conception	myomectomy
congenital anomaly	obstetrician
contraception	ovulation
contraction	Pap smear (Papanicolaou)
cystocele	placenta previa
dermoid cyst	preeclampsia
dyspareunia	rectocele
eclampsia	speculum
ectopic pregnancy	spontaneous abortion
fertilization	teratogenic
gestation	teratology
gravida	teratoma
hyperemesis gravidarum	urethrocele

Prefix	Definition
A	
a-, an-	not
ab-	away
ad-, af-	toward
ambi-	both
ambly-	dull
ante-	before
anti-	against
auto-	self
B	
bi-	two
brady-	slow
C	
cata-	down
circum-	around
con-	with, together
contra-	against
crypto-	hidden
D	
de-	down, away from
dia-	through
dipl-	double
dys-	bad
E	
e-	out
ec-	out
ecto-	outside
ef-	out
em-, en-	in, inside
endo-	in, inside
epi-	upon
eso-	inward
eu-	good, normal
ex-	out
exo-	outside
extra-	outside
H	
hemi-	half
hetero-	different
homo-	similar
hyper-	over
hypo-	under

Prefix	Definition
I	
idio-	private
inter-	between
intra-	in, inside
iso-	equal
M	
macro-	large
meta-	after, other, beyond
micro-	small
mono-	one
multi-	many
N	
neo-	new
O	
ob-	in the way
oligo-	few
ortho-	straight
P	
pan-	all
par-, para-	around, beside
per-	through
peri-	around
poly-	many
post-	after
pre-	before
presby-	old
pro-	before, on behalf of
pros-	to, toward
pseud-, pseudo-	false
R	
re-	again
S	
schizo-	divided
semi-	half
sub-	beneath
sym-, syn-	with, together
T	
tachy-	fast
trans-	through, across
U	
uni-	one

Suffix	Definition
A	
-acusis	hearing condition
-agon	to lead
-ant	agent
-arche	beginning
-asthenia	weakness
-ation	process, procedure
C	
-cide	to kill
-cision	cut
-clasia	breaking
-clasis	breaking
D	
-drome	run
E	
-ectasia	expansion, dilation
-ectasis	expansion, dilation
-ectomy	removal
-edema	swelling
-emia	blood condition
G	
-genic	beginning in, producing
-graft	transplant
I	
-iasis	presence
-icle	little
-ictal	seizure
-ive	agent
L	
-listhesis	slipping
-lith	stone
-loqui	speak
-luxation	dislocation
-lytic	break down
M	
-malacia	abnormal softening
-megaly	abnormal enlargement
O	
-opia	vision condition
-opsia	vision condition

Suffix	Definition
P	
-paresis	slight or partial paralysis
-pareunia	sexual intercourse
-pathy	disease/condition
-penia	deficiency
-phagia	eating
-philia	abnormal liking for or tendency toward
-phoria	carry condition
-plasia	formation
-plasm	formation
-plastic	formation
-plasty	surgical reconstruction
-plegia	paralysis
-pnea	breathing
-poesis	formation
-ptosis	drooping
-ptysis	cough
R	
-rrhage, -rrhagia	excessive flow
-rrhaphy	suture
-rrhea	flow
-rrhexis	rupture
S	
-sclerosis	hardening condition
-scope	instrument used to look
-scopy	process of looking
-spasm	involuntary contraction
-stenosis	narrowing
-stomy	creation of an opening
T	
-thesis	place
-tomy	incision
-toxic	poisonous
-toxin	a substance poisonous to
-tripsy	wear down procedure, surgical crushing
-trophy	nourishment condition
-tropin	stimulating hormone
U	
-ula	small
-uria	urine condition
Y	
-y	condition or process

appendix C: roots only mentioned in word analysis

Root	Definition
A	
acr/o	extremity, top, heights
aer/o	air
ambul/o	walk
B	
bi/o	life
C	
carcin/o	cancer
chem/o	chemical
chron/o	time
chyl/o	chyle
coni/o	dust
cry/o	cold
cyan/o	blue
D	
desicc/o	drying
dips/o	thirst
E	
electr/o	electricity
eury/o	wide
F	
fibr/o	fiber
G	
galact/o	milk
gen/o	generation/cause
gnosi/o	knowledge
graph/o	write
H	
hem/o, hemat/o	blood
hepat/o	liver
hydr/o	water
I	
isch/o	hold back
K	
kel/o	tumor
klept/o	theft
kyph/o	bent
L	
lex/o	reading
lord/o	bend backward

Root	Definition
M	
morph/o	change
muc/o	mucus
myc/o	fungus
N	
narc/o	sleep
necr/o	death
neur/o	nerve
noct/o	night
O	
orth/o	straight
osm/o	smelling
P	
path/o	suffering/disease
phag/o	eat
pharmac/o	drug
phas/o	speaking
phil/o	love
phon/o	sound/voice
plas/o	formation
poli/o	gray
por/o	pore
prosop/o	face
py/o	pus
pylor/o	gatekeeper
pyr/o	fire
S	
sarc/o	flesh
scler/o	hard
scoli/o	crooked
sept/i	rotting
sept/o	wall, partition
somat/o	body
son/o	sound
spin/o	spine
stigmat/o	point
stom/o	mouth
T	
tel/o	complete, end
thel/o	breast
thromb/o	clot
tom/o	cut
top/o	place
trich/o	hair

Root	Definition
trop/o	turn
troph/o	nourishment/development
tuss/o	cough
X	
xen/o	foreign
xer/o	dry

glossary

A

abdominocentesis (ab-DAW-min-oh-sin-TEE-sis) puncture of the abdomen (usually for the purpose of withdrawing fluid)

abdominoplasty (ab-DAW-min-oh-PLAS-tee) surgical reconstruction of the abdomen

abortifacient (ah-BOR-tih-FAY-shunt) drug or device that causes the termination of a pregnancy

abortion (ah-BOR-shun) termination of pregnancy

abrasion (ah-BRAY-zhun) a scraping away of skin

abruptio placentae (ah-BRUP-shee-oh plah-SIN-tee) separation of the placenta from the wall of the uterus

abscess (AB-ses) a localized collection of pus in the body

achondroplasia (AY-kawn-droh-PLAY-zhah) a defect in the formation of cartilage

acidemia (A-sih-DEE-mee-ah) abnormal acidity of the blood

acne vulgaris (AK-nee vul-GAR-is) common acne; an inflammation of the skin follicles

acoustic neuroma (ah-KOO-stik nir-OH-mah) a tumor on the acoustic nerve

acromegaly (AK-roh-MEH-gah-lee) abnormal enlargement of the extremities

acrophobia (AK-roh-FOH-bee-ah) fear of heights

actinic dermatitis (ak-TIN-ik der-mah-TAI-tis) inflammation of the skin caused by sun exposure

actinic keratosis (ak-TIN-ik keh-rah-TOH-sis) horny skin condition caused by sun exposure

adenalgia (AD-en-AL-jah) pain in a gland

adenectomy (AD-en-EK-toh-mee) removal of a gland

adenitis (AD-en-AI-tis) inflammation of a gland

adenocarcinoma (ad-EN-oh-KAR-sih-NOH-mah) cancerous tumor of a gland

adenocarcinoma of the breast (AD-en-oh-KAR-sih-NOH-mah) glandular tumor in the breast

adenoidectomy (a-din-oid-EK-toe-mee) removal of the adenoids

adenoma (AD-eh-NOH-mah) glandular tumor

adenomegaly (ah-DEN-oh-MEH-gah-lee) abnormal enlargement of a gland

adenopathy (AD-en-AW-pah-thee) gland disease

adenosis (AD-en-OH-sis) gland condition

adipocele (a-dih-poh-SEEL) hernia filled with fatty tissue

adrenal adenoma (ad-REE-nal AD-en-OH-mah) tumor of the adrenal gland

adrenal insufficiency (ad-REE-nal IN-suh-FIH-shun-see) condition in which the adrenal glands underproduce necessary hormones

adrenal virilism (ad-REE-nal VIR-il-izm) development of male secondary sexual characteristics caused by excessive secretion of the adrenal gland

adrenalectomy (ad-REE-nal-EK-toh-mee) removal of the adrenal gland

adrenaline (ad-REN-ah-lin) hormone secreted by the adrenal gland (from Latin; see also *epinephrine*)

adrenalitis (ad-REE-nah-LAI-tis) inflammation of the adrenal gland

adrenarche (AD-ren-AR-kay) beginning of adrenal secretion (at puberty)

adrenocortical carcinoma (ad-REE-noh-KOR-tih-kal KAR-sih-NOH-mah) cancerous tumor originating in the cortex of the adrenal gland

adrenocortical insufficiency (ad-REE-noh-KOR-tih-kal IN-suh-FIH-shun-see) condition in which the adrenal cortex underproduces necessary hormones

adrenocorticohyperplasia (ad-REE-noh-KOR-tih-koh-HAI-per-PLAY-zhah) overdevelopment of the cortex of the adrenal gland

adrenocorticotropic hormone (ACTH) (ah-DREH-noh-KOR-tih-koh-TROH-pik HOR-mohn) hormone secreted by the pituitary gland that stimulates the cortex of the adrenal gland

adrenomegaly (ad-REN-oh-MEH-gah-lee) abnormal enlargement of the adrenal gland

aerodontalgia (ER-oh-dawn-TAL-jah) tooth pain caused by exposure to air

aerotitis (AIR-oh-TAI-tis) inflammation of the ear caused by air

afferent nerve (A-fir-ent NIRV) a nerve that carries impulses toward the central nervous system

agnosia (AG-noh-zhah) inability to comprehend

agoraphobia (ah-GOR-ah-FOH-bee-ah) fear of outdoor spaces

akinetopsia (ah-KEE-nah-TOP-see-ah) the inability to see objects in motion

albinism (AL-bin-ism) lack of pigment in skin causing the patient to look white

albino (al-BAY-noh) a person afflicted with albinism

albuminuria (al-byoo-mih-NUR-ee-ah) protein in the urine

alkalemia (AL-kah-LEE-mee-ah) abnormal alkalinity (opposite of acidity) of the blood

allograft (A-loh-GRAFT) see *homograft*

alopecia (a-loh-PEE-sha) baldness

amastia (ay-MAS-tee-ah) absence of breasts

ambiopia (AM-bee-OH-pee-ah) double vision

amblyopia (AM-blih-OH-pee-ah) decreased vision (when it occurs in one eye, it is referred to as lazy eye)

amenorrhea (AY-men-oh-REE-ah) no menstruation

amniocentesis (AM-nee-oh-sin-TEE-sis) surgical puncture of the amnion

amniorrhea (AM-nee-oh-REE-ah) discharge of amniotic fluid

amniorrhexis (AM-nee-oh-REK-sis) rupture of the amniotic sac

amnioscope (AM-nee-oh-SKOHP) instrument for examining the amnion

amnioscopy (AM-nee-AW-skoh-pee) procedure for examining the amnion

amniotomy (AM-nee-AW-toh-mee) incision into the amnion

amytrophic lateral sclerosis (ALS) (a-MAI-aw-TROH-fik LAT-tih-ral skleh-ROH-sis) a degenerative disease of the central nervous system causing loss of muscle control; also known as Lou Gehrig's disease

anal fistula (AY-nal FIS-tyoo-la) abnormal opening between the rectum and the exterior perianal skin

analgesic (an-al-JEE-zik) a drug that relieves pain

anastomosis (ah-NAS-toh-moh-sis) creation of an opening; a surgical procedure connecting two previously unconnected hollow tubes

anemia (ah-NEE-mee-ah) reduction of red blood cells noticed by the patient by weakness and fatigue

anesthesiologist (A-neh-STHEE-zee-AW-loh-jist) doctor who specializes in anesthesiology

anesthetic (an-es-THET-ik) a drug that causes loss of sensation

aneurysm (AN-yir-IZ-um) bulge in a blood vessel

aneurysmectomy (AN-yir-IZ-um-EK-toh-mee) surgical removal of an aneurysm

angina pectoris (an-JAI-nah PEK-tor-is) oppressive pain in the chest caused by irregular blood flow to the heart

angiocarditis (AN-jee-oh-kar-DAI-tis) inflammation of the heart vessels

angioedema (AN-jee-oh-eh-DEE-mah) swelling of the blood vessels

angiogenesis (AN-jee-oh-JIN-eh-sis) development of blood vessels

angiogram (AN-jee-oh-GRAM) record of the blood vessels

angiography (AN-jee-AW-grah-fee) procedure to describe the blood vessels

angiolith (AN-jee-oh-LITH) stone forming in the wall of a blood vessel

angioma (AN-jee-OH-mah) blood vessel tumor

angioplasty (AN-jee-oh-PLAS-tee) surgical reconstruction of a vessel

angiopoiesis (AN-jee-oh-poh-EE-sis) formation of blood vessels

angiorrhaphy (AN-jee-OR-ah-fee) suture of a vessel

angiosclerosis (AN-jee-oh-skleh-ROH-sis) hardening of a blood vessel

angioscope (AN-jee-oh-SKOWP) device for looking into a blood vessel

anhidrosis (an-ih-DROH-sis) lack of sweating

aniridia (AN-ih-RIH-dee-ah) absence of an iris

anisocytosis (AN-ai-soh-SAI-toh-sis) condition characterized by a great inequality in the size of red blood cells

ankylosing spondylitis (an-kih-LOH-sing spawn-dih-LAI-tis) a stiffening inflammation of the vertebrae

ankylosis (an-kih-LOH-sis) joint stiffness

anophony (an-AW-foh-nee) sound from the anus

anoplasty (AN-noh-PLAS-tee) surgical reconstruction of the anus

anorchidism (an-OR-kih-DIZ-um) absence of a testicle

anorexia (a-noh-REK-see-ah) an eating disorder characterized by the patient's refusal to eat

anosigmoidoscopy (AN-oh-SIG-moid-AW-skoh-pee) procedure for looking at the anus and sigmoid colon

anosmia (an-AWZ-mee-ah) lack of a sense of smell

antacid (ant-AS-id) agent that neutralizes acid

antepartum (AN-tee-PAR-tum) time before birth

antianginal (AN-tee-AN-jih-nal) a drug that prevents or relieves the symptoms of angina pectoris

antiarrhythmic (AN-tee-a-RITH-mik) a drug that opposes an irregular heartbeat

antiarthritic (AN-tee-ar-THRIH-tik) a drug that opposes joint inflammation

antibiotic (an-tai-bai-OH-tik) a drug that destroys or opposes the growth of microorganisms

antibody (AN-tih-BAW-dee) substance produced by the body in response to an antigen

anticoagulant (AN-tee-coh-AG-yoo-lant) drug that prevents the coagulation of blood

anticonvulsant (AN-tee-kon-VUL-sant) a drug that opposes convulsions

antidepressant (AN-tee-deh-PREH-sant) a drug that opposes depression

antiemetic (AN-tih-EE-met-ik) agent that prevents/relieves nausea or vomiting

antigen (AN-tih-JIN) substance that causes the body to produce antibodies

antihistamine (an-tee-HIS-tah-meen) a drug that opposes the effects of histamine

antihypertensive (AN-tee-HAI-per-TEN-siv) drug that opposes high blood pressure

anti-inflammatory (AN-tee-in-FLA-mah-TOR-ee) a drug that opposes inflammation

antipruritic (an-tee-pruh-RIH-tik) a drug that prevents or relieves itching

antipsychotic (AN-tee-sai-KAW-tik) a drug that opposes psychosis

antipyretic (AN-tee-pir-ih-tik) a drug that opposes fever

antiseptic (an-tee-SEP-tik) a drug that prevents sepsis (rotting of flesh) by killing microorganisms

antispasmodic (AN-tee-spaz-MAW-dik) drug used to prevent spasms

antitussive (an-tee-TUSS-iv) a drug that prevents coughing

anuria (an-YUR-ee-ah) lack of urination

anxiolytic (ANG-zee-oh-LIH-tik) a drug that lessens anxiety

aortalgia (AY-or-TAL-jah) pain in the aorta

aortectasia (ay-OR-tek-TAY-zhah) dilation of the aorta

aortic aneurysm (ay-OR-tik AN-yir-IZ-um) bulging or swelling of the aorta

aortic regurgitation (ay-OR-tik ree-GIR-jih-TAY-shun) flow of blood backward from the aorta into the heart; caused by a weak heart valve

aortic stenosis (ay-OR-tik stih-NOH-sis) narrowing of the aorta

aortitis (ay-or-TAI-tis) inflammation of the aorta

aortogram (ay-OR-tah-GRAM) record of the aorta

aortolith (ay-OR-toh-LITH) stone deposit in the wall of the aorta

aortorrhaphy (ay-or-TOR-ah-fee) suture of the aorta

aortotomy (ay-or-TAW-toh-mee) incision into the aorta

apathy (A-pah-thee) lack of emotion

aphagia (a-FAY-jah) inability to eat

aphakia (ah-FAY-kee-ia) absence of a lens

aphasia (ah-FAY-zhah) inability to speak

apheresis (AH-fer-EE-sis) general term for a process, similar to dialysis, that draws blood, removes something from it, then returns the rest of the blood to the patient

aplastic anemia (AY-plas-tik ah-NEE-mee-ah) anemia caused by red blood cells not being formed in sufficient quantities

apnea (AP-nee-yah) cessation of breathing

arrhythmia (ay-RITH-mee-ah) irregular heartbeat

arteriectomy (ar-TER-ee-EK-toh-mee) surgical removal of an artery

arteriogram (ar-TER-ee-oh-GRAM) record of an artery

arteriolith (ar-TER-ee-oh-LITH) stone in an artery

arteriopathy (ar-TER-ee-AW-pah-thee) disease of the arteries

arterioplasty (ar-TER-ee-oh-PLAS-tee) surgical reconstruction of an artery

arteriorrhaphy (ar-TER-ee-OR-ah-fee) suture of an artery

arteriorrhexis (ar-TER-ee-oh-REK-sis) rupture of an artery

arteriosclerosis (ar-TER-ee-oh-skleh-ROH-sis) hardening of an artery

arteritis (AR-ter-AI-tis) inflammation of the arteries

arthralgia (ar-THRAL-jah) joint pain

arthrectomy (ar-THREK-toh-mee) removal of a joint

arthritis (ar-THRAI-tis) joint inflammation

arthrocele (AR-throh-seel) hernia of a joint

arthrocentesis (ar-throh-sin-TEE-sis) puncture of a joint

arthroclasia (AR-throh-KLAY-zhah) the therapeutic breaking of a joint to allow for increased mobility

arthrodesis (AR-throh-DEE-sis) the surgical fixation of a joint

arthrodynia (ar-throh-DAI-nee-ah) joint pain

arthrodysplasia (AR-throh-dis-PLAY-zhah) abnormal joint development

arthrogram (AR-throh-gram) visual record of a joint

arthrography (ar-THRAW-grah-fee) procedure used to examine a joint

arthrolysis (ar-THRAW-lih-sis) loosening a stiff joint

arthropathy (ar-THRAW-pah-thee) joint disease

arthroplasty (AR-throh-PLAS-tee) reconstruction of a joint

arthrosclerosis (AR-throh-skleh-ROH-sis) hardening of the joints

arthroscope (AR-throh-skohp) instrument for looking into a joint

arthroscopy (ar-THRAW-skoh-pee) procedure of looking into a joint

arthrotomy (ar-THRAW-toh-mee) incision into a joint

ascites (ah-SAI-teez) retention of fluid in the peritoneum

aspermia (ay-SPER-mee-ah) condition characterized by a lack of sperm

asplenia (ah-SPLEE-nee-ah) absence of a spleen or of spleen function

asthenopia (AS-then-OH-pee-ah) weak vision (i.e., eye strain)

asthma (AZ-ma) a disease caused by episodic narrowing and inflammation of the airway

astigmatism (ah-STIG-mah-TIZ-um) vision problem caused by the fact that light rays entering the eye aren't focused on a single point in the back of the eye

ataxia (ah-TAK-see-ah) lack of coordination

atelectasis (ah-tel-EK-ta-sis) incomplete expansion

atherectomy (A-ther-EK-toh-mee) surgical removal of fatty plaque within an artery

atherogenesis (A-ther-oh-JIN-eh-sis) formation of fatty plaque on the wall of an artery

atherosclerosis (A-ther-oh-skleh-ROH-sis) hardening of an artery due to build-up of fatty plaque

atopic dermatitis (AY-taw-pik der-mah-TAI-tis) an unusual inflammation of the skin (atopic usually means not in the right place)

atopognosis (AY-top-aw-GNOH-sis) inability to locate a sensation

atrial fibrillation (AY-tree-al FIB-rih-LAY-shun) quivering or spontaneous contraction of muscle fibers in the heart's atrium

atrial septal defect (AY-tree-al SEP-tal DEE-fekt) flaw in the septum that divides the two atria of the heart

atrophy (A-troh-fee) underdevelopment, decrease, or loss of muscle tissue

audiogram (AW-dee-oh-GRAM) record produced by an audiometer

audiologist (aw-dee-AW-loh-jist) hearing specialist

audiometer (aw-dee-AW-meh-ter) instrument for measuring hearing

audiometry (aw-dee-AW-meh-tree) procedure for measuring hearing

auditory prosthesis (AW-dih-TOR-ee praws-THEE-sis) hearing aid

aural (AW-ral) pertaining to the ear

auscultation (ah-skul-TAY-shun) from the Latin word *ausculto,* meaning "to listen"; a doctor using a stethoscope is performing an auscultation

autism (AH-tiz-um) a psychiatric disorder characterized by the withdrawal from communication with others. The patient is focused only on the self.

autograft (AW-toh-GRAFT) skin transplant taken from a different place on the patient's body

autoimmune disease (AW-toh-ih-MYOON dih-ZEEZ) a disease caused by the body's immune system attacking the body's own healthy tissue

azoospermia (ay-ZOH-aw-SPER-mee-ah) a condition characterized by lack of living sperm

azotemia (AZ-oh-TEE-mee-ah) excess nitrogen in the blood

azotorrhea (AZ-oh-toh-REE-ah) excessive discharge of nitrogen

azoturia (AZ-oh-TUR-ee-ah) excess nitrogen in the urine

B

balanitis (bal-ah-NAI-tis) inflammation of the penis

balanoplasty (BAL-ah-noh-PLAS-tee) surgical reconstruction of the penis

balanorrhea (BAL-ah-noh-REE-ah) discharge from the penis

bariatrics (BAR-ee-ah-triks) branch of medicine dealing with weight issues

basal cell carcinoma (BAY-zul SELL kar-sih-NOH-mah) cancerous tumor of basal skin cells

benign prostate hyperplasia (beh-NAIN PROS-tayt HAI-per-PLAY-zhah) noncancerous overdevelopment of the prostate; also known as enlarged prostate

benign prostate hypertrophy (beh-NAIN PROS-tayt hai-PER-troh-fee) another term for benign prostate hyperplasia

biligenesis (blh-lih-JIN-eh-sis) formation of bile

bilirubinemia (BIH-lee-ROO-bin-EE-mee-ah) the presence of bilirubin (red bile; a substance derived from red blood cells that have completed their life span) in the blood

binocular (bai-NAW-kyoo-lar) pertaining to both eyes

biopsy (BAI-op-see) removal of tissue in order to examine it

blepharedema (BLEF-ar-eh-DEE-mah) eyelid swelling

blepharitis (BLEF-ah-RAI-tis) eyelid inflammation

blepharoconjunctivitis (BLEF-ah-roh-con-JUNK-tih-VAI-tis) inflammation of the eyelid and conjunctiva

blepharoplasty (BLEF-ah-roh-PLAS-tee) surgical reconstruction of the eyelid

blepharoplegia (BLEF-ah-roh-PLEE-jah) paralysis of the eyelid

blepharoptosis (BLEF-ar-awp-TOH-sis) drooping eyelid

blepharopyorrhea (BLEF-ah-roh-PAI-oh-REE-ah) discharge of pus from the eyelid

blepharospasm (BLEF-ah-roh-SPAZ-um) involuntary contraction of an eyelid

blepharotomy (BLEF-ah-RAW-toh-mee) incision into the eyelid

blood pressure (BLUD PRESH-ir) force exerted by blood on the walls of blood vessels

blood urea nitrogen (BUN) (BLUD yoo-REE-ah NAI-troh-jun) nitrogen in the blood in the form of urea; it is the product of the breakdown of amino acids for energy

bradycardia (BRAY-dih-KAR-dee-ah) slow heartbeat

bradykinesia (bray-dih-kih-NEE-zhah) slow movement

bradypnea (brad-ip-NEE-ah) slow breathing

bradytocia (BRAY-dih-TOH-shee-ah) slow labor

Braxton Hicks contraction (BRAKS-ton HIKS con-TRAK-shun) sporadic contractions of the uterine muscles of women in labor; also known as false labor

bronchiectasis (bron-key-EK-ta-sis) expansion of the bronchi

bronchiogenic carcinoma (bron-kee-oh-JEN-ic car-si-NO-ma) a cancerous tumor originating in the bronchi

bronchiolitis (bron-kee-yo-LAI-tis) inflammation of the bronchiole

bronchioplasty (bron-koh-PLAS-tee) reconstruction of a bronchus

bronchitis (bron-KAI-tis) inflammation of the bronchi

bronchodilator (bron-koh-DAI-lay-tor) a drug that expands the walls of the bronchi

bronchorrhea (bron-koh-REE-ah) discharge from the bronchi

bronchoscopy (bron-KOS-koh-pee) a procedure to look inside the bronchi

bronchospasm (BRON-ko-spaz-um) involuntary contraction of the bronchia

bulimia (boo-LEE-mee-ah) an eating disorder characterized by overeating and usually followed by forced vomiting

bulla (BUL-lah) from Latin, for "bubble"; a large blister

bursectomy (bir-SEK-toh-mee) removal of a bursa

bursitis (bur-SAI-tis) inflammation of the bursa

bursolith (BIR-soh-lith) a stone in a bursa

bursopathy (bur-SAW-pah-thee) disease of the bursa

bursotomy (bir-SAW-toh-mee) incision into a bursa

C

calciuria (CAL-sih-YOO-ree-ah) calcium in the urine

capnography (cap-NAH-gra-fee) a procedure to record carbon dioxide levels

capnometer (cap-NOM-eh-ter) instrument to measure carbon dioxide levels

cardiac arrest (KAR-dee-ak ah-REST) cessation of functional circulation

cardiac catheterization (KAR-dee-ak KATH-eh-ter-ih-ZAY-shun) the process of inserting a tube (catheter) into the heart

cardiologist (KAR-dee-AW-loh-jist) heart specialist

cardiology (KAR-dee-AW-loh-jee) branch of medicine dealing with the heart

cardiomegaly (KAR-dee-oh-MEH-gah-lee) enlarged heart

cardiomyopathy (KAR-dee-oh-mai-AW-pah-thee) disease of the heart muscle

cardiomyotomy (KAR-dee-oh-mai-AW-toh-mee) incision into the heart muscle

cardiopulmonary bypass (KAR-dee-oh-PUL-mon-AR-ee BAI-pas) procedure that temporarily circulates and oxygenates a patient's blood during a portion of heart surgery where the heart is stopped

cardiopulmonary resuscitation (CPR) (KAR-dee-oh-PUL-mon-air-ee ree-sus-ih-TAY-shun) a method of artificially maintaining blood flow and airflow when breathing and pulse have stopped

cardiothoracic surgery (KAR-dee-oh-thoh-RA-sik SIR-jir-ee) surgery that involves cutting through the patient's chest to get to the heart

cardiotocograph (KAR-dee-oh-TOH-koh-GRAF) instrument for recording the fetal heart rate during labor

cardiotonic (KAR-dee-oh-TAW-nik) a drug that increases the strength of heart contractions

cardiotoxic (KAR-dee-oh-TOK-sik) poisonous to the heart

cardiovascular (KAR-dee-oh-VAS-kyoo-lar) pertaining to the heart and blood vessels

cardioversion (KAR-dee-oh-VER-zhun) returning a heart to normal rhythm

carditis (kar-DAI-tis) inflammation of the heart

carpectomy (kar-PEK-toh-mee) removal of all or part of the wrist

carpitis (kar-PAI-tis) wrist inflammation

caseous necrosis (KAYZ-ee-us ne-CROW-sis) the death of tissue with a cheeselike appearance

cataract (KAT-ah-RAKT) opacity (cloudiness) of the lens of the eye (from Latin, for "waterfall")

catatonia (KAT-ah-TOH-nee-ah) condition characterized by reduced muscle tone

cathartic (kah-THAR-tik) agent that produces bowel movements

causalgia (kaw-ZAL-jah) painful sensation of burning

celiomyositis (SEE-lee-oh-MAI-oh-sai-TOH-sis) inflammation of the abdominal muscle

celiopathy (see-lee-AW-pah-thee) disease of the abdomen

celiotomy (SEE-lee-AW-toh-mee) incision into the abdomen

cephalalgia (SEH-ful-AL-jah) head pain

cephalodynia (SEH-fah-loh-DAI-nee-ah) head pain

cephalopelvic disproportion (CPD) (SEE-fah-loh-PEL-vik DIS-proh-POR-shun) condition characterized by the inability of the mother's pelvis to allow the baby to pass through the birth canal

cerebellitis (ser-eh-bell-AI-tis) inflammation of the cerebellum

cerebral aneurysm (seh-REE-bral AN-yir-iz-um) the widening or abnormal dilation of a blood vessel in the brain

cerebral angiography (seh-REE-bral AN-gee-AW-grah-fee) procedure used to examine blood vessels in the brain

cerebral arteriosclerosis (seh-REE-bral ar-TIR-ee-oh-skleh-ROH-sis) the hardening of an artery in the brain

cerebral atherosclerosis (seh-REE-bral A-ther-oh-skleh-ROH-sis) the hardening of an artery in the brain caused by the buildup of fatty plaque

cerebral atrophy (seh-REE-bral A-troh-fee) wasting away of brain tissue

cerebral embolism (seh-REE-bral EM-boh-lih-zum) the blockage of a blood vessel in the brain caused by a foreign object (embolus) such as fat or bacteria

cerebral palsy (seh-REE-bral PAL-zee) paralysis caused by damage to the area of the brain responsible for movement

cerebral thrombosis (seh-REE-bral throm-BOH-sis) the blockage of a blood vessel in the brain caused by a clot

cerebromeningitis (seh-REE-broh-MEN-in-JAI-tis) inflammation of the brain and meninges

cerebrotomy (seh-ree-BRAW-toh-mee) incision into the brain

cerebrovascular accident (CVA) (seh-REE-broh-VAS-kyoo-lar AK-sih-dent) an accident involving the blood vessels of the brain

cerebrovascular disease (seh-REE-broh-VAS-kyoo-lar dih-ZEEZ) a disease of the blood vessels of the brain

cerumen impaction (SEH-roo-men im-PAK-shun) buildup of ear wax blocking the ear canal

ceruminolysis (seh-ROO-min-AW-lih-sis) breakdown of ear wax

ceruminolytic (seh-ROO-min-oh-LIH-tik) drug that aids in the breakdown of ear wax

ceruminoma (seh-ROO-min-OH-mah) benign tumor of the cerumen-secreting glands of the ear

ceruminosis (seh-ROO-min-OH-sis) excessive formation of ear wax

cervical dysplasia (SER-vih-kal dis-PLAY-zhah) bad formation of cervical cells

cervical intraepithelial neoplasia (SER-vih-kal IN-trah-EP-ih-THEE-lee-al NEE-oh-PLAY-zhah) abnormal growth of cervical cells

cervicectomy (SER-vih-SEK-toh-mee) surgical removal of the cervix

cervicitis (SER-vih-SAI-tis) inflammation of the cervix

cervicocolpitis (SER-vih-koh-kol-PAI-tis) inflammation of the cervix and vagina

cervicodynia (sir-vih-koh-DAI-nee-ah) neck pain

cervicography (SER-vih-KAW-grah-fee) procedure for imaging the cervix

cervicovaginitis (SER-vih-koh-VAJ-ih-NAI-tis) inflammation of the cervix and vagina

cesarean section (sih-SER-ee-an SEK-shun) delivery of a baby through an incision made in the uterus

chemosurgery (KEE-moh-SIR-juh-ree) removal of tissue that has been destroyed using chemicals

chemotherapy (KEE-moh-THER-ah-pee) treatment using chemicals

cherry angioma (CHEH-ree an-gee-OH-mah) a small blood vessel tumor

chloremia (klor-EE-mee-ah) increased chloride in the blood

cholangiogastrostomy (koh-LAN-jee-oh-gas-TRAWS-toh-mee) creation of an opening between the bile vessel (ducts) and the stomach

cholangiogram (koh-LAN-jee-oh-gram) record of the bile vessels (ducts)

cholangiography (koh-LAN-jee-AW-grah-fee) procedure for mapping the bile vessels (ducts)

cholangioma (koh-lan-jee-OH-mah) tumor of the bile vessels (ducts)

cholangiopancreatography (koh-LAN-jee-oh-PAN-kree-ah-TAW-grah-fee) procedure for mapping the bile vessels (ducts) and pancreas

cholangitis (KOH-lan-JAI-tis) inflammation of the bile vessels (ducts)

cholecystalgia (KOH-lay-sis-TAL-jah) pain in the gallbladder

cholecystectomy (KOH-lay-sis-TEK-toh-me) surgical removal of the bile (gall) bladder

cholecystitis (KOH-lay-sis-TAI-tis) inflammation of the bile (gall) bladder

cholecystogram (KOH-lay-SIS-toh-gram) record of the bile (gall) bladder

choledochocele (koh-lay-DOH-koh-seel) hernia of the (common) bile duct

choledocholithectomy (KOH-leh-DOH-koh-lih-THEK-toh-mee) surgical removal of a stone from the (common) bile duct

choledocholithiasis (koh-lay-DOH-koh-lith-AI-ah-sis) presence of a stone in the (common) bile duct

choledochotomy (KOH-leh-doh-KAW-toh-mee) incision into the (common) bile duct

cholelith (KOH-lay-lith) gallstone; literally, a stone in the bile

cholelithiasis (KOH-lay-lih-THAI-ah-sis) presence of a gallstone

cholelithotomy (KOH-lay-lih-THAW-toh-mee) incision to remove bile (gall) stones

cholelithotripsy (KOH-lay-lih-THOH-trip-see) crushing of bile (gall) stones

cholemesis (koh-LEM-eh-sis) vomiting bile

chondrectomy (kawn-DREK-toh-mee) removal of cartilage

chondroma (kawn-DROH-mah) a tumor-like growth of cartilage tissue

chondromalacia (KAWN-droh-mah-LAY-shah) abnormal softening of the cartilage

chondro-osteodystrophy (KAWN-droh-AW-stee-oh-DIH-stroh-fee) poor development of bones and cartilage

chondroplasty (KAWN-droh-PLAS-tee) reconstruction of cartilage

chorioamnionitis (KOR-ee-oh-AM-nee-oh-NAI-tis) inflammation of the chorion and amnion

chorioangioma (KOR-ee-oh-AN-jee-OH-mah) blood vessel tumor of the chorion

choriocarcinoma (KOR-ee-oh-KAR-sih-NOH-mah) cancerous tumor of the chorion

chorionitis (KOR-ee-aw-NAI-tis) inflammation of the chorion

chronic obstructive pulmonary disease (COPD) (KRON-ik ob-STRUKT-iv pul-mon-AIR-ee diz-EEZ) a lung disease caused by the continual blockage of lung passages

chylothorax (kai-low-THOR-aks) chyle in the chest

cicatrix (plural cicatrices) (SIK-ah-triks) from Latin, for "scar"; a scar

circulation (SIR-kyoo-LAY-shun) moving of blood from the heart through the vessels and back to the heart

circumcision (SIR-kum-SIH-zhun) surgical removal of the foreskin of the penis

cirrhosis (sir-OH-sis) liver disease named for the change of color in the liver

clonus (CLAH-nis) muscle spasm or twitching

closed reduction (KLOHZD ree-DUK-shun) returning bones to their proper position without the use of surgery

coagulopathy (coh-AG-yoo-LAW-pah-thee) any disease that deals with problems in blood coagulation

cochlear implant (KOH-klee-ar IM-plant) electronic device that stimulates the cochlea; it can give the sense of sound to those who are profoundly deaf

cochleitis (KOH-klee-AI-tis) inflammation of the cochlea

colectomy (koh-LEK-toh-mee) surgical removal of the colon

colitis (coh-LAI-tis) inflammation of the colon

colonoscopy (COH-lon-AW-skoh-pee) procedure for looking at the colon

colorectal carcinoma (COH-loh-REK-tal KAR-sih-NOH-mah) cancerous tumor of the colon or rectum

colostomy (koh-LAW-stoh-mee) creation of an opening in the colon

colovaginal fistula (COH-loh-VAJ-in-al FIS-tyoo-la) abnormal opening between the colon and vagina

colpitis (kol-PAI-tis) inflammation of the vagina

colpocystitis (KOL-poh-sis-TAI-tis) inflammation of the vagina and urinary bladder

colpopexy (KOL-poh-PEK-see) surgical fixation of the vagina

colpoplasty (KOL-poh-PLAS-tee) surgical reconstruction of the vagina

colpoptosis (KOL-pawp-TOH-sis) downward placement of the vagina

colposcope (KOL-poh-SKOHP) instrument used to examine the vagina

colposcopy (kol-PAW-skoh-pee) procedure for examining the vagina

colpostenosis (KOL-poh-steh-NOH-sis) narrowing in the vaginal opening

comedo (koh-MEE-doh) from Latin, for "to eat up"; a hair follicle plugged with sebum (blackhead, whitehead)

computed axial tomography (CAT or CT) (kom-PYOO-ted AK-see-al taw-MAW-grah-fee) imaging procedure using a computer to produce cross sections along an axis

computed tomography (kom-PYOO-ted tom-O-grah-fee) an imaging procedure using a computer to "cut" or view "slices" of a patient's organs

conductive hearing loss (con-DUK-tiv) sound does not get to the middle/inner ear (due to blockages)

congenital adrenal hyperplasia (kon-JEN-ih-tal ad-REE-nal HAI-per-PLAY-zhah) genetic disease in which the adrenal gland is overdeveloped, resulting in a deficiency of certain hormones and an overproduction of others

congenital anomaly (con-JIN-ih-tal ah-NAW-moh-lee) irregular condition that is present at the time of birth

congenital heart defect (con-JEN-ih-tal HART DEE-fekt) flaw in the structure of the heart, present at birth

congestive cardiomyopathy (con-JES-tiv KAR-dee-oh-mai-AW-pah-thee) heart cavity is unable to pump all the blood out of it (congestive) and becomes stretched (dilated), which causes weak/slow pumping of blood

congestive heart failure (con-JES-tiv HART FAYL-yir) heart failure characterized by the heart cavity being unable to pump all the blood out of it (congestive)

conjunctivitis (con-JUNK-tih-VAI-tis) inflammation of the conjunctiva (also known as pink eye)

constipation (KAWN-stih-PAY-shun) difficulty passing feces

continuous subcutaneous insulin infusion (kun-TIN-yoo-us SUB-koo-TAY-nee-us IN-suh-lin in-FYOO-zhun) continuous injection of insulin into the blood from a pump inserted under the skin

contraction (con-TRAK-shun) shortening or tightening of a muscle (during labor, uterine muscles contract)

corneal abrasion (KOR-nee-al a-BRAY-zhun) scratch on the cornea

corneal transplant (KOR-nee-al TRANZ-plant) replacement of damaged cornea with donated tissue

corneal xerosis (KOR-nee-al ZER-oh-sis) dryness of the cornea

coronary arterectomy (KOR-ah-NAR-ee AR-ter-EK-toh-mee) surgical removal of a coronary artery

coronary artery bypass graft (CABG) (KOR-ah-NAR-ee AR-ter-ee BAI-pas GRAFT) borrowed piece of blood vessel used to bypass a blocked artery in the heart

coronary artery bypass surgery (KOR-ah-NAR-ee AR-ter-ee BAI-pas SIR-jir-ee) surgery to bypass a blocked artery in the heart

coronary circulation (KOR-ah-NAR-ee SIR-kyoo-LAY-shun) circulation of blood from the heart to the heart muscle

coronary thrombosis (KOR-ah-NAR-ee throm-BOH-sis) obstruction of a coronary artery by a clot

corticotropin (KOR-tih-koh-TROH-pin) shorter name for adrenocorticotropic hormone

costalgia (kaws-TAL-jah) rib pain

costectomy (kaws-TEK-toh-mee) removal of a rib

costochondritis (KAW-stoh-kawn-DRAI-tis) inflammation of the cartilage of the rib

cranial hematoma (KRAY-nee-al HEE-mah-TOH-mah) a hematoma beneath the skull

craniectomy (KRAY-nee-EK-toh-mee) removal of a portion of the skull (bone is not replaced)

craniomalacia (KRAY-nee-oh-mah-LAY-shah) abnormal softening of the skull

craniosclerosis (KRAY-nee-oh-skleh-ROH-sis) abnormal hardening of the skull

craniostenosis (KRAY-nee-oh-steh-NOH-sis) abnormal narrowing of the skull

craniosynostosis (KRAY-nee-oh-SIN-aw-STOH-sis) the premature fusing of the skull bones

craniotomy (KRAY-nee-AW-toh-mee) removal of a portion of the skull (bone is later replaced)

crepitation (kreh-pih-TAY-shun) from Latin, for "rattle" or "creaking"; a crackling sound heard in joints

crust (KRUST) dried substance (i.e., blood, pus) on the skin

cryosurgery (KRAI-oh-SIR-juh-ree) destruction of tissue through freezing

cryptorchidism (krip-TOR-kih-DIZ-um) hidden testicle

culture & sensitivity (KUL-chur and sin-sih-TIH-vih-tee) growing microorganisms in isolation in order to determine which drugs it might respond to

cyanidrosis (sai-yan-ih-DROH-sis) blue sweat

cyanosis (SAI-ah-NOH-sis) a bluish appearance to the skin; a sign that the tissue isn't receiving enough oxygen

cyclokeratitis (SAI-cloh-keh-rah-TAI-tis) inflammation of the ciliary body and cornea

cycloplegia (SAI-kloh-PLEE-jah) paralysis of the ciliary body

cycloplegic (SAI-kloh-PLEE-jik) drug that paralyzes the ciliary body

cyclotomy (sai-KLAW-toh-mee) incision into the ciliary body

cystalgia (sis-TAL-jah) pain in the bladder

cystectomy (sis-TEK-toh-mee) surgical removal of the bladder

cystitis (sis-TAI-tis) inflammation of the bladder

cystocele (SIS-toh-seel) hernia of the bladder

cystodynia (SIS-toh-DAI-nee-ah) pain in the bladder

cystogram (SIS-toh-gram) image of the bladder

cystography (sis-TAW-grah-fee) process for recording/imaging the bladder

cystolith (SIS-toh-lith) stone in the bladder

cystolithectomy (sis-toh-lih-THEK-toh-mee) surgical removal of a stone in the bladder

cystoma (sis-TOH-mah) tumor of the bladder

cystoplegia (SIS-toh-PLEE-jah) bladder paralysis

cystoptosis (sis-TOP-toh-sis) downward displacement of the bladder

cystorrhexis (SIS-toh-REK-sis) rupture of the bladder

cystoscopy (sis-TAW-skoh-pee) process for examining the bladder

cystospasm (SIS-toh-SPAZ-um) involuntary contraction of the bladder

cystostomy (sis-TAW-stoh-mee) creation of an opening in the bladder

cystoureteritis (SIS-toh-yoo-REE-ter-AI-tis) inflammation of the bladder and urethra

cystourethrocele (SIS-toh-yoo-REE-throh-seel) hernia of the bladder and urethra

cytapheresis (SAI-tah-fer-EE-sis) apheresis to remove cellular material

D

dacryoadenalgia (DAK-ree-oh-AD-en-AL-jah) pain in the tear gland

dacryoadenectomy (DAK-ree-oh-AD-en-EK-toh-mee) removal of the tear gland

dacryoadenitis (DAK-ree-oh-AD-en-AI-tis) inflammation of the tear gland

dacryocystalgia (DAK-ree-oh-sis-TAL-jah) pain in the tear sac

dacryocystectomy (DAK-ree-oh-sis-TEK-toh-mee) removal of the tear sac

dacryocystitis (DA-kree-oh-sis-TAI-tis) inflammation of the tear sac

dacryocystorhinostomy (DAK-ree-oh-SIS-toh-rai-NAW-stoh-mee) creation of an opening between the tear sac and the nose

dacryocystotomy (DAK-ree-oh-sis-TAWT-oh-mee) incision into the tear sac

dacryohemorrhea (DAK-ree-oh-HIM-oh-REE-ah) discharge of blood in the tears

dacryolith (DAK-ree-oh-lith) hard formation (stone) in the tear system

dacryolithiasis (DAK-ree-oh-lih-THAI-ah-sis) presence of hard formations (stones) in the tear system

dacryopyorrhea (DAK-ree-oh-pai-REE-ah) discharge of pus in tears

dacryorrhea (DAK-ree-oh-REE-ah) excessive tearing

dacryostenosis (DAK-ree-oh-steh-NOH-sis) narrowing of the tear duct

dactylitis (DAK-tih-LAI-tis) finger inflammation

decubitus ulcer (deh-KYOO-bih-tus UL-sir) bed sore

deep vein thrombosis (DEEP VAYN throm-BOH-sis) the formation of a blood clot deep in the body, most commonly in the leg

delirium (deh-LEER-ee-um) brief loss of mental function

dementia (da-MEN-chah) loss/decline in mental function

dentalgia (den-TAL-jah) tooth pain

dentist (DEN-tist) specialist in teeth

dentistry (DEN-tis-tree) branch of medicine dealing with teeth

dentifrice (DEN-ti-fris) toothpaste

depigmentation (DE-pig-men-TAY-shun) loss of skin pigmentation

dermabrasion (der-mah-BRAY-zhun) rubbing or scraping away the outer surface of skin

dermatitis (der-mah-TAI-tis) inflammation of the skin

dermatoconiosis (der-ma-toh-COH-nee-oh-sis) a skin condition caused by dirt

dermatofibroma (der-MA-toh-fai-BROH-mah) a fibrous skin tumor

dermatolysis (der-mah-TAW-lih-sis) loss of skin

dermatomycosis (der-mah-toh-mai-KOH-sis) a fungal skin condition

dermatoscope (dir-MA-toh-SKOHP) instrument used to look at the skin

dermatosis (der-mah-TOH-sis) skin condition

dermoid cyst (DER-moyd SIST) ovarian cyst containing skin and sometimes hair, teeth, bone, or cartilage

dermopathy (der-MAW-pa-thee) skin disease

dermoscopy (der-MAW-skoh-pee) procedure for looking at the skin

diabetes mellitus (DAI-ah-BEE-teez MEH-lih-tis) metabolic disease characterized by excessive urination and hyperglycemia

diabetic ketoacidosis (DAI-ah-BEH-tik KEE-toh-ASS-ih-DOH-sis) acidity of the blood caused by the presence of ketone bodies produced when the body is unable to burn sugar; thus, it must burn fat for energy

diaphoresis (DAI-ah-for-EE-sis) profuse sweating

diaphragmatocele (dai-a-frag-MAT-o-seel) hernia of the diaphragm

diarrhea (DAI-ah-REE-ah) passing of fluid or unformed feces

diastolic pressure (DAI-ah-STAW-lik PRESH-ir) pressure exerted on blood vessels when the heart is relaxed

digital rectal exam (DIJ-ih-tal REK-tal ek-ZAM) examination of the prostate using a finger inserted into the rectum

dilated cardiomyopathy (DAI-lay-ted KAR-dee-oh-mai-AW-pah-thee) see *congestive cardiomyopathy*

diplopia (dih-PLOH-pee-ah) double vision

dipsogenic (DIP-soh-JIN-ik) creating thirst

diuresis (DAI-yur-EE-sis) excessive urination

diuretic (DAI-yur-IT-ik) agent that causes urination

duodenectomy (doo-AW-den-EK-toh-mee) surgical removal of the duodenum

duodenitis (doo-AH-den-AI-tis) inflammation of the duodenum

duritis (dur-AI-tis) inflammation of the dura

dysentery (DIS-en-TER-ee) another name for diarrhea

dysesthesia (DIS-es-THEE-zhah) bad feeling

dyskinesia (dis-kih-NEE-zhah) inability to control movement

dyslexia (dis-LEK-see-ah) difficulty reading

dysmenorrhea (DIS-men-oh-REE-ah) painful menstruation

dysmetabolic syndrome (DIS-meh-tah-BAW-lik SIN-drohm) combination of medical disorders associated with faulty metabolism

dyspareunia (dis-pah-ROO-nee-ah) painful sexual intercourse

dyspepsia (dis-PEP-see-ah) bad digestion

dysphasia (dis-FAY-zhah) difficulty speaking

dysphonia (dis-FON-ia) "bad voice condition"; hoarseness

dysphoria (dis-FOR-ee-ah) a negative emotional state

dysplastic nevus (dis-PLAS-tic NEE-vus) a mole with bad changes/formations (often precancerous)

dyspnea (disp-NEE-ah) difficulty breathing

dysrhythmia (dis-RITH-mee-ah) irregular heartbeat

dystaxia (dis-TAK-see-ah) poor coordination

dystocia (dis-TOH-shee-ah) difficult labor

dystonia (dis-TOH-nee-ah) poor muscle tone

dysuria (dis-YUR-ee-ah) painful urination

E

ear instillation (ear in-stil-AY-shun) ear drops

ear lavage (ear lah-VAJ) rinsing/washing the external ear canal (usually to remove ear wax); from Latin, for *to wash, bathe*

ecchymosis (eh-kih-MOH-sis) from Greek, for "to pour out"; a larger bruise

echocardiogram (EK-oh-KAR-dee-oh-GRAM) image of the heart produced using sound waves; it is the same procedure as an ultrasound performed on pregnant women, but done on the heart

echocardiography (EK-oh-KAR-dee-AW-grah-fee) use of sound waves to produce an image of the heart

echoencephalography (EH-koh-in-SEH-fah-LAW-grah-fee) procedure used to examine the brain using sound waves

eclampsia (eh-KLAMP-see-ah) severe, life-threatening complication of pregnancy characterized by seizures

ectopic pregnancy (ek-TOP-ik PREG-nan-see) implantation of a fertilized egg in a place other than the uterus

ectropion (ek-TROH-pee-on) outward turning of the eyelid, away from the eye

eczema (EK-zeh-mah) from Greek, for "to boil over"; a red, itchy rash that may weep or ooze, then become crusted and scaly

efferent nerve (EH-fir-ent NIRV) a nerve that carries impulses away from the central nervous system

effusion (ee-FYOO-zhun) fluid buildup

ejaculation (ee-JAK-yoo-LAY-shun) emission of semen from the urethra

electrocardiogram (eh-LEK-troh-KAR-dee-oh-GRAM) record of the electrical currents of the heart

electrocardiography (eh-LEK-troh-KAR-dee-AW-grah-fee) procedure for recording the electrical currents of the heart

electrocauterization (e-LEK-troh-KAW-ter-ai-ZAY-shun) using electricity to destroy tissue by burning it

electrodesiccation (e-LEK-troh-deh-sih-KAY-shun) using electricity to destroy tissue by drying it

electroencephalography (EEG) (eh-LEK-troh-in-SEH-fah-LAW-grah-fee) procedure used to examine the electrical activity of the brain

electromyogram (eh-lek-troh-MAI-o-gram) record of the electrical activity of a muscle

electromyography (eh-LEK-troh-mai-AW-grah-fee) procedure for measuring the electrical activity of a muscle

elliptocyte (ee-LIP-toh-SAIT) oval-shaped red blood cell

elliptocytosis (ee-LIP-toh-SAI-toh-sis) condition characterized by an increase in the number of oval-shaped red blood cells

embolectomy (EM-boh-LEK-toh-mee) surgical removal of an embolus

embolism (EM-boh-LIZ-um) blockage in a blood vessel caused by an embolus

embolus (EM-boh-lus) mass of matter present in the blood

emphysema (em-fi-ZEE-ma) a disease that causes the alveoli to lose their elasticity; patients can inhale but have difficulty exhaling

empyema (em-pie-EE-mah) pus inside (the chest)

encephalalgia (in-SE-ful-AL-jah) brain pain

encephalitis (in-SEF-ah-LAI-tis) inflammation of the brain

encephalmyeloneuropathy (in-SEF-ah-loh-MAI-el-oh-nir-AW-pah-thee) disease of the brain, spinal cord, and nerves

encephalocele (en-SEF-ah-loh-SEEL) hernia of the brain (normally through a defect in the skull)

encephalography (en-SEH-fah-LOH-grah-fee) procedure for studying the brain

encephalomyelitis (in-SEF-ah-loh-MAI-el-AI-tis) inflammation of the brain and spinal cord

encephalopathy (in-SEF-ah-LAW-pah-thee) disease of the brain

encephalopyosis (in-SEF-ah-loh-pai-OH-sis) a pus-filled abscess in the brain

endarterectomy (END-ar-ter-EK-toh-me) surgical removal of the inside of an artery

endocarditis (EN-doh-kar-DAI-tis) inflammation of the tissue lining the inside of the heart

endocardium (EN-doh-KAR-dee-um) tissue lining the inside of the heart

endocervicitis (EN-doh-SER-vih-SAI-tis) inflammation of the inside of the cervix

endocrine (EN-doh-krin) secrete internally (i.e., into the bloodstream)

endocrinologist (EN-doh-krih-NAW-loh-jist) specialist in internal secretions

endometriosis (EN-doh-MEE-tree-OH-sis) condition in which endometrium cells appear and grow outside the uterus

endometritis (EN-doh-meh-TRAI-tis) inflammation of the endometrium

endometrium (EN-doh-MEE-tree-um) inner layer of uterine tissue

endophthalmitis (EN-dof-thal-MAI-tis) inflammation of the inside of the eye (often a complication from intraocular surgery)

endoscope (EN-doh-SKOHP) instrument used to look inside

endoscopic retrograde cholangiopancreatography (EN-doh-SKAW-pik REH-troh-GRAYD KOHL-AN-jee-oh-PAN-kree-ah-TAW-grah-fee) procedure used to examine the bile ducts and pancreas in which an endoscope is passed backward from the digestive tract into the bile duct

endoscopy (en-DAW-skoh-pee) procedure of looking inside

endotracheal intubation (en-doh-TRAY-kee-al in-too-BAY-shun) insertion of a tube inside the trachea

endovascular neurosurgery (EN-doh-VAS-kyoo-lar NIR-oh-SIR-jir-ee) surgery on the nervous system performed by entering the body through blood vessels

enterectomy (en-ter-EK-toh-mee) surgical removal of the intestines

enterocele (EN-ter-oh-seel) hernia of the intestines

enterodynia (EN-ter-oh-DAI-nee-ah) pain in the intestines

enteropathy (EN-ter-AW-pah-thee) disease of the intestines

enterorrhaphy (en-ter-OR-ah-fee) suture of the intestines

enterotomy (en-ter-AW-toh-mee) incision into the intestines

entropion (en-TROH-pee-on) inward turning of the eyelid, toward the eye

enucleation (eh-NOO-clee-AY-shun) removal of an eye

enuresis (EN-yur-EE-sis) involuntary urination

epicardium (EH-pee-KAR-dee-um) tissue lining the outside of the heart

epidermal (eh-pi-DER-mal) pertaining to the skin

epidermal tumor (eh-pi-DER-mal TOO-mur) tumor on the skin

epididymectomy (EP-ih-DID-ih-MEK-toh-mee) surgical removal of the epididymis

epididymitis (EP-ih-DID-ih-MAI-tis) inflammation of the epididymis

epididymo-orchitis (EP-ih-DID-ih-moh-or-KAI-tis) inflammation of the testicles and epididymis

epididymotomy (EP-ih-DID-ih-MAW-toh-mee) incision into the epididymis

epidural anesthetic (eh-pih-DIR-al an-es-THET-ik) anesthetic applied in the dural region of the spinal cord

epidural hematoma (EH-pi-DIR-al HEE-mah-TOH-mah) a hematoma located on top of the dura

epigastric (eh-pee-GAS-trik) upper center portion of the abdomen

epilepsy (eh-pih-LEP-see) a disease marked by seizures

epinephrine (EH-pee-NEF-rin) hormone secreted by the adrenal gland (from Greek; see also *adrenaline*)

episiorrhaphy (eh-PEE-zee-OR-ah-fee) suture of the vulva

episiostenosis (eh-PEE-zee-oh-stih-NOH-sis) narrowing of the vulvar opening

episiotomy (eh-PEE-zee-AW-toh-mee) incision into the vulva

epistaxis (eh-pee-STAKS-is) nosebleed

erosion (ee-ROH-zhun) loss of skin

erythema (eh-rih-THEE-ma) from Greek, for "redness"; redness

erythrocyanosis (eh-RIH-throh-SAI-an-OH-sis) a red and/or blue discoloration of the skin

erythrocyte (eh-RIH-throh-SAIT) red blood cell

erythrocytosis (eh-RIH-throh-sai-TOH-sis) abnormal increase in the number of red blood cells

erythroderma (eh-RIH-throh-DER-ma) red skin

esophagalgia (eh-SAWF-ah-GAL-jah) pain in the esophagus

esophageal carcinoma (eh-SAWF-ah-JEE-al KAR-sih-NOH-mah) cancerous tumor of the esophagus

esophagectomy (eh-SAW-fah-JEK-toh-mee) surgical removal of the esophagus

esophagitis (eh-SAWF-ah-JAI-tis) inflammation of the esophagus

esophagogastroduodenoscopy (eh-SAW-fah-goh-GAS-stroh-DOO-aw-den-AW-skoh-pee) procedure for looking inside the esophagus, stomach, and duodenum

esophagogastroplasty (eh-SAW-fah-goh-GAS-troh-PLAS-tee) surgical reconstruction of the esophagus and stomach

esophagoscopy (eh-SAW-fah-GAW-skoh-pee) procedure for looking inside the esophagus

esotropia (AY-soh-TROH-pee-ah) inward turning of the eye, toward the nose

euglycemia (YOO-glai-SEE-mee-ah) good blood sugar

eupepsia (yoo-PEP-see-ah) good digestion

euphoria (yoo-FOR-ee-ah) a positive emotional state

eupnea (YOOP-nee-yah) good/normal breathing

euthyroid (YOO-thai-royd) a normal functioning thyroid

eutocia (yoo-TOH-shee-ah) normal labor

excisional biopsy (ek-SIH-zhun-al BAI-op-see) removal of an entire lesion for examination (to cut it out)

excoriation (eks-kor-ee-A-shun) a scratch

exocrine (EKS-oh-krin) secrete externally through ducts to the surface of an organ (i.e., sweat glands and salivary glands)

exophthalmos (EKS-of-THAL-mohs) protrusion of the eye out of the eye socket

exophthalmus (EKS-of-THAL-mus) protrusion of the eye out of the eye socket

exostosis (ek-saw-STOH-sis) an abnormal growth of bone out of another bone

exotropia (EK-soh-TROH-pee-ah) outward turning of the eye, away from the nose

expectorant (eks-PEK-tor-ant) a drug that encourages explusion of material from the lungs

expectoration (eks-pec-tor-A-shun) coughing or spitting material out of the lungs

external fixation (EKS-tir-nal fik-SAY-shun) a fixation of a fractured bone from the outside (i.e., using a cast or splint)

extracorporeal shock wave lithotripsy (ESWL) (EKS-trah-cor-POR-ee-al SHOK WAYV LIH-thoh-TRIP-see) breakdown of kidney stones using sound waves generated outside the body

F

fasciectomy (FA-shee-EK-toh-mee) removal of fascia

fasciitis (FA-shee-AI-tis) inflammation of the fascia

fasciodesis (FA-shoh-DEE-sis) binding of fascia

fascioplasty (FA-shoh-PLAS-tee) reconstruction of fascia

fasciorrhaphy (fah-SHOR-ah-fee) suturing of fascia

fasciotomy (FA-shee-AW-toh-mee) incision into fascia

fecal occult blood test (FOBT) (FEE-kal ah-KULT BLUD TEST) test of feces to discover blood not visibly apparent

fetometry (fee-TAW-meh-tree) procedure for measuring the fetus

fissure (FIH-zhur) from Latin, for a "split" or "divide"; a crack in the skin

fistula (FIS-tyoo-la) any abnormal passageway in the body that shouldn't be there

flatus (FLAH-tus) medical term for passing gas

fracture (FRAK-shur) from Latin, for "break"; a bone break

fulguration (FUL-gur-AY-shun) use of electric current to destroy tissue

G

galactorrhea (gah-LAK-toh-REE-ah) discharge of milk

gangliitis (GAN-glee-AI-tis) inflammation of the ganglion

ganglioma (GAN-glee-OH-mah) ganglion tumor

gastralgia (gas-TRAL-jah) stomach pain

gastrectomy (gas-TREK-toh-mee) surgical removal of the stomach

gastritis (gas-TRAI-tis) inflammation of the stomach

gastroduodenostomy (GAS-troh-doo-AH-den-AW-stoh-mee) creation of an opening between the stomach and the duodenum

gastrodynia (GAS-troh-DAI-nee-ah) stomach pain

gastroenteritis (GAS-troh-EN-ter-AI-tis) inflammation of the stomach and intestines

gastroenterocolitis (GAS-troh-EN-ter-oh-coh-LAI-tis) inflammation of the stomach, intestine, and colon

gastroenterologist (GAS-troh-EN-ter-AW-loh-jist) specialist in the stomach and intestines

gastroenterology (GAS-troh-EN-ter-AW-loh-jee) study of the stomach and intestines

gastroenterostomy (GAS-troh-EN-ter-AW-stoh-mee) creation of an opening between the stomach and the intestines

gastroesophageal reflux disease (GERD) (GAS-troh-eh-SOF-ah-JEE-al REE-fluks dih-ZEEZ) disease in which acid comes up from the stomach and damages the esophagus

gastrojejunostomy (GAS-troh-JEH-joo-NAW-stoh-mee) creation of an opening between the stomach and the jejunum

gastromalacia (GAS-troh-mah-LAY-shah) softening of the stomach

gastroparesis (GAS-troh-par-EE-sis) partial paralysis of the stomach

gastropexy (GAS-troh-PEK-see) surgical fixation of the stomach

gastroplasty (GAS-troh-PLAS-tee) surgical reconstruction of the stomach

gastroscope (GAS-troh-SKOHP) instrument for looking at the stomach

gastroscopy (gas-TRAW-skoh-pee) procedure for looking at the stomach

general anesthetic (JEH-nir-al an-es-THET-ik) anesthetic that causes complete loss of consciousness

genu valgum (JEH-noo VAL-gum) bow-legged

genu varum (JEH-noo VAH-rum) knock-kneed

gingival hyperplasia (JIN-jih-val HAI-per-PLAY-zhah) overformation of gum tissue

gingivalgia (JIN-jih-VAL-jah) gum pain

gingivectomy (JIN-jiv-EK-toh-mee) surgical removal of gum tissue

gingivitis (JIN-jih-VAI-tis) inflammation of the gums

gingivoglossitis (JIN-jih-voh-glaw-SAI-tis) inflammation of the gums and tongue

gingivoplasty (JIN-jiv-oh-PLAS-tee) surgical reconstruction of gum tissue

gingivostomatitis (JIN-jih-voh-STOH-mah-TAI-tis) inflammation of the mouth and gums

glomerulonephritis (gloh-MER-yoo-loh-neh-FRAI-tis) inflammation of the kidneys involving primarily the glomeruli

glomerulopathy (gloh-MER-yoo-LAW-pah-thee) disease of the kidney involving primarily the glomeruli

glomerulosclerosis (gloh-MER-yoo-loh-skleh-ROH-sis) hardening of the glomeruli

glossopathy (glaws-AW-pah-thee) disease of the tongue

glossoplasty (GLAWS-oh-PLAS-tee) surgical reconstruction of the tongue

glossoplegia (GLAW-soh-PLEE-jah) paralysis of the tongue

glossorrhaphy (glaws-OR-ah-fee) suture of the tongue

glossotomy (glaws-AW-toh-mee) incision into the tongue

glossotrichia (GLAWS-oh-TRIK-ee-ah) overdevelopment of bumps on the tongue, making the tongue appear to be hairy

glucagon (GLOO-kah-gawn) hormone secreted by the pancreas that stimulates the liver to increase blood sugar levels

glucocorticoid (GLOO-koh-KOR-tih-koyd) a hormone produced by the adrenal cortex with a role in carbohydrate metabolism

gluconeogenesis (GLOO-koh-NEE-oh-JIN-eh-sis) the formation of glucose from noncarbohydrate sources

glucosuria (GLOO-koh-SOO-ree-ah) sugar in the urine

glycemic index (glai-SEE-mik IN-deks) ranking of food based on the way it affects sugar levels in the blood

glycolysis (glai-KAW-lih-sis) breakdown of sugar

glycopenia (GLAI-koh-PEE-nee-ah) deficiency of sugar

glycosuria (GLAI-koh-shur-EE-ah) sugar in the urine

goiter (GOY-ter) swollen thyroid gland

gonadogenesis (goh-NAD-oh-JIN-eh-sis) creation/development of gonads

gonadotropin (goh-NAD-oh-TROH-pin) hormone that stimulates the gonads

gonads (GOH-nadz) the pair of organs used for sexual reproduction; testicles in males and ovaries in females

gonorrhea (GAW-noh-REE-ah) discharge from the gonads

graphospasm (gra-foh-SPAZ-um) writer's cramp

gravida (GRAH-vid-ah) another term for pregnant

gynecologist (GAI-neh-KAW-loh-jist) specialist in medical issues specific to women

gynecology (GAI-neh-KAW-loh-jee) study of medical issues specific to women

gynecomastia (GAI-neh-koh-MAS-tee-ah) development of breast tissue in males

H

hemarthrosis (hee-mar-THROH-sis) blood in a joint

hematemesis (HEM-at-EM-eh-sis) vomiting blood

hemathidrosis (heh-mat-ih-DROH-sis) sweating blood

hematocrit (hee-MAT-oh-krit) test to judge or separate the blood; used to determine the ratio of red blood cells to total blood volume

hematology (HEE-mah-TAW-loh-jee) study of the blood

hematoma (HEE-mah-TOH-mah) mass of blood within an organ, cavity, or tissue

hematopoiesis (heh-MAH-toh-poh-EE-sis) formation of blood cells

hematosalpinx (heh-MAT-oh-SAL-pinks) blockage in a fallopian tube caused by blood

hematuria (HEE-mah-TUR-ee-ah) bloody urination

hemianopsia (HEH-mee-an-OP-see-ah) blindness in half the visual field

hemicolectomy (HEH-mee-koh-LEK-toh-mee) surgical removal of half (a portion) of the colon

heminephrectomy (HEH-mee-neh-FREK-toh-mee) surgical removal of half a kidney

heminephroureterectomy (HEH-mee-NEH-froh-yoo-REE-ter-EK-toh-mee) surgical removal of half a kidney and a ureter

hemiparesis (HEH-mee-puh-REE-sis) partial paralysis on half of the body

hemiplegia (HEH-mee-PLEE-jah) paralysis on half the body

hemodialysis (HEE-moh-dai-AL-ah-sis) procedure for removing waste from the bloodstream

hemoglobin (HEE-moh-GLOH-bin) iron-containing pigment in red blood cells that carries oxygen to the cells

hemoglobinopathy (HEE-maw-GLOH-bin-AW-pah-thee) disease of the hemoglobin

hemolysis (hee-MAW-lih-sis) breakdown of blood cells

hemolytic anemia (HEE-moh-LIH-tik ah-NEE-mee-ah) anemia caused by the destruction of red blood cells

hemophilia (HEE-moh-FEE-lee-ah) condition in which the blood doesn't clot, thus causing excessive bleeding

hemoptysis (heem-op-TIS-is) coughing up blood

hemorrhage (HEM-oh-RIJ) excessive blood loss

hemorrhagic stroke (HEM-oh-RA-jik STROHK) a stroke where blood loss is caused by the rupture of a blood vessel

hemorrhoid (HEM-oh-ROID) inflammation of the veins surrounding the anus

hemorrhoidectomy (HEM-oh-roi-DEK-toh-mee) surgical removal of hemorrhoids

hemostatic (HEE-moh-STAT-ik) drug that stops the flow of blood

hemothorax (heem-o-THOR-aks) blood in the chest

hepatectomy (HEP-ah-TEK-toh-me) surgical removal of the liver

hepaticogastrostomy (heh-PAT-ih-koh-gas-TRAW-stoh-me) creation of an opening between the liver and the stomach

hepaticotomy (heh-PAT-ih-KAW-toh-me) incision into the liver

hepatitis (HEH-pah-TAI-tis) inflammation of the liver

hepatocarcinoma (heh-PAT-oh-KAR-sih-NOH-mah) cancerous tumor of the liver

hepatoma (HEH-pah-TOH-mah) tumor of the liver

hepatomalacia (heh-PAT-oh-mah-LAY-shah) softening of the liver

hepatomegaly (heh-PAT-oh-MEG-ah-lee) enlargement of the liver

hepatopexy (heh-PAT-oh-PEK-see) surgical fixation of the liver

hepatoptosis (heh-PAT-op-TOH-sis) downward displacement of the liver

hepatosclerosis (heh-PAT-oh-skleh-ROH-sis) hardening of the liver

hepatosplenitis (hih-PAT-oh-SPLEEN-ai-tis) inflammation of the liver and spleen

hepatosplenomegaly (heh-PAT-oh-SPLEE-noh-MEH-gah-lee) enlargement of the liver and spleen

hernia (HER-nee-ah) rupture or protrusion of an organ through the wall that normally contains it

herniorrhaphy (her-nee-OR-ah-fee) suture of a hernia

heterograft (HEH-ter-oh-GRAFT) skin transplant taken from a species other than the patient's

hidradenitis (hih-dra-deh-NAI-tis) inflammation of the sweat glands

hidradenoma (hih-dra-deh-NOH-mah) tumor of the sweat gland

hidropoiesis (hih-droh-poh-EE-sis) the formation of sweat

hirsutism (HIR-soo-tizm) excessive growth of facial and body hair in women

homograft (HOH-moh-GRAFT) skin transplant taken from another member of the patient's species

hydrarthrosis (hai-drar-THROH-sis) water (fluid) in a joint

hydrocele (HAI-droh-SEEL) fluid-filled mass in a testicle

hydrocelectomy (HAI-droh-seel-EK-toh-mee) surgical removal of a hydrocele

hydrocephaly (HAI-droh-SEH-fah-lee) abnormal accumulation of spinal fluid in the brain

hydronephrosis (HAI-droh-neh-FROH-sis) kidney condition caused by the obstruction of urine flow

hydrophobia (HAI-druh-FOH-bee-ah) fear of water

hydrosalpinx (HAI-droh-SAL-pinks) blockage in a fallopian tube caused by water (or any clear fluid)

hyperacusis (HAI-per-ah-KOO-sis) excessively sensitive hearing

hyperbilirubinemia (HAI-per-BIH-lee-ROO-bin-EE-mee-ah) excessive bilirubin in the blood

hypercalcemia (HAI-per-kal-SEE-mee-ah) excessive calcium in the blood

hypercapnia (hai-per-CAP-nee-yah) condition of having excessive carbon dioxide in the blood

hypercarbia (hai-per-CAR-bee-yah) excessive carbon dioxide

hypercholesterolemia (HAI-per-koh-LES-ter-aw-LEE-mee-ah) excessive cholesterol in the blood

hypercoagulability (HAI-per-koh-AG-yoo-lah-BIL-ih-tee) increased ability of the blood to coagulate

hyperemesis (HAI-per-EM-eh-sis) excessive vomiting

hyperemesis gravidarum (HAI-per-eh-MEE-sis GRAV-ih-DAR-um) excessive pregnancy-related vomiting; an extreme form of the more common morning sickness

hyperesthesia (HAI-per-es-THEE-zhah) increased sensation

hyperglycemia (HAI-per-glai-SEE-mee-ah) high blood sugar

hypergonadism (HAI-per-GOH-nad-izm) excessive secretion of the sex glands

hyperhidrosis (hai-per-hih-DROH-sis) excessive sweating

hyperkalemia (HAI-per-kah-LEE-mee-ah) excessive potassium in the blood

hyperkeratosis (hai-per-ker-ah-TOH-sis) excessive growth of horny skin

hyperkinesia (hai-per-kih-NEE-zhah) increase in muscle movement or activity

hyperlipidemia (HAI-per-lih-pih-DEE-mee-ah) excessive fat in the blood

hypermastia (HAI-per-MAS-tee-ah) excessively large breasts (can also refer to an abnormal number of breasts)

hypermelanosis (hai-per-mel-an-OH-sis) excessive melanin in the skin

hypernatremia (HAI-per-nah-TREE-mee-ah) excessive salt in the blood

hypernephroma (HAI-per-neh-FROH-mah) cancer of the kidneys; also called *renal cell carcinoma*

hyperopia (HAI-per-OH-pee-ah) farsightedness

hyperparathyroidism (HAI-per-PAR-ah-THAI-roid-IZM) overproduction by the parathyroid glands

hyperphosphatemia (HAI-per-FAWS-fay-TEE-mee-ah) excessive phosphate in the blood

hyperpigmentation (hai-per-pig-men-TAY-shun) excessive pigment in the skin

hyperpituitarism (HAI-per-pih-TOO-ih-tar-IZM) overfunctioning of the pituitary gland

hyperpnea (hai-perp-NEE-ah) heavy breathing

hypersplenism (HAI-per-SPLEE-nizm) increased spleen activity

hypertension (HAI-per-TEN-shun) high blood pressure

hyperthyroidism (HAI-per-THAI-roid-IZM) overproduction by the thyroid

hypertonia (hai-per-TOH-nee-yah) increased muscle tone or tightness

hypertrophic cardiomyopathy (HAI-per-TROH-fik KAR-dee-oh-mai-AW-pah-thee) heart muscle becomes enlarged and blocks blood flow

hypertrophic spondylitis (HAI-per-TROH-fik spon-dih-LAI-tis) overdevelopment of the vertebrae causing inflammation

hypertrophy (hai-PER-troh-fee) overdevelopment of muscle tissue

hyperventilation (hai-per-ven-ti-LAY-shun) overbreathing; condition of having too much air flowing into and out of the lungs; leads to hypocapnia

hypervolemia (HAI-per-voh-LEE-mee-ah) increased blood volume

hypnotic (hip-NAWT-ik) a drug that aids sleep

hypoacusis (HAI-poh-ah-KOO-sis) excessively insensitive hearing

hypocapnia (hai-po-CAP-nee-yah) insufficient carbon dioxide

hypocarbia (hai-po-CAR-bee-yah) insufficient carbon dioxide

hypochondriac (hai-poh-KON-dree-ak) upper side portions of the abdomen

hypodermia (hai-poh-DER-mia) pertaining to beneath the skin

hypogastric (hai-poh-GAS-trik) lower center portion of the abdomen

hypoglycemia (HAI-poh-glai-SEE-mee-ah) low blood sugar

hypoglycemic (HAI-poh-glai-SEE-mik) pertaining to low blood sugar

hypogonadism (HAI-poh-GOH-nad-izm) undersecretion of the sex glands

hypohidrosis (hai-poh-hih-DROH-sis) diminished sweating

hypokinesia (hai-poh-kih-NEE-zhah) decrease in muscle movement or activity

hypomagnesemia (HAI-poh-MAG-nee-SEE-mee-ah) deficient magnesium in the blood

hypomania (HAI-poh-MAY-nee-ah) a mental state just below mania

hypomastia (HAI-poh-MAS-tee-ah) abnormally small breasts

hypomelanosis (hai-poh-mel-an-OH-sis) diminished melanin in the skin

hyponatremia (HAI-poh-nah-TREE-mee-ah) low sodium in the blood

hypoparathyroidism (HAI-poh-PAR-ah-THAI-roid-IZM) underproduction by the parathyroid

hypoperfusion (HAI-poh-per-FYOO-zhun) inadequate flow of blood

hypophysectomy (hai-PAWF-is-EK-toh-mee) removal of the pituitary gland

hypophysitis (hai-PAWF-ih-SAI-tis) inflammation of the pituitary gland

hypopigmentation (hai-poh-pig-men-TAY-shun) diminished pigment in the skin

hypopituitarism (HAI-poh-pih-TOO-ih-tar-IZM) condition caused by the undersecretion of the pituitary gland

hypopnea (hai-POP-nee-ah) shallow breathing

hypospadias (HAI-poh-SPAY-dee-as) birth defect in which the opening of the urethra is on the underside, instead of the end, of the penis

hypotension (HAI-poh-TEN-shun) low blood pressure

hypothyroidism (HAI-poh-THAI-roid-IZM) underproduction by the thyroid

hypotonia (hai-poh-TOH-nee-yah) decrease in muscle tone or tightness

hypoventilation (hai-po-ven-ti-LAY-shun) underbreathing; condition of having too little air flowing into and out of the lungs; leads to hypercapnia

hypovolemia (HAI-poh-voh-LEE-mee-ah) decreased blood volume

hypoxemia (hai-poks-EEM-ee-yah) insufficient oxygen in the blood

hypoxia (hai-POKS-ee-yah) insufficient oxygen

hysteralgia (HIS-ter-AL-jah) pain in the uterus

hysterectomy (HIS-ter-EK-toh-mee) surgical removal of the uterus

hysterocele (HIS-ter-oh-SEEL) hernia of the uterus

hysterodynia (HIS-ter-oh-DAI-nee-ah) pain in the uterus

hysterography (HIS-ter-AW-grah-fee) procedure for imaging the uterus

hysteropexy (HIS-ter-oh-PEK-see) surgical fixation of the uterus

hysteroptosis (HIS-ter-awp-TOH-sis) downward displacement of the uterus into the vagina

hysterorrhexis (HIS-ter-oh-REK-sis) rupture of the uterus

hysterosalpingectomy (HIS-ter-oh-SAL-pin-JEK-toh-mee) surgical removal of the uterus and fallopian tube

hysterosalpingogram (HIS-ter-oh-sal-PIN-goh-gram) record of the uterus and fallopian tubes

hysteroscope (HIS-ter-oh-SKOHP) instrument for examining the uterus

hysteroscopy (HIS-ter-AW-skoh-pee) procedure for examining the uterus

hysterotomy (HIS-ter-AW-toh-mee) incision into the uterus

I

ichthyosis (ik-thee-OH-sis) a condition in which the skin is dry and scaly, resembling fish scales

icterus (IK-ter-us) see *jaundice*

idiopathic (IH-dee-oh-PAH-thik) having no known cause or origin

ileitis (IH-lee-AI-tis) inflammation of the ileum

ileocolitis (IH-lee-oh-koh-LAI-tis) inflammation of the ileum and colon

ileocolostomy (IH-lee-oh-koh-LAW-stoh-mee) creation of an opening between the ileum and colon

ileorrhaphy (IH-lee-OR-ah-fee) suture of the ileum

ileostomy (IH-lee-AW-stoh-mee) creation of an opening in the ileum

ileotomy (IH-lee-AW-toh-mee) incision into the ileum

immunocompromised (ih-MYOO-noh-COM-proh-MAIZD) having an immune system incapable of responding normally and completely to a pathogen or disease

immunodeficiency (ih-MYOO-noh-deh-FIH-shin-see) immune system with decreased or compromised response to disease-causing organisms

immunoglobulin (im-MYOO-noh-GLAW-byoo-lin) protein that provides protection (immunity) against disease

immunologist (IM-myoo-NAW-loh-jist) specialist in the immune system

immunology (IM-myoo-NAW-loh-jee) study of the immune system

immunosuppression (ih-MYOO-noh-suh-PREH-shun) reduction in the activity of the body's immune system

impetigo (im-peh-TAI-goh) from Latin, for "to attack"; a highly contagious bacterial infection of the skin

in vitro fertilization (in VEE-troh FER-tih-lih-ZAY-shun) fertilization of an egg done in a test tube

incision and drainage (I&D) (in-SIH-zhun and DRAY-nij) to cut into a wound to allow trapped infected liquid to drain

incisional biopsy (in-SIH-zhun-al BAI-op-see) removal of a portion of a lesion for examination (to cut into)

incontinence (in-CON-tih-nentz) inability to control urination

induced abortion (in-DOOST ah-BOR-shun) the intentional termination of pregnancy

inferior vena cava (in-FEER-ee-or VEE-nah CAY-vah) portion of the vena cava that gathers blood from the lower portion of the body

inguinal (IN-gwin-al) lower side portions of the abdomen

insomnia (in-SOM-nee-ah) inability to sleep

insulin (IN-suh-lin) hormone secreted by the pancreas that controls the metabolism and uptake of sugar and fats

insulinoma (IN-suh-lin-OH-mah) tumor that secretes insulin (found in the insulin-producing cells in the pancreas)

interictal (IN-ter-IK-tal) time between seizures

internal fixation (IN-tir-nal fik-SAY-shun) the fixation of a fractured bone from the inside (i.e., using screws, pins, plates, etc.)

intracerebral hematoma (IN-trah-seh-REE-bral HEE-mah-TOH-mah) a hematoma located inside the brain

intracerebral hemorrhage (IN-trah-seh-REE-bral HIH-moh-rij) excessive bleeding inside the brain

intracorporeal lithotripsy (IN-trah-cor-POR-ee-al LIH-thoh-TRIP-see) breakdown of kidney stones using a device placed inside the body

intradermal (in-tra-DER-mal) pertaining to inside the skin

intraocular lens implant (IN-trah-AW-kyoo-lar LENZ IM-plant) insertion of a new lens inside the eye

intrapartum (IN-trah-PAR-tum) time during birth

intravitreal antibiotic (IN-trah-VEE-tree-al AN-tai-bai-AW-tiks) antibiotic administered directly into the vitreous gel liquid

iridalgia (IH-rid-AL-jah) pain in the iris

iridectomy (EAR-id-EK-toh-mee) removal of the iris

iridemia (EAR-ih-DEE-mee-ah) bleeding from the iris

iridocyclectomy (EAR-ih-doh-sai-KLEK-toh-mee) removal of the iris and ciliary body

iridocyclitis (EAR-ih-doh-sai-KLAI-tis) inflammation of the iris and ciliary body

iridokeratitis (EAR-ih-doh-keh-rah-TAI-tis) inflammation of the iris and cornea

iridokinesis (IR-ih-doh-kin-EE-sis) movement of the iris

iridopathy (EAR-ih-DOP-ah-thee) disease of the iris

iridotomy (EAR-id-AW-toh-mee) incision into the iris

iritis (ai-RAI-tis) inflammation of the iris

iron deficiency anemia (AI-ern deh-FIH-shin-see ah-NEE-mee-ah) anemia caused by inadequate iron intake

ischemia (ih-SKEE-mee-ah) blockage of blood flow to an organ

ischemic stroke (ih-SKEE-mik STROHK) a stroke where blood loss is caused by a blockage

J

jaundice (JAWN-dis) yellowing of skin, tissue, and fluids caused by increased levels of bilirubin in the blood

jejunitis (JE-joo-NAI-tis) inflammation of the jejunum

jejunoileitis (je-JOO-noh-IH-lee-AI-tis) inflammation of the jejunum and ileum

jejunorrhaphy (JE-joo-NOR-ah-fee) suture of the jejunum

jejunostomy (JE-joo-NAW-stoh-mee) creation of an opening in the jejunum

jejunotomy (JE-joo-NAW-toh-mee) incision into the jejunum

K

keloid (KEE-loid) overgrowth of scar tissue

keratalgia (KEH-rah-TAL-jah) pain in the cornea

keratitis (KEH-rah-TAI-tis) inflammation of the cornea

keratogenic (keh-RA-toh-jen-ik) causing horny tissue development

keratomalacia (ker-AH-toh-mah-LAY-shah) abnormal softening of the cornea

keratopathy (KEH-rah-TOP-ah-thee) disease of the cornea

keratoplasty (ker-A-toh-PLAS-tee) surgical reconstruction of the cornea

keratosis (keh-rah-TOH-sis) horny tissue condition

keratotomy (KER-ah-TAW-toh-mee) incision into the cornea

ketogenesis (KEE-toh-JIN-eh-sis) creation of ketone bodies

ketogenic diet (KEE-toh-JIN-ik DAI-et) diet that aids in the production of ketones in the body

ketolysis (kee-TAW-lih-sis) breakdown of ketones

ketonuria (kee-toh-NUR-ee-ah) presence of ketones in the urine

ketosis (kee-TOH-sis) condition characterized by elevated levels of ketone bodies in the blood

kidney dialysis (KID-nee dai-AL-ah-sis) procedure for removing waste from the blood (a shorter name for hemodialysis)

kleptomania (KLEP-toh-MAY-nee-ah) desire to steal

kyphosis (kai-FOH-sis) humped back—abnormal forward curvature of the upper spine

L

labyrinthectomy (LAB-uh-rinth-EK-toh-mee) removal of the labyrinth

labyrinthitis (LAB-uh-rinth-AI-tis) inflammation of the labyrinth

labyrinthotomy (LAB-uh-rinth-AW-toh-mee) incision into the labyrinth

lacrimation (LAH-krih-MAY-shun) the formation of tears (i.e., crying)

lactation (lak-TAY-shun) production of milk

lactogenic (LAK-toh-JIN-ik) causing the formation of milk

lactorrhea (LAK-toh-REE-ah) discharge of milk

laparocele (LAP-ar-oh-seel) abdominal hernia

laparoenterostomy (LAP-ar-oh-EN-ter-AW-stoh-mee) creation of an opening between the abdomen and the intestines

laparonephrectomy (LAP-ah-roh-neh-FREK-toh-mee) surgical removal of a kidney through the abdomen

laparoscope (LAP-ar-oh-skohp) instrument for looking inside the abdomen

laparoscopic adrenalectomy (LAP-rah-SKAW-pik ad-REE-nal-EK-toh-mee) removal of an adrenal gland by means of a laparascope

laparoscopic surgery (LAP-rah-SKAW-pik SIR-jir-ee) use of a laparoscope to perform minimally invasive surgery

laparoscopy (LAP-ar-AW-skoh-pee) procedure for looking inside the abdomen

laparosplenectomy (LAP-ah-roh-splee-NEK-toh-mee) surgical removal of the spleen through the abdomen

laparotomy (LAP-ar-AW-toh-mee) incision into the abdomen

laryngectomy (la-rin-JEK-toe-mee) removal of the larynx

laryngitis (la-rin-JAI-tis) inflammation of the larynx

laryngoplasty (la-rin-GO-plas-tee) reconstruction of the larynx

laryngotracheobronchitis (la-rin-go-tray-key-o-bron-KAI-tis) inflammation of the larynx, trachea, and bronchi

leukemia (loo-KEE-mee-ah) cancer of the blood or bone marrow characterized by the abnormal increase in white blood cells

leukocyte (LOO-koh-sait) white blood cell

leukocytosis (LOO-koh-sai-TOH-sis) increase in the number of white blood cells

leukoderma (loo-koh-DER-mah) white skin

leukopenia (LOO-koh-PEE-nee-ah) deficiency in white blood cells

leukorrhea (LOO-koh-REE-ah) white vaginal discharge

lipectomy (lih-PEK-toh-mee) removal of fatty tissue

liposuction (LAI-poh-SUK-shun) removal of fatty tissue using a vacuum

lithectomy (lih-THEK-toh-mee) surgical removal of a stone in the bladder

lithocystotomy (LIH-thoh-SIS-TAW-toh-mee) incision into the bladder to remove a stone

lithonephritis (LIH-thoh-neh-FRAI-tis) inflammation of the kidneys caused by stones

lithonephrotomy (LIH-thoh-neh-FRAW-toh-mee) incision into a kidney to remove a stone

lithotripsy (LIH-thoh-TRIP-see) breakdown of a stone

lobectomy (loh-BEK-toh-mee) removal of a lobe

lobotomy (loh-BAW-toh-mee) incision into a lobe

local anesthetic (LOH-kal an-es-THET-ik) any anesthetic that does not affect consciousness

lordosis (lor-DOH-sis) swayback—abnormal forward curvature of the lower spine

lumbar (LUM-bar) middle side portions of the abdomen

lumbar puncture (LP) (LUM-bar PUNK-chir) inserting a needle into the lumbar region of the spine in order to collect spinal fluid

lymphadenectomy (lim-FAD-eh-NEK-toh-mee) surgical removal of a lymph gland (node)

lymphadenitis (LIM-fad-eh-NAI-tis) inflammation of a lymph gland (node)

lymphadenopathy (lim-FAD-eh-NAW-pah-thee) any disease of a lymph gland (node); used to refer to noticeably swollen lymph nodes, especially in the neck

lymphadenotomy (lim-FAD-eh-NAW-toh-mee) incision into a lymph gland (node)

lymphangiectasia (lim-FAN-jee-ek-TAY-zhah) dilation of a lymph vessel, normally noticed by swelling in the extremities

lymphangiogram (lim-FAN-jee-oh-GRAM) record of the study of lymph vessels

lymphangiography (lim-FAN-jee-AW-grah-fee) procedure to study the lymph vessels

lymphangitis (LIM-fan-JAI-tis) inflammation of the lymph vessels

lymphedema (LIM-fah-DEE-mah) swelling caused by abnormal accumulation of lymph

lymphocyte (LIM-foh-SAIT) lymph cell

lymphoma (lim-FOH-mah) tumor originating in lymphocytes

lymphopenia (LIM-foh-PEE-nee-ah) abnormal deficiency in lymph

M

macerate (MAS-ir-ayt) from Latin, for "to make soft"; to soften the skin

macrocephaly (MA-kroh-SEH-fah-lee) abnormally large head

macrocytosis (MAH-kroh-sai-TOH-sis) condition characterized by large red blood cells

macromastia (MAK-roh-MAS-tee-ah) abnormally large breasts

macrosomia (MAK-roh-SOH-mee-ah) baby with a large body

macrotia (mah-KROH-shee-ah) abnormally large ears

macule (MA-kyool) from Latin, for "spot" or "stain"; small, flat, discolored area (freckle)

magnetic resonance angiography (MRA) (mag-NET-ik REH-zawn-ants AN-gee-AW-grah-fee) procedure used to examine blood vessels

malignant cutaneous neoplasm (mah-LIG-nant kyoo-TAY-nee-us NEE-oh-plaz-um) a harmful new formation of the skin tissue (i.e., skin cancer)

malignant melanoma (ma-LIG-nant meh-lah-NOH-mah) a harmful tumor of melanin cell

mammogram (MAM-oh-GRAM) record of a breast exam

mammoplasty (MAM-oh-PLAS-tee) surgical reconstruction of a breast

manic depression (bipolar) (MAN-ik de-PREH-shun) a psychiatric disorder characterized by alternating bouts of excitement and depression

mastalgia (mas-TAL-jah) breast pain

mastectomy (mas-TEK-toh-mee) surgical removal of a breast

mastitis (mas-TAI-tis) inflammation of the breast

mastoidalgia (MAS-toid-AL-jah) pain in the mastoid

mastoidectomy (MAS-toy-DEK-toh-mee) removal of the mastoid

mastoiditis (MAS-toy-DAI-tis) inflammation of the mastoid

mastoidocentesis (mas-TOY-doh-sin-TEE-sis) puncture of the mastoid

mastopexy (MAS-toh-PEK-see) surgical fixation of a breast

mastoptosis (MAS-top-TOH-sis) downward displacement (drooping) of the breast

meatal stenosis (mee-AY-tal steh-NOH-sis) narrowing of the opening of the urethra

meatoplasty (mee-AH-toh-PLAS-tee) surgical reconstruction of the opening of the urethra

meatorrhaphy (MEE-ah-TOR-ah-fee) suture of the opening of the urethra

meatoscope (mee-AH-oh-SKOHP) instrument for examining the opening of the urethra

meatoscopy (MEE-ah-TAW-skoh-pee) process for examining the opening of the urethra

meatotomy (MEE-ah-TAW-toh-mee) incision into the opening of the urethra

menarche (MEN-ar-kee) beginning or first menstruation

meningioma (meh-NIN-jee-OH-mah) tumor of the meninges

meningitis (MEH-nin-JAI-tus) inflammation of the meninges

meningocele (meh-NIN-goh-seel) a hernia of the meninges

meningoencephalitis (meh-NIN-goh-in-SEF-ah-LAI-tis) inflammation of the meninges and brain

meningopathy (MEH-nin-GAW-pah-thee) disease of the meninges

menopause (MEN-oh-pawz) cessation of menstruation

menorrhagia (MEN-oh-RAY-jah) excessive menstrual flow

menorrhalgia (MEN-oh-RAL-jah) painful menstruation

metabolism (meh-TAB-oh-LIZM) breakdown of matter into energy

metacarpectomy (MEH-tah-kar-PEK-toh-mee) removal of a bone of the hand

metatarsalgia (meh-tah-tar-SAL-jah) pain in the bones of the foot

metrocolpocele (MEH-troh-KOL-poh-seel) hernia of the uterus and prolapse into the vagina

metromenorrhagia (MEH-troh-MEN-oh-RAY-jah) excessive menstrual bleeding at irregular intervals

metrophlebitis (MEH-troh-fleh-BAI-tis) inflammation of the blood vessels of the uterus

metrorrhagia (MEH-troh-RAY-jah) menstrual bleeding at irregular times

microcephalus (MAI-kroh-SEF-ah-lus) baby with a small head

microcephaly (MAI-kroh-SEH-fah-lee) abnormally small head

microcytosis (MAI-kroh-sai-TOH-sis) condition characterized by small red blood cells

micromastia (MAI-kroh-MAS-tee-ah) abnormally small breasts

microtia (mai-KROH-shee-ah) abnormally small ears

miosis (mai-OH-sis) abnormal contraction of the pupil (from Greek, for "to lessen")

miotic (mai-AW-tik) drug that causes the abnormal contraction of the pupil

mononucleosis (MAW-noh-NOO-klee-OH-sis) condition characterized by an abnormally large number of mononuclear leukocytes

monoparesis (MAW-noh-puh-REE-sis) partial paralysis of one limb

monoplegia (MAW-noh-PLEE-jah) paralysis of one limb

mucolytic (myoo-koh-LIT-ik) a drug that aids in the breakdown of mucus

murmur (MIR-mir) abnormal heart sound

muscular dystrophy (MUS-kyoo-lar DIS-troh-fee) disorder characterized by poor muscle development

myalgia (mai-AL-jah) muscle pain

myasthenia (mai-as-THEH-nee-ah) muscle weakness

mycodermatitis (mai-koh-der-mah-TAI-tis) inflammation of the skin caused by fungus

mycosis (mai-KOH-sis) fungus condition

mydriasis (mi-DRAI-ah-sis) abnormal dilation of the pupil

mydriatic (MID-ree-AT-ik) drug that causes the abnormal dilation of the pupil

myectomy (mai-EK-toh-mee) removal of muscle

myelitis (MAI-el-AI-tis) inflammation of the spinal cord

myelocele (MAI-el-oh-SEEL) a hernia of the spinal cord

myelodysplasia (MAI-el-oh-dis-PLAY-zhah) disease characterized by poor production of blood cells by the bone marrow

myelogram (MAI-el-oh-gram) image of the spinal cord, usually done using x-ray

myeloma (MAI-eh-LOH-mah) cancerous tumor of the bone marrow

myelomalacia (MAI-el-oh-mah-LAY-shah) abnormal softening of the spinal cord

myelomeningocele (MAI-el-oh-meh-NIN-goh-seel) a hernia of the spinal cord and meninges

myelopathy (MAI-el-AW-pah-thee) disease of the spinal cord

myelopoiesis (MAI-eh-loh-poh-EE-sis) formation of bone marrow

myocardial infarction (MAI-oh-KAR-dee-al in-FARK-shun) death of heart muscle tissue

myocardial ischemia (MAI-oh-KAR-dee-al ih-SKEE-mee-ah) blockage of blood to the heart muscle

myocarditis (MAI-oh-kar-DAI-tis) inflammation of the heart muscle

myocardium (MAI-oh-KAR-dee-um) heart muscle tissue

myocele (MAI-oh-seel) hernia of muscle tissue

myoclonus (mai-AWK-loh-nus) violent muscle contraction

myodesis (MAI-oh-DEE-sis) binding of muscle

myodynia (mai-oh-DAI-nee-ah) muscle pain

myofasciitis (MAI-oh-FA-shee-AI-tis) inflammation of the muscle and fascia

myography (mai-AW-grah-fee) procedure for studying muscles

myolysis (mai-AW-lih-sis) loss of muscle tissue

myoma (mai-OH-mah) a muscle tumor

myomalacia (mai-oh-mah-LAY-shah) softening of a muscle

myomectomy (MAI-oh-MEK-toh-mee) surgical removal of a tumor in the muscle (usually refers to the muscle of the uterine wall)

myometritis (MAI-oh-meh-TRAI-tis) inflammation of the myometrium

myometrium (MAI-oh-MEE-tree-um) the middle layer of uterine muscle tissue

myopathy (mai-AW-pah-thee) muscle disease

myopia (mai-OH-pee-ah) nearsightedness

myoplasty (MAI-oh-PLAS-tee) muscle reconstruction

myorrhaphy (mai-OR-ah-fee) muscle suture

myosarcoma (MAI-oh-sar-KOH-mah) a cancerous muscle tumor

myosclerosis (mai-oh-skleh-ROH-sis) hardening of a muscle

myositis (MAI-oh-SAI-tis) muscle inflammation

myospasm (MAI-oh-spaz-um) involuntary muscle contraction

myotasis (mai-AW-tah-sis) stretching of a muscle

myotomy (mai-AW-toh-mee) incision into muscle

myotonia (mai-oh-TOH-nee-ah) muscle tone

myringectomy (MIR-in-JEK-toh-mee) removal of the eardrum

myringitis (MIR-in-JAI-tis) inflammation of the eardrum

myringodermatitis (mir-IN-goh-DER-mah-TAI-tis) inflammation of the eardrum and surrounding skin

myringomycosis (mir-IN-goh-mai-KOH-sis) fungal condition of the eardrum

myringoplasty (mir-IN-goh-PLAS-tee) surgical reconstruction of the eardrum

myringotomy (mir-in-GAW-toh-mee) incision into the eardrum

myxedema (MIX-eh-DEE-mah) swelling of the skin caused by deposits under the skin

N

narcolepsy (NAR-coh-LEP-see) a disease characterized by sudden, uncontrolled sleepiness

nasogastric tube (NAY-zoh-GAS-trik TOOB) tube inserted through the nose into the stomach

nasolacrimal (NAY-zoh-LAH-krih-mal) pertaining to the nose and tear system

nasopharyngoscope (nay-zoh-fa-RIN-go-skohp) an instrument to look at the nose and throat

natal (NAY-tal) pertaining to birth

nebulizer (neh-byoo-LAI-zir) a machine that administers respiratory medication by creating a “cloud” or mist that is inhaled by the patient

necrosis (neh-KROH-sis) tissue death

necrotizing fasciitis (NEH-kroh-TAI-zing FA-shee-AI-tis) inflammation of the fascia causing the death of tissue

neonatal (NEE-oh-NAY-tal) pertaining to new birth (normally the first 28 days after birth)

neonatologist (NEE-oh-nay-TAW-loh-jist) specialist in the neonatal period

neonatology (NEE-oh-nay-TAW-loh-jee) study of the neonatal period

nephralgia (neh-FRAL-jah) pain in the kidney

nephrectomy (neh-FREK-toh-mee) surgical removal of a kidney

nephritis (neh-FRAI-tis) inflammation of the kidney

nephrocele (NEH-froh-seel) hernia of a kidney

nephrocystanastomosis (NEH-froh-SIST-ah-NAS-tah-MOH-sis) opening of a passageway between kidney and bladder

nephrogram (NEF-roh-gram) image of a kidney

nephrography (neh-FRAW-grah-fee) procedure for imaging a kidney

nephrohypertrophy (NEH-froh-hai-PER-troh-fee) overdevelopment of the kidney

nephrolithiasis (NEH-froh-lih-THAI-ah-sis) the presence of stones in the kidney

nephrolithotomy (NEH-froh-lih-THAW-toh-mee) incision into a kidney to remove a stone

nephrologist (neh-FRAW-loh-jist) specialist in the kidneys

nephrology (neh-FRAW-loh-jee) study of the kidneys

nephroma (neh-FROH-mah) kidney tumor

nephromalacia (NEH-froh-mah-LAY-shah) abnormal softening of a kidney

nephromegaly (NEH-froh-MEG-ah-lee) abnormal enlargement of a kidney

nephropathy (neh-FRAW-pah-thee) any kidney disease

nephropexy (NEH-froh-PEK-see) surgical fixation of a kidney

nephroptosis (nef-rop-TOH-sis) downward displacement of a kidney

nephrorrhaphy (neh-FROR-ah-fee) suture of a kidney

nephrosclerosis (NEH-froh-skleh-ROH-sis) abnormal hardening of a kidney

nephroscopy (neh-FRAW-skoh-pee) procedure for examining a kidney

nephrosis (neh-FROH-sis) kidney condition

nephrosonography (NEH-froh-soh-NAW-grah-fee) procedure for imaging a kidney using sound waves

nephrosplenopexy (NEH-froh-SPLEE-noh-PEK-see) surgical fixation of the spleen and a kidney

nephrostomy (neh-FRAW-stoh-mee) creation of an opening in a kidney

nephrotomy (neh-FRAW-toh-mee) incision into a kidney to remove a stone

nephrotoxin (NEH-froh-TOK-sin) an agent poisonous to the kidney

nephroureterectomy (NEH-froh-yoo-REE-ter-EK-toh-mee) surgical removal of a kidney and ureter

neuralgia (nir-AL-jah) nerve pain

neurasthenia (NIR-as-THEN-ee-ah) nerve weakness

neurectomy (nir-EK-toh-mee) removal of a nerve

neuritis (nir-AI-tis) nerve inflammation

neuroarthropathy (NIR-oh-ar-THRAW-pah-thee) disease of the joint associated with nerves

neurodynia (NIR-oh-DAI-nee-ah) nerve pain

neuroencephalomyelopathy (NIR-oh-in-SEF-ah-loh-MAI-el-AW-pah-thee) disease of the nerves, brain, and spinal cord

neurogenic (NIR-oh-JIN-ik) originating from/created by nerves

neuroglycopenia (NIR-oh-GLAI-koh-PEE-nee-ah) deficiency of sugar that interferes with normal brain activity

neurolysis (nir-AW-lih-sis) destruction of nerve tissue

neuroma (nir-OH-mah) a nerve tumor

neuropathy (nir-AW-pah-thee) disease of the nervous system

neuropharmacology (nir-oh-FAR-mah-KAW-loh-jee) the study of the effects of drugs on the nervous system

neuroplasty (NIR-oh-PLAS-tee) reconstruction of a nerve

neurorrhaphy (nir-OR-ah-fee) suturing of a nerve (often the severed ends of a nerve)

neurosclerosis (NIR-oh-skleh-ROH-sis) hardening of nerves

neurosis (nir-OH-sis) a nerve condition

neurotomy (nir-AW-toh-mee) incision into a nerve

neutropenia (NOO-troh-PEE-nee-ah) deficiency in neutrophil

nevus (NEE-vus) from Latin, for "birthmark" or "mole"; a mole

nocturia (nok-TIR-ee-ah) nighttime urination

nocturnal enuresis (nok-TIR-nal EN-yur-EE-sis) nighttime involuntary urination

nodule (NAWD-jyool) a solid mass that extends deeper into the skin

normocyte (NOR-moh-sait) normal-sized red blood cell

normotension (NOR-moh-TEN-shun) normal blood pressure

nystagmus (nih-STAG-mus) involuntary back-and-forth movement of the eyes (from Greek, for "to nod")

O

obstetrician (OB-steh-TRIH-shun) specialist in pregnancy, labor, and delivery of newborns

obstetrics (ob-STEH-triks) branch of medicine dealing with pregnancy, labor, and delivery of newborns

obstructive lung disorder (ob-STRUKT-iv) a lung disorder caused by a blockage

occlusion (oh-KLOO-zhun) closing or blockage of a passage

oculomycosis (AW-kyoo-loh-mai-KOH-sis) a fungal eye condition

oculopathy (AW-kyoo-LAW-pah-thee) disease of the eye

oculoplasty (AW-kyoo-loh-PLAS-tee) surgical reconstruction of the eye

odontalgia (OH-dawn-TAL-jah) tooth pain

odontectomy (oh-dawn-TEK-toh-mee) surgical removal of a tooth

odontoclasis (OH-dawn-TAWK-lah-sis) breaking of a tooth

odontodynia (oh-DAWN-toh-DAI-nee-ah) tooth pain

oligocythemia (AW-lih-goh-sih-THEE-mee-ah) deficiency in the number of red blood cells

oligohydramnios (AW-lih-goh-hai-DRAM-nee-ohs) not enough amniotic fluid

oligomenorrhea (AW-lih-goh-MEN-oh-REE-ah) infrequent or light menstrual periods

oligospermia (AW-lih-goh-SPER-mee-ah) condition characterized by low sperm production

oliguria (aw-lih-GYIR-ee-ah) low urine output

onychectomy (aw-nik-EK-toh-mee) removal of a nail

onychia (oh-NIK-ee-ah) a nail condition

onychocryptosis (AW-nih-koh-krip-TOH-sis) an ingrown nail

onychodystrophy (AW-nih-koh-DIS-troh-fee) poor nourishment (and development) of the nail

onycholysis (AW-nih-KAWL-is-is) the loss of a nail

onychomalacia (AW-nih-koh-mah-LAY-shah) abnormal softening of a nail

onychomycosis (AW-nih-koh-mai-KOH-sis) a fungal condition of the nail

onychopathy (aw-nik-AW-pah-thee) nail disease

onychophagia (aw-nih-koh-FAY-jah) eating (biting) the nail

onychotomy (aw-nih-KAW-toh-mee) incision into a nail

oophorectomy (OH-aw-for-EK-toh-mee) surgical removal of an ovary

oophoritis (OH-aw-for-AI-tis) inflammation of an ovary

oophorocystectomy (oh-AW-for-oh-sis-TEK-toh-mee) surgical removal of an ovarian cyst

oophorocystosis (OH-aw-FOR-oh-SIS-toh-sis) ovarian cysts

oophoroma (OH-aw-for-OH-mah) ovarian tumor

oophorotomy (oh-AW-for-AW-toh-mee) incision into an ovary

open reduction (OH-pen ree-DUK-shun) returning bones to their proper position through the use of surgery

ophthalmalgia (AWF-thal-MAL-jah) eye pain

ophthalmatrophy (AWF-thal-MAW-troh-fee) atrophy (wasting away) of the eye

ophthalmectomy (AWF-thal-MEK-toh-mee) removal of the eye

ophthalmic (awf-THAL-mik) pertaining to the eye

ophthalmitis (AWF-thal-MAI-tis) inflammation of the eye

ophthalmologist (AWF-thal-MAW-loh-jist) eye specialist

ophthalmomycosis (awf-THAL-moh-mai-KOH-sis) fungal eye condition

ophthalmomyitis (awf-THAL-moh-mai-AI-tis) inflammation of the eye muscles

ophthalmopathy (AWF-thal-MOH-pah-thee) eye disease

ophthalmoplegia (awf-THAL-moh-PLEE-jah) eye paralysis

ophthalmoscope (awf-THAL-mah-SKOHP) instrument for looking at the eye

optic (AWP-tik) pertaining to the eye

optic neuritis (AWP-tik nir-AI-tis) inflammation of the optic nerve

optokinetic (AWP-toh-kih-NEH-tik) pertaining to eye movement

optometrist (awp-TAW-meh-trist) specialist in measuring the eye

optomyometer (AWP-toh-MAI-oh-MEE-tir) device used to determine the strength of eye muscles

orchialgia (OR-kee-AL-jah) testicle pain

orchichorhea (OR-kee-kor-EE-ah) involuntary jerking movement of the testicles

orchidectomy (OR-kid-EK-toh-mee) surgical removal of a testicle

orchiditis (OR-kih-DAI-tis) inflammation of the testicles and epididymis

orchidopexy (OR-kid-oh-PEK-see) surgical fixation of a testicle

orchidoptosis (OR-kih-dop-TOH-sis) downward displacement of a testicle

orchidotomy (OR-kid-AW-toh-mee) incision into a testicle

orchiectomy (OR-kee-EK-toh-mee) surgical removal of a testicle

orchiepididymitis (OR-kee-EP-ih-DID-ih-MAI-tis) inflammation of the testicles and epididymis

orchiodynia (OR-kee-oh-DAI-nee-ah) testicle pain

orchiopathy (OR-kee-AW-pah-thee) disease of the testicles

orchiopexy (OR-kee-oh-PEK-see) surgical fixation of a testicle

orchioplasty (OR-kee-oh-PLAS-tee) surgical reconstruction of a testicle

orchitis (or-KAI-tis) inflammation of the testicles and epididymis

orthodontics (or-thoh-DAWN-tiks) branch of medicine dealing with the straightening of teeth

orthodontist (or-thoh-DAWN-tist) specialist in straightening teeth

orthopnea (or-thop-NEE-ah) able to breathe only in an upright position

orthotics (or-THAW-tiks) a device that aids in the straightening or stabilizing of a part of the body

ostalgia (aws-TAL-jah) bone pain

ostealgia (aws-tee-AL-jah) bone pain

ostectomy (aws-TEK-toh-mee) removal of a bone

osteectomy (aws-tee-EK-toh-mee) removal of a bone

osteitis (AW-stee-AI-tis) bone inflammation

osteoacusis (AW-stee-oh-ah-KOO-sis) hearing through bone

osteoarthritis (AW-stee-oh-ar-THRAI-tis) inflammation of the joints, specifically those that bear weight

osteocarcinoma (AW-stee-oh-KAR-sih-NOH-mah) bone cancer tumor

osteochondritis (AW-stee-oh-kon-DRAI-tis) inflammation of bone and cartilage

osteochondroma (AW-stee-oh-kon-DROH-mah) a tumor made up of bone and cartilage

osteodynia (aws-tee-oh-DAI-nee-ah) bone pain

osteodystrophy (aw-stee-oh-DIH-stroh-fee) poor bone development

osteogenesis imperfecta (AW-stee-oh-JIN-eh-sis IM-per-FEK-tah) a disease in which the bones do not develop correctly; also known as brittle bone disease

osteolysis (aw-stee-AW-lih-sis) bone loss

osteomalacia (AW-stee-oh-mah-LAY-shah) softening of the bone

osteometry (aw-stee-AW-meh-tree) procedure for measuring bone

osteomyelitis (AW-stee-oh-MAI-eh-LAI-tis) inflammation of the bone and bone marrow

osteonecrosis (aw-stee-oh-nih-KROH-sis) death of bone

osteopathy (AW-stee-AW-pah-thee) bone disease

osteopenia (AW-stee-oh-PEE-nee-yah) reduction in bone volume

osteoplasty (AWS-tee-oh-PLAS-tee) reconstruction of a bone

osteoporosis (AW-stee-oh-por-OH-sis) loss of bone density

osteosarcoma (AW-stee-oh-sar-KOH-mah) cancerous tumor arising out of bone cells

osteosclerosis (aw-stee-oh-skleh-ROH-sis) abnormal hardening of bone

osteotomy (AWS-tee-AW-toh-mee) incision into a bone

otalgia (oh-TAL-jah) ear pain

otitis externa (oh-TAI-tis eks-TERN-nah) inflammation of the outer ear

otitis media (oh-TAI-tis MEE-dee-ah) inflammation of the middle ear

otodynia (OH-toh-DAI-nee-ah) ear pain

otolaryngologist (OH-toh-LAH-rin-GAW-loh-jist) specialist in the ear and throat

otomycosis (oh-toh-mai-KOH-sis) a fungal ear condition

otoneurologist (OH-toh-nih-RAW-loh-jist) specialist in the nerve connections between the ear and brain

otoplasty (OH-toh-PLAS-tee) surgical reconstruction of the ear

otopyorrhea (OH-toh-PAI-oh-REE-ah) discharge of pus from the ears

otorhinolaryngologist (OH-toh-RAI-noh-LAH-rin-GAW-loh-jist) specialist in the ear, nose, and throat

otorrhea (OH-toh-REE-ah) discharge from the ear

otosclerosis (oh-toh-skleh-ROH-sis) hearing loss caused by the hardening of the bones of the middle ear

otoscope (OH-toh-SKOHP) instrument for looking in the ear

otoscopy (oh-TAW-skoh-pee) procedure for looking in the ear

otosteal (oh-TAWS-tee-all) pertaining to the bones of the ear

ototoxic (OH-toh-TOK-sik) drug that is damaging to the ear/hearing

ovaralgia (OH-var-AL-jah) pain in the ovaries

ovarialgia (oh-VAR-ee-AL-jah) pain in the ovaries

ovarian cystectomy (oh-VAR-ee-an sis-TEK-toh-mee) surgical removal of an ovarian cyst

ovariocentesis (oh-VAR-ee-oh-sin-TEE-sis) surgical puncture of an ovary

ovariocyesis (oh-VAR-ee-oh-sai-EE-sis) ectopic pregnancy in an ovary

ovariorrhexis (oh-VAR-ee-oh-REK-sis) rupture of an ovary

ovariostomy (oh-VAR-ee-AW-stoh-mee) creation of an opening into an ovary

ovaritis (OH-var-AI-tis) inflammation of an ovary

oximetry (ok-SIM-ah-tree) a procedure to measure oxygen levels

oxytocin (OK-see-TOH-sin) agent that stimulates uterine contractions and accelerates labor

P

pachyderma (pa-kih-DER-mah) tough skin

palatoplasy (pah-lah-toh-PLAS-tee) reconstruction of the palate

palpitation (PAL-pih-TAY-shun) rapid or irregular beating of the heart

pancreatalgia (PAN-kree-ah-TAL-jah) pain in the pancreas

pancreatectomy (PAN-kree-ah-TEK-toh-mee) surgical removal of the pancreas

pancreatic pseudocyst (PAN-kree-at-ik SOO-doh-sist) abnormally expanded area in the pancreas resembling a cyst

pancreatitis (PAN-kree-ah-TAI-tis) inflammation of the pancreas

pancreatoduodenectomy (PAN-kree-at-oh-DOO-aw-den-EK-toh-mee) surgical removal of the pancreas and duodenum

pancreatography (PAN-kree-ah-TAW-graw-FEE) procedure for mapping the pancreas

pancreatolith (PAN-kree-AT-oh-lith) stone in the pancreas

pancreatolithectomy (PAN-kree-ah-toh-lith-EK-toh-mee) removal of a stone in the pancreas

pancreatolithiasis (PAN-kree-at-oh-lih-THAI-ah-sis) presence of a stone in the pancreas

pancytopenia (PAN-SAI-toh-PEE-nee-ah) deficiency in all cellular components of the blood

panhypopituitarism (PAN-HAI-poh-pih-TOO-ih-tar-IZM) defective or absent function of the entire pituitary gland

pansinusitis (pan-sai-nus-AI-tis) inflammation of all sinuses

Pap (Papanicolaou) smear (PAP SMEER) test used to detect cancer cells, most commonly in the cervix

papilledema (PAH-pil-ah-DEE-mah) swelling of the optic nerve where it enters the retina

papule (PA-pyool) from Latin, for "pimple"; a small, solid mass

paralysis (puh-RAH-lu-sis) complete loss of sensation and motor function

parathyroidectomy (PAR-ah-THAI-roid EK-toh-mee) removal of the parathyroid

parathyroidoma (PAR-ah-THAI-roid-OH-mah) tumor of the parathyroid

paresis (puh-REE-sis) partial paralysis characterized by varying degrees of sensation and motor function

paresthesia (PAR-es-THEE-zhah) abnormal sensation (usually numbness or tingling in the skin)

paronychia (par-aw-NIH-kee-ah) a condition of the tissue around a nail

patch (pach) large, flat, discolored area

pectoralgia (PEK-tor-AL-jah) chest pain

pectoriloquy (pek-tor-IH-low-kwee) speaking from the chest; used as a means of finding masses in the lung

pectus carinatum (PEK-tus car-ee-NAH-tum) a chest that protrudes like the keel of a ship

pectus excavatum (PEK-tus eks-cuh-VAH-tum) a chest that is hollowed out

pelvic sonograph (PEL-vik SAW-noh-GRAF) instrument for imaging the pelvis using sound waves

pelvicephalometry (PEL-vih-SEF-eh-LAW-meh-tree) procedure for measuring the head size of the baby and the pelvis size of the mother

pelvimetry (pel-VIM-eh-tree) procedure for measuring the pelvis

percussion (per-KUH-shun) the body surface; in this context, to cause vibrations that can help locate fluid buildup in the chest

percutaneous (per-kyoo-TAY-nee-us) pertaining to through the skin

percutaneous coronary intervention (PER-kyoo-TAY-nee-us KOR-ah-NAR-ee IN-ter-VEN-shun) alternative treatment for the coronary artery that passes instruments up a patient's blood vessels into the heart

perfusion (per-FYOO-zhun) circulation of blood through tissue

pericardial effusion (PER-ee-KAR-dee-al ee-FYOO-zhun) fluid pouring out into the tissue around the heart

pericardiocentesis (PER-ee-KAR-dee-oh-sin-TEE-sis) puncture of the tissue around the heart

pericardiotomy (PER-ee-KAR-dee-AW-toh-mee) incision into the tissue around the heart

pericarditis (PER-ee-kar-DAI-tis) inflammation of the tissue around the heart

pericardium (PER-ee-KAR-dee-um) tissue around the heart

perimetritis (PEH-ree-meh-TRAI-tis) inflammation of the perimetrium

perimetrium (PEH-ree-MEE-tree-um) tissue on the outside of the uterus, the outer layer of the uterus

perinatal (PEH-ree-NAY-tal) time around birth (normally ranging from 28 weeks of pregnancy to 28 days after pregnancy)

perinatologist (PEH-ree-nay-TAW-loh-jist) specialist in the perinatal period

perinatology (PER-ee-nay-TAW-loh-jee) branch of medicine dealing with the perinatal period

perineocele (PER-ih-NEE-oh-seel) hernia in the perineum region

perineoplasty (PER-ih-NEE-oh-PLAS-tee) surgical reconstruction of the perineum

perineorrhaphy (PER-ih-nee-OR-ah-fee) suture of the perineum

perineotomy (PER-ih-nee-AW-toh-mee) incision into the perineum

periodontitis (PER-ee-OH-don-TAI-tis) inflammation of the region around the teeth

peritoneoscopy (PER-ih-TOH-nee-AW-skoh-pee) procedure for looking at the peritoneum

peritonitis (PER-ih-toh-NAI-tis) inflammation of the peritoneum

petechia (puh-TEE-kee-yah) small bruise

phacoemulsification (FAY-koh-ee-MUL-sih-fih-KAY-shun) fragmentation of an existing lens in order to remove and replace it

phacomalacia (FAH-koh-mah-LAY-shah) abnormal softening of the lens

phacosclerosis (FAH-koh-skleh-ROH-sis) abnormal hardening of the lens

phacoscope (FAY-koh-SKOHP) instrument for looking at the lens

phagocytosis (FAG-oh-sai-TOH-sis) process in which phagocytes (a type of white blood cell) destroy (or eat) foreign microorganisms or cell debris

phakitis (fah-KAI-tis) inflammation of the lens

phimosis (fih-MOH-sis) contraction of the foreskin of the penis, preventing it from being retracted

phlebalgia (fleh-BAL-jah) pain in a vein

phlebarteriectasia (FLEB-ar-TER-ee-ek-TAY-zhah) dilation of blood vessels

phlebectomy (fleb-EK-toh-mee) surgical removal of a vein

phlebitis (fleh-BAI-tis) inflammation of the veins

phlebologist (fleb-AW-loh-jist) specialist in veins

phlebology (fleb-AW-loh-jee) study of veins

phlebophlebostomy (FLEB-oh-fleb-AW-stoh-mee) procedure to create an opening between two veins

phlebosclerosis (FLEB-oh-skleh-ROH-sis) hardening of a vein

phlebostenosis (FLEB-oh-sten-OH-sis) narrowing of the veins

phlebotomist (fleh-BAW-toh-mist) specialist in drawing blood

phlebotomy (fleh-BAW-toh-mee) incision into a vein (another name for drawing blood)

photophobia (FOH-toh-FOH-bee-ah) excessive sensitivity to light

phrenoplegia (fre-no-PLEE-jah) paralysis of the diaphragm

phrenoptosis (fre-nop-TOE-sis) drooping of the diaphragm

phrenospasm (fre-no-SPAZ-um) involuntary contraction of the diaphragm

pituitary adenoma (pih-TOO-ih-TEH-ree AD-en-OH-mah) tumor on the pituitary gland

pituitary dwarfism (pih-TOO-ih-TER-ee DWAR-fizm) abnormally short height caused by undersecretions of growth hormone from the pituitary gland

pituitary gigantism (pih-TOO-ih-TER-ee jai-GAN-tizm) abnormally tall height caused by oversecretion of growth hormone from the pituitary gland

pituitary infarction (pih-TOO-ih-TEH-ree in-FARK-shun) death of the pituitary gland

placenta previa (plah-SIN-tah PREE-vee-ah) condition in which the placenta is attached to the uterus near the cervix

plaque (PLAK) a solid mass on the surface of the skin

plasmapheresis (PLAZ-mah-fer-EE-sis) apheresis to remove plasma

plateletpheresis (PLAYT-let-fer-EE-sis) apheresis to remove platelets (for the purpose of donating them to patients in need of platelets)

pleural effusion (PLUR-al ef-YOO-zhun) fluid pouring out into the pleura

pleuralgia (plur-AL-jah) pain in the pleura

pleurisy (PLUR-ih-see) inflammation of the pleura; another word for pleuritis

pleuritis (plur-AI-tis) inflammation of the pleura

pleurodynia (plur-oh-DAI-nee-ah) pain in the pleura

pleuropexy (ploo-rah-PEK-see) reattachment of the pleura

pneumatic otoscopy (new-MA-tik oh-TAW-skoh-pee) procedure for looking in the ear using air

pneumatocele (new-MAT-oh-seel) hernia of the lung

pneumoconiosis (new-moh-con-ai-OH-sis) a lung condition caused by dust

pneumohemothorax (new-moh-hee-moh-THOR-aks) air and blood in the chest

pneumonectomy (new-moh-NEK-toh-mee) removal of a lung

pneumonia (new-MOH-nee-yah) a lung condition

pneumonitis (new-moh-NAI-tis) inflammation of the lung

pneumothorax (new-moh-THOR-aks) air in the chest

poikilocytosis (POI-kih-loh-sai-TOH-sis) condition characterized by red blood cells in a variety of shapes

poliomyelitis (POH-lee-oh-MAI-el-AI-tis) inflammation of the gray matter of the spinal cord

polyadenopathy (PAW-lee-AD-en-AW-pah-thee) disease involving many glands

polycystic kidney disease (PAW-lee-SIS-tik KID-nee dih-ZEEZ) disease characterized by the formation of many fluid-filled cysts in the kidneys

polycythemia (PAW-lee-sih-THEE-mee-ah) excess of red blood cells

polydactyly (paw-lee-DAK-tih-lee) having more than the normal number of fingers (or toes)

polydipsia (PAW-lee-DIP-see-ah) excessive thirst

polyhydramnios (PAW-lee-hai-DRAM-nee-ohs) excessive amniotic fluid

polymenorrhea (PAW-lee-MEN-oh-REE-ah) menstrual periods occurring with greater than normal frequency

polymyositis (PAW-lee-MAI-oh-SAI-tis) inflammation of multiple muscles

polyneuritis (PAW-lee-nir-AI-tis) inflammation of multiple nerves

polyneuropathy (PAW-lee-nir-AW-pah-thee) disease affecting multiple nerves

polyphagia (PAW-lee-FAY-jah) excessive eating

polysomnography (paw-lee-som-NAH-graw-fee) recording multiple aspects of sleep

polyuria (PAW-lee-YOO-ree-ah) excessive urination

positron emission tomography (PET scan) (PAWZ-ih-trawn ee-MISH-un taw-MAW-graw-fee) an imaging procedure that uses radiation (positrons) to produce cross-sections of the brain

postictal (post-IK-tal) time after a seizure

postnatal (post-NAY-tal) pertaining to after birth

postpartum (post-PAR-tum) pertaining to after birth

postpartum alopecia (post-PAR-tum al-oh-PEE-shah) baldness experienced by women after a pregnancy

preeclampsia (PREE-eh-KLAMP-see-ah) condition characterized by high blood pressure and high levels of protein in the urine

preictal (pree-IK-tal) time before a seizure

prenatal (pree-NAY-tal) pertaining to before birth

presbycusis (PREZ-bih-KOO-sis) loss of hearing in old age

presbyopia (PREZ-bee-OH-pee-ah) decreased vision caused by old age

priapism (PREE-ap-izm) persistent and painful erection

proctitis (prok-TAI-tis) inflammation of the anus and rectum

proctologist (prok-TAW-loh-jist) specialist in the anus, rectum, and colon

proctology (prok-TAW-loh-jee) branch of medicine dealing with the anus, rectum, and colon

proctoplasty (PROK-toh-PLAS-tee) surgical reconstruction of the anus and rectum

proctoptosis (prok-TOP-toh-sis) downward displacement of the rectum and anus

proctoscope (PROK-toh-skohp) instrument for looking at the anus and rectum

proctoscopy (prok-TAW-skoh-pee) procedure for looking at the anus and rectum

prosopagnosia (PRAW-soh-pag-NOH-zhah) inability to recognize faces

prostatectomy (PROS-tat-TEK-toh-mee) surgical removal of the prostate

prostatitis (PROS-tah-TAI-tis) inflammation of the prostate

prostatocystitis (pros-tat-oh-sis-TAI-tis) inflammation of the prostate and bladder

prostatolith (pros-ta-toh-lith) a stone in the prostate

prostatolithotomy (pros-ta-toh-lih-THAW-toh-mee) incision into a prostate to remove a stone

prostatomegaly (pros-ta-toh-MEH-gah-lee) abnormal enlargement of the prostate

prostatorrhea (pros-ta-toh-REE-ah) discharge from the prostate

prostatovesiculectomy (pros-ta-toh-veh-SIK-yoo-LEK-toh-mee) surgical removal of the prostate and seminal vesicles

prostatovesiculitis (pros-ta-toh-veh-SIK-yoo-LAI-tis) inflammation of the prostate and seminal vesicles

prosthesis (pros-THEE-sis) a device that is added to a body to replace a missing part or lost function

pruritus (prur-AI-tis) from Latin, for "burning nettle"; swollen, raised, itchy areas of the skin

pseudocyesis (SOO-doh-sai-EE-sis) false pregnancy

pseudoesthesia (SOO-des-THEE-zhah) false sensation

psychiatrist (sai-KAI-ah-trist) doctor who specializes in treatment of the mind

psychiatry (sai-KAI-ah-tree) branch of medicine that focuses on the treatment of the mind

psychogenic (SAI-koh-JIN-ik) originating in/created by the mind

psychologist (sai-KAW-loh-jist) doctor who specializes in the study of the mind

psychology (sai-KAW-loh-jee) branch of medicine that focuses on the study of the mind

psychopathy (sai-KAW-pah-thee) a mental illness

psychopharmacology (SAI-koh-FAR-mah-KAW-loh-jee) the study of the effects of drugs on mental processes

psychosis (sai-KOH-sis) a mind condition (involves some sort of break with reality interfering with rational thought or daily functioning)

psychosomatic (SAI-koh-soh-MA-tik) pertaining to the relationship between the body and the mind

psychotropic (SAI-koh-TROH-pik) drugs that are able to turn the mind

pterygium (ter-IH-jee-um) winglike growth of conjunctival tissue extending to the cornea (from Greek, for "wing")

pulmonary angiography (pul-mon-AIR-ee an-jee-O-grah-fee) an imaging procedure for recording pulmonary blood vessel activity

pulmonary circulation (pul-mon-AIR-ee SIR-kyoo-LAY-shun) circulation of blood from the heart to the lungs

pulmonary edema (pul-mon-AIR-ee ah-DEE-ma) swelling in the lungs

pulmonary embolism (pul-mon-AIR-ee em-bol-IZ-um) blockage in the pulmonary blood supply

pulmonary function testing (pul-mon-AIR-ee FUNK-shun TES-ting) a group of tests used to evaluate the condition of the lungs

pulmonary neoplasm (pul-mon-AIR-ee nee-oh-PLAZ-sum) new growth (tumor) in the lung

pustule (PUS-tyool) from Latin, for "little blister"; a pus-filled blister

pyarthrosis (pai-ar-THROH-sis) pus in a joint

pyelitis (PAI-el-AI-tis) inflammation of the renal pelvis

pyelocystitis (PAI-el-oh-sis-TAI-tis) inflammation of the renal pelvis and bladder

pyelocystostomosis (PAI-el-oh-SIS-toh-staw-MOH-sis) creation of an opening between the renal pelvis and bladder

pyelogram (PAI-el-oh-GRAM) image of the renal pelvis

pyelolithotomy (PAI-el-oh-lih-THAW-toh-mee) incision into a renal pelvis to remove a stone

pyelonephritis (PAI-el-oh-neh-FRAI-tis) inflammation of the kidney and renal pelvis

pyelopathy (PAI-el-AW-pah-thee) disease of the renal pelvis

pyeloplasty (PAI-el-oh-PLAS-tee) surgical reconstruction of a renal pelvis

pyelostomy (PAI-el-AW-stoh-mee) creation of an opening in a renal pelvis

pyelotomy (PAI-el-AW-toh-mee) incision into a renal pelvis

pyeloureterectasia (PAI-el-oh-yoo-REE-ter-ek-TAY-zhah) dilation of the renal pelvis and ureter

pyloric stenosis (PAI-lor-ik steh-NOH-sis) narrowing of the sphincter at the base of the stomach

pyonephritis (PAI-oh-neh-FRAI-tis) inflammation of the kidney caused by pus

pyonephrolithiasis (PAI-oh-NEH-froh-lih-THAI-ah-sis) the presence of pus and stones in the kidney

pyopyeloectasis (PAI-oh-PAI-el-oh-EK-tah-sis) pus in a dilated renal pelvis

pyosalpinx (PAI-oh-SAL-pinks) blockage in a fallopian tube caused by pus

pyothorax (pai-oh-THOR-aks) pus in the chest

pyromania (PAI-roh-MAY-nee-ah) desire to set fires

pyuria (pai-YUR-ee-ah) pus in the urine

R

rectalgia (rek-TAL-jah) rectum pain

rectitis (rek-TAI-tis) inflammation of the rectum

rectocele (REK-toh-seel) hernia or protrusion of the rectum into the vagina

rectopexy (REK-toh-PEK-see) surgical fixation of the rectum

regional anesthetic (REE-jih-nal an-es-THET-ik) anesthetic that is injected into a nerve, causing loss of sensation over a particular area

renal angiogram (REE-nal AN-jee-oh-GRAM) image of a kidney blood vessel

renal angiography (REE-nal AN-jee-AW-grah-fee) process of imaging a kidney blood vessel

renal angioplasty (REE-nal AN-jee-oh-PLAS-tee) surgical reconstruction of a kidney blood vessel

renal arteriogram (REE-nal ar-TER-ee-oh-GRAM) image of a kidney artery

renal cell carcinoma (REE-nal SELL KAR-sih-NOH-mah) cancer of the kidneys; also known as *hypernephroma*

renal failure (REE-nal FAYL-yur) kidney failure

renal ischemia (REE-nal ih-SKEE-mee-ah) deficiency of blood in a kidney

reperfusion injury (REE-pir-FYOO-zhun IN-jir-ee) injury to tissue that occurs after blood flow is restored

resectoscope (rih-SEK-toh-SKOHP) instrument for examining and cutting (usually the prostate)

restrictive cardiomyopathy (ree-STRIK-tiv KAR-dee-oh-mai-AW-pah-thee) heart muscle hardens, restricting the expansion of the heart and thus limiting the amount of blood it can pump to the rest of the body

restrictive lung disorder (re-STRIKT-iv) a lung disorder caused by the limiting of air into the lungs

reticulocyte (reh-TIK-yoo-loh-SAIT) immature red blood cell

retinal (REH-tih-nal) pertaining to the retina

retinitis (REH-tih-NAI-tis) inflammation of the retina

retinopathy (REH-tih-NOP-ah-thee) disease of the retina

retinopexy (reh-TIH-noh-PEK-see) surgical fixation (reattachment) of a retina

retinoscope (RET-in-aw-SKOP) instrument for looking at the retina

retinoscopy (RET-in-AW-skoh-pee) procedure for looking at the retina

retinosis (REH-tih-NOH-sis) retinal condition

retinotomy (REH-tih-NAW-toh-mee) incision into the retina

retrograde pyelogram (REH-troh-grayd PAI-el-oh-GRAM) image of the renal pelvis produced by injecting a contrast dye from the bladder to the kidney

rheumatoid arthritis (ROO-mah-toyd ar-THRAI-tis) inflammation of the joint; called rheumatoid because its symptoms resemble those of rheumatic fever

rhinitis (rai-NAI-tis) inflammation of the nasal passages

rhinorrhagia (rai-no-RAY-jah) excessive blood flow from the nose (another term for nosebleed)

rhinorrhea (rai-no-REE-yah) runny nose

rhinosalpingitis (RAI-noh-SAL-pin-JAI-tis) inflammation of the nose and eustachian tubes

rhytidoplasty (rih-tih-doh-PLAS-tee) reconstruction of wrinkled skin

S

salpingectomy (SAL-pin-JEK-toh-mee) surgical removal of a fallopian tube

salpingitis (SAL-pin-JAI-tis) inflammation of a fallopian tube

salpingocyesis (sal-PING-goh-sai-EE-sis) ectopic pregnancy in a fallopian tube

salpingo-oophorectomy (sal-PING-goh-OH-aw-for-EK-toh-mee) surgical removal of a fallopian tube and ovary

salpingocele (sal-PING-goh-seel) hernia of a fallopian tube

salpingo-oophoritis (sal-PING-goh-OH-aw-for-AI-tis) inflammation of a fallopian tube and ovary

salpingopexy (sal-PING-goh-PEK-see) surgical fixation of a fallopian tube

salpingopharyngeal (sal-PING-goh-fah-RIN-jee-al) pertaining to the eustachian tubes and the throat

salpingoscope (sal-PING-goh-skohp) instrument for looking at the eustachian tubes

scale (SKAYL) skin flaking off

schizophrenia (SKIT-zoh-FREH-nee-ah) a mental illness characterized by delusions, hallucinations, and disordered speech

sclerectasia (SKLER-ek-TAY-zhah) overexpansion of the sclera

sclerodermatitis (skleh-roh-der-mah-TAI-tis) inflammation of the skin accompanied by thickening and hardening

scleroiritis (SKLER-oh-ai-RAI-tis) inflammation of the sclera and iris

sclerokeratitis (SKLER-oh-KEH-rah-TAI-tis) inflammation of the sclera and cornea

sclerokeratoiritis (SKLER-oh-KEH-ra-toh-ai-RAI-tis) inflammation of the sclera, cornea, and iris

scleromalacia (SKLEH-roh-mah-LAY-shah) abnormal softening of the sclera

scleronychia (skleh-raw-NIH-kee-ah) thickening and hardening of the nails

sclerosing cholangitis (skleh-ROH-sing KOH-lan-JAI-tis) inflammation and hardening of the bile vessels (ducts)

sclerotomy (skler-AW-toh-mee) incision into the sclera

scoliosis (SKOH-lee-OH-sis) crooked back, or abnormal lateral curvature of the spine

scotoma (skaw-TOH-mah) dark spot in the visual field

scotopia (skaw-TOH-pee-ah) the adjustment of the eye to seeing in darkness

seborrheic dermatitis (se-boh-RAY-ik der-mah-TAI-tis) inflammation of the skin caused by the discharge of oil (sebum)

seminoma (SEM-oh-NOH-mah) type of testicular cancer arising from sperm-forming tissue

sensorineural hearing loss (SEN-sor-ee-NIR-al) sound is not transmitted from the inner ear to the brain (due to problems with the sense organs or nerves)

septic arthritis (SEP-tik ar-THRAI-tis) inflammation of the joint caused by infection

septicemia (SEP-tih-SEE-mee-ah) presence of disease-causing microorganisms in the blood

septoplasty (sep-toh-PLAS-tee) reconstruction of a septum

sialagogic (sai-AL-ah-GAW-jik) agent that causes salivation

sialoadenectomy (sai-AL-oh-AD-en-EK-toh-mee) surgical removal of a salivary gland

sialoadenitis (sai-AL-oh-AD-en-AI-tis) inflammation of the salivary glands

sialoadenosis (sai-AL-oh-AD-en-OH-sis) condition of the salivary glands

sialoangiectasis (SAI-ah-loh-AN-jee-EK-tah-sis) overexpansion of the salivary vessels

sialolith (sai-AL-oh-lith) stone in the saliva

sialolithiasis (sai-AL-oh-lih-THAI-ah-sis) presence of salivary stones

sialolithotomy (sai-AL-oh-lih-THAW-toh-mee) incision to removal salivary stones

sialorrhea (SAI-ah-loh-REE-ah) excessive salivation

sialostenosis (SAI-ah-loh-steh-NOH-sis) narrowing of the salivary glands

sigmoidoscope (sig-MOY-doh-skohp) instrument for looking at the sigmoid colon

sigmoidoscopy (sig-moy-DAW-skoh-pee) procedure for looking at the sigmoid colon

sinusitis (sai-nus-AI-tis) inflammation of the sinus

sleep apnea (SLEEP AP-nee-ah) a condition where the patient ceases to breathe while asleep

somnambulism (sawm-NAM-byoo-liz-um) sleep walking

sonography (saw-NAW-grah-fee) use of sound waves to produce diagnostic images; also called an ultrasound

sonohysterography (SOH-noh-HIS-ter-AW-grah-fee) procedure using sound waves to examine the uterus

speculum (SPEH-kyoo-lum) device for examining a body cavity, most commonly the vagina

spermatocele (sper-MAT-oh-SEEL) hernia or distention of the epididymis caused by sperm cells

spermatogenesis (sper-MAT-oh-JIN-eh-sis) creation of sperm

spermatolysis (SPER-mah-TAW-lih-sis) destruction of sperm cells

spermicide (SPER-mih-sahyd) agent that kills sperm

spermolytic (SPER-moh-LIH-tik) agent that kills sperm

spherocyte (SFEE-roh-SAIT) red blood cell that assumes a spherical shape

spherocytosis (SFEER-oh-sai-TOH-sis) condition in which red blood cells assume a spherical shape

sphygmomanometer (SFIG-moh-mah-NAW-meh-ter) fancy name for the device used to measure blood pressure

spider angioma see *telangiectasia*

spinal stenosis (SPAI-nal stih-NOH-sis) abnormal narrowing of the spine

spirometry (speer-OH-meh-tree) a procedure to measure breathing

splenalgia (splee-NAL-jah) pain in the spleen

splenectomy (spleh-NEK-toh-mee) surgical removal of the spleen

splenectopy (splee-NEK-toh-pee) displacement of the spleen, sometimes called floating spleen

splenitis (splee-NAI-tis) inflammation of the spleen

splenodynia (SPLEE-noh-DAI-nee-ah) pain in the spleen

splenolysis (splee-NAW-lih-sis) breakdown (destruction) of spleen tissue

splenomalacia (SPLEE-noh-mah-LAY-shah) softening of the spleen

splenomegaly (SPLEE-noh-MEH-gah-lee) enlargement of the spleen

splenopathy (splee-NAW-pah-thee) any disease of the spleen

splenoptosis (SPLEE-nawp-TOH-sis) downward displacement (drooping) of the spleen

splenorrhexis (SPLEE-noh-REK-sis) rupture of the spleen

spondylitis (spawn-dih-LAI-tis) inflammation of the vertebra

spondyloarthropathy (SPAWN-dih-loh-ar-THRAW-pah-thee) joint disease of the vertebrae

spondylodynia (spawn-dih-loh-DAI-nee-ah) vertebra pain

spondylolisthesis (SPAWN-dih-loh-lis-THEE-sis) the slipping or dislocation of a vertebra

spondylolysis (SPAWN-dih-LO-li-sis) loss of vertebra structure

spondylomalacia (spawn-dih-loh-mah-LAY-shah) softening of the vertebra

spondylosis (SPAWN-dih-LOH-sis) vertebra condition

spondylosyndesis (SPAWN-dih-loh-sin-DEE-sis) fusing together of multiple vertebrae

spontaneous abortion (spawn-TAY-nee-is ah-BOR-shun) the naturally occurring termination of pregnancy; also known as a miscarriage

sputum (SPYOO-tum) mucus discharged from the lungs by coughing

squamous cell carcinoma (SKWAY-mus SELL kar-sih-NO-mah) cancerous tumor of squamous skin cells

steatitis (stay-ah-TAI-tis) inflammation of fat tissue

steatoma (STAY-ah-TOH-mah) a fatty tumor

steatorrhea (STAY-at-oh-REE-ah) excessive fat discharged in the feces

sternotomy (stir-NAW-toh-mee) incision into the sternum

stomatitis (STOH-mah-TAI-tis) inflammation of the mouth

stomatodynia (stoh-MAT-oh-DAI-nee-ah) mouth pain

stomatogastric (stoh-MAT-oh-GAS-trik) pertaining to the mouth and stomach

stomatomycosis (stoh-MAT-oh-mai-KOH-sis) fungus condition of the mouth

stomatoplasty (stoh-MAT-oh-PLAS-tee) surgical reconstruction of the mouth

stomatosis (STOH-mah-TOH-sis) mouth condition

strabismus (struh-BIZ-mus) condition where the eyes deviate when looking at the same object (from Latin, for "to squint")

stress electrocardiogram (STRES eh-LEK-troh-KAR-dee-oh-GRAM) image of the heart produced using sound waves while the patient experiences increases of exercise stress

stress urinary incontinence (SUI) (STRES YUR-ih-NAR-ee in-CON-tih-nentz) loss of bladder control caused by the application of external pressure

stroke (STROHK) loss of brain function caused by interruption of blood flow/supply to the brain

subcutaneous (sub-kyoo-TAY-nee-us) pertaining to beneath the skin

subdural hematoma (sub-DIR-al HEE-mah-TOH-mah) a hematoma located beneath the dura

subluxation (sub-luk-SAY-shun) partial dislocation of a joint

superior vena cava (soo-PEER-ee-or VEE-nah CAY-vah) portion of the vena cava that gathers blood from the upper portion of the body (head and arms)

syncope (SIN-koh-pee) fainting; losing consciousness due to temporary loss of blood flow to the brain

syndactyly (sin-DAK-tih-lee) fusion (sometimes called webbing) of fingers or toes

synesthesia (SIN-es-THEE-zhah) condition where one sensation is experienced as another

systemic circulation (sih-STEM-ik SIR-kyoo-LAY-shun) circulation of blood from the heart to the rest of the body

systolic pressure (sih-STAW-lik PRESH-ir) pressure exerted on blood vessels when the heart is contracting

T

tachycardia (TAK-ih-KAR-dee-ah) rapid heartbeat

tachypnea (ta-KIP-nee-yah) rapid breathing

tardive dyskinesia (TAR-div DIS-kin-EE-zhah) condition characterized by the loss of muscle control

tarsectomy (tar-SEK-toh-mee) removal of all or a portion of the ankle

tarsoclasia (TAR-soh-KLAY-zhah) the surgical fracture of the ankle (i.e., to treat clubfoot)

tarsoptosis (tar-sawp-TOH-sis) flat feet

telangiectasia (tel-an-jee-ek-TAY-zhuh) the overexpansion of the blood vessel, sometimes called a spider angioma because of how it looks on the skin

tenalgia (ten-AL-jah) tendon pain

tendectomy (ten-DEK-toh-mee) removal of a tendon

tendonitis (TEN-dah-NAI-tis) tendon inflammation

tendoplasty (TEN-doh-PLAS-tee) reconstruction of a tendon

tenodesis (TEN-oh-DEE-sis) binding of a tendon

tenolysis (ten-AW-lih-sis) freeing/loosening a tendon

tenonectomy (TEN-oh-NEK-toh-mee) removal of a tendon

tenoplasty (TEN-oh-PLAS-tee) reconstruction of a tendon

tenorrhaphy (ten-OR-ah-fee) suture of a tendon

tenotomy (ten-AW-toh-mee) incision into a tendon

teratogenic (TER-ah-toh-JIN-ik) causing the formation of birth defects

teratology (TER-ah-TAW-loh-jee) branch of medicine dealing with the study of birth defects and their causes

teratoma (TER-ah-TOH-mah) see *dermoid cyst*

testicular carcinoma (tes-TIK-yoo-lar KAR-sih-NOH-mah) testicular cancer

testitis (tes-TAI-tis) inflammation of the testicles and epididymis

thelarche (thee-LAR-kay) beginning of breast development

thoracalgia (thor-a-KAL-jah) chest pain

thoracentesis (thor-a-sin-TEE-sis) puncture of the chest

thoracocentesis (thor-a-koh-sin-TEE-sis) puncture of the chest

thoracoplasty (thor-a-koh-PLAS-tee) reconstruction of the chest

thoracoscopy (thor-a-KOS-koh-pee) examination of the chest

thoracostomy (thor-a-KOS-toh-mee) creation of an opening in the chest

thoracotomy (thor-a-KAH-toh-mee) incision into the chest

thrombocyte (THROM-boh-sait) cell that helps blood clot (also known as a platelet)

thrombocytopenia (THROM-boh-SAI-toh-PEE-nee-ah) deficiency in the number of platelets (clot cells)

thrombocytosis (THROM-boh-sai-TOH-sis) increase in the number of platelets (clot cells)

thromboembolism (THROM-boh-EM-boh-LIZ-um) blockage of a vessel (embolism) caused by a clot that has broken off from where it formed

thrombogenic (THROM-boh-JIN-ik) capable of producing a blood clot

thrombolytic (THROM-boh-LIH-tik) drug that breaks down blood clots

thrombophlebitis (THROM-boh-fleh-BAI-tis) inflammation of a vein caused by a clot

thrombosis (throm-BOH-sis) formation of a blood clot

thrombus (THROM-bus) blood clot

thymectomy (thai-MEK-toh-mee) surgical removal of the thymus

thymic hyperplasia (THAI-mik HAI-per-PLAY-zhah) overdevelopment of the thymus

thymoma (thai-MOH-mah) tumor of the thymus

thymopathy (thai-MAW-pah-thee) disease of the thymus

thyrocele (THAI-roh-seel) see *goiter*

thyroid function tests (THAI-roid FUNK-shun TESTS) tests performed to evaluate the function of the thyroid

thyroidectomy (THAI-roid-EK-toh-mee) removal of the thyroid

thyroiditis (THAI-roid-AI-tis) inflammation of the thyroid

thyroidotomy (THAI-roid-AW-toh-mee) incision into the thyroid

thyroidotoxin (thai-ROI-doh-TOK-sin) substance poisonous to the thyroid gland

thyromegaly (THAI-roh-MEH-gah-lee) enlargement of the thyroid

thyroparathyroidectomy (THAI-roh-PAR-ah-THAI-roid-EK-toh-mee) removal of the thyroid and parathyroid glands

thyroptosis (THAI-rop-TOH-sis) downward displacement (drooping) of the thyroid

thyrotoxicosis (THAI-roh-TOKS-ih-KOH-sis) condition caused by the exposure of body tissue to excessive levels of thyroid hormone (an extreme version of this is known as "thyroid storm")

thyrotropin (THAI-roh-TROH-pin) hormone that stimulates the thyroid

tibialgia (tih-bee-AL-ja) tibia (shin) pain

tinnitus (tih-NAI-tis) ringing in the ears (from Latin, for "to ring" or "jingle")

tocodynagraph (TOH-koh-DAI-nah-GRAF) instrument for recording the strength of labor contractions

tocography (toh-KAW-grah-fee) procedure for recording the strength of labor contractions

tocolytic (TOH-koh-LIH-tik) agent that stops or delays premature labor and contractions

tonic (TAW-nik) pertaining to muscle tone (normally weak or unresponsive)

tonic-clonic seizure (TAW-nik CLAH-nik SEE-zhir) a seizure characterized by both a tonic and a clonic phase

tonometer (TOH-naw-MEE-tir) instrument for measuring tension or pressure in the eye (intraocular pressure)

tonsillectomy (TON-sil-EK-toh-mee) surgical removal of a tonsil

tonsillitis (TON-sil-AI-tis) inflammation of a tonsil

topical anesthetic (TAW-pih-kal an-es-THET-ik) local anesthesia applied to the surface of the area to be anesthetized

tracheitis (tray-kee-AI-tis) inflammation of the trachea

tracheomalacia (tray-kee-oh-mah-LAY-shah) softening of the trachea

tracheostenosis (tray-kee-oh-sten-OH-sis) narrowing of the trachea

tracheostomy (tray-kee-AH-stoh-mee) creation of an opening in the trachea

tracheotomy (tray-kee-AH-toh-mee) incision into the trachea

transcranial Doppler sonography (tranz-KRAY-nee-al DAW-plir saw-NAW-grah-fee) an imaging technique that produces an image of the brain using sound waves sent through the skull

transdermal (trans-DER-mal) pertaining to through the skin

transesophageal electrocardiogram (TRANZ-eh-SOF-ah-JEE-al EK-oh-KAR-dee-oh-GRAM) record of the heart using sound waves performed by inserting the sonograph into the esophagus

transfusion (tranz-FYOO-zhun) infusion into a patient of blood from another source

transient ischemic attack (TIA) (TRAN-zee-ent ih-SKEE-mik ah-TAK) a mini-stroke caused by the blockage of a blood vessel that resolves (goes away) within 24 hours

transrectal ultrasonography (TRANZ-REK-tal UL-trah-soh-NAW-grah-fee) procedure involving a probe inserted into the rectum using high-frequency sound waves to scan through the rectum to nearby tissue (most commonly, the prostate)

transurethral resection of the prostate (TURP) (TRANS-yoo-REE-thral ree-SEK-shun of the PROS-tayt) procedure of removing all or part of the prostate by the insertion of a resectoscope into the urethra

transvaginal sonography (TRANZ-VAJ-ih-nal soh-NAW-grah-fee) imaging procedure using sound waves emitted from device inserted in the vagina

trichiasis (trih-KAI-ah-sis) condition caused by eyelashes growing backward and coming in contact with the eye

trichomycosis (trik-koh-mai-KOH-sis) a fungal condition of the hair

tumor (TOO-mur) a larger solid mass

tympanic perforation (tim-PAN-ik per-fer-AY-shun) tear or hole in the eardrum

tympanocentesis (tim-PAN-oh-sin-TEE-sis) puncture of the eardrum

tympanolabyrinthopexy (tim-PAN-oh-lab-uh-rinth-oh-PEK-see) surgical fixation of the eardrum to the labyrinth

tympanometry (tim-pan-AW-meh-tree) procedure for measuring the eardrum

tympanoplasty (tim-PAN-oh-PLAS-tee) surgical reconstruction of the eardrum

tympanosclerosis (tim-PAN-oh-skleh-ROH-sis) hardening of the eardrum

tympanostomy (TIM-pan-AW-stoh-mee) creation of an opening in the eardrum

U

ulcer (UL-sir) from Latin, for *sore;* a sore

ultrasonography (UL-trah-soh-NAW-grah-fee) imaging procedure using high-frequency sound waves

umbilical (um-BIL-ih-kal) middle center portion of the abdomen

uremia (yoo-REE-mee-ah) presence of urinary waste in the blood

ureteralgia (yur-EE-ter-AL-jah) pain in the ureter

ureteritis (yoo-REE-ter-AI-tis) inflammation of a ureter

ureterocele (yoo-REE-ter-oh-SEEL) hernia of the ureter

ureteroileostomy (yoo-REE-ter-oh-IL-ee-AW-stoh-mee) creation of an opening between a ureter and the ileum, a portion of the small intestine

ureterolithiasis (yoo-REE-ter-oh-lih-THAI-ah-sis) presence of stones in a ureter

ureteronephrectomy (yoo-REE-ter-oh-neh-FREK-toh-mee) surgical removal of a kidney and ureter

ureteroplasty (yoo-REE-ter-oh-PLAS-tee) surgical reconstruction of a ureter

ureteropyelitis (yoo-REE-ter-oh-PAI-el-AI-tis) inflammation of a ureter and renal pelvis

ureteropyelonephritis (yoo-REE-ter-oh-PAI-el-oh-neh-FRAI-tis) inflammation of a kidney, renal pelvis, and ureter

ureterorrhaphy (yoo-REE-ter-OR-ah-fee) suture of the ureter

ureteroscopy (yoo-REE-ter-AW-skoh-pee) process of examining a ureter

ureterostenosis (yoo-REE-ter-oh-steh-NOH-sis) narrowing of a ureter

urethrectomy (yoo-ree-THREK-toh-mee) surgical removal of the urethra

urethritis (yoo-ree-THRAI-tis) inflammation of the urethra

urethrocele (yoo-REE-throh-seel) hernia or prolapse of the urethra into the vagina

urethrocystitis (yoo-REE-throh-sis-TAI-tis) inflammation of the urethra and bladder

urethrodynia (yoo-REE-throh-DAI-nee-ah) pain in the urethra

urethrogram (yoo-REE-throh-GRAM) image of the urethra

urethropexy (yoo-REE-throh-PEK-see) surgical fixation of the urethra

urethroplasty (yoo-REE-throh-PLAS-tee) surgical reconstruction of the urethra

urethrorrhea (yoo-REE-throh-REE-ah) discharge from the urethra

urethroscope (yoo-REE-throh-SKOHP) instrument for examining the urethra

urethroscopy (yoo-ree-THRAW-skoh-pee) process of examining the urethra

urethrospasm (yoo-REE-throh-SPAZ-um) involuntary contraction of the urethra

urethrostenosis (yoo-REE-throh-steh-NOH-sis) narrowing of the urethra

urethrotomy (yoo-ree-THRAW-toh-mee) incision into the urethra

urinalysis (YUR-ih-NAL-ih-sis) analysis of the urine

urinary catheterization (YUR-ih-NAR-ee KATH-eh-ter-ih-ZAY-shun) insertion of a catheter into the bladder to drain urine

urinary tract infection (UTI) (YUR-ih-NAR-ee TRAKT in-FEK-shun) infection of the urinary tract

urocyanosis (YUR-oh-SAI-ah-NOH-sis) blue urine

urodynia (YUR-oh-DAI-nee-ah) painful urination

urologist (yur-AW-loh-jist) specialist in the urinary tract

urology (yur-AW-loh-jee) study of the urinary tract

uropathy (yur-AW-pah-thee) disease of the urinary tract

uropoesis (YUR-oh-poh-EE-sis) formation of urine

urostomy (yur-AW-stoh-mee) creation of an opening in the urinary tract, normally to divert urine flow away from a diseased bladder

uroxanthin (YUR-oh-ZAN-thin) substance in urine that makes it yellow

uterine prolapse (YOO-ter-in PROH-laps) downward displacement of the uterus into the vagina

V

vaginitis (VAJ-ih-NAI-tis) inflammation of the vagina

vaginodynia (VAJ-ih-noh-DAI-nee-ah) vaginal pain

vaginomycosis (VAJ-ih-noh-MAI-koh-sis) fungal condition of the vagina

vaginoperineoplasty (VAJ-ih-noh-PER-ih-NEE-oh-PLAS-tee) suture of the vagina and perineum

vaginoperineorrhaphy (VAJ-ih-noh-PER-ih-nee-OR-ah-fee) suture of the vagina and perineum

vaginoperineotomy (VAJ-ih-noh-PER-ih-nee-AW-toh-mee) incision into the vagina and perineum

vaginoplasty (vah-JI-noh-PLAS-tee) surgical reconstruction of the vagina

vaginoscope (VAJ-ih-noh-SKOHP) instrument used to examine the vagina

vaginosis (VAJ-ih-NOH-sis) condition of the vagina

valvectomy (val-VEK-toh-mee) surgical removal of a heart valve

valvotomy (val-VAW-toh-mee) incision into a heart valve

valvulitis (VAL-vyoo-LAI-tis) inflammation of a heart valve

valvuloplasty (VAL-vyoo-loh-PLAS-tee) surgical reconstruction of a heart valve

varicocele (VAR-ih-koh-SEEL) overexpansion of the blood vessels of the testicles, leading to a soft tumor

varicose veins (VAR-ih-kohs VAYNS) enlarged, dilated vein toward the surface of the skin

varicotomy (VAR-ih-KAW-toh-mee) surgical removal of a varicose vein

vas deferens (VAS DEH-frenz) vessel carrying sperm from the testicles

vascular endoscopy (VAS-kyoo-lar en-DAW-skoh-pee) procedure to look inside a blood vessel

vascular lesion (VAS-kyoo-lar LEE-zhun) wounds related to blood vessels

vasculitis (VAS-kyoo-LAI-tis) inflammation of blood vessels

vasectomy (vah-SEK-toh-mee) surgical removal of the vas deferens

vasoconstrictor (VAS-oh-kin-STRIK-tor) drug that constricts or narrows the diameter of a blood vessel

vasodilator (VAS-oh-DAI-lay-tor) drug that causes the relaxation or expansion of a blood vessel

vasopressor (VAS-oh-PRES-or) drug that constricts or narrows the diameter of a blood vessel

vasospasm (VAS-oh-SPAZ-um) involuntary contraction of a blood vessel

vasovasostomy (VAS-oh-vah-SAW-stoh-mee) creation of an opening between two vessels; technical term for a vasectomy reversal

vena cava (VEE-nah CAY-vah) large-diameter vein that gathers blood from the body and returns it to the heart

venectomy (vee-NEK-toh-mee) surgical removal of a vein

venogram (VEE-noh-gram) record of a vein

venosclerosis (VEE-noh-skleh-ROH-sis) hardening of a vein

venospasm (VEE-noh-SPAZ-um) involuntary contraction of a vein

venostasis (VEE-noh-STA-sis) trapping of blood in an extremity due to compression

ventilation–perfusion scan (ven-ti-LAY-shun–per-FYOO-shun SKAN) a scan that tests whether a problem in the lungs is caused by airflow (ventilation) or blood flow (perfusion)

ventricular septal defect (VSD) (ven-TRIK-yoo-lar SEP-tal DEE-fekt) flaw in the septum that divides the two ventricles of the heart

ventriculotomy (ven-TRIK-yoo-LAW-toh-mee) incision into a ventricle

vertigo (VER-tih-goh) sensation of moving through space (while stationary); from Latin, for "to whirl around"

verucca (vah-ROO-kah) from Latin, for "wart"; a wart

vesicle (VEH-sih-kul) from Latin, for "little bladder" a small blister

vesicocele (VES-ih-koh-SEEL) hernia of the bladder

vesicostomy (VEH-sih-KAW-stoh-mee) creation of an opening in the bladder

vesicotomy (VEH-sih-KAW-toh-mee) incision into the bladder

vesicoureteral reflux (VUR) (VES-ih-koh-yoo-REE-ter-al REE-fluks) abnormal flow of urine from the bladder back into the ureters

vesicovaginal fistula (VES-ih-koh-VAJ-ih-nal FIS-tyoo-lah) abnormal opening between the urinary bladder and the vagina

vesiculectomy (veh-SIK-yoo-LEK-toh-mee) surgical removal of the seminal vesicles

vestibular neuritis (ves-TIH-byoo-lar nir-AI-tis) inflammation of the vestibular nerve

vestibulitis (ves-TIH-byoo-LAI-tis) inflammation of the vestibule

vestibulotomy (ves-TIH-byoo-LAW-toh-mee) incision into the vestibule

vitiligo (vih-tih-LAI-goh) see *patch*

vitrectomy (vih-TREK-toh-mee) the removal of the vitreous liquid from the eye

voiding (VOI-ding) another term for urination

voiding cystourethrogram (VOI-ding SIS-toh-yoo-REE-throh-GRAM) imaging procedure of the bladder and urethra produced during urination

vulvitis (vul-VAI-tis) inflammation of the vulva

vulvodynia (VUL-voh-DAI-nee-ah) pain in the vulva

vulvovaginitis (VUL-voh-VAJ-ih-NAI-tis) inflammation of the vulva and vagina

xanthoderma (zan-thoh-DER-mah) yellow skin

xanthoma (zan-THOH-mah) a yellow tumor

xanthosis (zan-THOH-sis) yellowing of the skin

xenograft (ZEE-noh-graft) see *heterograft*

xeroderma (zeh-roh-DER-mah) dry skin

xerophthalmia (ZER-off-THAL-mee-ah) dry eyes

xerosis (ze-ROH-sis) condition of dryness

A

B

C

D

E

F

G

H

I

J

K

L

M

N

O

P

Q

R

S

T

U

V

W

X

Y

Z